Register Now for Online Your Book!

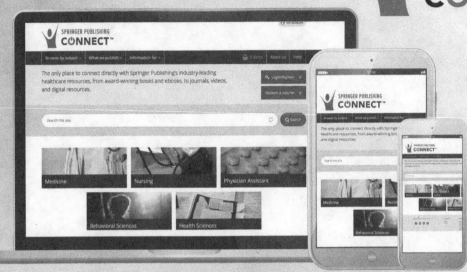

SPRINGER PUBLISHING
C⏻NNECT™

Your print purchase of *Adult-Gerontology Acute Care Practice Guidelines, Second Edition,* **includes online access to the contents of your book**—increasing accessibility, portability, and searchability!

Access today at:
http://connect.springerpub.com/content/book/978-0-8261-7618-9
or scan the QR code at the right with your smartphone. Log in or register, then click "Redeem a voucher" and use the code below.

SRDBE6SN

Scan here for quick access.

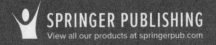

SPRINGER PUBLISHING
View all our products at springerpub.com

ADULT-GERONTOLOGY ACUTE
CARE PRACTICE GUIDELINES

Catherine Harris, PhD, MBA, AGACNP, is an associate professor of graduate programs and a faculty member in the Acute Care Nurse Practitioner Program at Thomas Jefferson University in Philadelphia. She earned her PhD in nursing at the University of Pennsylvania and an MBA from Drexel University before becoming credentialed as an acute care nurse practitioner at Thomas Jefferson University in Philadelphia. Dr. Harris specializes in neurocritical care, having presented extensively on ischemic and hemorrhagic stroke. She has been a mentee for the Fellows of the American Association of Nurse Practitioners Mentorship Program and has won numerous research grants in neurocritical care and global health.

ADULT-GERONTOLOGY ACUTE CARE PRACTICE GUIDELINES

SECOND EDITION

Catherine Harris, PhD, MBA, AGACNP

Editor

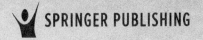

SPRINGER PUBLISHING

Springer Publishing Company, LLC
11 West 42nd Street, New York, NY 10036
www.springerpub.com

Acquisitions Editor: Elizabeth Nieginski
Compositor: diacriTech

ISBN: 978-0-8261-7617-2
ebook ISBN: 978-0-8261-7618-9
DOI: 10.1891/9780826176189

23 24 25 26 / 5 4 3 2 1

The author and the publisher of this Work have made every effort to provide information that is accurate and compatible with the standards generally accepted at the time of publication. Because medical science is continually advancing, our knowledge base continues to expand. Therefore, as new information becomes available, changes in procedures become necessary. The reader should always consult current research and specific institutional policies before performing any clinical procedure or delivering any medication. The author and publisher shall not be liable for any special, consequential, or exemplary damages resulting, in whole or in part, from the readers' use of, or reliance on, the information contained herein.

Library of Congress Control Number: 2023930850

Contact sales@springerpub.com to receive discount rates on bulk purchases.

Publisher's Note: **New and used products purchased from third-party sellers are not guaranteed for quality, authenticity, or access to any included digital components.**

Printed in the United States of America.

To Matthew,

    My beautiful little boy, you are always in my heart, and I am so proud of you!

Mom and Dad,

    Thank you for your encouragement and always being there for me.

CONTENTS

SECTION I: ACUTE CARE GUIDELINES BY SYSTEM

SECTION IV: SPECIAL TOPICS

CONTRIBUTORS

Melissa Barnett, PA-C
Physician Assistant, Department of Stem
Cell Transplant and Cellular Therapy
University of Texas, MD Anderson Cancer
Center
Houston, Texas

Suzanne Barron, MSN, RN, CRNP, FNP
Adult and Gerontology Acute Care Nurse
Practitioner
Thomas Jefferson University
Philadelphia, Pennsylvania

David J. Bergamo, PA-C
Physician Assistant, Infectious Disease
Associates
Infectious Disease, Christiana Hospital
Newark, Delaware;
Physician Assistant, Urgent Care
Florida Medical Clinic
Zephyrhills, Florida

Amy Blake, MSN, FNP-BC
TeamHealth Acute and Post Acute Care
Knoxville, Tennessee

Ann E. Burke, MSN, CRNP, FNP-BC
Nurse Practitioner
Thomas Jefferson University Hospital
Philadelphia, Pennsylvania

Dawn Carpenter, DNP, ACNP-BC, CCRN
Nurse Practitioner
Guthrie Healthcare System, Trauma/
Surgical Critical Care
Sayre, Pennsylvania;
Associate Professor
University of Massachusetts Chan
Medical School
Tan Chingfen Graduate School of Nursing
Worcester, Massachusetts

**E. Moneé Carter-Griffin, DNP, MAOL,
APRN, ACNP-BC**
Director of Education, Advanced Practice
Providers
Dallas Pulmonary and Critical Care
Dallas, Texas;
Clinical Assistant Professor, Department
of Graduate Nursing
University of Texas at Arlington
Arlington, Texas

**Nicole Cavaliere, DNP, CRNP,
AGACNP-BC**
Critical Care Nurse Practitioner
Thomas Jefferson University Hospital,
Faculty, Adult-Gerontology Acute Care
Nurse Practitioner Program
Jefferson College of Nursing
Philadelphia, Pennsylvania

**Christine Chmielewski, MS, CRNP,
ANP-BC, CNN-NP**
Nephrology Nurse Practitioner
Jefferson Renal Associates
Thomas Jefferson University Hospital
Philadelphia, Pennsylvania

**Jennifer Coates, DNP, MBA, ACNPC,
ACNP-BC**
Director, Adult Gerontology Acute Care
Nurse Practitioner Program
Associate Clinical Professor
College of Nursing and Health Professions
Drexel University
Philadelphia, Pennsylvania

Kathleen L. Collins, MD
Resident Physician, Department of
Orthopaedic Surgery
University of Pennsylvania
Philadelphia, Pennsylvania

Jennifer Creed, MD, PhD
Neurointensivist, Department of
Neurocritical Care Specialists
Christiana Care Health System
Newark, Delaware

**Jo Ann M. Davidson, MSN, CRNP,
FNP-BC**
Nurse Practitioner
Milton S. Hershey Medical Center, Penn
State Cancer Center
Hershey, Pennsylvania

**Michele DeCastro, MSN, CRNP,
AHNP-BC, AGACNP-BC**
Nurse Practitioner
Division of Hospital Medicine, Thomas
Jefferson University
Philadelphia, Pennsylvania

Pamela B. Dudkiewicz, DNP, APRN, FNP-BC, AOCNP
University of Miami Sylvester Comprehensive Cancer Center
Department of Medicine, Division of Hematology
Miami, Florida

William A. Edwards, Jr., DNP, APN, CRNA, AGACNP-BC, PMH-BC
Adjunct Professor, Thomas Jefferson University
Philadelphia, Pennsylvania;
Certified Registered Nurse Anesthesiologist, Hackensack Meridian Health System
Hackensack, New Jersey;
Certified Registered Nurse Anesthesiologist
RWJ Barnabas Healthcare System
New Brunswick, New Jersey

Kathryn Evans Kreider, DNP, APRN, FNP-BC, BC-ADM, FAANP
Associate Clinical Professor
Duke University School of Nursing
Durham, North Carolina

Abimbola Farinde, PhD
Columbia Southern University
College of Business
Orange Beach, Alabama

Diann C. Fernandez, MSN, APRN
Instructor, Division of Gynecologic Oncology
Department of Obstetrics, Gynecology and Reproductive Sciences
University of Miami Miller School of Medicine
Sylvester Comprehensive Cancer Center
Miami, Florida

Lauren M. Franker, DNP, APRN, ACNP-BC
Rush Copley Medical Center
Advanced Practice Registered Nurse
Neuroscience Institute
Aurora, Illinois

Susan F. Galiczynski, RN, MSN, ANP-BC, AGACNP-BC
Trauma Nurse Practitioner
Crozer-Chester Medical Center
Upland, Pennsylvania

Alexis C. Geppner, MLS, CTTS, MPAS, PA-C
Physician Assistant, Leukemia,
University of Texas, MD Anderson Cancer Center
Houston, Texas

Debra J. Hain, PhD, ARNP, AGPCNP-BC, FAAN, FAANP, FNKF
Professor and DNP Program Director
Florida Atlantic University, Christine E Lynn College of Nursing
Boca Raton, Florida

Catherine Harris, PhD, MBA, AGACNP
Associate Professor, Graduate Programs
Thomas Jefferson University
Philadelphia, Pennsylvania

Carey Heck, PhD, CRNP, AGACNP-BC, CCRN-K, CNRN
Associate Professor, Director Adult-Gerontology Acute Care Nurse Practitioner Program
Thomas Jefferson University, College of Nursing
Philadelphia, Pennsylvania

Shannon Holloway, MHS, PA-C
Physician Assistant, Infectious Diseases
MD Anderson Cancer Center
Houston, Texas

Sara Hollstein, MSN, AOCNP, ACHPN, ANP-BC
Nurse Informaticist, Senior Business Analyst
DaVita Kidney Care, Clinical Intelligence
Denver, Colorado

Eric Jacala, PA-C
Orthopaedic Surgical Physician Assistant
Department of Penn Orthopaedics, Pennsylvania Hospital
Philadelphia, Pennsylvania

Elizabeth Jordan, CRNP, PMHNP-BC
Thomas Jefferson University College of Nursing
Philadelphia, Pennsylvania

Lewis J. Kaplan, MD, FACS, FCCP, FCCM
Professor of Surgery
Perelman School of Medicine, University of Pennsylvania
Division of Trauma, Surgical Critical Care and Emergency Surgery;
Section Chief, Surgical Critical Care
Director, Surgical Intensive Care Unit
Corporal Michael J Crescenz VA Medical Center
Philadelphia, Pennsylvania

Allison Koblitz, MSN, CRNP, FNP-BC
Nurse Practitioner, Hematology/Oncology
Penn State Milton S. Hershey Medical Center
Hershey, Pennsylvania

Aparna Kumar, PhD, MPH, CRNP
Assistant Professor/Program Director
Psychiatric Mental Health Nurse
  Practitioner Program
Thomas Jefferson University College of
  Nursing
Philadelphia, Pennsylvania

Monique Lambert, DNP, APRN
Northshore University Health System
Evanston, Illinois

Sarah L. Livesay, DNP, APRN, FNCS, FAAN
Rush University College of Nursing
Chicago, Illinois

Marissa E. Luft, MSN, CRNP, AGACNP-BC, ACHPN
Adjunct Professor
Thomas Jefferson University College of
  Nursing
Philadelphia, Pennsylvania

Shawn Mangan, MSN, RNFA, ANP-C, AGACNP-BC
Enterprise Surgery Service Line Lead
  Advanced Practice Provider
Surgical Intensive Care Unit Lead
  Advanced Practice Provider
Thomas Jefferson University
Philadelphia, Pennsylvania

Rose Milano, DNP, ACNP-BC
Assistant Professor
Department of Adult Health and
  Gerontologic Nursing
Rush University College of Nursing
Chicago, Illinois

Robin Miller, MSN, FNP-BC, AGACNP-BC
Nurse Practitioner
Thomas Jefferson University Hospital
Philadelphia, Pennsylvania

Divya Monga, MD
Division of Nephrology
University of Mississippi Medical Center
Jackson, Mississippi

Caitlyn Moore, DNP, MS, CRNP, AGACNP-BC, ACHPN
Assistant Professor of Nursing
Thomas Jefferson University, College of
  Nursing
Philadelphia, Pennsylvania;
Palliative Care and Hospice Nurse
  Practitioner, Main Line Health
Radnor, Pennsylvania

Dominick Osipowicz, MSN, APRN, AGACNP-BC
Nurse Practitioner, Neurocritical Care
  Unit
Christiana Care Health System
Newark, Delaware

Jennifer W. Parker, BSN, MSN, PhD
Nurse Practitioner and Hospitalist
Valley View Hospital
Glenwood Springs, Colorado

Joanne Elaine Pechar, MSN, ANP-C, AGACNP-BC
Lead Orthopedic Surgery Nurse
  Practitioner
Department of Penn Orthopedics,
  Pennsylvania Hospital
Philadelphia, Pennsylvania

Cheryl Pfennig, MSN, RN, NP-C, AOCNP
Advanced Practice Registered Nurse,
  Surgical Oncology
MD Anderson Cancer Center
Houston, Texas

Timothy Ray, DNP, CNP, CNN-NP
Cleveland Kidney and Hypertension
  Consultants
Euclid, Ohio

Rae Brana Reynolds, PhD, RN, ACNP-BC
Manager, Advanced Practice
  Providers
MD Anderson Cancer Center
Houston, Texas

Monica Richey, MSN, ANP-BC
Nurse Practitioner/Clinical Instructor
Northwell Health
Hofstra School of Nursing
New York, New York

Courtney Robb, RN, MS, CRNFA, FNP-C
Advanced Practice Registered Nurse,
  Department of Thoracic and
  Cardiovascular Surgery
MD Anderson Cancer Center
Houston, Texas

Alycia Rosendale, MS, PA-C
Lead APP Outpatient Hematology/
  Oncology
Penn State Cancer Institute
Penn State Hershey Medical Center
Hershey, Pennsylvania

Krista M. Rubin, MS, FNP-BC
Nurse Practitioner
Center for Melanoma, MGH Cancer
 Center
Boston, Massachusetts

Allison Rusgo, MHS, MPH, PA-C
Drexel University, College of Nursing and
 Health Professions
Physician Assistant Department
Philadelphia, Pennsylvania

Kelley Scott, DNP, FNP-BC, ENP-BC
Drexel University
Philadelphia, Pennsylvania

Lori Sheneman, MPAS, PA-C
Physician Assistant, Hematology/
 Oncology
Penn State Cancer Institute
Hershey, Pennsylvania

**Cara M. Staley, MSN, RN-BC,
 AGACNP-BC**
Vascular Surgery Nurse Practitioner
Vascular Surgery, Thomas Jefferson
 University Hospital
Philadelphia, Pennsylvania

**Kristen L. Talvacchia, MSN, CRNP,
 ACNP-BC, CCRN**
Acute Care Nurse Practitioner
Corporal Michael J Crescenz VA Medical
 Center, Department of Surgery
Philadelphia, Pennsylvania

Megan C. Thomas Hebdon
University of Texas at Austin
Austin, Texas

Yvonne Tumbali, DNP, APRN, ACNP-BC
Director, Adult Gerontology Acute Care
 Nurse Practitioner Program
Assistant Professor, Department of Adult
 Gerontology
Rush University, College of Nursing
Chicago, Illinois

**Sara Van Craeynest, MSN, CRNP,
 AGACNP-BC**
Nurse Practitioner
Thomas Jefferson University
Philadelphia, Pennsylvania

Steven H. Wei, EdD, MPH, PA-C
Supervisor, Advanced Practice Providers,
 Department of Surgical Oncology
MD Anderson Cancer Center
Houston, Texas

**Catherine Wells, DNP, ACNP, CNN-NP,
 FNKF**
Assistant Professor
Division of Nephrology, University of
 Mississippi Medical Center
Jackson, Mississippi

**Mary L. Wilby, PhD, MSN, MPH, CRNP,
 ANP-BC**
Associate Professor, Adult Gerontology
 Nurse Practitioner Track Coordinator
La Salle University School of Nursing and
 Health Sciences
Philadelphia, Pennsylvania

Dolores Diana Zollo, MSPA, PA-C
Penn Medicine Advanced Practice
 Physician Assistant
Norristown, Pennsylvania

REVIEWERS

Dennis Absher Taylor, DNP, NP
Atrium Health, Wake Forest Baptist
Winston-Salem, North Carolina

Elizabeth Bell, RN, MSN, FNP-C
Nurse Practitioner
Duke University Health System
Durham, North Carolina

Brennan Bowker, MHS, PA-C, CPAAPA
Physician Assistant; Part-Time Clinical
 Assistant Professor of Physician
 Assistant Studies
Yale New Haven Hospital Department
 of Surgery; Quinnipiac University
 Department of Physician Assistant
 Studies
New Haven, Connecticut

**Courtney Cawthon, MPH, MSN,
 AGACNP**
Lead Advanced Practice Provider for
 Palliative Care
Emory Healthcare
Atlanta, Georgia

**Kathleen O. Chennell, MS, CNS,
 ACNP-BC, CCRN**
Adult-Gerontology Acute Care Nurse
 Practitioner
Division of Nephrology, University of
 Cincinnati
Cincinnati, Ohio

**Carolina Dimsdale Tennyson, DNP,
 ACNP-BC, AACC**
Nurse Practitioner, Clinical Associate
 Faculty
Duke University School of Nursing
Durham, North Carolina

Donna Gullette, NP
Clinical Professor at University of
 Arkansas for Medical Sciences
Little Rock, Arkansas

**Stefanie La Manna, PhD, MPH, APRN,
 FNP-C, AGACNP-BC**
Associate Professor and Assistant/
 Associate Dean of Graduate Programs
Nova Southeastern University
Palm Beach Gardens, Florida

Alexander Menard, DNP, AGACNP-BC
Surgical Critical Care, Staff Nurse
 Practitioner
University of Massachusetts Chan
 Medical School, Tan Chingfen Graduate
 School of Nursing
University of Massachusetts Memorial
 Medical Center
Worcester, Massachusetts

Brianna Miller, DNP, NP
Atrium Health, Wake Forest Baptist
Winston-Salem, North Carolina

**Caitlyn Moore, DNP, MS, CRNP,
 AGACNP-BC, ACHPN**
Assistant Professor of Nursing
Thomas Jefferson University, College of
 Nursing
Philadelphia, Pennsylvania;
Palliative Care and Hospice Nurse
 Practitioner, Main Line Health
Radnor, Pennsylvania

PREFACE

The need for an acute care textbook has been growing. Although outpatient practices have long seen the value of utilizing advanced practice providers (APPs), the surge in acute care providers has been relatively recent. I remember when I was a registered nurse back in the 1990s, I had no idea there was such a role as a nurse practitioner (NP) or a physician assistant (PA) in the hospital, despite the fact they have been around since the 1960s!

I was immediately fascinated and intrigued by the role of APPs. It was not long before I found myself enrolled in an NP program. When I graduated, I was one of the first NPs on the neurosurgery service in the facility where I practiced. The service appreciated the help, but they did not really know what to do with me. It took many months for me to garner the trust of the surgeons, and to show them the true capacity of what APPs could do and how we could really become essential parts of the team.

APPs have come a long way over the years. I have seen the role of NPs and PAs expand tremendously since I first began practicing in this role. I have seen the negative terms to describe us, such as midlevels, physician extenders, and helpers, evolve into advanced practice providers.

I have also seen collaborative growth and mutual respect grow between NPs and PAs, a relationship that was previously more isolated. I respect my PA colleagues, and as an NP I have learned quite a bit from their struggles with role and identity. I find that I personally relate to these struggles in how I practice and how I see my own role on the healthcare team. I have also learned the value of combining resources and focusing on how we are similar, rather than different.

It was important to write this textbook with PAs and NPs together. Both groups have immense knowledge, resources, and experience to share with each other.

Finally, it was essential to write this textbook because it fills a void in the marketplace. Countless times my students have asked if there were an acute care textbook that they could use. I have tried many different textbooks, but either I found them to be too cumbersome or the information provided was just too scant.

This final iteration of the textbook came about as a result of those experiences and discussions with students about what they needed and they wanted. We all suffer from information overload and overwhelm, so the focus of this textbook was to provide the minimum of what new graduate students need to know in order to be competent when they start practice.

We are now in our second edition of this book and the value of it has been an incredible resource. This edition has added new sections to cover COVID and to update best practices for a variety of conditions. In addition, we have added case studies and quiz questions to help the reader to best synthesize the material and prep for the board.

ORGANIZATION

This book is organized into four major sections.

Section I: Acute Care Guidelines by System—In Section I, the APP is exposed to the most common medical conditions organized by system. Although it is by no means comprehensive or inclusive of every medical condition, the section is meant to provide APP students with an overview of very common medical conditions that they should focus on during their studies. In my teachings, I have found students tend to gravitate toward understanding the "zebras" in medicine, or those conditions that are unusual, instead of diagnosing common problems or unusual variants of common problems. This phenomenon might have to do with the common practice of testing on zebras or the student perception that we (as academic institutions) are out to trick them on a test. By not introducing zebras into the context of this book, the students can maintain focus on the most common disease states.

Section II: Perioperative Considerations—Section II contains an operative overview. Again, this section is not a comprehensive review of the operating room, but it does provide APP students an overview of what they should know regardless of where they work. In the acute care setting, operative procedures are very common. It does not matter if acute care practitioners work directly or indirectly with patients in the perioperative period. A review of the common issues is mandatory.

Section III: Procedures—Not all APPs will perform procedures, but students frequently feel a sense of accomplishment in being able to do something tangible. It is difficult to measure the progress of one's own critical thinking, but if a student can perform a procedure, their confidence level goes up quickly. In this section, some of the more common procedures are listed.

Section IV: Special Topics—There are many issues that we will deal with as APPs; however, these issues do not all fall neatly into predefined categories. This section was created for select topics that could not be defined by systems but were equally important to address. These topics include end-of-life issues, palliative care, health promotion, hemodynamic monitoring devices, telemedicine, transitions of care, and acute care billing. All APPs will deal with these issues during the course of their careers. These topics will also continue to evolve as we conduct more research and clinical studies and as technology improves.

WHAT IS DIFFERENT ABOUT THIS BOOK

This book was created for APP students in the acute care setting. In talking to students about their wants and needs in a textbook, I found students were not able to absorb and assimilate information in heavy, dense textbooks that we had been using. I also found myself telling my students not to bother with a large portion of the textbook because it was not immediately relevant to their basic knowledge. Students struggled to understand what to focus on and what they needed to know versus what was nice to know.

No one can memorize everything they need to know about medicine. As students specialize in various fields, they will learn in-depth information about their specialties that is beyond the scope of this book. However, there is a body of knowledge that every APP should know, and I have done my best to include those topics in this book.

Catherine Harris

ACKNOWLEDGMENTS

I have so many people to acknowledge in the creation of this textbook, particularly Dr. Ksenia Zukowsky, Dr. Carey Heck, and Dr. Jack Jallo. Dr. Zukowsky saw so much potential in my plans. She pushed me to do things I was scared to do, and she made them seem possible. Her incredible stories have inspired me over the years, and she remains a powerful influence in my life.

Dr. Heck has been an incredible colleague. As the director of the Acute Care Nurse Practitioner Program at Thomas Jefferson University, she has entertained my "big" ideas and helped me implement them. She has been a rock of support and has contributed massively to the publication of this book as well as the profession.

Dr. Jallo has been my main physician support over the years in neurocritical care and neurosurgery. He never told me something could not be done, and he has made me believe that more was always possible.

I want to acknowledge all the people who contributed to my growth as a nurse and an academic, especially Dr. Bob Hess. Dr. Hess knew me as a little girl. He was my neighbor across the street. Then, he was my teacher when I went to undergraduate nursing school at the University of Pennsylvania. Then he became my employer when I picked up extra time doing some editing work at the nursing magazine that he edited. Finally, he became my colleague and friend who encouraged me to keep rising through the ranks.

Of course, I would not be the clinician, academic, and nurse I am today without my students, fellow faculty, friends, and family. I want to express my gratitude to so many people, but it is not possible to list them all here. From my first nursing job to where I am today, I am thankful for everyone in my life who has taught me so much.

It has been an absolute pleasure to work with Springer Publishing Company. I worked most closely with Elizabeth Nieginski and Jennifer Ehlers. Their talent, expertise, and encouragement were the guiding light for me through this entire process.

I need to acknowledge all the work done by the editing team. What you produced is absolutely amazing. I really appreciate everything you have done in the editorial process.

INTRODUCTION

INFORMATION OVERLOAD

No book can serve all the needs of students, nor should that be the goal. This book was specifically designed to provide a foundation of basic information about acute care that students or any advanced practice provider (APP) should know about a body system. Acute care is defined as treatment that is received in the short term for an injury, emergency, or episode of illness. Acute care can be delivered in the hospital setting, EDs, or even outpatient clinics and includes a vast array of conditions and issues. However, patients also come to the acute care setting with chronic problems that APPs need to address, and the table of contents was developed with this in mind. The table of contents is divided into four sections to accommodate the large scope of acute care. Videos demonstrating arterial line placement, digital block, and lumbar puncture procedures are available at https://connect.springerpub.com/content/reference-book/978-0-8261-7618-9.

Section IV is designed to address special issues that are unique to the acute care setting. The topics addressed are transitional care, end-of-life issues, palliative care, health promotion, hemodynamic monitoring devices, telemedicine, and acute care billing. When a patient comes into the acute care setting, it is an opportunity for all healthcare providers to address health promotion. Not everyone sees healthcare providers on a regular basis or gets evaluated for routine screening. Therefore, it is essential for all acute care providers to be well-versed on the types of health promotion that are necessary based on a patient's age and other demographic factors.

Telemedicine is also addressed because it is becoming increasingly prevalent. The ICUs in rural areas can now be monitored by intensivists and APPs in central regions. There is a burgeoning role for APPs in this area. Transitional care is the point at which a patient either comes into the acute care setting or returns to the outpatient community. This period of transition is the most vulnerable time for patients. Careful attention must be devoted to updating and informing the accepting provider on patient status and the management plan. Finally, end-of-life and palliative care issues are often addressed in the hospital system after an acute episode. Knowledge of these issues is essential to practice.

This edition includes all-new Knowledge Check review questions at the end of selected chapters. The answer keys for the review questions are available at the end of the chapters; just turn the page to see the correct answers with rationales. New case scenarios with review questions are also provided for selected conditions. The answer key for the case scenario review questions can be found in Appendix A.

Appendix B provides normal lab values as a reference tool for APPs. There may be slight variations from institution to institution that may be attributed to different vendors. Please use these values as guides for quick reference, but defer to your institutional normal reference range.

Medicine is clearly and overwhelmingly a vast body of knowledge. Students who try to take it all on at once make learning seem like an insurmountable task. The brain can only absorb so much information at once. When students pick up a dense textbook and see there are hundreds of conditions that could exist within just one body system, it makes it difficult for them to focus on the relatively few conditions that we treat most commonly. The goal of this book is to deconstruct large topics into focused, core conditions. Students will not learn everything they need to know about a topic by using this book, but they will get what they need to know as a new graduate. Practicing APPs can refer to this resource as a quick review of what they need to know. Continuing to strive for more learning is a lifelong duty as an APP. Furthering the learning process far beyond graduate school and continuing to seek out information that is unfamiliar is essential.

In this day and age, the internet is a quick and easy resource to utilize. Patients use it as well. While no one expects any one person to know everything at all times, there is an expectation that the providers are resourceful and will know how to find the information.

IMPOSTER SYNDROME

At the end of the day, students will never feel like they know enough to get started, and much of this anxiety can be attributed to what we know about *imposter syndrome*. Going from the role of an expert in one area to a novice is extremely challenging, and creates feelings of uneasiness. This is a completely natural transition mode. In fact, I would be more concerned about a student who thinks they know everything than a student who feels like their peers just have not yet "figured out" that they do not belong.

This unease and uncertainty of feeling like an imposter will help students be cautious and humble when they enter the healthcare system as an acute care provider. Developing clinical judgment is an art that is guided by science, and occurs over time and through experiential learning. Being unsure will motivate new graduates to consult evidence-based materials to search for answers.

Frequently textbooks, articles, and case studies provide classic presentations that are useful for learning a concept. However, in practice, the APP quickly discovers that didactic content in a lecture or a book does not account for the number of variables that are present in real clinical situations. Hence, textbook learning has limitations that can only be remedied with practice. A student in the novice stage of a new role would be best advised to spend as much time as possible with patients, practicing active, focused listening, and asking questions. This practice will help the new graduate APP gain confidence quickly.

ROLE OF ADVANCED PRACTICE PROVIDERS

The role of APPs continues to evolve and expand in the healthcare system. New opportunities open up as the healthcare system begins to depend heavily on the utilization of APPs, particularly in the acute care system. It was not too long ago that most nurse practitioners (NPs) and physician assistants (PAs) worked primarily in primary care settings. Now, NPs and PAs work in primary care, all aspects of the acute care system, and beyond.

More and more collaborative efforts are being established between NPs and PAs as we move away from contrasting how we are different and focus on achieving the same goals.

Both NPs and PAs struggle with practice issues, prescribing issues, and levels of autonomy. However, many legislative advancements have been achieved over the past 10 years that have created a growing demand for APPs. As the roles and responsibilities of APPs continue to expand, the stronger the collaboration between them needs to be. This book is one step forward in developing and creating these collaborative efforts for NPs and PAs.

FUTURE OPPORTUNITIES

There are many opportunities for APPs. One of the major next steps I see for APPs is acute care billing. Billing provides visibility of the extent of work that is truly being done by APPs. Billing can also be leveraged for improved working conditions and better pay. In the current system where APP billing is absorbed by physician groups, APPs are left with basically nothing to show for their efforts. How can a hospital administration effectively determine if more or fewer APPs are needed in a particular department? How can a practice group determine if an APP is exceeding expectations in their work or even underperforming? How can an APP justify a raise for themselves when there is nothing quantifiable to show the value of what has been done?

Billing is more than just sending off charges to insurance companies to get paid. Billing provides visibility, which in turn comes with responsibilities and challenges. At the time of the writing of this book, there were no models (or too few to use) of acute care billing for APPs to devote an entire section to the issue; however, it is definitely coming. Insurance companies and compliance programs are taking steps to implement a structure that recognizes the contribution of the APP to the patient's care.

Acute care billing is going to be a controversial issue in the years to come, and APPs would be well-advised to keep on top of how it is implemented, and to participate in any committees that are designated to discuss such planning. See the last chapter in this book for information on acute care billing, which is new to this edition.

FINAL NOTE

Being an APP is an exciting and excellent career choice that has countless opportunities. Learning about disease states and management of patients is one aspect of the role of the APP. There is so much to learn, and it can be incredibly overwhelming. My advice to students, new graduates, and even seasoned APPs would be this: Acknowledge that there is a massive amount of information to be learned . . . *over time*. Accept that you have roles and responsibilities to the healthcare system and your community that extend beyond treating disease states. And accelerate your learning curve by being present with your patients, collaborating with your team, and staying involved in your profession.

Best of luck in this amazing profession as an APP.

LIST OF VIDEOS

Three procedures in Part III of this book include a corresponding video narrated by Catherine Harris. Subtitles are available for each video. To access the videos, use the QR codes provided and enter the voucher code on the first page of this book.

ARTERIAL LINES

Video 1. Arterial Line Placement
Guest: Dominick Osipowicz

DIGITAL NERVE BLOCKS

Video 2. Digital Nerve Block
Guest: Dominick Osipowicz

LUMBAR PUNCTURE

Video 3. Lumbar Puncture
Guest: Dominick Osipowicz

SECTION ▌I

ACUTE CARE GUIDELINES BY SYSTEM

1. Ear, Nose, and Throat Guidelines
2. Pulmonary Guidelines
3. Cardiac Guidelines
4. Gastrointestinal Guidelines
5. Nephrology Guidelines
6. Neurology Guidelines
7. Temperature Management Guidelines in Acute Brain Injury
8. Endocrine Guidelines
9. Psychiatric Guidelines
10. Infection Guidelines
11. Peripheral Vascular Guidelines
12. Hematology Guidelines
13. Oncology Guidelines
14. Immune System, Connective Tissue, and Joints Guidelines
15. Dermatology Guidelines
16. Geriatric Guidelines
17. Trauma Guidelines

CHAPTER 1

EAR, NOSE, AND THROAT GUIDELINES

Carey Heck

CONJUNCTIVITIS

DEFINITION
A. Inflammation of the conjunctiva, a thin transparent membrane that lines the inside of the eyelids and covers the sclera.
B. Commonly called "pink eye."

INCIDENCE
A. Allergic conjunctivitis.
   1. Most common cause of conjunctivitis (15%–40% of the population).
   2. Most frequently occurs in spring and summer.
B. Viral conjunctivitis.
   1. Most common cause of infectious conjunctivitis.
   2. Most common type in adults.
   3. More frequently occurs in the summer months.
C. Bacterial conjunctivitis.
   1. Most common cause of infectious conjunctivitis in children.
   2. Most frequently occurs in the winter and early spring months.

PATHOGENESIS
A. Allergic: Caused by allergens that come in contact with the eye.
   1. Not contagious.
   2. Common in individuals with other signs of allergic disease.
   3. Reaction to allergic triggers.
B. Infectious.
   1. Bacterial: Caused by bacteria spread through contact with infected eye secretions.
      a. Highly contagious.
      b. Most common causative agents.
         i. *Staphylococcus aureus*.
         ii. *Haemophilus influenzae*.
         iii. *Streptococcus pneumoniae*.
         iv. *Moraxella catarrhalis*.
   2. Viral: Caused by common viruses. May occur alone or with general cold symptoms.
      a. Highly contagious.
      b. Most common causative agents.
         i. Adenoviruses.
         ii. Rubella virus.
         iii. Rubeola virus.
         iv. Herpes viruses.

C. Noninfectious: Not caused by infection, allergy, or toxin.
   1. Dry eye.
   2. Foreign body.
   3. Irrigation after environmental exposure.
D. Toxic.
   1. Environmental irritants.
   2. Medications.
   3. Chemicals.

PREDISPOSING FACTORS
A. Exposure to allergens.
B. Exposure to environmental irritants.
C. Contact lens wearers.
D. Use of ophthalmic drops.
E. Expired makeup products.
F. Occupational exposure to chemicals.

SUBJECTIVE DATA
A. Common complaints/symptoms (will vary depending on the type of conjunctivitis).
   1. Redness.
   2. Discharge.
      a. From the eye.
      b. Matted eyelids that stick together, especially after sleep.
   3. Itching and burning.
   4. Increased tearing.
   5. Blurred vision.
   6. Painless.
   7. Feeling of foreign body in the eye.
B. Common/typical scenario.
   1. Specific presentation varies depending on the type of conjunctivitis.
   2. Symptoms of eye redness and discharge are common regardless of specific cause.
   3. Contributing history and appearance of discharge often determine the diagnosis.
C. Family and social history.
   1. Review of symptoms.
      a. Elicit the onset and duration of symptoms.
      b. Determine if the patient or close contacts have any systemic illnesses.
      c. Assess the patient for any risk factors.
      d. Associated symptoms.
         i. Rhinorrhea.
         ii. Earache.

iii. Sore throat.
iv. Rash.
e. Unilateral or bilateral eye involvement.
2. Medical history.
a. Recent illnesses.
b. Sick contacts.
c. Allergies.
d. Possible occupational exposure history.
e. Sexual history.
f. Contact lens use.
D. Review of systems.
1. Recent illnesses.
a. Determine the onset and duration of symptoms
i. Abrupt or gradual onset.
b. Determine if the patient or close contacts have any systemic illnesses.
2. Allergies.
3. Possible occupational exposure history.
4. Sexual history: History of sexually transmitted infection (STI) may increase the likelihood of gonococcal conjunctivitis.
5. Pertinent systems review.
a. Head, ear, eyes, nose, and throat (HEENT).
i. Headache.
ii. Vision loss.
iii. Eye pain.
iv. Eye discharge.
v. Ear pain.
vi. Rhinorrhea.
vii. Nasal congestion.
viii. Cough.
b. Integumentary.
i. Rash.
ii. Lesions.
iii. Irritations.

PHYSICAL EXAMINATION

A. Perform examination of lymph nodes, especially preauricular.
B. Perform examination of integument.
1. Note any rashes, lesions, or irritations, especially on the face.
C. Perform an eye examination, assessing for vision loss and eye discharge.
1. Appearance of eyes.
a. Allergic: Typically both eyes are infected.
b. Bacterial: Typically one eye is infected but may spread to the other eye.
c. Viral: Typically both eyes are infected.
d. Toxin: There is unilateral or bilateral involvement depending on exposure.
2. Discharge.
a. Allergic: Stringy.
b. Bacterial: Mucopurulent.
i. Copious yellow-green discharge is consistent with gonorrheal infection.
c. Viral: Watery.
3. Visual acuity.
4. Corneal opacity.
5. Pupil size and shape.

6. Eyelid swelling.
7. Presence of proptosis.
D. Red flags.
1. Reduction of visual acuity.
2. Ciliary flush.
3. Photophobia.
4. Severe foreign body sensation.
5. Corneal opacity.
6. Fixed pupil.
7. Severe headache with nausea.
8. Dendriform lesion indicative of herpes simplex virus (HSV).

DIAGNOSTIC TESTS

A. Diagnosis is made with history and physical examination in most cases.
B. Imaging studies are not indicated unless underlying condition is suspected.
C. Culture should be considered.
1. In severe cases.
2. In patients who wear contact lenses.
3. In patient unresponsive to initial treatment.
4. If STI is suspected.

DIFFERENTIAL DIAGNOSIS

A. Conjunctivitis.
1. Allergic: Likely with accompanying allergic symptoms and contributing history.
2. Bacterial: Likely with thick, yellow-green discharge.
3. Viral: Likely with accompanying cold or respiratory symptoms and watery discharge from the eye. Often accompanied by preauricular lymphadenopathy.
B. Corneal abrasion.
1. Different from conjunctivitis in that there is a subjective complaint of severe pain that worsens over time.
C. Foreign body in the eye.
D. Keratitis.
E. Varicella zoster ophthalmicus.
F. Glaucoma.

EVALUATION AND MANAGEMENT PLAN

A. General plan.
1. Symptomatic relief is the first step for all forms of conjunctivitis.
a. Most symptoms resolve without treatment.
b. Supportive care.
i. Medications.
1) Topical over-the-counter (OTC) medications effective for symptomatic relief in allergic conjunctivitis when symptoms are primarily ocular. Multiple formulations are available.
2) Systemic antihistamines may be helpful when rhinoconjunctivitis symptoms are present.
ii. Moist cold compress to the eyes.
iii. Avoidance of allergic triggers.

2. Antibiotics are not indicated in most cases of bacterial conjunctivitis.

  a. Return to work or school requirements. These may necessitate initiation of antibiotic for confirmed cases of bacterial conjunctivitis.

   i. Antibiotics initiated within the first 2 to 5 days can hasten the resolution of symptoms.

   ii. Initiation of antibiotics after 5 days of the start of symptoms has a minimal effect, and use is not recommended.

  b. Indications for antibiotic therapy.

   i. Cases caused by gonorrhea infection.

   ii. Cases caused by chlamydia infection.

   iii. Contact lens wearers.

    1) Consider *Pseudomonas* infection.

B. Patient/family teaching points.

  1. Frequent hand hygiene to prevent spread.

  2. Avoid touching the eyes.

  3. Instruct patients to dispose of current contact lenses and to avoid wearing contact lenses until irritation/infection is cleared.

  4. Instruct patients to dispose of all eye makeup.

C. Pharmacotherapy.

  1. Allergic.

   a. Artificial tears.

   b. Topical antihistamine/decongestant drops (OTC).

   c. Topical mast cell stabilizer/antihistamine drops (OTC).

   d. Nonsteroidal anti-inflammatory drugs.

   e. Topical corticosteroid therapy (should be prescribed only under the care of an ophthalmologist).

  2. Viral.

   a. Antibiotics not indicated.

   b. Antihistamine/decongestant drops (OTC).

   c. Artificial tears (OTC).

   d. Nonsteroidal anti-inflammatory drugs

   e. Viral therapy for HSV infection.

  3. Bacterial conjunctivitis.

   a. Mild bacterial conjunctivitis is usually self-limiting and does not require treatment.

   b. Superiority of any topical antibiotic agent is not supported in the literature.

   c. Topical (eye drops or ointment) antibiotic therapy.

    i. Erythromycin 5 mg/g ophthalmic ointment: ½ in. (1.25 cm) QID for 5 to 7 days.

    ii. Ciprofloxacin 0.3% ophthalmic drops (preferred agent in contact lens wearer): 1 to 2 drops QID for 5 to 7 days.

   d. Systemic antibiotics indicated for gonorrhea and chlamydia infections.

    i. Ceftriaxone 500 mg intramuscularly (IM), single dose. If chlamydia has not been excluded, addition of doxycycline 100 mg orally BID for 7 days is recommended.

D. Discharge instructions.

  1. Symptoms should resolve in 5 to 7 days.

  2. If symptoms continue or different symptoms appear, then follow-up is recommended.

FOLLOW-UP

A. Instruct patients with acute bacterial conjunctivitis to follow up in 1 to 2 days if symptoms worsen or do not improve.

B. Instruct patients with other forms of conjunctivitis to follow up within 2 weeks if symptoms worsen or do not improve.

CONSULTATION/REFERRAL

A. Consider referral to an allergy specialist for allergen testing in severe cases of allergic conjunctivitis.

B. Referral to an ophthalmologist for cases that are resistant to initial treatment.

C. Urgent referral to an ophthalmologist due to increased risk of vision loss.

  1. Hyperacute bacterial conjunctivitis.

  2. Keratitis.

  3. Varicella zoster ophthalmicus.

SPECIAL/GERIATRIC CONSIDERATIONS

A. Infants (highly susceptible to conjunctivitis).

  1. At risk for more serious complications.

  2. Prophylactically treated with optic antibiotics at birth.

  3. Conjunctival cultures are indicated in all suspected infectious neonatal cases.

B. Geriatric.

  1. Varicella zoster ophthalmicus can be sight-threatening.

  2. Vaccination against herpes zoster strongly recommended for adults starting at 50 years of age.

  3. Treatment options may be limited by comorbidities and drug interactions.

C. Contact lens wearers.

  1. Higher risk for keratitis: Careful evaluation to rule out keratitis is essential before diagnosis of conjunctivitis is made.

  2. Discontinue use until the eye has healed. Use can begin again when the eye is white and the patient has no discharge for 24 hours after completion of antibiotics.

D. Returning to school or work. This is appropriate 24 hours after antibiotics have been initiated or there is no discharge.

E. Awareness of local board of health reporting laws for sexually transmitted diseases (STDs). This is essential when the diagnosis of conjunctivitis is made in the setting of gonorrhea and chlamydia.

BIBLIOGRAPHY

Alfonso, S. A., Fawley, J. D., & Lu, X. A. (2015). Conjunctivitis. *Primary Care: Clinics in Office Practice*, 42(3), 325–345. https://doi.org/10.1016/j.pop.2015.05.001

Bielory, L. D., Delgado, L., Katelaris, C.H., Leonardi, A., Rosario, N., & Vichyanoud, P. (2020). ICON: Diagnosis and management of allergic conjunctivitis. *Annals of Allergy, Asthma & Immunology*, 124(2), 118–134. https://doi.org/10.1016/j.anai.2019.11.014

Chasco, G. C., Carreras-Castaner, X., Zboromyrska, Y., Pitart, C., Palma-Carvajal, F., Bosch, J., & Figueroa-Vercellino, J. P. (2021). Adult gonococcal conjunctivitis: Prevalence, clinical features and complications. *Journal of Medical Microbiology*, 70(9), 1–5. https://doi.org/10.1099/jmm.0.001416

Leonardi, A., Silva, D., Formigo, D. P., Bozkurt, B., Sharma, V., Allegri, P., Rondon, C., Calder, V., Ryan, D., Kowalski, M. L., Delgado, L., Doan, S., & Fauquert, J. L. (2019). Management of ocular allergy. *Allergy*, 74, 1611–1630. https://doi.org/10.1111/all.13786

McAnena, L., Knowles, S. J., Curry, A. S., & Cassidy, L. (2015). Prevalence of gonococcal conjunctivitis in adults and neonates. *Eye*, 29(7), 875–880. https://doi.org/10.1038/eye.2015.57

Varu, D. M., Rhee, M. K., Akpek, E. K., Amescua, G., Farid, M., Garcia-Ferrer, F. J., Lin, A., Musch, D. C., Mah, F. S., & Dunn, S. P. (2019). Conjunctivitis preferred practice pattern. *Ophthalmology*, 126, 94–169. https://doi.org/10.1016/j.ophtha.2018.10.020

PHARYNGITIS

DEFINITION
A. Inflammation of the pharynx.
B. Commonly referred to as a "sore throat."

INCIDENCE
A. Acute pharyngitis accounts for more than 12 million office and emergency/urgent care visits in the United States annually.
B. Viral pharyngitis occurs most frequently with 80% of the cases due to viruses. It occurs more frequently in the adult population.
C. Bacterial pharyngitis occurs more frequently in children and adolescents.
  1. Particularly the group A beta-hemolytic streptococci (GAS).
    a. Peak incidence occurs in 5 to 15 years age group.
    b. Only 5% to 15% of adults present with GAS.
  2. Bacterial pharyngitis occurs most frequently in late winter and early spring months.
D. Fungal etiologies account for a small percentage of the cases of pharyngitis.

PATHOGENESIS
A. Infectious.
  1. Viral.
    a. Adenoviruses and rhinoviruses responsible for most cases of viral pharyngitis.
    b. Other causes include:
      i. Herpes simplex virus (HSV) 1 and 2.
      ii. Coxsackievirus.
      iii. Human herpes virus 4 (Epstein–Barr virus [EBV]).
      iv. Human herpes virus 5 (cytomegalovirus).
      v. HIV.
  2. Bacterial.
    a. The most important causative agent is the GAS. It is the most common cause of bacterial pharyngitis.
      i. Severe complications of GAS warrant prompt identification and treatment.
    b. Other causes include:
      i. Group C streptococci.
      ii. *Neisseria gonorrhoeae.*
      iii. *Corynebacterium diphtheriae.*
      iv. *Treponema pallidum.*
      v. Mixed anaerobes.
  3. Fungal.
    a. Infrequent cause of pharyngitis.
    b. *Candida albicans* most common organism.
B. Noninfectious.
  1. Allergy.
  2. Irritants.
  3. Gastrointestinal reflux.

PREDISPOSING FACTORS
A. Exposure to infectious agents.
  1. Bacteria.
  2. Viruses.
  3. Fungi.
B. Exposure to allergens.
C. Exposure to environmental irritants.
D. History of gastrointestinal reflux.
E. History of immunosuppression.

SUBJECTIVE DATA
A. Common complaints/symptoms.
  1. "Sore throat."
  2. Difficulty swallowing.
  3. Nasal congestion.
  4. Sinus tenderness.
  5. Cough.
  6. Malaise.
  7. Headache.
  8. Distinguishing features of pharyngitis associated with GAS.
    a. Absent cough.
    b. Fever.
    c. Tonsillar exudates.
    d. Anterior cervical lymphadenopathy.
B. Common/typical scenario.
  1. Patients typically complain of sore or scratchy throat, fever, and general malaise. Symptom overlap is often present. Correct identification of pharyngitis type is essential to avoid more serious complications associated with bacterial or fungal pharyngitis.
C. Review of systems.
  1. Medical history.
    a. Recent illnesses.
      i. Determine the onset and duration of symptoms.
        1) Abrupt or gradual onset.
        2) Duration longer than 3 weeks unlikely to be pharyngitis.
    b. Sick contacts.
      i. Determine if the patient or close contacts have any systemic illnesses.
    c. Assess the patient for any risk factors.
  2. Allergies.
  3. Possible occupational exposure history.
  4. Travel history.
  5. Sexual history.
  6. Pertinent systems review.
    a. Constitutional.
      i. Fever.
      ii. Malaise.
    b. Head, ear, eyes, nose, and throat (HEENT).
      i. Sore throat.
      ii. Cough.
      iii. Rhinorrhea.

    iv. Nasal congestion.
    v. Headache.
    vi. Sinus tenderness/pain.
  c. Integumentary.
    i. Rash.
    ii. Lesions.

PHYSICAL EXAMINATION
A. Appearance of the pharynx.
  1. Pale to red.
  2. Mild erythema to profound edema.
  3. Vesicular lesions.
    a. HSV.
    b. Coxsackievirus.
B. Appearance of tonsils.
  1. Redness.
  2. Edema.
  3. Exudates.
    a. White (oropharyngeal candidiasis, GAS).
    b. Grayish membrane (diphtheria).
C. Lymph nodes.
  1. Cervical lymphadenopathy.
  2. Tonsillar lymphadenopathy.
D. Integumentary.
  1. Scarlatiniform rash may be present in GAS infections.
  2. Palatine petechiae may be present in GAS infection.
E. Red flags: All necessitate transfer to higher level of care with emergent airway protection.
  1. "Hot potato" voice.
    a. Garbled speech due to pharyngeal edema.
    b. Suggestive of peritonsillar abscess.
  2. Unilateral neck swelling.
  3. Difficulties with secretion management.
    a. Drooling.
    b. Compromised airway.
      i. Tonsillar pillars touching.
      ii. "Kissing tonsils."
  4. Uvula deviation.
    a. Indicative of peritonsillar abscess.

DIAGNOSTIC TESTS
A. Clinical examination: The modified Centor criteria is an algorithmic approach to facilitate decision-making in patients presenting with signs and symptoms of pharyngitis.
  1. Scoring system developed to quickly diagnose the likelihood of streptococcal pharyngitis.
  2. One point assigned for each of the following clinical findings: History of fever, tonsillar exudates, anterior cervical lymphadenopathy, and absence of cough (Figure 1.1).
  3. Empiric treatment based on symptoms, and higher Centor score is no longer recommended to prevent overprescribing of antibiotics.
B. Rapid antigen detection test (RADT).
  1. Indicated because clinical examination alone cannot always differentiate between viral and bacterial pharyngitis.
  2. Generally not necessary if overt viral symptoms are present (e.g., cough, rhinorrhea).

C. Throat culture.
  1. Pediatric.
    a. Indicated in children with negative RADT and clinical symptoms supportive of bacterial pharyngitis.
  2. Adults.
    a. Not necessary in adults with negative RADT due to low incidence of GAS in adults.
    b. Possibly indicated:
      i. In adults with negative RADT if there is high suspicion for GAS.
      ii. In adults at high risk for infection (immunocompromised or other comorbidities).
      iii. Those who are in close contact with high-risk populations.

DIFFERENTIAL DIAGNOSIS
A. Viral pharyngitis.
B. Bacterial pharyngitis.
C. Oropharyngeal candidiasis (thrush).
  1. Immunocompromised patients.
  2. Patients receiving broad-spectrum antibiotics or corticosteroids.
D. Gonococci.
  1. Possible in patients engaging in orogenital sex.
E. Diphtheria.
F. Mononucleosis.

EVALUATION AND MANAGEMENT PLAN
A. General plan.
  1. Pain relief.
    a. Over-the-counter (OTC) oral analgesics.
      i. Nonsteroidal anti-inflammatory drugs.
      ii. Acetaminophen.
      iii. Aspirin.
    b. Topical therapies.
      i. Lozenges.
      ii. Sprays.
      iii. Fluids (e.g., tea, honey).
    c. Environmental measures.
      i. Humidified air.
      ii. Avoidance of irritants.
    d. Glucocorticoid.
      i. Not recommended for routine use.
      ii. Limited role in patients with extreme sore throat and inability to swallow.
  2. Antibiotics only for confirmed bacterial infection.
B. Patient/family teaching points.
  1. Frequent hand hygiene to prevent spread.
C. Pharmacotherapy.
  1. Avoidance of empiric antibiotics.
    a. Overprescribing contributes to antibiotic resistance.
    b. Antimicrobial therapy generally does not benefit bacterial pharyngitis caused by infection other than streptococcal bacteria.
    c. Infections due to other organisms are possible but tend to be the exception.
      i. *N. gonorrhoeae.*
      ii. *C. diphtheriae.*

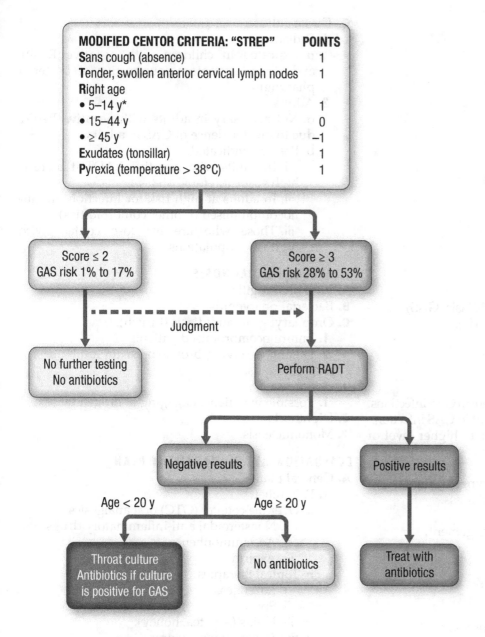

MODIFIED CENTOR CRITERIA: "STREP"	POINTS
Sans cough (absence)	1
Tender, swollen anterior cervical lymph nodes	1
Right age	
• 5–14 y*	1
• 15–44 y	0
• ≥ 45 y	–1
Exudates (tonsillar)	1
Pyrexia (temperature > 38°C)	1

Score ≤ 2
GAS risk 1% to 17%

Score ≥ 3
GAS risk 28% to 53%

Judgment

No further testing
No antibiotics

Perform RADT

Negative results

Positive results

Age < 20 y

Age ≥ 20 y

Throat culture
Antibiotics if culture
is positive for GAS

No antibiotics

Treat with
antibiotics

FIGURE 1.1 Modified Centor criteria for pharyngitis.

Source: From Sykes, E. A., Wu, V., Beyea, M. M., Simpson, M., & Beyea, J. A. (2020). Pharyngitis: Approach to diagnosis and treatment. *Canadian family physician Medecin de famille canadien, 66*(4), 251–257. https://www.ncbi.nlm.nih.gov/pmc/articles/PMC7145142/.

*The decision matrix has been defined for ages 5-14 y, because those younger than 3 y require backup validation with throat culture regardless of scoring.

GAS, group A beta-hemolytic streptococci; RADT, rapid antigen detection test.

2. Bacterial pharyngitis.
   a. Penicillin is the antibiotic of choice for GAS pharyngitis.
      i. 10-day course recommended.
   b. First-generation cephalosporin for penicillin allergies.
   c. Alternatively, a 5-day course of azithromycin is acceptable.
      i. Local and regional resistance has increasingly been reported.
3. Viral pharyngitis.
   a. Supportive care.
D. Discharge instructions.
   1. Follow-up is recommended if symptoms do not improve in 3 to 4 days.

FOLLOW-UP
A. Instruct patients to follow up if pharyngitis does not improve in 5 to 7 days.

B. Further evaluation indicated if no improvement or worsening of symptoms.
   1. Possible suppurative complication.
   2. Alternative diagnosis.

CONSULTATION/REFERRAL
A. Urgent referral to an otolaryngologist for suppurative complications.
   1. Peritonsillar abscess.
   2. Retropharyngeal abscess.
   3. Epiglottitis.

SPECIAL/GERIATRIC CONSIDERATIONS
A. Suppurative complications.
   1. Rare but potentially life-threatening complications of GAS pharyngitis.
   2. Early recognition and appropriate treatment essential to avoid associated morbidity and mortality.
   3. Complications include:

a. Peritonsillar abscess.

b. Retropharyngeal abscess.

c. Streptococcal bacteremia.

d. Epiglottitis.

B. Nonsuppurative complications.

  1. Rheumatic fever.

    a. Rare in developed countries.

  2. Poststreptococcal glomerulonephritis.

C. Other considerations.

  1. Morbilliform rash may develop in patients with pharyngitis caused by EBV who have been treated with penicillin or amoxicillin.

BIBLIOGRAPHY

Gunnarsson, R., Orda, U., Elliott, B., Heal, C., & Del Mar, C. (2022). What is the optimal strategy for managing primary care patients with an uncomplicated acute sore throat? Comparing the consequences of nine different strategies using a compilation of previous studies. *BMJ Open, 12*(4), e059069. https://doi.org/10.1136/bmjopen-2021-059069

McIsaac, W. J., White, D., Tannenbaum, D., & Low, D. E. (1998). A clinical score to reduce unnecessary antibiotic use in patients with sore throat. *Canadian Medical Association Journal, 158*(1), 75–83.

Ressner, R. (2020). Hidden harms in managing adult pharyngitis. *Military Medicine, 185*, e1385–1386. https://web.p.ebscohost.com/ehost/pdfviewer/pdfviewer?vid=0&sid=6e5a4bae-ff14-4b31-8bea-ad506d302d45%40redis

Shapiro, D., Lindgren, C., Neuman, M., & Fine, A. (2017). Viral features and testing for streptococcal pharyngitis. *Pediatrics, 139*(5), e20163403. https://doi.org/10.1542/peds.2016-3403

Sykes, E. A., Wu, V., Beyea, M. M., Simpson, M., & Beyea, J. A. (2020). Pharyngitis: Approach to diagnosis and treatment. *Canadian family physician Medecin de famille canadien, 66*(4), 251–257. https://www.ncbi.nlm.nih.gov/pmc/articles/PMC7145142/

van Driel, M. L., De Sutter, A. I. M., Thorning, S., & Christiaens, T. (2021). Different antibiotic treatments for group a streptococcal pharyngitis. *Cochrane Database of Systematic Reviews, 3*. https://doi.org/10.1002/14651858.CD004406.pub5

RHINOSINUSITIS

DEFINITION

A. Inflammation of the nasal cavity and paranasal sinuses.

B. Preferred terminology: "Rhinosinusitis" rather than "sinusitis" since inflammation of the sinuses rarely occurs without inflammation of the nasal mucosa as well.

C. Classification.

  1. Acute rhinosinusitis (ARS; Figure 1.2).

    a. Acute viral rhinosinusitis (AVRS; common cold): Lasts up to 10 days.

    b. Postviral (postviral ARS): Symptoms persisting past 10 days or worsening after 5 days.

  2. Bacteria (acute bacterial rhinosinusitis [ABRS]): Three or more clinical findings on physical exam.

    a. Fever >100.4°F/38°C.

    b. Severe local pain.

    c. Worsening symptoms after period of improvement (double sickening).

    d. Unilateral symptoms with purulent nasal discharge.

    e. Elevated erythrocyte sedimentation rate (ESR)/C-reactive protein (CRP) ratio.

  3. Chronic rhinosinusitis (CRS): Symptoms lasting greater than 12 weeks.

INCIDENCE

A. Viral infection due to rhinopharyngitis (common cold) is the most common cause of ARS.

B. Annually, one in seven to eight persons in the United States will experience an episode of ARS.

C. More frequent in women.

D. Higher in the 45- to 64-year-old age group.

E. ABRS accounts for less than 2% of cases of ARS.

PATHOGENESIS

A. Viral.

  1. Rhinovirus.

  2. Influenza virus.

  3. Parainfluenza virus.

B. Bacterial.

  1. *Streptococcus pneumoniae.*

  2. *Haemophilus influenzae.*

  3. *Moraxella catarrhalis.*

PREDISPOSING FACTORS

A. Older age.

B. Smoking.

C. Air travel.

D. Exposure to changes in atmospheric pressure.

E. Asthma and allergies.

  1. May be a predisposing factor but is controversial.

  2. ARS has been reported to be higher in patients with allergic rhinitis (AR) but studies were not conclusive.

  3. History may help distinguish between AR and ARS.

F. Swimming.

G. Dental disease.

H. Immunodeficiency.

SUBJECTIVE DATA

A. Common complaints/symptoms.

  1. Posterior rhinorrhea: One of the most common symptoms in adults.

  2. Hyposmia (reduced sense of smell): One of the most common symptoms in adults.

  3. Cough: Most common symptom in children.

  4. Nasal congestion.

  5. Nasal discharge, oftentimes thick yellow.

  6. Facial pressure or feeling of fullness, particularly when bending forward.

B. Other complaints.

  1. Fatigue.

  2. Headache.

  3. Difficulty sleeping.

  4. Toothache.

  5. Ear pain or fullness.

C. Family and social history.

  1. Family and social history is noncontributory.

D. Common/typical scenario.

  1. Common complaints.

    a. Fever.

    b. Sore throat.

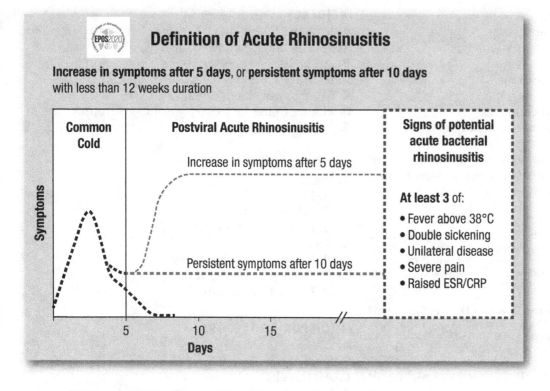

Definition of Acute Rhinosinusitis

Increase in symptoms after 5 days, or **persistent symptoms after 10 days** with less than 12 weeks duration

| Common Cold | Postviral Acute Rhinosinusitis | Signs of potential acute bacterial rhinosinusitis |

Increase in symptoms after 5 days

Persistent symptoms after 10 days

At least 3 of:
- Fever above 38°C
- Double sickening
- Unilateral disease
- Severe pain
- Raised ESR/CRP

Symptoms (y-axis) — *Days* (x-axis: 5, 10, 15)

FIGURE 1.2 Acute rhinosinusitis.

Source: From Jaume, F., Valls-Mateus, M., & Mullol, J. (2020). Common cold and acute rhinosinusitis: Up-to-date management in 2020. *Current Allergy and Asthma Reports,* *20*(7), 28. https://doi.org/10.1 007/s11882-020-00917-5

CRP, C-reactive protein; ESR, erythrocyte sedimentation rate.

c. Nasal discharge.
d. Facial pain.
e. Frontal pain or pressure that worsens when the patient bends forward.
2. Patients frequently complain of headaches.
E. Review of systems.
1. Medical history.
 a. Recent illnesses.
  i. Elicit onset and duration of symptoms.
 b. Sick contacts.
  i. Determine if the patient or close contacts have any systemic illnesses.
 c. Asthma.
2. Allergies.
3. Possible occupational exposure history.
4. Travel history.
5. Pertinent systems review.
 a. Constitutional.
  i. Fever.
  ii. Malaise.
 b. Head, ear, eyes, nose, and throat (HEENT).
  i. Sinus pain/tenderness.
  ii. Headache.
  iii. Nasal congestion.
  iv. Cough.
  v. Rhinorrhea.
  vi. Purulent discharge with bacterial infection.

PHYSICAL EXAMINATION
A. Appearance.
1. Erythema and/or edema of involved cheek.
2. Erythema and/or edema of periorbital area.

B. Drainage.
1. Mucopurulent: More likely ABRS.
2. Clear: More likely viral ARS.
C. Percussion.
1. Increased pain or tenderness of sinuses.
2. Not specific or sensitive test for diagnosis of rhinosinusitis.
D. Transillumination of frontal and maxillary sinuses.
1. Limited diagnostic value.
2. Not specific or sensitive test for diagnosis of rhinosinusitis.
E. Nasal examination.
1. Diffuse mucosal edema.
2. Narrowing of middle meatus.
3. Inferior turbinate hypertrophy.
4. Presence or absence of polyps.
 a. Presence may indicate anatomic risk for development of ABRS.

DIAGNOSTIC TESTS
A. Generally not indicated for uncomplicated cases of rhinosinusitis.
B. Nasal cultures are not useful in the diagnosis of ABRS.
C. Sinus aspiration is the definitive diagnostic test for organism identification.
1. Reserved for complicated cases.
2. Referral to otolaryngologist.
D. CT.
1. Persistent symptoms.
2. Recurrent symptoms.
3. Complicated ABRS.
4. Planning for sinus surgery.

DIFFERENTIAL DIAGNOSIS
A. Rhinosinusitis.
B. AR.
C. Rhinopharyngitis.
D. Headache.

EVALUATION AND MANAGEMENT PLAN
A. General plan.
  1. Use pain relief: Over-the-counter (OTC) analgesics and antipyretics.
  2. Reduce mucosal inflammation: Topical nasal corticosteroids.
  3. Enhance sinus drainage: Saline irrigation.
  4. Modulate environmental triggers.
    a. Treat concurrent AR symptoms if present with OTC antihistamines and allergy therapy as needed.
  5. Eradicate infection indicated for ABRS.
B. Patient/family teaching points.
  1. Frequent hand hygiene to prevent spread.
C. Pharmacotherapy.
  1. Acute sinusitis.
    a. Most cases of acute sinusitis are viral, and pharmacotherapy is targeted to symptomatic relief.
      i. OTC analgesics and antipyretics.
      ii. Saline nasal irrigation.
        1) Mechanical irrigation of nasal passages.
        2) Use only sterile or bottled water irrigants to avoid risk of rare amebic encephalitis complication with use of tap water irrigants.
      iii. Intranasal corticosteroids.
        1) Most beneficial in patients with concomitant symptoms of AR.
        2) Increased symptom improvement achieved with higher corticosteroid dose.
        3) Useful when combined with nasal saline sprays.
      iv. Intranasal sprays.
        1) Moistens and loosens secretions in nasal passages.
        2) May temporarily increase nasal passage patency.
        3) Ensure saline sprays are sterile.
      v. Intranasal decongestants.
        1) May provide subjective relief of symptoms.
        2) No evidence to support use.
        3) Use not to exceed 3 to 5 days to avoid rebound congestion.
      vi. Antihistamines.
        1) No clinical studies support use in viral sinusitis.
      vii. Expectorants and cough suppressants.
        1) Clinical studies do not support efficacy in use for ARS.
    b. Suspected bacterial sinusitis.
      i. Classic progression is mild symptoms that begin to resolve and then suddenly become worse.
      ii. Watchful waiting: Plan to follow up if symptoms worsen or do not improve in 10 days. The majority of cases of uncomplicated ABRS resolve within 14 days. Given the rise in antibiotic resistance, antibiotics should be reserved for use in vulnerable populations such as pediatrics, immunosuppressed, cases of severe rhinosinusitis, or those with persistent symptoms. Referral to an otolaryngologist is recommended.
      iii. Nonmacrolide therapy.
        1) Amoxicillin/clavulanate 875/125 mg orally BID for 5 to 7 days.
        2) Doxycycline 200 mg orally daily for 5 to 7 days for penicillin (PCN) allergies.
      iv. OTC analgesics and antipyretics.
      v. Saline irrigation.
        1) Use as adjuvant to corticosteroids in chronic sinusitis.
      vi. Intranasal corticosteroid spray.
        1) Increased symptom improvement achieved with higher corticosteroid dose.
        2) Useful when combined with nasal saline sprays.
  2. Chronic sinusitis.
    a. Initial management is intranasal corticosteroid spray. Spray should be used on a routine basis and not as a rescue medication.
    b. Saline irrigation can be used alone or in addition to intranasal corticosteroid sprays. Irrigation should be performed prior to intranasal corticosteroid spray.
    c. Consider a short course of nonmacrolide therapy if active mucopurulence is present on examination.
    d. For patients with persistent symptoms.
      i. Systemic corticosteroids are not recommended due to potential side effects.
      ii. Macrolide therapy is a treatment option due to its immunomodulatory effects.
    e. Topical antibiotics and antifungals are not recommended in the treatment of chronic sinusitis.

FOLLOW-UP
A. Patients should be instructed to follow up if symptoms do not improve in 7 days.
B. Further evaluation is indicated if no improvement or worsening of symptoms.

CONSULTATION/REFERRAL
A. Persistent cases should be referred to otolaryngology.
  1. Endoscopic nasal evaluation.
  2. Endoscopic nasal surgery.

SPECIAL/GERIATRIC CONSIDERATIONS
A. Long-term use of nasogastric tubes can put patients at risk for developing sinusitis.

BIBLIOGRAPHY

Carter, A., Dattani, N., & Hannan, S. A. (2019). Chronic rhinosinusitis. *BMJ*, *364*(l131). https://doi.org/10.1136/bmj.l131

Cevc, G. (2017). Differential diagnosis and proper treatment of acute rhinosinusitis: Guidance based on historical data analysis. *Allergy & Rhinology*, *8*(2), e45–e52. Advance online publication. https://doi.org/10.2500/ar.2017.8.0206

Jaume, F., Valls-Mateus, M., & Mullol, J. (2020). Common cold and acute rhinosinusitis: Up-to-Date management in 2020. *Current Allergy and Asthma Reports*, *20*(7), 28. https://doi.org/10.1007/s11882-020-00917-5

Lees, K. A., Orlandi, R. R., Oakley, G., & Alt, J.A. (2020). The role of macrolides and doxycycline in chronic rhinosinusitis. *Immunology and Allergy Clinics of North America*, *40*(2), 303–315. https://doi.org/10.1016/j.iac.2019.12.005

Lemiengre, M. B., van Driel, M. L., Merenstein, D., Liira, H., Mäkelä, M., & De Sutter, A. I. M. (2018). Antibiotics for acute rhinosinusitis in adults. *Cochrane Database of Systematic Reviews*, *9*. https://www.cochranelibrary.com/cdsr/doi/10.1002/14651858.CD006089.pub5/full

KNOWLEDGE CHECK: CHAPTER 1

1. A 25-year-old patient reports right eye redness and discharge for the past 2 days. The patient states that their eye is "stuck together" upon awakening in the morning, with a yellow crust, and that the discharge thins as the day progresses. There is no report of pain, but the patient states that their eye is itchy. The patient denies any vision changes, photophobia, foreign body sensation, or recent trauma. The patient does not wear contact lenses. The recommended treatment for the presumed diagnosis is:

   A. Ceftriaxone 50 mg intramuscularly (IM) once plus doxycycline 100 mg BID for 7 days.
   B. Ciprofloxacin 0.3% ophthalmic drops 1 to 2 drops QID for 5 to 7 days.
   C. Ganciclovir 0.15% ophthalmic gel Q3H, 5 times daily.
   D. Ketotifen 0.025% (Alaway OTC, Zaditor) 1 to 2 drops in each eye BID.

2. A 17-year-old patient presents to the urgent care setting reporting sore throat, fever of 101.12°F/38.4°C, and malaise. The patient denies any cough, nausea, or vomiting. They work as a server at a local restaurant and report that their coworker has the same symptoms. On physical exam, the patient has cervical lymphadenopathy and the tonsils are inflamed with a white exudate. Which of the following is the best course of action for this patient?

   A. Admit to hospital with urgent referral to otolaryngology.
   B. Begin empiric antibiotics to avoid suppurative complications.
   C. Obtain a rapid antigen detection test (RADT).
   D. Order topical anesthetic spray and antipyretic medication.

3. The pathogens responsible for the majority of bacterial pharyngitis cases are:

   A. Adenoviruses.
   B. Group A *Streptococcus*.
   C. *Neisseria gonorrhoeae*.
   D. *Treponema pallidum*.

4. A 45-year-old patient is referred from their primary care provider to the otolaryngology office for evaluation of a 2-week history of unilateral sinus pain, mucopurulent nasal discharge, fever, and hyposmia. What is the most likely diagnosis for this patient?

   A. Acute bacterial rhinosinusitis
   B. Acute viral rhinosinusitis
   C. Chronic bacterial rhinosinusitis
   D. Postviral acute rhinosinusitis

5. Initial treatment of the patient with chronic rhinosinusitis (CRS) should include:

   A. Intranasal corticosteroids.
   B. Nonmacrolide therapy.
   C. Sinus surgery.
   D. Systemic corticosteroids.

(See answers next page.)

1. **D) Ketotifen 0.025% (Alaway OTC, Zaditor) 1 to 2 drops in each eye BID**
Presentation is consistent with allergic conjunctivitis. Treatment is supportive mast cell stabilizers, which can be obtained over the counter. Topical antihistamines can also be applied for symptomatic relief. Ceftriaxone 50 mg is the systemic treatment for gonorrhea and chlamydia and would be indicated for gonococcal conjunctivitis. Ciprofloxacin 0.3% ophthalmic drops are the treatment for bacterial conjunctivitis. Ganciclovir 0.15% ophthalmic gel is the treatment for herpes simplex keratitis.

2. **C) Obtain a rapid antigen detection test (RADT).**
The patient's modified Centor score is 4. Her symptoms are strongly suggestive of group A beta-hemolytic streptococcal infection. An RADT is indicated. Empiric antibiotics are no longer recommended to avoid antibiotic resistance and overprescribing. Only if the RADT is positive should antibiotics (10-day course of PCN) be started. If RADT is negative, throat cultures are recommended in patients younger than 20 years. If throat cultures are positive, antibiotics should be started; if they are negative, supportive care is indicated. The patient does not exhibit symptoms of airway compromise and thus does not need to be admitted or need an otolaryngology consult.

3. **B) Group A *Streptococcus***
Group A *Streptococcus* is the most common pathogen responsible for bacterial pharyngitis. Adenoviruses are the most common pathogens responsible for viral pharyngitis. *Neisseria gonorrhoeae* and *Treponema pallidum* are less frequent causes of bacterial pharyngitis.

4. **A) Acute bacterial rhinosinusitis**
The patient's symptoms are consistent with acute bacterial rhinosinusitis (ABRS). Bacterial symptoms are present. Viral symptoms would be unlikely to include fever or unilateral pain. Discharge is expected to be clear rather than mucopurulent.

5. **A) Intranasal corticosteroids**
The initial treatment in chronic rhinosinusitis (CRS) includes intranasal corticosteroids with or without saline irrigation. Systemic corticosteroids are not recommended and have no role in the treatment of CRS. Nonmacrolide therapy is indicated for acute bacterial rhinosinusitis, but with CRS macrolide therapy is a treatment option.

CHAPTER 2

PULMONARY GUIDELINES

E. Moneé Carter-Griffin

ACUTE RESPIRATORY DISTRESS SYNDROME

DEFINITION

A. Acute respiratory distress syndrome (ARDS) is a life-threatening syndrome resulting in acute, severe lung injury characterized by inflammation, hypoxemia, and diffuse lung involvement.
B. ARDS is defined by three variables using the Berlin definition.
    1. Bilateral opacities on imaging not fully explained by cardiac failure or volume overload.
    2. Onset within 7 days of a clinical event or worsening respiratory symptoms.
    3. Hypoxemia defined by the PF ratio (PaO_2/FiO_2) and a minimum positive end-expiratory pressure greater than or equal to 5 cm H_2O.
C. ARDS severity is classified based on the degree of hypoxemia (PF ratio) and identified as mild, moderate, or severe.
    1. Mild ARDS: Less than or equal to 300 mmHg.
    2. Moderate ARDS: Less than or equal to 200 mmHg.
    3. Severe ARDS: Less than or equal to 100 mmHg.

INCIDENCE

A. It is difficult to obtain an accurate incidence due to variations in the definition used to identify or describe ARDS.
B. An estimated 190,000 to 200,000 cases of ARDS occur each year in the United States.
C. The incidence increases with advancing age.
D. ARDS has not been shown to occur more in one sex than the other; however, males have been shown to have a higher average ARDS-related mortality rate.
E. Mortality and morbidity are associated with worsening of the PF ratio.
F. Morality rates have improved; however, the rates remain as high as 40% in those with severe ARDS.
G. Literature demonstrates relative race disparities in mortality rates.

PATHOGENESIS

A. An indirect or direct insult causes an inflammatory response and accumulation of proinflammatory mediators in the lung microcirculation. Injury occurs to the microvascular endothelium and alveolar epithelium. Endothelium injury leads to capillary permeability and migration of protein-rich fluid into the alveolar space. Due to injury of the alveolar epithelium, pulmonary edema forms and damage occurs to the cells lining the alveoli.
B. Damage to type I and II cells leads to decreased clearance of fluid in the pleural space, increased fluid entry into the alveoli, and decreased surfactant production resulting in decreased alveolar compliance and alveoli collapse.
C. An influx of fibroblasts leads to collagen deposition and possibly fibrosis.

PREDISPOSING FACTORS

A. Aspiration, including gastric content and drowning.
B. Sepsis.
C. Pneumonia.
D. Massive transfusions.
E. Pancreatitis.
F. Burns.
G. Trauma, including cases with and without pulmonary injury.
H. Underlying interstitial lung disease.
I. Drug toxicity, especially inhalation.
J. Coronavirus disease 2019 (COVID-19).

SUBJECTIVE DATA

A. Common complaints/symptoms.
    1. Severe dyspnea.
    2. Chest discomfort.
    3. Tachypnea.
B. Common/typical scenario.
    1. Onset is typically 12 to 48 hours after the insult.
    2. History shows progressive worsening symptoms.
    3. Extrapulmonary complaints may have led to the development of ARDS.

PHYSICAL EXAMINATION

A. Dyspnea (Figure 2.1).
B. Tachypnea.
C. Abdominal retractions; obvious respiratory distress.
D. Hypoxia and possibly cyanosis.
E. Tachycardia.
F. Altered mental status, agitation, or confusion.
G. Rales during auscultation.
H. Additional findings that may relate to the underlying etiology of ARDS (e.g., febrile, hypotension, an acute abdomen, nausea and vomiting seen in pancreatitis).

DIAGNOSTIC TESTS

A. Chest x-ray (CXR).
    1. Patchy infiltrates rapidly evolve and progress to diffuse, bilateral infiltrates.

Obtain the History

Quality/sensation, timing, precipitating factors, alleviating factors, any associated factors.
- Gradual or sudden onset?
- Continuous or episodic?
- Occur with exertion or at rest?
- Positional?

Physical Examination

General: Positioning? Accessory muscle use? Paradoxical abdominal movement? Overt distress? Able to speak in full sentences? Audible stridor?
Vital signs: Tachycardia? Tachypnea? Pulsus paradoxus? Oxygen desaturations?
Cardiac: Elevated JVD? Murmur? S3 or S4 gallop? Edema?
Respiratory: Adventitious breath sounds such as crackles/rales, wheezes, or diminished? Chest shape? Dullness or hyperresonance on percussion? Respiratory pattern? Symmetrical chest movement?
Extremities: Cyanosis? Edema? Clubbing?

The physical exam should always focus on airway, breathing, circulation first. Proceed with a full exam in the stable patient

Initial Diagnostics

Chest x-ray: Evidence of pulmonary edema? Pneumonia? Pleural effusion? Hyperinflation of the lungs suggestive of obstructive disease? Heart size? Lung volumes? Elevation of hemidiaphragm?
EKG: To assess for myocardial injury or ischemia.

Respiratory

ABG: Assess for hypercapnia or hypoxemia
D-dimer, age-adjusted: Can aid in ruling out a pulmonary embolus.
Chest CT/Angiography: Assess for pneumonia, emphysematous changes, fluid, honeycombing suggestive of fibrosis, pulmonary embolus.
Pulmonary function testing: Assess for obstructive or restrictive disease.

Cardiovascular

Echocardiogram: Assess heart size, function, valves, pulmonary pressures, pericardial effusion, and so forth.
NT-proBNP: Can aid in the diagnosis of heart failure in the appropriate clinical context.

Additional Testing

Thyroid studies: Assess for hyperthyroidism (high cardiac output state).
Hemoglobin/Hematocrit: Assess for anemia.
Cardiopulmonary exercise test: Can help distinguish between the two by indicating ischemic changes on EKG (cardiac), bronchospasm during exercise (respiratory), and so forth.

FIGURE 2.1 Algorithm for the evaluation of dyspnea.

ABG, arterial blood gas; JVD, jugular venous distention; NT-proBNP, N-terminal probrain natriuretic peptide.

2. Daily CXRs may be required, especially for patients on mechanical ventilation.
B. Arterial blood gas (ABG).
1. Regular ABGs may or may not be required to evaluate management pending the severity of ARDS, associated medical treatment (e.g., mechanical ventilation), and/or changes in medical management.
2. Initially, patients may present with respiratory alkalosis (increased pH and decreased CO_2).
3. As the ARDS progressively worsens, respiratory acidosis develops (decreased pH and rising CO_2).
4. Hypoxemia is defined by the PF ratio.
C. Complete blood count (CBC).
1. Evaluate the white blood cell count and platelets.
D. Comprehensive metabolic panel.
1. Evaluate renal and liver function.

2. Magnesium and phosphorus: Strict electrolyte repletion is necessary for cardiac stability and prevention of arrhythmias, especially in the setting of profound tissue hypoxia and/or septic shock, which is often concomitant.
E. Coagulation studies.
1. Prothrombin time and international normalized ratio (INR).
2. Fibrinogen level.
3. Fibrin degradation products.
F. N-terminal probrain natriuretic peptide (NT-proBNP) level.
1. This is used to assess for heart failure causing or contributing to the bilateral infiltrates and hypoxemia.
2. It is important for the clinician to note this value may be elevated secondary to etiologies other than heart failure, such as sepsis and renal failure.

G. Blood cultures.

    1. Evaluate infective etiology as a source of ARDS development.

H. Systemic infection markers.

    1. Lactic acid: Measure the level of tissue hypoxia and dysfunction. Trending the lactic acid may be appropriate pending the suspected or actual etiology for ARDS.

    2. Procalcitonin: Consider trending every 48 to 72 hours as an adjunct to the overall clinical evaluation and as a strategy to aid with antibiotic discontinuation in select patient populations.

I. Urinalysis and urine culture.

    1. Evaluate infective etiology as source of ARDS development.

J. Sputum culture.

    1. Evaluate infective etiology as a source of ARDS development.

DIFFERENTIAL DIAGNOSIS

A. Asthma.

B. Chronic obstructive pulmonary disease (COPD).

C. Congestive heart failure (CHF).

D. Acute eosinophilic pneumonia.

E. Diffuse alveolar hemorrhage.

F. Pneumonia.

EVALUATION AND MANAGEMENT PLAN

A. Treatment is dependent on the severity of ARDS.

    1. Oxygen therapy (e.g., high-flow nasal cannula, noninvasive positive pressure ventilation, invasive mechanical ventilation).

    a. In acute hypoxemic respiratory failure, high-flow nasal cannula may be necessary. It results in improved mortality at 90 days compared with non-invasive and invasive mechanical ventilation.

    b. Lung protective ventilation is the primary aim of invasive mechanical ventilatory support.

       i. Lung protective ventilation aims to prevent overdistention of the lung alveoli. Overdistention of the alveoli has been shown to disrupt the pulmonary endothelium and epithelium, resulting in the release of inflammatory mediators, further inflammation, and hypoxemia.

       ii. Lung protective ventilation is aimed at low tidal volumes based on the predicted body weight (PBW), use of positive end expiratory pressure (PEEP), and low plateau pressures.

    c. Invasive mechanical ventilation: Recommended tidal volume of 4 to 8 mL/kg PBW and maintaining plateau pressures less than 30 cm H_2O.

       i. Ideally, the initial tidal volume should be set at 6 mL/kg PBW.

       ii. Lower tidal volumes of 4 to 5 mL/kg PBW may be required if one is unable to obtain a plateau pressures less than 30 cm H_2O.

       iii. Plateau pressures less than 30 cm H_2O may not be attainable in obese patients.

       iv. Low tidal volumes usually result in hypoventilation. Permissive hypercapnia is typically accepted to a pH of 7.20.

    d. PEEP is an integral part of mechanical ventilation in ARDS.

       i. Multiple titration strategies have been used in the literature with varying results on patient outcomes.

       ii. PEEP of at least 5 cm H_2O is recommended.

       iii. Higher PEEP levels may be warranted in patients with moderate to severe ARDS.

       iv. Dynamic PEEP adjustment may be required to ensure low plateau pressures and adequate oxygenation that align with an overall lung protective strategy.

    e. Targeting an oxygen saturation of 88% or greater is sufficient for ARDS management.

       i. No indication of targeting a higher oxygen saturation (e.g., greater than 95%) improves outcomes.

    f. Weaning from mechanical ventilation is typically initiated once the patient requires 50% or less FiO_2, physiologic levels of PEEP, hemodynamically stable, assessed neurological status, and so forth.

    2. Positioning.

    a. Studies have shown prone positioning results in decreased mortality and improved oxygenation.

       i. Recommended to start early in those with moderate to severe and severe ARDS.

       ii. Prone positioning ideally should occur for greater than 12 hours per day before supine positioning.

    b. Prone positioning requires the patient to be hemodynamically stable while proning, adequate sedation and paralytics, well-trained staff to care for the patient, and adequate space for the equipment (if used).

    c. Consider cessation of prone positioning in those with a PF ratio consistently above 150 mmHg in the supine position.

    3. Conservative fluid management.

    a. Increased ventilator-free days but no difference in mortality.

    b. Initial fluid resuscitation depends on the underlying etiology of the development of ARDS. Conditions such as hemorrhagic shock and pancreatitis initially require more aggressive fluid management.

    c. Guidelines for fluid resuscitation should be followed for certain diagnoses, such as sepsis, pancreatitis, and so forth.

B. Pharmacotherapy.

    1. Neuromuscular blockades and sedatives.

    a. Minimizing sedation to achieve compliance with ventilation and early mobilization show improved outcomes in the ICU setting when clinically appropriate in mild–moderate ARDS.

b. Daily sedation vacation and ventilator liberation procedures should be initiated when oxygen requirements are compatible with extubation.

c. Neuromuscular blockades should be administered in combination with sedatives.

i. Paralytics should be considered with ventilatory dyssynchrony and difficulty with ventilation such as poor airway compliance.

ii. Early administration in severe ARDS has not been associated with increased muscle weakness.

iii. Associated with decreased risk of barotrauma and improved oxygenation after 48 hours.

iv. Should be administered early in ARDS and by continuous infusion with daily evaluation for need.

v. A commonly used paralytic is cisatracurium.

2. Corticosteroids: Evidence is lacking to recommend for or against steroid use in ARDS.

a. Steroids may be appropriate for conditions (e.g., diffuse alveolar hemorrhage) mimicking ARDS.

3. Antibiotics are indicated in patients with an infective etiology.

4. Inhaled nitric oxide has not shown to improve outcomes and has been associated with renal dysfunction.

5. Deep vein thrombosis (DVT) and stress ulcer prophylaxis is required.

a. Heparin or enoxaparin (Lovenox) is used for DVT prophylaxis. The renal function will dictate the use of heparin versus enoxaparin.

b. DVT prophylaxis is often held in patients with significant coagulopathies.

c. Proton pump inhibitors (e.g., pantoprazole) or H2 receptor antagonists (e.g., famotidine) are for stress ulcer prophylaxis.

C. Other treatment methods.

1. High-frequency ventilation: Has not shown to improve outcomes and some evidence suggests it may increase mortality.

2. Venovenous extracorporeal membrane oxygenation (VV ECMO).

a. Not recommended for all patients with ARDS.

i. May be appropriate for select patients with severe ARDS.

b. Limited evidence to support regular use and no guidelines for widespread use.

c. Limited to certain institutions, and patient selection criteria may vary.

d. Associated with improved outcomes if used earlier in ARDS.

FOLLOW-UP

A. This is dependent on the patient's clinical course, outcomes, and length of hospital stay.

CONSULTATION/REFERRAL

A. Consultation with a pulmonologist and/or intensivist is ideal for management of mechanical ventilation and critical care needs.

B. Additional consultation may be required depending on the underlying etiology of ARDS (e.g., trauma, infectious disease).

C. Ancillary staff (e.g., physical therapy, nutrition) may be required pending the severity of ARDS and subsequent patient needs.

SPECIAL/GERIATRIC CONSIDERATIONS

A. Open communication with the family is required.

B. Nutritional support is recommended. The preferred route is enteral.

C. Patients with prolonged mechanical ventilation—typically greater than 14 days—should undergo tracheostomy placement.

BIBLIOGRAPHY

Adhikari, N. K., Dellinger, R. P., Lundin, S., Payen, D., Vallet, B., Gerlack, H., Park, K. W., Mehta, S., Slutsky, A. S., & Friedrich, J. O. (2014). Inhaled nitric oxide does not reduce mortality in patients with acute respiratory distress syndrome regardless of severity: Systematic review and meta-analysis. *Critical Care Medicine, 42*, 404–412. https://doi.org/10.1097/CCM.0b013e3182a27909

Cavalcanti, A. B., Suzumura, R. A., Laranjeira, L. N., de Mores Paisani, D., Damiani, L. P., Guimaraes, H. P., Romano, E. R., Regenga, M. M., Taniguchi, L. N. T., Teixeira, C., Oliveira, R. P., Machado, F. R., Diaz-Quijano, F. A., Filho, M. S. A., Maia, I. S., Caser, E. B., Filho, W. O., Borges, M. C., Martins, M. A. ... Ribeiro de Carvalho, C. R. (2017). Effect of lung recruitment and titrated positive end-expiratory-pressure (peep) vs low peep on mortality in patients with acute respiratory distress syndrome: A randomized clinical trial. *Journal of American Medical Association, 318*, 1335–1345. https://doi.org/10.1001/jama.2017.14171

Cochi, S. E., Kempker, J. A., Annangi, S., Kramer, M. R., & Martin, G. S. (2016). Mortality trends of acute respiratory distress syndrome in the United States from 1999 to 2013. *Annals of the American Thoracic Society, 13*, 1742–1751. https://doi.org/10.1513/AnnalsATS.201512-841OC

Evans, L., Rhodes, A., Alhazzani, W., Antonelli, M., Coopersmith, C. M., French, C., Machado, F. R., Mcintyre, L., Ostermann, M., Prescott, H. C., Schorr, C., Simpson, S., Wiersinga, W. J., Alshamsi, F., Angus, D. C., Arabi, Y., Azevedo, L., Beale, R., Beilman, G. ... Levy, M. (2021). Surviving sepsis campaign: International guidelines for management of sepsis and septic shock 2021. *Critical Care Medicine, 49*, e1063–e1143. https://doi.org/10.1097/CCM.0000000000005337

Fan, E., Del Sorbo, L., Goligher, E. C., Hodgson, C. L., Munshi, L., Walkey, A. J., Adhikari, N. K. J., Amato, M. B. P., Branson, R., Brower, R. G., Ferguson, N. D., Gajic, O., Gattinoni, L., Hess, D., Mancebo, J., Meade, M. O., McAuley, D. F., Pesenti, A., Ranieri, V. M. ... Brochard, L. J. (2017). An official American Thoracic Society/European Society of Intensive Care Medicine/Society of Critical Care Medicine clinical practice guideline: Mechanical ventilation in adult patients with acute respiratory distress syndrome. *American Journal of Respiratory and Critical Care Medicine, 195*, 1253–1263. https://doi.org/10.1164/rccm.201703-0548ST

Ferguson, N. D., Fan, E., Camporota, L., Antonelli, M., Anzueto, A., Beale, R., & Ranieri, V. M. (2012). The Berlin definition of ARDS: An expanded rationale, justification, and supplementary material. *Intensive Care Medicine, 38*, 1573–1582. https://doi.org/10.1007/s00134-012-2682-1

Fernando, S. M., Ferreyro, B. L., Urner, M., Munshi, L., & Fan, E. (2021). Diagnosis and management of acute respiratory distress syndrome. *Canadian Medical Association Journal, 193*, E761–E768. https://doi.org/10.1503/cmaj.202661

Frat, J. P., Thille, A. W., Mercat, A., Girault, C., Ragot, S., Perbet, S., & Robert, R. (2015). High-flow oxygen through nasal cannula in acute hypoxemic respiratory failure. *New England Journal of Medicine, 372*, 2185–2196. https://doi.org/10.1056/NEJMoa1503326

Griffiths, M. J. D., McAuley, D. F., Perkins, G. D., Barrett, N., Blackwood, B., Boyle, A., Chee, N., Connolly, B., Dark, P., Finney, S., Salam, A., Silversides, J., Tarmey, N., Wise, M. P., & Baudoin, S. V. (2019). Guidelines on the management of acute respiratory distress syndrome. *BMJ Open Respiratory Research, 6*, 1–27. https://doi.org/10.1136/bmjresp-2019-000420

Guerin, C., Reignier, J., Richard, J. C., Beuret, P., Gacouin, A., Boulain, T., Mercier, E., Badet, M., Mercat, A., Baudin, O., Clavel, M., Chatellier, D., Jaber, S., Rosselli, S., Mancebo, J., Sirodot, M., Hilbert, G., Bengler, C., Richecoeur, J. … Ayzac, L. (2013). Prone positioning in severe acute respiratory distress syndrome. *New England Journal of Medicine, 368*, 2159–2168. https://doi.org/10.1056/NEJMoa1214103

Liaqat, A., Mason, M., Foster, B. J., Kulkarni, S., Barlas, A., Farooq, A. M., Patak, P., Liaqat, H., Basso, R. G., Zaman, M. S., & Pau, D. (2022). Evidence-based mechanical ventilatory strategies in ards. *Journal of Clinical Medicine, 11*, 1–12. https://doi.org/10.3390/jcm11020319

Papaziana, L., Aubron, C., Brochard, L., Chiche, J. D., Combes, A., Dreyfuss, D., Forel, J. M., Guerin, C., Jaber, S., Mekontso-Dessap, A., Mercat, A., Richard, J. C., Roux, D., Viellard-Baron, A., & Faure, H. (2019). Formal guidelines: Management of acute respiratory distress syndrome. *Annals of Intensive Care, 9*, 1–18. https://doi.org/10.1186/s13613-019-0540-9

Saguil, A., & Fargo, M. V. (2020). Acute respiratory distress syndrome: Diagnosis and management. *American Family Physician, 101*, 730–738. https://www.aafp.org/afp/2020/0615/p730.html

ASTHMA

DEFINITION
A. A chronic airway inflammatory disease defined by a variation in expiratory airflow limitation and history of respiratory symptoms that vary in intensity over time. There are various asthma phenotypes, such as allergic asthma and late-onset asthma.

INCIDENCE
A. Approximately 25 million people in the United States currently have asthma.
B. It is estimated that 20 million adults currently have asthma.
C. Asthma accounts for greater than 183,000 hospitalizations, 1.6 million ED visits, and approximately 7 million office visits.
D. The prevalence in adults is highest in women and African Americans.

PATHOGENESIS
A. Interplay among host factors and environmental exposures, resulting in airway inflammation, airflow obstruction, and bronchial hyperresponsiveness.
  1. Immune response to antigen, causing activation of T-lymphocytes.
  2. Release of cytokines and interleukins, leading to a release of mast cells, eosinophils, and basophils.
  3. Subsequent release of inflammatory mediators (e.g., histamine, prostaglandins) that cause airway inflammation and mucus secretion.
B. Resulting development of airway hyperplasia, airway obstruction, and bronchial hyperresponsiveness.

PREDISPOSING FACTORS
A. Direct and indirect exposure to tobacco smoke.
B. Allergens (e.g., animals such as cats and dogs, dust mites, pollen).
C. Occupational exposures or irritants (e.g., paint, sprays).
D. Pollution.
E. Respiratory infections.
F. Exercise.
G. Stress.
H. Gastroesophageal reflux disease (GERD).
I. Obesity.
J. Sex (more likely in female adults).
K. Viral infections.

SUBJECTIVE DATA
A. Common complaints/symptoms.
  1. Respiratory symptoms (e.g., wheezing, dyspnea, chest tightness, cough).
  2. Possible extrapulmonary manifestations (e.g., allergic skin conditions, conjunctival irritation).
B. History of the present illness.
  1. Onset of asthma and/or symptoms.
  2. Precipitating factors.
  3. Asthma symptom control such as frequency of reliever inhaler use.
  4. Comorbid conditions (e.g., rhinosinusitis, obstructive sleep apnea) that may contribute to the patient to developing poor asthma control, symptoms, and/or poor quality of life.
  5. Number of exacerbations in the past year.
  6. History of ED visits, hospitalizations, and intubations related to asthma.
C. Family and social history.
  1. Family history of asthma.
  2. Social history such as smoking and inhaled illicit drug use.
  3. Employment/environmental factors (e.g., working outside, mining operations, military service).

PHYSICAL EXAMINATION
A. The physical examination may vary depending on the severity of the asthma and if the patient is having an exacerbation.
B. Expiratory wheezing on auscultation may be audible (Figure 2.2). Expiratory wheezing may also be audible without auscultation.
C. Dyspnea may be evident (see Figure 2.1).
D. Changes in mentation (e.g., confusion, lethargy) may be apparent.10
E. Patients with moderate to severe asthma exacerbations may be in a tripod position and have tachypnea, absent breath sounds (silent chest) on auscultation, accessory muscle use (e.g., intercostal), and tachycardia.
F. Some patients may have extrapulmonary symptoms such as dermatitis, conjunctival irritation, and a swollen nasal mucosa.

DIAGNOSTIC TESTS
A. Lung function. Initial diagnosis is based on a history of a characteristic pattern of variable respiratory symptoms (e.g., wheezing, dyspnea) and confirmed variation in expiratory airflow limitation. Lung function can vary between normal to complete obstruction.

Obtain the History

Onset, quality, precipitating factors, alleviating factors, any associated factors.
- Acute or gradual onset?
- Associated with other symptoms such as dyspnea, cough, hoarseness, flushing, pruritus, chest discomfort/tightness, and so forth?
- Triggers such as exercise, fumes/smoke, allergens, and so forth?
- Medication or food allergies? Initiation of new medications?
- Comorbid conditions such as asthma, COPD, heart failure, myocardial infarction, GERD, and so forth?
- Recent respiratory infections?
- Current or history of smoking?
- Prior intubations? History of throat or neck cancer, surgeries, and so forth?
- Aspiration?

Completed in the stable patient with wheezing

Physical Examination

General: Accessory muscle use? Diaphoresis? Flushing?
Vital signs: Febrile? Tachypnea? Tachycardia? Oxygen desaturations?
HEENT: Facial or lip/oropharynx swelling? Central cyanosis? Rhinorrhea? Redness and/or watery eyes? Assessment of voice quality?
Neck: Surgical scars? Old tracheostomy sites? Swelling? Goiter? Tracheal deviation? High pitched noises or stridor on auscultation?
Cardiac: Elevated JVD? Murmur? S3 or S4 gallop? Edema?
Respiratory: Inspiratory or expiratory wheezing? Other adventitious breath sounds such as crackles? Diminished breath sounds? Chest shape? Respiratory pattern? Retractions? Dullness or hyperresonance on percussion?
Extremities: Cyanosis? Edema? Clubbing?
Skin: Rash? Hives? Noted insect stings or bites?

Diagnostics

Pulse oximetry: Assess oxygen saturations
ABG: Assess oxygenation and ventilation
Chest x-ray: Assess for lung mass, consolidation/infiltrate, pulmonary edema, or hyperinflation
Pulmonary function testing: Assess for obstructive or restrictive disease
Chest CT/Angiography: Assess for pneumonia, changes associated with obstructive disease, fluid, fibrosis, pulmonary embolus, mass, tracheal narrowing/stenosis, and so forth
Allergy testing
Respiratory viral testing: Such as RSV
Bronchoscopy: Assess for tracheomalacia, tracheal narrowing/stenosis, foreign objects, masses/tumors
Echocardiogram: To evaluate for heart failure
Esophagram/barium swallow: Assess for reflux disease or aspiration

FIGURE 2.2 Algorithm for the evaluation of wheezing.

ABG, arterial blood gas; COPD, chronic obstructive pulmonary disease; GERD, gastroesophageal reflux disease; HEENT, head, ear, eyes, nose, and throat; JVD, jugular venous distention; RSV, respiratory syncytial virus.

---

1. Evidence of obstruction with reduction in the forced expiratory volume in 1 second/forced vital capacity (FEV_1/FVC) when the FEV_1 is also low.

2. One or more tests documented with excessive variability in lung function.

  a. Positive bronchodilator reversibility test with a greater than 12% and 200 mL increase from baseline in the FEV_1.

  b. Excessive variability of greater than 10% in twice-daily peak expiratory flow (PEF) over 2 weeks.

  c. Positive exercise challenge test with decrease in FEV_1 of greater than 10% and 200 mL from baseline.

  d. Positive bronchial challenge test.

  e. Increase in the FEV_1 by greater than 12% and 200 mL *OR* a greater than 20% increase in the PEF from baseline after 4 weeks of treatment.

  f. Variation of lung function between office visits.

  i. Increase in FEV_1 greater than 12% and 200 mL that is not related to a respiratory infection.

B. PEF.

  1. Short-term monitoring can be used to assess treatment responsiveness, evaluate triggers, and/or establish a baseline.

  2. Long-term monitoring is usually only recommended in severe asthma.

  3. A patient will usually reach their personal best PEF within 2 weeks after being on an inhaled corticosteroid (ICS).

  4. Significant variations in the PEF may indicate poor asthma control and increase exacerbation risk.

  5. Repeat values compared with personal best or predicted value by patients.

  6. Typically, severe symptoms at or less than 50% predicted.

C. Allergy skin testing.

  1. Positive allergen test: Allergen not necessarily causing asthma symptoms.

2. Essential to account for the timing of symptoms in relation to allergen exposure and the patient's history.

D. Chest x-ray (CXR).

  1. Usually normal in patients with asthma but may reveal hyperinflation.

  2. If a patient has a fever and infiltrates in conjunction with respiratory symptoms: may be diagnostic of pneumonia.

E. Pulse oximetry and arterial blood gas (ABG).

  1. Used to evaluate for hypoxemia.

  2. ABG can also be used to evaluate for hypercapnia and respiratory acidosis, especially in patients presenting with an acute exacerbation.

DIFFERENTIAL DIAGNOSIS

A. Chronic obstructive pulmonary disease (COPD).

B. Pulmonary embolism (PE).

C. Congestive heart failure (CHF).

D. Chronic rhinosinusitis.

E. Alpha-1 antitrypsin deficiency.

EVALUATION AND MANAGEMENT PLAN

A. General plan.

  1. A patient with asthma should be assessed for asthma control, including symptom control and risk for adverse events.

    a. Asthma symptom control is assessed by evaluating symptoms (e.g., daytime asthma symptoms more than twice/week, night waking due to asthma) in the preceding 4 weeks.

    b. Modifiable risk factors include high use of a short-acting beta$_2$ agonist (SABA), inadequate or failure to be prescribed an ICS, poor medication adherence, improper inhaler technique, obesity, exposure to smoke or other allergens, and so forth.

    c. The goal is to control symptoms and minimize the risk of asthma exacerbations, asthma-related mortality, persistent airflow limitation, and treatment side effects.

  2. Treatment includes assessment (e.g., symptom control, inhaler technique), adjustment of pharmacologic and nonpharmacologic treatment, and response review (e.g., symptoms, exacerbations).

  3. Emergency treatment: Patients with progressively worsening symptoms may present to the ED.

    a. Evaluation of ABCs, PEF, and physical assessment are necessary.

    b. Medication management consists of a SABA via continuous nebulizer or a metered-dose inhaler, corticosteroids, oxygen therapy, and ipratropium bromide.

    c. Patients with a more severe exacerbation as demonstrated by a PEF less than 50% will receive intravenous (IV) instead of oral corticosteroids (OCS) and possibly IV magnesium sulfate.

    d. Posttreatment, PEF should be reassessed.

    e. Patients with an alteration in mental status (e.g., somnolence, confusion), absent breath sounds, worsening hypoxemia or hypercapnia, and hemodynamic instability should be placed on invasive mechanical ventilation and admitted to the ICU.

B. Patient/family teaching points.

  1. Nonpharmacologic interventions should be addressed, such as smoking cessation, engagement in regular physical activity, and avoidance of known occupational exposures and allergen triggers.

  2. Patients should be provided with self-management education to reduce morbidity. Essential components included in self-management are:

    a. Self-monitoring of symptoms and/or PEF.

    b. A written action plan that includes recognition and response to worsening asthma symptoms.

    c. Regular review of asthma control and treatment by a healthcare provider.

C. Pharmacotherapy.

  1. Asthma pharmacologic treatment has two tracks:

    a. Track 1, which is the preferred approach to asthma treatment, is use of an ICS as the reliever and controller inhaler.

     i. A reliever inhaler is an ICS combined with a long-acting beta$_2$ agonist (LABA).

    b. Track 2 is use of a reliever inhaler as needed utilizing a SABA.

     i. This is not a recommended approach and patients should be assessed for their ability to be adherent to a controller inhaler with an ICS.

     ii. Use of SABA without an ICS is correlated with an increased risk of asthma exacerbations.

  2. The decision to start a controller inhaler versus a reliever inhaler is based on the presenting symptoms, frequency of symptoms, and asthma control.

  3. Early treatment with an ICS has been shown to improve lung function, improve asthma control, decrease asthma exacerbations, and reduce hospitalizations.

    a. A controller treatment is not indicated in patients with symptoms less than 4 to 5 days in a week.

    b. An ICS (controller treatment) is recommended in patients with symptoms most days in the week or awakening with asthma symptoms at least once a week.

  4. A stepwise approach is used for treatment adjustment. See Table 2.1 for commonly used medications in asthma management.

    a. Steps 1 and 2 (preferred): Low-dose ICS and LABA combination as needed.

     i. Step 1 (alternative): SABA as needed for reliever inhaler plus the patient would take the ICS when taking the SABA.

     ii. Step 2 (alternative): Low-dose ICS as a controller inhaler plus SABA as a reliever inhaler.

TABLE 2.1   ASTHMA MEDICATIONS

Beta₂ Agonists
SABA
Levalbuterol
Salbutamol (albuterol)
Terbutaline
Anticholinergics/Antimuscarinics
SAMA
Ipratropium bromide (reduces risk of admissions in acute asthma; less effective in the long term)
LAMA
Tiotropium (add-on option in patients with history of exacerbations on controller medications)
ICS
Beclometasone dipropionate
Budesonide
Ciclesonide
Fluticasone furoate
Fluticasone propionate
Mometasone furoate
Combination ICS Plus LABA
ICS/LABA
Beclometasone/formoterol
Budesonide/formoterol
Fluticasone furoate/vilanterol
Fluticasone propionate/formoterol
Fluticasone propionate/salmeterol
Mometasone/formoterol
Systemic Corticosteroids
Prednisone (oral)
Methylprednisolone (intravenous)
LTRA
Montelukast
Pranlukast
Zafirlukast
Zileuton

ICS, inhaled corticosteroid; LABA, long-acting beta₂ agonist; LAMA, long-acting muscarinic antagonist; LTRA, leukotriene receptor antagonist; SABA, short-acting beta₂ agonist; SAMA, short-acting muscarinic antagonist.

b. Step 3 (preferred): Low-dose ICS/LABA as a controller inhaler plus low-dose ICS/LABA as the reliever inhaler.
   i. Step 3 (alternative): Low-dose ICS/LABA as controller inhaler plus SABA as a reliever inhaler.
c. Step 4 (preferred): Medium-dose ICS/LABA as controller inhaler plus low-dose ICS/LABA as a reliever inhaler.
   i. Step 4 (alternative): Medium- or high-dose ICS/LABA as controller inhaler plus SABA as a reliever inhaler.
   ii. A short course of OCS may be needed for those presenting with severely uncontrolled asthma.
d. Step 5 (preferred): Addition of LAMA to current medical management and consideration of adding a high-dose ICS/LABA plus a low-dose ICS/LABA as a reliever inhaler.
   i. Step 5 (alternative): Addition of long-acting muscarinic antagonist (LAMA) and consideration of adding a high-dose ICS/LABA plus a SABA as a reliever inhaler.
   ii. Refer to specialist for further assessment and evaluation of asthma.
e. Leukotriene receptor antagonist (LTRA) can be added to the treatment regimen to aid with symptom control.

5. With the stepwise approach, the treatment regimen can be adjusted up or down by the provider based on the frequency and severity of asthma symptoms.

6. Asthma exacerbations are characterized by an increase or worsening of respiratory symptoms and lung function compared with the patient's baseline.
   a. The patient requires a change in their treatment.
   b. Common triggers resulting in an exacerbation include viral respiratory infections, allergens, air pollution, poor ICS adherence, and/or season changes.
   c. It is important for the provider to identify factors that increase the risk of asthma-related death, such as history of mechanical ventilation, hospitalization and/or ED visit in the past year, and not currently on or poor adherence with an ICS.

7. Patients with acute exacerbations and an asthma action plan in place can increase their usual inhaler, a low ICS/LABA or SABA, as well as their maintenance controller inhaler. OCS can be added for patients with a PEF or FEV₁ less than 60% predicted of their personal best or no improvement in symptoms after 48 hours (see Exhibit 2.1).

8. Patients with severe exacerbations may need to present to an acute care facility.
   a. The initial assessment should include airway, breathing, and circulation. Additionally, the provider should assess for mental status changes (e.g., drowsiness and confusion) and silent chest.
      i. Those with mental status or a silent chest should receive an ICU consult, immediately ▶

EXHIBIT 2.1   Stepwise Approach for Managing Asthma Long Term

The stepwise approach tailors the selection of medication to the level of asthma severity or asthma control. The stepwise approach is meant to help, not replace, the clinical decision-making needed to meet individual patient needs.

ASSESS CONTROL:

STEP UP IF NEEDED (first, check medication adherence, inhaler technique, environmental control, and comorbidities)

STEP DOWN IF POSSIBLE (and asthma is well controlled for at least 3 months)

	STEP 1	STEP 2	STEP 3	STEP 4	STEP 5	STEP 6

At each step: Patient education, environmental control, and management of comorbidities

0–4 years of age

	Intermittent Asthma	Persistent Asthma: Daily Medication — Consult with asthma specialist if step 3 care or higher is required. Consider consultation at step 2.				
Preferred Treatment[†]	SABA* as needed	low-dose ICS*	medium-dose ICS*	medium-dose ICS* + either LABA* or montelukast	high-dose ICS* + either LABA* or montelukast	high-dose ICS* + either LABA* or montelukast + oral corticosteroids
Alternative Treatment[†,‡]		cromolyn or montelukast				

If clear benefit is not observed in 4–6 weeks, and medication technique and adherence are satisfactory, consider adjusting therapy or alternate diagnoses.

Quick-Relief Medication	■ SABA* as needed for symptoms; intensity of treatment depends on severity of symptoms. ■ With viral respiratory symptoms: SABA every 4–6 hours up to 24 hours (longer with physician consult). Consider short course of oral systemic corticosteroids if asthma exacerbation is severe or patient has history of severe exacerbations. ■ Caution: Frequent use of SABA may indicate the need to step up treatment.

5–11 years of age

	Intermittent Asthma	Persistent Asthma: Daily Medication — Consult with asthma specialist if step 4 care or higher is required. Consider consultation at step 3.				
Preferred Treatment[†]	SABA* as needed	low-dose ICS*	low-dose ICS* + either LABA,* LTRA,* or theophylline[(b)] OR medium-dose ICS	medium-dose ICS* + LABA*	high-dose ICS* + LABA*	high-dose ICS* + LABA* + oral corticosteroids
Alternative Treatment[†,‡]		cromolyn, LTRA,* or theophylline[§]		medium-dose ICS* + either LTRA* or theophylline[§]	high-dose ICS* + either LTRA* or theophylline[§]	high-dose ICS* + either LTRA* or theophylline[§] + oral corticosteroids

Consider subcutaneous allergen immunotherapy for patients who have persistent, allergic asthma.**

Quick-Relief Medication	■ SABA* as needed for symptoms. The intensity of treatment depends on severity of symptoms: up to 3 treatments every 20 minutes as needed. Short course of oral systemic corticosteroids may be needed. ■ Caution: Increasing use of SABA or use >2 days/week for symptom relief (not to prevent EIB*) generally indicates inadequate control and the need to step up treatment.

≥12 years of age

	Intermittent Asthma	Persistent Asthma: Daily Medication — Consult with asthma specialist if step 4 care or higher is required. Consider consultation at step 3.				
Preferred Treatment[†]	SABA* as needed	low-dose ICS*	low-dose ICS* + LABA* OR medium-dose ICS*	medium-dose ICS* + LABA*	high-dose ICS* + LABA* AND consider omalizumab for patients who have allergies[††]	high-dose ICS* + LABA* + oral corticosteroid[§§] AND consider omalizumab for patients who have allergies[††]
Alternative Treatment[†,‡]		cromolyn, LTRA,* or theophylline[§]	low-dose ICS* + either LTRA,* theophylline,[§] or zileuton[‡]	medium-dose ICS* + either LTRA,* theophylline,[§] or zileuton[‡]		

Consider subcutaneous allergen immunotherapy for patients who have persistent, allergic asthma.**

Quick-Relief Medication	■ SABA* as needed for symptoms. The intensity of treatment depends on severity of symptoms: up to 3 treatments every 20 minutes as needed. Short course of oral systemic corticosteroids may be needed. ■ Caution: Use of SABA >2 days/week for symptom relief (not to prevent EIB*) generally indicates inadequate control and the need to step up treatment.

* **Abbreviations:** EIB, exercise-induced bronchospasm; ICS, inhaled corticosteroid; LABA, inhaled long-acting beta$_2$-agonist; LTRA, leukotriene receptor antagonist; SABA, inhaled short-acting beta$_2$-agonist.
† Treatment options are listed in alphabetical order, if more than one.
‡ If alternative treatment is used and response is inadequate, discontinue and use preferred treatment before stepping up.
§ Theophylline is a less desirable alternative because of the need to monitor serum concentration levels.
** Based on evidence for dust mites, animal dander, and pollen; evidence is weak or lacking for molds and cockroaches. Evidence is strongest for immunotherapy with single allergens. The role of allergy in asthma is greater in children than in adults.
†† Clinicians who administer immunotherapy or omalizumab should be prepared to treat anaphylaxis that may occur.
‡ Zileuton is less desirable because of limited studies as adjunctive therapy and the need to monitor liver function.
§§ Before oral corticosteroids are introduced, a trial of high-dose ICS + LABA + either LTRA, theophylline, or zileuton, may be considered, although this approach has not been studied in clinical trials.

Source: From the U.S. Department of Health and Human Services. (2012). *Asthma care quick reference: Diagnosing and managing asthma.* https://www.nhlbi.nih.gov/ les/docs/guidelines/asthma_qrg.pdf.

started on a SABA, oxygen administration, and possible preparation for intubation.

b. Those with a mild to moderate exacerbation may present with an increased respiratory rate, no accessory muscle use, tachycardia with a heart rate of 100 to 120 beats per minute, ability to talk in phrases, oxygen saturation greater than 90% on room air, and PEF greater than 50% predicted.

   i. Treatment for these patients consist of SABAs, OCS, and oxygen therapy to maintain oxygen saturations at 93% to 95%. The provider may consider ipratropium bromide.

   ii. The provider should reassess frequently and an hour after initial treatment.

c. Those with a severe exacerbation may present hunched over with the ability to only talk in words, agitated, a respiratory rate greater than 30 breaths per minute, accessory muscle use, tachycardia with a heart rate greater than 120 beats per minute, oxygen saturation less than 90% on room air, and a PEF equal to or less than 50% predicted.

   i. Treatment for these patients consists of SABAs, ipratropium bromide, oxygen therapy to maintain oxygen saturations at 93% to 95%, oral or IV corticosteroids, and consideration of IV magnesium and high-dose ICS.

d. For patients with any signs of clinical deterioration, ICU admission should be considered.

D. Discharge instructions.

1. Discharge criteria. Patients should:

   a. Show improvement in symptoms such as resolution of accessory muscle use and dyspnea, improved respiratory rate, and oxygen saturation greater than 93% on room air.

   b. Improved PEF of greater than 60% predicted or personal best.

   c. Have adequate home resources.

2. Diet.

   a. Restrictions: specific diet is based on whether the patient has underlying comorbid conditions, such as diabetes or renal disease.

   b. No restrictions: The patient can resume regular diet.

3. Medications.

   a. OCS: Usually prescribed for 5 to 7 days.

   b. SABA-only treatment should be avoided and is no longer recommended.

   c. Resume reliever inhaler with the addition of an ICS.

   d. ICS-containing medication prior to discharge.

      i. If the patient is already on an ICS-containing medication, increase the dose for 2 to 4 weeks.

   e. Medication reconciliation and continuation of appropriate medications for comorbid conditions.

4. Treatment plan.

   a. Identification of risk factors that contribute to exacerbations.

   b. Individualized written asthma action plan.

c. Evaluation of maintenance therapy understanding.

d. Assessment of inhaler technique.

e. Assessment of PEF meter technique if applicable outside of an acute exacerbation.

f. Smoking cessation counseling.

g. Immunizations such as influenza. Influenza can trigger acute and severe asthma exacerbations that could potentially result in necessitating ventilatory support.

h. Management of comorbid conditions.

5. Discuss with the patient.

   a. Importance of medication compliance and proper inhaler technique to reduce symptoms and exacerbations.

   b. As previously stated, avoidance of known risk factors that worsen asthma symptoms or lead to exacerbations, such as smoking or other known allergens.

   c. Signs and symptoms of an impending exacerbation, such as increasing reliever inhaler use, frequent awakening at night with coughing or dyspnea, and PEF less than 60% of predicted or personal best.

FOLLOW-UP

A. Regular follow-up is dependent on symptom control and exacerbation risk, but should occur 2 to 3 months after treatment initiation and every 3 to 12 months once stabilized.

B. Patients should see their primary care provider or pulmonologist 1 to 2 weeks after self-management of an exacerbation.

C. Patients should see their primary care provider or asthma specialist/pulmonologist within 2 to 7 days of discharge from the ED or hospital.

CONSULTATION/REFERRAL

A. Patients with progressively worsening asthma despite increasing treatment may require a referral to a pulmonologist or allergist.

B. A pulmonologist and/or intensivist consultation is indicated for patients with a moderate to severe exacerbation necessitating ICU admission and/or noninvasive and invasive mechanical ventilation.

SPECIAL/GERIATRIC CONSIDERATIONS

A. Poor inhaler technique needs to be considered in patients with persistent symptoms.

B. Comorbid conditions may contribute and complicate asthma management.

C. The severity of asthma is evaluated retrospectively, and it is important to distinguish between uncontrolled asthma versus severe asthma.

1. Ideally, the severity of asthma should be assessed after the patient has been placed on the appropriate treatment needed to control symptoms and exacerbations.

D. Routine CXRs and antibiotic therapy are not indicated in asthma management.

E. In the older adult population, asthma can be under-diagnosed or overdiagnosed due to varying assumptions and perceptions over dyspnea.

BIBLIOGRAPHY

Centers for Disease Control and Prevention. (2021). Asthma surveillance: United states, 2006-2018. *Morbidity and Mortality Weekly Report*, 70, 1–36. https://www.cdc.gov/mmwr/volumes/70/ss/pdfs/ss7005a1-H.pdf

Global Initiative for Asthma. (2021). *Global strategy for asthma management and prevention*. https://ginasthma.org/wp-content/uploads/2021/05/GINA-Main-Report-2021-V2-WMS.pdf

CHRONIC OBSTRUCTIVE PULMONARY DISEASE

DEFINITION
A. A chronic and progressive respiratory disease characterized by persistent respiratory symptoms and expiratory airflow limitation.

INCIDENCE
A. Chronic obstructive pulmonary disease (COPD) is a leading cause of death in the United States and the third leading cause of disability.
B. The incidence is much higher in smokers and ex-smokers compared with nonsmokers.
C. It is more prevalent in individuals greater than 40 years, with the greatest prevalence in those greater than 65 years.
D. Women are expected to disproportionately represent those with COPD and expected to have higher direct costs when compared with men.

PATHOGENESIS
A. The pathogenesis of COPD is the result of small airway disease and lung parenchymal destruction.
B. The lungs are exposed to a stimulus (e.g., smoking, fumes) that causes inflammation of the airways. Neutrophils and various other immune cells are recruited to the airways leading to breakdown of elastic fibers and increasing oxidative stress.
  1. This inflammation becomes chronic, leading to structural changes, small airway narrowing, decreased elastic recoil, and loss of alveoli attachments.
C. Ultimately, there is destruction of alveolar walls, decreased repair of the alveoli, fibrosis, and bronchiolar wall thickening, leading to further narrowed airways and airflow limitation, mucociliary dysfunction, impaired gas exchange, and enlarged air spaces.

PREDISPOSING FACTORS
A. Tobacco smoke: Leading environmental risk factor.
B. Individuals greater than 40 years.
C. Occupational exposures to lung irritants (e.g., dust, chemical agents, fumes).
D. Alpha-1 antitrypsin is a genetic condition leading to COPD that should be tested in a new diagnosis of COPD.
E. Airway hyperresponsiveness (e.g., asthma).
F. Low socioeconomic status is associated with an increased risk of COPD but unclear if this is the result of increased exposure to lung irritants, infections, or other factors related to the individual's socioeconomic status.
G. Recurrent respiratory infections, especially if there is history of severe respiratory infections in childhood.

SUBJECTIVE DATA
A. Common complaints/symptoms.
  1. Dyspnea (see Figure 2.1): Chronic and progressive; this is a cardinal symptom.
  2. Cough (Figure 2.3) with or without sputum production and may be intermittent.
  3. Chronic sputum production.
    a. Not uncommon for individuals to produce small amounts of sputum.
    b. Increasing sputum production with change in color may indicate bacterial infection.
  4. Wheezing (see Figure 2.2) and/or chest tightness.
  5. Severe COPD: Possible fatigue, weight loss, and anorexia.
B. Family and social history.
  1. Inquire about environmental and/or occupational risk factors and family history of COPD or other chronic respiratory diseases.
  2. Inquire about smoking because it can accelerate or exacerbate COPD symptoms.
C. Review of symptoms.
  1. Evaluate for symptom onset, duration, severity, associated symptoms (e.g., increased wheezing or sputum), and aggravating and alleviating factors.
  2. Inquire about early onset of COPD.

PHYSICAL EXAMINATION
A. The physical examination for COPD is rarely diagnostic. Physical signs of COPD may or may not be present, depending on the severity of disease. However, it is still important to assess for respiratory and systemic symptoms that may be associated with COPD.
B. General examination.
  1. Assess the respiratory rate. It may be normal or increased.
  2. Assess the patient's posture. Leaning forward with outstretched palms of the knees is associated with an attempt to relieve dyspnea.
  3. Check breathing. In advanced disease or severe dyspnea, pursed-lip breathing is possible.
  4. Inspect for clubbing.
  5. In more severe disease, cyanosis, elevated jugular venous pressure, and peripheral edema may be present.
C. Respiratory examination.
  1. Inspect the chest.
    a. Check for an increased anteroposterior chest diameter due to hyperinflation of the lungs, giving a barrel chest shape.
    b. Assess for use of accessory muscles (e.g., sternocleidomastoids, scalenes, intercostals).

Obtain the History
Onset, timing, description of cough, alleviating factors, any associated factors.
- Acute (<3 weeks), subacute (3–8 weeks), or chronic (>8 weeks)?
- Associated with other symptoms such as dyspnea, wheezing, chest tightness, or hemoptysis?
- Recent respiratory infection?
- Occupational or environmental exposures?
- Medications such as ACE inhibitors?
- Known comorbid conditions such as asthma, COPD, GERD, and so forth.
- Current or history of smoking?
- Occurrence of cough? Upon awakening? Lying down? During exercise?

Physical Examination
The initial physical exam focuses on clues suggestive of cardiopulmonary disease. A thorough full exam should follow because a cough may be a manifestation of a more systemic disease process.
General: Weight loss? Fatigue?
Vital signs: Usually normal unless associated with another disease process. May have tachypnea, tachycardia, oxygen desaturations, and/or fever.
HEENT: Red and/or watery eyes? Fluid behind eardrum? Boggy, swollen, and/or pale mucus membranes? Nasal polyps? Thin, watery, or purulent secretions? Congestion? Throat redness? Hoarseness?
Respiratory: Adventitious breath sounds such as crackles or wheezing? Chest shape? Respiratory pattern? Dullness or hyperresonance on percussion?
Extremities: Clubbing? Edema?

Initial Diagnostic
Chest x-ray:
- All individuals with a chronic cough.
- All individuals with an acute cough AND dyspnea, chest pain, fever, hemoptysis, or weight loss.

Acute/Subacute
Usually does not require further testing.

Additional testing focuses on a suspected etiology.
- **Allergy testing.**
- **Chest CT/Angiography:** Assess for pneumonia, changes associated with obstructive disease, fluid, fibrosis, pulmonary embolus.
- **Pulmonary function testing:** Assess for obstructive or restrictive disease.
- **Tuberculosis skin testing.**
- **Pertussis testing.**

Chronic
Pulmonary function testing: Assess for obstructive or restrictive disease
Additional work-up may follow after empirical treatment for disorders such as GERD.
Bronchoscopy: To evaluate for chronic inflammation
Sinus imaging
High-resolution Chest CT: Used in cough with atypical presentations and concern for chronic pulmonary disease
Esophagram or swallow evaluation: Assess for reflux disease or aspiration
Echocardiogram: To evaluate for heart failure or elevated pulmonary pressures

FIGURE 2.3 Algorithm for the evaluation of cough.

ACE, angiotensin-converting enzyme; COPD, chronic obstructive pulmonary disease; GERD, gastroesophageal reflux disease; HEENT, head, ear, eyes, nose, and throat.

2. Percuss the chest wall.
  a. Observe for hyperresonance due to overinflation of the lungs.
3. Auscultate bilaterally.
  a. Diminished breath sounds throughout.
  b. Occasional expiratory wheezing.
  c. Prolonged expiratory phase.
  d. Coarse rhonchi throughout the respiratory phase, especially during times of increased sputum production.

DIAGNOSTIC TESTS
A. Pulmonary function test: Spirometry.
  1. Objective measurement of airflow limitation.
  2. Ratio between the volume of air forcibly exhaled after maximal inspiration (forced vital capacity [FVC]) and the volume of air forcibly exhaled during the first second (forced expiratory volume in 1 second [FEV$_1$]). A ratio less than 0.7 after bronchodilator testing indicates obstruction.
  3. Reduced FEV$_1$ (reduction in expiratory flow rates).
  4. Possibly reduced FVC, usually to a lesser extent than the FEV$_1$.
  5. Spirometry evaluation is based on a comparison of appropriate reference values based on the patient's age, height, sex, and race.
B. Chest x-ray (CXR; see Figure 2.3).
  1. Hyperinflation, as evidenced by a flattened diaphragm and increased retrosternal air space.
  2. Hyperlucency of the lungs.
  3. Rapid tapering of the vascular markings.
C. Arterial blood gas (ABG).
  1. May reveal hypercapnia and/or hypoxemia.

a. Early or mild COPD: Typically normal.

b. Worsening as COPD progresses. Individuals with moderate to severe disease may have a chronic respiratory acidosis often with metabolic compensation as evidenced by increased serum bicarbonate.

2. Can provide clues to the acuteness and severity of COPD in individuals with an exacerbation.

D. Pulse oximetry.

1. Used to assess arterial oxygen saturation. If the pulse oximetry is less than 92%, then an ABG is warranted.

E. Exercise testing (e.g., 6-minute walking distance).

1. Objectively measures functional capacity by evaluating whether the individual has a reduction in walking distance.

2. Useful for disability assessment, risk of mortality, and indicator of impairment of health status.

F. Laboratory evaluation.

1. Alpha-1 antitrypsin screening: should be assessed in individuals with a family history of COPD at an early age and less than 45 years.

DIFFERENTIAL DIAGNOSIS

A. Lung carcinoma.

B. Chronic cough.

C. Congestive heart failure (CHF).

D. Interstitial lung disease.

E. Asthma.

F. Bronchiectasis.

EVALUATION AND MANAGEMENT PLAN

A. General plan.

1. The interventions listed in the following are part of the general plan for a COPD patient. We should incorporate these interventions in all COPD patients who meet the criteria.

2. Specific interventions.

a. Smoking cessation.

i. Literature has indicated that counseling from healthcare professionals increases cessation rates compared with self-initiated strategies.

ii. A five-step program initiated by healthcare providers offers a helpful framework for cessation.

iii. Nicotine replacement (e.g., gum, lozenge, transdermal patch) can increase long-term cessation rates.

iv. Pharmacologic agents, such as varenicline and bupropion, can increase long-term cessation rates but should be used as an adjunct to an intervention program.

b. Individuals should receive the influenza and pneumococcal vaccine. The Centers for Disease Control and Prevention (CDC) also recommends the SARS-CoV-2 vaccine.

c. Reduction of risk factors, such as avoidance of occupational irritants can help.

d. Pulmonary rehabilitation lasting from 6 to 8 weeks has been shown to improve dyspnea, health status, exercise intolerance, and hospitalizations

in patients with a recent exacerbation. This requires collaboration among multiple healthcare professionals.

e. Treatment recommendations should consider the symptomatic assessment (ABCD group) and the individual's spirometric classification (GOLD 1–4). In addition, they should consider comorbid conditions and other medications.

f. The GOLD categories 1 to 4 (spirometric grade) are used to classify the degree or severity of airflow limitation, which is identified using the following:

i. GOLD 1: Mild, FEV_1 80% or greater than the predicted.

ii. GOLD 2: Moderate, FEV_1 greater than or equal to 50% predicted but less than 80% predicted.

iii. GOLD 3: Severe, FEV_1 greater than or equal to 30% predicted but less than 50% predicted.

iv. GOLD 4: Very severe, FEV_1 is less than 30% predicted.

v. The GOLD grade is assigned after identification of an airflow limitation, as evidenced by an FEV_1/FVC ratio less than 0.70 postbronchodilator testing.

g. Symptom assessment can be evaluated using the COPD Assessment Test (CAT) or the modified British Medical Research Council (mMRC) Questionnaire. The CAT or mMRC is commonly used in the clinical setting in conjunction with the GOLD grade and exacerbation history to guide therapy.

h. The ABCD Assessment Tool (groups A–D) is a measure of the individual's symptoms and risk of exacerbations.

i. Groups A and B indicate the individual has no more than one exacerbation with no hospitalizations and a CAT score less than 10 or greater than or equal to 10, respectively, in the past year.

ii. Groups C and D indicate the individual has two or more exacerbations or one or more exacerbations leading to hospitalization and a CAT score less than 10 or greater than or equal to 10, respectively, in the past year.

3. Management of stable COPD.

a. Treatment should be individualized based on symptoms and risk for exacerbations.

4. Goals of treatment.

a. Symptom relief.

b. Increased exercise tolerance.

c. Improved health status.

d. Reduction of mortality.

e. Prevention of disease progression and exacerbations.

f. Management should include pharmacologic and nonpharmacologic interventions.

g. Smoking cessation and avoidance of occupational irritants are important.

h. Treatment should include a review of symptoms and exacerbations; assessment of inhaler ▶

technique, adherence, and nonpharmacologic management; and adjustment of pharmacologic management, including escalation and de-escalation.

5. Management of exacerbations.

a. Acute worsening in symptoms from baseline resulting in additional therapy.

    i. Increased sputum, including purulence, increased dyspnea, and increased cough and/or wheezing.

b. Can be classified as:

    i. Mild: Treatment with short-acting bronchodilators.

    ii. Moderate: Treatment with short-acting bronchodilators plus antibiotics and/or oral steroids.

    iii. Severe: Requires hospitalization or ED visits.

c. Symptoms can last 7 to 10 days and contribute to disease progression, negatively impact health status, and increase the rate of hospitalizations.

d. Most exacerbations are triggered by respiratory viral infections; however, bacterial infections, pollution, allergens, and temperature changes can also lead to an exacerbation.

e. Indications for hospitalization include severe symptoms (e.g., mental status changes, worsening dyspnea at rest), acute respiratory failure, physical signs (e.g., cyanosis), initial exacerbation treatment failure, and so forth.

f. In hospitalized patients, the severity of exacerbation is based on the individual's symptoms and whether respiratory failure is present.

    i. No respiratory failure: Respiratory rate 20 to 30 per minute; no accessory muscle use, mental status change, or elevation in $PaCO_2$; hypoxemia improved with less than 35% of inspired oxygen.

    ii. Acute respiratory failure, non-life-threatening: Respiratory rate greater than 30 per minute; use of accessory muscles, no change in mental status, $PaCO_2$ above baseline or 50 to 60 mmHg; hypoxemia improved with greater than 35% inspired oxygen.

    iii. Acute respiratory failure, life-threatening: Respiratory rate greater than 30 per minute; accessory muscle use, acute mental status changes, $PaCO_2$ above baseline or greater than 60 mmHg or presence of a respiratory acidosis with a pH less than 7.25; hypoxemia requiring greater than 40% of inspired oxygen or not improving with supplemental oxygen.

B. Pharmacotherapy.

1. See Table 2.2.

2. Adequate pharmacotherapy can reduce symptoms, reduce the frequency and severity of exacerbations, and improve overall health status.

3. Most medications are inhaled. It is essential that individuals receive education on proper technique.

TABLE 2.2   COPD MEDICATIONS
Beta₂ Agonists (Inhaled)
SABA
Fenoterol
Levalbuterol
Salbutamol (albuterol)
Terbutaline
LABA
Arformoterol
Formoterol
Salmeterol
Anticholinergics/Antimuscarinics (Inhaled)
SAMA
Ipratropium bromide
Oxitropium bromide
LAMA
Aclidinium bromide
Glycopyrronium bromide
Tiotropium
Combination SABA Plus Short-Acting Anticholinergic (Inhaled)
SABA/SAMA
Fenoterol/ipratropium
Salbutamol/ipratropium
Combination LABA Plus Long-Acting Anticholinergic (Inhaled)
LABA/LAMA
Formoterol/aclidinium
Formoterol/glycopyrronium
Combination LABA Plus ICS (Inhaled)
LABA/ICS
Formoterol/budesonide
Formoterol/mometasone
Salmeterol/fluticasone propionate
Vilanterol/fluticasone furoate
Methylxanthines (Oral and Intravenous)
Theophylline (SR)

(continued)

TABLE 2.2 COPD MEDICATIONS (CONTINUED)

Systemic Corticosteroids
Prednisone (oral)
Methylprednisolone (intravenous)
Phosphodiesterase-4 Inhibitors (Oral)
Roflumilast
Antibiotics (Oral)
Azithromycin
Erythromycin
Mucolytics
Carbocysteine
N-acetylcysteine

COPD, chronic obstructive pulmonary disease; ICS, inhaled corticosteroid; LABA, long-acting beta-2 agonist; LAMA, long-acting antimuscarinics; SABA, short-acting beta$_2$ agonist; SAMA, short-acting antimuscarinics; SR, sustained release.

4. Bronchodilators.
   a. Often prescribed in COPD to prevent or reduce symptoms.
   b. Central to symptom management.
   c. Inhaled beta-2 agonists.
      i. Functional antagonism to bronchoconstriction by relaxing airway smooth muscle.
      ii. Short-acting beta-2 agonist (SABA) and long-acting beta-2 agonist (LABA).
         1) SABAs: Typically last 4 to 6 hours; shown with regular use to improve symptoms and FEV$_1$ in COPD.
         2) LABAs: Duration of 12 hours or more; shown to improve lung function, dyspnea, and reduce exacerbations.
   d. Anticholinergics/antimuscarinics.
      i. Blockage of acetylcholine on muscarinic receptors leading to relaxation of airway smooth muscle.
      ii. Short-acting (SAMA) and long-acting (LAMA) antimuscarinics.
         1) SAMAs: Shown to improve symptoms and FEV$_1$ with regular or as-needed use.
         2) LAMAs: Shown to improve lung function, dyspnea, and health status. Literature has shown that LAMAs compared with LABAs reduce exacerbations and decrease hospitalizations.
   e. Methylxanthines.
      i. Theophylline most commonly used.
      ii. Literature has not consistently demonstrated methylxanthines, such as theophylline, reduce COPD exacerbations.
      iii. Theophylline has shown to have a small bronchodilator effect in stable COPD.

   f. Inhaled corticosteroid (ICS).
      i. No mortality benefit or modification in the long-term decline of FEV$_1$ with ICS monotherapy.
      ii. Severe COPD and regular use of ICS: increased risk for pneumonia.
   g. Combination inhaled therapy.
      i. Combination of SABA and SAMA: Superior in improving symptoms compared with either medication used alone.
      ii. Combination of LABA and LAMA: Improves FEV$_1$ and reduces symptoms and exacerbations compared with either medication used alone or compared with those individuals treated with a combination of ICS and LABA.
      iii. Combination therapy with ICS and LABA compared with monotherapy with either medication: improves lung function and health status, as well as reduces exacerbations.
      iv. Triple inhaled therapy with LABA/LAMA/ICS: shown to improve lung function and reduce exacerbations when compared with LABA/ICS, LABA/LAMA, or monotherapy with a LAMA.
   h. Oral glucocorticoids.
      i. Long-term risks: Preclude use in stable COPD.
      ii. In acute exacerbations in hospitalized patients: Decreased treatment failure and relapse, as well as improved lung function.
   i. Phosphodiesterase-4 inhibitors.
      i. Only one approved drug, roflumilast: Used for patients with chronic bronchitis, history of exacerbations, and severe to very severe COPD.
      ii. Has been shown to improve lung function and decrease moderate to severe exacerbations.
      iii. Requires caution in those with depression and those who are underweight.
   j. Antibiotics.
      i. Reduced exacerbations: Azithromycin 250 mg daily or 500 mg three times a week OR erythromycin 500 mg BID for 1 year.
         1) Use of azithromycin: Association with increased antibiotic resistance.
      ii. No data indicating efficacy of chronic antibiotic therapy beyond 1 year.
   k. Mucolytics.
      i. Reduced risk of exacerbation in select populations.
5. Pharmacologic treatment using the ABCD Assessment Tool.
   a. Use of an algorithm based on ABCD Assessment Tool groups A to D.
      i. Group A.
         1) Should be placed on a bronchodilator, either short-acting or long-acting.
         2) The provider should evaluate drug effectiveness and decide to continue, stop, or try an alternative bronchodilator class. ▶

ii. Group B.
   1) Should be initiated on a long-acting bronchodilator. Choice of long-acting bronchodilator should be based on symptom relief.
   2) Two bronchodilators are recommended for individuals with persistent dyspnea.
iii. Group C.
   1) Should be initiated on a bronchodilator; preferred choice is a LAMA secondary to superior exacerbation prevention.
iv. Group D.
   1) Should be initiated on a bronchodilator; preferred choice is a LAMA secondary to superior exacerbation prevention and effects on breathlessness.
   2) Individuals with severe symptoms may be started on LABA/LAMA secondary to superior results compared with monotherapy with either drug.
   3) LAMA/ICS may be an appropriate initial therapy for those with eosinophilia or asthma–COPD overlap.
   4) For continued exacerbations:
      a) On monotherapy with a long-acting bronchodilator, escalate the treatment regimen to LABA/LAMA or LABA/ICS (in select patient populations).
      b) Despite being on LABA/LAMA, escalate the treatment regimen to LABA/LAMA/ICS in those with eosinophilia OR add roflumilast or azithromycin.
      c) Despite being on LABA/ICS, escalate the treatment regimen to triple therapy or switch to LABA/LAMA.
      d) Despite triple inhaled therapy, add roflumilast; add a macrolide, specifically azithromycin; and/or stop the ICS.
6. Hospital medication management and medical therapy of COPD exacerbations.
   a. Combination of SABA and anticholinergics.
   b. Possible systemic steroids.
      i. Have been shown to shorten recovery time, improve oxygenation, and improve the risk of early relapse and treatment failure.
      ii. Oral prednisone recommended at 40 mg daily for 5 days.
   c. Consideration of oral antibiotics when signs of bacterial infection are present.
   d. Possible oxygen therapy and noninvasive ventilation.
      i. Noninvasive ventilation has been shown to reduce intubation rates, mortality, and hospital length of stay.
7. Invasive mechanical ventilation.
   a. Warranted in patients who are unable to undergo or who fail noninvasive ventilation, are hemodynamically unstable, status post arrest, profound hypoxemia in patients not able to tolerate noninvasive ventilation, massive aspiration, and significant changes in levels of consciousness.

C. Discharge instructions.
1. Be aware that these vary based on the severity of the underlying COPD and exacerbation.
2. Review all clinical (e.g., improved dyspnea, sputum production, cognition) and laboratory data.
3. Assess continual need for oxygen therapy. Patients on chronic home oxygen should resume their baseline oxygen requirements.
4. Check functional status.
5. Ensure adequate home resources.
6. Activity.
   a. Pulmonary rehabilitation.
      i. Shown to reduce hospitalizations, as well as improve dyspnea and health status.
      ii. Indicated in all patients with symptoms and/or high risk for exacerbation.
      iii. Early rehabilitation has been associated with improved mortality.
   b. Regular physical activity.
      i. Combination of interval training with strength training.
      ii. Strong predictor of mortality.
7. Diet.
   a. May vary depending on underlying comorbid conditions, such as diabetes, heart failure, or renal disease.
   b. Nutritional supplementation: recommended; should be considered in malnourished COPD patients.
8. Medications (see "Pharmacotherapy").
   a. Bronchodilators.
      i. Most patients are likely to receive two long-acting bronchodilators (LABA/LAMA) or a long-acting bronchodilator and ICS (LABA/ICS).
   b. Additional agent: The provider may choose to initiate a long-term macrolide or roflumilast in patients who meet the criteria and continue to have exacerbations despite multimedication inhaled therapy.
   c. Other drugs: Medication reconciliation and continuation of medications for comorbid conditions are necessary.
9. Treatment plan.
   a. Evaluation of psychosocial needs and home resources, such as availability of home oxygen.
   b. Inclusion of family in the treatment and education plan.
   c. Evaluation maintenance therapy understanding.
   d. Ensuring understanding of withdrawal medications prescribed for an acute exacerbation, such as steroids.
   e. Assessment of inhaler technique.
   f. Pulmonary hygiene (e.g., deep breathing).
   g. Smoking cessation counseling.
   h. Encouragement of pneumococcal and influenza vaccinations.
      i. Setting up pulmonary rehabilitation.
      j. Management of comorbid conditions such as gastroesophageal reflux disease (GERD) and heart failure.

▶

10. Discuss with the patient.

a. Discuss signs and symptoms associated with infection and/or exacerbations, such as fever, chills, increased dyspnea, and increasing sputum production or change in sputum color.

b. Instruct patients on the importance of medication compliance and physical activity to reduce the occurrence of exacerbations, reduce symptoms, and improve quality of life.

FOLLOW-UP

A. Follow up with a primary care physician or pulmonologist, ideally within 1 to 4 weeks of discharge.

1. Especially during initiation, escalation, and de-escalation in therapy.

2. With new or worsening symptoms.

3. Posthospitalization.

B. Association of early follow-up with fewer readmissions.

CONSULTATION/REFERRAL

A. Consultation with a pulmonologist: In patients with progressively worsening symptoms, severe or very severe COPD, frequent exacerbations, and respiratory failure.

SPECIAL/GERIATRIC CONSIDERATIONS

A. Chronic use of oxygen is indicated for patients with severe hypoxemia at rest and chronic respiratory failure.

B. Patients should be evaluated and treated for comorbid conditions such as heart failure, obstructive sleep apnea, obesity, hypoventilation syndrome, and so forth.

C. Education alone has not been shown to change behaviors; however, education and self-management with a case manager may prevent exacerbation complications.

D. Physical activity is highly encouraged given its strong mortality prediction.

E. Nutritional supplements may be indicated in malnourished patients.

F. Patients should be considered for lung volume reduction surgery if they have upper-lobe predominance emphysema.

G. Patients with very severe COPD and advanced systemic symptoms may be considered for lung transplantation.

H. Discussions with patients and families regarding palliative and end-of-life care should take place in the event the patient becomes critically ill.

BIBLIOGRAPHY

Bollmeier, S. G., & Hartmann, A. P. (2020). Management of chronic obstructive pulmonary disease: A review focusing on exacerbations. *American Journal of Health-System Pharmacists, 77*, 259–268. https://doi.org/10.1093/ajhp/zxz306

Global Initiative for Chronic Obstructive Lung Disease. (2022). *Global strategy for the diagnosis, management, and prevention of chronic obstructive pulmonary disease*. https://www.goldcopd.org

National Heart, Lung, and Blood Institute. (2021). *COPD national action plan*. https://www.nhlbi.nih.gov/health-topics/education-and-awareness/COPD-national-action-plan

Nici, L., Mammen, M. J., Charbek, E., Alexander, P. E., Au, D. H., Boyd, C. M., Criner, G. J., Donaldson, G. C., Dreher, M., Fan, V. S., Gershon, A. S., Han, M. K., Krishnan, J. A., Martinez, F. J., Meek, P. M., Morgan, M., Polkey, M. I., Puhan, M. A., Sadatsafavi, M. ... Aaron, S. D. (2020). Pharmacologic management of chronic obstructive pulmonary disease: An official American Thoracic Society Clinical Practice Guideline. *American Journal of Respiratory and Critical Care Medicine, 201*, e56–e69. https://doi.org/10.1164/rccm.202003-0625ST

PLEURAL EFFUSIONS

DEFINITION

A. Result of excess fluid production or decreased absorption of fluid in the pleural space.

INCIDENCE

A. There are an estimated 1 to 1.5 million cases annually.

B. In general, the incidence is similar in both males and females. However, certain causes are more likely in males or females.

PATHOGENESIS

A. Pleural effusions are a manifestation of an underlying disease process.

B. Effusions can be transudative or exudative.

1. Transudative effusions are typically due to imbalance that occurs between the hydrostatic pressure and oncotic pressure.

2. Exudative effusions are the result of an alteration of the pleural surface, such as pleural or lung inflammation, impairment of lymphatic drainage, and so forth.

PREDISPOSING FACTORS

A. Any disease that may lead to accumulation of pleural fluid. The most common causes of pleural effusions are heart failure, malignancy, and pneumonia.

B. Diseases that can predispose a patient to a transudative effusion.

1. Heart failure.

2. Cirrhosis.

3. Nephrotic syndrome.

C. Diseases that can predispose a patient to an exudative effusion.

1. Pneumonia (parapneumonic effusion or empyema).

2. Malignancy.

3. Pancreatitis/pancreatic disease.

4. Trauma.

SUBJECTIVE DATA

A. Common complaints/symptoms.

1. Patients may have complaints of cough, pleuritic chest pain, and dyspnea.

2. Patients may have additional symptoms or clinical manifestations secondary to the underlying etiology of the pleural effusion.

B. Review of systems.

1. Depending on the suspected etiology of the effusion, the provider may want to inquire about heart ▶

failure, known liver disease or chronic alcoholism, recent trauma, history of cancer, occupational exposures, recent signs and symptoms of respiratory infection, and so forth.

PHYSICAL EXAMINATION
A. Typically, no physical findings when the pleural effusion is less than 300 mL.
B. Other findings.
   1. Diminished breath sounds.
   2. Dullness on percussion.
   3. Pleural friction rub.
   4. Decreased tactile fremitus.
C. Possible other findings such as fever and edema, depending on the etiology.

DIAGNOSTIC TESTS
A. Chest x-ray (CXR; Figure 2.4).
   1. Blunting of costophrenic angle in upright posteroanterior x-ray when 175 mL or more is present.
B. Smaller pleural effusions observed in lateral decubitus x-rays.
C. Failure of a pleural effusion to layer on a lateral decubitus x-ray. This may indicate a loculated pleural effusion.
D. Chest CT: Possible for evaluation of a loculated pleural effusion.
E. Ultrasonography: Can be used to evaluate the size of the pleural effusion and location.
F. Diagnostic thoracentesis.
   1. Should be performed in patients whose etiology is unclear and who fail to respond to therapy.
   2. Pleural fluid for diagnosis. Send for glucose, lactate dehydrogenase (LDH), pH, cell count, protein, and culture to aid with a possible diagnosis. Serum blood levels of LDH, total protein, and glucose are needed for comparison.
   3. Light's criteria: Used to differentiate between transudative and exudative pleural effusions.
      a. Exudative if one of the following is present:

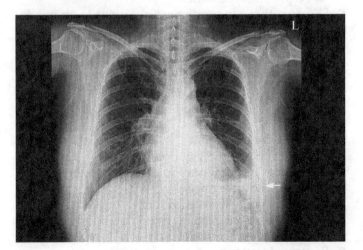

FIGURE 2.4 Chest x-ray of a left pleural effusion.

      i. Ratio of pleural fluid to serum protein is greater than 0.5.
      ii. Ratio of pleural fluid to serum LDH is greater than 0.6.
      iii. Pleural fluid LDH is greater than two-thirds the normal serum LDH.
   4. Additional testing may be indicated when trying to identify the etiology.

DIFFERENTIAL DIAGNOSIS
A. First, it is important to determine if the pleural effusion is transudate or exudate using Light's criteria in order to establish a differential diagnosis.
B. Transudate pleural effusion.
   1. Congestive heart failure (CHF).
   2. Cirrhosis.
   3. Exudate pleural effusion.
   4. Pneumonia.
   5. Cancer.
   6. Tuberculosis.
   7. Pulmonary embolism (PE).

EVALUATION AND MANAGEMENT PLAN
A. General plan.
   1. For transudative effusions, manage the underlying disease process, such as diuretics for patients with effusions due to heart failure.
   2. Specific interventions.
      a. Monitoring of CXRs: As needed pending the size, symptoms associated with the effusion, and following treatment to evaluate for reaccumulating fluid.
      b. Therapeutic thoracentesis: Used for patients with refractory, large pleural effusions and/or severe respiratory compromise to relieve symptoms. Diagnostic evaluation may be required if concerned for malignancy, infectious process, and so forth.
        i. Patients with malignant pleural effusions may require more than one thoracentesis due to reaccumulating fluid.
        ii. Patients who need frequent thoracentesis may require a pleurodesis or indwelling tunneled pleural catheter for home drainage. The patient and family will require teaching about home use of the tunneled pleural catheter.
      c. Chest tube.
        i. Required for a parapneumonic effusion or an empyema, but ultimately the patient will need to be treated with antibiotics and possible surgical intervention.
        ii. Required for patients with a hemothorax (bloody pleural effusion).
B. Patient/family teaching points.
   1. Teach patients that it may help to cough or take a deep breath by holding a pillow against your chest to prevent pain.

2. Practice smoking cessation and avoid second-hand smoke.

3. Keep hydrated.

4. Use an incentive spirometer for frequent deep breathing and coughing exercises.

C. Pharmacotherapy (depends on the etiology of pleural effusion).

    1. Antibiotics.

        a. For use in parapneumonic effusions, empyemas, and abscesses.

        b. Use empiric coverage and consider the patient's age, comorbidities, and clinical picture before tailoring the final selection of antibiotics.

        c. In general, the antimicrobial coverage should cover anaerobic organisms.

    2. Vasodilators and diuretics: For use in pleural effusions related to CHF and pulmonary edema.

    3. Anticoagulants: For use in pleural effusions due to pulmonary emboli.

D. Discharge instructions.

    1. Instruct patients to report any increased work in breathing, fevers, and pain that does not go away or gets worse. Take medications as prescribed.

FOLLOW-UP

A. For patients in the hospital, monitor with CXRs as needed and/or based on their symptoms.

B. The etiology of the effusion determines the course and frequency of outpatient follow-up.

CONSULTATION/REFERRAL

A. Thoracentesis: This can be completed by a hospitalist, pulmonologist, or interventional radiologist. If a more invasive procedure such as a surgical intervention is indicated, then a cardiothoracic surgeon will need to be consulted.

B. Further referrals may be indicated depending on the etiology of the effusion. If the effusion is malignant, then oncology will need to be consulted.

BIBLIOGRAPHY

Bedawi, E. O., Hassan, M., & Rahman, N. M. (2018). Recent developments in the management of pleural infection: A comprehensive review. *The Clinical Respiratory Journal, 12*, 2309–2320. https://doi.org/10.1111/crj.12941

Bhatnagar, R., & Maskell, N. (2015). The modern diagnosis and management of pleural effusions. *British Medical Journal, 351*, 26–30. https://doi.org/10.1136/bmj.h4520

Bintcliffe, O. J., Lee, G. Y. C., Rahman, N. M., & Maskell, N. A. (2016). The management of benign non-infective pleural effusions. *European Respiratory Review, 25*, 303–316. https://doi.org/10.1183/16000617.0026-2016

Kummerfeldt, C. E., Pastis, N. J., & Huggins, J. T. (2017). Pleural diseases. In S. C. McKean, J. J. Ross, D. D. Dressler, & D. B. Scheurer (Eds.), *Principles and practice of hospital medicine* (2nd ed., pp. 1923–1932). McGraw-Hill.

Saguil, A., Wyrick, K., & Hallgren, J. (2014). Diagnostic approach to pleural effusion. *American Family Physician, 90*, 99–104. https://www.aafp.org/afp/2014/0715/p99.html

PNEUMONIA

DEFINITION

A. An infection of the lungs that can have varying degrees of severity.

B. Caused by bacteria, viruses, or fungi.

C. Can be further divided into three types: community-acquired pneumonia (CAP), hospital-acquired pneumonia (HAP), and ventilator-associated pneumonia (VAP).

INCIDENCE

A. Pneumonia (combined with influenza) is the eighth leading cause of mortality in the United States, accounting for approximately 50,000 deaths annually.

B. Older adults are at an increased risk of acquiring pneumonia and more likely to die from pneumonia. Pneumonia is a leading cause of hospital admissions.

C. It accounts for one of the top 10 most costly conditions in the United States, with approximately $9.5 billion spent for 960,000 hospital stays.

D. It is the most common cause of sepsis and septic shock.

PATHOGENESIS

A. A pathogenic microorganism invades the lung parenchyma. Neutrophils aggregate to the site of invasion and begin to phagocytize the microorganisms and release an extracellular trap.

B. The immune response is activated. Inflammatory mediators are released, causing the capillaries to become permeable and an exudative fluid to be formed. The protein-rich fluid containing neutrophils, bacteria, fibrin, and so forth fills the alveoli, leading to a lung consolidation.

C. Inflammatory mediators lead to harm of the lung parenchyma resulting in systemic inflammation, which leads to extrapulmonary symptoms (e.g., fever, chills, fatigue).

PREDISPOSING FACTORS

A. An impaired immune response and/or dysfunction of the body's defense mechanism, HIV.

B. Advanced age.

C. Smoking.

D. Chronic lung disease (e.g., chronic obstructive pulmonary disease [COPD], asthma).

E. Other chronic comorbid conditions (e.g., heart failure, diabetes).

F. Recent respiratory viral infection.

G. Excessive alcohol consumption.

SUBJECTIVE DATA

A. Common complaints/symptoms:

    1. Cough with sputum production (see Figure 2.3).

    2. Fever.

    3. Chills.

4. Altered mental status or confusion, especially in older adults.

5. Pleuritic chest pain.

B. Common/typical scenario.

1. Patients typically present with sudden onset of symptoms, such as shortness of breath, productive cough, and fever. They may also complain of chills and malaise.

C. Family and social history.

1. May be more prevalent in smokers, among older adults, and in the chronically ill.

D. Review of symptoms.

1. Symptoms may vary depending on age, activity level, and underlying comorbid conditions. Older adults typically present differently from younger adults, in part due to the normal physiologic changes of aging.

2. The provider should inquire about onset, severity, and associated symptoms.

3. Assessment of recent respiratory viral illnesses is important, especially given the correlation of pneumonia following influenza.

4. It may help to inquire about recent sick contacts.

PHYSICAL EXAMINATION

A. General: Vital signs.

1. Fever, which may or may not be present.

2. Tachycardia, which may or may not be present.

3. Possibly high respiratory rate, which may be normal or increased.

B. Neurologic.

1. More likely to see changes in the older adult. Patients can be described as having confusion, decreased interactions, and/or is "acting differently."

C. Respiratory.

1. Rales/crackles on auscultation in the affected area. Patients may also have rhonchi.

2. Dullness on percussion in the affected area.

3. Increased tactile fremitus in the affected area.

4. Possible pleural friction rub.

5. Decreased breath sounds.

D. Other possible findings.

1. Cyanosis, respiratory failure, and septic shock in patients with a more virulent type of pneumonia, multilobar pneumonia, and/or comorbid conditions.

DIAGNOSTIC TESTS

A. Chest x-ray (CXR).

1. Evidence of an infiltrate, which can be patchy or a dense consolidation of a lobe or segment.

B. Sputum culture and Gram stain.

1. Used to identify the microorganism responsible for the pneumonia.

2. Only recommended in those with severe disease and/or those receiving empiric treatment for a possible drug-resistant pneumonia.

3. Most sensitive if the patient can provide an adequate specimen and has not recently been treated or is not currently receiving treatment with antibiotics.

4. For intubated patients, obtain an endotracheal aspirate.

C. Blood cultures.

1. Usually indicated for patients with more severe forms of pneumonia.

D. Urinary antigen testing.

1. Used to assess for pneumococcal pneumonia, mycoplasma pneumonia, and Legionnaires' disease.

2. Rapid and simple; however, it does not provide information for narrowing of antibiotics.

3. Usually recommended for patients with severe disease.

E. Serum procalcitonin.

1. Can assist the provider with antibiotic duration in conjunction with the patient's clinical presentation.

2. Procalcitonin should not be used to determine the need for initial antibiotic therapy.

3. No recommended use of procalcitonin in patients with HAP or VAP according to the Infectious Diseases Society of America and the American Thoracic Society guidelines.

F. Comprehensive metabolic panel.

1. Can assist with risk stratification and sequela of pneumonia.

G. Complete blood count (CBC).

1. Assessment of a leukocytosis or leukopenia.

H. Arterial blood gas (ABG).

1. May be indicated in more severe presentations, such as cyanosis or respiratory failure, to evaluate for hypoxemia and/or hypercapnia.

I. Chest CT scan.

1. Not typically indicated, especially if one is able to obtain a good-quality CXR.

DIFFERENTIAL DIAGNOSIS

A. COPD.

B. Asthma.

C. Pulmonary edema.

D. Bronchiectasis.

E. Lung cancer.

F. Pulmonary embolism (PE).

G. Bronchitis.

H. Less common infectious causes of pneumonia include histoplasmosis, *Pneumocystis jirovecii* pneumonia (PJP).

EVALUATION AND MANAGEMENT PLAN

A. General plan.

1. Management of pneumonia is dependent on the severity of the disease, classification or type of pneumonia (e.g., CAP vs. HAP), and pathogens involved.

2. Supportive care, such as oxygen therapy or other methods of respiratory support (e.g., noninvasive ventilation, invasive mechanical ventilation), should be considered in patients with hypoxemia and/or respiratory failure.

3. Patients presenting with sepsis due to pneumonia should receive care in accordance with the sepsis guidelines.

4. Guidelines suggest that antimicrobial therapy be tailored to the individual's clinical picture, suspected organism, severity, and so forth, rather than fixed therapy.

5. Transitioning to oral therapy is appropriate once patients' clinical status has improved and they are hemodynamically stable.

6. In patients with coexisting influenza A, early treatment with oseltamivir or zanamivir is appropriate.

7. Systemic corticosteroids: Current guidelines recommend against use of corticosteroids; however, they may be considered in patients with refractory shock.

  a. CAP.

    i. Clinical prediction tools, specifically the Pneumonia Severity Index (PSI), combined with clinical judgment can be used to identify patients who can be treated as outpatient versus inpatient. These prediction tools should not be used to determine higher levels of inpatient care.

    ii. Severe CAP can be defined using the validated definition developed by the Infectious Diseases Society of America and the American Thoracic Society.

      1) Minor criteria: Respiratory rate greater than or equal to 30 breaths per minute, PF (PaO_2/FiO_2) ratio less than or equal to 250, multilobar infiltrates, confusion, uremia, leukopenia, thrombocytopenia, hypothermia (less than 96.8°F/36°C), and hypotension requiring aggressive fluid resuscitation.

      2) Major criteria: Septic shock and respiratory failure requiring mechanical ventilation.

      3) Three or more minor criteria OR one major criteria is defined as severe CAP.

    iii. Duration of treatment: Patients should receive a minimum of 5 days of treatment and literature suggests that more than 7 days is typically not needed.

    iv. Antibiotic therapy focuses on the likely pathogen and severity.

      1) The most common outpatient pathogens are *Streptococcus pneumoniae*, *Haemophilus influenzae*, *Mycoplasma pneumoniae*, *Chlamydia pneumoniae*, *Legionella*, and respiratory viruses.

        a) Patients with no comorbidities or risk factors (e.g., recent hospitalization and parenteral antibiotics in the last 90 days) for methicillin-resistant *Staphylococcus aureus* (MRSA) or *Pseudomonas aeruginosa* can be initiated on amoxicillin, doxycycline, or a macrolide.

        b) Patients with chronic comorbid conditions (e.g., heart failure, lung, liver, or renal disease, diabetes) should be started on combination therapy with amoxicillin–clavulanate or cephalosporin (e.g., cefpodoxime, cefuroxime) *AND* a macrolide or doxycycline *OR* monotherapy with a respiratory fluoroquinolone (e.g., moxifloxacin, levofloxacin, or gemifloxacin).

      2) The most common inpatient, non-ICU pathogens are *S. pneumoniae*, *M. pneumoniae*,

C. pneumoniae, *H. influenzae*, *Legionella* species, aspiration, and respiratory viruses.

      3) The most common inpatient, ICU pathogens are *S. pneumoniae*, *S. aureus*, *Legionella* species, gram-negative bacilli, and *H. influenzae*.

      4) Patients with non-severe inpatient pneumonia should be treated with a respiratory fluoroquinolone *OR* a beta-lactam (e.g., ceftriaxone, cefotaxime, or ampicillin/sulbactam) *plus* a macrolide.

      5) Patients with severe inpatient pneumonia should be started on a beta-lactam (e.g., cefotaxime, ceftriaxone, or ampicillin-sulbactam) *plus* a macrolide (e.g., azithromycin) *OR* a beta-lactam plus a respiratory fluoroquinolone.

      6) For patients with CAP and risk factors for MRSA and *P. aeruginosa*, treatment should consist of:

        a) MRSA coverage: Vancomycin or linezolid.

        b) *P. aeruginosa* coverage: Piperacillin–tazobactam, cefepime, ceftazidime, or meropenem.

  b. HAP.

    i. Develops 2 or more days after admission to the hospital.

    ii. Use of a local antibiogram tailored to HAP pathogens and susceptibilities for empiric coverage as recommended by guidelines.

    iii. Antibiotic treatment: Recommended 7-day course.

      1) Empiric coverage depends on the patient's mortality risk and suspicion for multidrug-resistant (MDR) pathogens.

        a) A risk factor for MDR pathogens in HAP include prior intravenous (IV) antibiotic use within 90 days.

        b) Septic shock and/or mechanical ventilation due to HAP are associated with a high risk of mortality.

      2) Patients not at high risk for mortality or likelihood of MDR pathogens can be placed on piperacillin–tazobactam (Zosyn) *OR* cefepime *OR* levofloxacin.

      3) Patients not at high risk for mortality but who have factors that may increase their likelihood of MRSA should be placed on piperacillin–tazobactam, cefepime *OR* levofloxacin *OR* meropenem *OR* aztreonam *plus* vancomycin or linezolid (second line due to toxic effects if vancomycin cannot be used).

      4) Patients with a high mortality risk or who have received IV antibiotics in the prior 90 days should be started on:

        a) Piperacillin–tazobactam (Zosyn) *OR* cefepime *OR* levofloxacin *OR* meropenem *OR* amikacin/gentamicin/tobramycin *OR* aztreonam *plus* vancomycin or linezolid.

b) Providers should cover for MRSA and pick two additional medications while avoiding prescribing two beta-lactams.

c. VAP.

i. A pneumonia that develops more than 2 days after intubation and mechanical ventilation.

ii. Use of a local antibiogram tailored to the ICU population, VAP pathogens, and susceptibilities for adequate coverage as recommended per guidelines.

iii. Antibiotic treatment: Recommended 7-day course.

1) *S. aureus, Pseudomonas,* and other gram-negative bacilli coverage should be included in all empiric regimens.

2) Patients with risk factors for MRSA should receive empiric coverage with vancomycin or linezolid.

3) For patients with no known risk factors for MRSA and suspected of methicillin-susceptible *Staphylococcus aureus* (MSSA), the suggested regimen includes piperacillin–tazobactam, cefepime, levofloxacin, or meropenem. If the patient has proven MSSA, then the preferred agents are cefazolin or nafcillin.

4) Patients with risk factors for gram-negative infection, including *Pseudomonas* and resistant microorganisms, should receive treatment with two antipseudomonal drugs.

a) Piperacillin–tazobactam. *OR*

b) Cefepime. *OR*

c) Meropenem. *OR*

d) Aztreonam. *OR*

e) Ciprofloxacin.

5) Guidelines recommend against the routine use of aminoglycosides and colistin if adequate coverage is available with alternative antibiotics.

B. Discharge instructions.

1. Discharge criteria. These primarily focus on improvement in clinical status/condition.

a. Resolution of fever (e.g., <100.4°F/38°C).

b. Improving symptoms (e.g., dyspnea, cough, sputum production).

c. Heart rate less than 100 beats per minute.

d. Respiratory rate less than 24 per minute.

e. Oxygen saturation greater than 90%.

f. Diminishing leukocytosis.

g. Maintaining oral intake.

h. Systolic blood pressure greater than 90 mmHg.

i. Return to baseline mentation.

2. Activity.

a. Regular or baseline activity as tolerated.

3. Diet.

a. Comorbid conditions such as diabetes, heart failure, or renal disease: May vary.

b. No underlying comorbid conditions: Resumption of regular diet.

4. Medications.

a. Antibiotics: Duration of 7 days, including the days the patient received antibiotics while hospitalized.

b. Other drugs: Medication reconciliation and continuation of medications for comorbid conditions.

5. Treatment plan.

a. Important for patients to complete the full course of antibiotics even if feeling better.

b. Coughing with sputum production: Normal and should improve over time.

c. Vaccinations such as influenza annually and pneumococcal disease necessary for those at risk.

d. Pulmonary hygiene (e.g., deep breathing).

e. Smoking cessation counseling.

f. Remaining hydrated.

g. Managing comorbid conditions.

6. Discuss with the patient.

a. Stress that patients should contact their provider if they develop fever or worsening symptoms, such as increased cough and dyspnea despite antibiotic therapy, decreased appetite, nausea, and mentation changes.

b. Reemphasize the importance of completing antibiotic therapy to reduce reoccurrence and avoid resistance emergence.

FOLLOW-UP

A. Follow-up is highly dependent on the type and severity of pneumonia, as well as functional status and comorbid conditions.

B. Patients in the outpatient setting typically see improvement in symptoms within 3 to 7 days, so failure to see improvement or clinical deterioration should be dealt with immediately.

C. Patients discharged from the hospital should be seen 1 to 2 weeks after discharge.

CONSULTATION/REFERRAL

A. Outpatient management typically does not require a referral unless the patient's clinical status worsens, in which case the patient should be sent to the hospital.

B. Inpatient management may include a pulmonologist and infectious disease pending the severity of the pneumonia and the patient's condition.

SPECIAL/GERIATRIC CONSIDERATIONS

A. Older adults should be instructed to receive pneumococcal and influenza vaccinations.

B. All patients should be counseled regarding smoking cessation.

BIBLIOGRAPHY

American Thoracic Society. (2019). *Top 20 pneumonia facts.* https://www.thoracic.org/patients/patient-resources/resources/top-pneumonia-facts.pdf

Kalil, A. C., Metersky, M. L., Klompas, M., Muscedere, J., Sweeney, D. A., Palmer, L. B., & Brozek, J. L. (2016). Management of adults with hospital-acquired and ventilator-associated pneumonia: 2016 clinical practice guidelines by the Infectious Diseases Society of America and the American Thoracic Society. *Clinical Infectious Diseases, 63*, e61–e111. https://doi.org/10.1093/cid/ciw353

Klompas, M. (2017). Health care and hospital-acquired pneumonia. In S. C. McKean, J. J. Ross, D. D. Dressler, & D. B. Scheurer (Eds.), *Principles and practice of hospital medicine* (2nd ed., pp. 1514–1518). McGraw-Hill.

Metlay, J. P., Waterer, G. W., Long, A. C., Anzueto, A., Brozek, J., Crothers, K., Cooley, L. A., Dean, N. C., Fine, M. J., Flanders, S. A., Griffin, M. R., Meterksy, M. L., Musher, D. M., Restrepo, M. I., & Whitney, C. G. (2019). Diagnosis and treatment of adults with community-acquired pneumonia: An official clinical practice guideline of the American Thoracic Society and Infectious Diseases Society of America. *American Journal of Respiratory and Critical Care Medicine, 200*, e45–e67. https://doi.org/10.1164/rccm.201908-1581ST

Musher, D. M. (2017). Community-acquired pneumonia. In S. C. McKean, J. J. Ross, D. D. Dressler, & D. B. Scheurer (Eds.), *Principles and practice of hospital medicine* (2nd ed., pp. 1503–1513). McGraw-Hill.

Rider, A. C., & Frazee, B. W. (2018). Community-acquired pneumonia. *Emergency Medicine Clinics of North America, 36*, 665–683. https://doi.org/10.1016/j.emc.2018.07.001

PULMONARY EMBOLISM

DEFINITION
A. A blockage of one or more of the pulmonary arteries. Most commonly, pulmonary embolism (PE) is the result of an embolic thrombus formation elsewhere in the body (e.g., lower extremity).
B. PE can be classified into different subgroups: based on presentation (e.g., acute, subacute, chronic), hemodynamic status (e.g., massive PE, submassive PE, low-risk PE), and anatomic location (e.g., saddle, lobar, segmental, subsegmental).

INCIDENCE
A. PE is more common in patients with deep vein thrombosis (DVT).
B. It is considered the third most common cause of cardiovascular death, with an estimated mortality of 60,000 to 100,000 deaths annually.
C. In those who present with sudden cardiac death, it is speculated that up to 25% have a PE.
D. Approximately one-third of patients will have a recurrence within 10 years.

PATHOGENESIS
A. A thrombus forms secondary to a hypercoagulable state, injury to the vascular endothelium, and venostasis, which concentrates blood clotting factors at the site of vessel injury. Clot formation occurs as a result of blood pooling.
B. The clot can dislodge from the extremity, travel through the venous system, move through the right side of the heart, and obstruct a pulmonary artery. Obstructions that are large enough can prevent blood flow to the affected area, creating a ventilation/perfusion (V/Q) mismatch leading to respiratory failure and/or increase the pulmonary artery pressure, resulting in right-sided heart failure.
C. Ultimately, an acute PE impacts circulation and gas exchange.

PREDISPOSING FACTORS
A. Factor V mutation.
B. Protein C or S deficiency.
C. Malignancy.
D. Immobility.
E. Trauma.
F. Surgery, especially a hip or knee replacement.
G. Smoking.
H. Obesity.
I. Prior PE.
J. Chronic diseases such as heart failure and chronic obstructive pulmonary disease (COPD).
K. Prolonged travel.
L. Lower limb fracture.

SUBJECTIVE DATA
A. Common complaints/symptoms.
  1. These can vary depending on the degree of clot burden.
  2. Patients may be asymptomatic, especially in the setting of a small segmental branch PE. The condition is usually found incidentally in these cases.
  3. Symptoms may include:
    a. Pleuritic chest pain.
    b. Dyspnea/tachypnea.
    c. Hypoxia.
    d. Cough with possible blood-tinged sputum production.
    e. Tachycardia.
    f. Dizziness or syncope.
    g. Hypotension/shock with a massive PE.
    h. Cardiac collapse, with the patient presenting in cardiac arrest.
    i. Heart failure, specifically right-sided heart failure.
    j. Recent symptoms associated with a DVT (e.g., extremity pain, warmth, erythema, edema).
B. Family and social history.
  1. It is important for the provider to assess for family history of hypercoagulable states, clot formation, and/or known factor deficiencies.
  2. The provider should assess symptom onset and any associated risk factors for PE development, such as history or current malignancy, decreased mobility, travel, recent surgeries, and so forth.

PHYSICAL EXAMINATION
A. Findings depend on the degree of clot burden.
B. Perform a general examination, which may reveal diaphoresis, fever, and tachycardia. On presentation, most patients are hemodynamically stable unless significant clot burden resulting in increased right ventricular (RV) afterload, RV failure, and subsequent decreased left ventricular (LV) preload and decreased cardiac output resulting in hypotension/shock.
C. Assess neurologic status. Patients may present with syncope, altered mentation, or agitation, especially those presenting with hypoxemia and shock.

D. Assess respiratory rate. In more significant PEs, the rate will be increased. Auscultation of breath sounds may reveal rales or crackles.

E. Perform a cardiac examination. Patients may have a murmur, accentuated second heart sound, or S3/S4 gallop.

F. Extremities may reveal signs of a DVT, such as pain, edema, or erythema.

DIAGNOSTIC TESTS

A. D-dimer (age-adjusted).

   1. High sensitivity: With negative results indicating a low probability of a PE.

   2. Most reliable in young patients with no comorbid conditions and short symptom onset.

   3. Can have nonspecific elevations in those with malignancy, severe infection and/or inflammatory disease, and hospitalized patients.

B. Chest CT angiography (CTA).

   1. Allows for direct visualization of the emboli within the pulmonary arteries.

   2. Considered the standard of care for diagnosing patients with high probability of a PE or low/intermediate probability but positive D-dimer.

   3. RV dilation: Associated with short-term adverse outcomes.

C. V/Q lung scan.

   1. An alternative to the chest CTA, especially in the setting of contraindications such as renal failure.

   2. Evaluates for perfusion defects, which are nonspecific and only present in one-third of patients with PE.

   3. Inconclusive results in 50% of cases and unable to provide alternative diagnosis if PE is excluded.

D. Echocardiography.

   1. Often indirectly helps diagnose PE in conjunction with the patient's clinical presentation.

   2. Can also be used for risk stratification and as a prognostic factor in PE.

   3. Possible findings consistent with a PE: Acute RV enlargement and in some cases dysfunction, evidence of pulmonary hypertension with elevated RV systolic pressures, and possible flattening of the septum.

   4. May be able to visualize an intracardiac thrombi.

   5. RV dilation: Associated with an increased risk for adverse outcomes.

E. Ultrasonography.

   1. Typically, used to identify an etiology for PE and/or assist with diagnosis of PE when other diagnostics (e.g., angiography) cannot be utilized.

F. Additional diagnostics for acute risk stratification.

   1. Pulmonary Embolism Severity Index (PESI).

      a. Used to predict the 30-day outcomes/mortality in patients with acute PE.

      b. Score greater than 106 on the original PESI: High risk for morbidity and mortality.

      c. Score greater than or equal to 1 on the simplified PESI: High risk for morbidity and mortality.

   2. Troponin.

      a. Elevated troponin levels in patients presenting or receiving treatment for PE: Associated with adverse outcomes.

   3. N-terminal probrain natriuretic peptide (NT-proBNP).

      a. Similar to cardiac troponins, elevated NT-proBNP levels are associated with adverse outcomes.

DIFFERENTIAL DIAGNOSIS

A. Pericarditis.

B. Pleuritis.

C. Musculoskeletal pain.

EVALUATION AND MANAGEMENT PLAN

A. General plan.

   1. Diagnosis of a PE requires the provider to account for the patient's clinical presentation as well as evaluating the diagnostic tests.

   2. Treatment recommendations are highly dependent on the patient's clinical status, including respiratory and hemodynamic stability at the time of presentation.

   3. In the clinical setting and literature, PEs have been described as low risk, submassive, and massive.

      a. Low-risk PEs: Patients with hemodynamic stability, no elevation in biomarkers, and no evidence of RV dysfunction on imaging.

         i. Those with low-risk PEs are initiated on direct oral anticoagulants (DOACs), such as apixaban, dabigatran, or rivaroxaban.

         ii. These patients can be assessed for early discharge.

      b. Submassive PEs (intermediate risk): Patients with hemodynamic stability but evidence of RV dysfunction on imaging and/or biomarker elevation.

         i. Those with intermediate-risk PEs can be admitted for intravenous (IV) anticoagulation or may be a candidate for catheter-directed thrombolysis.

         ii. These patients will need to be discharged home on a DOAC.

      c. Massive PEs (high risk): Patients with hemodynamic instability, elevation in biomarkers, and evidence of RV dysfunction.

         i. Those with high-risk PEs with no contraindications may be a candidate for systemic thrombolysis.

         ii. Those with high-risk PEs may need further supportive therapy such as mechanical circulatory support in patients with cardiac collapse, oxygen and/or mechanical ventilation, and vasopressors to support their hemodynamic status while definitive treatment is being employed.

   4. Ideally, patients should have pretest clinical assessment, diagnostics with consideration of risk stratification, and initiation of treatment. ▶

5. Low to intermediate probability of PE.
   a. Pretest clinical assessment.
      i. Wells Clinical Prediction Rule for PE. Patients are evaluated using seven variables in which they can receive 1 to 3 points. A score of 2 to 6 points indicates an intermediate risk and a score greater than or equal to 6 indicates high risk.
      ii. Revised Geneva Score. Patients are evaluated using eight variables in which they can receive 1 to 5 points. A score of 4 to 10 points indicates an intermediate risk and a score greater than or equal to 11 indicates high risk.
      iii. Appropriate for patients who are hemodynamically stable. Patients with a high probability of PE should proceed immediately to diagnostic testing.
   b. Age-adjusted D-dimer.
      i. If negative, no further imaging needed.
      ii. If positive, further imaging needed.
      iii. It is important that the provider use an age-adjusted scale due to decreased specificity in the older adult. Using the appropriate scale can reduce the number of false-positive results.
   c. Chest CTA versus V/Q lung scan.
      i. If no contraindications to CTA, chest CTA is preferred.
   d. Treatment: Anticoagulation therapy.
6. High probability of PE.
   a. Patients may be hemodynamically unstable; pretest clinical assessment not appropriate.
   b. Immediate chest CTA: If unable to obtain a chest CTA due to hemodynamic instability/ uncontrolled hypotension, then findings consistent with a PE on echocardiography may be a suitable alternative.
B. Pharmacotherapy.
   1. Decision about medication management should consider whether the PE was provoked (caused by an identifiable risk factor such as cancer) versus unprovoked, as well as the duration of therapy.
   2. Patients should be routinely reevaluated for anticoagulation needs if receiving extended therapy.
   3. Treatment with dabigatran, rivaroxaban, apixaban, or edoxaban is recommended over a vitamin K antagonist in patients with a PE.
   4. A vitamin K antagonist is recommended for patients with an unprovoked PE if not receiving treatment with dabigatran, rivaroxaban, apixaban, or edoxaban.
   5. It is suggested that a provider treating a patient with a PE and cancer use a low molecular weight heparin (LMWH). It is also recommended that patients receive extended therapy (e.g., no stop date) depending on their bleeding risk.
   6. Anticoagulation is recommended for 3 months in patients with a PE provoked by surgery or transient risk factors.
   7. For patients with an unprovoked PE at a low or moderate bleeding risk, initiation of extended anticoagulation therapy (e.g., no stop date) is suggested.

For patients with a high bleeding risk, it is recommended to initiate anticoagulation for 3 months.
   8. Surveillance is suggested in patients with a distal (subsegmental) PE who have no proximal DVTs and a low risk for recurrent venous thromboembolism (VTE).
   9. Systemic thrombolytic therapy is suggested for hemodynamically unstable patients.
   10. Additional management: Catheter-directed thrombolysis may be appropriate in select patient populations but require a multidisciplinary approach and additional provider consultation.
C. Patient/family teaching points.
   1. Prevent more blood clots from forming by taking the medication as prescribed.
   2. Be sure to follow up with lab tests as directed.
   3. Encourage patients to get up and be active.
   4. Smoking cessation.
   5. On long trips, make frequent stops to get out and move about.
   6. On airplane rides, perform exercises that keep your legs, feet, and toes moving.
D. Discharge instructions.
   1. Call your healthcare provider if there is any increase in symptoms.

FOLLOW-UP

A. Patient follow-up is variable in the literature primarily due to the type of medication, cause of PE, and severity of illness due to the PE.
B. A vitamin K antagonist requires that the patient follow up 2 to 3 days postdischarge for international normalized ratio (INR) evaluation.

CONSULTATION/REFERRAL

A. Pulmonologist may be consulted due to the pulmonary symptoms associated with a PE.
B. Hematologist may be warranted especially if concerned for a procoagulant defect.
C. An interventional radiologist or interventional cardiologist may be consulted for catheter-directed thrombolysis.
D. Critical care may be needed if the patient is admitted to the ICU or becomes hemodynamically unstable.

SPECIAL/GERIATRIC CONSIDERATIONS

A. An inferior vena cava (IVC) filter may be appropriate in patients with absolute contraindications to anticoagulation and in patients with recurrent PE.
B. IV anticoagulation therapy should be started prior to administering dabigatran and edoxaban.

BIBLIOGRAPHY

Bernal, A. G., Fanola, C., & Bartos, J. A. (2020). *Management of PE.* https://www.acc.org/latest-in-cardiology/articles/2020/01/27/07/42/management-of-pe
Faluk, M., Hasan, S. M., Chacko, J. J., Abdelmaseih, R., & Patel, J. (2021). Evolution of acute pulmonary embolism management: Review article. *Current Problems in Cardiology, 46,* 1–11. https://doi.org/10.1016/j.cpcardiol.2020.10051
Kearon, C., Akl, E. A., Ornelas, J., Blaivas, A., Jimenez, D., Bounameaux, H., Huisman, M., & Moores, C. L. (2016). Antithrombotic therapy for

VTE disease: CHEST guideline and expert panel report. *Chest, 149,* 315–352. https://doi.org/10.1016/j.chest.2015.11.026

Konstantinides, S. V., Barco, S., Lankeit, M., & Meyer, G. (2016). Management of pulmonary embolism: An update. *Journal of the American College of Cardiology, 67,* 976–990. https://doi.org/10.1016/j.jacc.2015.11.061

Konstantinides, S. V., Meyer, G., Becattini, C., Bueno, H., Geersing, G., Harjola, V., Huisman, M. V., Humbert, M., Jennings, C. S., Jimenez, D., Kucher, N., Lang, I. M., Lankeit, M., Lorusso, R., Mazzolai, L., Meneveau, N., Ainle, F. N., Prandoni, P., Pruszczyk, P. … Zamorano, J. L. (2020). 2019 ESC guidelines for the diagnosis and management of acute pulmonary embolism developed in collaboration with the European Respiratory Society (ERS). *European Heart Journal, 41,* 543–603. https://doi.org/10.1093/eurheartj/ehz405

Martinez-Licha, C. R., McCurdy, C. M., Maldonado, S. M., & Lee, L. S. (2020). Current management of acute pulmonary embolism. *Annals of Thoracic and Cardiovascular Surgery, 26,* 65–71. https://doi.org/10.5761/atcs.ra.19-00158

Ortel, T. L., Neumann, I., Ageno, W., Beyth, R., Clark, N. P., Cuker, A., Hutten, B. A., Jaff, M. R., Manja, V., Schulman, S., Thurston, C., Vedantham, S., Verhamme, P., Witt, D. M., Florez, I. D., Izcovich, A., Nieuwlaat, R., Ross, S., Schunemann, H. J. … Zhang, Y. (2020). American society of hematology 2020 guidelines for management of venous thromboembolism: Treatment of deep vein thrombosis and pulmonary embolism. *Blood Advances, 4,* 4693–473. https://doi.org/10.1182/bloodadvances.2020001830

Yamamoto, T. (2018). Management of patients with high risk pulmonary embolism: A narrative review. *Journal of Intensive Care, 6,* 1–9. https://doi.org/10.1186/s40560-018-0286-8

RESTRICTIVE LUNG DISEASE

DEFINITION

A. A reduction in the total lung capacity (TLC) secondary to a decrease in lung elasticity or disease of the chest wall, pleura, or neuromuscular etiology. Disorders can be classified as intrinsic or extrinsic.

   1. Intrinsic disorders (pulmonary parenchymal disease) include interstitial lung diseases (ILDs) such as idiopathic pulmonary fibrosis (IPF), interstitial pneumonia, medication-induced pulmonary fibrosis, and so forth.

      a. ILDs are a heterogeneous group of pulmonary disorders.

      b. Extrinsic disorders (extrapulmonary disease) include obesity and neuromuscular disorders (e.g., muscular dystrophy, amyotrophic lateral sclerosis).

INCIDENCE

A. The incidence is highly variable and dependent on the etiology of restriction.
B. The incidence of some disorders is not well known.
C. ILDs, although rare, are a cause of restrictive lung disease affecting approximately 650,000 individuals each year and resulting in 21,000 deaths.
D. Nonidiopathic and IPF (type of ILD) are a common cause of restrictive lung disease.
E. Approximately 30 per 100,000 cases of restrictive lung disease are due to IPF.
F. The prevalence of disease increases with age, especially in those over 75 years.

G. The frequency of occurrence is typically higher in men, especially among older adults.
H. Black Americans have a higher incidence of restrictive lung disease compared with White Americans.

PATHOGENESIS

A. Intrinsic disease.

   1. An exogenous or endogenous stimulus causes repetitive injury to the lung parenchyma, leading to epithelial and endothelial damage. Activation of local and systemic factors (e.g., fibroblasts, growth factors, clotting, factors, cytokines) occurs.

   2. A provisional matrix is formed. There is a dysregulation of the intricate network and lack of matrix degradation, leading to aberrant wound healing and progressive lung remodeling, ultimately causing pulmonary fibrosis.

   3. The diffuse lung parenchymal destruction results in reduced lung volumes and expiratory airflow.
B. Extrinsic disease.

   1. The mechanism for extrapulmonary form varies greatly compared with intrinsic etiologies. Extrapulmonary etiologies result in altered mechanical function that may be the result of rib deformities and/or underlying neurologic or muscular pathologies.

PREDISPOSING FACTORS

A. Predisposing factors depend on the etiology of the restrictive lung disease.
B. Risk factors include:

   1. Obesity.
   2. Kyphoscoliosis.
   3. Muscular dystrophy.
   4. Chronic pleural disease (e.g., trapped lung).
   5. Autoimmune disease (e.g., scleroderma, systemic lupus erythematosus).
   6. Occupational exposures.
   7. Medications such as amiodarone, bleomycin, and methotrexate.
   8. Idiopathic lung disease such as pulmonary fibrosis: more common in older adults and men.
   9. Sarcoidosis.

SUBJECTIVE DATA

A. Common complaints/symptoms.

   1. Symptoms and complaints may vary depending on the underlying cause of the restrictive lung disease.
   2. Dyspnea (see Figure 2.1): Most common complaint and usually insidious. It can be present with exercise or at rest as the disease progresses.
   3. Possible chronic cough (see Figure 2.3), wheezing (see Figure 2.2), or chest discomfort.
   4. Possible hemoptysis.
   5. Fatigue.
B. Duration of illness (e.g., acute onset, chronic).

   1. The duration of illness and/or symptom onset can aid with identifying the etiology and understanding ▶

the likely progression of the disease. For example, acute interstitial pneumonitis has an acute onset that usually lasts for days to weeks.
C. Family and social history.
  1. Smoking history.
  2. Occupational and/or environmental history or exposures.
  3. Family history of lung disease known to cause restrictive lung diseases (e.g., IPF, sarcoidosis).
D. Review of symptoms.
  1. Neurologic:aAny confusion, fatigue, and muscle weakness.
  2. Respiratory: Shortness of breath at rest and on exertion, or that is progressive; dry cough; bloody sputum; pain on inspiration; and recent or frequent colds.
  3. Use of medications such as nitrofurantoin, amiodarone, methotrexate, or others that have the potential to cause lung disease.

PHYSICAL EXAMINATION
A. Dyspnea, which may be more evident with activity.
B. Tachypnea.
C. Cyanosis or oxygen desaturation with activity.
D. Possible bibasilar inspiratory crackles, scattered inspiratory rhonchi, or wheezing.
E. Digital clubbing.
F. Obese.
G. Other disease-specific signs and symptoms (e.g., rash, Raynaud, muscle weakness), depending on the underlying etiology.

DIAGNOSTIC TESTS
A. Laboratory studies.
  1. Usually nonspecific.
  2. Serologic testing: This may be appropriate in patients suspected of having an underlying disorder or connective tissue disease causing a restrictive disease such as rheumatoid arthritis.
B. Chest x-ray (CXR).
  1. Typically nonspecific findings, which may vary with the type of restrictive disease.
  2. Possible evidence of increased interstitial markings, bibasilar reticular pattern, or a nodular pattern.
  3. Honeycombing, which is typically noted as a late or advanced finding.
  4. If an extrinsic factor is suspected, then imaging may reveal a trapped lung, pleural effusion, and so forth.
C. Chest CT.
  1. More sensitive and better assessment of the extent of disease compared with a CXR.
  2. May reveal findings characteristic of specific restrictive diseases. Some restrictive diseases such as IPF can be diagnosed solely with a chest CT.
  3. If an extrinsic factor is suspected, then imaging may reveal a trapped lung, pleural effusion, and so forth.
D. Pulmonary function testing.

  1. Valuable in assessing response to therapy and monitoring disease progression.
  2. Does not diagnose a specific disease but does indicate restrictive lung disease pattern, if present.
  3. Characteristic findings include reduced TLC, functional residual capacity (FRC), and residual volume (RV).
  4. The forced expiratory volume in 1 second (FEV_1) and forced vital capacity (FVC) ratio is usually normal or increased.
  5. The diffusing capacity of carbon monoxide (DLCO) is reduced in patients with an intrinsic etiology of restrictive disease. If the diffusing capacity is normal, then the etiology of restrictive disease is an extrinsic factor such as neuromuscular disease.
E. Arterial blood gas (ABG).
  1. May be normal or indicate hypoxemia and a respiratory alkalosis.
  2. May reveal an increased alveolar–arterial gradient.
F. Bronchoscopy and/or lung biopsy.
  1. Beneficial for identifying diseases associated with intrinsic factors or the lung parenchyma, especially if there is suspicion for IPF but imaging is indeterminate.
  2. A bronchoalveolar lavage (BAL) may be useful in narrowing the differential diagnoses.
    a. The clinical usefulness of BAL has not been well-established.
    b. BAL has shown little value in its ability to discriminate between the various types of ILD.
  3. A lung biopsy can confirm the diagnosis, evaluate disease activity, and exclude other diagnoses. A lung biopsy is not recommended in those with IPF confirmed via CT chest.
    a. Open thoracotomy.
    b. Video-assisted thoracoscopic lung biopsy.
    c. Transbronchial lung biopsy via bronchoscopy.
G. Additional imaging or testing may be warranted to assess for complications resulting from restrictive diseases, such as an echocardiogram to evaluate for pulmonary hypertension or right-sided heart failure.
  1. Patients may also undergo diagnostics such as the 6-minute walk test to assess functional status.

EVALUATION AND MANAGEMENT PLAN
A. Treatment varies depending on the underlying etiology of the restrictive disease.
B. Patients should receive smoking cessation counseling.
C. Avoidance of environmental and/or occupational exposures.
D. Medications suspected of causing restrictive disease should be stopped immediately.
E. Supplemental oxygen therapy should be administered in all patients with oxygen saturations less than 88% on room air at rest or on exertion.
F. Pulmonary rehabilitation or regular activity/exercise should be encouraged because it has been shown to improve endurance and quality of life.
G. Patients should receive vaccinations for influenza and pneumococcal.

H. Treatment regimens for intrinsic causes usually include:

1. Corticosteroid therapy.
   a. Use of corticosteroids is generally accepted; however, timing, dosing, and continuation versus discontinuation of treatment are highly variable and dependent on the intrinsic cause of the restrictive disease as well as patient responsiveness.
   b. The long-term effects of corticosteroid therapy must be considered.
   c. Pulse high-dose corticosteroids are typically used for acute exacerbations.
2. Immunosuppressive agents (e.g., cyclosporine, azathioprine) may be used in certain diagnoses and in those with corticosteroid treatment failure. These medications should not be routinely or empirically used without a definitive diagnosis.
3. If worsening respiratory symptoms, patients may require invasive mechanical ventilation.
4. Patients with refractory disease to treatment and progressive worsening may be a candidate for lung transplantation and should be referred to a lung transplant specialist and center.

I. Treatment for extrinsic causes include:

1. Weight loss counseling and plan for patients with obesity.
2. Noninvasive positive pressure ventilation for patients who have impaired gas exchange.
3. Identification of the extrinsic disorder and treatment accordingly.
4. For patients with a trapped lung, chronic effusion, or empyema, a decortication may be required.

FOLLOW-UP

A. Follow-up is variable and dependent on the patient's symptoms and medical management. It should be individualized.

B. Posthospital discharge: Patients will follow up with their provider in 1 week.

CONSULTATION/REFERRAL

A. Patients with restrictive lung disease should be referred to a pulmonologist for diagnosis and management. Patients may require a specialist on their specific restrictive lung disease within the pulmonary discipline.

B. Patients with an extrinsic etiology for the restrictive disease, such as muscular dystrophy, should be referred to a neurologist or the appropriate consultant for the disorder.

INDIVIDUAL/SPECIAL/GERIATRIC CONSIDERATIONS

A. To adequately assess responsiveness to immunosuppressive medications, the provider should note it may not be evident until 8 to 12 weeks after therapy initiation.

B. Patients with progressive disease are typically discharged on home oxygen therapy. Increased oxygen requirements may be necessary to maintain a goal saturation greater than 88%. The patient and the family are instructed that oxygen therapy may be tailored to maintain oxygen saturations at rest and with exertion. If the patient is requiring increased oxygen therapy from baseline, then an immediate follow-up appointment with their pulmonologist or hospital admission may be warranted.

BIBLIOGRAPHY

Garibaldi, B. T., & Danoff, S. K. (2017). Interstitial lung disease/diffuse parenchymal lung diseases. In S. C. McKean, J. J. Ross, D. D. Dressler, & D. B. Scheurer (Eds.), *Principles and practice of hospital medicine* (pp. 1898–1903). McGraw Hill.

GBD Chronic Respiratory Disease Collaborators. (2020). Prevalence and attributable health burden of chronic respiratory disease, 1990-2017: A systematic analysis for the global burden of disease study 2017. *The Lancet Respiratory Medicine, 8*, 585–596. https://doi.org/10.1016/S2213-2600(20)30105-3

Jeganathan, N., & Sathananthan, M. (2022). The prevalence and burden of interstitial lung disease in the US. *ERJ Open Research.* https://doi.org/10.1183/23120541.00630-2021 8

King Jr., T. E. (2017). Interstitial lung disease. In J. Loscalzo (Ed.), *Harrison's pulmonary and critical care medicine* (pp. 204–218). McGraw Hill.

Martinez-Pitre, P. J., Sabbula, B. R., & Cascella, M. (2022). *Restrictive lung disease.* StatPearls Publishing. https://www.ncbi.nlm.nih.gov/books/NBK560880/#_NBK560880_pubdet_

Raghu, G., Remy-Jardin, M., Myers, J. L., Richeldi, L., Ryerson, C. J., Lederer, D. J., Behr, J., Cottin, V., Danoff, S. K., Morell, F., Flaherty, K. R., Wells, A., Martinez, F. J., Azuma, A., Bice, T. J., Bouros, D., Brown, K. K., Collard, H. R., Duggal, A. … Wilson, K. C. (2018). Diagnosis of idiopathic pulmonary fibrosis: An official ATS/ERS/JRS/ALAT clinical practice guideline. *American Journal of Respiratory and Critical Care Medicine, 198*, e44–e68. https://doi.org/10.1164/rccm.201807-1255ST

CHAPTER 3

CARDIAC GUIDELINES

Allison Rusgo

ACUTE CORONARY SYNDROMES

DEFINITION

A. Umbrella term encompassing unstable angina (UA), non-ST-segment elevation myocardial infarction (NSTEMI), and ST-segment elevation myocardial infarction (STEMI).

B. UA: no cardiac damage as defined by a lack of myocyte necrosis, no elevation in cardiac laboratory biomarkers, and no ST-segment elevation on EKG, but may show transient ST-segment changes and/or T-wave inversions, flattening, or peaking.

1. Indicates narrowing of coronary arteries secondary to thrombosis, hemorrhage, or plaque rupture.

2. Represents a temporary mismatch in myocardial oxygen supply and demand; most notably, the available blood supply is decreased due to overall reduced coronary blood flow.

C. NSTEMI: Evidence of cardiac damage, evidence of elevation in cardiac laboratory biomarkers, and no ST-segment elevation on EKG (but may show ST-segment depression and T-wave abnormalities, including peaking, inversions, or flattening).

1. Indicates partial blockage of coronary artery secondary to atherosclerotic narrowing.

2. Cardiac damage/myocyte necrosis at the area of the heart supplied by the partially blocked artery.

D. STEMI: Evidence of cardiac damage, evidence of elevation in cardiac biomarkers, and positive ST-segment elevation on EKG. Infarction may produce Q-waves which, in the setting of ischemia, is representative of necrosis.

1. Indicates complete blockage of an artery, damaging the area of the heart supplied by the completely occluded vessel.

E. Important note: Patients with stable coronary artery disease (CAD) can have acute coronary syndrome (ACS) without atherosclerotic plaque rupture where physiologic stress (e.g., trauma, acute blood loss anemia, fever/infection, thyrotoxicosis) increases the myocardial oxygen demand of the heart.

INCIDENCE

A. Ischemic heart disease is the leading cause of death worldwide and in the United States; it is estimated to affect 1.26 million adults (~1.72% of the world's population) globally and 18.2 million adults in the United States.

B. According to the Centers for Disease Control and Prevention, ischemic heart disease results in approximately 659,000 deaths per year in the United States.

C. Ischemic heart disease is also more common among individuals from certain racial/ethnic groups, including those who identify as Black/African American, Hispanic, and Asian American/Pacific Islander.

PATHOGENESIS

A. Mismatch between myocardial oxygen supply and demand, where supply is affected by coronary artery blood flow and oxygen-carrying capacity of the blood.

B. Overall oxygen-carrying capacity determined by hemoglobin level and oxygen saturation.

C. Coronary artery blood flow: Connection between peripheral vascular resistance and ability of the heart to relax during diastole.

D. Primary cardiac ischemia caused by atherosclerotic narrowing of the coronary vasculature.

E. Secondary cardiac ischemia (less common) can occur in the setting of stable or fixed coronary artery obstructions as a result of etiologies that are unrelated to atherosclerotic narrowing of the coronary vasculature.

1. Increased myocardial oxygen demand (e.g., infection, tachyarrhythmias, thyrotoxicosis).

2. Decreased blood flow (e.g., hypotension, septic shock).

3. Decreased oxygen availability (e.g., severe anemia).

F. Atherosclerotic-related ACS: Coronary arteries undergo a cascade of reactions leading to increased plaque accumulation, resulting in plaque rupture and finally artery blockage.

1. Vascular injury: Triggered by factors such as tobacco by-products, elevated blood pressure (BP), elevated glucose, and oxidized low-density lipoproteins (LDL).

2. Results in increased vascular permeability and inflammation.

3. Inflammatory mediators (macrophages and smooth muscle cells) activated: Create "fatty streaks" in vasculature.

4. "Fatty streaks": Transformed into foam cells (i.e., plaque), which form fibrous caps.

5. When the top layer of the thin fibrous cap ruptures, platelets are activated.

6. Platelet response: Consists of adhesion, aggregation, and activation; potentiates further damage to affected artery via platelet-laden thrombi, ▶

hemorrhage, and inflammation (overall blood flow decreased).

7. Immediate onset of the artery blockage created by ischemia secondary to rapid decrease in blood flow.

8. Amount and duration of the myocardial oxygen supply and demand mismatch related to whether there is reversible ischemia (UA) or irreversible damage with myocardial death (STEMI or NSTEMI).

PREDISPOSING FACTORS

A. Hypertension (HTN).
B. Hyperlipidemia (HLD).
C. Diabetes mellitus (DM).
D. Metabolic syndrome.
E. Obesity and sedentary lifestyle.
F. Tobacco use.
G. Family history of cardiovascular disease.
H. Medications/toxins (cocaine, ergonovine, serotonin).
I. Homocystinuria (inherited autosomal recessive generic disorder).
J. Psychological stress.

SUBJECTIVE DATA

A. Common complaints/symptoms.
1. Chest discomfort (vise-like pressure, tightness/squeezing, or burning); less likely sharp/stabbing.
   a. Reproducible chest tenderness in some cases (less common).
   b. Classic: Left-sided or substernal chest discomfort that radiates to the jaw or left arm, especially the ulnar surfaces of the forearm and hand.
   c. Can also radiate to the upper abdomen, back (intrascapular area), or shoulders, but rarely affects the trapezius muscles.
2. Nausea/vomiting.
3. Diaphoresis.
4. Palpitations.
5. Dyspnea.
6. Lightheadedness or syncope.
7. Feelings of anxiety.
8. Women, older adults persons, and those with DM are more likely to experience the following anginal equivalents:
   a. Fatigue.
   b. Weakness.
   c. Generalized malaise.
   d. Nonspecific chest or back discomfort.
   e. Decreased exercise tolerance.
   f. Altered mental status (older adults) or depressive symptoms (women).
   g. Gastrointestinal symptoms.
   h. No pain.
B. History of the present illness.
1. Information regarding onset, provoking and alleviating factors, duration, quality, severity, and timing of chest discomfort.
   a. Compared with stable angina or UA, myocardial infarctions (MIs) cause more severe chest discomfort that is prolonged (>20 minutes) and unrelieved by nitroglycerin.

   b. Can be potentiated by exposure to cold, physical activity, or emotional stress.
   c. Possible history of angina and any recent changes in anginal symptoms over the past several months.
   d. Possible recent decrease in activity level due to decreased tolerance.
2. More likely to experience associated symptoms with MIs as opposed to angina (i.e., nausea, dyspnea, fatigue, diaphoresis).
C. Family and social history.
1. Family history of premature CAD or MI in first-degree relative (males <45 years and females <55 years).
2. Tobacco or illegal substance use, especially cocaine.
3. Lifestyle factors, including level of exercise and dietary habits.
D. Review of systems.
1. General: Fatigue and diaphoresis.
2. Cardiovascular: Chest pain/discomfort (with radiation) and palpitations.
3. Pulmonary: Dyspnea (at rest, during sleep, and/or on exertion) and shortness of breath (SOB).
4. Abdominal: Epigastric discomfort, indigestion, nausea, and vomiting.
5. Neurologic: Dizziness, lightheadedness, near-syncope/syncope, and mental status changes.

PHYSICAL EXAMINATION

A. General appearance (one of the following):
1. Unremarkable and appearing well without any signs of distress, resting calmly.
2. Mild respiratory distress, anxiousness, and/or restlessness.
3. Cyanotic (central or peripheral) and in respiratory distress.
B. Vital signs: Assess pulse, BP, respirations, oxygen saturation, and temperature.
1. Pulse: Can be regular, irregular, tachycardic, or bradycardic (bradycardia can occur with anterior or inferior wall MIs).
2. BP: Can be elevated (due to anxiety, pain, underlying HTN, catecholamine surge) or decreased (indicates ventricular dysfunction, which is especially common in inferior wall MIs secondary to ventricular infarction).
C. Skin: Diaphoresis, cool/clammy skin (concern for cardiogenic shock), peripheral edema, and diminished peripheral pulses (secondary to accompanying peripheral vascular disease [PVD]).
D. Neck: Possible jugular venous distention (JVD), carotid bruits.
E. Cardiac.
1. Inspect for lifts, heaves, and pulsations.
2. Palpate for possible chest wall tenderness.
3. Auscultate.
   a. Extra heart sounds. S3 is present in approximately 15% of cases and indicates acute MI with heart failure (HF).

b. A new systolic murmur. This is concerning for papillary muscle dysfunction, ventricular septal defect, or new mitral regurgitation (MR) from a flail segment of the valve.

F. Pulmonary: Auscultate lung sounds for evidence of rales/crackles; concern for pulmonary edema or congestive heart failure (CHF).

G. Abdominal: Inspect, auscultate for bruits, and palpate for tenderness and evidence of pulsatile abdominal mass (concern for abdominal aortic aneurysm).

DIAGNOSTIC TESTS

A. EKG: Should be performed within 10 minutes of presentation to healthcare provider. Note that a normal EKG or one unchanged from the patient's baseline does not rule out the possibility of ischemic cardiac damage.

   1. Fixed ST-segment elevations (indicating an STEMI).

   2. Fixed ST-segment depressions (indicating ischemia).

   3. T-wave inversions, flattening, and/or peaking (can indicate ischemia).

   4. Transient ST-segment elevations (consider pericarditis, Prinzmetal angina, left ventricular aneurysm).

B. Cardiac biomarkers.

   1. Serial troponins (troponin I [cTnI] or troponin T [cTnT]): sensitive and specific for ACS diagnosis (biomarker of choice); recommended as set of three drawn approximately 4 to 6 hours apart.

   2. Consider use of creatine kinase-MB (CK-MB) and myoglobin in clinical settings where troponins are unavailable or to detect reinfarction several days after an initial ACS event, as these biomarkers return to baseline in days where troponins can remain elevated for up to 2 weeks.

C. Complete blood count: Useful for baseline information and ruling out anemia as cause of ACS.

D. Basic metabolic panel.

   1. To assess electrolytes, especially magnesium and potassium (causes of cardiac arrhythmias).

   2. To assess renal function: Important if going to use angiotensin-converting enzyme (ACE) inhibitors for future therapy and/or contrast dye during catheterization (want to avoid contrast-induced nephropathy).

E. Chest radiography: To assess for pulmonary edema and cardiomegaly, and rule out other causes of chest pain such as pneumonia or thoracic aneurysm.

F. Cardiac echocardiography: Can be especially helpful if diagnosis is questionable. It is used to:

   1. Assess left ventricular function.

   2. Evaluate for regional wall motion abnormalities.

   3. Check for pericardial effusions or valvular abnormalities (i.e., acute MR).

G. CT coronary angiography (CTCA)/CT coronary artery calcium (CAC) scoring.

   1. Noninvasive diagnostic studies: Aid in early CAD diagnosis and risk stratification considerations; not for use in evaluation of emergent/acute ACS.

   2. CTCA: Uses contrast dye to evaluate the integrity of coronary arteries (can also evaluate previously implanted stents and bypass grafts for patency).

   3. CT CAC: Useful for low- or intermediate-risk ACS patients (no contrast dye and low radiation levels); evaluation of calcium in coronary arteries, which is related to atherosclerotic burden.

DIFFERENTIAL DIAGNOSIS

A. MIs (STEMI, NSTEMI).

B. Stable or UA.

C. Pericarditis.

D. Myocarditis.

E. Esophagitis/gastritis/ruptured peptic ulcer.

F. Hypertensive emergency.

G. Anxiety/panic attack.

H. Ruptured thoracic or abdominal aortic aneurysm.

I. Pulmonary embolus.

J. Pneumonia.

EVALUATION AND MANAGEMENT PLAN

A. General plan.

   1. Management based on patient presentations, characteristics of symptoms, medical history, physical examination findings, and diagnostic results.

   2. Goal: To limit necrosis and overall cardiac damage.

   3. Risk stratification: Imperative when designing treatment plan. One option is the Thrombosis in Myocardial Infarction (TIMI) Score (Table 3.1).

      a. Instrument for determining risk of all-cause morbidity, new or recurrent MI, or need for emergent revascularization within 14 to 30 days of presentation of NSTEMI or UA.

      b. Each of the seven items on the checklist is equivalent to 1 point; the higher the score, the higher the patient's risk.

B. Management of STEMI.

   1. Aspirin 324 mg in ED (or prehospital).

TABLE 3.1 THROMBOSIS IN MYOCARDIAL INFARCTION SCORE

Age >65 years	1 point
≥3 CAD risk factors (HTN, hyperlipidemia, DM, tobacco use, family history of CAD)	1 point
Known CAD with stenosis ≥50%	1 point
Acetylsalicylic acid (aspirin) use in the past 7 days	1 point
At least two episodes of severe angina in the past 24 hours	1 point
ST changes on EKG 0.5 mm above baseline	1 point
Positive cardiac biomarkers	1 point

CAD, coronary artery disease; DM, diabetes mellitus; HTN, hypertension.
Source: From About TIMI. TIMI Study Group. Published October 18, 2019. https://timi.org/about-timi/.

2. Loading dose of antiplatelet agent (i.e., clopidogrel, 300–600 mg).

3. Supplemental oxygen if hypoxemia.

4. Antithrombolytic agent (unfractionated or low-molecular weight heparin).

5. Nitrates: Provide symptomatic relief; do not improve mortality.

    a. Strong risk of hypotension: Causes decreased coronary perfusion.

    b. Should not be given if patient has hypotension, known right ventricular infarction, large pericardial effusion, recent use of 5-phosphodiesterase inhibitor, or severe aortic stenosis (AS).

6. Beta-blockers.

    a. Caution if decreased systolic BP, cardiogenic shock, severe asthma, decompensated CHF, or severe bradycardia.

7. Goal: Reperfusion therapy.

    a. Obtained via percutaneous coronary intervention (PCI) with or without stent placement.

        i. Should be achieved within 90 minutes of patient arrival at PCI-capable hospital.

        ii. If hospital is without PCI capabilities, goal is patient transfer to PCI center within 120 minutes of patient arrival.

    b. PCI options.

        i. Coronary angioplasty with or without stent placement.

        ii. Balloon angioplasty stretches inner layer of the coronary artery.

        iii. Drug-eluting stents (DES) or bare metal stents (BMS): Wire mesh cage implanted in the blocked vessel for structure and patency.

        iv. BMS preferable if unable to utilize dual antiplatelet therapy (DAPT) for a minimum of 6 months; minimum duration of DAPT is one-month in patients with stable ischemic heart disease who receive a BMS.

    c. If PCI is not achievable in these time parameters, fibrinolytics should be administered within 30 minutes of patient arrival to hospital.

        i. Indicated if symptom onset is within 6 to 12 hours; 1 mm ST-segment elevation in more than two anatomically contiguous EKG leads.

        ii. Aims to dissolve existing clot, improve left ventricular function, and decrease mortality.

        iii. Examples: Tissue plasminogen factor, streptokinase, or tenecteplase.

        iv. Major risk: Bleeding such as intracranial hemorrhage (ICH).

    d. At discretion of cardiothoracic surgeon and interventional cardiologist, consider coronary artery bypass grafting (CABG) if cardiac catheterization yields extensive stenosis and/or stenosis not amenable to stenting/balloon options.

    e. For unconscious STEMI patients with prehospital cardiac arrest caused by ventricular fibrillation (VF) or pulseless ventricular tachycardia (VT), obtain immediate cardiology consultation regarding the usage of targeted temperature management (therapeutic hypothermia).

C. Management of NSTEMI and/or UA.

  1. Monitoring during inpatient hospitalization for serial EKGs, biomarker elevation, and symptom evolution.

  2. Early invasive therapy (PCI) in NSTEMI or UA: Recommended only if refractory angina; high risk for cardiac events or hemodynamic instability.

  3. American Heart Association (AHA) and American College of Cardiology (ACC) recommendations for early (within 48 hours) PCI intervention in NSTEMI/UA if: Refractory angina, elevated biomarkers, new ST-changes, positive stress test results, decreased left ventricular function, or hemodynamic instability.

  4. NSTEMI/UA patients requiring PCI should receive similar medications to STEMI management.

    a. Aspirin 324 mg initially followed by daily dose of 81 mg.

    b. Antiplatelet agent (clopidogrel).

    c. Supplemental oxygen if evidence of hypoxemia.

    d. Nitrates.

    e. Anticoagulant agents (unfractionated or low-molecular weight heparin).

    f. Beta-blockers if not contraindicated.

  5. Patients admitted for ACS evaluations with normal serial EKGs, normal biomarkers, and complete resolution of symptoms can undergo stress testing or CTCA prior to discharge or within 72 hours of discharge if deemed appropriate by cardiologist. The following is for patients discharged prior to definitive diagnostic testing.

    a. Prescribe aspirin, short-acting nitroglycerin, and beta-blockers (if appropriate).

    b. Provide instructions regarding lifestyle modification (e.g., no physical activity until evaluated by cardiologist), tobacco cessation, and cardiac healthy diet.

  6. Helpful flow chart for evaluation of patients with ACS (Figure 3.1).

D. Patient/family teaching points.

  1. Knowledge of ACS/angina symptoms: Decreases time before presenting for medical care (decreases door to PCI time, if STEMI).

  2. Tobacco cessation.

  3. Importance of regular cardiovascular physical activity.

  4. Use of heart-healthy (low fat, low cholesterol, low sodium) diet.

  5. Adherence with all medications (especially aspirin and antiplatelet agent) and clinic follow-up visits.

E. Pharmacotherapy.

  1. Antiplatelet drugs.

    a. Aspirin: To prevent platelet aggregation.

        i. Immediate administration of 324 mg aspirin if STEMI, NSTEMI, or UA.

        ii. Daily use of aspirin to reduce cardiac mortality; for patients with high risk for ICH, a ▶

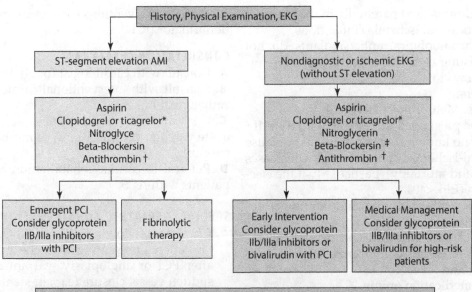

FIGURE 3.1 Algorithm for evaluation of patients with acute coronary syndrome.

Source: From Hollander, J. E., & Diercks, D. B. (2016). Acute coronary syndromes. In J. E. Tintinalli, J. Stapczynski, O. Ma, D. M. Yealy, G. D. Meckler, & D. M. Cline (Eds.), *Tintinalli's emergency medicine: A comprehensive study guide* (8th ed., pp. 332–348). McGraw-Hill.

lower aspirin dose of 81 to 160 mg should be considered.
iii. Can be combined with other antiplatelets for DAPT.
iv. Consider use of proton pump inhibitor or H2 receptor block to prevent gastrointestinal irritation.
b. Adenosine diphosphate receptor antagonists.
i. Examples: Prasugrel, clopidogrel, or ticagrelor.
ii. Overall function: Platelet inhibition via complex pharmacologic mechanisms.
iii. Major risk: Bleeding—The U.S. Food and Drug Administration issued a boxed warning for prasugrel (not for use in those with prior cerebrovascular accident [CVA]/transient ischemic attack [TIA] or bleeding disorders).
iv. Can be combined with aspirin for DAPT.
v. If elective CABG planned: Recommended to hold clopidogrel for 5 days to reduce the risk of bleeding and improve morbidity/mortality.

vi. Specific agent chosen by cardiologist/interventional cardiologist and continued for at least several months post-PCI.
c. Glycoprotein IIB/IIIA inhibitors.
i. Examples: Abciximab and tirofiban.
ii. Routine administration in ED not recommended due to timing of PCI and risk of bleeding.
iii. During hospitalization, can be used in combination with aspirin for high-risk ACS patients and those likely to undergo PCI.
2. Thrombolytics.
a. Examples: streptokinase, urokinase, and alteplase.
b. Used in the management of MIs when access to PCI is limited.
c. The goal of therapy is to rapidly dissolve the thrombus, restore coronary blood flow, and mitigate myocardial damage.
3. Anticoagulants.
a. Examples: Unfractionated heparin, low-molecular weight heparin.

b. Can be administered parentally in the management of myocardial ischemia/infarctions.

c. Unlike thrombolytics, anticoagulants do not dissolve existing clots but rather prevent the formation of new clots.

4. Beta-blockers.

a. Examples: Metoprolol, bisoprolol.

b. Should be prescribed in patients with STEMI/NSTEMI (if no known contraindications) because of their anti-ischemic characteristics (decreases infarct size and mortality), particularly if the ejection fraction (EF) <40%.

c. Maintains antiarrhythmic and antihypertensive properties.

d. Reduces cardiac afterload and overall cardiac stress (helps to equalize myocardial oxygen supply and demand levels).

5. Additional medication options.

a. ACE inhibitors: For those with left ventricular EF less than 40% and/or HTN, DM, or stable chronic kidney disease (CKD; can consider angiotensin receptor blockers if ACE-intolerant).

b. High-intensity statin (if no contraindications; as tolerated) with ongoing lipid panel and side effect monitoring.

c. Nondihydropyridine calcium channel blockers: Can be used if intolerance or contraindication to beta-blockers as long as there is no left ventricular dysfunction, known prolonged PR interval on EKG, or second- or third-degree heart block.

F. Discharge instructions.

1. Prior to hospital discharge.

a. Ensure all required prescriptions have been given based on cardiac status and interventions performed during hospitalization.

b. Emphasize lifestyle modifications via teach-back method regarding tobacco cessation, cardiac rehabilitation for exercise program, and eating heart-healthy diet.

2. Verify that the patient has appropriate follow-up with cardiologist/interventional cardiologist, primary care provider, and cardiac rehabilitation.

3. For patients discharged with instructions to follow up with cardiologist for stress testing, ensure appointment occurs within 72 hours after discharge with instructions for no physical activity prior to appointment.

4. Ensure patients understand all reasons to return to ED regarding cardiac-related symptoms.

FOLLOW-UP

A. Patients should have regular monitoring by their primary care provider and/or cardiologist to address medication compliance; adherence to lifestyle changes; and monitoring laboratory markers, including lipid and metabolic panels.

B. Cardiologist may consider follow-up echocardiogram to assess left ventricular function (EF percentage) at 40 days post-MI; this will help determine the need

for further interventions such as an implantable cardiac defibrillator (ICD).

CONSULTATION/REFERRAL

A. Consult with cardiologist for all ACS.

B. Consult with interventional cardiologist for cardiac catheterization.

C. Consult with cardiothoracic surgeon for CABG, acute valvular complications, or mechanical circulatory support.

D. Referral to cardiac rehabilitation recommended for patients with ACS.

SPECIAL/GERIATRIC CONSIDERATIONS

A. Chest pain following PCI or CABG.

1. Patients presenting with chest pain immediately after PCI or angioplasty warrant consideration for sudden vessel closure (e.g., in-stent stenosis, in-stent thrombosis, or stent failure).

a. Treat aggressively for ACS and immediately consult a cardiologist.

b. Use of BMS is more likely to lead to restenosis in the short term, while the use of DES is more likely to lead to restenosis within 9 to 12 months (after cessation of daily antiplatelet such as clopidogrel).

2. Chest pain after CABG may indicate possible graft failure; immediate consultation with cardiologist and cardiothoracic surgeon is necessary.

3. Consider other etiologies such as post-MI pericarditis.

B. Chest pain secondary to cocaine intoxication.

1. MI occurs in approximately 6% of patients after cocaine use.

2. Use of cardiac biomarkers is imperative for diagnosis.

3. Treatment involves aspirin, nitrates, and benzodiazepines (no beta-blockers for the first 24 hours).

4. For STEMI secondary to cocaine, patients typically undergo PCI with antithrombolytic and antiplatelet agents per cardiologist and interventional cardiologist.

C. Geriatric considerations.

1. Recognize that nontraditional symptoms are common (confusion, malaise, weakness, fatigue).

2. Considerations must be made regarding the use of the most beneficial diagnostic testing.

a. Age-related cardiac changes (specifically, if unable to reach target heart rate (HR) during exercise stress testing) can mask diagnosis.

b. Older adult patients may be unable to walk on treadmill due to orthopedic comorbidities (nuclear or pharmacologic stress testing is often preferred).

c. Coronary atherosclerosis is more diffuse and more calcified combined with decreased diastolic filling.

d. Risk versus benefit analysis should be done with regard to the use of multiple antiplatelet and anticoagulant agents due to increased risk of bleeding.

e. Overall health status, cognitive abilities, and comorbidities should be considered before using invasive clinical or surgical interventions.

BIBLIOGRAPHY

About TIMI.(2019, October 18). *TIMI STUDY GROUP.* https://timi.org/about-timi/

Agabegi, S. S., & Agabegi, E. D. (2019). *Step-up to medicine* (5th ed.). Wolters Kluwer.

The American College of Cardiology Foundation and the American Heart Association, Inc. (2022). ACC/AHA/SCAI guideline for coronary artery revascularization. *Journal of the American College of Cardiology, 79*(2). Elsevier.

Antman, E. M., & Loscalzo, J. (2018). Ischemic heart disease. In J. Jameson, A. S. Fauci, D. L. Kasper, S. L. Hauser, D. L. Longo, & J. Loscalzo (Eds.), *Harrison's principles of internal medicine* (20th ed.). McGraw Hill.

Baik, A. H., & Dhruva, S. S. (2021). Coronary artery disease. In L. C. Walter, A. Chang, P. Chen, G. Harper, J. Rivera, R. Conant, D. Lo, & M. Yukawa (Eds.), *Current diagnosis & Treatment Geriatrics* (3rd ed.). McGraw Hill.

Bayés de Luna, A., Goldwasser, D., Fiol, M., & Bayés-Genis, A. (2017). Surface electrocardiography. In V. Fuster, R. A. Harrington, J. Narula, & Z. J. Eapen (Eds.), *Hurst's the heart* (14th ed.). McGraw Hill.

Centers for Disease Control and Prevention. (2022, February 7). *Heart disease facts.* Author. https://www.cdc.gov/heartdisease/facts.htm

Chyu, K., & Shah, P. K. (2017). Unstable angina/non-st elevation myocardial infarction. In M. H. Crawford (Ed.), *Current diagnosis & treatment: Cardiology* (5th ed.). McGraw Hill.

Giugliano, R. P., Cannon, C. P., & Braunwald, E. (2018). Non-st-segment elevation acute coronary syndrome (non-st-segment elevation myocardial infarction and unstable angina). In J. Jameson, A. S. Fauci, D. L. Kasper, S. L. Hauser, D. L. Longo, & J. Loscalzo (Eds.), *Harrison's principles of internal medicine* (20th ed.). McGraw Hill.

Khan, M. A., Hashim, M. J., Mustafa, H., Baniyas, M. Y., Al Suwaidi, S., AlKatheeri, R., Alblooshi, F., Almatrooshi, M., Alzaabi, M., Al Darmaki, R. S., & Lootah, S. (2020). Global epidemiology of ischemic heart disease: Results from the Global Burden of Disease Study. *Cureus, 12*(7), e9349. https://doi.org/10.7759/cureus.9349

Libby, P. (2018). Atlas of atherosclerosis. In J. Jameson, A. S. Fauci, D. L. Kasper, S. L. Hauser, D. L. Longo, & J. Loscalzo (Eds.), *Harrison's principles of internal medicine* (20th ed.). McGraw Hill.

Malakar, A. K., Choudhury, D., Halder, B., Paul, P., Uddin, A., & Chakraborty, S. (2019). A review on coronary artery disease, its risk factors, and therapeutics. *Journal of Cellular Physiology, 234*(10), 16812–16823. https://doi.org/10.1002/jcp.28350

Weitz, J. I. (2018). Antiplatelet, anticoagulant, and fibrinolytic drugs. In J. Jameson, A. S. Fauci, D. L. Kasper, S. L. Hauser, D. L. Longo, & J. Loscalzo (Eds.), *Harrison's principles of internal medicine* (20th ed.). McGraw Hill.

ANGINA

DEFINITION
A. Cardiac symptoms produced by myocardial ischemia.
B. Three types.
  1. Stable angina.
    a. Secondary to fixed atherosclerotic plaques that narrow coronary vasculature.
    b. Occurs because of an imbalance between myocardial blood supply and oxygen demand.
  2. Unstable angina (UA).
    a. Progression from stable angina, leading to total vessel occlusion.
    b. Indication that narrowing of coronary vasculature has increased via thrombosis, hemorrhage, or plaque rupture.
    c. Myocardial oxygen demand unchanged, but blood supply decreased due to reduced coronary flow.
  3. Prinzmetal variant (or vasospastic) angina.
    a. Transient focal spasms of an epicardial coronary artery in the setting of fixed atherosclerosis (75% of cases) or healthy coronary arteries.

INCIDENCE
A. Estimated 3.4 million Americans age ≥40 years old experience angina pectoris.
B. The age-adjusted prevalence of angina is higher in females than in males.
C. Annual incidence rates are highest among individuals from lower resourced communities secondary to insufficient access to preventive healthcare.
D. Incidence and prevalence of angina and coronary artery disease (CAD) increase with age.
E. Epidemiologically, there is evidence of a decline in the rate of deaths secondary to ischemic heart disease due to risk factor modification and efficacious treatment modalities.

PATHOGENESIS
A. Coronary atherosclerosis causes narrowing of the coronary arteries, thereby reducing blood flow through the system.
B. Myocardial ischemia (damage) results when the amount of blood flow through the coronary arteries is insufficient to meet myocardial oxygen demand.
  1. Normally, the myocardium senses the body's required oxygen needs and directs the proper amount of blood to the heart, thus preventing ischemia or hyperperfusion.
  2. The major components of myocardial oxygen consumption (MVO_2) are heart rate (HR), contractility, and myocardial wall tension.
  3. To supply the myocardium with a sufficient level of oxygen to meet the body's demands, an appropriate level of oxygen-carrying capacity of the blood and coronary blood flow is needed.

PREDISPOSING FACTORS
A. Diabetes mellitus (DM).
B. Hyperlipidemia (HLD; elevated low-density lipoprotein [LDL], low high-density lipoprotein [HDL], or elevated triglycerides [TGs]).
C. Hypertension (HTN).
D. Tobacco use.
E. Increased age (males >45 years and females >55 years).
F. Family history of premature CAD or myocardial infarction (MI) in first-degree relative (males <45 years and females <55 years).
G. Obesity or metabolic syndrome.
H. Sedentary lifestyle.
I. Underlying valvular heart disease (VHD).

SUBJECTIVE DATA

A. Common complaints/symptoms.

   1. Chest discomfort is the most common symptom of acute coronary syndrome (ACS), but not all chest discomfort is cardiac; chest pain should be described as "cardiac" or "noncardiac." Multiple less common anginal equivalents include dyspnea, abdominal pain, or neck/facial pain.

   2. Stable angina.

      a. Retrosternal chest discomfort: Described as pressure, heaviness, burning, squeezing.

      b. Can be located in central chest, epigastrium, neck, upper back, or shoulders (pain below the mandible or epigastrium is rarely angina).

      c. Can radiate to the jaw, left arm, or shoulders (typically spares the trapezius muscles).

      d. Typically preceded by exertion (e.g., exercise, sexual activity), eating, cold exposure, or emotional upset.

      e. Usually does not change with positions or respiration.

      f. Typically lasts 1 to 5 minutes and relieved by rest or use of nitroglycerin.

   3. Differentiating features of UA.

      a. Symptoms occur at rest or with minimal excretion.

      b. Any new-onset (typically within the previous 2 weeks) angina or change in usual stable anginal symptoms; most commonly described as attacks that are more severe, increasing in frequency or lasting longer.

      c. Angina unrelieved by rest or nitroglycerin.

      d. Typically lasts longer than stable angina (i.e., ≥10 minutes).

B. History of the present illness.

   1. Obtain information regarding the nature, onset and duration, location and radiation, severity, precipitating and relieving factors, and associated symptoms.

      a. Of note, relief of discomfort with nitroglycerin is not necessarily diagnostic of myocardial ischemia and should not be used as a diagnostic criteria.

      b. Localized or positional chest pain is typically nonischemic (e.g., musculoskeletal).

   2. Associated symptoms may include:

      a. Fatigue.

      b. Diaphoresis.

      c. Shortness of breath (SOB).

      d. Decreased exercise tolerance.

      e. Nausea/vomiting.

      f. Palpitations.

      g. Presyncope or syncope.

C. Family and social history.

   1. Family history of premature CAD, MI, or sudden cardiac death in first-degree relative (males <45 and females <55 years).

   2. Tobacco use, alcohol consumption, and illicit substance use (especially cocaine).

   3. Lifestyle, including exercise and dietary habits.

D. Review of systems.

   1. General: Fatigue or diaphoresis.

   2. Cardiovascular: Chest pain or palpitations.

   3. Pulmonary: Dyspnea on exertion or SOB.

   4. Abdominal: Epigastric discomfort, nausea, or vomiting.

   5. Peripheral vascular: Claudication or skin changes related to venous stasis and HTN.

PHYSICAL EXAMINATION

A. Unremarkable in most patients with stable angina.

B. Vital signs: Assess heart rate (HR) and rhythm, blood pressure (BP), oxygen saturation, and respiration rate.

C. General: Observe the patient's level of distress.

   1. Levine sign: Fist clenched over the sternum is suggestive of angina.

D. Skin: Diaphoresis and evidence of poor lipid metabolism (xanthoma) are possible.

E. Neck: Carotid bruits and increased jugular venous pressure are possible.

F. Cardiovascular: Inspect, palpate (pain on chest wall palpation is not usually cardiac in nature), and auscultate (partially audible S3, S4 due to left ventricular dysfunction and/or murmur of mitral regurgitation (MR) as sign of papillary muscle dysfunction). Evaluate for signs or symptoms of low cardiac output (cool skin, diaphoresis, jugular venous distention [JVD]).

G. Pulmonary: Auscultate the lungs for evidence of rales/crackles (concern for pulmonary edema related to left ventricular function insult).

H. Abdomen: Auscultate for bruits, palpate for discomfort, and assess for a pulsatile abdominal mass.

I. Peripheral vascular: Assess peripheral pulses, possible venous stasis changes, and peripheral edema.

DIAGNOSTIC TESTS

A. 12-lead EKG: Usually normal in patients with stable angina. If there are ST-segment elevations, activate the clinical decision pathway for acute MI.

B. Chest radiograph: Usually normal but evaluate for cardiomegaly, pulmonary edema, and pericardial effusion.

C. Blood serum tests.

   1. Cardiac biomarkers: Serial troponins, troponin T (cTnT), and troponin I (cTnI) to evaluate for MI. High-sensitivity cardiac troponin (cTn) is the preferred biomarker because it enables a more rapid detection or exclusion of myocardial injury.

   2. Lipid panel to assess for risk of atherosclerosis.

   3. Complete blood count to assess for underlying exacerbating cardiac factors such as evidence of anemia.

   4. Complete metabolic panel to assess electrolytes (metabolic dysfunction can lead to arrhythmias) and kidney function (important if cardiac catheterization with contrast dye is needed).

D. For intermediate-risk patients with acute chest pain, a transthoracic echocardiogram (TTE) is recommended ▶

to establish baseline ventricular and valvular function, evaluate for wall motion abnormalities, and to assess for pericardial effusion.

E. Stress testing.

    1. For a positive stress test and when deemed appropriate by the cardiologist and interventional cardiologist, a cardiac catheterization with coronary angiography is performed. During this intervention, contrast dye is injected into the coronary vasculature to aid in the visualization and revascularization of the affected vessel(s).

    2. Exercise stress testing.

        a. Stress EKG: An EKG is performed before, during, and after treadmill exercise. The test is 75% sensitive if heart rate (HR) reaches 85% of maximum predicted value for age. Exercise-induced ischemia results in subendocardial ischemia (ST-segment depression on EKG); can also see hypotension or ventricular arrhythmias.

        b. Stress echocardiography: Cardiac echocardiography is performed before and after exercise.

            i. Exercise-induced ischemia is detected by cardiac wall-motion abnormalities not present at rest.

            ii. It is more sensitive for detecting ischemia than stress EKG and beneficial for determining left ventricular function.

    3. Pharmacologic stress testing (for patients unable to walk on treadmill, achieve a high enough level of exercise, or have abnormal baseline EKGs).

        a. Intravenous (IV) adenosine or dobutamine can be used to replace treadmill activity.

        b. These agents create cardiac stress, and they can be combined with an EKG, echocardiogram, or nuclear imaging.

    4. Nuclear stress testing.

        a. Thallium or technetium 99m sestamibi is used in patients with baseline EKG abnormalities to localize ischemia.

        b. Areas of damage will be ill-perfused on imaging.

F. Other cardiac diagnostic testing.

    1. CT coronary angiography (CTCA).

        a. Relatively new test.

        b. Uses electron-beam or multidetector CT imaging to evaluate specific coronary arteries (i.e. left main, left anterior descending, left circumflex, and right coronary) for level of calcium (coronary artery calcium [CAC] or Agatston score).

        c. Useful in select patient populations, particularly those with persistent pain despite negative imaging studies and/or individuals who are asymptomatic with intermediate-level risk factors.

        d. Can function as an objective measurement of CAD and assist in identifying patients who would benefit from aggressive risk factor/lifestyle modifications.

G. The flow chart in Figure 3.2 can help with diagnosis and risk stratification in angina.

DIFFERENTIAL DIAGNOSIS

A. MI.
B. Coronary vasospasm.
C. Pulmonary embolus.
D. Pericarditis.
E. Congestive heart failure (CHF).
F. Acute gastritis.
G. Cholecystitis.
H. Ruptured abdominal or thoracic aortic aneurysm.
I. Anxiety/panic attack disorders.
J. Gastroesophageal reflux/peptic ulcer disease.
K. Cocaine toxicity.
L. Hypertensive urgency or emergency.
M. Valvular abnormalities.
N. Hiatal hernia.
O. Costochondritis.

EVALUATION AND MANAGEMENT PLAN

A. General plan.

    1. Prevention of MIs and reduction of angina-type symptoms; can consider the **ABCDE** mnemonic.

        a. **A**spirin and antianginal agents.

        b. **B**eta-blockers and BP management.

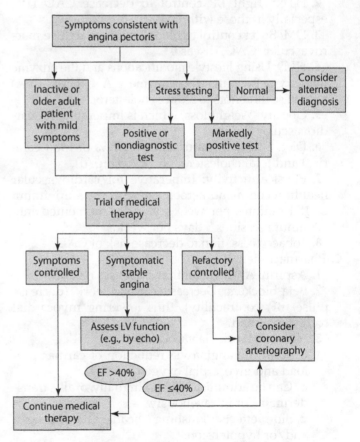

FIGURE 3.2 Diagnosis and risk stratification in angina.

Source: From Kasper, D. L., Fauci, A. S., Hauser, S. L., Longo, D. L., Jameson, J. L., & Loscalzo, J. (Eds.). (2015). Chronic stable angina. *Harrison's principles of internal medicine* (19th ed.). McGraw-Hill. EF, ejection fraction; LV, left ventricular.

c. **C**holesterol management and cigarette smoking abstinence.
d. **D**iet and diabetic management.
e. Education and exercise.
2. Treatment using risk stratification considerations.
a. Mild disease (normal cardiac function and mild angina): Aspirin, nitrates, and beta-blockers (possibly calcium channel blockers).
b. Moderate disease (moderate angina, normal cardiac function, two-vessel coronary disease): Use of medications for mild disease and cardiac catheterization for revascularization.
c. Severe disease (decreased cardiac function, three-vessel/left main/left anterior artery disease with severe angina): Pharmacologic and consideration of coronary artery bypass grafting (CABG).
3. Evaluation of patients with anginal symptoms for acute cardiac ischemia (ST-elevation MI or non-ST-segment elevation MI).
4. For patients with UA, hospitalization for monitoring, stabilization, and possible cardiac catheterization (or stress testing if determined safe by cardiologist).
B. Patient/family teaching points.
1. Compliance with medications and primary care provider appointments.
2. HTN: Tight BP control to decrease CAD risk, especially in those with DM.
3. DM: Strict control of blood sugars to reduce macrovascular (CAD) disease.
4. HLD: Using lifestyle modifications and the enzyme hydroxymethylglutaryl-coenzyme A (HMG-CoA) reductase inhibitors to reduce cholesterol.
5. Obesity: Weight loss, which is imperative for cardiovascular health.
6. Diet: Reducing saturated fat (<7% of total calories) and total cholesterol (TC <200 mg/d).
7. Physical activity: Imperative for cardiovascular health; recommend aerobic exercise for a minimum of 150 minutes per week, typically segmented into 30 minute sessions 5 days per week.
8. Tobacco cessation to decrease risk of CAD.
C. Pharmacotherapy.
1. Aspirin: Antiplatelet that decreases risk of MI.
2. Beta-blockers: Decrease cardiac work (decrease pulse, BP, contractility), thus lowering myocardial oxygen demand.
3. Nitrates: Work via vasodilation.
a. Alleviate angina via reduction of cardiac preload and myocardial oxygen demand.
b. Can be administered sublingually, orally, transdermally, or intravenously.
c. Side effects: Flushing, headache, dizziness, and/or hypotension.
4. Phosphodiesterase inhibitors: Caution necessary with medications such as sildenafil, tadalafil, and vardenafil; risk of hypotension.
5. Calcium channel blockers: Decrease cardiac afterload and cause coronary vasodilation to increase coronary blood flow.
6. Lipid-lowering agents: HMG-CoA reductase inhibitors to decrease atherosclerosis and risk of MIs.

FOLLOW-UP
A. Important issues during follow-up visits for patients with angina.
1. Increased or decreased exercise tolerance.
2. Any change in anginal symptoms.
3. Problems with medication adherence.
4. Any changes in modifiable risk factors (diet, activity level, tobacco cessation).
5. Monitoring of management of comorbid conditions that contribute to CAD.
B. Additional recommendations.
1. Annual treadmill stress testing for patients with stable CAD.
2. Stress imaging in patients with change in CAD status or who underwent initial stress imaging due to known risk factors.
3. Use of echocardiography to evaluate left ventricular function and wall motion in CAD patients with worsening heart failure (HF) or recent MI.

CONSULTATION/REFERRAL
A. Consult with a cardiologist in patients with angina/CAD for proper risk stratification, diagnostic testing, treatment regimen planning, and ongoing monitoring.
B. Consult with an interventional cardiologist for patients requiring cardiac catheterization.
C. Consult with a cardiothoracic surgeon for patients requiring CABG, valvular disease requiring repair/replacement, or mechanical circulatory support.

SPECIAL/GERIATRIC CONSIDERATIONS
A. Prinzmetal variant (or vasospastic) angina.
1. Secondary to coronary vasospasms.
2. Rare diagnosis: Usually occurs in patients 40 to 60 years of age.
3. Can be provoked by factors such as cold exposure, tobacco/marijuana use, cocaine use, emotional stress, excessive alcohol use, and certain medications (histamine, serotonin, pseudoephedrine, sumatriptan).
4. Chest pain episodes: Very painful; last approximately 15 minutes and usually occur at rest.
5. Can mimic symptoms of MIs; very difficult to differentiate on history and physical examination.
6. Hallmark: transient ST-segment changes (elevation or depression) or new negative U-waves in at least two contiguous leads on EKG during chest pain episodes.
7. Coronary angiography is test of choice: Can see evidence of spontaneous coronary vasospasms or provoke their occurrence via medications such as acetylcholine or ergonovine.
8. Can be relieved by antianginal medications.
9. Use of calcium channel blockers and nitrates can be helpful for treatment.
B. Geriatric considerations.
1. Age: Not a limitation for evaluation and treatment of CAD.
2. Presentation: May have nontraditional symptoms.

3. Higher incidence of multivessel coronary disease.

4. Greater prevalence of renal impairment (concern for use of contrast dye during catheterization).

5. Higher incidence of polypharmacy: Potential drug interactions and medication adherence.

6. Possibly too risky for surgical intervention, thus requiring only conservative (medical) management.

7. Important to assess baseline cognitive status and comorbidities when discussing treatment plan and to involve family when necessary.

BIBLIOGRAPHY

Agabegi, S. S., & Agabegi, E. D. (2019). *Step-up to medicine* (5th ed.). Wolters Kluwer.

Antman, E. M., & Loscalzo, J. (2018). Ischemic heart disease. In J. Jameson, A. S. Fauci, D. L. Kasper, S. L. Hauser, D. L. Longo, & J. Loscalzo (Eds.), *Harrison's principles of internal medicine* (20th ed.). McGraw Hill.

Barile, M. F., & Jacobson, F. L. (2017). Advanced cardiothoracic imaging. In S. C. McKean, J. J. Ross, D. D. Dressler, & D. B. Scheurer (Eds.), *Principles and practice of hospital medicine* (2nd ed.). McGraw Hill.

Giugliano, R. P., Cannon, C. P., & Braunwald, E. (2018). Non-st-segment elevation acute coronary syndrome (non-st-segment elevation myocardial infarction and unstable angina). In J. Jameson, A. S. Fauci, D. L. Kasper, S. L. Hauser, D. L. Longo, & J. Loscalzo (Eds.), *Harrison's principles of internal medicine* (20th ed.). McGraw Hill.

Gulati, M., Levy, P. D., Mukherjee, D., Amsterdam, E., Bhatt, D. L., Birtcher, K. K., Blankstein, R., Boyd, J., Bullock-Palmer, R. P., Conejo, T., Diercks, D. B., Gentile, F., Greenwood, J. P., Hess, E. P., Hollenberg, S. M., Jaber, W. A., Jneid, H., Joglar, J. A., Morrow, D. A. ... Shaw, L. J. (2021). AHA/ACC/ASE/CHEST/SAEM/SCCT/SCMR guideline for the evaluation and diagnosis of chest pain: A report of the American College of Cardiology/American Heart Association Joint Committee on Clinical Practice Guidelines. *Journal of the American College of Cardiology, 78*(22), e187–e285.

Thomas, G. S., & Ellestad, M. H. (2017). Electrocardiographic exercise testing. In V. Fuster, R. A. Harrington, J. Narula, & Z. J Eapen (Eds.), *Hurst's the heart* (14th ed.). McGraw Hill.

ARRHYTHMIAS

DEFINITION

A. Any change from the normal electrical cardiac conduction: Can result in impulses that occur too quickly, too slowly, or erratically.

B. Divided into two categories: Ventricular and supraventricular.

1. Ventricular abnormalities begin in the ventricles.

2. Supraventricular disorders originate above the ventricles (in the atria).

C. Can result in tachycardias or bradycardias.

1. Bradycardia is defined as a ventricular rate less than 60 beats per minute.

2. Conduction system causes of bradycardia: Sick sinus syndrome (SSS) or heart block (first-degree atrioventricular [AV] block, second-degree AV block types 1 and 2, and third-degree AV block).

INCIDENCE

A. Atrial fibrillation (AF) is the most common sustained cardiac arrhythmia where prevalence increases with age, most notably after 65 years old. It affects three to six million U.S. adults, with a prevalence of approximately 1% to 2%.

1. AF is estimated to occur in 1% of the population <60 years old.

2. Approximately 12% of those diagnosed with AF are between 75 and 84 years old and more than 33% of those with AF are ≥80 years old.

3. AF affects different racial/ethnic groups differently: The incidence and prevalence are lowest among those who identify as Asian or African American/Black and highest among those of European descent.

a. According to the Multi-Ethnic Study of Atherosclerosis (MESA), the incidence of AF (>65 years old) is 45% to 65% lower in Hispanic, Asian, and Black/African American persons as compared with non-Hispanic White persons.

B. Approximately 50% of patients experience sudden cardiac death as an initial clinical presentation of a cardiac arrhythmia.

1. The arrhythmias most likely to cause sudden cardiac death are ventricular fibrillation (VF) or ventricular tachycardia (VT), with approximately 300,000 deaths per year.

2. VT is more commonly seen in males secondary to underlying coronary artery disease (CAD).

C. Supraventricular tachycardias: Specifically, paroxysmal supraventricular tachycardia (PSVT) affects approximately 1 in every 300 U.S. adults, with the highest rates noted among women and older adults.

PATHOGENESIS

A. The pathophysiology of arrhythmias can be complex and vary based on type of abnormality.

B. Overall, there is an abnormality in the normal activation sequence of the cardiac fibers within the myocardium. There are three primary mechanisms.

1. Increased or decreased automaticity: Increased automaticity can result in atrial or ventricular arrhythmia.

2. Triggered activity.

3. Dysfunction in circulatory pathways: Specifically notable for reentry conduction pathways.

C. The pathogenesis of AF occurs due to three underlying factors: Electrical, structural, and contractile dysfunction.

1. In the simplest terms, AF's irregularly irregular tachycardic rhythm arises because of the multiple foci within the atria (principally around the orifices of the pulmonary arteries) that send chaotic impulses through the heart's electrical system.

2. This causes the atria to quiver or "fibrillate" instead of contract normally.

3. Typically, the atrial rate is greater than 400 beats per minute, but some impulses are successfully blocked by the AV node. Thus, a ventricular (or calculated pulse) rate of 75 to 175 beats per minute is appreciated.

D. Atrial flutter is a variation of AF where there is one primary automatic focus in the atria that fires between 250 and 350 beats per minute. The ventricular rate is typically one-half to one-third the atrial rate due to a refractory period of the AV node.

E. PSVT occurs due to AV nodal reentry tachycardia.

1. Two pathways within the AV node: Fast and slow.

2. Reentrant circuit revolving around the AV node.

F. Ventricular arrhythmias.

1. VT originates below the bundle of His and occurs due to quick and constant firing of three or more premature ventricular contractions (PVCs) at a rate of 100 to 250 beats per minute.

2. PVCs are defined as a heartbeat that fires on its own accord from a specific focus in one ventricle and proceeds to simulate the other ventricle.

3. VF occurs when there are multiple foci within the ventricles that are functioning on overdrive. This leads to irregular quivering of the ventricles and results in no cardiac output.

G. Bradycardias.

1. SSS: Typically occurs due to spontaneous persistent bradycardia.

2. First-degree AV block: Noted to have a conduction delay at the AV node that results in decreased pulse.

3. Second-degree AV block.

a. Type 1: Occurs because of a block within the AV node to cause bradycardia.

b. Type 2: Occurs because of a block within the bundle of His–Purkinje fibers to cause bradycardia (this can also progress to third-degree AV block).

4. Third-degree AV block: Complete dissociation between the atria and ventricles. There is no continuation of cardiac impulses between the two structures; results in significant bradycardia, typically 25 to 40 beats per minute.

PREDISPOSING FACTORS

A. AF.

1. Underlying CAD/previous myocardial infarction (MI).

2. Hypertension (HTN).

3. Valvular heart disease (VHD).

4. Endocrine disorders such as hyperthyroidism.

5. Postoperative physiologic stress.

6. Systemic illnesses such as sepsis or cancers.

7. Excess alcohol consumption (known as "holiday heart syndrome").

8. Age.

B. Atrial flutter.

1. Chronic obstructive pulmonary disease (COPD; most common cause).

2. Comorbid CAD.

3. Congestive heart failure (CHF).

4. Atrial septal defects or rheumatic heart disease.

C. PSVT.

1. Acute cardiac ischemia.

2. Medications: The most common is digoxin toxicity (causes paroxysmal atrial tachycardia with 2:1 block).

3. Atrial flutter with rapid ventricular response.

4. Excess caffeine, stimulant, or alcohol consumption.

D. VT.

1. Comorbid MI and CAD (most common causes).

2. Acute cardiac ischemia or hypotension.

3. Cardiomyopathy.

4. Congenital heart defects.

5. History of long QT syndrome.

E. VF.

1. Ischemic cardiac damage (most common cause).

2. Medications: Multiple drug classes prolong the QT interval; many antiarrhythmics, selective serotonin reuptake inhibitors (SSRIs), central nervous system (CNS) stimulants, and tricyclics.

SUBJECTIVE DATA

A. Common complaints/symptoms.

1. Fatigue.

2. Dyspnea on exertion (or at rest).

3. Chest discomfort.

4. Palpitations or "heart fluttering."

5. Dizziness, lightheadedness, syncope, or near-syncope.

6. Diaphoresis.

B. History of the present illness.

1. Recognize that patient presentation varies based on the type and degree of arrhythmia.

a. For example, SSS can present with dizziness, fatigue, and change in mental status, while VT can present asymptomatically as sudden cardiac death (if rate is slow enough).

2. Understand the onset, provoking/palliative factors, quality, severity, and timing of symptoms.

3. Obtain information regarding a patient's medical history, specifically regarding the aforementioned conditions, that can predispose them to abnormal heart rhythms.

C. Family and social history.

1. Determine any family history of CAD, HTN, hyperlipidemia (HLD), VHD, congenital heart defects, or arrhythmias.

2. Obtain information on sleep habits (AF maintains a strong association with obstructive sleep apnea), tobacco use, alcohol/caffeine consumption, and other substance use (especially stimulants).

D. Review of systems.

1. General: Fatigue, malaise, fevers, and chills.

2. Cardiac: Angina, racing heartbeat, palpitations, decreased exercise tolerance, and peripheral edema.

3. Pulmonary: Shortness of breath (SOB) and dyspnea on exertion.

4. Neurologic: Lightheadedness, dizziness, syncope, and near-syncope.

PHYSICAL EXAMINATION

A. Evaluate patients for signs and symptoms of heart failure (HF), as arrhythmias frequently decrease cardiac output.

B. Vital signs: Assess ventricular rate, blood pressure (BP), respiration, temperature, and oxygen saturation.

1. Important to note temperature, as an underlying febrile illness can exacerbate underlying AF.

2. In VF/VT, it is likely that the patient will be unconscious with no pulse and unmeasurable BP.

C. Neck: Jugular venous distention (JVD).

D. Pulmonary: Possible rales or crackles (sign of increased fluid accumulation as related to underlying CHF).

E. Cardiac: Inspection and palpation for thrills and auscultation.

    1. Auscultation.

      a. Assess rate (tachycardic or bradycardic).

      b. Rhythm (regular, irregularly irregular, or irregularly regular).

      c. Extra heart sounds (S3 and S4).

      d. Murmurs consistent with underlying VHD.

F. Peripheral vascular: Assess peripheral pulses, possible peripheral edema (sign of fluid overload and concomitant CHF).

G. Neurologic: Mental status examination (if mental status changes) or complete neurologic examination if there is concern for associated syncope/near-syncope.

DIAGNOSTIC TESTS

A. EKG.

    1. AF: Tachycardia rate (110–180 beats per minute), irregularly irregular rhythm (irregularly spaced R-R intervals) with no discernable P-waves.

    2. Atrial flutter: Tachycardic rate with a "saw-tooth" (F-wave) baseline pattern; best seen in leads VI, II, III, and augmented vector foot (aVF), where the QRS complex appears after several "saw-tooth" P-waves (number of F-waves can vary depending on atrioventricular node [AVN] blockade).

    3. VF: Irregular rhythm, no identifiable P-waves, or QRS complexes.

    4. VT: Tachycardic rate (150–250 beats per minute) and wide QRS complexes (can have identical morphologies in monomorphic VT or different ones in polymorphic VT).

    5. PSVT (most common etiology of reentry conduction): Tachycardic rate, narrow QRS complexes with no discernable P-waves (P-waves are buried within the QRS complexes secondary to simultaneous rapid firing of the atria and ventricles).

    6. First-degree heart block: The hallmark is a PR interval greater than 0.20 seconds where a QRS complex follows each P-wave.

    7. Second-degree heart block.

      a. Type 1 (Mobitz type I or Wenckebach): The hallmark is progressive prolongation of the PR interval with a nonconducted P-wave, with the longest PR interval preceding the dropped QRS and the shortest immediately after.

      b. Type 2 (Mobitz Type II): The hallmark is an intermittent nonconducted P-wave without progressive prolongation, but immediate PR interval to dropped QRS is prolonged.

    8. Third-degree heart block: Bradycardic rate, with no discernable pattern or connection between P-waves and QRS complexes.

B. Laboratory tests.

    1. Complete blood count with differential: Determine if an anemia is contributing to the arrhythmia.

    2. Complete metabolic panel: Determine if an electrolyte disturbance or renal dysfunction is contributing to the arrhythmia.

    3. Thyroid panel: Hypothyroidism or hyperthyroidism can be an underlying etiology for arrhythmias (i.e., thyrotoxicosis can trigger AF).

    4. Cardiac biomarkers: These should be obtained in any patient with chest discomfort or evidence of an arrhythmia; they evaluate for the possibility of underlying MI.

    5. Digitalis level (if clinically indicated): Supratherapeutic levels can lead to various arrhythmias, including PSVT and AF with rapid ventricular response.

    6. Toxicology screening (if clinically indicated): Illicit substances, especially stimulants, can precipitate arrhythmias.

    7. D-dimer: This can help rule out a pulmonary embolus, which can occur in the setting of AF.

C. Chest x-ray: Checks for underlying cardiomegaly, pulmonary edema, or pulmonary infections such as pneumonia, or pneumothorax, which can exacerbate or precipitate arrhythmias.

D. Exercise stress testing: Helps provide an overall understanding of one's cardiovascular health and evaluate for underlying ischemia.

E. Holter monitor or loop recorder: Can be helpful in monitoring patients on a continuous basis when an arrhythmia is suspected but unable to be captured via EKG; can also be helpful in patients with vague or nonspecific cardiac symptoms.

F. Transesophageal echocardiogram (TEE): Especially important for new-onset arrhythmias to evaluate overall cardiac function (ejection fraction [EF]), identify VHD, rule out intracardiac thrombus (particularly within the left atrial appendage), and measure atria and ventricle sizes.

DIFFERENTIAL DIAGNOSIS

A. AF.

B. Atrial flutter.

C. VF.

D. Ventricular flutter.

E. Atrial tachycardia.

F. PSVT.

G. SSS.

H. First-degree heart block.

I. Second-degree heart block types 1 and 2.

J. Third-degree heart block.

EVALUATION AND MANAGEMENT PLAN

A. General plan.

    1. Diagnose the arrhythmia and determine the patient's clinical symptoms.

    2. Stabilize heart rate (HR) and rhythm based on clinical scenario using pharmacologic or procedural methods such as electrocardioversion or transcutaneous/transvenous pacing.

    3. Evaluate underlying cardiac status and comorbidities to guide treatment plan.

4. Determine if arrhythmia is secondary to an underlying etiology that requires additional management (e.g., sepsis, thyrotoxicosis, intoxication, MI, cerebrovascular accident [CVA]).

5. Consult with a cardiologist (and electrophysiologist) if device implantation or ablation procedures are required.

6. For arrhythmias requiring anticoagulation (AC) for thromboembolic prophylaxis, such as AF, complete risk stratification assessment, and discuss the risks and benefits of these medications with patients and families.

   a. Use the CHA$_2$DS$_2$-VASc score to determine the risk of thromboembolic strokes (Table 3.2).

   b. For patients with a score of 2+, oral AC is recommended using a vitamin K antagonist (e.g., warfarin with an international normalized ratio [INR] goal of 2.0–3.0) or a novel anticoagulant (e.g., dabigatran, rivaroxaban, edoxaban, or apixaban).

   c. For patients with a score of "0" in males or "1" in females, no therapy is recommended.

B. Patient/family teaching points.

1. Educate regarding specific arrhythmia and symptoms that can precipitate recurrence (if clinically relevant).

2. Educate on reasons to return to the ED, specifically those that signal worsening cardiac status or development of a life-threatening arrhythmia.

3. Educate on the importance of medication compliance and regular follow-up appointments with a cardiologist/electrophysiologist.

4. For patients using warfarin for AC, it is important to discuss dietary restrictions. It is also essential to educate patients on any anticoagulant regarding risk of bleeding.

5. For implantable devices, ensure patients understand the purpose of their device, the importance of device maintenance, who to contact if there is an equipment malfunction, and how device monitoring will occur.

C. Pharmacotherapy.

1. Acute AF/atrial flutter.

   a. Rate control: The target ventricular rate is 60 to 100 beats per minute.

      i. Calcium channel and beta-blockers are first-line therapies.

      ii. Caution in patients with HF: Many rate and rhythm control agents decrease contractility and cardiac output. Consider digoxin or amiodarone for patients with low output HF who require rate control.

      iii. Patients with chronic AF can use calcium channel blockers or beta-blockers for long-term rate control.

   b. Rhythm control.

      i. Can use electrical, surgical, or pharmacologic methods (electrical cardioversion is preferred). AF ablation has shown to be useful in patients with HF.

      ii. If pharmacologic conversion, consider options such as sotalol, flecainide, amiodarone, and dofetilide.

   c. AC: Assess the need based on risk stratification tools and comorbidities.

      i. If a patient is hemodynamically unstable, initiate immediate electrical cardioversion to convert to normal sinus rhythm regardless of AC considerations.

      ii. If a patient is hemodynamically stable and AF is under hypothermic conditions, gradual slow rewarming via a warming blanket is recommended.

      iii. If AF is present for greater than 48 hours (or unknown period of time), there is high risk of stroke if electrical cardioversion is performed immediately; recommend AC for 3 weeks before and at least 4 weeks after successful cardioversion (INR goal of 2.0–3.0 if using warfarin).

      iv. To expedite cardioversion timing, obtain TEE to rule out thrombus in the left atrial appendage, administer intravenous (IV) heparin, cardiovert within 24 hours, and then use oral AC agent for 1 month.

      v. If a patient is hemodynamically stable and AF is present for less than 48 hours, electrical cardioversion without prior AC or TEE can occur at the discretion of the cardiologist and must take into account the patient's CHA$_2$DS$_2$-VASc score. If the procedure is completed, postprocedure AC is also utilized for 1 month.

      vi. If a patient is in hemodynamically unstable AF (regardless of duration), electrocardioversion should be performed immediately without the need for prior AC or TEE.

2. PSVT.

   a. If hemodynamically stable, first attempt vagal maneuvers such as Valsalva, breath-holding, or immersion of the head in cold water.

TABLE 3.2 CHA$_2$DS$_2$.VASc SCORE FOR RISK ASSESSMENT IN ATRIAL FIBRILLATION

	Criteria	Score
C	Congestive heart failure	1
H	Hypertension history	1
A$_2$	Age ≥75 years	2
D	Diabetes mellitus	1
S$_2$	Prior stroke, transient ischemic attack, or history of thromboembolism	2
V	Vascular disease (e.g., peripheral artery disease, myocardial infarction, aortic plaque)	1
A	Age 65–74 years	1
Sc	Sex (i.e., female)	1

b. If nonpharmacologic maneuvers are unsuccessful, administer IV adenosine (drug of choice) to reduce sinoatrial (SA) and AV node activity.

c. If adenosine is unsuccessful in converting acute PSVT to normal sinus rhythm, the most common IV alternatives are beta-blockers (e.g., metoprolol, propranolol, esmolol) or calcium channel blockers (e.g., verapamil, diltiazem) for patients without left ventricular dysfunction; for individuals with HF or structural heart disease, IV amiodarone can be used.

d. If pharmacologic methods are unsuccessful or the patient is hemodynamically unstable, perform electrical cardioversion (almost always successful).

e. For long-term rate control, beta-blockers and calcium channel blockers are used. Digoxin can also be used in the setting of HF; if symptoms are recurrent and persistent, refer to an electrophysiologist for ablation.

3. VT.

a. Described by type (monomorphic or polymorphic), duration (sustained or nonsustained) and heart rate (HR). Identify the patient's clinical response to the arrhythmia to determine the next steps.

  i. If sustained VT (lasts longer than 30 seconds, usually symptomatic and with hemodynamic instability), initiate immediate electrical cardioversion and then IV amiodarone to maintain sinus rhythm. Follow the Advanced Cardiac Life Support (ACLS) VT algorithm.

  ii. If sustained VT without hemodynamic compromise and mild symptoms, consider IV medications such as sotalol, procainamide, or lidocaine.

  iii. If sustained VT and abnormal EF, placement of implantable cardiac defibrillator (ICD) for long-term management will likely be required.

b. If nonsustained VT (brief asymptomatic episodes of VT) without cardiac comorbidities, do not treat (no increased risk of morbidity).

  i. If nonsustained VT with underlying cardiac disease, consider ICD as first-line long-term management.

4. VF.

a. Medical emergency that requires immediate CPR and defibrillation per the ACLS VF algorithm.

b. Follow ACLS algorithm for pharmacologic management.

5. Bradycardic rhythms.

a. Defined as a ventricular rate <60 beat per minute. Bradycardia is common in athletes and patients on beta-blockade. For several types of bradycardias, including SSS, second-degree heart block type 2, and third-degree heart block, pacemaker implantation is the most effective long-term monitoring strategy.

b. Pharmacologic interventions.

  i. Atropine: Can be used for acute symptomatic bradycardia (if reversible cause not identified).

  ii. Dopamine: Second-line drug for symptomatic bradycardia if atropine is ineffective.

  iii. Epinephrine: Can be utilized as an infusion for symptomatic bradycardia if atropine or pacing methods are unsuccessful.

D. Discharge instructions.

1. Ensure patients receive all appropriate prescriptions prior to discharge.

2. Ensure patients have prearranged follow-up appointments with a cardiologist/electrophysiologist.

3. For patients with newly implanted devices, ensure information is provided regarding the device, clinic follow-up, and home monitoring systems (if indicated).

a. Educate on proper wound care of incision site for a newly implanted device and reasons to return to a healthcare provider for signs of infection (e.g., erythema, edema, worsening pain, drainage, dehiscence, systemic symptoms).

4. Understand that it is important that patients understand limitations regarding physical activity, depending on the type and degree of arrhythmia and their cardiac status.

FOLLOW-UP

A. Ensure patient adherence with all medications, particularly with respect to antiarrhythmic or AC therapy.

1. Patients on antiarrhythmic therapy should have close follow-up with a cardiologist or electrophysiologist to minimize adverse effects.

a. Patients using amiodarone should have a clear understanding of its side effects and monitor closely for amiodarone-induced liver, lung, thyroid, and other organ toxicities.

2. Patients on AC therapy with warfarin should understand their follow-up plan with regard to frequency of INR monitoring and how dosing adjustments will be communicated.

B. Outpatient oral medication choices for arrhythmias depend on the degree of ventricular dysfunction, type of arrhythmia, and comorbidities.

C. Patients should have close monitoring of their electrolytes to reduce the risk of arrhythmias secondary to electrolyte imbalances.

D. Patients with ICDs and pacemakers require regular outpatient device follow-up at electrophysiology clinics where their devices are monitored for lead integrity and battery life.

CONSULTATION/REFERRAL

A. Consult with a cardiologist to further evaluate arrhythmia and underlying cardiac status.

B. Consult with an electrophysiologist for in-depth electrophysiologic diagnostics and ablative procedures.

SPECIAL/GERIATRIC CONSIDERATIONS

A. Additional device considerations.

1. Temporary pacemakers.

a. Transcutaneous pacing.

   i. Used for symptomatic bradycardias if the patient fails to respond to atropine, dopamine, or epinephrine (can also be utilized in the setting of tachyarrhythmias to break the conduction disturbance).

   ii. Should be started immediately if the patient is hemodynamically unstable, especially in those with second-degree heart block type II or third-degree heart block.

   iii. Can be painful; use analgesia and sedation for pain control.

   iv. Use transvenous pacing if transcutaneous pacing is unsuccessful (cardiologist or electrophysiologist should be consulted prior to initiation).

2. Permanent pacemakers.

a. Single-chamber pacemakers: Stimulate either the atria or (more commonly) the ventricle.

b. Dual-chamber pacemakers: Send electrical impulses to both the atrium and the ventricle; provides synchronization that closely mimics the natural heartbeat (commonly used for bradycardias).

c. Biventricular pacemakers: Pace the rhythm of the ventricles so that the chambers contract simultaneously; used in patients with HF and conduction abnormalities.

d. Combination pacemaker: Have pacemaker and defibrillation functions.

3. ICD: Surgically placed and functions by detecting lethal cardiac arrhythmias and delivering electrical shocks until the rhythm normalizes; indicated in VF and/or VT that are uncontrolled with medication (important prevention for sudden cardiac death).

B. Geriatric considerations.

1. The aging process is associated with the development of arrhythmias, particularly AF.

2. Degenerative changes of the cardiac conduction system (i.e., SA and AV nodes) are more common in older adult patients, who are more likely to experience heart blocks due to conduction delays.

3. Older adult patients are more likely to have ventricular heart disease and thus a higher risk of arrhythmias secondary to structural abnormalities (especially within the aortic and mitral valves).

4. During the physiologic aging process, the PR interval can be prolonged.

5. Geriatric patients can report vague complaints (e.g., weakness, fatigue, malaise) as presenting symptoms for an arrhythmia. It can be difficult to separate these from the normal aging process.

6. The frequency of PVCs also increases with age.

7. If considering a device for geriatric patients, it is important to address comorbidities, life span, impact on quality of life, maintenance of device, and occurrence of unnecessary shocks during end-of-life care.

8. The use of anticoagulants in the geriatric population should be carefully reviewed with patients (and family members, if necessary) to ensure that the risks versus benefits of these medications are evaluated.

a. Cognitive status (important for medication compliance).

b. Comorbidities (e.g., is the patient already utilizing other antiplatelet or anticoagulant agents, thus increasing the risk of bleeding events?).

c. Overall functional status: Important to address the risk of falls and bleeding complications.

BIBLIOGRAPHY

Agabegi, S. S., & Agabegi, E. D. (2019). *Step-up to medicine* (5th ed.). Wolters Kluwer.

Bashore, T. M., Granger, C. B., Jackson, K. P., & Patel, M. R. (2022). Atrial fibrillation. In M. A. Papadakis, S. J. McPhee, M. W. Rabow, & K. R. McQuaid (Eds.), *Current medical diagnosis & treatment 2022*. McGraw Hill.

Centers for Disease Control and Prevention. (2021, September 27). *Atrial fibrillation. Centers for disease control and prevention.* https://www.cdc.gov/heartdisease/atrial_fibrillation.htm

Elmoselhi, A., & Seif, M. (2017). *Electrophysiology of the heart.* In A. Elmoselhi (Ed.), *Cardiology: An integrated approach.* McGraw Hill.

Hindricks, G., Potpara, T., Dagres, N., Arbelo, E., Bax, J. J., Blomström-Lundqvist, C., Boriani, G., Castella, M., Dan, G.-A., Dilaveris, P. E., Fauchier, L., Filippatos, G., Kalman, J. M., Meir, M. L., Lane, D. A., Lebeau, J.-P., Lettino, M., Lip, G. Y. H., Pinto, F. J. … ESC Scientific Document Group. (2021). 2020 ESC Guidelines for the diagnosis and management of atrial fibrillation developed in collaboration with the European Association for Cardio-Thoracic Surgery (EACTS): The Task Force for the diagnosis and management of atrial fibrillation of the European Society of Cardiology (ESC) Developed with the special contribution of the European Heart Rhythm Association (EHRA) of the ESC, *European Heart Journal*, 42(5), 373–498. https://doi.org/10.1093/eurheartj/ehaa612

Hsu, J., & Scheinman, M. M. (2017). Atrial fibrillation. In M. H. Crawford M.H (Ed.), *Current diagnosis & treatment: Cardiology* (5th ed.). McGraw Hill.

Kornej, J., Börschel, C. S., Benjamin, E. J., & Schnabel, R. B. (2020). Epidemiology of atrial fibrillation in the 21st century: Novel methods and new insights. *Circulation Research*, 127(1), 4–20. https://doi.org/10.1161/circresaha.120.316340

Michaud, G. F., & Stevenson, W. G. (2018). Paroxysmal supraventricular tachycardias. In J. Jameson, A. S. Fauci, D. L. Kasper, S. L. Hauser, D. L. Longo, & J. Loscalzo (Eds.), *Harrison's principles of internal medicine* (20th ed.). McGraw Hill.

Panchal, A. R., Bartos, J. A., Cabañas, J. G., Donnino, M. W., Drennan, I. R., Hirsch, K. G., Kudenchuk, P. J., Kurz, M. C., Lavonas, E. J., Morley, P. T., O'Neil, B. J., Peberdy, M. A., Rittenberger, J. C., Rodriguez, A. J., Sawyer, K. N., Berg, K. M., Arafeh, J., Benoit, J. L., Chase, M., & D. J, … Magid. (2020). Part 3: Adult basic and advanced life support: 2020 American Heart Association guidelines for cardiopulmonary resuscitation and emergency cardiovascular care. *Circulation*, 142(16_suppl_2), S366–S468. https://doi.org/10.1161/CIR.0000000000000916

Rehorn, M., Sacks, N. C., Emden, M. R., Healey, B., Preib, M. T., Cyr, P. L., & Pokorney, S. D. (2021). Prevalence and incidence of patients with paroxysmal supraventricular tachycardia in the United States. *Journal of Cardiovascular Electrophysiology*, 32(8), 2199–2206. https://doi.org/10.1111/jce.15109

Upadhyay, G. A., & Singh, J. P. (2017). Pacemakers and defibrillators. In V. Fuster, R. A. Harrington, J. Narula, & Z. J. Eapen (Eds.), *Hurst's the heart* (14th ed.). McGraw Hill.

DYSLIPIDEMIA

DEFINITION

A. Hyperlipidemia (HLD): elevation of cholesterol levels, which includes total cholesterol (TC) and its components, low-density lipoprotein cholesterol (LDL-C) and high-density lipoprotein cholesterol (HDL-C); can ▶

also occur in the setting of elevated triglycerides (TGs; hypertriglyceridemia).

1. HLD can be inherited (familial) or caused by secondary diagnoses.

2. It increases the risk of atherosclerosis, leading to stroke and heart disease.

B. Dyslipidemia: Elevation of plasma cholesterol, TGs, or both, or a decreased HDL level that augments atherosclerosis.

INCIDENCE

A. The Framingham Heart Study noted an epidemiologic link between elevated cholesterol and atherosclerotic cardiovascular disease (ASCVD).

B. Current epidemiologic data show that approximately 100 million (53%) U.S. adults have increased LDL-C levels, where only 50% of these individuals are receiving appropriate pharmacotherapy and less than 35% have LDL-C levels showing control.

C. Approximately 31 million U.S. adults have TC levels >240 mg/dL, which doubles their risk of developing ischemic heart disease when compared with those with normal cholesterol levels.

PATHOGENESIS

A. Disease process starts in the gastrointestinal tract with hydroxymethylglutaryl-coenzyme A (HMG-CoA).

B. HMG-CoA is a precursor that undergoes complex biochemical reactions to produce cholesterol.

C. Once synthesized, cholesterol travels through the plasma.

D. The liver also plays a role, converting very low-density lipoprotein (VLDL) to LDL, which moves through the plasma.

E. Also, dietary cholesterol that moves from the small intestines to the liver through the serum with LDLs must be considered.

F. Cholesterol is an important organic molecule for cell membrane integrity and serves as a precursor to steroid hormones, vitamin D, and bile acid. However, with increased levels of cholesterol, the concern is for atherosclerosis.

G. Atherosclerosis is an inflammatory process where various cells and mediators undergo a cascade of reactions to form plaques in the vasculature.

1. Various factors trigger inflammation, such as elevated glucose, tobacco by-products, elevated blood pressure (BP), and oxidized LDLs.

2. With increased inflammation, there is increased permeability and injury to the vessel walls. The result is increased accumulation of LDLs within the tunica intima layer of the vasculature.

3. The inflammation causes increased activation of inflammatory mediators (e.g., monocytes and macrophages).

4. Inflammatory mediators uptake the oxidized LDLs, leading to transformation of macrophages into foam cells, also known as "fatty streaks" within the vasculature.

5. Foam cells eventually result in plaque formation with fibrous caps; when the thin top layer of these caps

dislodges, exposing highly thrombotic necrotic contents, platelet aggregation and cardiac ischemia can result.

PREDISPOSING FACTORS

A. Hereditary: Genetic component for the metabolism of LDL.

1. Familial hypercholesterolemia (FH): A group of autosomal dominant pathologies (localized to chromosome 19) that result in increased levels of LDL-C.

a. FH affects approximately 1 in 500 people in the United States and maintains a global prevalence of approximately 10 million, yet fewer than 15% are diagnosed and treated properly.

b. As a result of elevated LDL-C levels, those affected are at an increased risk of developing atherosclerotic heart disease and strokes at a relatively young age and its complications.

c. Individuals diagnosed with FH will typically have TC levels >200 mg/dL (<40 years old) or >250 mg/dL (>40 years old).

B. Diet: Foods high in saturated fat and cholesterol.

C. Lifestyle: Physical inactivity, which can lead to increased cholesterol levels.

D. Comorbidities.

1. Secondary causes of HLD: Hypothyroidism, diabetes mellitus (DM), nephrotic syndrome, Cushing disease, chronic kidney disease (CKD), and medications (oral contraceptives, diuretics).

2. Secondary causes of elevated TGs: Obesity, DM, alcohol use, CKD, and medications (estrogen).

3. Concern for metabolic syndrome: Large waist circumference, elevated TGs, low HDL level, elevated BP, and elevated glucose levels.

SUBJECTIVE DATA

A. Common complaints/symptoms.

1. Rarely any complaints from HLD alone.

2. Concern exists from its sequelae, such as cardiovascular disease, peripheral vascular disease (PVD) secondary to claudication, and neurologic diseases (e.g., transient ischemic attack [TIA] and cerebrovascular accident [CVA]).

B. History of the present illness.

1. Determine the duration of patients' HLD diagnosis and how the diagnosis occurred (e.g., detected during routine screening vs. after an acute event such as a myocardial infarction [MI] or CVA/TIA).

2. Assess patients' routine monitoring of cholesterol: When levels were last checked and how they have evolved over time.

3. Assess patients' medical history for associated comorbidities such as hypertension (HTN), MI, peripheral artery disease (PAD)/PVD, coronary artery disease (CAD), carotid artery stenosis, or DM type 2. It is also important to assess for any underlying liver disease, which can be a contraindication to statin use.

4. If a patient is using lipid-lowering medication, assess for side effects, such as myopathies that are commonly appreciated in statin use. If a patient is utilizing nonpharmacologic interventions, such as diet and exercise, those interventions should also be reviewed. ▶

5. Determine if a patient is experiencing any cardiovascular or neurologic complaints as a result of the HLD.

C. Family and social history.

1. Assess for family history of HLD, dyslipidemia, CAD, DM type 2, PVD, PAD, and neurologic complications (CVA, TIA).

2. Understand dietary routine, exercise/activity levels, and use of tobacco and alcohol consumption.

D. Review of systems.

1. Evidence of weight gain.

2. Skin changes: Yellow deposits (xanthomas) which can occur around the eyelids or attached to certain tendons (tendon xanthomas) like the Achilles, the latter of which is most commonly seen in patients with FH.

3. Cardiac symptoms: Chest pain, palpitations, decreased exercise tolerance, shortness of breath (SOB), and dyspnea on exertion.

4. Peripheral vascular status: Claudication.

5. Neurologic (if concern for CVA or TIA): Changes in mental status, vision, speech, sensation, and strength.

PHYSICAL EXAMINATION

A. Vital signs: Determine body mass index (BMI) and consider comorbid HTN.

B. Skin: Check for xanthomas.

C. Ophthalmologic: Perform funduscopic examination and check for possible corneal arcus, which will appear as a white ring at the scleral–iris junction.

D. Neck: Auscultate carotid arteries and evaluate for carotid bruits.

E. Cardiovascular: Inspect for lifts/heaves/visible pulsations, assess point of maximum impulse (PMI), palpate for thrills, and auscultate using diaphragm and bell for murmurs and extra heart sounds.

F. If there is concern for CVA/TIA, consider complete neurologic examination.

DIAGNOSTIC TESTS

A. For the evaluation of dyslipidemia, obtain a fasting (9–12 hours fast) lipid panel for TC, LDL-C, and HDL-C (Table 3.3).

B. For secondary causes of dyslipidemia, workup should include a complete blood count, complete metabolic panel, fasting glucose, thyroid-stimulating hormone (TSH), and urinary protein.

C. Lipid measurement should be accompanied by evaluation for other cardiovascular risk factors, including an EKG, stress testing, and echocardiogram.

DIFFERENTIAL DIAGNOSIS

A. The focus of the differential diagnosis in dyslipidemia is on primary versus secondary causes.

1. Primary causes: Inherited disorder.

2. Secondary causes.

   a. Hypothyroidism.

   b. Medications (e.g., corticosteroids diuretics, protease inhibitors).

   c. Alcoholism.

   d. Smoking.

TABLE 3.3 DIAGNOSTIC INTERPRETATION OF FASTING LIPID PANEL

LDL Cholesterol (mg/dL)	
<100	Optimal
100–129	Near optimal
130–159	Borderline high
160–189	High
>190	Very high

HDL Cholesterol (mg/dL)	
<40	Low (risk factor for atherosclerotic heart disease)
>60	High (protective against atherosclerotic heart disease)

TC (mg/dL)	
<200	Preferable
200–239	Borderline high
>240	High

HDL, high-density lipoprotein; LDL, low-density lipoprotein; TC, total cholesterol.
Source: From MedlinePlus. Bethesda (MD): National Library of Medicine (US); Cholesterol Levels; [updated 2020 July 30]. https://medlineplus.gov/heartattack.html.

   e. Obstructive liver/biliary disease.

   f. Renal failure.

   g. Uncontrolled diabetes.

   h. Nephrotic syndrome.

EVALUATION AND MANAGEMENT PLAN

A. General plan.

1. The National Cholesterol Education Program (NCEP) and Adult Treatment Panel (ATP) III have created a process for management of elevated cholesterol.

2. Determine LDL-C, TC, and HDL-C levels.

3. Identify any comorbidities, including cardiovascular disease or its equivalents (DM, PAD, abdominal aortic aneurysm).

4. Identify modifiable and unmodifiable risk factors: Low HDL, tobacco use, HTN, age (males >45 years and females >55 years), and family history of CAD.

5. Assess overall cardiovascular risk and determine LDL-C goal using tools such as the American College of Cardiology (ACC) and American Heart Association (AHA) ASCVD risk calculator; this tool is most reliable for use in non-Hispanic White and Black/African American adults ages 40 to 79 years old.

6. Initiate the Therapeutic Lifestyle Changes (TLC) plan if LDL is higher than the goal: Consists of increased physical activity, weight management, and low trans fat and low cholesterol diet.

7. Utilize medications if LDL remains above goal. ▶

8. Assess for metabolic syndrome and evaluate TGs.

9. Treat low HDL-C and elevated TGs if required.

B. Patient/family teaching points.

1. Emphasize medication compliance, use of TLC plan, and elimination of modifiable risk factors (e.g., tobacco cessation, reduction of alcohol consumption).

2. Stress the importance of compliance with clinician appointments.

C. Pharmacotherapy.

1. Lipid management.

a. Statins (HMG-CoA reductase inhibitor).

i. Important considerations regarding side effects of statins.

ii. Elevation in liver enzymes (usually alanine aminotransferase [ALT]).

iii. Myalgia: Occurs in approximately 10% of patients and can be dose-dependent; switching to a different statin can help relieve symptoms.

iv. Rhabdomyolysis: Myalgias plus creatine kinase (CK) levels greater than 10,000 U/L can result in renal failure.

v. Myositis: Myalgias with CK less than 10,000 U/L.

vi. Anticoagulants: Caution with concomitant use of most statins and anticoagulants; a dose reduction in the anticoagulant is advised.

vii. Statins are contraindicated in pregnancy.

b. Bile acid sequestrants.

c. Cholesterol absorption inhibitors.

d. Injectable medications (monoclonal antibodies termed proprotein convertase subtilisin/kexin type 9 [PCSK9] inhibitors): Works by allowing the liver to absorb increased level of cholesterol, thus decreasing circulating plasma cholesterol.

2. Medications for high TG.

a. Fibrates.

b. Niacin.

c. Omega-3 fatty acids supplements.

FOLLOW-UP

A. Check lipid levels per ACC and AHA recommendations, which stipulate checking levels at 4 to 12 weeks after initiating (or changing) statin therapy and then every 3 to 12 months thereafter.

B. Obtain baseline liver and CK levels before initiating statin therapy (routine monitoring not required).

C. Monitor patients for the development of modifiable risk factors, noting that the U.S. Preventive Task Force (USPSTF) recommends (level B evidence) the initiation of a low- to moderate-intensity statin as primary prevention in adults (ages 40–75 years old) without heart disease who have at least one cardiovascular risk factor (e.g., dyslipidemia, tobacco use, HTN, DM type 2) and a ≥10% risk of a cardiovascular event within the next 10 years per the ACC and AHA ASCVD risk calculator.

CONSULTATION/REFERRAL

A. Consult with a lipidologist in the following situations:

1. Suspicion for primary genetic disorder.

2. Unsuccessful treatment plans despite optimal therapy and patient compliance.

3. Comorbid liver disease if limiting therapeutic options.

4. Young adults in whom long-term therapy and monitoring is a consideration.

SPECIAL/GERIATRIC CONSIDERATIONS

A. Patients with statin intolerance. Use the following:

1. Lower intensity statin or nondaily moderate intensity statin.

2. Low-dose statin with selective cholesterol absorption therapy (ezetimibe), bile acid sequestrants, or niacin.

3. Nonstatin monotherapy with a goal of 30% reduction in LDL levels.

B. Geriatric considerations.

1. For patients *at least* 65 to younger than 80 years of age with ASCVD or DM, consider moderate- or high-intensity statin once risks/benefits have been assessed by the provider and the patient).

2. For secondary cardiovascular prevention in patients 80 years of age or older, consider moderate-intensity statin once risks/benefits have been assessed by the provider and the patient.

BIBLIOGRAPHY

Grundy, S. M., Stone, N. J., Bailey, A. L., Beam, C., Birtcher, K. K., Blumenthal, R. S., Braun, L. T., Ferranti, S., Faiella-Tommasino, J., Forman, D. E., Goldberg, R., Heidenreich, P. A., Hlatky, M. A., Jones, D. W., Lloyd-Jones, D., Lopez-Pajares, N., … Yeboah, J. (2019). AHA/ACC/AACVPR/AAPA/ABC/ACPM/ADA/AGS/APhA/ASPC/NLA/PCNA guideline on the management of blood cholesterol: A report of the American college of cardiology/American heart association task force on clinical practice guidelines. *Journal of the American College of Cardiology, 73*(24), e285–e350. https://doi.org/10.1016/j.jacc.2018.11.003

Karr, S. (2017). Epidemiology and management of hyperlipidemia. *The American Journal of Managed Care, 23*(9 Suppl), S139–S148.

MedlinePlus. (2020). *Heart attack.* National Library of Medicine (US); Cholesterol Levels. https://medlineplus.gov/heartattack.html

Pyeritz, R. E. (2022). Familial hypercholesterolemia. In M. A. Papadakis, S. J. McPhee, M. W. Rabow, & K. R. McQuaid (Eds.), *Current medical diagnosis & treatment 2022.* McGraw Hill.

Rader, D. J., & Kathiresan, S. (2018). Disorders of lipoprotein metabolism. In J. Jameson, A. S. Fauci, D. L. Kasper, S. L. Hauser, D. L. Longo, & J. Loscalzo (Eds.), *Harrison's principles of internal medicine* (20th ed.). McGraw Hill.

Ramlee, R. A., Subramaniam, S. K., Yaakob, S. B., Rahman, A. S. F., & Saad, N. M. (2020). Corneal arcus classification for hyperlipidemia detection using gray level co-occurrence matrix features. *Journal of Physics: Conference Series, 1432*(1), 012084. https://doi.org/10.1088/1742-6596/1432/1/012084

US Preventive Services Task Force., Bibbins-Domingo, K., Grossman, D. C., Curry, S. J., Davidson, K. W., Epling, J. W. Jr., García, F. A. R., Gillman, M. W., Kemper, A. R., Krist, A. H., Kurth, A. E., Landefeld, C. S., LeFevre, M. L., Mangione, C. M., Phillips, W. R., Owens, D. R., Phipps, M. G., & Pignone, M. P. (2016). Statin use for the primary prevention of cardiovascular disease in adults: US Preventive Services Task Force recommendation statement. *JAMA, 316*(19), 1997–2007. https://doi.org/10.1001/jama.2016.15450

Virani, S. S., Morris, P. B., Agarwala, A., Ballantyne, C. M., Birtcher, K. K., Kris-Etherton, P. M., Ladden-Stirling, A. B., Miller, M. Orringer., E, C., & Stone, N. J. (2021). ACC expert consensus decision pathway on the management of ASCVD risk reduction in patients with persistent hypertriglyceridemia: A report of the American college of cardiology solution set oversight committee. *Journal of the American College of Cardiology, 78*(9), 960–993. https://doi.org/10.1016/j.jacc.2021.06.011

HEART FAILURE

DEFINITION

A. Inability of the heart to meet the metabolic demands of the body.

B. Left-sided heart failure (HF): Further classified by the functional capacity of the left ventricle via ejection fraction (EF).

　1. Heart failure with preserved ejection fraction (HFpEF).

　　a. EF ≥50% (those with EFs between 40% and 50% are considered to have borderline EF).

　　b. Occurs when the ventricle is unable to properly fill during diastole (muscle has stiffened).

　　c. Amount of available blood for circulation is decreased.

　2. Heart failure with reduced ejection fraction (HFrEF).

　　a. EF <50%.

　　b. Occurs when the ventricle has lost its normal contractile ability.

　　c. Force/amount of blood pumped during systole is decreased.

C. Right-sided HF: A subtype of HF; usually occurs secondary to HFrEF, but also seen in HFpEF, idiopathic pulmonary arterial hypertension (IPAH), and chronic obstructive pulmonary disease (COPD).

　1. Left ventricular dysfunction causes an increase in fluid pressure that travels into the lungs and affects the right ventricle (RV).

　2. This results in fluid accumulation in the peripheral system.

D. High-output HF: A subtype of HF where there is an increase in the body's oxygen demands (e.g., chronic anemia, pregnancy, hyperthyroidism).

　1. Increased demand forces the heart to work harder to meet these needs.

　2. This eventually results in decreased cardiac function.

E. HF can be defined by the New York Heart Association (NYHA) classification, which is a method to categorize the severity of HF based on patient symptoms (Table 3.4).

INCIDENCE

A. HF affects approximately 20 million people globally and the prevalence in high-resourced countries is 2%.

B. The prevalence of HF increases with age, where the lifetime risk of developing HF in North America or Europe is one in five for a 40-year-old.

C. HF is the leading cause of hospital admissions for patients older than 65 years of age.

D. HF is the second most common cardiovascular diagnosis evaluated during outpatient primary care visits.

E. In the United States, the annual median cost of medical care for HF was approximately $24,383 per patient between 2014 and 2020.

PATHOGENESIS

A. During the aging process, the heart develops a decreased ability to respond appropriately to normal

TABLE 3.4   NEW YORK HEART ASSOCIATION CLASSIFICATION OF HEART FAILURE

Class I	Evidence of cardiac disease but nearly asymptomatic; can experience HF symptoms (fatigue, angina, palpitations, dyspnea) with vigorous activity
Class II	Slight limitation of physical activity secondary to cardiac disease where ordinary activities (i.e., climbing steps) cause HF symptoms; asymptomatic at rest
Class III	Marked limitation of physical activity secondary to cardiac disease where basic activity (e.g., walking on a flat surface) causes HF symptoms; asymptomatic at rest
Class IV	Unable to perform any activity without symptoms of HF; symptoms also present at rest, disease is incapacitating, as any activity results in discomfort

HF, heart failure.

stressors (e.g., physical activity) or disease states (e.g., hypertension [HTN] or myocardial infarction [MI]).

B. Four major pathophysiologic changes have been identified.

　1. Decreased ability to reach maximum heart rate (HR) and contractility under stressful conditions (secondary to impaired beta-adrenergic activity).

　2. Increased stiffness of coronary and peripheral vasculature: This affects EF and causes increased afterload.

　3. Altered diastolic filling ability.

　4. Insufficient amount of energy production (on a cellular level) to meet the needs of the heart under stressful physiologic and/or pathophysiologic conditions.

PREDISPOSING FACTORS

A. Coronary artery disease (CAD; MI/ischemic cardiomyopathy).

B. HTN/hyperlipidemia (HLD).

C. Valvular heart disease (VHD; atrial stenosis [AS], atrial regurgitation [AR], mitral stenosis [MS], mitral regurgitation [MR]).

D. Peripheral vascular disease (PVD).

E. Connective tissue diseases (e.g., sarcoidosis).

F. Arrhythmias (new-onset/persistent atrial fibrillation [AF], ventricular arrhythmias, bradyarrhythmias).

G. Cardiomyopathies (alcohol-related; nonischemic, restrictive, or hypertrophic; medication-related).

H. Infectious (myocarditis, pericarditis, endocarditis).

I. High-output HF (anemia of chronic disease, pregnancy, hyperthyroidism, thiamine deficiency, atrioventricular [AV] shunting).

J. Noncardiac etiologies: Pulmonary embolus, pneumonia, and exacerbation of COPD.

SUBJECTIVE DATA

A. Common complaints/symptoms.

　1. Shortness of breath (SOB) or dyspnea (during activity or rest).

2. Fatigue or generalized weakness.

3. Decreased exercise tolerance.

4. Orthopnea: Manifests as difficulty breathing while supine; relieved with head elevation using pillows.

5. Paroxysmal nocturnal dyspnea (PND): Sudden awakening during sleep due to acute SOB, usually 1 to 3 hours after retiring, that manifests as coughing or wheezing; this is secondary to increased pressure in the bronchial arteries and interstitial pulmonary edema.

6. Nonproductive cough (worse at night).

7. Confusion/change in mental status: Due to inadequate cerebral perfusion in the late stages of HF.

8. Peripheral edema: Secondary to volume overload.

B. History of the present illness.

1. Determine chief complaint that is associated with HF and evaluate the onset, provoking factors, palliative factors, quality, and severity and timing of the symptoms.

2. Determine if this is an initial presentation or exacerbation of a previously diagnosed HF.

3. Evaluate medical history for known HF, previous MI, HTN, HLD, diabetes mellitus (DM), cardiomyopathies, congenital heart defects, sleep apnea, renal disease, or collagen vascular diseases.

4. Determine if a previous cardiac evaluation was performed (e.g., EKG, stress test, echocardiogram, cardiac catheterization).

C. Family and social history.

1. Determine past and present tobacco use, alcohol consumption, and use of illegal substances.

2. Review daily diet and nutrition information.

3. Determine the frequency and degree of physical activity routines.

4. Evaluate family history for cardiac diseases such as HF, MI, HTN, HLD, CAD, and cardiovascular equivalents (e.g., DM).

   a. If there is evidence of cardiomyopathy, the Heart Failure Society of America recommends an in-depth, three-generation family history evaluation for cardiovascular diseases, especially those related to cardiomyopathies.

D. Review of systems.

1. General: Fatigue, malaise, weight changes, appetite changes, and generalized weakness.

2. Skin/nails: Changes in nail shape (e.g., clubbing).

3. Cardiac: Chest discomfort, palpitations, decreased exercise tolerance, and peripheral edema.

4. Pulmonary: Nonproductive cough, SOB, dyspnea on exertion, orthopnea, and PND.

5. Gastrointestinal: Anorexia, early satiety, bloating, and nausea.

6. Genitourinary: Oliguria and nocturia.

7. Neurologic: Syncope, near-syncope, confusion, memory impairment, sleep disturbances, and headaches.

8. Psychological: Anxiety and irritability.

PHYSICAL EXAMINATION

A. Assessment of HF patients can vary based on stage of disease and underlying comorbidities.

B. The most common physical examination findings are based on severity (Table 3.5).

DIAGNOSTIC TESTS

A. The American Heart Association (AHA), American College of Cardiology (ACC), and Heart Failure Society of America recommend the following tests in the evaluation of HF:

1. Complete blood count: Identifies anemias or infections as underlying factors of HF.

2. Complete metabolic panel: Identifies electrolyte imbalances (especially important for patients using diuretics).

3. Renal function test: Identifies underlying kidney dysfunction (decreased renal perfusion) as a marker of HF.

4. Fasting glucose: Helps identify underlying DM as a contributing factor to overall cardiovascular health.

5. Natriuretic peptides (brain natriuretic peptide [BNP] or pro-BNP): Help evaluate ventricular pressure and volume status; clinically useful in situations

TABLE 3.5   COMMON PHYSICAL FINDINGS IN HEART FAILURE (GROUPED BY SEVERITY)

Mild	Crackles in lung bases • S3 gallop (best heard at the apex with bell) • S4 gallop (best heard at the left sternal border with bell), more commonly appreciated in patients with diastolic dysfunction • Jugular vein distention • Generalized weakness • Peripheral pitting edema • Weight gain/increased abdominal girth • Prolonged, widened, and laterally displaced point of maximal impulse
Moderate	In addition to earlier findings: Nonproductive cough • JVD and/or HJR • Right ventricular heave • Loud pulmonic component of the second heart sound (best heard at the left sternal border due to pulmonary hypertension) • Crackles in lung bases • Dullness to percussion of lung bases and decreased tactile fremitus (secondary to pleural effusions) • Tachypnea (especially at rest and results in conversational dyspnea and/or fragmented speech) • Tachycardia • Hepatomegaly/ascites/HJR • Edema (extremities, sacral, and scrotal)
Severe	Ascites • Cheyne–Stokes respiration • Central and peripheral cyanosis with accompanying cool extremities • Decreased level of consciousness • Frothy sputum and/or pink sputum • Hypotension • Murmurs of mitral and/or tricuspid regurgitation

HJR, hepatojugular reflex; JVD, jugular venous distention.

of diagnostic uncertainty and when determining disease severity/prognosis.

6. Liver function panel: Evaluates aspartate aminotransferase (AST) and alanine aminotransferase (ALT), which can be elevated in cardiac cirrhosis or congestive hepatomegaly as a result of long-standing HF.

7. Urinalysis: Evaluates for proteinuria, which is a marker of cardiovascular disease.

8. EKG: Somewhat nonspecific but can be useful to detect left ventricular hypertrophy (LVH), underlying cardiac disease (denoted by Q-waves) or arrhythmias.

9. Chest x-ray: Important evaluation tool for size and shape of the cardiac silhouette and presence of effusions.

a. Can appreciate cardiomegaly.

b. May show Kerley B lines: Short, thin horizontal lines that are noted near the border of the lung and extend outward as a marker of increased interstitial pulmonary fluid.

c. Can appreciate interstitial or pulmonary edema.

10. Three-dimensional (3D) echocardiogram: Diagnostic test of choice for suspected HF.

a. Used to determine right and left heart function, valvular abnormalities, presence of wall motion abnormalities, and pericardial effusions.

b. Useful for determining the EF, where a value less than 40% can help delineate between HF with preserved versus reduced EF.

c. A stress echocardiogram can assess underlying cardiac ischemia/CAD.

11. Coronary angiography via cardiac catheterization.

a. Useful in the following scenarios:

i. Evaluation for percutaneous coronary intervention (PCI) if there is suspicion that ischemia is inducing HF (angina, wall motion abnormalities on echocardiogram, nuclear evidence of reversible ischemia).

ii. To define coronary anatomy prior to cardiac surgery, cardiac transplant, or device implantation.

12. Hemodynamic assessment.

a. Can be performed in ICU or cardiac catheterization lab.

b. Swan–Ganz catheter is inserted percutaneously and guided intravascularly through the right heart and to the pulmonary artery.

c. Measurements include right atrial pressure, pulmonary artery pressure, pulmonary artery pulsatility index, cardiac output, and ventricular filling pressures.

d. Benefits of these data include diagnosing shock states and evaluating congestion and pulmonary pressures.

DIFFERENTIAL DIAGNOSIS

A. Acute respiratory distress syndrome (ARDS).

B. COPD.

C. Pulmonary edema.

D. Cirrhosis.

E. Idiopathic pulmonary fibrosis.

F. Pulmonary embolus.

G. MI.

H. Nephrotic syndrome.

I. Acute kidney injury/insufficiency.

EVALUATION AND MANAGEMENT PLAN

A. General plan.

1. Use pharmacologic and nonpharmacologic mechanisms to achieve the following goals:

a. Improve overall quality of life.

b. Decrease the frequency of HF exacerbations and need for hospitalizations.

c. Extend patient survival.

d. Increase exercise/functional capacity and enhance overall patient well-being.

2. Treat underlying comorbidities that may contribute to HF (e.g., cardiac revascularization for ischemia, valvular replacement for compromising VHD, and treatment of HTN).

B. Patient/family teaching points.

1. Strong focus on nonpharmacologic modalities.

a. Emphasize the importance of medication and clinic appointment compliance.

b. Discuss the signs and symptoms of worsening HF and when to seek medical care.

c. Design a daily weight chart for patients with specific instructions regarding weight parameters and when to seek medical care.

d. Educate on dietary guidelines.

i. Sodium: Less than 2.3 g/d.

ii. Fluid restriction: Less than 2.0 L/d.

iii. Low-fat and low-cholesterol diet.

e. Ensure patients have close follow-up via inperson and phone contact with providers.

f. Educate on tobacco cessation and decreased alcohol intake (if indicated).

g. Collaborate with cardiac rehabilitation specialist to design HF-focused exercise program.

i. Should contain flexibility, strengthening, and aerobic activities.

ii. Encourage daily low to moderate activity with gradual increased intensity over weeks to months with heart monitoring (for most patients).

C. Pharmacotherapy.

1. Guideline-directed medical therapy (GDMT) should be prescribed as soon as possible after a diagnosis of HF as it has been shown to improve mortality, hospitalization rate, and patient symptoms. GDMT refers to the concomitant use of the following four drug classes:

a. Angiotensin-converting enzyme (ACE) inhibitors.

i. Work by increasing preload and afterload via vascular dilatation; known to decrease morbidity and hospitalizations while alleviating HF-related symptoms and improving quality of life.

ii. It is recommended that all patients regardless of symptoms receive an ACE inhibitor.

iii. Important to monitor blood pressure (BP), renal function, and electrolytes.

iv. Advise to start at low dose and titrate.

v. Caution to avoid nonsteroidal anti-inflammatory drugs (NSAIDs) in combination with ACE inhibitors because NSAIDs are ACE inhibitor antagonists and will decrease ACE inhibitor effectiveness; in addition, NSAIDs promote sodium and water retention.

vi. Typically, combination of an ACE inhibitor and diuretic: First-line therapy for most HF patients.

1) Patients who cannot tolerate ACE inhibitors should use angiotensin II receptor blockers (ARBs).

2) Can also consider the use of an angiotensin receptor-neprilysin inhibitor in patients with NYHA class II to IV HFrEF.

3) Patients intolerant to ACE and ARB therapy can use a combination of hydralazine and oral or topical nitrates for similar benefits.

b. Beta-blockers.

i. Proven to decrease mortality in post-MI HF patients.

ii. In the United States, carvedilol and metoprolol succinate are approved for treatment of NYHA HF classes I, II, and III.

iii. Several contraindications to beta-blocker therapy include NYHA class IV HF, significant pulmonary disease, marked bradycardia, baseline hypotension, and all heart blocks except first degree.

c. Mineralocorticoid antagonists.

i. Most commonly used: Spironolactone.

ii. Function as a potassium-sparing diuretic that affects aldosterone.

iii. Recommended in NYHA HF classes II to IV HF with EF less than 35% or an EF less than 40% in post-MI HF.

iv. Contraindicated in patients with renal dysfunction (creatinine (Cr) >2.5 mg/dL) or known hyperkalemia.

v. Caution: In the geriatric population, many patients with underlying renal dysfunction are predisposed to electrolyte abnormalities.

d. Sodium-glucose transport protein 2 (SGLT2) inhibitors.

i. Emerging data show improvement in mortality and hospitalization rates with SGLT2 inhibition use in patients with HFpEF or HFrEF with or without DM type 2. This is the first medication found to benefit patients with preserved EF.

ii. Initially thought to be glucose-lowering agents, studies show that there are cardio-metabolic-renal benefits from this drug class for patients with HF and chronic kidney disease (CKD). SGLT2 inhibitors reduce

inflammation, oxidative stress, intraglomerular HTN, and sympathetic nervous system activation. These mechanisms provide metabolic, cardioprotective, and nephroprotective effects.

iii. It is believed that all SGLT2 inhibitors have class effects, so an SGLT2 inhibitor that is available for the institution and the patient should be prescribed.

iv. When prescribing an SGLT2 inhibitor, consider downtitration of any existing insulin and diuretic regimen and collaborate with primary care providers to monitor patients' responses.

2. Symptom management.

a. Diuretics.

i. Diuretics are the most effective pharmacologic treatment for fluid balance and decreasing symptoms of edema; however, they have no proven morbidity/mortality benefits.

ii. Either thiazide (less potent) or loop diuretics (more potent) can be used. Common loop diuretics include furosemide, torsemide, and bumetanide.

iii. If the patient is unresponsive to loop or thiazide diuretics, consider the addition of metolazone for enhanced results (caution with metolazone in older adults, as small doses can result in life-threatening hyponatremia).

iv. The most important side effect of diuretics is electrolyte imbalance, particularly hypokalemia, hyponatremia, hypomagnesemia, and increased bicarbonate.

v. All patients, but especially geriatric individuals, utilizing these medications should have routine electrolyte monitoring and should be counseled to weigh themselves daily.

b. Digoxin.

i. Has a positive ionotropic effect.

ii. Beneficial in HF patients with EF less than 30%, NYHA HF class IV, or concomitant AF.

iii. Has not been shown to decrease morbidity/mortality.

iv. Careful monitoring of digoxin levels necessary.

v. Can be added to preexisting therapy with diuretics, ACE inhibitors, or ARBs in patients with severe disease.

D. Additional treatment options.

1. Implantable cardiac defibrillator (ICD) placement reduces mortality rate from sudden cardiac death in patients with NYHA class II and III HF and an EF less than 35% (primary prevention) or following cardiac arrest secondary to ventricular arrhythmias (secondary prevention).

a. Note that ICDs help prevent sudden cardiac death but do not improve quality of life.

2. Cardiac resynchronization therapy (CRT) is used in patients with systolic (decreased EF) HF to improve clinical symptoms, exercise tolerance, and overall survival.

▶

a. Procedure requires placement of a biventricular pacemaker (one lead in RV and one lead in the left ventricle via the coronary sinus vein) to assist in pacing the left ventricle. This helps by improving cardiac contractile ability.

b. Works by increasing stroke volume, EF, and cardiac output.

c. Indicated in patients with NYHA HF classes II to IV, EF less than 35%, and QRS duration greater than 150 msec on EKG.

3. Advanced HF: Inotropes and mechanical circulatory support. Advanced structural heart disease and marked HF symptoms at rest, repeated exacerbations/ hospitalizations, or progressive decline in EF despite optimal medical therapy requires a consult to an advanced HF center to evaluate for inotrope, left ventricular assistive device (LVAD), or cardiac transplant.

a. Consider additional supportive devices such as LVADs, right ventricular supportive devices (RVADs), or biventricular assistive devices (BIVADs).

b. Can also consider advanced intravenous (IV) ionotropic therapy to increase cardiac output and strength of contractility (e.g., dobutamine or milrinone).

c. Extracorporeal membrane oxygenation (ECMO) is a temporary full circulatory support pump that can be deployed emergently in settings of circulatory collapse, and is indicated in persistent NYHA class IV HF as potential bridge to advanced HF therapies.

4. Cardiac transplantation: Gold standard for treatment of severe, chronic HF. Can be a consideration in patients with refractory cardiogenic shock, constant dependency on IV ionotropic therapy, or persistent NYHA class IV HF with oxygen consumption less than 10 mL/kg/min.

a. However, many contraindications to transplant exist.

b. In-depth evaluation and dedicated cardiac transplant treatment team are necessary.

E. Discharge instructions.

1. Ensure proper transition from inpatient to outpatient management of underlying comorbidities that can exacerbate HF (DM, HTN, and HLD).

2. Ensure adequate understanding of modifiable cardiovascular risk factors (e.g., smoking cessation, weight loss, and diet/activity restrictions).

3. Prior to discharge:

a. Ensure that the patient is at optimal volume status with proper transition from IV to oral diuretic therapy.

b. Ensure that the patient has had echocardiogram with documented EF.

c. Ensure that the patient has been stable on all oral cardiac medications for 24 hours.

d. Ensure that the patient is receiving optimal oral pharmacologic therapy including an ACE inhibitor and beta-blocker (if decreased EF); if optimal therapy is not prescribed, must document reasoning for deviation from accepted practice guidelines.

e. Consult with physical therapy (and occupational therapy) to ensure patient is stable with ambulation and activities of daily living prior to discharge.

f. Ensure that the patient has follow-up with outpatient cardiologist scheduled for 7 to 10 days postdischarge.

g. Based on the patient's functional status and degree of HF, consider home health nursing or short-term rehabilitation facilities (or long-term care).

FOLLOW-UP

A. Ensure effective coordination of care between primary care physician and cardiologist. If recent hospitalization:

1. Follow up within 7 days of discharge, then 1 to 2 weeks until patient is asymptomatic and then every 3 to 6 months thereafter.

2. All providers should ensure efficient communication regarding a patient's current clinical status, medication regimen, diagnostic test results, and goals of care.

B. Encourage medication adherence and emphasize the importance of all clinic visits.

C. Create patient-centered exercise plan: Consider referral to cardiac rehabilitation.

D. Provide instruction about daily home weight monitoring.

1. If weight gain is more than 2 lb in 24 hours or 5 lb above target in 1 week, notify healthcare provider.

2. Discuss weight loss if indicated (body mass index [BMI] ≥30 kg/m^2).

3. Consider fluid restriction.

E. Educate on proper dietary habits, including low fat, low cholesterol, and low sodium (<2,000 mg/d).

F. Provide smoking cessation and decreased alcohol consumption information, if necessary.

G. Ensure patient understanding regarding symptoms of worsening HF (cough, weight gain, worsening or rest dyspnea, orthopnea, and edema) and importance of seeking early medical care.

CONSULTATION/REFERRAL

A. Recommend consultation with cardiologist and HF specialist.

B. Refer to interventional cardiologist and cardiothoracic surgeon for device implantation or if cardiac catheterization/revascularization is needed. Consider referral to transplant surgeon for evaluation of transplant candidacy.

C. Recommend consultation with nutritionist to assist with dietary restrictions of HF.

D. Recommend referral to cardiac rehabilitation for assistance with physical activity plan (newly approved for NYHA classes II to IV, EF less than 35%, and on optimal medical therapy for at least 6 weeks).

E. Consider consultation with physical therapy, occupational therapy, and case manager during hospitalization to evaluate patients' functional capacity and assist with discharge planning.

F. Refer to palliative/hospice care for end-stage HF.

SPECIAL/GERIATRIC CONSIDERATIONS

A. Additional considerations for HF.

   1. Considerations for hospitalization.

      a. Hypotension or other hemodynamic instability.

      b. Worsening renal function or significant electrolyte disturbance.

      c. Change in mental status.

      d. Dyspnea at rest (resting tachypnea) or oxygen saturation less than 90%.

      e. New-onset or worsening arrhythmia such as AF or a ventricular arrhythmia.

      f. Evidence of worsening pulmonary congestion on physical examination (rales, jugular venous distention [JVD]) despite changes in oral diuretic regimen.

B. Geriatric considerations.

   1. HF in the geriatric population can manifest with nondescript symptoms.

      a. Malaise.

      b. Weight loss.

      c. Decreased exercise tolerance.

      d. Changes in mental status (confusion, changes in mood/irritability, sleep disturbances).

      e. Gastrointestinal dysfunction (nausea, abdominal pain, anorexia, alterations in bowel habits).

   2. Note that geriatric patients also experience typical HF symptoms, especially orthopnea; inquire about sleeping in a recliner (to alleviate SOB) and elevated JVD (noted on physical examination).

   3. The mnemonic **DEFEAT** (**D**iagnosis, **E**tiology, **F**luid volume status, **E**jection fr**A**ction, and **T**reatment) may be useful in the geriatric population.

      a. The general principle for the treatment of HF in older adults is similar to that of younger adults: Divided between symptom-relieving and disease-modifying treatment.

      b. All geriatric HF patients should receive an ACE inhibitor or an ARB; can also utilize a low-dose beta-blocker such as metoprolol.

      c. Can also utilize an aldosterone antagonist (e.g., spironolactone) in advanced HF; however, use caution in those with impaired renal function (common in geriatric population) due to risk of hyperkalemia.

      d. Recommend to avoid digoxin in geriatric patients but could consider in low doses if the patient remains symptomatic despite maximal medical therapy with other pharmacologic classes.

      e. Diuretics should be used to achieve euvolemia using the lowest dose possible with careful monitoring of electrolytes.

      f. Realize that HF is a debilitating condition in the geriatric population. Fewer than 25% will survive greater than 5 years. It is important to:

         i. Have comprehensive discussions with patients and families regarding end-of-life wishes and ensure that appropriate referrals to palliative care and hospice are made when the patient's condition declines.

         ii. Understand patients' and family members' wishes regarding aggressiveness of clinical interventions before designing treatment plans.

            1) Recommend that risk versus benefit analysis for geriatric patients be considered with regard to device implantation.

            2) Understand that patients with low life expectancies (12–18 months) are unlikely to benefit from ICDs and patients older than 80 years of age are likely to experience major complications following device placement.

BIBLIOGRAPHY

Agabegi, S. S., & Agabegi, E. D. (2019). *Step-up to medicine* (5th ed.). Wolters Kluwer.

Bashore, T. M., Granger, C. B., Jackson, K. P., & Patel, M. R. (2022). Heart failure. In M. A. Papadakis, S. J. McPhee, M. W. Rabow, & K. R. McQuaid (Eds.), *Current medical diagnosis & treatment 2022*. McGraw Hill.

Maddox, T. M., Januzzi, J. L., Allen, L. A., Breathett, K., Butler, J., Davis, L. L., Fonarow, G. C., Ibrahim, N. E., Lindenfeld, J., Masoudi, F. A., Motiwala, S. R., Oliveros, E., Patterson, J. H., Walsh, M. N., Wasserman, A., Yancy, C. W., & Youmans, Q. R. (2021). 2021 update to the 2017 ACC expert consensus decision pathway for optimization of heart failure treatment: answers to 10 pivotal issues about heart failure with reduced ejection fraction. *Journal of the American College of Cardiology*, 77(6), 772–810. https://doi.org/10.1016/j.jacc.2020.11.022

Mann, D. L., & Chakinala, M. (2018). Heart failure: pathophysiology and diagnosis. In J. Jameson, A. S. Fauci, D. L. Kasper, S. L. Hauser, D. L. Longo, & J. Loscalzo (Eds.), *Harrison's principles of internal medicine* (20th ed.). McGraw Hill.

McGuire, D. K., Shih, W. J., Cosentino, F., Charbonnel, B., Cherney, D. Z. I., Dagogo-Jack, S., Pratley, R., Greenberg, M., Wang, S., Huyck, S., Gantz, I., Terra, S. G., Masiukiewicz, U., & Cannon, C. P. (2021). Association of SGLT2 inhibitors with cardiovascular and kidney outcomes in patients with type 2 diabetes: A meta-analysis. *JAMA Cardiology*, 6(2), 148–158. https://doi.org/10.1001/jamacardio.2020.4511

McMurray, J. J. V., Solomon, S. D., Inzucchi, S. E., Køber, L., Kosiborod, M. N., Martinez, F. A., Ponikowski, P., Sabatine, M. S., Anand, I. S., Bělohlávek, J., Böhm, M., Chiang, C.-E., Chopra, V. K., de Boer, R. A., Desai, A. S., Diez, M., Drozdz, J., Dukát, A., Ge, J. … Langkilde, A. (2019). Dapagliflozin in patients with heart failure and reduced ejection fraction. *The New England Journal of Medicine*, 381(21), 1995–2008. https://doi.org/10.1056/NEJMoa1911303

Mehra, M. R. (2018). Heart failure: Management. In J. Jameson, A. S. Fauci, D. L. Kasper, S. L. Hauser, D. L. Longo, & J. Loscalzo (Eds.), *Harrison's principles of internal medicine* (20th ed.). McGraw Hill.

Packer, D. L., Piccini, J. P., Monahan, K. H., Al-Khalidi, H. R., Silverstein, A. P., Noseworthy, P. A., Poole, J. E., Bahnson, T. D., Lee, K. L., & Mark, D. B. (2021). Ablation versus drug therapy for atrial fibrillation in heart failure. *Circulation*, 143(14), 1377–1390. https://doi.org/10.1161/CIRCULATIONAHA.120.050991

Urbich, M., Globe, G., Pantiri, K., Heisen, M., Bennison, C., Wirtz, H. S., & Di, Tanna. G. L. (2020). A systematic review of medical costs associated with heart failure in the USA (2014-2020). *Pharmacoeconomics*, 38(11), 1219–1236. https://doi.org/10.1007/s40273-020-00952-0

HYPERTENSION

DEFINITION

A. According to the American College of Cardiology (ACC) and American Heart Association (AHA) guidelines, a normal blood pressure (BP) is defined as a systolic blood pressure (SBP) less than 120 mmHg and a diastolic blood pressure (DBP) less than 80 mmHg. An elevated BP is now defined as an SBP between 120 and 129 mmHg *and* a DBP less than 80 mmHg. Stage I hypertension (HTN) is now defined as an SBP between 130 and 139 mmHg *or* a DBP between 80 and 90 mmHg.

Stage II HTN is any SBP of 140 mmHg or more *or* a DBP of 90 mmHg or more.

B. HTN applies to a person whose BP is found to be elevated (per the guidelines above) by two or more readings (averaged) on two or more occasions. Patients can also use home and/or ambulatory monitoring—compare those readings with those obtained in the clinic.

INCIDENCE

A. According to the National Health and Nutrition Examination Survey (NHANES), 45% of U.S. adults (age ≥20 years) have a BP greater than 140/90 mmHg or receive treatment for HTN.

B. Majority of patients (95%) are diagnosed with primary (idiopathic) HTN.

C. According to the World Health Organization, an estimated 1.28 billion adults (ages 30–79 years old) are affected by HTN yet only 46% are aware of their diagnosis.

D. Globally, African Americans maintain the highest prevalence rate of HTN and experience the highest mortality rates from associated complications, including cardiovascular disease, end-stage renal disease, and cerebrovascular accident (CVA).

PATHOGENESIS

A. Believed to be multifactorial, with many sites of target organ damage.

   1. Cardiac: left ventricular hypertrophy (LVH), myocardial infarction (MI), congestive heart failure (CHF), and acceleration of atherosclerosis.

   2. Central nervous system (CNS): CVA and transient ischemic attack (TIA).

   3. Renal: chronic kidney disease (CKD).

   4. Vascular: peripheral vascular disease (PVD).

   5. Ophthalmologic: Retinopathy.

B. In increased systemic vascular resistance (cardiac afterload), concentric LVH, and decreased left ventricular function secondary to left ventricular dilatation: leads to a weakened heart muscle and eventual CHF.

C. Decreased stroke volume and cardiac output.

D. Endothelial cell dysfunction due to altered renin–aldosterone–angiotensin cascade.

PREDISPOSING FACTORS

A. Nonmodifiable risk factors.

   1. Age: Both SBP and DBP increase with age.

   2. Sex.

      a. Until age 45, more males are affected than females.

      b. From ages 45 to 64, males and females are affected equally.

      c. After age 65, more females are affected than males.

   3. Race and ethnicity: Most common in African Americans.

   4. Hereditary: Heritable component between 33% and 57% according to the Framingham Heart Study.

B. Modifiable risk factors.

   1. Sedentary lifestyle; obesity (body mass index [BMI] ≥30 kg/m^2).

   2. Increased sodium intake.

   3. Increased alcohol consumption (8 oz. wine or 24 oz. beer per day).

   4. Tobacco use.

   5. Hyperlipidemia (HLD): Elevated low-density lipoprotein (LDL) cholesterol (or total cholesterol [TC] ≥240 mg/dL) or low high-density lipoprotein (HDL) cholesterol.

   6. Diabetes mellitus (DM) as a component of metabolic syndrome.

SUBJECTIVE DATA

A. Common complaints/symptoms.

   1. Headache (particularly headache upon awakening) and dizziness.

   2. Visual changes; subconjunctival hemorrhages.

   3. Epistaxis.

B. History of the present illness.

   1. Documented elevated BP on two or more occasions.

      a. Based on average of two or more readings at each follow-up visit after initial screening.

   2. HTN-related comorbidities and evidence of target end-organ damage.

   3. Possible evaluation for secondary causes of HTN based on patients' symptomatology.

      a. Pheochromocytoma: Headache, pallor, markedly elevated BP, palpitations, and diaphoresis (episodic in nature lasting minutes to hours).

      b. Hypothyroidism: Cold intolerance, lethargy, and bradycardia.

      c. Hyperthyroidism: Heat intolerance, tachycardia, and diaphoresis.

      d. Obstructive sleep apnea: Snoring and daytime sleepiness.

      e. Hyperparathyroidism: Nephrolithiasis, gastrointestinal symptoms, and osteitis fibrosa cystica.

      f. Cushing disease: Weight gain, hirsutism, and abdominal striae.

C. Family and social history.

   1. Family history of HTN and premature history of cardiovascular disease (males <55 years and females <65 years).

   2. Use of alcohol, tobacco, anabolic steroids, and illicit drugs, particularly cocaine and amphetamines.

   3. Diet (sodium, fat, caloric intake), exercise, and life stressors.

D. Review of systems (focus should be on target organ damage).

   1. General: Weight gain/obesity.

   2. Integumentary: Edema and ulcerations.

   3. Neurologic: Headache, dizziness, lightheadedness, syncope/near-syncope, and weakness.

   4. Ophthalmologic: Visual changes.

   5. Cardiovascular and respiratory: Chest pain, palpitations, tachycardia, shortness of breath (SOB), and dyspnea on exertion.

   6. Gastrointestinal/genitourinary: Abdominal pain and changes in urinary habits.

PHYSICAL EXAMINATION

A. Measure accurate BP: Average of two readings taken 2 minutes apart; on first visit, BP should be taken in both arms and (can be taken) in one leg to evaluate ▶

for coarctation of aorta and subclavian artery stenosis, respectively.

B. Evaluate pulse, oxygen saturation, respiratory rate, and temperature.

C. Assess skin for changes related to venous stasis: Brawny appearance with red/blue discoloration and possible venous stasis ulcerations.

D. Check the following body systems:

1. Ophthalmologic: Perform visual acuity; funduscopic examination for arteriovenous nicking, copper/silver wiring, exudates, retinal hemorrhages, and papilledema.

2. Neck: Evaluate thyroid, carotid bruits, and jugular venous distention (JVD).

3. Respiratory: Auscultate all lung fields.

4. Cardiac: Assess for a left ventricular heave, point of maximum impulse (PMI) displacement, sustained/enlarged apical impulse, presence of S3 or S4, evidence of murmurs, rubs or gallops, femoral pulse abnormalities, and peripheral edema.

5. Abdomen: Evaluate for pulsatile abdominal mass over aorta, presence of bruits (aortic, renal, femoral, and iliac), and assess for radial–femoral delay, which can indicate coarctation of the aorta.

6. Neurologic: Perform complete mental status examination.

DIAGNOSTIC TESTS

A. BP measurement (diagnostic criteria): Two or more DBP measurements on at least two subsequent visits of greater than or equal to 90 mmHg or when the average of SBP readings on two or more subsequent visits is consistently greater than or equal to 140 mmHg.

B. Initial laboratory evaluation.

1. Complete blood count.

2. Complete metabolic panel, including renal function and glomerular filtration rate (GFR).

3. Fasting lipid panel.

4. Hemoglobin A1C.

5. Urinalysis (microalbumin levels correlate with clinical BP readings).

6. Serum uric acid (hyperuricemia can be a contraindication for some diuretic medications).

7. Can also consider EKG (looking for a "strain" pattern of ST-T wave changes), echocardiogram, and stress testing to further evaluate cardiac status.

C. Additional diagnostic tests for secondary causes of HTN.

1. Pheochromocytoma: 20-hour urinary metanephrine level (can also appreciate hyperglycemia).

2. Primary aldosteronism: Plasma aldosterone to renin activity ratio.

3. Renal artery stenosis (RAS): Doppler flow ultrasound or CT angiography (CTA).

4. Obstructive sleep apnea: Sleep study with oxygen saturation measurements.

5. Thyroid and parathyroid disease: Thyroid and parathyroid hormone levels.

6. Cushing disease: Dexamethasone suppression test.

7. Coarctation of the aorta: CTA.

DIFFERENTIAL DIAGNOSIS

A. Primary idiopathic HTN.

B. Secondary HTN.

1. Drug/toxin: Nicotine, alcohol, cocaine, amphetamines, ephedrine-containing decongestants, herbal supplements containing licorice, nonsteroidal anti-inflammatory drugs (NSAIDs), and oral contraceptives.

2. Cardiovascular: MI and CHF.

3. Endocrine: Primary hyperaldosteronism, Cushing disease, pheochromocytoma, hyperthyroidism or hypothyroidism, and hyperparathyroidism.

4. Neurologic: CVA, TIA, obstructive sleep apnea, intracranial HTN, brain tumor, and serotonin syndrome.

5. Vascular: Coarctation of aorta, vasculitis, collagen vascular diseases, and subclavian artery stenosis.

6. Renal: CKD, polycystic kidney disease (PCKD), and RAS.

EVALUATION AND MANAGEMENT PLAN

A. General plan.

1. Lifestyle modification.

a. Diet modification: Dietary Approaches to Stop Hypertension (DASH) diet; no-added-salt diet (4 g/d) or low-sodium diet (2 g/d).

b. Limit alcohol and encourage tobacco cessation.

c. Exercise regularly (30 min/d for 5–7 days per week).

d. Engage in stress reduction activities.

e. Discontinue unnecessary medications that can raise BP.

B. Patient/family teaching points.

1. Encourage family support with regard to lifestyle modifications and medication compliance.

C. Pharmacotherapy.

1. Appropriate medications.

a. Thiazide diuretics: Initial medication of choice (first-line therapy in African Americans without coexisting heart failure [HF] or CKD).

b. Angiotensin-converting enzyme (ACE) inhibitors: Preferred in patients with DM due to its renal protective properties (can use angiotensin II receptor blocker (ARB) if the patient is intolerant to ACE inhibitor).

c. Beta-blockers: Decrease heart rate (HR), cardiac output, and renin release.

d. Calcium channel blockers: Work by vasodilation of atrial vasculature.

2. Patients with HTN and DM often require two medications for control.

3. If BP is greater than 20/10 mmHg above goal, consider use of two agents, one of which is usually a thiazide diuretic.

4. Often a combination drug of a thiazide with either an ACE inhibitor or ARB is used because thiazides increase the effectiveness of other antihypertensive medications.

5. Note that if the patient has poor response to one medication, experts recommend changing to another first-line agent in an alternative class before adding a second agent.

6. Medications such as hydralazine and minoxidil are not commonly used; if initiated, it is typically done with beta-blockers or diuretics for resistant HTN.

7. Caution: With clonidine, it is important to educate about not stopping abruptly due to risk of rebound HTN.

FOLLOW-UP

A. Encourage patients to monitor BP at home and keep a log.

B. Emphasize medication compliance and clinic appointment follow-up with a cardiologist or primary care provider.

CONSULTATION/REFERRAL

A. Consider consultation with a cardiologist for patients with multiple cardiovascular risk factors and/or comorbidities.

B. Consider consultation with a nephrologist for patients with resistant HTN and/or comorbid renal disease.

C. Based on the etiology of secondary HTN, consultation with an appropriate specialist is advised.

SPECIAL/GERIATRIC CONSIDERATIONS

A. BP goals for special populations.
   1. Renal insufficiency: Less than 130/80 mmHg.
   2. DM: Less than 130/80 mmHg.
   3. Older patients: Current ACC/AHA guidelines for this population suggest the use of antihypertensives when SBP ≥130 mmHg (no DBP threshold reported).
   4. HTN/CHF: Less than 130/80 mmHg.

B. Complications.
   1. Thoracic and abdominal aortic aneurysms.
   2. MI.
   3. Hypertensive urgency (asymptomatic HTN) and emergency.
   4. CVA and TIA.
   5. Target end-organ damage (eyes, kidneys, nervous system).

C. Urgent and emergent hypertensive situations.
   1. Hypertensive urgency: This term was previously used to describe asymptomatic patients with severely elevated blood BP without any diagnostic evidence of end-organ damage. While still used by some, this categorization is now more commonly described as asymptomatic HTN.
    a. Patients should seek immediate evaluation and treatment as they are at risk for end-organ damage if BP continues to worsen.
    b. Avoid rapid lowering of BP to prevent neurologic complications; initiate treatment of BP using oral agents for gradual reduction of BP over 24 to 48 hours.
    c. Ensure close follow-up and BP monitoring in addition to regulation of antihypertensive medications to prevent future recurrence.
   2. Hypertensive emergency: Best defined as patients with elevated BPs and evidence of end-organ damage.
    a. Goal is to decrease BP safely, typically reducing it by 25% within the first hour of presentation.

This process reverses target organ damage without iatrogenic malperfusion. If the patient tolerates this reduction, BP to normalization can occur over the subsequent 24 hours.
    b. Hypertensive emergency in pregnancy is defined as acute onset, with BP greater than 160/110 mmHg persisting more than 15 minutes.
    c. Patients should be monitored in the ICU with use of intravenous (IV) antihypertensive medications until stabilized.
   3. It should be noted that the use of specific numerical parameters to define both asymptomatic HTN (i.e., hypertensive urgency) and hypertensive emergency is no longer emphasized, as the values are too patient-specific to provide meaningful generalizable conclusions.

D. Geriatric considerations: Structural changes due to aging.
   1. Changes in venous system due to aging.
    a. Reflex alterations in venous vasomotor tone.
    b. Vasoconstriction.
    c. Stiffness and loss of elasticity of valves in veins which can result in falsely elevated BPs via sphygmomanometry.
   2. Arterial changes due to aging.
    a. Thickening of the intimal and medial layers of the vasculature.
    b. Lipid deposits.
    c. Over time, the intimal and medial layers of the arteries acquire collagen deposits that subsequently decrease their elasticity and cause hardening of the vasculature walls.

BIBLIOGRAPHY

Agabegi, S. S., & Agabegi, E. D. (2019). *Step-up to medicine* (5th ed.). Wolters Kluwer.

Benham, M. D., & Fannell, M. W. (2017). Cardiac emergencies. In C. Stone & R. L. Humphries (Eds.), *Current diagnosis & treatment: Emergency medicine* (8th ed.). McGraw Hill.

Flack, J. M., & Adekola, B. (2020). Blood pressure and the new ACC/AHA hypertension guidelines. *Trends in Cardiovascular Medicine*, 30(3), 160–164. https://doi.org/10.1016/j.tcm.2019.05.003

Sutters, M. (2022). Approach to hypertension. In M. A. Papadakis, S. J. McPhee, M. W. Rabow, & K. R. McQuaid (Eds.), *Current medical diagnosis & treatment 2022*. McGraw Hill.

Sutters, M. (2022). How is blood pressure measured & hypertension diagnosed? In M. A. Papadakis, S. J. McPhee, M. W. Rabow, & K. R. McQuaid (Eds.), *Current medical diagnosis & treatment 2022*. McGraw Hill.

Sutters, M. (2022). Overview: Systemic hypertension. In M. A. Papadakis, S. J. McPhee, M. W. Rabow, & K. R. McQuaid (Eds.), *Current medical diagnosis & treatment 2022*. McGraw Hill.

World Health Organization. (2021, August 25). *Hypertension. Who.int.* https://www.who.int/news-room/fact-sheets/detail/hypertension

PERICARDIAL EFFUSIONS

DEFINITION

A. An abnormal amount or type of fluid within the pericardium of the heart secondary to various etiologies.

B. Can be acute or chronic, pathologic or idiopathic, or symptomatic or asymptomatic.

C. Arise when there is an increase in production or a decrease in drainage of pericardial fluid; both mechanisms lead to an overabundance of fluid within the pericardial space. The excess fluid leads to inflammation and irritation of the pericardium, which is termed pericarditis.

INCIDENCE

A. Data from the Framingham Heart Study ($n = 5,652$) showed that 6.5% of adults had benign pericardial effusions and prevalence was shown to increase with age.

B. Pericardial effusions are common after surgeries involving cardiotomy, including valve replacement procedures (self-limiting).

C. It is common for patients with underlying hematologic/oncologic malignancies to have malignant pericardial effusions (21%).

   1. Lung cancer (37%), breast cancer (22%), and leukemia/lymphoma (17%) are the most common cancers that cause pericardial effusions.

D. Evidence of HIV or AIDS increases the risk of pericardial effusions (prevalence between 5% and 43%, depending on the study's inclusion criteria).

PATHOGENESIS

A. The pericardium is a double-walled sac that surrounds the heart. Its two layers work together to evenly distribute pressure and volume forces across the heart, allowing for stretching of the myocardium and uniform contractions. The layers are:

   1. Visceral pericardium (closer to the heart): Composed of ultrafiltered plasma (pericardial fluid is thought to come from this layer).

   2. Parietal pericardium (farther from the heart): Contributes to diastolic pressure and pressure within the right side of the heart.

B. The pericardium normally contains 15 to 50 mL of pericardial fluid, which is used for lubrication for each of the pericardial layers.

C. Clinical manifestations of pericardial effusions differ based on the rate of accumulation of the fluid. For example:

   1. Instant accumulation of less than 80 mL of fluid can cause significant cardiac compromise.

   2. Slow accumulation (months–years) requires more than 2 L of fluid before symptoms arise.

   3. Acute pericarditis typically involves accumulation of 150 to 200 mL of fluid when symptoms occur.

D. Pericardium has an important role during inspiration.

   1. As the right atrium and ventricle fill, the pericardium prevents the left atrium and ventricle from expanding.

   2. This process stretches the atrial and ventricular septum, decreases left ventricular filling volumes, and reduces cardiac output.

   3. If there is a significant accumulation of fluid within the pericardial space, the pressure within the pericardial spaces increases, stroke volume declines, and a life-threatening cardiac tamponade can result.

PREDISPOSING FACTORS

A. Postprocedures (coronary artery bypass grafting [CABG], cardiac device implantation, or valve replacement).

B. Post-myocardial infarction (MI), termed Dressler syndrome.

C. Neoplastic status.

   1. Benign: Atrial myxoma.

   2. Primary malignancy: Mesothelioma.

   3. Metastatic malignancy: Lung cancer or breast cancer.

   4. Hematologic malignancy: Leukemia or lymphoma.

D. Congestive heart failure (CHF) as a result of rheumatic heart disease, cor pulmonale, or cardiomyopathies.

E. Connective tissue disorders: Rheumatoid arthritis, systemic lupus erythematosus, or scleroderma.

F. Chronic renal disease (secondary to uremia) or nephrotic syndrome.

G. Severe hypothyroidism with myxedema coma.

H. Medications: Procainamide, hydralazine, or status post radiation therapy.

I. Infectious pericarditis (most common is viral).

   1. HIV/AIDS: Secondary bacterial infection, opportunistic infections, or Kaposi sarcomas.

   2. Viral: Coxsackievirus A and B, adenovirus, influenza, and some forms of hepatitis.

   3. Fungal: *Candida*, histoplasmosis, or coccidioidomycosis.

   4. Protozoal.

   5. Parasitic.

   6. Pyogenic: Streptococci, pneumococci, *Neisseria*, *Legionella*, or staphylococci.

   7. Tuberculosis.

   8. Syphilitic.

J. Trauma (blunt or penetrating).

SUBJECTIVE DATA

A. Common complaints/symptoms.

   1. Chest pain/discomfort: Can be relieved by leaning forward and worsened by lying supine.

   2. Palpitations.

   3. Syncope/lightheadedness.

   4. Cough/hoarseness.

   5. Dyspnea.

   6. Anorexia.

   7. Anxiety.

   8. Confusion/change in mental status.

B. History of the present illness.

   1. Inquire about the onset, provoking/alleviating factors, quality, severity, and timing of symptoms.

      a. Especially important regarding chest pain and positioning for pericarditis (sitting up/leaning forward improves symptoms, while lying flat worsens discomfort).

      b. Chest discomfort often described as pleuritic (worse with inspiration) and sharp/stabbing.

   2. Discuss medical history, particularly recent viral illnesses connective tissue disorders; neoplastic diseases; cardiac comorbidities; and infectious diseases such as HIV/AIDS, tuberculosis, or hepatitis.

▶

C. Family and social history.

1. Review family history for connective tissue disorders, cardiac diseases, neoplastic diseases, or renal failure.

2. Determine use of tobacco, alcohol, or illegal substances.

3. Obtain information regarding medications, especially procainamide or hydralazine.

4. Ensure vaccinations and screenings are current.

   a. Influenza vaccine.

   b. Tuberculosis purified protein derivative (PPD), HIV/AIDS, and sexually transmitted infection testing (e.g., gonorrhea and syphilis).

   c. Cancer screenings.

5. Assess for recent travel to wooded areas (exposure to tickborne illnesses).

D. Review of systems.

1. General: Fevers, chills, weight changes, appetite changes, or malaise.

2. Cardiac: Chest pain/discomfort, or palpitations.

3. Pulmonary: Shortness of breath (SOB), dyspnea, cough, or hoarseness/change in voice quality.

4. Gastrointestinal: Singultus (hiccoughs).

5. Neurologic: Syncope, lightheadedness, confusion, or change in mental status.

6. Psychiatric: Anxiety.

PHYSICAL EXAMINATION

A. Vital signs: Pulse, blood pressure (BP), respirations, temperature, oxygen saturation, and weight.

1. Necessary to assess; possible hypotension, pulsus paradoxus, fever, tachycardia, or tachypnea.

B. General: Variable based on patient status; could be asymptomatic or in hemodynamic compromise if positive cardiac tamponade.

C. Neck: Possible hepatojugular reflux or jugular venous distention (JVD).

D. Pulmonary: Possible tachypnea, decreased breath sounds, Ewart sign (dullness to percussion below the left scapula secondary to pericardial fluid near the left lung).

E. Cardiac: Possible tachycardia, S1 and S2, murmurs, rubs, extra heart sounds (i.e., S3 and S4), pericardial friction rub, and muffled heart sounds. Also assess for increased JVD, hypotension, and muffled heart sounds (Beck triad), which is the hallmark for cardiac tamponade.

F. Peripheral vascular: Possible peripheral edema, decreased pulses, or cyanosis.

G. Gastrointestinal: Possible hepatosplenomegaly.

H. Neurologic: Mental status examination (if necessitated by patient status).

DIAGNOSTIC TESTS

A. EKG (abnormal in 90% of cases).

1. Low-voltage QRS.

2. Diffuse nonspecific ST-wave changes (can see T-wave flattening) and/or electrical alternans, which is defined as alternating QRS amplitudes in any/all leads (electrical alternans is usually a sign of a massive effusion).

B. Echocardiography (imaging test of choice): Used to assess overall cardiac function and amount of pericardial fluid present; can detect as little as 20 mL of fluid.

C. Chest x-ray.

1. Can show a "water-bottle"-shaped cardiac silhouette and/or pericardial fat stripe.

2. Can show an associated pleural effusion.

D. CT or MRI: Can be helpful in some instances for small effusions or loculated effusions.

E. Laboratory studies.

1. Complete metabolic panel: Assess electrolytes and renal function.

2. Complete blood count: Assess for leukocytosis and/or underlying HIV/AIDS or malignant process.

3. Cardiac biomarkers: Can see minimal elevation.

4. Thyroid-stimulating hormone (TSH): Assess for hypothyroidism as a cause for pericardial effusion.

5. Rheumatoid factor and/or antinuclear antibody (ANA): Obtain if there is concern for underlying rheumatologic etiology.

6. HIV/AIDS screening: Obtain if clinically suggested.

7. Rickettsial antibody tests: Obtain if clinically indicated.

8. Throat swab for influenza and adenovirus virus.

9. Blood cultures: Obtain if febrile and clinically indicated.

10. Tuberculin skin testing: Perform if indicated.

F. Pericardial fluid analysis.

1. Currently under debate: Usually done if poor prognosis, likelihood of purulent effusion, pericardial tamponade, or recurrent and/or large effusions (especially conditions that do not resolve with medical management).

2. Can send fluid for a variety of laboratory studies.

   a. Cell count and differential.

   b. Protein and lactate dehydrogenase.

   c. Glucose.

   d. Gram stain.

   e. Cultures: Bacterial, fungal, acid-fast stain, and culture.

   f. Tumor cytology.

   g. Rheumatoid factor and ANA if collagen vascular disease is suspected.

DIFFERENTIAL DIAGNOSIS

A. Acute pericarditis.

B. Chronic pericarditis.

C. MI (Dressler syndrome is defined as pericarditis after an MI).

D. Pulmonary embolus.

E. Cardiac tamponade.

F. Constrictive pericarditis.

G. Cardiogenic pulmonary edema.

H. Dilated cardiomyopathy.

EVALUATION AND MANAGEMENT PLAN

A. General plan.

1. The goal is to determine the underlying etiology and treat accordingly. It is also important to determine level of care that the patient requires (intensive care, inpatient, or outpatient).

2. If positive cardiac tamponade or significant hemodynamic compromise, ICU admission is required.

3. Pericardiocentesis is required if hemodynamically unstable; recommended for large effusions or those secondary to bacterial infections or cancerous processes.

   a. This procedure is considered to be diagnostic and therapeutic.

      i. Done via open surgical procedure or catheter drainage.

      ii. Catheter drainage via fluoroscopy, echocardiography, or CT guidance is the most common method.

   b. Following the procedure, an in-dwelling catheter can be placed to prevent fluid reaccumulation. This is removed or replaced within 72 hours.

   c. A sclerosing agent (e.g., tetracycline or bleomycin) within the pericardium can also be used to prevent reaccumulation.

   d. Other options to prevent recurrence are surgical intervention (pericardial window, thoracotomy or video-assisted thoracic surgery, or balloon pericardiotomy).

   e. If constrictive pericarditis, surgical resection is always indicated.

4. Pharmacologic treatments (see "Pharmacotherapy").

B. Patient/family teaching points.

1. Educate regarding symptoms of cardiac compromise and signs and symptoms of worsening effusions; especially important if the patient is treated as an outpatient.

2. Educate regarding the importance of medication compliance and follow-up visits with provider.

3. Explain to patients that despite proper diagnostic testing, an underlying etiology remains undiscovered in 50% of cases.

C. Pharmacotherapy.

1. Aspirin or nonsteroidal anti-inflammatory drugs (NSAIDs): Can be used for acute idiopathic or viral pericarditis.

   a. Aspirin is preferred for post-MI pericarditis.

   b. NSAIDs are preferred for viral pericarditis (avoid indomethacin in those with coronary artery disease [CAD]).

   c. Concomitant gastroprotection via proton pump inhibitor therapy is also recommended during NSAID/aspirin use.

2. Colchicine: Can be used for acute pericarditis in combination with aspirin or NSAIDs.

   a. Avoid in asymptomatic postoperative pericarditis.

   b. Discuss with patients regarding side effects: The most common is diarrhea.

   c. Contraindicated in patients with hepatic or renal dysfunction.

3. Steroids: If used early in acute pericarditis, there is an increased risk of reoccurrence once steroids are tapered.

   a. Consider in recurrent disease that is unresponsive to NSAIDs and colchicine.

   b. Consider for patients with comorbid connective tissue disorder, uremic pericarditis, or autoreactive pericarditis.

   c. Recommend use of full-dose steroids for 2 to 4 days followed by a taper.

4. Antibiotics.

   a. If purulent pericardial fluid and bacterial infection, combine urgent drainage and aggressive intravenous (IV) antibiotics (e.g., vancomycin, ceftriaxone, and ciprofloxacin).

D. Discharge instructions.

1. Educate regarding pericardial effusions and pericarditis.

2. Educate on reasons to return to the ED: Specifically signs of hemodynamic instability, cardiac compromise, or worsening infection (if etiology is bacterial or viral).

3. Educate on the importance of medication and clinic follow-up compliance.

FOLLOW-UP

A. Patients will require close monitoring until pericardial effusion and symptoms resolve.

B. Patients should have repeat echocardiography to ensure effusion resolution and no evidence of constrictive pericarditis (usually within 4 weeks of diagnosis).

C. Pericardial effusions usually resolve with treatment and when the underlying illness is treated; often reoccur with comorbid conditions such as neoplasms.

CONSULTATION/REFERRAL

A. Consult with cardiologist.

B. Consult with interventional cardiologist (if cardiac catheterization or minimally invasive pericardiocentesis is indicated).

C. Consult with cardiothoracic surgeon (if invasive procedure is required or the patient is status post cardiothoracic surgery).

D. Consult with infectious disease specialist (if indicated).

E. Consult with rheumatologist (if indicated).

F. Consult with interventional radiologist (if pericardial drainage procedure via fluoroscopy is indicated).

G. Consult with hematologist/oncologist (if indicated).

SPECIAL/GERIATRIC CONSIDERATIONS

A. It is important to assess the cognitive status and comorbidities of geriatric patients, especially if invasive procedures may be required.

B. Studies have shown that in older adult patients undergoing echocardiography for other purposes, those with ▶

incidental small asymptomatic pericardial effusions had a higher mortality than those without effusions.

C. Older adult patients may present with more vague symptoms (generalized malaise, confusion).

D. As with many other diagnoses, older adult patients with pericarditis and pericardial effusions have poorer outcomes as compared with younger patients with the same disease process.

BIBLIOGRAPHY

Agabegi, S. S., & Agabegi, E. D. (2019). *Step-up to medicine* (5th ed.). Wolters Kluwer.

Bashore, T. M., Granger, C. B., Jackson, K. P., & Patel, M. R. (2021). Pericardial effusion & tamponade. In M. A. Papadakis, S. J. McPhee, & M. W. Rabow (Eds.), *Current medical diagnosis & treatment 2021*. McGraw Hill.

Braunwald, E. (2018). Pericardial disease. In J. Jameson, A. S. Fauci, D. L. Kasper, S. L. Hauser, D. L. Longo, & J. Loscalzo (Eds.), *Harrison's principles of internal medicine* (20th ed.). McGraw Hill.

VALVULAR HEART DISEASE

DEFINITION

A. Damage or defect in one of the four heart valves: Mitral, aortic, tricuspid, or pulmonary.

B. Two most common abnormalities: Regurgitation and stenosis of the aortic and mitral valves.

1. Regurgitation or insufficiency: Occurs when the valve leaflets do not close tightly; blood leaks backward into the respective chamber instead of flowing forward through the proper circulatory path.

2. Stenosis: Occurs due to stiffening and narrowing of the valve leaflets.

a. This prevents the valve from opening properly; the result is not enough blood flowing through the valve and circulatory path, which leads to an outflow-type obstruction during systole.

b. Mitral stenosis (MS) results in an increase in left atrial, pulmonary artery, and right ventricular pressures.

c. Mitral regurgitation (MR) leads to a backflow (or reversal) of blood from the left ventricle to the left atrium during systole; it can be primary or secondary and acute or chronic.

i. Acute MR: Typically occurs due to endocarditis or myocardial infarction (MI) with structural cardiac damage (papillary muscle rupture, chordae rupture).

ii. Chronic MR: Can be primary or secondary.

iii. Causes of primary MR: Mitral valve prolapse (MVP; subtype of MR where the mitral valve leaflets close improperly and bulge into the left atrium during systole), rheumatic heart disease, MI with resultant structural cardiac damage, or endocarditis.

iv. Causes of secondary MR: Left ventricular dysfunction.

INCIDENCE

A. The global prevalence of valvular heart disease (VHD) is estimated at 2.5%.

1. Rheumatic fever, secondary to group A streptococcal pharyngitis, is the most common cause of VHD in developing countries, accounting for 12% to 65% of hospital admissions; its mortality and prevalence rates vary within countries and geographic regions according to the availability of resources to treat group A streptococcal pharyngitis.

B. The prevalence of VHD increases in individuals older than 65 years of age, particularly in those with atrial stenosis (AS) or MR. More than 33% of those older than age 75 have moderate to severe VHD.

C. AS is the leading cause of clinically significant VHD in geriatric patients (severe AS is estimated to affect 2%–3% of adults >65 years old).

D. Acute aortic regurgitation (AR) is a rare and life-threatening condition. Chronic AR is common in geriatric patients (prevalence of 20%–30% in geriatric patients).

E. MS is more common in females as compared with males and usually occurs due to rheumatic heart disease (97%).

1. MS caused by rheumatic heart disease typically presents in the fourth or fifth decade but can occur in individuals older than 65 years of age.

2. Only 60% of patients with MS secondary to rheumatic heart disease can recall a history of the infection.

3. Among geriatric patients with nonrheumatic heart disease-related MS, the etiology is typically due to age-related calcifications that narrow the valve.

4. Approximately 50% to 80% of patients diagnosed with MS will develop paroxysmal or chronic atrial fibrillation (AF).

F. MR occurs equally in males and females, with a prevalence of 2%.

1. The most common cause of MR is MVP.

2. MVP can be spontaneous or genetically linked.

3. Can be asymptomatic for years (or lifetime).

PATHOGENESIS

A. Stenosis.

1. Senile AS or MS.

a. The exact mechanism is still not entirely understood; it is thought to be secondary to a buildup of calcifications within the valve.

b. Very similar to the process of atherosclerosis.

c. Increase in lipids, inflammation, and calcification of the valve.

2. Bicuspid AS.

a. Secondary to an inherited congenital condition (affecting 0.5%–1.4% of the general population) where two (of the normally structured three) leaflets of the aortic valve are fused together.

b. This improper fusion of the two valve leaflets results in a bicuspid aortic valve instead of a tricuspid-shaped valve.

c. The result is an increase in calcification formation and outflow obstruction.

3. Rheumatic heart disease-related AS or MS.

a. Can affect the aortic or mitral valves via fusion of the leaflets to create narrowing and outflow obstruction.

B. Regurgitation.

1. Acute MR: Results in increase in preload and decrease in afterload.

a. This causes an increase in end-diastolic volume (EDV) and decrease in end-systolic volume (ESV).

b. Thus, stroke volume and left atrial pressures are increased.

2. Chronic MR: Slow deterioration of the valve allows the left atrium and left ventricle to adjust (dilate) to the increased backflow of blood.

a. Left atrial pressure is usually normal or slightly elevated; end-diastolic pressure is also within an acceptable range.

b. Over time, the left ventricle will continue to dilate, further damaging the mitral valve leaflets and worsening the MR.

3. Acute AR: Increased volume in the left ventricle during diastole; the ventricle does not have sufficient time to dilate appropriately to accommodate the sudden increase in fluid.

a. EDV increases quickly, which causes an elevation in pulmonary artery pressures, affecting coronary and pulmonary circulation.

b. With this increase in volume and pressures, patients develop symptoms consistent with pulmonary congestion (e.g., dyspnea).

4. Chronic AR: Results in slow progressing fluid overload within the left ventricle.

a. This condition causes the left ventricle to dilate over time, resulting in left ventricular hypertrophy (LVH).

b. Initially, the hypertrophy helps mitigate the increased pressure and volume that occurs within the left ventricle.

c. In early phase, cardiac contractility (or ejection fraction [EF]) remains normal via compensation mechanisms.

d. As the disease progresses and the ventricle continues to dilate, it reaches maximal stretch capacity; beyond this threshold there is an increase in end-diastolic pressures and decrease in perfusion of the coronary system.

e. As the left ventricle structure and function worsen, the EF decreases and symptoms (e.g., dyspnea) ensue.

PREDISPOSING FACTORS

A. Recent MI with resultant structural damage of valve leaflets, chordae, and papillary muscles.

B. Most common risk factors for MR: MVP, rheumatic heart disease, infective endocarditis, known coronary artery disease (CAD), and cardiomyopathies. Note the following:

1. Rheumatic heart disease most commonly causes regurgitation of the mitral valve followed by the aortic valve (rarely affects tricuspid or pulmonary valves).

2. Infective endocarditis can technically affect any valve: It most commonly targets the tricuspid but also affects the aortic and mitral valves.

C. Possible cause of MS: Age-related degenerative changes or more rare etiologies, including congenital malformations and intracardiac tumors (myxoma).

D. AS: Age-related changes, bicuspid aortic valves, and rheumatic heart disease.

E. Advanced hypertension (HTN) and atherosclerosis, which can affect valvular function.

F. Conditions that can lead to VHD: Autoimmune and connective tissue processes such as systemic lupus erythematous and Marfan syndrome.

G. Other conditions that increase risk: Tobacco use, insulin resistance/diabetes mellitus (DM), obesity, and a family history of VHD.

H. Acute aortic dissection, which can result in acute life-threatening AR.

SUBJECTIVE DATA

A. Common complaints/symptoms.

1. AS.

a. Angina, syncope, and findings associated with heart failure (HF; i.e., fatigue, orthopnea, paroxysmal nocturnal dyspnea [PND], shortness of breath [SOB], decreased exercise tolerance, dyspnea on exertion).

2. AR.

a. Acute AR: Dramatic presentation of cardiogenic shock (secondary to infective endocarditis or aortic dissection).

b. Chronic AR: Palpitations, angina, HF presentation (dyspnea on exertion, peripheral edema, fatigue, PND).

3. MS.

a. Often presents with new-onset AF (e.g., fatigue, chest discomfort, palpitations, lightheadedness, dizziness).

b. Rarely presents with Ortner syndrome: Occurs with MS where there is compression of the left recurrent laryngeal nerve due to an enlarged left atrium; results in hoarseness.

4. MR.

A. New-onset AF (similar to MS), anxiety, chest discomfort, dyspnea, fatigue, and/or signs of volume overload consistent with HF.

B. History of the present illness.

1. Obtain information regarding specific symptom: Onset, provoking/palliative, quality, severity, radiation (if applicable), and timing.

2. Review the patient's medical history: Particularly, recent MIs, known CAD, HTN, or hyperlipidemia (HLD); congenital cardiac abnormalities, previous rheumatic fever, connective tissue disorders, cardiomyopathies, or congestive heart failure (CHF).

3. Determine if the patient ever had a previous cardiac evaluation, especially an echocardiogram, or learned about a heart murmur.

4. Understand that patient scenarios will vary based on the valve affected, type of dysfunction (stenosis or regurgitation), and underlying etiology.

C. Family and social history.

1. Gather information regarding family history of VHD (especially bicuspid aortic valves or MVP), HTN, HLD, CHF, arrhythmias (i.e., atrial fibrillation [AF]), or connective tissue disorders.

2. Obtain social history information, especially regarding tobacco use, alcohol use, and illegal substance use (very important to document any intravenous [IV] drug use due to high risk of infective endocarditis).

D. Review of systems.

1. General: Fatigue, malaise, fevers, chills, weight changes, and appetite changes.

2. Skin/nails: Painful red-purple nodules on hands/feet (Osler nodes of infective endocarditis) and painless red areas on palms/soles (Janeway lesions of infective endocarditis).

3. Head, ear, eyes, nose, and throat (HEENT): Hoarseness.

4. Cardiac: Chest discomfort, palpitations, racing heartbeat, decreased exercise tolerance, peripheral edema, and uncomfortable awareness of heartbeat (associated with AR).

5. Pulmonary: Cough, SOB, dyspnea on exertion, orthopnea, PND, and hemoptysis (rare but associated with MS).

6. Gastrointestinal: Increasing abdominal girth.

7. Neurologic: Lightheadedness, dizziness, syncope, and near-syncope.

8. Psychological: Anxiety.

PHYSICAL EXAMINATION

A. Vital signs: Assess pulse rate and rhythm, blood pressure (BP), respirations, temperature, and oxygen saturation.

1. Possible tachycardia or bradycardia.

2. Possible irregularly irregular pulse (consistent with AF).

3. Possible hyperthermia (concern for infection) or hypothermia (in geriatric patients with infections who cannot mount fevers).

4. Decreased oxygen saturation (concern for signs of CHF).

5. Possible HTN (acute or long-standing) or hypotension (concern for cardiogenic shock).

6. Widened pulse pressure (associated with AR).

7. Mayne sign: Decrease in BP with arm elevation (associated with AR).

8. Hill sign: Higher BP in lower as compared with upper extremity (associated with AR).

B. General survey: Determine if the patient is in acute distress or asymptomatic.

C. Skin/nails: Assess for Osler nodes (painful erythematous lesions on hands/feet) and Janeway lesions (painless

irregularly hemorrhagic shaped macules on palms/soles) that are associated with infective endocarditis.

D. Head: Possible evidence of head bobbing with each heartbeat (de Musset sign of AR).

E. Neck.

1. Consider possible jugular venous distention (JVD; concern for CHF).

2. Evaluate carotids.

a. "Pulsus parvus et tardus" (associated with AS) where there is a weakened and delayed pulse with late carotid upstroke.

b. Brisk carotid upstroke (associated with MR).

F. Pulmonary: Possible rales or crackles (sign of increased fluid accumulation).

G. Gastrointestinal: Possible ascites or hepatomegaly (concern for worsening HF).

H. Cardiac.

1. Inspect for lifts/heaves (concern for ventricular enlargement).

2. Palpate for thrills (grade IV to VI murmurs) and the point of maximum impulse (PMI; if displaced, concern for ventricular hypertrophy).

3. Auscultate for S1, S2, and evidence of extra heart sounds (S3 and S4) and murmurs.

a. AS: Harsh, late-peaking crescendo–decrescendo systolic murmur that radiates to the carotids and best heard over the right second intercostal space (ICS); can also have paradoxical splitting of the second heart sound.

b. AR: PMI often displaced toward the axilla, possible S3, diastolic low-pitched rumbling murmur best heard at the left sternal border; can also hear an Austin Flint murmur (severe AR: Low-pitched, rumbling, mid-diastolic murmur; heard best at the apex).

c. MS: Loud first heart sound, positive high-pitched opening snap after A2 heart sound; nonradiating mid-diastolic murmur best heard at the apex.

d. MR: Decreased S1, wide splitting of S2, high-pitched holosystolic (can be early systole in acute MR) best heard at cardiac apex and radiates to the left axilla.

i. MVP: If there is concern for MVP (associated with MR), murmur is usually in late systole and associated with the hallmark mid-systolic click that precedes that MR murmur.

I. Peripheral vascular: Possible bounding peripheral pulses (water hammer pulse associated with AR), possible peripheral edema.

J. Neurologic: Mental status examination (if positive mental status changes) and complete neurologic examination if there is concern for associated syncope/near-syncope.

DIAGNOSTIC TESTS

A. MS.

1. Routine laboratory studies: Complete blood count, electrolytes, renal function, and liver function.

2. Chest x-ray: Can see left atrial enlargement, prominent pulmonary vasculature, and interstitial edema (Kerley A and B lines).

3. EKG: If severe MS, signs of left atrial enlargement, AF, and right ventricular hypertrophy.

4. Transthoracic echocardiogram (TTE) to assess overall cardiac function, left ventricular dysfunction, and degree of stenosis.

    a. Mild: Valve area greater than 1.5 cm².

    b. Moderate: Valve area of 1.0 to 1.5 cm².

    c. Severe: Valve area less than 1.0 cm².

    d. Consider transesophageal echocardiogram (TEE) if TTE does not produce quality images; there is question of a left atrial thrombus or prior to surgical intervention.

5. Cardiac catheterization is not routine, but can be considered in several circumstances.

    a. If discrepancy between physical examination and echocardiogram results.

    b. Patients with severe underlying lung disease and pulmonary HTN who require further evaluation.

    c. Geriatric patients with severe MS to rule out comorbid CAD.

B. AS.

1. Routine laboratory studies: Complete blood count, electrolytes, cardiac biomarkers, renal function, and liver function.

2. EKG: Could be normal, possible LVH pattern, and possible AF.

3. TTE.

    a. Follow recommendations of American Heart Association (AHA) for evaluation of grade 3 AS murmurs via TTE.

    b. Consider stress echocardiogram in asymptomatic patients with severe AS to determine need for clinical intervention.

    c. Perhaps consider TEE if there is concern for bicuspid aortic valve.

4. Cardiac catheterization.

    a. Use if discrepancy between patient presentation and echocardiogram results.

    b. Consider in patients older than 35 years of age with AS requiring surgical intervention to evaluate for CAD.

5. Exercise stress testing: Absolutely contraindicated in severe symptomatic AS (can be considered in those with asymptomatic severe AS under strict surveillance of a cardiologist).

6. CT angiography: Can be used in patients for whom transcatheter aortic valve replacement (TAVR) is being considered.

7. Chest x-ray: Findings vary based on severity of AS.

    a. In severe AS: May appreciate aortic valve calcifications, left atrial enlargement, right-sided heart enlargement, and pulmonary congestion.

C. AR: Evaluation is based on clinical scenario and suspected underlying etiology.

1. Laboratory studies.

    a. For infective endocarditis: Complete blood count, electrolytes, renal function, kidney function, blood cultures, lactate levels, prothrombin time (PT)/partial thromboplastin time (PTT), and international normalized ratio (INR).

    b. For connective tissue disorders: Consider serologic tests (antinuclear antibody [ANA], anti-dsDNA).

2. TTE: Assesses valve structure and degree of dysfunction, overall left ventricular function, EF percentage, size of aortic root, and presence of vegetations (TEE may be required if there is evidence of vegetation on TTE).

3. Cardiac catheterization: Obtain if surgical intervention is a consideration, especially if there is concern for underlying CAD.

D. MR.

1. Chest x-ray: Possible left ventricular enlargement and increased pulmonary venous congestion (if concomitant CHF).

2. TTE.

    a. The American College of Cardiology (ACC) and American Heart Association (AHA) recommend TTE for several reasons.

      i. Evaluate left ventricular size and function.

      ii. Determine right ventricular (RV) and left atrial size, pulmonary artery pressure, and severity of MR.

      iii. Monitor EF of symptomatic patients with moderate-to-severe MR.

      iv. Determine the etiology of MR.

      v. Monitor EF and left ventricular size and function if the patient has change in clinical status.

      vi. Evaluate MR integrity and left ventricular function in patients with mitral valve repair or replacement.

    b. Consider TEE if TTE is nondiagnostic or prior to surgical repair/replacement.

DIFFERENTIAL DIAGNOSIS

A. MS.

B. MR.

C. MVP.

D. AS.

E. AR.

F. Pulmonic stenosis.

G. Acute coronary syndrome (ACS).

H. Tricuspid stenosis.

I. Tricuspid regurgitation.

J. Infective endocarditis.

EVALUATION AND MANAGEMENT PLAN

A. General plan.

1. Determine the etiology of given VHD and treat accordingly.

2. Monitor patients for symptoms of worsening VHD.

3. Evaluate patients to determine management: Medical versus surgical (open approach vs. percutaneous approach, such as TAVR).

4. Manage symptoms associated with given VHD (e.g., CHF).

5. Treat underlying comorbidities that contribute to worsening VHD (e.g., HTN, HLD, DM).

B. Patient/family teaching points.

1. Explain the underlying etiology and the specific type of VHD.

2. Discuss the course of therapy: Medical versus surgical and the importance of ongoing monitoring.

3. Emphasize the importance of compliance with follow-up appointments and medications.

    a. If using anticoagulation (AC) agents, ensure patients understand not to discontinue drugs prior to any procedures without consulting a cardiologist.

    b. If clinically indicated, educate regarding preinvasive procedure prophylactic antibiotics.

4. Geriatric patients: Consider involving family members to help determine the best course of treatment.

5. For patients at high risk for endocarditis, discuss use of preprocedure prophylactic antibiotics.

6. Ensure understanding regarding reasons for urgent return to ED, such as hemodynamic instability, new or worsening chest discomfort, palpitations, new or worsening difficulty breathing, syncope/near-syncope, or mental status changes.

C. Management of specific valvular diseases.

  1. AR.

    a. Surgical intervention via valve replacement: If there is angina, evidence of CHF, or ventricular failure.

    b. Medical management: Typically reserved for patients who are not surgical candidates (due to comorbidities) because conservative management of symptomatic patients is rarely successful.

      i. There is conflicting evidence with regard to use of medical management for asymptomatic patients with AR.

      ii. With medications: The goal is to reduce afterload via vasodilators such as calcium channel blockers or angiotensin-converting enzyme [ACE] inhibitors); beta-blockers are not first-line drugs (due to bradycardia) but could benefit patients with significant left ventricular dysfunction.

  2. AS.

    a. According to the AHA, there is no acceptable medical management to alleviate AS.

    b. Available medical therapy is only used to alleviate symptoms and manage comorbidities (diuretics are not indicated due to the possibility of a decrease in cardiac output).

      i. Beta-blockers (help with HTN and CAD).

      ii. ACE inhibitors (help with HTN, DM, and left ventricular fibrosis).

    c. Once patients are symptomatic, considerations should be made for surgery.

      i. Surgery is recommended in patients <65 years old with a life expectancy >20 years.

      ii. If patient is not a candidate for surgical (traditional) aortic valve replacement (SAVR), consider TAVR, which is less invasive.

  3. MS.

    a. Medical management may be useful, although it cannot ameliorate the narrowing of the mitral valve.

    b. Several classes of medications can be used to assist with symptoms.

      i. Beta-blockers: Decrease heart rate (HR) and improve dyspnea on exertion.

      ii. Diuretics: Decrease pulmonary edema.

    c. Symptomatic patients will require surgical intervention. There are several options.

      i. Percutaneous mitral valvuloplasty: Typically used in younger patients and those with mild MS (contraindicated in moderate to severe disease).

      ii. Surgical procedures: Open repair with commissurotomy or valve replacement with mechanical or bioprosthetic valve (considered high-risk procedures; mortality >20% in geriatric population with multiple comorbidities).

4. MR.

    a. Asymptomatic patients with normal BPs and no left ventricular dysfunction do not require treatment.

    b. Medical therapy can be used for symptom management (e.g., vasodilators and diuretics to manage BP).

    c. Symptomatic patients should be considered for surgical repair/replacement.

      i. If possible, valve repair is preferred to replacement: Eliminates requirement for long-term AC, improves symptoms, and increases postoperative survival rates.

      ii. Surgical management indicated if New York Heart Association (NYHA) class II to IV CHF, severe MR regardless of cardiac size and function, or asymptomatic patients with MR and AF, pulmonary HTN, or left ventricular dysfunction.

      iii. Various percutaneous options are in the development process.

D. Additional pharmacologic considerations.

  1. Outpatient AC.

    a. INR monitoring is recommended in patients with mechanical prosthetic valves.

    b. The goal is INR of 2.0 to 3.0 in patients with mechanical aortic valve replacement (AVR) and no other risk of thromboembolism.

    c. The goal is INR 2.5 to 3.5 in patients with a mechanical AVR, mitral valve replacement (MVR), and additional risk factors for thromboembolisms (e.g., AF, previous thromboembolism).

    d. Low-dose daily aspirin is recommended in addition to AC in patients with a mechanical valve prosthesis.

    e. Low-dose daily aspirin can be used in patients with a bioprosthetic aortic or mitral valve.

    f. AC can be used for the first 3 months after bioprosthetic MVR or AVR or repair to achieve an INR of 2.5.

    g. Can consider clopidogrel 75 mg daily for the first 6 months after TAVR in addition to daily lifelong aspirin.

  2. AC with bridging.

    a. Continuation of AC with a therapeutic INR is recommended in patients with mechanical heart valves undergoing minor procedures (e.g., dental ▶

extractions or cataract removal) where bleeding is easily controlled.

b. Bridging AC with heparin is recommended for invasive procedures when the INR is subtherapeutic preoperatively in those with a mechanical AVR, any thromboembolism risk factor, older generation mechanical AVRs, or a mechanical MVR.

E. Discharge instructions.

1. Ensure patients receive all prescriptions prior to discharge.

2. Arrange timely follow-up appointments with a cardiologist.

3. Educate patients about reasons to return to ED with regard to worsening symptoms of VHD.

4. Based on clinical scenario and degree of VHD, provide patients with information regarding physical activity restrictions.

FOLLOW-UP

A. Patients require monitoring via history/physical examinations and echocardiography based on clinical scenario, degree of VHD, and overall cardiac status (e.g., EF and left ventricular function). In AS, for example:

1. If mild disease, echocardiograms every 3 to 5 years.

2. If moderate disease, echocardiograms every 1 to 2 years.

3. If severe disease, echocardiograms every 6 months to 1 year.

CONSULTATION/REFERRAL

A. Consult with cardiologist for VHD.

B. Consult with infectious disease specialist (if there is concern for underlying infective endocarditis).

C. Consult with rheumatologist (if there is concern for underlying connective tissue disorder).

D. Consult with cardiothoracic surgeon (if surgical repair is a consideration).

E. Consult with interventional cardiologist (if consideration for TAVR).

F. Refer to cardiac rehabilitation following invasive valve repair/replacement procedure.

SPECIAL/GERIATRIC CONSIDERATIONS

A. Antibiotic prophylaxis.

1. According to AHA, preinvasive procedure prophylactic antibiotics (against *Streptococcus viridans*) should be used in certain populations and scenarios with risk of infective endocarditis.

a. Prosthetic heart valve.

b. History of infective endocarditis.

c. Congenital heart disease (CHD) that is unrepaired and cyanotic, repaired CHD using prosthetic material/device for 6 months, or repaired CHD with a residual defect.

d. Cardiac transplant patients with VHD.

e. Recommended for patients with MVP or moderate to severe primary MR.

f. Procedures: Dental (if manipulation of gingiva, perforation of oral mucosa, or significant teeth manipulation) or respiratory (e.g., tonsillectomy, adenoidectomy). Amoxicillin (2 g 1 hour preprocedure), clindamycin (600 mg 1 hour preprocedure), or cephalexin (2 g 1 hour preprocedure) may be used.

B. Geriatric considerations.

1. Aortic valve disease is the most common type of VHD in this demographic.

2. If surgical intervention is a consideration, it is important to assess underlying CAD risk, cognitive status, and overall health status.

3. For older adult patients with severe AS who are not surgical candidates, consultation should be obtained for TAVR, which is minimally invasive (recommended in patients >80 years old).

4. If valve replacement procedure is indicated, it is necessary to assess risk versus benefit regarding use of AC.

5. It is important to remember that VHD symptoms in this population can be vague (e.g., fatigue and dyspnea) and difficult to differentiate from normal aging.

CASE SCENARIO: CARDIAC CARE

A 50-year-old man presents to the ED with episodic chest pain for the past 3 hours. He describes the discomfort as a pressure or vice-like sensation that radiates to his left arm, and reports that that it worsens with physical activity but improves with rest. The patient denies any associated symptoms, including nausea/vomiting, dizziness, or diaphoresis, and explains that he has never experienced chest pain before. He denies any significant medical history but reports a history of early-onset coronary artery disease in his father and smokes one pack of cigarettes per day (20 pack-year history). The patient denies any allergies to medication. On arrival, his vital signs include a temperature of 98.6°F/37°C, blood pressure of 100/72, pulse rate of 88 beats per minute, respiratory rate of 12 breaths per minute, and oxygen saturation of 96% on room air. Physical examination of the neck does not reveal any jugular venous distention or carotid bruits and lungs are clear to auscultation bilaterally. The cardiovascular exam does not reveal any lifts, heaves, abnormalities of the point of maximum impulse or thrills, S1 and S2 appreciated without any murmurs, rubs, or gallops, and there is no evidence of peripheral edema. An EKG is obtained which reveals a normal sinus rhythm with ST-segment depressions in leads II, III, and aVF, and an initial troponin is elevated.

1. Which of the following is a modifiable risk factor for atherosclerotic heart disease in this patient's history?
A. Age of 50 years
B. Male sex
C. Use of tobacco
D. Family history of early-onset cardiovascular disease

2. Which of the following, if appreciated on this patient's physical examination, would be an ominous sign of impending cardiovascular compromise?
A. Carotid bruit
B. Xanthoma
C. New systolic murmur
D. Corneal arcus

3. Which of the following best describes this patient's most likely diagnosis?
  A. ST-segment elevation myocardial infarction (STEMI)
  B. Non-ST-segment elevation myocardial infarction (NSTEMI)
  C. Unstable angina
  D. Acute pericarditis

4. Which of the following classes of medication should the patient receive first?
  A. Antiplatelet
  B. Vasodilator
  C. Fibrinolytic
  D. Opioid

BIBLIOGRAPHY

Bashore, T.M., Granger, C.B., Jackson, K.P., & Patel, M.R. (2022). Aortic stenosis. In M. A. Papadakis, S. J. McPhee, M. W. Rabow, & K. R. McQuaid (Eds.), *Current medical diagnosis & treatment 2022*. McGraw Hill.

Bashore, T. M., Granger, C. B., Jackson, K.P., & Patel, M. R. (2022). Valvular heart disease. In M. A. Papadakis, S. J. McPhee, M. W. Rabow, & K. R. McQuaid (Eds.), *Current medical diagnosis & treatment 2022*. McGraw Hill.

Bashore, T. M., Granger, C. B., Jackson, K. P., & Patel, M. R. (2022). Mitral stenosis. In M. A. Papadakis, S. J. McPhee, M. W. Rabow, & K. R. McQuaid (Eds.), *Current medical diagnosis & treatment 2022*. McGraw Hill.

Bashore, T. M., Granger, C. B., Jackson, K. P., & Patel, M. R. (2022). Mitral regurgitation. In M. A. Papadakis, S. J. McPhee, M. W. Rabow, & K. R. McQuaid (Eds.), *Current medical diagnosis & treatment 2022*. McGraw Hill.

Bashore, T. M., Granger, C. B., Jackson, K. P., & Patel, M. R. (2022). Management of anticoagulation for patients with prosthetic heart valves. In M. A. Papadakis, S. J. McPhee, M. W. Rabow, & K. R. McQuaid (Eds.), *Current medical diagnosis & treatment 2022*. McGraw Hill.

Bashore, T. M., Granger, C. B., Jackson, K. P., & Patel, M. R. (2022). Aortic regurgitation. In M. A. Papadakis, S. J. McPhee, M. W. Rabow, & K. R. McQuaid (Eds.), *Current medical diagnosis & treatment 2022*. McGraw Hill.

O'Gara, P. T., & Loscalzo, J. (2018). Aortic regurgitation. In J. Jameson, A. S. Fauci, D. L. Kasper, S. L. Hauser, D. L. Longo, & J. Loscalzo (Eds.), *Harrison's principles of internal medicine* (20th ed.). McGraw Hill.

O'Gara, P. T., & Loscalzo, J. (2018). Aortic valve disease. In J. Jameson, A. S. Fauci, D. L. Kasper, S. L. Hauser, D. L. Longo, & J. Loscalzo (Eds.), *Harrison's principles of internal medicine* (20th ed.). McGraw Hill.

O'Gara, P. T., & Loscalzo, J. (2018). Mitral regurgitation. In J. Jameson, A. S. Fauci, D. L. Kasper, S. L. Hauser, D. L. Longo, & J. Loscalzo (Eds.), *Harrison's principles of internal medicine* (20th ed.). McGraw Hill.

O'Gara, P. T., & Loscalzo, J. (2018). Mitral stenosis. In J. Jameson, A. S. Fauci, D. L. Kasper, S. L. Hauser, D. L. Longo, & J. Loscalzo (Eds.), *Harrison's principles of internal medicine* (20th ed.). McGraw Hill.

KNOWLEDGE CHECK: CHAPTER 3

1. When considering secondary causes of cardiac ischemia, which of the following best describes the underlying pathophysiologic mechanism associated with a tachyarrhythmia-like atrial fibrillation?

   A. Increased myocardial oxygen demand
   B. Decrease in coronary artery blood flow
   C. Decreased oxygen availability
   D. Narrowing of the vasculature secondary to atherosclerotic lesions

2. Which of the following laboratory tests is the most sensitive and specific when diagnosing an acute coronary syndrome?

   A. Creatine kinase-MB (CK-MB)
   B. Myoglobin
   C. Troponins
   D. Complete metabolic panel

3. When providing education to patients with a diagnosis of angina secondary to coronary artery disease, which of the following should be recommended?

   A. Increase physical activity.
   B. Increase daily fluid intake.
   C. Follow a diet that is high in animal protein.
   D. Increase red wine consumption to two glasses nightly.

4. Which of the following best describes unstable angina?

   A. Gradual onset of chest discomfort that occurs with activity and relieved with rest lasting 1 to 2 minutes
   B. Sudden onset of chest discomfort that occurs with rest and unrelieved with medication
   C. Sudden onset of reproduceable chest discomfort that is worsened by deep breathing
   D. Chronic chest discomfort that is worse when lying supine and associated with shortness of breath

5. When evaluating a patient with stable anginal symptoms, which of the following is most commonly seen on EKG?

   A. Normal EKG
   B. ST-segment depressions in two contiguous leads
   C. ST-segment elevations in three contiguous leads
   D. Peaked T-waves

6. Which of the following best describes the EKG pattern that is most commonly seen in atrial flutter?

   A. Tachycardic rate with a "saw-tooth" baseline pattern
   B. Irregularly irregular rhythm (irregularly spaced R-R intervals) with no discernable P-waves
   C. Tachycardic rate and narrow QRS complexes with no discernable P-waves
   D. Bradycardic rate, with no discernable pattern or connection between P-waves and QRS complexes

7. Which of the following diagnostic modalities is beneficial when evaluating a patient for a suspected arrhythmia that is undetected via EKG or conventional in-hospital telemetry monitoring?

   A. Chest x-ray
   B. Nuclear stress test
   C. Holter monitor
   D. Transesophageal echocardiogram

8. Which of the following best describes the components of the Therapeutic Lifestyle Change plan, which is an important aspect in managing hyperlipidemia?

   A. Increased physical activity, weight management, low-trans fat/cholesterol diet
   B. Decreased physical activity, low-salt diet, elimination of alcohol products
   C. Increased physical activity, low-sugar diet, smoking cessation
   D. Increased daily fluid intake, weight management, decreased stress levels

9. When providing follow-up care to a patient with atherosclerosis who was just started on statin therapy, which of the following is the time frame for rechecking fasting lipid levels?

   A. 1 week
   B. 6 weeks
   C. 8 months
   D. 1 year

(See answers next page.)

1. A) Increased myocardial oxygen demand
In the setting of a prolonged tachyarrhythmia-like atrial fibrillation with rapid ventricular response, pathophysiologically, there is a supply demand mismatch. This occurs due to an increased myocardial oxygen demand combined with a lack of available oxygen-rich blood to supply the heart.

2. C) Troponins
Troponins are the most sensitive and specific laboratory test that should be used in the diagnosis of acute coronary syndrome. These biomarkers should be drawn as a set of three, 6 hours apart relative to a patient's initial presentation. Troponins generally begin to rise within 2 to 3 hours of the onset of pain, peak between 12 and 48 hours, and then fall (back to normal) within 1 to 2 weeks.

3. A) Increase physical activity.
Patients with coronary artery disease should participate in aerobic exercise for a minimum of 150 minutes per week. Most commonly, this is accomplished in 30-minute sessions 5 days per week.

4. B) Sudden onset of chest discomfort that occurs with rest and unrelieved with medication
Unstable angina is defined as a sudden onset of chest discomfort at rest that is unrelieved with medications such as antiplatelets (e.g., aspirin) or vasodilators (e.g., nitroglycerine).

5. A) Normal EKG
In patients with stable angina, EKG results can often be normal. In patients with unstable angina or myocardial infarctions, one would expect ST-segment depressions or elevations, respectively; peaked T-waves are most commonly seen in the setting of hyperkalemia.

6. A) Tachycardic rate with a "saw-tooth" baseline pattern
On EKG, atrial flutter produces a "saw-tooth" appearance at baseline with an accompanying tachycardic rate. This rhythm is often confused with atrial fibrillation, which results in irregularly spaced R-R intervals (secondary to the irregularly irregular rhythm) with no discernable P-waves.

7. C) Holter monitor
In patients for whom an arrhythmia is suspected but unable to be confirmed via an EKG or telemetry monitoring, the use of a Holter monitor is advantageous. This device can evaluate patients' heart rhythm continuously for the duration of its use, where the results are sent electronically to a cardiologist or an electrophysiologist. This modality can also be helpful when evaluating patients with vague or nonspecific cardiac symptom for whom an underlying arrhythmia is plausible.

8. A) Increased physical activity, weight management, low-trans fat/cholesterol diet
As designed by the National Institutes of Health, the Therapeutic Lifestyle Change (TLC) plan is a three-pronged approach to help patients lower their cholesterol. The plan focuses on increasing aerobic physical activity, weight loss/management, and the use of foods that are low in trans fat, saturated fat, and total cholesterol.

9. A) 1 week
According to the guidelines from the American College of Cardiology (ACC) and American Heart Association (AHA), providers should check a fasting lipid panel between 4 and 12 weeks after beginning (or changing) statin therapy and then every 3 to 12 months thereafter to monitor patients' progress.

10. Which of the following diagnostic tests can be used to assess ventricular pressure and overall volume status in a patient with suspected congestive heart failure?

    A. EKG
    B. Troponins
    C. Brain natriuretic peptide
    D. Urinalysis

11. Which of the following classes of medications are key in the treatment of congestive heart failure given their ability to increase preload and afterload via vascular dilatation thereby alleviating heart failure (HF) symptoms?

    A. Sodium-glucose transport protein 2 (SGLT2) inhibitors
    B. Thiazide diuretics
    C. Calcium channel blockers
    D. Angiotensin-converting enzyme inhibitors

12. Which of the following best describes the recommended strategy for diagnosing a patient with primary hypertension (HTN)?

    A. Two elevated blood pressure readings (averaged) taken at one clinic visit
    B. One elevated blood pressure reading taken at two separate clinic visits
    C. A month of consistently elevated blood pressure readings via home monitoring
    D. Two elevated blood pressure readings (averaged) at two clinic visits

13. Which of the following signs/symptoms is a marker of end-organ damage in a patient who is presenting with a hypertensive emergency?

    A. Retinal copper wiring
    B. Persistent chest pain
    C. Nonproductive cough
    D. Radial-femoral delay

14. Which of the following best describes the development of a pericardial effusion that would raise the most cause for concern as it relates to hemodynamic instability?

    A. A slow accumulation of a large amount of fluid
    B. A slow accumulation of a small amount of fluid
    C. A fast accumulation of a small amount of fluid
    D. A fast accumulation of a large amount of fluid

15. Which of the following is the most common EKG finding associated with a pericardial effusion?

    A. Low-voltage QRS
    B. Progressive prolongation of the PR interval
    C. Intermittent nonconducted P-wave without progressive prolongation
    D. Sinus tachycardia

16. Which of the following best describes the murmur of aortic stenosis?

    A. Systolic crescendo–decrescendo murmur that radiates to the carotids and best heard at the right second intercostal space
    B. Diastolic low-pitched rumbling murmur best heard at the left sternal border
    C. Mid-diastolic nonradiating murmur best heard at the apex
    D. Holosystolic high-pitched murmur that radiates to the left axilla and best heard at the cardiac apex

17. Which of the following is the most likely diagnosis in a patient presenting with painful lesions on their hands/feet, painless macules on their palms/soles, and a new holosystolic murmur best heard at the cardiac apex and radiates to the left axilla?

    A. Rheumatic fever
    B. Infective endocarditis
    C. Atrial myxoma
    D. Systemic lupus erythematous

(See answers next page.)

10. C) Brain natriuretic peptide

When evaluating a patient with suspected heart failure (HF), it can be helpful to order a brain natriuretic peptide (BNP or pro-BNP) level. When cardiac cells are forced to stretch due to fluid overload (commonly appreciated in HF), they produce and secrete the prohormone pro-BNP, and through an enzymatic cascade BNP is produced; elevations in these markers can signal acute HF.

11. D) Angiotensin-converting enzyme inhibitors

The use of angiotensin-converting enzyme inhibitors (ACEIs) is paramount in the treatment of congestive heart failure (HF). Pharmacokinetically, the medications increase cardiac preload and afterload via vascular dilatation and lessens patients' HF-related symptoms. Additionally, ACEIs have been shown to decrease morbidity and rate of hospitalizations, which improves patients' overall quality of life.

12. D) Two elevated blood pressure readings (averaged) at two clinic visits

According to the current guidelines of the American College of Cardiology (ACC)/American Heart Association (AHA), a diagnosis of hypertension (HTN) can be made by obtaining (at least) two elevated blood pressure (BP) readings (averaged) on at least two clinic visits. Patients can use home monitoring to compare their readings with those obtained in a healthcare setting, but this adjunctive method cannot be used as the sole method to diagnose HTN.

13. B) Persistent chest pain

In the setting of hypertensive urgency, a hallmark symptom of end-organ damage is chest pain, as this can signify a myocardial infarction and necrosis.

14. D) A fast accumulation of a large amount of fluid

In the development of a pericardial effusion, the speed at which the effusion develops is of utmost importance, as the resultant clinical manifestations directly correlate to the rate of fluid accumulation in conjunction with the amount of fluid that collects. When an effusion develops quickly with a large accumulation, this scenario is cause for concern. Pathophysiologically, the pressure within the pericardial spaces increases and stroke volume decreases and this can result in cardiovascular compromise via cardiac tamponade.

15. A) Low-voltage QRS

The most common EKG finding in the setting of a pericardial effusion is low-voltage QRS, where the amplitude is <5 mm in the limb leads and <10 mm in the precordial leads. This occurs due to the increased amount of fluid that has collected between the heart and the EKG electrode when trying to measure the electrical activity of the heart.

16. A) Systolic crescendo–decrescendo murmur that radiates to the carotids and best heard at the right second intercostal space

The murmur of aortic stenosis, which is often termed a systolic ejection murmur (SEM), is appreciated during systole. It is described as harsh with a crescendo–decrescendo pattern that is loudest over the right intercostal space (ICS; anatomically closet to the aortic valve) and can radiate toward the carotid arteries.

17. B) Infective endocarditis

This patient's most likely diagnosis is infective endocarditis secondary to the presence of Osler nodes (painful lesions on the hands/feet), Janeway lesions (painless macules on the palms/soles), and a new murmur of mitral regurgitation, which is a common valvular abnormality that can develop as a result of this infection attacking the mitral valve.

CHAPTER 4

GASTROINTESTINAL GUIDELINES

ACUTE ABDOMEN

Shawn Mangan

DEFINITION

A. Acute abdomen is defined as pain which arises suddenly and is usually less than 48 hours in duration. Acute abdomen sometimes requires urgent surgical intervention, but not always.

B. Nontraumatic pain in the abdominal region with an onset of less than a few days and has worsened progressively until presentation.

C. Conditions categorized under acute abdomen:
1. Abdominal aortic aneurysm (AAA).
2. Acute cholecystitis.
3. Acute mesenteric ischemia.
4. Acute pancreatitis.
5. Appendicitis.
6. Diverticulitis.
7. Ectopic pregnancy/ovarian torsion.
8. Intestinal obstruction.
9. Perforated duodenal ulcer.

INCIDENCE

A. Acute abdomen accounts for approximately 5% to 10% of all ED visits.

B. Approximately 20% of these patients will have small bowel obstruction, 14% will be diagnosed with appendicitis, 5% with cholecystitis, and less than 1% with perforated peptic ulcer. Another 25% will not be diagnosed and will be discharged from the ED.

PATHOGENESIS

A. Acute abdomen depends on the origin of the pain: Ischemia, distention, obstruction, ulceration, or inflammation in the affected area.

PREDISPOSING FACTORS

A. Previous abdominal surgery.
B. Diverticulitis.
C. Constipation.
D. History of gallstones.
E. Abdominal cancers.
F. Peptic/duodenal ulcers.
G. Crohn's disease or ulcerative colitis.
H. Severe endometriosis or ectopic pregnancy.
I. Medications, including nonsteroidal anti-inflammatory drugs (NSAIDs) and steroids.

J. Alcohol abuse.
K. Age older than 50 years.

SUBJECTIVE DATA

A. Common complaints/symptoms.
1. Right upper quadrant (RUQ).
   a. Cholecystitis: Colicky, intermittent waves of pain that come and go. The pain may radiate to back, cause nausea, and worsen after a fatty meal. Pain improves with rest.
   b. Peptic ulcer disease (PUD): Pain worsens after a meal.
   c. Pancreatitis: Diffuse, burrowing, stabbing pain radiates to the midback.
2. Right lower quadrant (RLQ).
   a. Appendicitis: Starts in the midabdomen, becoming more acute in the RLQ. Sometimes nausea and vomiting occur.
3. Left lower quadrant (LLQ).
   a. Diverticulitis.

B. Common/typical scenario.
1. AAA: If ruptured, patients who do not die immediately present with abdominal or back pain, hypotension, and tachycardia. They may have a recent history of straining (such as lifting a heavy object), and most will also have a history of tobacco use.
2. Acute cholecystitis: Abrupt, severe, constant, aching pain in the RUQ with radiation to the back and right shoulder lasting 24 hours or more, associated with nausea and vomiting.
3. Acute mesenteric ischemia: Patients are usually greater than 50 years old.
   a. Arterial: Sudden onset of severe pain out of proportion to physical findings (abdomen soft; little or no tenderness) in patients at risk (coronary artery disease, atrial fibrillation, generalized atherosclerosis, low-flow states). Patients may have a history of postprandial pain, suggesting intestinal angina. However, many patients have no identifiable risk factors.
   b. Venous (10% of all cases): Similar symptoms to arterial, but with a more gradual onset.
4. Acute pancreatitis: Steady, piercing, upper abdominal pain severe enough to require intravenous (IV) opioid pain management. Pain radiates to the back in some patients. Patients may find pain reduction by sitting up and leaning forward. Nausea and vomiting ▶

may be present. Pain develops suddenly in gallstone pancreatitis. In alcoholic pancreatitis, pain usually develops over several days.

5. Appendicitis: In about 50% of patients, epigastric or periumbilical pain is followed by nausea and vomiting, then pain shifts to the RLQ. Direct and rebound tenderness at McBurney's point is present. In other patients, pain may not be localized or may be diffuse.

6. Diverticulitis: Pain or tenderness in the LLQ with fever. Rebound or guarding, nausea, vomiting, and abdominal distention occur if concurrent bowel obstruction is present.

7. Ectopic pregnancy: Sudden, severe pelvic pain and/or vaginal bleeding followed by syncope and signs of hemorrhagic shock in females of reproductive age.

8. Intestinal obstruction.

a. Small bowel: Cramping near the epigastrium, vomiting (with some relief in pain), and, if complete obstruction, obstipation. Range of bowel sounds (BS) on auscultation from high-pitched peristalsis in early presentation to no BS in later presentations.

b. Large bowel: Gradual development of constipation, then abdominal distention, lower abdominal cramps, and borborygmi (loud prolonged BS).

9. Perforated duodenal ulcer: Sudden, agonizing pain usually in patients with history of PUD or NSAID therapy. Frequently occurs in older adults (60–70 years age group). Pain occurs initially in the upper abdomen, then becomes diffuse. Patients lie still, in a knee to chest position, breathe shallowly, and are tachycardic. Hypotension and fever are late findings. Abdomen appears nondistended, with board-like rigidity.

C. Family and social history.

1. Smoking.

2. Alcohol abuse.

3. Low-fiber or high-fat diet.

4. Obesity.

5. Family history may increase risk.

D. Review of systems.

1. SOCRATES acronym.

a. **S**ite: Ask about the location of pain.

b. **O**nset: Inquire about the exact time and mode of pain. Did it occur suddenly or gradually?

c. **C**haracter: How is the pain characterized? Is it confined to one area or all around? Is the pain dull or sharp?

d. **R**adiation or referral of pain: Does the pain stay in one place or does it move around?

e. **A**ssociated symptoms: Is there any weight loss, nausea, vomiting, diarrhea, constipation, pain on urinating, skin discoloration, and vaginal bleeding?

f. **T**ime course: Is the pain continuous or intermittent?

g. **E**xacerbating/relieving factors: Does it hurt to cough, eat, or does it feel better to vomit?

h. **S**everity: Can the pain be measured on a scale from 1 to 10, 10 being the worst pain ever felt?

PHYSICAL EXAMINATION

A. Vital signs: Check postural vital signs to assess for hypovolemia or bleeding.

B. Inspection: From nipples to knees.

1. Distention.

2. Scars.

3. Ecchymosis, such as Grey Turner sign.

C. Auscultation.

1. BS (hyperactive/hypoactive/absent?).

2. Bruit.

D. Palpation.

1. Rebound tenderness.

2. Ask the patient to cough to ascertain peritonitis.

3. Guarding.

4. Organomegaly.

5. Hernia.

6. Rectal, pelvic, and testicular examination.

E. Diagnosis: Specific findings.

1. AAA.

a. Abdomen rigid or distended, very tender.

b. Shock-like symptoms (pallor, diaphoresis, tachycardia).

2. Ectopic pregnancy.

a. Appears toxic and shock-like symptoms.

b. Lower abdominal tenderness.

3. Appendicitis: Guarding and rebound tenderness, prefers fetal position.

4. Diverticulitis: LLQ pain.

5. Biliary colic cholecystitis: RUQ pain with Murphy sign.

6. Renal colic: Severe pain, costovertebral angle tenderness on the affected side.

7. Pancreatitis.

a. Epigastric tenderness, abdominal distention, fever, and tachycardia.

b. Signs of jaundice.

c. May develop Cullen or Grey Turner sign.

8. Special abdominal examination maneuvers: Prior to the advent of radiologic imaging, several clinical maneuvers were utilized to differentiate abdominal pain diagnoses. While most of these tests will be followed by imaging studies today to confirm findings, they are still utilized.

a. Iliopsoas sign: Have the patient roll on their left side and hyperextend the right hip joint. If pain is present, the test is positive and suggests irritation of the iliopsoas muscle by appendicitis.

b. Obturator sign: With the patient supine, passively flex the thigh and rotate inward. If pain is elicited, the obturator muscle is inflamed due ▶

to a pathology such as appendicitis, diverticulitis, pelvic inflammatory disease (PID), or ectopic pregnancy.

c. Rovsing sign: Apply pressure to the LLQ. If pain is referred to the McBurney's point (RLQ), the test is positive and appendicitis is suspected.

d. Murphy sign: Ask the patient to take a deep breath while palpating the RUQ. If the patient abruptly stops inspiration, the sign is positive and suggests acute cholecystitis.

e. Cullen and Grey Turner signs: Both Cullen and Grey Turner signs are associated with ecchymosis on the abdomen.

  i. Cullen sign is superficial edema and bruising in the subcutaneous tissue around the umbilicus. This is associated with ruptured ectopic pregnancies but can be seen in other conditions as well, such as pancreatitis or trauma.

  ii. Grey Turner sign is bruising along the flank associated with retroperitoneal bleeding or intra-abdominal bleeding.

DIAGNOSTIC TESTS

A. Ordered based on differential diagnosis, but can include the following:

1. In all women of childbearing age, assume the patient is pregnant unless proven otherwise; use human chorionic gonadotropin (HCG) test, or possibly transvaginal ultrasound (US).

2. Complete blood count (CBC) with differential.

3. Metabolic panel.

4. Electrolytes.

5. Amylase and lipase.

6. Consider blood culture in older adults with fever or hypothermia for suspected sepsis.

7. Urinalysis.

8. Abdominal x-ray.

9. Chest x-ray.

10. EKG to rule out cardiac cause of pain.

11. Consider abdominal US.

12. Consider CT abdomen with PO and IV contrast.

13. Consider endoscopic retrograde cholangiopancreatography (ERCP) to visualize distal common bile duct.

14. *Helicobacter pylori* testing.

15. Endoscopy.

16. Stool guaiac.

17. Colonoscopy.

DIFFERENTIAL DIAGNOSIS

A. Location and duration of abdominal pain can often help in narrowing.

1. RUQ pain.

a. Acute cholecystitis and biliary colic.

  i. Biliary tract: Increased serum amylase.

  ii. Ascending cholangitis presents with fever and jaundice.

  iii. In acute cholecystitis, pain radiates to the scapula and is associated with nausea, vomiting, and fever. Murphy sign (inspiratory arrest in response to deep RUQ palpation) may be seen.

b. Perforated duodenal ulcer: Accompanied by increased serum amylase.

c. Acute pancreatitis.

  i. Bilateral right and left upper quadrant pain.

  ii. Accompanied by increased serum amylase.

d. Myocardial infarction.

e. Pulmonary pathology.

2. RLQ pain.

a. Appendicitis: Dull, steady periumbilical pain and nausea, which then localize to the RLQ at the McBurney's point.

b. Abdominal aneurysm.

c. Ruptured ectopic pregnancy/ovarian cyst.

d. Incarcerated inguinal hernia.

e. Diverticulitis.

3. Left upper quadrant (LUQ) pain.

a. Acute pancreatitis: Epigastric pain which radiates to the back and is associated with nausea.

b. Splenic enlargement infarction or aneurysm.

c. Myocardial ischemia.

d. Left lower lobe pneumonia.

4. LLQ pain.

a. Diverticulitis.

b. Aortic aneurysm.

c. Ruptured ectopic pregnancy/ovarian cyst.

B. Must-not-miss diagnoses:

1. Small bowel obstruction.

2. Large bowel obstruction.

3. Nonspecific bowel pain.

a. Appendicitis.

b. Perforated ulcer.

c. Acute cholecystitis.

C. Common abdominal pain culprits:

1. Acute pancreatitis.

2. Diverticulitis.

3. Acute pyelonephritis.

EVALUATION AND MANAGEMENT PLAN

A. General plan.

1. Determine if patient is hemodynamically stable and if peritoneal signs are present.

2. Obtain imaging studies and treat based on suspected condition.

a. AAA.

  i. If rupture is suspected, attempts at hemodynamic stability are begun as the patient is optimized for surgery. A US provides bedside results to assist in diagnosis (without treatment, mortality rate approaches 100%).

  ii. Patients who present in shock will need fluid resuscitation, but mean arterial pressure should not exceed 65 mmHg to prevent further bleeding. ▶

iii. If patient is stable, abdominal CT or CT angiography (CTA) can more precisely characterize aneurysm size and anatomy to assist with surgical intervention if necessary.

iv. Surgical options include endovascular stent grafting versus open repair.

v. Medical management if AAA is less than 5 mm includes repeat US imaging every 6 to 12 months to monitor for size increase of greater than 5 mm or to assess for rapid growth. Both are indications for elective surgical repair.

b. Acute cholecystitis.

i. On examination, RUQ pain to palpation with inspiratory arrest (positive Murphy sign).

ii. US (showing presence of stones, gallbladder wall thickening, or enlargement) is the study of choice and can often establish the diagnosis.

iii. Management.

1) Medical: Single episode may not warrant surgery. Counsel the patient to avoid fatty foods, fasting, or starvation diets, and to see their provider for recurrent pain. Tylenol as needed for pain. Actigall decreases the amount of cholesterol produced by the liver and absorbed by intestines and may be helpful.

2) Surgical management: Laparoscopic cholecystectomy. Conversion to open procedure occurs approximately 5% of the time.

3) Surgical cases need their liver and pancreatic enzyme levels assessed, as elevated levels may show common duct stones.

c. Acute mesenteric ischemia.

i. Clinical diagnosis is more important than testing due to time delay. Increased mortality is observed once intestinal infarction occurs. Intestinal infarction can occur as soon as 10 hours after the onset of symptoms. Untreated, mortality approaches 90%.

ii. For patients with peritoneal signs, proceed directly to surgery for diagnosis and treatment. CTA is used if diagnosis is unclear.

iii. Support blood pressure (BP) with IV fluids (avoid vasopressors), adequate oxygenation, broad-spectrum antibiotics, and adequate pain control. Consider anticoagulation.

iv. Treatment involves surgical embolectomy and revascularization with possible bowel resection. Angiographic vasodilators (papaverine) or thrombolytics may be used.

v. Depending on the severity of bowel ischemia, patient may require long inpatient hospital stay, maintaining a *nil per os* (NPO)

status, and supporting nutrition with total parenteral nutrition.

vi. Find and treat predisposing causes.

vii. Plan for long-term anticoagulation.

d. Acute pancreatitis.

i. Condition ranges from mild abdominal pain and vomiting to severe with systemic inflammatory response syndrome (SIRS) response, shock, and multiorgan failure.

ii. Mortality rates are as high as 40% to 50% of cases. It is important to assess the severity of illness on admission using tools (Ranson criteria, others) that predict mortality risk. Early recognition of severe pancreatitis improves outcomes by risk stratification and correct admission placement of the patient.

iii. Diagnose based on clinical suspicion, especially in patients with a history of gallstones or chronic heavy alcohol abuse, and noting elevated amylase and lipase.

iv. Urine dipstick for trypsinogen-2 has sensitivity and specificity of greater than 90%. White blood cell (WBC) elevation range is 12 to 20,000. Imaging with plain abdominal film shows calcifications within pancreatic ducts and gallstones. Obtain US if gallstone pancreatitis is suspected. CT of the abdomen with contrast is usually done to identify necrosis, fluid collection, or cysts once condition is diagnosed.

v. Treatment includes fluid resuscitation (up to 8 L/d), maintaining NPO status (until tenderness subsides, amylase within normal limits), pain control, antibiotic therapy for pancreatic necrosis, and drainage of collections. Some recent recommendations reverse the need to maintain NPO, unless there is a clear reason, such as nausea/vomiting.

e. Appendicitis.

i. Surgical management: Appendectomy.

ii. Medical management: Antibiotics may be used to treat uncomplicated, nonsurgical appendicitis; however, there are recurrences. More studies need to be done in order to determine the efficacy of antibiotic therapy alone.

f. Diverticulitis.

i. Typical presentation is with LLQ pain with or without peritonitic findings, an absence of vomiting, fever, and leukocytosis with left shift. May also complain of back pain, flatulence, borborygmi (loud prolonged BS), diarrhea, or constipation.

ii. A C-reactive protein greater than 50 mg/L, along with LLQ pain and absence of vomiting, is highly predictive of acute colonic diverticulosis.

iii. CT scan of the abdomen and pelvis is the current gold standard in confirming the diagnosis of acute diverticulitis if the clinical picture is unclear.

iv. US is fast becoming an additional modality in the diagnosis of the disease.

v. Management.

   1) Medical: Bowel rest (NPO). Nasogastric (NG) tube placement to low-suction, IV fluid replacement therapy. Antimicrobial therapy covering gram-negative organisms and anaerobes should be initiated when associated with systemic manifestations of infection. If relapse, same regimen for 1 month.

   2) Surgical resection for abscess, peritonitis, obstruction, fistula, failure to improve after several days, or recurrence.

   3) Nonsurgical cases should be referred for a colonoscopy 4 to 6 weeks after the event.

g. Ectopic pregnancy.

  i. Urine pregnancy test (beta-HCG) is 99% sensitive for ectopic and uterine pregnancy. If positive, follow with serum beta-HCG and transvaginal pelvic US. Diagnostic laparoscopy may be necessary for confirmation.

  ii. Surgical resection is usually necessary to treat. If possible, salpingotomy is done to conserve the tube. Salpingectomy indicates when ectopic pregnancies are greater than 5 cm, when tubes are severely damaged, or when no future childbearing is planned.

  iii. Resuscitate if hemodynamically unstable or in hemorrhagic shock and prepare for immediate surgery.

  iv. Methotrexate may be an option if unruptured tubal pregnancy is less than 3 cm, no fetal heart activity is heard, and beta-HCG level is less than 5,000. Follow up within 1 week for repeat beta-HCG level.

h. Intestinal obstruction.

  i. Supine and, if possible, upright abdominal x-rays are usually adequate to diagnose obstruction, showing a "coiled spring" sign in a series of distended small bowel loops or right colon. Large bowel obstruction shows distention of the colon proximal to the obstruction.

  ii. Treatment for both small and large bowel obstruction includes NG decompression and resuscitation with IV crystalloid fluid administration and IV antibiotics covering gram-negative and anaerobes if bowel ischemia is suspected.

  iii. Complete obstruction of small bowel is treated with early laparotomy.

  iv. Obstructing colon cancers can be treated with resection and anastomosis, with or without a colostomy or ileostomy.

i. Perforated duodenal ulcer.

  i. Upright chest x-ray reveals free air. Upper gastrointestinal (GI) film with water-soluble contrast is also helpful to diagnose perforation and if it has healed spontaneously.

  ii. Leukocytosis and elevated amylase usually present.

  iii. In approximately 50% of cases, the perforation self-heals. Those who are poor surgical candidates or who present more than 24 hours after perforation and who are stable may be admitted. Provide careful observation for clinical deterioration, IV fluids, NG suction, and broad-spectrum antibiotics. Low threshold for surgical repair if condition deteriorates.

   1) *H. pylori* infection is implicated in 70% to 90% of all perforated ulcers. Medical therapy for PUD includes the combination of omeprazole 20 mg BID, plus clarithromycin 500 mg BID, plus metronidazole 500 mg TID for 14 days, for non-penicillin allergic patients.

B. Patient/family teaching points.

  1. Do not take laxatives, use enemas, or take medications, food, or liquids until a healthcare provider has been consulted for suspected abdominal pain and with the following:

   a. Increased or unusual-looking vomit or stool.

   b. Hard, swollen abdomen.

   c. Lump in scrotum, groin, or lower abdomen.

   d. Missed period or suspected pregnancy.

  2. Engage in activity as tolerated. Abdominal pain with nausea and vomiting, fever, or pain that lasts more than 3 hours and which halts daily activities should be reported to a healthcare provider.

  3. Eat regular foods as tolerated. Do not eat food or drink liquids until a healthcare provider has been consulted if pain occurs with nausea and vomiting, fever is present, or pain lasts longer than 3 hours.

C. Pharmacotherapy.

  1. Regardless of the cause, early use of analgesia before diagnosis is associated with improved diagnosis and treatment.

   a. Acetaminophen 1,000 g IV is recommended regardless of pain severity.

   b. IV narcotic analgesics can be added depending on the severity of pain. Morphine and opioids such as fentanyl can be considered in cases of acute abdomen.

   c. NSAIDs are effective for colic of biliary tract and ureteral stones; caution in older adults.

  2. If abdominal infections are suspected, blood cultures should be obtained and antimicrobial agents administered (within 1 hour in cases of suspected septic shock). Coverage of gram-negative organisms is prudent. Broad antibiotic coverage is used if there is concern for sepsis.

  3. When surgery is necessary, antimicrobial agents should be given just prior to the start of surgery (ideally within 30 minutes), which significantly reduces the risk of surgical site infection.

D. Discharge instructions.

  1. Surgery instructions depend on the procedure and surgeon preference, if applicable.

  2. Stress the importance of follow-up and adherence to prescription instructions, and to call the healthcare provider with questions.

FOLLOW-UP

A. If surgical intervention, perform as per surgeon instructions.

CONSULTATION/REFERRAL

A. Consultation/referral depends on the underlying cause of acute abdomen.
1. Surgery.
2. Medicine (anticoagulation, antibiotic therapy management).
3. Nutrition.
4. Oncology.
5. Gynecology.
6. Counseling.
7. Geriatric medicine.

SPECIAL/GERIATRIC CONSIDERATIONS

A. Consider that obesity distorts the abdominal examination, making organ palpation or pelvic examination difficult.
B. Men over 40 and women over 50 should warrant a high suspicion of cardiac origin of pain when epigastric.
C. Geriatrics.
1. Geriatric patients have a higher incidence of:
   a. Biliary disease.
   b. Ischemic disease.
   c. Mortality.
   d. Hospital admission and complication rates.
2. Reliable history and physical can be difficult as findings in other age groups are often absent in older adults.
3. Older adults may have a vague or atypical presentation of pain, varying in location, severity, and presentation of fever or nonspecific findings. Classic presentation of peritonitis rebound tenderness and local rigidity occurs less often. Urinary tract infection (UTI) symptoms are more likely to be frequency, dysuria, or urgency. Abdominal pathology may advance to a dangerous point prior to symptom development, and altered mental status may play a role in the assessment.
4. AAA occurs most often in older adults: Maintain a high level of suspicion in patients presenting with symptoms suggestive of renal colic or musculoskeletal back pain (approximately 65% of men older than 65 years have AAA).
5. Patients older than 65 have a 30% to 50% risk of gallstones and may not present with significant pain.
6. Fever and elevated WBC count occur in less than half of older adult patients with diverticulitis.
7. Presence of PUD is more common in older adults due to NSAIDs. The most common presenting symptom of PUD in older adults is melena.

CASE SCENARIO: ACUTE ABDOMEN

Mr. N is a 28-year-old patient who presents with diffuse abdominal pain. He felt fine until several hours prior to presentation when he started to perceive "pressure" in his mid/upper abdomen. He denies feeling this sensation prior. He denies fever, nausea, vomiting, constipation, or diarrhea. Currently he has no appetite. He denies urinary symptoms such as frequency, dysuria, or hematuria. He reports no history of nonsteroidal anti-inflammatory drug, aspirin, or alcohol abuse. He denies history of gallstones or abdominal surgery. He also denies any previous medical history. Physical exam reveals temperature of 98.78°F/37.1°C, respiratory rate of 18, blood pressure of 112/70, and heart rate of 84. His head, ear, eyes, nose, and throat (HEENT), cardiac, and pulmonary exams are normal. Abdominal exam reveals a flat abdomen with positive (but hypoactive) bowel sounds. He has no rebound or guarding, but admits to mild diffuse tenderness, with no focal tenderness. No hepatosplenomegaly is noted. Rectal exam is nontender, and stool is guaiac-negative.

1. What is the differential diagnosis for this patient?
   A. Bowel obstruction
   B. Appendicitis
   C. Pancreatitis
   D. All of the above

2. What tests need to be performed?
   A. Complete blood count (CBC) and CT abdomen
   B. Blood glucose and chest x-ray
   C. Basic metabolic panel (BMP) and abdominal x-ray
   D. Hepatitis panel and liver ultrasound

3. The complete blood count (CBC) reveals white blood cell (WBC) of 7,800 mcL (88% neutrophils, 0% bands) and a hematocrit test (HCT) of 43%. On reexamination, the patient complains of pain migrating to the right lower quadrant (RLQ), and he is moderately tender but without rebound or guarding. He is waiting to go to CT. What is the next step?
   A. Order pain medication and suggest the patient take some.
   B. Discharge the patient to home.
   C. Consult cardiology.
   D. Notify surgery of the exam findings.

4. How would the approach differ if this patient were a woman?
   A. It should not differ.
   B. Chest x-ray would be imperative.
   C. Expand differential to consider pregnancy, pelvic inflammatory disease (PID), and ovarian pathology.
   D. Expand differential to consider myocardial infarction.

BIBLIOGRAPHY

Barkely, T. W., & Meyers, C. M. (2021). *Practice Considerations for adult gerontology acute care nurse practitioners* (3rd ed.). Barkley & Associates.
Cash, J. C., & Glass, C. A. (2017). *Family practice guidelines* (4th ed.). Springer Publishing Company.
Chey, W. D., Leontiadis, G. I., Howden, C. W., & Moss, S. F. (2017). ACG clinical guideline: Treatment of *Helicobacter pylori* infection. *American Journal of Gastroenterology*, 112, 212–239. https://journals.lww.com/ajg/Abstract/2017/02000/ACT_Clinical_Guideline__Treatment_of_Helicobacter.12.aspx
Di Saverio, S., Podda, M., de Simone, B., Ceresoli, M., Augustin, G., Gori, A., Boermeester, M., Sartelli, M., Coccolini, F., Tarasconi, A., de'Angelis, N., Weber, G. D., Tolonen, M., Birindelli, A., Biffl, W., Moore, E. E., Kelly, M., Soreide, K., Kashuk, J., . . . Davies, R. J. (2020). Diagnosis and treatment of acute appendicitis: 2020 update of the WSES Jerusalem guidelines. *World Journal of Emergency Surgery*, 15(1), 27–27. https://doi.org/10.1186/s13017-020-00306-3
DuBose, J., & Seehusen, D. A. (2021). Diagnosis and initial management of acute colonic diverticulitis. *American Family Physician*, 104(2), 195–197.

Kendal, J. L., & Moreira, M. (2018). *Evaluation of the adult with abdominal pain in the emergency department*. In J. Grayzel (Ed.), *UpToDate* https://www.uptodate.com/contents/evaluation-of-the-adult-with-abdominal-pain-in-the-emergency-department

Kühn, F., Schiergens, T. S., & Klar, E. (2020). Acute mesenteric Ischemia. *Visceral Medicine, 36*, 256–263. https://doi.org/10.1159/000508739

McGee. (2020). Abdominal pain in primary care. *Journal for Nurse Practitioners, 16*(10), e185–e188. https://doi.org/10.1016/j.nurpra.2020.06.005

Morrison. (2019). Point of care ultrasound utilization for the evaluation of ectopic pregnancy in the emergency department. *Journal of Emergency Nursing, 45*(6), 707–711. https://doi.org/10.1016/j.jen.2019.07.015

Samarasekera, E., Mahammed, S., Carlisle, S., & Charnley, R. (2018). Pancreatitis: Summary of NICE guidance. *BMJ (Online), 362*, k3443–k3443. https://doi.org/10.1136/bmj.k3443

Schwarze, V., Marschner, C., Schulz, C., & Streitparth, F. (2019). Acute abdomen - gastrointestinal causes. *Radiologe, 59*(2), 114–125. https://doi.org/10.1007/s00117-019-0491-z

Sotelo. (2019). Ovarian ectopic pregnancy: A clinical analysis. *Journal for Nurse Practitioners, 15*(3), 224–227. https://doi.org/10.1016/j.nurpra.2018.12.020

Stack, S. W. (2020). *Approach to the patient with abdominal pain - case 1*. In S. C. Stern, A. S. Cifu & D. Altkorn (Eds.), *Symptom to diagnosis: An evidence-based guide* (4th ed.). *McGraw Hill*. https://accessmedicine.mhmedical.com/content.aspx?bookid=2715&sectionid=249057775

Tarafdar, S. A., & Gannon, M. X. (2017). Abdominal aortic aneurysm. *InnovAiT, 10*(5), 290–296. https://doi.org/10.1177/1755738017693654

Vaghef-Davari, F., Ahmadi-Amoli, H., Sharifi, A., Teymouri, F., & Paprouschi, N. (2019). Approach to acute abdominal pain: Practical algorithms. *Advanced Journal of Emergency Medicine, 4*(2), e29. https://doi.org/10.22114/ajem.v0i0.272

Ward, A., Bell, J., Campbell, E., & Gray, K. (2021). A 24-Year-old woman with acute abdominal pain. *Journal for Nurse Practitioners, 17*(3), 354–356. https://doi.org/10.1016/j.nurpra.2020.11.010

CIRRHOSIS

Ann Burke and Robin Miller

DEFINITION
A. Chronic inflammation leading to fibrosis/scarring of the liver. Causes of injury may be viral, autoimmune, metabolic, drug-induced, alcohol, and/or fat.
   1. Compensated: Mild portal hypertension but normal synthetic function (bilirubin, prothrombin time [PT], albumin, creatinine).
   2. Decompensated: Progression of disease due to complications of portal hypertension, which include variceal hemorrhage, hepatic encephalopathy, ascites, and spontaneous bacterial peritonitis (SBP).
      a. Median survival in decompensated cirrhosis is 6 months or less.
      b. Model for End-Stage Liver Disease (MELD) score: Model to predict prognosis in patients with cirrhosis using the bilirubin, creatinine, and international normalized ratio (INR).

INCIDENCE
A. The Centers for Disease Control and Prevention (CDC) data from 2018 report 4.5 million people in the United States with cirrhosis.
B. The National Institute of Health (NIH) reports cirrhosis is the 12th leading cause of death in the United States.

PATHOGENESIS
A. The most common causes of cirrhosis in the United States include alcoholic liver disease and nonalcoholic fatty liver disease (NAFLD).
B. Other less common causes include viral hepatitis B and C, hemochromatosis, autoimmune, primary biliary cholangitis (PBC), primary sclerosing cholangitis (PSC), drug-induced liver injury (DILI), Wilson disease, alpha-1 antitrypsin deficiency, celiac disease, polycystic liver disease, sarcoidosis, and right-sided heart failure.

PREDISPOSING FACTORS
A. Combination of more than one factor may lead to an accelerated progression to fibrosis.
   1. Heavy alcohol use.
   2. Viral hepatitis.
   3. Fatty liver disease.
   4. Genetic or metabolic disorder (e.g., Wilson disease, alpha-1 antitrypsin, hemochromatosis).
   5. Autoimmune disease.
   6. Hepatic congestion (e.g., heart failure).

SUBJECTIVE DATA
A. Common complaints/symptoms.
   1. Nonspecific: Anorexia, weight loss, and fatigue.
   2. Decompensated: Jaundice, abdominal distention, confusion, and gastrointestinal (GI) bleeding.
B. Common history of the present illness.
   1. May be incidental finding on lab tests or imaging without any symptoms.
   2. There may be an acute presentation with hepatic decompensation.
C. Family and social history.
   1. Detailed history of alcohol use, drug use, sex partners, body piercings, and tattoos.
   2. Inquire about family history of autoimmune disease, liver disease, and liver cancer.
   3. Living situation: Household contacts with infected individuals with viral hepatitis.
   4. Occupation: Potential exposure to viral hepatitis.
   5. Travel: Recent travel or country of origin.
D. Review of systems.
   1. May present with jaundice, pruritus, easy bruising, hematemesis, melena, hematochezia, ascites, lower extremity edema, confusion, and sleep disturbances.

PHYSICAL EXAMINATION
A. May have no physical findings.
B. In cirrhosis, may see:
   1. Jaundice.
   2. Spider angiomas on the neck or chest.
   3. Gynecomastia.
   4. Ascites: Associated with edema in the scrotum and/or lower extremities.
   5. Firm nodular liver.
   6. Splenomegaly.
   7. Palmar erythema.
   8. Digital clubbing.
   9. Asterixis: Bilateral flapping of dorsiflexed hands.
   10. Low blood pressure (BP).

DIAGNOSTIC TESTS
A. Labs: Complete blood count (CBC), comprehensive metabolic panel (CMP), PT, and INR.

1. All liver tests may be abnormal. In decompensated disease, rising bilirubin, low albumin, and elevated INR and creatinine indicate synthetic dysfunction and progression of cirrhosis.

2. Thrombocytopenia: Related to portal hypertension and splenomegaly; platelets <150.

3. Anemia: Due to GI blood loss, chronic disease, renal disease, bone marrow suppression, and hemolysis.

4. Leukopenia: Secondary to hypersplenism.

5. Hyponatremia: Inability to excrete free water.

B. Imaging.

1. Ultrasound (US): Shrunken nodular liver with or without splenomegaly/ascites.

2. US with Doppler: Portal hypertension, portal vein thrombosis, and collateral flow may be present.

3. MRI: Can identify cirrhosis, hepatocellular carcinoma (HCC), or other liver masses. It is the preferred study for cancer surveillance and staging.

C. Liver biopsy.

1. It is the gold standard to diagnose or identify the cause of cirrhosis.

2. FibroScan is a noninvasive tool to stage fibrosis.

DIFFERENTIAL DIAGNOSIS

A. Cirrhosis related to chronic hepatic inflammation due to:

1. Viral: Hepatitis A, B, and C.

2. Alcohol.

3. Fatty liver.

4. Autoimmune: Autoimmune hepatitis, celiac, PBC, and PSC.

5. Genetic/metabolic: Wilson disease, hemochromatosis, alpha-1 antitrypsin, and polycystic liver disease.

B. Extrahepatic causes of cirrhosis.

1. Congestive heart failure.

2. Sarcoidosis.

3. Budd–Chiari syndrome.

4. Portal and splenic vein thrombosis.

EVALUATION AND MANAGEMENT OF COMPLICATIONS

A. Ascites and SBP.

1. General plan and definitions.

a. Ascites: Abdominal accumulation of fluid due to high portal pressures. It is typically treated with sodium restriction and diuretics. Refractory cases require paracentesis or transjugular intrahepatic portosystemic shunt (TIPS).

b. SBP is an infection of the ascitic fluid. Cultures will show high absolute polymorphonuclear leukocyte counts greater than 250 cells/mm.

2. Patient/family teaching points.

a. Ascitic fluid may reaccumulate despite diuretic therapy and will likely require multiple paracenteses to manage fluids and mitigate side effects such as shortness of breath and edema.

b. Daily weights.

c. 2,000 mg sodium restricted diet.

d. Laboratory monitoring of electrolytes and renal function for safe dosing of diuretics.

e. Report any fever, abdominal pain, and altered mental status, which may indicate SBP.

f. Prophylactic antibiotics for SBP is a lifelong therapy or until transplant.

3. Pharmacotherapy.

a. Combination diuretics, usually Lasix and Aldactone, to balance potassium. Diuretic starting dose is 20 mg Lasix with 50 mg Aldactone, then increased using the same ratio.

b. SBP is typically treated with third-generation cephalosporin, such as ceftriaxone or cefotaxime, typically for 5 days. At discharge, switch to long-term prophylaxis using Cipro 500 mg PO daily or Bactrim DS one tablet daily.

4. Discharge instructions.

a. Low-sodium diet.

b. Diuretics as prescribed.

c. Lab testing as recommended.

d. Follow up with hepatologist.

e. Call office or report to ED with abdominal pain, distention, shortness of breath, fever, and altered mental status.

B. Encephalopathy.

1. General plan and definitions.

a. Impairment in cognitive and neuromuscular function associated with decompensated cirrhosis. Manifestations range from mild confusion to severe somnolence and coma. Treatment is based on underlying cause/trigger (e.g., GI bleeding, infection, dehydration, medication noncompliance).

2. Patient/family teaching points.

a. Review with family/caregiver to be alert for confusion, memory lapses, mood changes, speech abnormalities, slowed movements, gait disturbance, or day/night reversal.

b. Clearance of neurotoxins such as ammonia is important. This is primarily achieved through the stool. Medications for treatment target that means of clearance through promotion of several bowel movements daily.

3. Pharmacotherapy.

a. Lactulose: Synthetic disaccharide which is a mainstay of therapy and causes a purging of ammonia through the bowels. This has been shown to improve symptoms in 70% to 80% of patients. Typical dose of 30 to 45 mL orally, two to four times per day. Dose is titrated to achieve two to three bowel movements per day. If patient is comatose, it may be given as an enema.

b. Xifaxan: Also known as rifaximin. A nonabsorbable antibiotic that reduces the risk of hepatic encephalopathy recurrence. This is usually added to lactulose therapy or for patients who are intolerant of lactulose side effects. Dose is usually 550 mg orally BID.

c. Benzodiazepines are contraindicated in cirrhotic patients who have encephalopathy.

4. Discharge instructions.

   a. Medication compliance is reinforced.

   b. Encourage two to three bowel movements daily for control of encephalopathy.

   c. Call the office or report to the ED with worsening confusion, fever, slurred speech, or lethargy.

   d. Follow up with hepatologist.

C. GI bleeding.

  1. General plan and definition.

   a. Definition: Acute variceal hemorrhage is the result of portal hypertension and usually occurs in the upper GI tracts. Other causes of GI bleeding in patients with liver disease include peptic ulcers, portal hypertensive gastropathy, and gastric antral vascular ectasias (GAVE).

   b. Plan: Stabilization of patient.

   c. Blood and blood products: Goal of hemoglobin of 7 to 9 g/dL.

   d. Restoration of intravascular volume: Intravenous (IV) fluids and pressors.

   e. Treatment with endoscopic evaluation and interventions to stop the bleeding. Epinephrine, banding, argon plasma coagulation, and clipping may be used alone or in combination.

   f. Patients at high risk of rebleeding may be considered a candidate for TIPS.

   g. Bleeding that is refractory to traditional measures may require esophageal tamponade (short term only).

   h. Prevention and management of complications (e.g., sepsis, renal failure, aspiration pneumonia).

  2. Patient/family teaching points.

   a. High risk of recurrent bleeding within 6 weeks of the initial episode.

   b. If banding was performed, expect a sore throat for a few days. Soft diet recommended.

   c. Review signs of bleeding: Vomiting blood or coffee ground emesis, black tarry or maroon-colored stools, weakness, and lightheadedness.

   d. If TIPS was placed, worsening encephalopathy may be seen.

   e. Avoid NSAIDs.

  3. Pharmacotherapy.

   a. Vasoactive medication: Initiated at the time of presentation to decrease portal blood flow (e.g., octreotide). Usually given for 2 to 5 days.

   b. Proton pump inhibitor (PPI).

   c. Prophylactic antibiotics: Broad-spectrum antibiotics such as ceftriaxone 1 g IV daily for 7 days to prevent bacterial infections, which can occur in 20% of hospitalized cirrhotic patients (e.g., urinary tract infection [UTI], bacteremia, respiratory infections).

   d. A nonselective beta-blocker is often prescribed to reduce portal pressures for prevention of rebleeding after vasoactive medication has been discontinued. Titrate dose to a heart rate of 60 beats per minute. Propranolol and nadolol are commonly used.

4. Discharge instructions.

   a. If esophageal band ligation was performed, the patient will need repeat esophagogastroduodenoscopy (EGD) every 4 weeks until eradicated.

   b. Medication compliance with beta-blockers.

   c. Monitor CBC.

   d. Follow-up visit with hepatology.

D. Hepatorenal syndrome (HRS).

  1. General plan and definitions.

   a. Definition: Chronic or acute kidney injury (AKI) related to advanced hepatic failure and portal hypertension. Must exclude other causes, that is, shock, nephrotoxic drugs, and dehydration. Can be precipitated by an acute insult, such as SBP or GI bleeding. Without therapy, most patients with HRS die within weeks of onset of renal impairment.

    i. Type I HRS: More severe with rapid onset and poor prognosis. May reverse if cause of hepatic disease is treatable, that is, alcohol cessation and antiviral therapy.

    ii. Type II HRS: Less rapid progression.

   b. Plan.

    i. Correction of underlying hepatic cause, if able.

    ii. Medications to raise the mean arterial pressure and improve renal perfusion.

    iii. Monitor fluid status closely.

    iv. Dialysis as a bridge to transplant or renal recovery.

    v. May need dual renal/liver transplant.

  2. Patient/family teaching points.

   a. Avoid nephrotoxic drugs.

   b. Stop diuretic therapy.

   c. May require dialysis while awaiting transplant.

   d. Teaching subcutaneous (SQ) injections for home therapy (e.g., octreotide).

  3. Pharmacotherapy: Combined therapy with the goal to improve renal and systemic hemodynamics.

   a. Midodrine: Selective alpha-1 adrenergic agonist, 7.5 to 15 mg orally TID.

   b. Octreotide: Somatostatin analog, IV infusion 50 mcg/hr or SQ 100 mcg TID.

   c. Albumin: Volume expander, IV bolus, 1 g per kilogram of body weight per day.

  4. Discharge instructions.

   a. Compliance with medical regimen of dialysis and medications.

   b. Close monitoring of electrolytes and renal function.

   c. Follow up with hepatology.

FOLLOW-UP

A. Follow up with hepatology.

B. Patients will need HCC and esophageal varices screening.

  1. Imaging every 6 months: Alternating US and MRI of the abdomen.

  2. Variceal surveillance: EGD every 2 to 3 years.

C. Labs every 3 months: CBC, CMP, INR, and alpha fetoprotein (AFP).

D. Will need vaccination for hepatitis A and B if not immune.

CONSULTATION/REFERRAL

A. MELD score of 10 or higher will be referred to a transplant center.

B. If alcohol-related cirrhosis, must complete a substance use program.

C. Social services may need to help with insurance coverage if transplant is indicated.

SPECIAL CONSIDERATIONS

A. Transplant eligibility varies between centers, but usually age >70 years is contraindicated.

B. Cirrhosis is considered a high risk for abdominal, cardiac, or orthopedic surgeries due to high portal pressures and coagulopathies. It is usually determined by the surgeon on a case-by-case basis.

BIBLIOGRAPHY

Bajaj, J. S., & Sanyal, A. J. (2017, May 5). *Methods to achieve hemostasis in patients with acute variceal hemorrhage.* https://www.uptodate.com/contents/methods-to-achieve-hemostasis-in-patients-with-acute-variceal-hemorrhage

Centers for Disease Control and Prevention. (2016, October 6). *Chronic liver disease and cirrhosis.* https://www.cdc.gov/nchs/fastats/liver-disease.htm

Ferenci, P. (2017, August 17). *Hepatic encephalopathy in adults: Treatment.* https://www.uptodate.com/contents/hepatic-encephalopathy-in-adults-treatment

Garcia-Tsao, G., Abraldes, J. G., Berzigotti, A., & Bosch, J. (2017). Portal hypertensive bleeding in cirrhosis: Risk stratification, diagnosis, and management: 2016 practice guidance by the American Association for the study of liver diseases. *Hepatology, 65*(1), 310–335.

Goldberg, E., & Chopra, S. (2016, August 15). *Cirrhosis in adults: Etiologies, clinical manifestations, and diagnosis.* https://www.uptodate.com/contents/cirrhosis-in-adults-etiologies-clinical-manifestations-and-diagnosis

Goldberg, E., & Chopra, S. (2017, March 7). *Cirrhosis in adults: Overview of complications, general management, and complications.* https://www.uptodate.com/contents/cirrhosis-in-adults-overview-of-complications-general-management-and-prognosis

Runyon, B. A. (2016, January 4). *Spontaneous bacterial peritonitis in adults: Treatment and prophylaxis.* https://www.uptodate.com/contents/spontaneous-bacterial-peritonitis-in-adults-treatment-and-prophylaxis

Runyon, B. A. (2017, November 8). *Hepatorenal syndrome.* https://www.uptodate.com/contents/hepatorenal-syndrome

Sanyal, A. J. (2017, February 21). *General principles of the management of variceal hemorrhage.* https://www.uptodate.com/contents/general-principles-of-the-management-of-variceal-hemorrhage

Such, J., & Runyon, B. A. (2017, June 28). *Ascites in adults with cirrhosis: Initial therapy.* https://www.uptodate.com/contents/ascites-in-adults-with-cirrhosis-initial-therapy

DRUG-INDUCED LIVER INJURY

Ann Burke and Robin Miller

DEFINITION

A. Liver injury due to prescription medications, over-the-counter (OTC) medications, and herbal supplements.

INCIDENCE

A. The estimated annual incidence is 10% of all cases of acute hepatitis. It is the most common cause of acute liver failure in the United States.

PATHOGENESIS

A. Over 1,000 medications and herbal products have been implicated in the development of drug-induced liver injury (DILI).

B. The most common drug in acute DILI in the United States is acetaminophen.

PREDISPOSING FACTORS

A. Women are more susceptible due to smaller body size.

B. Alcohol abuse.

C. Malnutrition.

SUBJECTIVE DATA

A. Common complaints.
1. Itching.
2. Jaundice.
3. Malaise.
4. Low-grade fever.
5. Nausea and vomiting.
6. Right upper quadrant (RUQ) pain.
7. Dark urine.
8. Clay-colored stools.

B. Common history of the present illness.
1. Patients may be asymptomatic with incidental findings of elevated liver tests.
2. Ask patients about recent antibiotic use, herbal supplements, weight loss products, or OTC medications.
3. Thorough medication reconciliation.

C. Social history.
1. Be culturally sensitive to nontraditional medicine and the patient's use of herbal products.
2. Alcohol use.

D. Review of systems.
1. Same as common complaints.
2. Rash.
3. Pruritus.
4. Weight loss.

PHYSICAL EXAMINATION

A. Depending on the severity, no physical findings or the following:
1. Scleral icterus.
2. Generalized jaundice.
3. Skin excoriations from scratching.
4. RUQ tenderness.
5. Hepatomegaly.

DIAGNOSTIC TESTS

A. Lab workup includes complete blood count (CBC), comprehensive metabolic panel (CMP), international normalized ratio (INR), hepatitis A, B, and C serologies, antinuclear antibody (ANA), antimitochondrial antibody (AMA), anti-smooth muscle antibody (ASMA), kidney microsomal 1 antibody (LKM1), ceruloplasmin (Wilson disease), iron, ferritin (hemochromatosis), and alpha-1 antitrypsin.

B. Hepatic function panel will show cholestatic, hepatocellular, or mixed pattern of injury.

C. Imaging: Ultrasound (US) and MRI.

D. Liver biopsy: If labs and imaging are nondiagnostic, biopsy may be considered.

DIFFERENTIAL DIAGNOSIS

A. Acute viral hepatitis.

B. Alcoholic liver disease.

C. Nonalcoholic fatty liver disease.

D. Autoimmune hepatitis.
E. Wilson disease.
F. Biliary obstruction: Primary biliary cholangitis (PBC) or primary sclerosing cholangitis (PSC).

EVALUATION AND MANAGEMENT PLAN
A. General plan.
   1. Obtain a careful drug history and rule out other causes.
   2. Monitor for improvement of symptoms and serologic markers after stopping the offending drug.
B. Patient/family teaching points.
   1. Regular liver tests at recommended interval to monitor for improvement.
   2. Avoid alcohol.
   3. Normalization of liver tests may take several months.
   4. Do not start any new medications or OTC supplements.
   5. Teach signs and symptoms associated with hepatic injury.
   6. Follow up with gastroenterology or hepatology.
C. Pharmacotherapy.
   1. Primary treatment is withdrawal of the offending drug. Recovery will occur in the majority of patients once the medication is stopped.
D. Discharge instructions.
   1. Monitor labs.
   2. Follow up with gastroenterologist or hepatologist.

FOLLOW-UP
A. Gastroenterologist/hepatologist should be monitoring labs and seeing the patient on a regular basis.

CONSULTATION/REFERRAL
A. May refer for liver transplant if there is no recovery of liver function.

BIBLIOGRAPHY
Larson, A. M. (2017, July 10). *Drug-induced liver injury*. https://www.uptodate.com/contents/drug-induced-liver-injury

HEPATITIS: ALCOHOLIC

Ann Burke and Robin Miller

DEFINITION
A. Syndrome of progressive inflammatory liver injury associated with long-term heavy intake of alcohol.
B. Alcohol abuse is the most common cause of serious liver disease in Western society.

INCIDENCE
A. In the United States, alcoholic liver disease affects more than two million people. The true prevalence of alcoholic hepatitis is unknown as the patient may be asymptomatic or never seek medical attention.

PATHOGENESIS
A. Although the pathogenesis is not known, genetic, environmental, nutrition, metabolic, and immunologic factors may play a role.

PREDISPOSING FACTORS
A. Majority of patients have a history of heavy alcohol use for two or more decades. Heavy use is defined as greater than 100 g/d.
B. Women are more susceptible than men.
C. Peak age is 40 to 50 years old.
D. Alcoholic liver disease is more common in minority groups, particularly among Native Americans.

SUBJECTIVE DATA
A. Common complaints.
   1. Anorexia.
   2. Fever.
   3. Right upper quadrant (RUQ) pain.
   4. Abdominal distention.
   5. Dark urine.
   6. Clay-colored stools.
B. Common history of the present illness.
   1. History of daily alcohol use.
   2. Stressful life events may trigger increased intake.
   3. It is common for patients to cease alcohol intake several weeks prior to presentation due to feeling more ill.
C. Social history.
   1. It is essential that the healthcare provider take a careful alcohol history.
   2. May need to elicit a more accurate history by including family members.
   3. Drinking patterns may vary. Heavy drinking can be intermittent (e.g., weekends only) or hidden from family members.
   4. A standard drink is defined as 14 g of alcohol:
      a. 12 oz of beer.
      b. 5 oz of wine.
      c. 1.5 oz of distilled spirits.
      d. 8 to 9 oz of malt liquor.
D. Review of systems.
   1. Cognitive changes (encephalopathy).
   2. Jaundice.
   3. Anorexia.
   4. Fever.
   5. RUQ/epigastric pain.
   6. Abdominal distention.

PHYSICAL EXAMINATION
A. Temporal wasting.
B. Scleral icterus.
C. Generalized jaundice.
D. Hepatomegaly.
E. Ascites.
F. Spider angiomas, palmar erythema, and gynecomastia suggest advanced disease.
G. Lower extremity edema.

DIAGNOSTIC TESTS
A. Lab tests.
   1. Hepatic function panel: Aspartate aminotransferase (AST) to alanine aminotransferase (ALT) ratio is 2:1.
   2. Complete blood count (CBC): Elevated white blood cell (WBC).

3. International normalized ratio (INR): Elevated.

4. Testing for hepatitis A, B, and C; autoimmune markers (ANA, AMA, ASMA, LKM1).

B. Imaging.

1. Abdominal ultrasound (US) with Doppler to rule out biliary obstruction, Budd–Chiari malformation, or cirrhosis.

C. Liver biopsy.

D. If labs and imaging are nondiagnostic, biopsy may be considered.

DIFFERENTIAL DIAGNOSIS

A. Acute viral hepatitis.

B. Autoimmune hepatitis.

C. Drug-induced liver injury (DILI).

D. Shock liver.

E. Ischemic hepatitis.

F. Budd–Chiari syndrome.

G. Wilson disease.

H. Alpha-1 antitrypsin deficiency.

I. Toxin-induced hepatitis (e.g., mushroom poisoning).

EVALUATION AND MANAGEMENT PLAN

A. General plan.

1. Admission to ICU in patients who are unstable (e.g., encephalopathic).

2. Fluid management and nutritional support.

3. Acuity of illness based on Maddrey Discriminant Function (DF) score and need for glucocorticoid therapy. DF is a calculation using bilirubin and prothrombin time (PT).

4. Alcohol withdrawal protocol per institutional guidelines.

5. Infectious workup to rule out other causes of mental status change.

6. Prophylaxis against gastrointestinal (GI) bleeding.

B. Patient/family teaching points.

1. Referral for substance use counseling.

2. Length of sobriety to meet transplant candidacy requirement per institution policy.

3. Steroid tapering schedule.

C. Pharmacotherapy.

1. GI prophylaxis: proton pump inhibitor (PPI) or H2 blocker.

2. Stop nonselective beta-blocker during acute crisis due to risk of acute kidney injury (AKI). May resume later.

3. Nutritional support: Adequate calories and protein; vitamins, thiamine, and folate.

4. Glucocorticoids.

a. Severe cases with DF >32 receive prednisone/prednisolone for 28 days.

b. Discontinue if no improvement after 7 days. This is based on the Lille score, a predictor of response to steroid treatment.

5. Lactulose or trial of Xifaxan therapy for encephalopathy.

D. Discharge instructions.

1. Review tapering schedule of steroids if applicable.

2. Set up outpatient substance abuse counseling or inpatient rehab.

3. Repeat lab tests in 1 week.

4. Close follow-up with hepatologist.

FOLLOW-UP

A. As per discharge instructions, close follow-up with hepatologist and transplant center, if appropriate.

CONSULTATION/REFERRAL

A. Psychiatry: Addiction specialist.

B. Transplant center.

SPECIAL CONSIDERATIONS

A. HELLP (hemolysis, elevated liver enzymes, low platelet count in the setting of pregnancy).

BIBLIOGRAPHY

Friedman, S. L. (2016, December 15). *Alcoholic hepatitis: Clinical manifestations and diagnosis.* https://www.uptodate.com/contents/alcoholic-hepatitis-clinical-manifestations-and-diagnosis

Friedman, S. L. (2016, October 18). *Management and prognosis of alcoholic hepatitis.* https://www.uptodate.com/contents/management-and-prognosis-of-alcoholic-hepatitis

Heuman, D. M. (2016). *Alcoholic hepatitis: Overview.* https://emedicine.medscape.com/article/170539-overview

National Institute on Alcohol Abuse and Alcoholism. (2017, November). *What is a standard drink?* https://www.niaaa.nih.gov/alcohol-health/overview-alcohol-consumption/what-standard-drink

HEPATITIS: AUTOIMMUNE

Ann Burke and Robin Miller

DEFINITION

A. Chronic inflammatory condition of the liver characterized by transaminase elevation in the presence of autoantibodies.

1. Chronic illness: Clinical or biochemical evidence of liver disease greater than 6 months in duration.

INCIDENCE

A. The exact prevalence in the United States is unknown but is estimated to be 1.1 per 100,000 persons per year.

B. Female predominance, but occurs in both sexes and all age groups.

PATHOGENESIS

A. Thought to result from an environmental trigger in a genetically predisposed individual.

PREDISPOSING FACTORS

A. Strong genetic association with other autoimmune diseases from 26% to 49%.

SUBJECTIVE DATA

A. Common complaints.

1. The presentation can vary from asymptomatic (up to 25%) to fulminant hepatic failure (rare).

2. May see anorexia, arthralgia, rash, and fatigue.

3. Fulminant illness: Onset of liver failure as manifested by encephalopathy and synthetic dysfunction within 8 weeks of the recognition of liver disease.

B. Common history of the present illness.

   1. Insidious onset with constitutional symptoms as listed above. Asymptomatic patients will be diagnosed incidentally with laboratory testing.

C. Social history.

   1. Not applicable.

D. Review of systems.

   1. Flu-like symptoms of nausea, anorexia, fatigue, lethargy, malaise, abdominal pain, itching, and arthralgia.

PHYSICAL EXAMINATION

A. Ranges from a normal physical exam to evidence of advanced disease, that is, hepatomegaly, splenomegaly, jaundice, temporal wasting, and spider angiomas.

DIAGNOSTIC TESTS

A. Lab workup includes complete blood count (CBC), comprehensive metabolic panel (CMP), international normalized ratio (INR), hepatitis B and C serologies, ANA, AMA, ASMA, LKM1, quantitative immunoglobulins, ceruloplasmin (Wilson disease), iron, ferritin (hemochromatosis), and alpha-1 antitrypsin.

B. Lab abnormalities include elevated aspartate aminotransferase (AST)/alanine aminotransferase (ALT; 5–10 times the upper limit), elevated immunoglobulin G (IgG), positive ANA, ASMA, or LKM1.

C. Imaging: Abdominal ultrasound (US) and MRI/ magnetic resonance cholangiopancreatography (MRCP) to rule out other biliary disorders.

D. Liver biopsy: Gold standard to confirm diagnosis and severity of disease.

DIFFERENTIAL DIAGNOSIS

A. Hepatitis A, B, and C.

B. Primary biliary cholangitis (PBC).

C. Primary sclerosing cholangitis (PSC).

D. Wilson disease.

E. Hemochromatosis.

F. Alpha-1 antitrypsin deficiency.

G. Fatty liver disease.

H. Drug-induced liver injury (DILI).

I. Alcohol use.

EVALUATION AND MANAGEMENT PLAN

A. General plan: The decision to treat a patient is based on severity of symptoms, magnitude of AST/ALT elevations, histologic findings, and the potential for side effects.

   1. Supportive care.

   2. Monitor liver function tests (LFTs).

   3. Glucocorticoid monotherapy or in combination with azathioprine.

B. Patient/family teaching points.

   1. Avoid alcohol or over-the-counter (OTC) supplements.

   2. Discuss side effect management of steroid therapy.

   3. Discuss importance of steroid tapering schedule; do not stop abruptly.

C. Pharmacotherapy.

   1. Glucocorticoids: The goal of therapy is to achieve quick remission and taper off steroids to minimize potential side effects.

      a. Moderate to severe activity: Prednisolone intravenous (IV) or oral prednisone starting at 60 mg daily.

      b. Mild activity: Lower dose of prednisone starting at 20 mg daily.

   2. Nonsteroidal immunosuppressant: Imuran or 6 mercaptopurine (6MP) in combination with steroids that are continued long term after steroid taper. This may also be appropriate for populations that are steroid-sensitive. Thiopurine methyltransferase (TPMT) should be obtained prior to starting Imuran or 6MP. It measures the enzyme that breaks down azathioprine and helps guide dosing and risk of potential side effects.

D. Teaching points.

   1. As listed above.

E. Discharge instructions.

   1. Avoid alcohol or OTC supplements.

   2. Discuss side effect management of steroid therapy.

   3. Discuss the importance of steroid tapering schedule; do not stop abruptly.

   4. Weekly CBC, glucose, and liver tests.

   5. Follow up with gastroenterologist or hepatologist.

FOLLOW-UP

A. Get baseline bone density scan.

B. Follow up with primary care provider (PCP) for lab monitoring.

C. Follow up with gastroenterologist or hepatologist within 1 month.

CONSULTATION/REFERRAL

A. Refer to transplant center. Of patients with autoimmune hepatitis, 10% to 20% will require a liver transplant for acute liver failure, decompensated cirrhosis, and hepatocellular carcinoma (HCC).

SPECIAL CONSIDERATIONS

A. Patients at increased risk for glucocorticoid side effects:

   1. Prediabetes, diabetes.

   2. Osteoporosis.

   3. Emotional liability.

   4. Sleep disturbance.

BIBLIOGRAPHY

Fialho, A., Fialho, A., & Carey, W. (2015, July). *Autoimmune hepatitis*. http://www.clevelandclinicmeded.com/medicalpubs/diseasemanagement/hepatology/chronic-autoimmune-hepatitis/

Heneghan, M.A. (2017, September 27). *Autoimmune hepatitis: Treatment*. https://www.uptodate.com/contents/autoimmune-hepatitis-treatment

HEPATITIS A

Ann Burke and Robin Miller

DEFINITION

A. Inflammation of the liver.

B. Vaccine-preventable, communicable disease of the liver caused by the hepatitis A virus.

C. Self-limited disease that does not result in chronic infection.

   1. Acute illness: Clinical or biochemical evidence of liver disease less than 6 months.

INCIDENCE

A. Most common form of acute viral hepatitis in the world.

B. In the United States, the estimated number of new infections in 2019 was 37,700 people (a 1,325% increase in incidence since 2015).

PATHOGENESIS

A. Transmitted person to person by the fecal–oral route or consumption of contaminated food or water.

PREDISPOSING FACTORS

A. International travel to developing countries.
B. Day-care employees and children.
C. Poor hygiene practices at restaurants/cafeterias.
D. Living with an infected person.
E. Men who have sex with men.

SUBJECTIVE DATA

A. Common complaints.
  1. Fatigue.
  2. Fever.
  3. Malaise.
  4. Headache.
  5. Nausea.
  6. Right upper quadrant (RUQ) pain.
  7. Loss of appetite.
  8. Itching.
  9. Myalgia.
B. Common history of the present illness (HPI).
  1. Onset of symptoms.
  2. Vaccination history.
  3. Recent travel.
  4. Food history.
C. Social history.
  1. Living situation.
  2. Sexual practices.
D. Review of systems.
  1. Dark urine.
  2. Light-colored stool.
  3. Jaundice.

PHYSICAL EXAMINATION

A. Jaundice.
B. Scleral icterus.
C. Fever up to 104°F/40°C.
D. RUQ tenderness.
E. Hepatomegaly.

DIAGNOSTIC TESTS

A. Workup includes complete blood count (CBC), comprehensive metabolic panel (CMP), international normalized ratio (INR), hepatitis A immunoglobulin M (IgM) and IgG antibodies, hepatitis B serologies (Hep B surface antibody, Hep B surface antigen, Hep B core antibody), hepatitis C antibody screen, and hepatitis E antibody.

B. Lab abnormalities include elevations of aspartate aminotransferase (AST)/alanine aminotransferase (ALT) often greater than 1,000 IU/L, followed by elevations of bilirubin up to 10 mg/dL.

C. Ultrasound (US) of the abdomen.

DIFFERENTIAL DIAGNOSIS

A. Hepatitis E.
B. Alcoholic hepatitis.
C. Autoimmune hepatitis.
D. Acute drug-induced liver injury (DILI).
E. Acute HIV infection.
F. Cytomegalovirus (CMV) infection.
G. Epstein–Barr virus (EBV).
H. Herpes simplex virus (HSV).

EVALUATION AND MANAGEMENT PLAN

A. General plan.
  1. Supportive care: Intravenous (IV) fluids and antiemetic medications.
B. Patient/family teaching points.
  1. Vaccination of close contacts.
  2. Safe sex practices.
  3. Good hand hygiene.
C. Pharmacotherapy.
  1. Acetaminophen may be cautiously administered but limited to 2 g/d.
  2. Administration of immunoglobulin within 14 days of exposure to achieve passive immunization and reduce severity of illness.
D. Discharge instructions.
  1. Rest.
  2. Return to work should be delayed for 10 days after onset of jaundice.
  3. Follow up with primary care provider (PCP).

FOLLOW-UP

A. Primary care doctor visit: Repeat liver tests.
B. Vaccination for hepatitis B, if not immune.
C. Most people have a full recovery; infection confers lifelong immunity (positive hepatitis A antibody).
D. Up to 10% of patients experience a relapse of symptoms during the 6 months after acute illness.

CONSULTATION/REFERRAL

A. Hepatologist for chronic elevated liver tests post infection.

SPECIAL CONSIDERATIONS

A. Liver transplant should be considered in fulminant disease. This occurs in less than 1% of patients and is most common in individuals older than 50 years or with any other chronic liver disease.
  1. Fulminant: Onset of liver failure as manifested by encephalopathy and synthetic dysfunction within 8 weeks of the recognition of liver disease.

BIBLIOGRAPHY

Centers for Disease Control and Prevention. (2017, September 29). *Hepatitis a information*. https://www.cdc.gov/hepatitis/hav/havfaq.htm

Gilroy, R. K. (2017, October 16). *Hepatitis A*. https://emedicine.medscape.com/article/177484-overview

Lai, M., & Chopra, S. (2017, October 27). *Hepatitis A virus infection in adults: An overview*. https://www.uptodate.com/contents/hepatitis-a-virus-infection-in-adults-an-overview

Mayo Clinic. (2017, October). *Hepatitis A*. https://www.mayoclinic.org/diseases-conditions/hepatitis-a/symptoms-causes/syc-20367007

HEPATITIS B

Ann Burke and Robin Miller

DEFINITION
A. Inflammation of the liver.
B. Vaccine-preventable, communicable disease of the liver caused by the hepatitis B virus.
C. Global health problem.
D. Acute or chronic forms.
   1. Acute illness: Clinical or biochemical evidence of liver disease less than 6 months.
   2. Chronic illness: Clinical or biochemical evidence of liver disease greater than 6 months in duration.

INCIDENCE
A. More than 257 carriers worldwide.
B. 820,000 deaths annually in the world.
C. In the United States, the rate of hepatitis B-related hospitalizations, cancer, and death has doubled in the last decade.

PATHOGENESIS
A. Transmission through activities that involve percutaneous or mucosal contact with infectious blood or body fluids.

PREDISPOSING FACTORS
A. Intravenous (IV) drug use that involves sharing of needles.
B. Birth to an infected patient (vertical transmission).
C. Needlesticks (healthcare worker).
D. Sex with an infected partner.
E. Travel to a region that has high infection rates (e.g., Asia, Pacific islands, Africa, Eastern Europe).

SUBJECTIVE DATA
A. Common complaints.
   1. Fever.
   2. Fatigue.
   3. Malaise.
   4. Headache.
   5. Nausea.
   6. Vomiting.
   7. Right upper quadrant (RUQ) pain.
   8. Loss of appetite.
   9. Itching.
   10. Myalgias.
B. Common history of the present illness.
   1. Onset of symptoms.
   2. Vaccination history.
   3. Recent travel.
   4. Food history.
C. Social history.
   1. Sexual activity (unprotected intercourse, multiple partners).
   2. IV drug use.
   3. Alcohol use.
   4. Living situation (infected roommate or partner).
   5. Family history of hepatitis B.
   6. Dialysis.
D. Review of systems.
   1. See common complaints (jaundice, dark urine, clay-colored stool).

PHYSICAL EXAMINATION
A. Acute illness.
   1. Jaundice.
   2. Scleral icterus.
   3. Fever: low grade.
   4. RUQ tenderness.
B. Chronic illness.
   1. Fatigue.
   2. Anorexia.
   3. Nausea.
   4. Mild RUQ tenderness.
C. Fulminant illness (onset of liver failure as manifested by encephalopathy and synthetic dysfunction within 8 weeks of the recognition of liver disease).
   1. Ascites.
   2. Hepatic encephalopathy.
   3. Gastrointestinal (GI) bleeding.

DIAGNOSTIC TESTS
A. Lab tests.
   1. Hepatitis B surface antigen, surface antibody, core antibody, and immunoglobulin M (IgM) antibody.
   2. Antibodies for hepatitis A, C, D, and E.
   3. HIV.
   4. Complete blood count (CBC).
   5. International normalized ratio (INR).
   6. Liver function tests (LFTs).
   7. Iron studies.
   8. AFP.
B. Imaging.
   1. Abdominal ultrasound (US).
   2. Abdominal MRI.
C. Liver biopsy if indicated.

DIFFERENTIAL DIAGNOSIS
A. Hepatitis A, C, D, and E.
B. Alcoholic hepatitis.
C. Autoimmune hepatitis.
D. Acute drug-induced liver injury (DILI).
E. Hemochromatosis.
F. Wilson disease.

EVALUATION AND MANAGEMENT PLAN
A. General plan.
   1. Supportive.
   2. The likelihood of liver failure from acute hepatitis B is less than 1% and the likelihood of progression to chronic hepatitis B is less than 5% in an immunocompetent adult.

B. Patient/family teaching points.

  1. Vaccination of close contacts and safe sex practices.

C. Pharmacotherapy.

  1. Antiviral medication: Tenofovir or entecavir for patients with acute liver failure or severe disease (elevated bilirubin, coagulopathic).

  2. Fulminant hepatitis: Refer for liver transplant.

D. Discharge instructions.

  1. Follow up with primary care provider (PCP) or hepatologist.

  2. Avoid alcohol or drugs that could harm the liver.

  3. Do not share toothbrush, razor, or needle.

  4. Limit sexual partners and practice safe sex.

  5. Call for fever, vomiting, bloody or black stool, dark urine, jaundice, and ascites.

FOLLOW-UP

A. See PCP if mild course.

B. Antiviral medication as prescribed.

C. Repeat lab tests to monitor recovery.

D. Vaccination for hepatitis A if indicated.

CONSULTATION/REFERRAL

A. Hepatologist to manage if becomes chronic hepatitis B.

B. Transplant center per hepatologist.

SPECIAL CONSIDERATIONS

A. Hepatitis D coinfection requires the presence of hepatitis B virus for infection. Should be treated by a hepatologist with peg interferon.

B. Pregnancy: Neonate born to a patient with hepatitis B receives immunoglobulin as well as vaccination after delivery.

C. Fulminant failure: Consider for transplant.

BIBLIOGRAPHY

Centers for Disease Control and Prevention. (2015, May 31). *Hepatitis B information*. https://www.cdc.gov/hepatitis/hbv/hbvfaq.htm

Lok, A. (2017, September 29). *Hepatitis B virus: Overview and management*. https://www.uptodate.com/contents/hepatitis-b-virus-overview-of-management

Mayo Clinic. (2017, October 27). *Hepatitis B*. https://www.mayoclinic.org/diseases-conditions/hepatitis-b/symptoms-causes/syc-20366802

Pyrsopoulos, N. T. (2017, September 22). *Hepatitis B Workup*. https://emedicine.medscape.com/article/177632-workup

HEPATITIS C

Ann Burke and Robin Miller

DEFINITION

A. Inflammation of the liver.

B. One of the most common liver diseases.

C. Bloodborne disease of the liver caused by the hepatitis C virus (HCV).

D. 70% to 85% of those infected develop chronic illness.

  1. Chronic illness: Clinical or biochemical evidence of liver disease greater than 6 months in duration.

INCIDENCE

A. According to the Centers for Disease Control and Prevention (CDC), new hepatitis C infections from 2018 were estimated at 36,000 in the United States.

B. The estimated prevalence is approximately 2.4 million people in United States.

C. It accounts for 14,242 deaths each year in the United States.

D. Infection rates have dramatically increased among young adults (age 20–39 years) in the past decade due to opioid epidemic.

PATHOGENESIS

A. Transmission through blood from contaminated individual or blood products.

B. After 1990, blood and blood products began to undergo screening.

PREDISPOSING FACTORS

A. Intravenous (IV) drug use and needle sharing.

B. Healthcare worker.

C. Transfusion before 1990.

D. Body piercing and tattoos.

E. Shared razors.

F. Born between 1945 and 1965.

G. Dialysis patient.

H. Maternal history of HCV: The rate of vertical transmission is 5%.

SUBJECTIVE DATA

A. Common complaints.

  1. Most people have no symptoms.

  2. Among those who do have symptoms, they complain of fatigue, muscle and joint pain, pruritus, nausea, loss of appetite, weakness, and weight loss.

B. Common history of the present illness.

  1. Incidental diagnosis for elevated liver tests, insurance screening, or primary care provider (PCP) following the CDC recommendations.

C. Social history.

  1. Injection drug use.

  2. Sexual or household contact.

  3. Incarceration.

D. Review of systems.

  1. In chronic illness, there are very few symptoms unless advanced to cirrhosis.

PHYSICAL EXAMINATION

A. Generally there are no obvious features of chronic hepatitis C unless cirrhosis is present.

DIAGNOSTIC TESTS

A. Hepatitis C antibody.

  1. CDC recommends at least once in a lifetime hepatitis C screening for all adults aged 18 years and older.

B. Hepatitis C viral RNA quantitative level and genotype.

C. Screening tests to rule out coinfection for HIV and hepatitis B.

D. Complete blood count (CBC), comprehensive metabolic panel (CMP), thyroid-stimulating hormone (TSH), and drug and alcohol screen.

E. Imaging: Ultrasound (US) or MRI if advanced disease present.

F. Procedure to assess the degree of fibrosis: Elastography and liver biopsy.

DIFFERENTIAL DIAGNOSIS

A. Autoimmune hepatitis.

B. Cholangitis.

C. Hepatitis A, B, D, and E.

EVALUATION AND MANAGEMENT PLAN

A. General plan.

　1. Treatment with antiviral therapy is well-tolerated and effective in curing the disease.

　2. The decision to treat is based on genotype, the person's overall health and comorbidities, and stage of fibrosis.

B. Patient/family teaching points.

　1. If the decision is made to pursue antiviral treatment, medication adherence is essential to achieve optimal outcomes.

　2. Skipping doses may lead to resistant strains and impact success of therapy.

　3. Alcohol is prohibited, as well as herbal supplements.

　4. Successful treatment can mitigate progression to cirrhosis.

C. Pharmacotherapy.

　1. Antiviral therapy: Must be ordered by a specialist. Drug options include Harvoni, Epclusa, Vosevi, Mavyret, Zepatier, and ribavirin.

　2. Common side effects: Usually mild and may include fatigue, headaches, and nausea.

D. Discharge instructions.

　1. Follow up with gastroenterologist/hepatologist.

　2. Will need vaccinations for hepatitis A and B if indicated.

　3. Avoid alcohol or any over-the-counter (OTC) supplements.

FOLLOW-UP

A. Gastroenterologist/hepatologist to initiate treatment and monitor therapy and side effects.

B. For the cirrhotic patient, biannual imaging of the liver to screen for hepatocellular cancer.

CONSULTATION/REFERRAL

A. Gastroenterologist/hepatologist.

B. If patient has hepatocellular carcinoma (HCC), will be referred to interventional radiology or oncology.

C. Consider transplant for any patient with decompensated cirrhosis or HCC.

SPECIAL CONSIDERATIONS

A. Decision to treat any dialysis patient is undertaken on a case-by-case basis.

B. A patient with HIV/hepatitis C coinfection may require changes in their highly active antiretroviral therapy (HAART) due to drug interactions with hepatitis C treatment.

C. Pregnancy is contraindicated for treatment.

BIBLIOGRAPHY

Centers for Disease Control and Prevention. (2015, May 31). *Hepatitis C Information*. https://www.cdc.gov/hepatitis/hcv/index.htm

Chopra, S., & Pockros, P. J. (2017, August 7). *Overview of the management of chronic hepatitis C virus infection*. https://www.uptodate.com/contents/overview-of-the-management-of-chronic-hepatitis-c-virus-infection

Dhawan, V. K. (2016, March 28). *Hepatitis C clinical presentation*. https://emedicine.medscape.com/article/177792-clinical

NONALCOHOLIC FATTY LIVER DISEASE

Ann Burke and Robin Miller

DEFINITION

A. Medical condition characterized by fatty infiltration in the liver without a history of alcohol use. Two types exist based on presence of inflammation.

　1. Nonalcoholic fatty liver disease (NAFLD): Benign condition without inflammation.

　2. Nonalcoholic steatohepatitis (NASH): Inflammation is present, which leads to scarring. May progress to cirrhosis in 20% of the population.

INCIDENCE

A. The most common liver disease in Western industrialized countries.

B. In the United States, the prevalence of NAFLD is estimated at 10% to 46%.

C. The incidence is as high as 50% to 75% in patients with obesity.

PATHOGENESIS

A. Cause is not fully understood but thought to be linked to insulin resistance and oxidative stress in an individual with risk factors.

PREDISPOSING FACTORS

A. Male sex assigned at birth.

B. Higher prevalence in Hispanic people.

C. Commonly diagnosed at age 40 to 50 years.

D. Metabolic syndrome is present with one or more of the following:

　1. Obesity.

　2. Diabetes.

　3. Hypertension.

　4. Dyslipidemia.

E. Other disorders that may be associated include polycystic ovarian syndrome (PCOS), sleep apnea, and hypothyroidism.

SUBJECTIVE DATA

A. Common complaints.

　1. Most patients are usually asymptomatic.

　2. May have fatigue, malaise, and right upper quadrant (RUQ) discomfort.

B. Common history of the present illness.

    1. Incidental findings of elevated alanine amino-transferase (ALT) on lab testing or imaging suggestive of fatty infiltration.

C. Social history.

    1. Take a detailed history of alcohol intake to rule out alcohol-related liver disease.

    2. Diet and weight history.

D. Review of systems.

    1. There are very few symptoms.

    2. In advanced liver disease, patients may have evidence of synthetic dysfunction.

PHYSICAL EXAMINATION

A. Most patients have obesity.

B. Hepatomegaly.

C. In cirrhosis, may have stigmata of chronic liver disease.

DIAGNOSTIC TESTS

A. Diagnosis made after exclusion of other causes and positive findings of fatty infiltration on imaging or biopsy.

B. Labs: Complete blood count (CBC), comprehensive metabolic panel (CMP), cholesterol, iron studies, ferritin, thyroid-stimulating hormone (TSH), and celiac antibody.

C. Hepatitis A, B, and C serologies.

D. Autoimmune markers ANA, AMA, and ASMA.

E. Ceruloplasmin, alpha-1 antitrypsin, and HFE gene for hemochromatosis.

F. Imaging: Ultrasound (US) or MRI.

G. Liver biopsy.

DIFFERENTIAL DIAGNOSIS

A. Viral hepatitis.

B. Autoimmune disease.

C. Wilson disease.

D. Alpha-1 antitrypsin deficiency.

E. Hemochromatosis.

F. Alcohol-related hepatitis.

G. Celiac disease.

H. Thyroid disease.

I. Medication-induced: Amiodarone, methotrexate, tamoxifen, steroids, and antiretrovirals.

EVALUATION AND MANAGEMENT PLAN

A. General plan.

    1. If no biopsy performed, consider noninvasive testing to assess the degree of fibrosis (i.e., FibroScan).

    2. Lifestyle modifications: Weight loss, diet, and exercise.

    3. Control of sugars.

    4. Treatment of hyperlipidemia and hypertension.

    5. Monitor liver tests every 3 months.

    6. Bariatric surgery may be considered if appropriate.

B. Patient/family teaching points.

    1. In general, control of risk factors contributing to metabolic syndrome.

    2. Weight loss of 7% to 10% of current weight to improve fibrosis.

    3. Avoid alcohol.

    4. Good glucose control.

    5. Vitamin E not recommended if patient has heart disease or diabetes.

    6. Reassure the patient that NAFLD is a chronic condition. Most people will not develop advanced liver disease.

C. Pharmacotherapy.

    1. Vitamin E: Improves liver histology. 800 IU/d is recommended.

    2. Statin therapy.

    3. Clinical trials: Obeticholic acid (OCA) shows promise for future therapy.

D. Discharge instructions.

    1. Follow up with gastroenterologist/hepatologist, primary care provider (PCP), and endocrinologist.

    2. Lifestyle modifications of diet and exercise.

    3. Avoid alcohol.

    4. Do not take any new medications/supplements without consulting your doctor.

FOLLOW-UP

A. As noted in discharge instructions, follow up with PCP, gastroenterology/hepatology, and endocrinology.

B. Patients with NASH cirrhosis will need hepatocellular carcinoma (HCC) screening and esophageal varices screening under the supervision of a hepatologist.

CONSULTATION/REFERRAL

A. Dietitian.

B. Endocrinologist.

C. Bariatric surgeon.

D. Cardiologist.

SPECIAL CONSIDERATIONS

A. Another cause of hepatic steatosis is acute fatty liver of pregnancy. This is a rare condition and typically occurs in the third trimester in mothers with multiple gestation pregnancies. Early diagnosis and prompt delivery are primary treatments.

BIBLIOGRAPHY

Chalasani, N., Younossi, Z., Lavine, J. E., Charlton, M., Cusi, K., Rinella, M., Harrison, S. A., Brunt, E. M., & Sanyal, A. J. (2018). The diagnosis and management of nonalcoholic fatty liver disease: Practice guidance from the American Association for the Study of Liver Diseases. *Hepatology*, 67(2), 328–357.

Sheth, S. G., & Chopra, S. (2016, November 8). *Natural history and management of nonalcoholic fatty liver disease in adults.* https://www.uptodate.com/contents/natural-history-and-management-of-nonalcoholic-fatty-liver-disease-in-adults

Sheth, S. G., & Chopra, S. (2017, November). *Epidemiology, clinical features, and diagnosis of nonalcoholic fatty liver disease in adults.* https://www.uptodate.com/contents/epidemiology-clinical-features-and-diagnosis-of-nonalcoholic-fatty-liver-disease-in-adults

Tendler, D. A. (2016, March 9). *Pathogenesis of nonalcoholic fatty liver disease.* https://www.uptodate.com/contents/pathogenesis-of-nonalcoholic-fatty-liver-disease

PANCREATITIS

Catherine Harris

DEFINITION
A. Acute pancreatitis is a sudden inflammation of the pancreas.

INCIDENCE
A. The incidence of acute pancreatitis ranges from 4.9 to 13 every 100,000 persons.
B. Leading gastrointestinal (GI) cause of hospitalization, with more than 300,000 admissions per year.
C. 16.5% to 25% of patients experience recurrent episodes in the first several years post diagnosis.
D. Acute pancreatitis is frequently an isolated event, but may develop into chronic pancreatitis, particularly in the setting of chronic alcoholism.
E. 60% to 90% of patients with pancreatitis have a history of chronic alcohol consumption; however, only a minority of alcoholics develop the disease.
F. Mortality rate for acute pancreatitis has remained the same over the past decade at 10%.
G. Optimal outcomes depend on recognition of acute pancreatitis as quickly as possible.

PATHOGENESIS
A. Gallstones and alcohol account for about 80% of all cases of acute pancreatitis.
B. Other causes of acute pancreatitis can be related to medications and very rarely to infections, trauma, or surgery of the abdomen. About 10% of cases are idiopathic.
  1. Gallstones.
    a. Gallstones can lodge in the common bile duct and cause obstruction of the pancreatic fluid by impinging on the main pancreatic duct.
    b. The mechanism is not completely understood.
  2. Alcohol.
    a. Alcohol is metabolized by the pancreas and is thought to have a toxic effect on key cells.
    b. Alcohol may also cause the production of excess collagen, which contributes to fibrosis.
    c. Large amounts of alcohol (80 g/d; approximately 10–11 drinks) for 6 to 12 years are required to produce symptomatic pancreatitis.
  3. Medications.
    a. Very rare and not well-understood mechanism of how medications induce acute pancreatitis.
    b. Possible theories include pancreatic duct constriction, cytotoxic, and metabolic effects.
    c. Medications associated with acute pancreatitis:
      i. Angiotensin-converting enzyme inhibitors.
      ii. Statins.
      iii. Oral contraceptives.
      iv. Diuretics.
      v. Valproic acid.
      vi. Glucagon-like peptide 1 (GLP-1) hypoglycemic agents.

  4. Trauma or surgery.
    a. Injury to the pancreas from trauma or surgery typically occurs from hemorrhage and sepsis related to primary injury.
    b. Least commonly injured organ in abdominal trauma due in part to its location.

PREDISPOSING FACTORS
A. Choledocholithiasis.
B. Chronic alcoholism.
C. Hypertriglyceridemia (greater than 1,000 mg/dL).
D. Cigarette smoking.
E. Obesity.
F. Diabetes.

SUBJECTIVE DATA
A. Common complaints/symptoms.
  1. Severe abdominal pain.
  2. Nausea and vomiting.
  3. Diarrhea.
B. Common/typical scenario.
  1. Patients may start with sudden-onset dull pain in the abdomen that becomes increasingly more severe.
  2. Pain localizes to the upper abdomen and may radiate to the back.
  3. Usually associated with nausea and vomiting.
  4. Patients usually restless and bending forward to try to alleviate the constant pain.
C. Family and social history.
  1. Alcoholism.
  2. Familial history of hypertriglyceridemia.
  3. Recent abdominal surgery or trauma.
D. Review of systems.
  1. Constitutional: Ask about any fever.
  2. Cardiovascular: May have rapid heartbeat or feel lightheaded.
  3. Respiratory: Ask about any difficulty breathing or trouble getting air in.
  4. GI: Ask about nausea, vomiting, diarrhea, pain location and intensity, and if any radiation.
  5. Weight loss.8

PHYSICAL EXAMINATION
A. GI: Abdominal tenderness, distention, guarding, bowel sounds (BS) may be diminished or absent, and may have jaundice.
B. Respiratory: Dyspnea from diaphragmatic inflammation.
C. Cardiovascular: Hemodynamic instability in severe acute pancreatitis; assess for signs and symptoms of shock.
D. Skin: Physical findings consistent with severe necrotizing pancreatitis.
  1. Cullen sign: Periumbilical bluish discoloration.
  2. Grey Turner sign: Reddish brown discoloration along the flanks consistent with extravasated pancreatic exudate.

DIAGNOSTIC TESTS

A. Lab studies.

1. Amylase and lipase are routinely ordered and will be elevated at least three times above the normal reference range in acute pancreatitis. The serum level of amylase or lipase does not correlate with severity.

a. Amylase: Half-life is short (less than 12 hours) and will return to normal; not specific to acute pancreatitis.

b. Lipase elevations support the diagnosis of acute pancreatitis and more specific than amylase to the pancreas.

2. Liver function tests (LFTs).

a. Alkaline phosphatase.

b. Total bilirubin.

c. Aspartate aminotransferase (AST).

d. Alanine aminotransferase (ALT) greater than 150 U/L suggests gallstone pancreatitis.

3. Basic metabolic panel (BMP), electrolytes, cholesterol, and triglycerides.

a. Hypertriglyceridemia (greater than 1,000 mg/dL).

4. C-reactive protein.

a. Higher levels (greater than 10 mg/dL) associated with severe pancreatitis, but not specific for pancreatitis.

5. Lactic dehydrogenase (LDH) should be checked to provide prognosis based on the Ranson criteria (see "Evaluation and Management Plan").

6. Immunoglobulin G4 (IgG4) if there is concern for autoimmune pancreatitis.

B. Imaging studies.

1. Ultrasound (US).

a. Good screening test for determining the etiology of pancreatitis and the standard of care for detecting gallstones.

b. Cannot measure severity of disease.

2. Endoscopic ultrasonography.

a. High-frequency US can provide more detailed imagery.

3. Contrast-enhanced CT or MRI only necessary if a diagnosis is uncertain with clinical presentation and laboratory data.

C. Endoscopic retrograde cholangiopancreatography (ERCP).

1. Endoscopic procedure used in patients with severe acute pancreatitis with suspected gallstones or biliary pancreatitis with worsening clinical examination.

2. Not used routinely in patients with acute pancreatitis and should be used with caution and only in cases where gallstones are suspected to be the underlying etiology.

DIFFERENTIAL DIAGNOSIS

A. Cholecystitis.

B. Acute abdomen.

C. Pneumonia.

D. Peptic ulcer disease (PUD).

E. Hepatitis.

F. Irritable bowel syndrome.

G. Myocardial infarction.

H. Chronic pancreatitis.

I. Gastroenteritis.

J. Peritonitis.

EVALUATION AND MANAGEMENT PLAN

A. General plan.

1. Stage acute pancreatitis to determine prognosis using the 11-point Ranson criteria within 48 hours. Each criteria is 1 point. Ranson score 0 to 2: minimal mortality; Ranson score 3 to 5: 10% to 20% mortality; Ranson score greater than 5 after 48 hours has a mortality rate greater than 50%. The Ranson score is broken up into criteria present on admission and develops within 48 hours.

a. Present on admission.

i. Patient older than 55 years.

ii. White blood cell (WBC) count higher than 16,000 mcL.

iii. Blood glucose higher than 200 mg/dL.

iv. Serum LDH level higher than 350 IU/L.

v. AST level higher than 250 IU/L.

b. Develops within 48 hours.

i. Drop of hematocrit more than 10%.

ii. Blood urea nitrogen (BUN) increases more than 8 mg/dL.

iii. Fluid retention greater than 6 L.

iv. Base deficit greater than 4 mEq/L.

v. PaO_2 less than 60 mmHg.

vi. Serum calcium less than 8 mg/dL.

2. Supportive medical care.

a. Early return to eating as long as food is tolerated.

b. Nutritional support with dextrose 5% in water for mild pancreatitis.

c. In moderate to severe pancreatitis, start nasojejunal feeds with low-fat formulation.

d. Parenteral nutrition should be avoided except in very severe cases in order to minimize the risk of infections.

e. Pain management.

f. Aggressive rehydration with IV fluids within the first 12 to 24 hours of symptom onset: Monitor patients with cardiovascular and renal comorbidities very closely.

3. Surgical therapy.

a. ERCP within 24 hours of admission if patient has concurrent acute cholangitis.

b. Gallstones may require surgical intervention.

c. Resection of necrotic tissue if necrotizing pancreatitis or abscess.

d. Sphincteroplasty may be performed if sphincter dysfunction is found.

4. Monitor for complications associated with severe acute pancreatitis.

a. Shock.

b. Pulmonary complications.

c. Inflammatory changes.

i. Kidney dysfunction.

    ii. GI bleeding.

    iii. Colitis.

    iv. Splenic vein thrombosis.

  d. Localized complications are more likely to occur in patients with alcoholic and biliary pancreatitis.

    i. Fluid collection.

    ii. Ascites.

    iii. Pseudocysts.

B. Patient/family teaching points.

1. Acute pancreatitis is typically relieved after a couple days but can become severe.

2. Avoid binge drinking.

3. Smoking cessation is thought to exacerbate episodes of acute pancreatitis but the studies are not conclusive.

4. Recurrence of acute pancreatitis may occur and prevention depends on the cause.

  a. If gallstones caused acute pancreatitis, patient may need to have their gallbladder removed.

  b. If alcohol is the cause, patient should stop drinking.

5. Diet changes may be required in people with high fat intake.

6. Medication changes may be necessary if acute pancreatitis is associated with a particular drug.

7. Some patients may develop chronic pancreatitis, but acute pancreatitis is more frequently a one-off event, especially if the underlying cause is treated.

C. Pharmacotherapy.

1. No specific pharmacologic therapy for acute pancreatitis.

2. Supportive fluid resuscitation and management of pain.

3. Antibiotic therapy only in cases of suspected infection.

D. Discharge instructions.

1. Eliminate alcohol from diet.

2. Eat small, frequent meals.

3. Reduce fat in diet.

4. Do not smoke.

5. Follow up with the gastroenterologist.

FOLLOW-UP

A. No guidelines established for long-term follow-up.

B. Depending on the etiology, may need follow-up imaging or lab monitoring.

CONSULTATION/REFERRAL

A. Gastroenterology should evaluate all cases of pancreatitis.

B. Surgical consult for acute pancreatitis related to gallstones.

C. Endocrinology consult if patient has hyperparathyroidism, hypertriglyceridemia, or hypercalcemia-induced pancreatitis.

D. Refer patients to social work if alcohol abuse suspected.

SPECIAL/GERIATRIC CONSIDERATIONS

A. Gallstone pancreatitis is much more likely in older adults and pregnant persons.

B. Presenting abdominal pain may be more vague in older adults.

C. Acute pancreatitis is rare during pregnancy but typically occurs in the third trimester and is mostly due to gallstones, which can cause preterm labor or in utero fetal demise.

CASE SCENARIO: PANCREATITIS

A 52-year-old patient presents with sudden-onset midabdominal pain radiating to his back. The pain woke him from sleep and he vomited several times. Emesis did not relieve his pain. He has a history of mild hypertension and has been told he has prediabetes, but otherwise his history is insignificant. On examination his blood pressure is 110/60, heart rate is 110 beats per minute, respiratory rate is 22, and temperature is 100.4°F/38°C. His abdomen is tender, and he is guarding. No bowel sounds are heard.

1. Which of the following is NOT part of the Ranson score present on admission?

A. Age >55 years

B. White blood cell (WBC) >16,000/mm²

C. Calcium <8 mg/dL

D. Aspartate aminotransferase (AST) >250 IU/L

2. The natural history of acute pancreatitis includes all of the following EXCEPT:

A. Most cases are mild and self-limiting.

B. Nearly 25% of all attacks are severe.

C. Obesity is a major risk factor for severe pancreatitis.

D. The overall mortality is less than 1%.

BIBLIOGRAPHY

Balthazar, E. J. (2002). Staging of acute pancreatitis. *Radiologic Clinics*, 40(6), 1199–1209. https://doi.org/10.1016/S0033-8389(02)00047-7

Banks, P. A., Bollen, T. L., Dervenis, C., Gooszen, H. G., Johnson, C. D., Sarr, M. G., Tsiotos, G. G., Vege, S. S., & Acute Pancreatitis Classification Working Group. (2013). Classification of acute pancreatitis—2012: Revision of the Atlanta classification and definitions by international consensus. *Gut*, 62(1), 102–111. https://doi.org/10.1136/gutjnl-2012-302779

Crockett, S., Wani, S., Gardner, T., Falck-Ytter, Y., & Barkun, A. (2018). American gastroenterological association institute clinical guidelines committee. American gastroenterological association institute guideline on initial management of acute pancreatitis. *Gastroenterology*, 154(4), 1096–1101.

Ducarme, G., Maire, F., Chate, P., Luton, D., & Hammel, P. (2014). Acute pancreatitis during pregnancy: A review. *Journal of Perinatology*, 34, 87–94. https://doi.org/10.1038/jp.2013.161

Imrie, C. W. (2003). Prognostic indicators in acute pancreatitis. *Canadian Journal of Gastroenterology*, 17(5), 325–358. https://doi.org/10.1155/2003/250815

Jones, M., Hall, O., Kaye, A. M., & Kaye, A. D. (2015). Drug-induced acute pancreatitis: A review. *Ochsner Journal*, 15(1), 45–51. http://www.ochsnerjournal.org/content/15/1/45

Ranson, J., Rifkind, K., Roses, D., Fink, S., Eng, K., & Spencer, F. Prognostic signs and the role of operative management in acute pancreatitis. *Surgery Gynecology Obstetrics*, 139(1), 69–81.

Strate, T., Yekebas, E., Knoefel, W., Bloechle, C., & Izbicki, J. (2002). Pathogenesis and the natural course of chronic pancreatitis. *European Journal of Gastroenterology & Hepatology*, 14(9), 929–934. https://journals.lww.com/eurojgh/Fulltext/2002/09000/Pathogenesis_and_the_natural_course_of_chronic.2.aspx

Tenner, S., Baillie, J., DeWitt, J., & Vege, S. S. (2013). American College of gastroenterology guideline: Management of acute pancreatitis. *The*

American Journal of Gastroenterology, 108(9), 1400–1416. https://journals.lww.com/ajg/Abstract/2013/09000/American_College_of_Gastro enterology_Guideline_.6.aspx

Vege, S. S., Ziring, B., Jain, R., & Moayyedi, P. (2015). American Gastroenterological Association institute guideline on the diagnosis and management of asymptomatic neoplastic pancreatic cysts. *Gastroenterology*, 148(4), 819–822. https://doi.org/10.1053/j.gastro.20 15.01.015

Whitcomb, D. C. (2006). Clinical practice. Acute pancreatitis. *New England Journal of Medicine*, 354(20), 2142–2150. https://doi.org/10.1056/NEJ Mcp054958

Whitcomb, D. C., Yadav, D., Adam, S., Hawes, R. H., Brand, R. E., Anderson, M. A., Money, M. E., Banks, P. A., Bishop, M. D., Baillie, J., Sherman, S., DiSario, J., Burton, F. R., Gardner, T. B., Amann, S. T., Gelrud, A., Lo, S. K., DeMeo, M. T., Steinberg, W. M., . . . Barmada, M. M. (2008). Multicenter approach to recurrent acute and chronic pancreatitis in the United States: The North American Pancreatitis Study 2 (NAPS2). *Pancreatology*, 8(4-5), 520–531. https://doi.org/10.1159/000152001

PEPTIC ULCER DISEASE

Catherine Harris

DEFINITION

A. An ulcer that forms in the lining of the esophagus, stomach, or small intestine.

INCIDENCE

A. 10% of the population are thought to have evidence of peptic ulcer disease (PUD).
B. Similar occurrence in males and females.
C. Mortality rate due to hemorrhagic ulcer is approximately 5%.

PATHOGENESIS

A. Defect of mucosal lining of digestive tract; frequently occurs when there is an imbalance between gastric acid secretion and degradation of the mucosal defense mechanism caused by use of anti-inflammatory drugs, *Helicobacter pylori* infection, alcohol, acid, and pepsin.
B. *H. pylori* infection can colonize the gastric mucosa and cause inflammation.
C. Nonsteroidal anti-inflammatory drug (NSAID) use can disrupt the mucosal barrier.
D. Alcohol is a gastric mucosal irritant.
E. Stress ulceration can occur and is associated with serious systemic illnesses.
F. Brain injury or tumors are associated with high gastric acid output.
G. Hypersecretory states can also cause PUD, most notably Zollinger–Ellison syndrome.
H. Three types of ulcers (location-based):
  1. Gastric ulcers.
  2. Esophageal ulcers.
  3. Duodenal ulcers.
I. Major risk of perforation, which carries a mortality rate of up to 30%.

PREDISPOSING FACTORS

A. Taking NSAIDs, including ibuprofen, and aspirin.
B. Smoking.
C. Excessive alcohol.
D. Excess stress.
E. Obesity.
F. Zollinger–Ellison disease.

SUBJECTIVE DATA

A. Common complaints/symptoms.
  1. Gnawing or burning sensation that occurs shortly after meals (gastric ulcers) or at 2 to 3 hours (duodenal ulcers).
  2. Heartburn.
  3. Belching.
  4. Bloating.
  5. Distention.
B. Common/typical scenario.
  1. Gastric and duodenal ulcers typically cannot be differentiated with history alone, but there are some differences.
    a. Most patients regardless of type of PUD complain of epigastric pain.
    b. Patients with gastric ulcers typically complain of pain shortly after meals.
    c. In patients with duodenal ulcers:
      i. Antacid use commonly ineffective.
      ii. Complaints of pain 2 to 3 hours after a meal.
      iii. Frequent night waking.
C. Family and social history.
  1. Ask about smoking and alcohol use.
  2. Ask about family history of any type of gastric cancer.
D. Review of systems.
  1. Evaluate for dysphagia, nausea, vomiting, or blood in stool.
  2. Evaluate pain intensity, timing, and duration.
  3. Inquire about back pain (which may indicate gallstones or pancreatitis).

PHYSICAL EXAMINATION

A. Gastrointestinal (GI) focus.
  1. Epigastric tenderness.
  2. Typically pain will be vague and nonlocalizing.
  3. Melena may be present.
B. If the ulcer perforates.
  1. Sudden onset of severe abdominal pain that is generalized and worsens with movement.
  2. Rebound abdominal tenderness.
  3. Guarding.
  4. Rigidity.
  5. May have signs of shock, including:
    a. Tachycardia.
    b. Hypotension.
    c. Anuria.

DIAGNOSTIC TESTS

A. Obtain complete blood count (CBC) and liver function tests (LFTs) in all suspected cases of PUD.
B. Use amylase or lipase to rule out other causes of epigastric pain.
C. Test for *H. pylori*.
  1. Serologic testing.

2. Urea breath test.

3. Measured antibodies to *H. pylori*.

D. Esophagogastroduodenoscopy (EGD) is the gold standard diagnostic test in PUD.

    1. Differentiates gastric and duodenal ulcers.

    2. Allows for biopsy if indicated.

E. Angiography may be needed in cases with massive GI bleeding.

F. If Zollinger–Ellison syndrome is suspected, obtain serum gastrin level: If inconclusive, order secretin stimulation test.

G. Biopsy if there is concern for cancer.

DIFFERENTIAL DIAGNOSIS

A. Gastritis.

B. Gastroesophageal reflux disease (GERD).

C. Inflammatory bowel disease.

D. Cholecystitis.

E. Coronary artery disease.

F. Esophageal rupture.

G. Diverticulitis.

H. Pancreatitis.

I. Viral hepatitis.

J. Mesenteric vasculitis.

EVALUATION AND MANAGEMENT PLAN

A. General plan.

    1. Gastric ulcers can be staged according to Johnson classification.

        a. Type I: Normal or decreased gastric acid secretion.

        b. Type II: Combination of stomach and duodenal ulcers with normal or increased gastric acid secretion.

        c. Type III: Prepyloric associated with normal or increased gastric acid secretion.

        d. Type IV: Near gastroesophageal junction with normal or decreased gastric acid secretion.

    2. Treatment plans vary on the location of the peptic ulcer and clinical presentation.

    3. Typical treatment options include:

        a. Empiric antisecretory therapy.

        b. Triple therapy for *H. pylori* infection.

        c. Endoscopy 6 to 8 weeks after diagnosis to document healing of ulcers.

        d. Document *H. pylori* cure with noninvasive test.

            i. Urea breath test.

            ii. Fecal antigen test (complicated ulcers).

B. Patient/family teaching points.

    1. Avoid NSAIDs and aspirin.

    2. Reduce or eliminate alcohol.

    3. Smoking cessation.

    4. Reduce or eliminate caffeine from diet.

    5. Weight loss.

    6. Stress reduction.

C. Pharmacotherapy.

    1. *H. pylori* infection.

        a. Option 1: 10 to 14 days of quadruple therapy.

            i. Bismuth to facilitate killing of the *H. pylori*, along with antibiotics

            ii. Proton pump inhibitor (PPI).

            iii. Two antibiotics such as amoxicillin, tetracycline, tinidazole, metronidazole, and clarithromycin.

        b. Option 2: 10 to 14 days.

            i. PPI.

            ii. Clarithromycin.

            iii. Amoxicillin.

            iv. Nitroimidazole.

        c. Option 3: 10 to 14 days of triple therapy (no previous macrolide exposure and clarithromycin resistance low).

            i. Clarithromycin.

            ii. PPI.

            iii. Amoxicillin or metronidazole.

        d. Other suggested options per guidelines.

    2. *H. pylori* infection persists.

        a. Up to 20% of *H. pylori* infections persist after 2 weeks.

        b. Avoid previously used antibiotics.

        c. Choose a new option from the aforementioned list.

D. Discharge instructions.

    1. Follow up with primary care provider (PCP) for long-term monitoring and further evaluation.

FOLLOW-UP

A. Follow up routinely with PCP to assure proper maintenance therapy is initiated and symptoms are controlled.

B. If *H. pylori* eradication is not achieved, antisecretory therapy should be recommended.

CONSULTATION/REFERRAL

A. Consult gastroenterology for bleeding (hematemesis or melena), anemia, unexplained weight loss, associated vomiting, or family history of GI cancer.

B. Surgical consultation for all bleeding ulcers or suspected perforations.

C. Urgent referral for sudden and severe onset of symptoms, which may indicate perforation.

D. Failure of medical management.

SPECIAL/GERIATRIC CONSIDERATIONS

A. NSAID-induced PUD may not be overtly symptomatic in older adult patients.

B. Older adults may also present with significantly less profound signs and symptoms of shock in the case of perforated ulcers.

CASE SCENARIO: PEPTIC ULCER DISEASE

A 63-year-old patient complains of discomfort and unintentional weight loss of 10 lb in 2 months due to feeling consistently bloated. This morning she had some black stool, which was new for her. For the last 2 months, she has had burning epigastric abdominal pain that also occurred in the chest area and radiated to the back. Taking aspirin and drinking coffee made the pain worse. The pain was relieved after taking antacids. She also reports nausea and vomiting. Her concern was that the food appeared undigested when she vomited.

She routinely takes nonsteroidal anti-inflammatory drugs for back pain and has increased those recently. The patient looks exhausted when she comes in. Her blood pressure is 140/82, heart rate is 98 beats per minute, respiratory rate is 20, temperature is 97.52°F/36.4°C, and oxygen is 99%.

1. Which of the following is the gold standard diagnostic test for evaluating peptic ulcer disease (PUD)?

A. *Helicobacter pylori* testing

B. Esophagogastroduodenoscopy (EGD)

C. CT angiogram of the abdomen

D. Barium swallow

2. Which of the following is NOT part of *Helicobacter pylori* treatment protocol?

A. Use of a combination of antibiotics

B. Antacids

C. Nonsteroidal anti-inflammatory drugs (NSAIDs)

D. Bismuth

BIBLIOGRAPHY

Chey, W. D., Leontiadis, G. I., Howden, C. W., & Moss, S. F. (2017). ACG clinical guideline: Treatment of *Helicobacter pylori* infection. *The American Journal of Gastroenterology*, 112, 212–238. https://journals.lww.com/ajg/Abstract/2017/02000/ACG_Clinical_ Guideline__Treatment_of_Helicobacter.12.aspx

Ford, A. C., Marwaha, A., Lim, A., & Moayyedi, P. (2010). What is the prevalence of clinically significant endoscopic findings in subjects with dyspepsia? Systematic review and meta-analysis. *Clinical Gastroenterology and Hepatology*, 8(10), 830–837. e2. https://doi.org/10.1016/j.cgh.2010.05.031

Lanas, A., & Chan, F. (2017). Peptic ulcer disease. *Lancet*, 390(10094), 613–623.

Leontiadis, G. I., Sreedharan, A., Dorward, S., Barton, P., Delaney, B., Howden, C. W., Orhewere, M., Gisbert, J., Sharma, V. K., Rostom, A., Moayyedi, P., & Forman, D. (2007). Systematic reviews of the clinical effectiveness and cost-effectiveness of proton pump inhibitors in acute upper gastrointestinal bleeding. *Health Technology Assessment*, 11(51), 1–164. https://doi.org/10.3310/hta11510

Malik, T., Gnanapandithan, K., & Singh, K. (2021). Peptic ulcer disease. In *StatPearls [Internet]*. StatPearls Publishing. https://www.ncbi.nlm.nih.gov/books/NBK534792/

Narayanan, M., Reddy, K., & Marsicano, E. (2018). Peptic ulcer disease and *Helicobacter pylori* infection. *Missouri Medicine*, 115(3), 219–224. https://www.ncbi.nlm.nih.gov/pmc/articles/PMC6140150/

Strand, D., Kim, D., & Peura, D. (2017). 25 years of proton pump inhibitors: A comprehensive review. *Gut and Liver*, 11(1), 27–37.

Sung, J. J., Tsoi, K. K., Ma, T. K., Yung, M.-Y., Lau, J. Y., & Chiu, P. W. (2010). Causes of mortality in patients with peptic ulcer bleeding: A prospective cohort study of 10,428 cases. *The American Journal of Gastroenterology*, 105(1), 84–89. https://journals.lww.com/ajg/Abstract/2010/01000/Causes_of_Mortality_in_Patients_With_ Peptic_Ulcer.15.aspx

CHAPTER 5

NEPHROLOGY GUIDELINES

Christine Chmielewski

DEFINITION

A. A sudden but potentially reversible loss of kidney function, usually occurring in less than 1 day. The time course is identified as occurring over a few hours to 1 week and prompt diagnosis is important.

   1. It is diagnosed by an increase in serum creatinine (SCr) and/or by a decrease in urine output (UO).

   2. SCr and UO are surrogate markers of the estimated glomerular filtration rate (eGFR). However, both have limitations.

   a. SCr is affected by altered production (age, diet, muscle mass), dilution (fluid administration), elimination (underlying kidney dysfunction), and secretion (medications).

   b. UO is affected by volume status, hemodynamic status, and the use of diuretics.

   c. Cystatin C has been used to estimate glomerular filtration rate (GFR). It is less affected by muscle mass and dietary intake.

   i. Using SCr and cystatin C together has been found to provide a better estimate of GFR.

B. Kidney Disease: Improving Global Outcomes (KDIGO) definition and stages: The stages are defined by the maximum change of either the SCr or the UO.

   1. Acute kidney injury (AKI) stage 1.
   a. SCr 1.5 to 1.9 times the baseline value. *OR*
   b. UO <0.5 mL/kg/hr (6–12 hours).

   2. AKI stage 2.
   a. SCr 2.0 to 2.9 times the baseline value. *OR*
   b. UO <0.5 mL/kg/hr (≥12 hours).

   3. AKI stage 3.
   a. SCr 3.0 times the baseline value. *OR*
   b. UO <0.5 mL/kg/hr (≥24 hours) *OR* anuria ≥12 hours.

INCIDENCE

A. The true incidence of AKI is difficult to determine due to variations in clinical presentations and in the diagnostic criteria.

   1. Mortality increases with the severity of AKI, for example, the need for kidney replacement therapy (KRT) and the duration of AKI.

B. The incidence is estimated to be ~5% to 7% in hospitalized patients.

C. The incidence is estimated to be ~30% to 70% in critically ill patients.

D. Short-term outcomes of AKI include:
   1. Increased hospital length of stay.
   2. Increased healthcare costs.
   3. Increased mortality.

E. Long-term outcomes of AKI include:
   1. Increased risk of cardiovascular disease (CVD; hypertension [HTN], heart failure [HF], myocardial infarction [MI], cerebrovascular accident [CVA]).
   2. Recurrent episodes of AKI.
   3. Progression to chronic kidney disease (CKD).
   4. Long-term mortality (CVD, hematologic and genitourinary [GU] cancers).

F. Major adverse kidney events (MAKE).
   1. Clinically meaningful endpoints that include impaired kidney function, new hemodialysis, and death.

PATHOGENESIS

A. AKI is multifactorial but is categorized into three broad categories:

   1. Prerenal AKI results from reduced blood flow and hypoperfusion of the kidneys.
   a. It is often due to hypovolemia, impaired cardiac function, systemic vasodilation, and/or increased vascular resistance.
   b. It accounts for up to 60% of AKI.

   2. Intrinsic AKI results from structural damage to the tubular, glomerular, interstitial, and/or vascular components of the kidney.
   a. It is often due to direct insults to the renal parenchyma.
   b. It accounts for up to 40% of AKI.

   3. Obstructive AKI results from increased tubular pressure from urinary obstruction.
   a. It is often due to more easily identifiable and potentially reversible causes.
   b. It occurs much less frequently.

PREDISPOSING FACTORS

A. Prerenal AKI results from the functional adaptation to hypoperfusion of structurally normal kidneys.

   1. Hypovolemia (fluid loss, blood loss, third spacing).
   2. Impaired cardiac function (HF, cardiogenic shock, massive pulmonary embolus).
   3. Systemic vasodilation (septic shock, cirrhosis, anaphylaxis).

4. Increased vascular resistance (nonsteroidal anti-inflammatory drugs [NSAIDs], renin–angiotensin–aldosterone system [RAAS] inhibitors).
B. Intrinsic AKI results from structural damage to any component of the renal parenchyma.
  1. Tubular (renal ischemia, nephrotoxic drugs, toxins).
  2. Glomerular (glomerulonephritis, lupus nephritis.
  3. Interstitial (infections, medications).
  4. Vascular (large vessel disease, small vessel disease).
C. Postrenal AKI results from a shift in filtration forces caused by urinary tract obstruction.
  1. Extrarenal obstruction (prostate hypertrophy, bladder cancer).
  2. Intrarenal obstruction (nephrolithiasis, papillary necrosis).

SUBJECTIVE DATA
A. Common complaints/symptoms.
  1. AKI is not associated with specific symptoms and is therefore often asymptomatic.
    a. Patients may experience symptoms related to the underlying cause of AKI (see "Differential Diagnosis").
  2. If symptomatic, patients may complain of:
    a. Edema.
    b. Decreased UO.
    c. Nausea and vomiting.
    d. Diarrhea.
    e. Dizziness.
B. Family and social history.
  1. May not be relevant.
  2. Family history of CKD.
  3. Social history.
    a. Tobacco.
      i. Acute renal ischemia (nicotine).
    b. Alcohol.
      i. Dehydration (binge drinking).
      ii. Alcohol poisoning.
    c. Drug use.
      i. Methamphetamines.
        1) Rhabdomyolysis.
      ii. Bath salts.
        1) Rhabdomyolysis, hyperuricemia, and acute tubular necrosis (ATN).
      iii. NMDA (N-methyl-D-aspartate) receptor antagonists.
        1) Rhabdomyolysis (phencyclidine).
        2) Lower urinary tract dysfunction (Ketamine).
C. Review of systems.
  1. Ask patient about the presence of:
    a. Any new medications, especially:
      i. Statins (rhabdomyolysis).
      ii. Antibiotics (nephrotoxicity).
      iii. RAAS inhibitors (decreased renal perfusion).
      iv. NSAIDs (decreased renal perfusion, nephrotoxicity).

b. Chemotherapy treatment (tumor lysis).
c. Exposure to toxic substances such as ethyl alcohol or ethylene glycol.
d. Changes in blood pressure (BP) or BP management (prerenal hypoperfusion).
e. Blood loss or transfusion.
f. History of liver disease (cirrhosis—prerenal).
g. Recent or past history of thromboembolic disease (prerenal—renal artery thrombosis).
h. History of renal artery stenosis.
i. Recent history of infectious disease (ID; postinfectious glomerulonephritis).
j. Recent procedures or diagnostic examinations (use of intravenous [IV] contrast).
k. Extreme exercise or trauma (rhabdomyolysis).
l. History of multiple myeloma.
m. History of kidney stones or gout (intratubular crystal deposition, postrenal obstruction).
n. Rash (vasculitis).

PHYSICAL EXAMINATION
A. Skin.
  1. Livedo reticularis (systemic vasculitis).
    a. Digital ischemia.
    b. Butterfly rash.
    c. Palpable purpura.
  2. Maculopapular rash (allergic interstitial nephritis).
  3. Track marks (intravenous drug abuse).
  4. Mucosal or cartilaginous lesions (Wegener granulomatosis).
  5. Skin turgor (hypovolemia).
B. Ophthalmic examination.
  1. Conjunctival jaundice (liver disease).
  2. Band keratopathy (hypercalcemia, multiple myeloma).
  3. Papilledema or flame-shaped hemorrhages (malignant hypertension).
  4. Atheroemboli (cholesterol microemboli)
  5. Uveitis (vasculitis).
  6. Ocular palsy (ethylene glycol poisoning).
C. Ears.
  1. Hearing acuity/hearing loss (aminoglycoside toxicity, Alport disease).
D. Cardiovascular system.
  1. Assessment of volume status (intra- and extravascular volume).
    a. BP and pulse: Sitting and standing.
    b. Jugular vein distention (volume overload, heart failure).
    c. S3 heart sounds (HF).
    d. Peripheral/dependent edema.
    e. Hourly intake and output records.
    f. Daily weight.
  2. Heart rate/rhythm.
    a. Atrial fibrillation (thromboembolism, decreased cardiac output).
    b. Murmurs (endocarditis).
    c. Pericardial friction rub (pericarditis).

▶

E. Pulmonary system.
   1. Auscultation of lung sounds.
      a. Pulmonary vascular congestion (volume overload, congestive heart failure [CHF]).
      b. Crackles (pulmonary edema, volume overload, pulmonary infection, pulmonary-renal syndromes).
   2. Hemoptysis (antineutrophil cytoplasmic antibodies [ANCA] vasculitis, anti-glomerular basement membrane [anti-GBM] syndrome, Goodpasture syndrome).
   3. Respiratory rate and effort (CHF, volume overload).
F. Abdomen.
   1. Pulsatile mass or bruit (atheroemboli, renal artery stenosis).
   2. Abdominal or costovertebral angle tenderness (CVAT; nephrolithiasis, renal artery thrombosis, renal vein thrombosis).
   3. Abdominal fluid wave (ascites, cirrhosis, or elevated intra-abdominal pressure).
   4. Signs of urinary obstruction (pelvic/rectal masses, prostatic hypertrophy, distended bladder).

DIAGNOSTIC TESTS

A. Comprehensive blood chemistry panel.
   1. Kidney function tests.
   2. Electrolytes.
   3. Glucose level.
   4. Liver function tests.
B. Complete blood count (CBC).
   1. Anemia.
C. Renal ultrasound.
   1. Rule out hydronephrosis.
   2. Assess kidney size.
D. 24-hour urine for creatinine clearance.
   1. Gives an accurate assessment of current renal clearance.
   2. SCr is a later indicator of renal dysfunction.
E. Urinalysis with microscopy.
   1. Granular, muddy casts (ATN).
   2. Oxalate crystals (ATN).
   3. Eosinophils (interstitial nephritis).
F. Urine sodium and osmolality.
   1. Fractional excretion of sodium (FENa).
      a. FENa helps differentiate the cause of AKI in the presence of oliguria.
         i. FENa less than 1% is usually prerenal AKI.
         ii. FENa greater than 1% is usually ATN.
G. Urine albumin to creatinine ratio (UACR).
H. Hourly UO.
   1. Nonoliguric AKI.
   2. Oliguric AKI.
   3. Anuric AKI.
I. Chest x-ray.
   1. Volume overload.
   2. Infectious process.
   3. Vasculitis.
J. Renal biopsy.
   1. May be indicated if the cause cannot be determined, renal function does not return for a prolonged period of time, and/or results guide the course of treatment.
I. Further testing depends on the suspected cause of AKI.
   1. ANCA.
   2. Anti-GBM antibodies.
   3. Antinuclear antibodies (ANA).
   4. Anti-double-stranded DNA (anti-dsDNA) antibodies.
   5. Complement factors.
   6. Rheumatoid factor.
   7. Cryoglobulins.
   8. Serum and urine protein electrophoresis (SPEP, UPEP).
   9. Immunoglobulins.
   10. Serum free light chains.
   11. Hepatitis B and C and HIV serologies.

DIFFERENTIAL DIAGNOSIS

A. Prerenal.
   1. Hypovolemia.
      a. Volume depletion.
      b. Hemorrhage.
      c. Renal fluid loss (overdiuresis).
      d. Gastrointestinal (GI) fluid losses (vomiting, diarrhea).
      e. Third spacing (muscle trauma, burns, peritonitis).
   2. Impaired cardiac function.
      a. HF.
      b. Acute coronary syndrome.
      c. Massive pulmonary embolus.
      d. Cardiogenic shock.
   3. Systemic vasodilation.
      a. Antihypertensive medications.
      b. Gram-negative bacteremia.
      c. Cirrhosis.
      d. Septic shock.
      e. Anaphylaxis.
   4. Increased vascular resistance.
      a. NSAIDs.
      b. RAAS inhibitors.
      c. Anesthesia.
      d. Hepatorenal syndrome.
B. Intrarenal AKI results from structural damage to any component of the renal parenchyma.
   1. Tubular.
      a. Renal ischemia.
      b. Nephrotoxic drugs.
      c. Endogenous toxins.
      d. Exogenous toxins.
   2. Glomerular.
      a. Glomerulonephritis (e.g., postinfectious).
      b. Lupus nephritis.
      c. Anti-GBM disease.
   3. Interstitial.
      a. Infections.
         i. Bacterial.
         ii. Viral.

b. Medications.
  i. NSAIDs.
  ii. Antibiotics.
  iii. Diuretics.
4. Vascular.
  a. Large vessel.
    i. Renal artery stenosis (bilateral).
    ii. Renal vein thrombosis (bilateral).
  b. Small vessel.
    i. Vasculitis.
    ii. Thrombotic emboli.
    iii. Hemolytic uremic syndrome (HUS).
    iv. Thrombotic thrombocytopenic purpura (TTP).

C. Postrenal AKI results from a shift in filtration forces caused by urinary tract obstruction.
  1. Extrarenal obstruction.
    a. Prostate hypertrophy.
    b. Cancer.
      i. Bladder.
      ii. Prostate.
      iii. Cervical.
  2. Intrarenal obstruction.
    a. Nephrolithiasis.
    b. Papillary necrosis.
    c. Blood clots.
    d. Medications.
      i. Acyclovir.
      ii. Methotrexate.

EVALUATION AND MANAGEMENT PLAN

A. Identify at-risk patients.
  1. CKD history.
  2. BP assessment.
  3. SCr level.
  4. Urine dipstick.
  5. Medication review/reconciliation.
B. Correct hypovolemia.
  1. Individualized fluid therapy.
  2. Monitor fluid balance.
  3. Isotonic saline.
  4. Albumin.

C. Maintain blood pressure (mean arterial pressure >65 mmHg).
  1. Vasopressor support.
D. Discontinue/adjust medication.
  1. NSAIDs.
  2. RAAS inhibitors.
  3. IV contrast.
  4. Metformin.
  5. Aminoglycosides.
  6. Vancomycin.
E. KRT.
  1. Indications.
    a. Include anuria, severe/refractory hyperkalemia, severe/refractory metabolic acidosis, and refractory volume overload.
  2. Type of KRT.
    a. Patient status, treatment availability, staff availability, and expertise.
    b. Continuous renal/kidney replacement therapy (CRRT/CKRT).
    c. Most common therapy in critical care setting.
    d. Intermittent hemodialysis (IHD).
    e. Peritoneal dialysis (PD).
F. General plan.
  1. Use the ABCDE-IT mnemonic to quickly determine a treatment plan (Box 5.1).
  2. Determine the stage of AKI using the KDIGO criteria and manage accordingly.
  3. Monitor SCr.
  4. Avoid further renal insult.
  5. Ensure that BP is in the target range (patient's age and comorbidities, BP guidelines).
  6. Correct fluid overload to achieve volume homeostasis.
  7. Correct any acidosis or electrolyte abnormalities.
G. Patient/family teaching points.
  1. Signs/symptoms to monitor: Edema, headache, dizziness, or syncope.
  2. Common occurrences: Hypotension or hypertension.
  3. Readmission concerns.
    a. Recurrent AKI due to secondary renal insult that is often due to inappropriate resumption ▶

BOX 5.1 ACUTE KIDNEY INJURY ABCDE-IT MNEMONIC

Assess for acute complications (high potassium, acidosis, fluid overload)
BP check (if systolic BP <110, consider fluid challenge)
Catheterize (to eliminate postbladder obstructive process and monitor intake and output)
Drugs; stop/avoid nephrotoxins, hold ACE RAAS inhibitors
Exclude obstruction (renal US)
Investigations; urinalysis with microscopy, for stage 2/3 AKI add ANCA, Anti-GBM Ab, dsDNA, ANA, immunoglobulin, serum and protein electrophoresis
Treat the cause

Ab, antibodies; ACE, angiotensin-converting enzyme; AKI, acute kidney injury; ANA, antinuclear antibody; ANCA; antineutrophil cytoplasmic antibodies; BP, blood pressure; dsDNA, double-stranded DNA; GBM, glomerular basement membrane; RAAS, renin–angiotensin–aldosterone system; US, ultrasound.

of medications (RAAS inhibitors, NSAIDs) or hypotension/hypertension.

b. Patients should be clear about which medications to hold/restart after discharge and check home BP. If the patient is able to check home BP, provide high and low parameters for reporting readings.

c. These parameters will vary according to the clinical context, comorbidities, and risk factors for both CV disease and recurrent AKI.

d. Renal vasculature is sensitive to BP fluctuations in the recovery phase of AKI, and hypotension or hypertension can precipitate further renal injury.

H. Pharmacotherapy.

1. No pharmacotherapy treatment in AKI. The primary cause must be reversed.

2. IV isotonic sodium chloride solution should be used to maintain euvolemia as clinically indicated.

3. Medications.

a. Hold RAAS inhibitors, NSAIDs, and any other medications associated with renal insult (e.g., nephrotoxic chemotherapy, aminoglycoside, and beta-lactam antibiotics) until patient's SCr has stabilized.

I. Discharge instructions.

1. Based on the trajectory of AKI and kidney function.

a. Has returned to baseline. *OR*

b. Continues to improve. *OR*

c. Remains in acute kidney disease (AKD).

i. Acute or subacute damage and/or loss of kidney function.

ii. Duration between 7 and 90 days after exposure of AKI-initiating event has progressed to CKD.

iii. The persistence of kidney damage for a period of longer than 90 days.

FOLLOW-UP

A. Nephrology appointment postdischarge.

1. Timing of follow-up appointment depends on:

a. Cause of AKI.

b. Severity of AKI.

c. Trajectory of kidney function.

i. Recovery.

ii. AKD.

iii. CKD.

iv. End-stage kidney disease (ESKD).

B. Monitor.

1. Kidney function.

a. Renal function panel.

i. SCr and eGFR.

ii. Electrolytes.

b. Check creatinine within 1 to 2 weeks after discharge to confirm improvement.

c. SCr at 3 months postdischarge may be a better indicator of renal recovery.

d. Urine studies.

i. Albuminuria/proteinuria.

ii. UACR.

e. Medication review/reconciliation.

i. Determine if/when medications should be restarted.

ii. Adjust medications per eGFR.

f. Prevent recurrent AKI episode.

i. Identify patients at risk.

e. Prevent CKD progression.

i. Kidney function at time of discharge.

1) AKI recovery.

2) AKD.

3) CKD.

a) CKD stage.

b) Clinical action plan.

C. Pursue other follow-up as indicated specific to the underlying cause(s) of the AKI, AKI-associated complications, patient's comorbidities, and risk factors for recurrent AKI.

CONSULTATION/REFFERAL

A. Early nephrology consultation should occur after hospitalization.

SPECIAL/GERIATRIC CONSIDERATIONS

A. Geriatric considerations.

1. Kidney function declines with age-related changes within the kidneys.

a. Changes in the older kidney include loss of renal reserve and decline in GFR.

b. Age is an independent risk factor for AKI and for both short- and long-term adverse outcomes.

2. Older patients have comorbidities that increase their risk for AKI, for example, HTN, diabetes mellitus (DM), and CVD.

3. They are at high risk for AKI from medications used to treat comorbidities (RAAS inhibitors, diuretics, sodium-glucose cotransporter inhibitors, NSAIDs) as well as from polypharmacy.

4. SCr in older patients with diminished muscle mass underestimates the extent of renal impairment.

CASE SCENARIO: ACUTE KIDNEY INJURY

A 58-year-old male presents to the ED with gradual worsening of generalized weakness over the past 2 weeks. He reports muscle aches in both legs, increased fatigue, and dyspnea on exertion. He also noticed decreased urine output (UO) and increased swelling in his legs. His medical history includes hypertension, hypercholesterolemia, and chronic low back pain. He saw his primary care provider approximately 4 weeks ago. At that visit, his blood pressure (BP) medication dose was increased, he was started on medication for his cholesterol, and he was given a 10-day course of a muscle relaxant. He denies nausea, vomiting, chest discomfort, or shortness of breath at rest. His vital signs include temperature of 97.1°F/36.1°C, BP of 181/90, pulse rate of 108 beats per minute, and respiratory rate of 18 breaths per minute. Pulse oximeter is 97% on room air. Cardiovascular, pulmonary, and abdominal examinations are normal. Musculoskeletal exam shows evidence of bilateral lower extremity weakness, with the patient showing difficulty when trying to stand from a sitting position. The patient's current medications include lisinopril (Zestril) 10 mg PO daily, cyclobenzaprine (Flexeril) 5 mg PO TID PRN, ezetimibe (Zetia) 10 mg PO daily, rosuvastatin (Crestor) 20 mg PO daily, and ibuprofen (Motrin) 400 mg PO Q8H PRN. His laboratory results show sodium of 132 mEq/L, potassium of 4.0 mEq/L, chloride of 85 mEq/L, carbon dioxide of 14 mEq/L, blood urea nitrogen (BUN) of 82 mg/dL, creatinine of 9.23 mg/dL, creatine kinase (CK) of 86,000 U/L, and serum myoglobin of 453,120 ng/mL. Urinalysis is positive for blood with 0 to 2 red blood cells (RBCs) on microscopy. He is diagnosed with acute kidney injury (AKI) secondary to rhabdomyolysis and admitted to the hospital.

1. Based on the patient's history and findings, the MOST likely etiology of the patient's acute kidney injury (AKI) is:

A. Lisinopril.

B. Ibuprofen.

C. Cyclobenzaprine.

D. Rosuvastatin.

BIBLIOGRAPHY

Andonovic, M., Traynor, J. P., Shaw, M., Sim, M. A. B., Mark, P. B., & Puxty, K. A. (2022). Short- and long-term outcomes of intensive care patients with acute kidney disease. *EClinicalMedicine, 44*, 101291. https://doi.org/10.1016/j.eclinm.2022101291

Chen, Y. S., Chou, C. Y., & Chen, A. L. P. (2020). Early prediction of acquiring acute kidney injury for older inpatients using most effective laboratory test results. *BMC Medical Informatics and Decision Making, 20*(1), 36. https://doi.org/10.1186/s12911-020-1050-2

Forde, C., McCaughan, J., & Leonard, N. (2012). Acute kidney injury: It's as easy as ABCDE. *BMJ Quality Improvement Reports, 1*(1), u200370. w326. https://doi.org/10.1136/bmjquality.u200370.w326

Gameiro, J., Fonseco, J. A., Outerelo, C., & Lopes, J. A. (2020). Acute kidney injury: From diagnosis to treatment strategies. *Journal of Clinical Medicine, 9*(6), 1704. https://doi.org/10.3390/jcm9061704

Ivica, J., Sanmugalingham, G., & Selvaratnam, R. (2022). Alerting to acute kidney injury—Challenges, benefits, and strategies. *Practical Laboratory Medicine, 30*, e00270. https://doi.org/10.1016/j.plabm.2022.e00270

Jamme, M., Legrand, M., & Geri, G. (2021). Outcome of acute kidney injury: How to make a difference. *Annals of Intensive Care, 11*(1), 60. https://doi.org/10.1186/s13613-021-00849-x

Kashani, K., Rosner, M. H., Haase, M., Lewington, A., O'Donoghue, D. J., Wilson, F. P., Nadim, M. K., Siver, S. A., Zarbock, A., Ostermann, M., Mehta, R. L., Kane-Gill, S. L., Ding, X., Pickkers, P., Bihorac, A., Siew, E. D., Barreto, E. F., Macedo, E., Kellum, J. A., . . . Wu, V. C. (2019). Quality improvement goals for acute kidney injury. *Clinical Journal of the American Society of Nephrology, 14*(6), 941–953. https://doi.org/10.2215/CJN.01250119

Kellum, J. A., Romagnani, P., Ashuntantang, G., Ronco, C., Zarbock, A., & Anders, H. J. (2021). Acute kidney injury. *Nature Reviews Disease Primers, 7*(1), 52. https://doi.org/10.1038/s41572-021-00284-z

Kidney Disease: Improving Global Outcomes (KDIGO) Acute Kidney Injury Work Group. (2012). KDIGO clinical practice guideline for acute kidney injury. *Kidney International Supplement, 2*(1), 1–138. https://doi.org/10.1038/kisup.2012.1

Koyner, J. L., Topf, J. M., & Lerma, E. V. (2021). *Handbook of critical care nephrology.* Wolters Kluwer.

Lamiere, N. (2022). Reflections on the KDIGO definition of acute kidney injury and its integration in the concept of acute diseases and disorders and chronic kidney disease. *Kidney and Dialysis, 2*, 68–79. https://doi.org/10.3390/kidneydial2010008

Lamiere, N. H., Levin, A., Kellum, J. A., Cheung, M., Jadoul, M., Winkelmayer, W. C., & Stevens, P. E. (2021). Harmonizing acute and chronic kidney disease definition and classification: Report of a Kidney Disease: Improving Global Outcomes (KDIGO) consensus conference. *Kidney International, 100*(3), 516–526. https://doi.org/10.1016/j.kint.2021.06.028

Levey, A. S. (2022). Defining AKD: The spectrum of AKI, AKD, and CKD. *Nephron, 146*(3), 302–305. https://doi.org/10.1159/000516647

Liu, K. D., Forni, L. G., Heung, M., Wu, V. C., Kellum, J. A., Mehta, R. L., Ronco, C., Kashani, K., Rosner, M. H., Haase, M., Koyner, J. L., & Acute Disease Quality Initiative Investigators. (2020). Quality of care for acute kidney disease: Current knowledge gaps and future directions. *Kidney International Reports, 5*(10), 1634–1642. https://doi.org/10.1016/j.ekir.2020.07.031

Liu, K. D., Goldstein, S. L., Vijayan, A., Parikh, C. R., Kashani, K., Okusa, M. D., Agarwal, A., & Cerda, J., & AKI!Now Initiative of the American Society of Nephrology. (2020). *AKI!Now* initiative: Recommendations for awareness, recognition, and management of AKI. *Clinical Journal of the American Society of Nephrology, 15*(12), 1838–1847. https://doi.org/10.2215/CJN.15611219

Mansoor, K., Kheetan, M., Shahnawaz, S., Shapiro, A. P., Patton-Tackett, E., Dial, L., Rankin, G., Santhanam, P., Tzamaloukas, A. H., Nadasdy, T., Shapiron, J. I., & Khitan, Z. J. (2017). Systematic review of nephrotoxicity of drugs of abuse, 2005–2016. *BMC Nephrology, 18*, 379. https://doi.org/10.1186/s12882-017-0794-0

Ostermann, M., Bellomo, R., Burdmann, E. A., Doi, K., Endre, Z. H., Goldstein, S. L., Kane-Gill, S. L., Liu, K. D., Prowle, J. R., Shaw, A. D., Srisawat, N., Cheung, M., Jadoul, M., Winkelmayer, W. C., Kellum, J. A., & Conference Participants. (2020). Controversies in acute kidney injury: Conclusions from a Kidney Disease: Improving Global Outcomes (KDIGO) conference. *Kidney International, 98*(2), 294–309. https://doi.org/10.1016/j.kint.2020.04.020

Pickkers, P., Darmon, M., Hoste, E., Joannidis, M., Legrand, M., Ostermann, M., Prowle, J. R., Schneider, A., & Schetz, M. (2021). Acute kidney injury in the critically ill: An updated review on pathophysiology and management. *Intensive Care Medicine, 47*(8), 835–850. https://doi.org/10.1007/s00134-021-06454-7

Tsang, J. Y., Murray, J., Kingdon, E., Tomson, C., Hallas, K., Campbell, S., & Blakeman, T. (2020). Guidance for post-discharge care following acute kidney injury: An appropriateness ratings evaluation. *BJGP Open, 4*(3), bjgopen20X10154. https://doi.org/10.3399/bjgpopen20X101054

Workeneh, B. T., & Batman, V. (2022). *Acute kidney injury (AKI)* emedicine.medscape.com https://emedicine.medscape.com/article/243492-print

Wu, M. J., Huang, S. C., Chen, C. H., Cheng, C. Y., & Tsai, S. F. (2022). An early warning system for the differential diagnosis of in-hospital acute kidney injury for better patient outcome: Study of quality improvement imitative. *International Journal of Environmental Research and Public Health, 19*(6), 3704. https://doi.org/10.3390/ijerph19063704

BENIGN PROSTATIC HYPERTROPHY

Suzanne Barron

DEFINITION

A. A histologic change that develops within the prostate gland which may lead to the presence of an enlarged prostate gland and associated lower urinary tract symptoms (LUTS).

INCIDENCE

A. The prevalence of benign prostatic hypertrophy (BPH) increases with age.

　1. BPH begins to develop before age 30, with almost 10% of men having BPH by 40 years of age and 50% of men showing evidence by age 60.

　2. Nearly 80% of men will develop BPH, with 30% of men receiving treatment for symptoms.

PATHOGENESIS

A. There is abnormal microscopic hyperplasia and macroscopic growth.

B. The detrusor muscle generates higher pressures, leading to frequency, urgency, and nocturia.

▶

C. BPH may lead to bladder decompensation, with the bladder muscle no longer able to provide enough pressure to urinate.

D. The role of hormonal involvement in the development of BPH is still poorly understood, but there is evidence that the hormone androgen, which becomes dihydrotestosterone (DHT), plays a critical role in the growth of prostatic tissue.

PREDISPOSING FACTORS

A. Advancing age.

B. Family history of BPH.

C. Ethnic background.

  1. The risk of BPH is higher in Black and Hispanic men than in White and Asian men.

D. Diabetes and heart disease: Possible increased incidence in BPH.

E. Obesity: Possible association with increased prostate volume and LUTS.

SUBJECTIVE DATA

A. Common complaints/symptoms.

  1. LUTS.

    a. Storage symptoms or irritative voiding symptoms: Frequency, nocturia, dysuria, decreased volume, urgency, or urge incontinence.

    b. Voiding symptoms or obstructive voiding symptoms: Weak stream, intermittent stream, hesitancy, retention, abdominal straining, incomplete emptying, or postvoid dribbling.

B. Common/typical scenario.

  1. Onset is gradual, with symptoms increasing over time.

  2. Symptoms are often aggravated at night with significant nocturia, which may often cause difficulty sleeping.

  3. Symptoms may be aggravated by cough/cold medications (antihistamines, pseudoephedrine).

C. Family and social history.

  1. Increased likelihood if father or brother have history of BPH.

  2. Increased physical activity: Possible protection against BPH.

D. Review of systems.

  1. Constitutional: Weight loss or insomnia.

  2. Neurologic: Dizziness, weakness, tremors, or other signs that may indicate a neurologic condition, such as multiple sclerosis or Parkinson disease.

  3. Genitourinary (GU): LUTS; usually no flank pain.

    a. Possible report of suprapubic fullness/tenderness.

    b. Hematuria: Possible indication of GU malignancy (bladder cancer).

  4. Cardiovascular: Lower extremity edema that may indicate heart failure or diuretic use.

  5. Endocrine: Polyuria, polyphagia, or polydipsia that may indicate diabetes mellitus or diabetes insipidus (DI).

PHYSICAL EXAMINATION

A. Neurologic.

  1. Evaluate for musculoskeletal weakness, especially lower extremity motor and sensory function.

  2. Evaluate gait.

B. Digital rectal examination (DRE).

  1. To estimate prostate size, assess for prostatitis or evaluate prostate nodules that may indicate prostate cancer.

  2. Assess for anal sphincter tone; if absent or decreased, possible neurologic disorder.

C. Abdominal.

  1. Palpate for masses that may be pressing on the bladder.

D. GU.

  1. Assess for costovertebral angle tenderness (CVAT).

  2. Assess for obvious urethral strictures and phimosis.

DIAGNOSTIC TESTS

A. Urinalysis to exclude hematuria or possible infection.

B. Bloodwork.

  1. Prostate-specific antigen (PSA), especially if prostatic nodules are palpated on DRE or there is high concern for prostate cancer.

  2. Basic metabolic panel to assess for renal function, electrolyte abnormalities, and hyperglycemia.

C. Imaging: CT or MRI generally not indicated.

D. Uroflowmetry: Measures the volume/time of urine accumulation.

E. Postvoid residual: Volume of urine remaining in the bladder after voiding.

  1. Obtain from bladder ultrasound/bladder scan if possible.

  2. Straight catheterization if bladder ultrasound not available.

F. Urodynamic study to differentiate between bladder outlet obstruction and hypocontractile bladder. This may be necessary prior to surgical intervention for BPH.

DIFFERENTIAL DIAGNOSIS

A. Foreign body in urethra/bladder (stone or retained ureteral stents).

B. Meatal stenosis.

C. Urethral stricture.

D. Detrusor sphincter dyssynergia.

E. Neurogenic bladder (e.g., multiple sclerosis, Parkinson disease).

F. Bladder cancer.

G. Prostate cancer.

H. Overactive bladder.

I. Interstitial cystitis.

J. Infectious source: Acute cystitis, acute prostatitis/chronic prostatitis, or prostatic abscess.

K. Pelvic floor dysfunction.

L. Radiation cystitis.

M. DI causing polyuria.

N. Diabetes mellitus causing polyuria.

EVALUATION AND MANAGEMENT PLAN

A. General plan.

   1. Obtain urinalysis/urine culture.

   2. Obtain PSA if there is concern for prostate cancer.

   3. Determine the severity of LUTS and its impact on the quality of life with questionnaires such as the International Prostate Symptom Score (IPSS).

   4. Place Foley catheter for urinary retention or teach patient how to perform clean intermittent catheterization.

   5. Observe for postobstructive diuresis with urinary retention.

   6. Advise watchful waiting, with no treatment for men with mild symptoms and good quality of life.

   7. Use pharmacotherapy: Alpha-blockers or 5-alpha-reductase inhibitors (5-ARIs).

   8. Obtain prostate biopsy if elevated PSA or prostatic nodule.

   9. Order uroflowmetry/postvoid residual.

   10. Order urodynamic study if indicated.

   11. Referral to urology for surgery if indicated.

B. Patient/family teaching points.

   1. Have a thorough discussion with patient and family about the usefulness of PSA screening test in detecting prostate cancer.

   a. If the PSA is elevated, this will prompt prostate biopsy and possible treatment for prostate cancer, which may be a slow-growing disease.

   b. In 2010, the U.S. Preventive Services Task Force recommended against PSA screening, stating that the test has no net benefit and that the harms outweigh the benefits. The American Urological Association in 2013 also started to recommend against routine cancer screening.

   2. Discuss keeping a voiding diary.

   3. Discuss possible side effects of medical therapy, including orthostatic hypotension, dizziness, and retrograde ejaculation.

   4. Educate the patient with retention on how to perform clean intermittent catheterization because this is a better alternative to an indwelling Foley catheter.

   5. Avoid becoming constipated because this aggravates symptoms.

C. Pharmacotherapy.

   1. First-line therapy: Alpha-1-adrenergic receptor blockers (alpha-blockers); medication will rapidly relax the smooth muscles of the bladder neck and prostate without impairing bladder body contractility.

   a. Most commonly used: Tamsulosin 0.4 mg daily (max 0.8 mg daily).

   b. Side effects include hypotension, dizziness, retrograde ejaculation, ejaculatory dysfunction, and floppy iris syndrome (occurs in patients undergoing cataract surgery).

   2. 5-ARIs; medication works by shrinking the prostate by decreasing the production of the DHT hormone.

   a. Best for larger prostate glands (>40 mL).

   b. Most commonly used: Finasteride 5 mg.

   c. May take up to 6 months to see full effect. Prostate can regrow as soon as medication is stopped.

   d. Normally used in combination with alpha-blockers as combination therapy has greater efficacy in reducing the risk of urinary retention and the need for prostate-related surgery.

   e. Side effects include decreased libido, gynecomastia, and erectile dysfunction.

   3. Antimuscarinic agents, which help with bladder overactivity.

   a. Most commonly used: Oxybutynin 5 mg TID.

   4. Phosphodiesterase-5 inhibitor, tadalafil (Cialis), which is Food and Drug Administration (FDA)-approved for LUTS secondary to BPH.

   a. Can be used as initial therapy if patient has erectile dysfunction.

   b. Tadalafil (Cialis): 2.5 to 5 mg; contraindicated in men taking nitrates, nonselective alpha-blockers, and cytochrome P450 inhibitors.

D. Discharge instructions.

   1. Advise patients to limit caffeine, fluids, and alcohol. These may increase LUTS.

   2. Advise them to avoid cold medications, antihistamines, and pseudoephedrine.

   3. Advise them to seek medical attention if they are unable to void or have flank pain, gross hematuria, or passage of clots.

   4. Advise them to discontinue alpha-blockers with dizziness, lightheadedness, or falls.

FOLLOW-UP

A. Monitor response to treatment with uroflowmetry, postvoid residual, and presence of symptoms.

B. Advise that urodynamic studies may be indicated if there is no improvement of symptoms with medical therapy.

C. Advise that surgery may provide relief in the case of excessive symptoms refractory to medical management. Some of the more common options include:

   1. Transurethral resection of the prostate (TURP).

   2. Holmium laser enucleation of the prostate (HoLEP).

   3. Simple prostatectomy for large prostates greater than 100 mL.

CONSULTATION/REFFERAL

A. Urology.

   1. Urinary retention.

   2. Hematuria/clot retention.

   3. PSA elevation will need prostate biopsy.

   4. Suspected GU malignancy.

   5. Failed medical treatment with moderate to severe symptoms.

B. Neurology.

   1. With any concern for neurologic condition that may be causing LUTS.

C. Endocrinology.

   1. For hyperglycemia.

   2. Concern for DI.

SPECIAL/GERIATRIC CONSIDERATIONS

A. Many patients limit fluids due to symptoms; this may lead to dehydration, especially in geriatric individuals. Assess for dehydration and provide education to maintain normal fluid intake.

B. Monitor the geriatric population for medication side effects.

  1. Alpha-blockers: Hypotension and dizziness.

  2. Antimuscarinic agents: Dry mouth, constipation, and mental status changes.

    a. Monitor for polypharmacy with other possible anticholinergic medications that patients may be prescribed or taking over the counter.

    b. Studies have shown that transdermal oxybutynin and the newer anticholinergics may be better tolerated.

CASE SCENARIO: BENIGN PROSTATIC HYPERTROPHY

A 65-year-old African American male is s/p left total knee replacement yesterday. His past medical history (PMH) includes coronary artery disease with percutaneous transluminal coronary angioplasty (PTCA) with stents about 2 years ago, sleep apnea, and lumbar disc disease. Postoperatively, the patient required intermittent straight catheterization due to urinary retention. He is taking narcotic pain medication and reports constipation. He has not had a bowel movement in over 5 days. Prior to admission for surgery, the patient reports that he has significant nocturia and wakes up about five times at night to void. He denies urinary incontinence, hematuria, flank pain, fevers, or erectile dysfunction. He states he had a prostate-specific antigen (PSA) taken about 6 months ago and it was within normal limits. He also reports that his primary care provider performed a digital rectal examination and that he had an enlarged, smooth prostate without nodules. A urinalysis was sent yesterday and was within normal limits. Urine culture is pending. The patient is stable for discharge home otherwise and the orthopedic team is planning on discharging the patient home with a Foley catheter, with plans to see urology in the next week.

1. What medication should be considered first in treating this patient?

  A. Beta-blocker such as Tenormin

  B. Alpha-blocker such as tamsulosin

  C. Stool softener and laxative such as docusate sodium and senna

  D. Phosophodiesterase-5 inhibitor such as sildenafil

BIBLIOGRAPHY

Deters, L. A. (2019, January 15). Benign prostatic hypertrophy (BPH) differential diagnoses. In E. D. Kim (Ed.), *Medscape* http://emedicine.medscape.com/article/437359-differential

Kim, E. H., Larson, J. A., & Andriole, G. L. (2016). Management of benign prostatic hyperplasia. *Annual Review of Medicine, 67*, 137–151. https://doi.org/10.1146/annurev-med-063014-123902

Nicholson, T., & Ricke, W. (2011 November–December). Androgens and estrogens in benign prostatic hyperplasia, past, present and future. *National Institutes of Health, 82*(4–5), 184–189. https://www.ncbi.nlm.nih.gov/pmc/articles/PMC3179830

Siddiqui, M. (2022, January). *Medical student curriculum: Benign prostatic hypertrophy (BPH)–American Urological Association.* https://www.auanet.org/education/auauniversity/for-medical-students/medical-students-curriculym/medical-student-curriculum/bph

Yu, Z., Yan, H., Xu, F., Chao, H., Deng, L., Xu, X., Huang, J., & Zeng, T. (2020, May). Efficacy and side effects of drugs commonly used for the treatment of lower urinary tract symptoms with benign prostatic hyperplasia. *Frontiers in Pharmacology.* https://doi.org/10.3389/fphar2020.00658

CHRONIC KIDNEY DISEASE

Christine Chmielewski

DEFINITION

A. Reduction of kidney function: An estimated glomerular filtration rate (eGFR) less than 60 mL/min/1.73 m² for greater than 3 months. *OR*

B. Evidence of kidney damage, including persistent albuminuria, defined as greater than 30 mg of urine albumin per gram of urine creatinine for greater than 3 months.

  1. Anatomic abnormalities including, but not limited to, polycystic kidneys, kidney transplant, and genetic abnormalities.

  2. Chronic kidney disease (CKD) versus acute kidney injury (AKI). A 3-month time frame is used to distinguish CKD from AKI.

C. Classification.

  1. CKD stages are defined by presence of albuminuria and the eGFR (Table 5.1).

  2. The preferred equation is the 2021 Chronic Kidney Disease Epidemiology (CKD-EPI) creatinine equation.

    a. Variables include sex, age, and serum creatinine (SCr).

      i. https://www.uptodate.com/contents/calculator-glomerular-filtration-rate-gfr-by-ckd-epi-equation-in-adults.

    b. Race is no longer included in the equation.

INCIDENCE

A. It is estimated that approximately 15% of adults in the United States have CKD (CDC, 2021).

B. Approximately 9 out of 10 adults with CKD are unaware that they have CKD.

C. Approximately 2 out of 5 adults with severely reduced kidney function are unaware that they have CKD.

D. Approximately 786,000 individuals in the United States have end-stage renal disease (ESRD); of these, 71% are on dialysis and 29% have a functioning kidney transplant.

PATHOGENESIS

A. Initial kidney injury or insult leads to loss of functioning nephrons (nephron loss).

B. Hyperfiltration of the remaining intact nephrons occurs (glomerular hypertrophy/adaptive hyperfiltration).

C. Initially beneficial, adaptive hyperfiltration leads to ongoing damage (interstitial inflammation, fibrosis, and endothelial/vascular injury).

D. This injury eventually leads to further nephron loss (disease progression).

TABLE 5.1   STAGES OF CKD WITH MONITORING RECOMMENDATIONS

CKD classified based on: • GFR (G) • Albuminuria (A) KDIGO 2012				Albuminuria Categories: Description and Range		
				A1	**A2**	**A3**
				Normal to Mildly Increased	**Moderately Increased**	**Severely Increased**
				<30 mg/g **<3 mg/mmol**	**30–299 mg/g** **3–29 mg/mmol**	**≥300 mg/g** **≥30 mg/mmol**
GFR Categories (/min/1.73 m²): Description and Range	G1	Normal or high	≥90	Monitor 1	Monitor 1	Refer* 2
	G2	Mildly decreased	60–90	Monitor 1	Monitor 1	Refer* 2
	G3a	Mildly to moderately decreased	45–59	Monitor 1	Monitor 2	Refer 3
	G3b	Moderately to severely decreased	30–44	Monitor 2	Monitor 3	Refer 3
	G4	Severely decreased	15–29	Referᵃ 3	Referᵃ 3	Referᵃ 4+
	G5	Kidney failure	<15	Referᵃ 4+	Referᵃ 4+	Referᵃ 4+

Shades: Represents the risk for progression, morbidity, and mortality by shades, from best to worst. **White:** Low risk (if no other markers of kidney disease, no CKD). **Light gray:** Moderately increased risk. **Medium gray:** High risk. **Dark gray:** Very high risk. **Black:** High risk +4 times per year. The numbers represent a recommendation for the number of times per year the patient should be monitored. *Refer* indicates that nephrology referral and services are recommended.
ᵃReferring clinicians may wish to discuss with their nephrology service depending on local arrangements regarding monitoring or referral.
CKD, chronic kidney disease; GFR, glomerular filtration rate; KDIGO, Kidney Disease: Improving Global Outcomes.
Source: Modified with permission from KDIGO. (2012). Clinical practice guideline for the evaluation and management of chronic kidney disease. *Kidney International, 2013*(Suppl. 3), 1–150.

PREDISPOSING FACTORS
A. General risk factors.
  1. Diabetes mellitus.
  2. Hypertension.
  3. Cardiovascular disease (CVD).
  4. History of kidney disease.
  5. Family history of CKD.
  6. Race/ethnicity.
    a. African American.
    b. Hispanic.
    c. Native American.
    d. Asian.
  7. AKI.
  8. Older age.
  9. Smoking.
  10. Exposure to nephrotoxins.
  11. Obesity.
B. Risk factors for progression of CKD to next stage.
  1. Male sex.
  2. African American race.
  3. Diabetes mellitus.
  4. Hypertension.
  5. Proteinuria.
  6. Prior trajectory of kidney function.

SUBJECTIVE DATA
A. Common complaints/symptoms.
  1. Often silent.
  2. Lethargy/fatigue due to low hemoglobin.
  3. Metallic taste (dysgeusia)/anorexia due to uremia.
  4. Increased incidence of confusion with uremia.
  5. Edema.
B. Medication history.
  1. Medication review.
    a. Prescription drugs.
    b. Over-the-counter drugs.
    c. Herbal supplements.
  2. Medication-associated risk.
    a. Clearance by kidneys.
    b. Narrow therapeutic window.
    c. High risk in older population.
      i. Increased adverse events.
    d. Drug dosing data availability.
      i. Nephrotoxicity.
        1) Discontinue/avoid nephrotoxins.
      ii. Renal clearance.
        1) Adjust dose.
        2) Adjust administration schedule.
C. Review of systems.
  1. Constitutional: Change in activity and appetite changes.
  2. Head, ear, eyes, nose, and throat (HEENT): Changes in vision, facial swelling, and nosebleeds.
  3. Cardiovascular: Any pain in the chest, palpitations, irregular heart rate, and lower extremity swelling.
  4. Respiratory: Difficulty breathing and cough.
  5. Gastrointestinal (GI): Nausea or vomiting, loss of appetite, metallic taste, hiccups, and blood in stool.

6. Genitourinary (GU): Difficulty urinating, pain on urination, blood in urine, foam in urine, decreased urine volume, and nocturia.

7. Musculoskeletal: Back pain and muscle cramps.

8. Neurologic: Dizziness, weakness, peripheral neuropathy, and balance problems.

9. Integumentary: Dry skin, itching, and rash.

10. Psychiatric: Confusion or difficulty concentrating and sleep disturbance.

11. Endocrine: Cold intolerance.

12. Hematologic: Bruising easily and bleeding.

PHYSICAL EXAMINATION

A. Vital signs, including orthostatic signs.

B. Constitutional.

C. Eyes: Funduscopic examination.

  1. Changes secondary to diabetes mellitus and hypertension.

D. Cardiovascular: Rate, rhythm, heart sounds (S3 and S4, murmurs, rubs), distal pulses, lower extremity edema, carotid bruit, and jugular venous distension (JVD).

E. Pulmonary: Breath sounds and effort (use of accessory muscles).

F. Abdominal: Abdominal palpation, bowel sounds, and melena.

G. GU: Flank pain, proteinuria, hematuria, oliguria, and anuria.

H. Musculoskeletal: Gait disturbances.

I. Integumentary/nails: Rash and pale.

J. Neurologic: Confusion and asterixis.

K. Endocrine: Polydipsia, polyphagia, and polyuria.

L. Hematologic/lymphatic: Bruising, petechiae, and ecchymosis.

DIAGNOSTIC TESTS

A. Renal function panel.

B. Complete blood count (CBC) with differential.

C. Serum albumin.

D. Fasting lipid panel.

E. Urinalysis.

F. Urine albumin to creatinine ratio (UACR).

G. Urine culture and sensitivity (if indicated).

H. Renal ultrasound with postvoid residual.

I. Specialty serologic studies as indicated: Antinuclear antibodies (ANA), C3, C4, and hepatitis B and C serologies.

J. CKD-MBD (mineral bone disorder): Calcium, phosphorus, intact parathyroid hormone (iPTH), and 25(OH) vitamin D (25-dihydroxy-vitamin D).

K. Anemia.

  1. Microcytic:

    a. Mean corpuscular volume (MCV) <80 fL.

      i. Iron studies (iron, total iron-binding capacity [TIBC], percent transferrin saturation, ferritin).

  2. Macrocytic:

    a. MCV >100 fL.

      i. Folate and B_{12} levels.

L. Multiple myeloma/monoclonal gammopathy of unknown significance (MGUS)/paraprotein.

  1. Serum and urine protein electrophoresis (SPEP and UPEP).

  2. Serum and urine for immunoelectrophoresis.

  3. Serum for free light chains.

M. Renal biopsy: Reserved when the cause of CKD is unclear and findings will guide the course of treatment.

DIFFERENTIAL DIAGNOSIS

A. AKI.

  1. Prerenal.

  2. Intrarenal/intrinsic.

  3. Postrenal.

B. Multiple myeloma.

C. Nephrolithiasis.

D. Diabetic nephropathy.

E. Glomerulonephritis.

EVALUATION AND MANAGEMENT PLAN

A. General plan.

  1. Identify and treat reversible cause(s).

  2. Prevent or slow progression of CKD.

  3. Prevent or treat complications of CKD.

  4. Discontinue or adjust medications based on eGFR.

  5. Prepare for kidney replacement therapy (KRT).

  6. Determine CKD stage (see Table 5.1).

B. Specific plan.

  1. CKD stage 1.

    a. Manage comorbid conditions.

    b. Identify CVD risk factors.

    c. Slow progression of CKD.

  2. CKD stage 2.

    a. Monitor CKD trajectory.

    b. Slow progression of CKD.

    c. Manage comorbidities.

  3. CKD stages 3a and 3b.

    a. As above, for stage 2.

    b. Identify and treat CKD complications.

  4. CKD stage 4.

    a. As above, for stages 3a and 3b.

    b. Refer to nephrology.

      i. Discuss KRT.

  5. CKD stage 5.

    a. As above for stage 4.

    b. Prepare for/start KRT.

C. Manage complications.

  1. Metabolic acidosis.

    a. Medication therapy, for example, sodium bicarbonate.

  2. Anemia.

    a. Anemia of chronic disease (ACD).

    b. Iron deficiency anemia (IDA).

    c. Laboratory evaluation.

      i. CBC with differential and red blood cell (RBC) indices.

      ii. Absolute reticulocyte count.

      iii. Iron studies (serum iron, TIBC, percent transferrin saturation, serum ferritin) and count. ▶

iv. B_{12} and folate levels (MCV >100 fL).

v. Fecal occult blood test.

3. Hypertension.

a. Slow the progression of proteinuria.

b. Decrease cardiovascular complications.

c. Blood pressure (BP) goal <130/80.

4. Hyperkalemia.

a. Low potassium diet.

b. Avoid medications that contribute to hyperkalemia, for example, nonsteroidal anti-inflammatory drugs (NSAIDs).

c. Potassium binders.

i. Patiromer (Veltassa).

ii. Sodium zirconium cyclosilicate (SZC; Lokelma).

iii. Veltassa.

5. CKD-MBD.

a. Hypocalcemia.

i. Calcitriol.

ii. Calcium supplementation, only if indicated.

b. Hyperphosphatemia.

i. Low phosphorus diet.

ii. Phosphorus binders.

   1) Calcium-based binders.

   2) Noncalcium-based binders.

c. Secondary hyperparathyroidism.

i. Elevated iPTH.

ii. Calcitriol or vitamin D analog.

6. Dyslipidemia.

a. Diet therapy.

b. Medication therapy.

D. Indications for initiation of dialysis.

1. Hyperkalemia.

2. Uremic pericarditis.

3. Refractory metabolic acidosis.

4. Volume overload.

5. Pulmonary edema.

6. Uremic encephalopathy.

7. Persistent nausea and vomiting.

8. Blood urea nitrogen (BUN) greater than 100 mg/dL.

E. Patient/family teaching points.

1. Patient-centered educational efforts: A conceptual model.

a. Prevent CKD.

i. Awareness of risk.

ii. Knowledge of prevention strategies.

b. Identify CKD.

i. Awareness of diagnosis.

ii. Knowledge of health implications.

c. Manage CKD.

i. Knowledge of management goals and how to achieve them.

d. Comprehensive conservative care for ESRD.

i. Knowledge of treatments, risks, benefits, and management goals.

2. Dietary modifications.

a. Sodium intake: Less than 2 g/d.

b. Potassium intake: 2 g/d.

c. Protein intake.

i. Avoid high protein intake.

ii. Lower protein intake to 0.8 g/kg/d in adults with diabetes or without diabetes and a glomerular filtration rate (GFR) less than 30 mL/min/1.73 m^2.

d. Phosphorus intake: 800 to 1,000 mg/d.

e. Diabetes dietary guidelines: Target hemoglobin A1C (A1C) of 7.0%.

f. Target A1C can be extended above 7.0% in individuals with comorbidities or limited life expectancy and risk of hypoglycemia.

g. Hyperlipidemia dietary modifications.

i. Decrease intake of saturated and trans fat foods.

ii. Substitute with monounsaturated fats and moderate intake of polyunsaturated fats.

F. Pharmacotherapy (to prevent/treat complications).

1. Metabolic acidosis.

a. Maintain carbon dioxide/bicarbonate level.

b. Sodium bicarbonate/sodium citrate.

2. Anemia.

a. Monitor iron studies to determine iron supplementation plan.

i. Oral iron.

ii. Intravenous (IV) iron infusion.

b. Monitor hemoglobin to guide erythropoiesis-stimulating agents (ESA) therapy.

c. Ferrous sulfate tablets.

d. Folic acid replacement tablets.

e. Cobalamin for vitamin B_{12} replacement/supplementation.

f. ESA.

3. Hypertension: CKD with or without diabetes.

a. Use a renin–angiotensin–aldosterone system (RAAS) inhibitor.

i. Angiotensin-converting enzyme (ACE) inhibitor or angiotensin receptor blocker (ARB).

   1) Obtain a baseline SCr and serum potassium and follow.

   2) Recheck those levels in 1 to 2 weeks after starting or increasing dose to evaluate changes in eGFR (decreased) and/or serum potassium (increased).

4. CKD-MBD: Monitor serum calcium, phosphorus, and iPTH.

a. Phosphate binders.

i. Administered with food to bind with phosphorus in the GI tract.

ii. Calcium-based and noncalcium-based binders.

b. Vitamin D replacement.

i. Cholecalciferol.

ii. Ergocalciferol.

c. Bisphosphonates (avoid in CKD with GFR less than 30 mL/min/1.73 m^2).

5. Dyslipidemia: Lipid-lowering agent.

i. Statin therapy.

ii. Atorvastatin.

▶

1) Hepatic clearance.
2) No renal dose adjustments.
6. Diabetic complications.
  a. Keep A1C 7%.
7. Malnutrition.
  a. High biologic value (HBV) protein intake.
  b. Oral nutritional supplements (ONS).
8. Proteinuria.
  a. RAAS inhibitor (ACE inhibitor or ARB). *OR*
  b. Nondihydropyridine calcium channel blocker (diltiazem, verapamil).
  c. Sodium-glucose cotransporter 2 (SGLT2) inhibitors.

FOLLOW-UP
A. Follow-up in CKD is important to slow progression of disease and to manage risk factors that may contribute to worsening of the patient's clinical health.
B. A nephrologist should be consulted.
C. Regular visits with a primary provider are essential for long-term health maintenance.

CONSULTATION/REFERRAL
A. Consult nephrology in the acute care setting for patients with the following:
  1. An eGFR less than 30 mL/min/1.73 m².
  2. Significant albuminuria or overt proteinuria.
  3. An abrupt decrease in eGFR/acute rise in SCr.
  4. Evidence of worsening kidney function/CKD progression.
  5. Persistent hematuria.
  6. Resistant hypertension.

SPECIAL/GERIATRIC CONSIDERATIONS
A. CVD is the primary cause of morbidity and mortality in patients with CKD.
  1. The incidence of cardiovascular death increases with each stage of CKD.
  2. Individuals are more likely to die than to reach the next stage of CKD.
  3. The incidence of death related to cardiovascular procedures increases with CKD stage.
B. The incidence of hospitalization increases with CKD stage.
C. It is important to identify CKD in hospitalized patients.
  1. Prevent complications.
  2. Reduce mortality, length of stay, and readmission.
D. The incidence of CKD and AKI increases with age.
  1. Polypharmacy is more common in older individuals.
    a. Review medications regularly.
      i. Identify medications that are actual or potential nephrotoxins.
      ii. Identify medications that require dose or schedule changes.
E. Older individuals have an increased prevalence of decreased eGFR and increased albumin:creatinine ratio (ACR).

1. There is a debate concerning whether decreased GFR or increased UACR in older individuals represents disease or normal aging.

CASE SCENARIO: CHRONIC KIDNEY DISEASE

A 52-year-old male is admitted to the hospital with an infected right great toe. His medical history includes type 2 diabetes mellitus, hypertension, and hypercholesterolemia. He said he has not seen a healthcare provider in over 6 months because he felt good and had no problems until now. He admits to recently running out of his medications. His vital signs include a temperature of 98.2°F/36.7°C, blood pressure (BP) of 178/92, pulse rate of 92, and respiratory rate of 20. Cardiovascular and respiratory examinations are normal. Lower extremities have trace edema. Right great toe is red, warm, and edematous without drainage. Laboratory results include white blood cell (WBC) of 13,800, hematocrit and hemoglobin (H&H) of 10.2 g/dL and 30%, serum creatinine (SCr) of 1.97 mg/dL, estimated glomerular filtration rate (eGFR) of 40, potassium of 4.9 mEq/L, phosphorus (PO4) of 4.3 mg/dL, glucose of 268 mg/dL, A1C of 10.1%, vitamin D of 15 ng/mL, total cholesterol of 207 mg/dL, triglycerides of 162 mg/dL, and urine microalbumin of 245 mg/g.

1. The patient is diagnosed with chronic kidney disease (CKD). Based on the estimated glomerular filtration rate (eGFR), he is diagnosed as what CKD stage?
  A. 2
  B. 3a
  C. 3b
  D. 4

2. Studies have shown which of the following medications to be effective in slowing the progression of chronic kidney disease?
  A. Erythropoiesis-stimulating agents (ESA) and iron supplement
  B. Statin and fibrate
  C. Vitamin D and calcium supplement
  D. Renin–angiotensin–aldosterone system (RAAS) inhibitor and sodium-glucose cotransporter 2 (SGLT2) inhibitor

BIBLIOGRAPHY
Chen, T. K., Sperati, C. J., Thavarajah, S., & Grams, M. E. (2021). Reducing kidney function decline in patients with CKD: Core Curriculum 2021. *American Journal of Kidney Diseases: The Official Journal of the National Kidney Foundation, 77*(6), 969–983. https://doi.org/10.1053/j.ajkd.2020.12.022
Delgado, C., Baweja, M., Crews, D. C., Eneanya, N. D., Gadegbeku, C. A., Inker, L. A., Mendu, M. L., Miller, W. G., Moxey-Mims, M. M., Roberts, G. V., St Peter, W. L., Warfield, C., & Powe, N. R. (2022). A Unifying Approach for GFR Estimation: Recommendations of the NKF-ASN Task force on reassessing the inclusion of race in diagnosing kidney disease. *American Journal of Kidney Diseases: The Official Journal of the National Kidney Foundation, 79*(2), 268–288.e1. https://doi.org/10.1053/j.ajkd.2021.08.003
Freidin, N., O'Hare, A. M., & Wong, S. (2019). Person-centered care for older adults with kidney disease: Core curriculum 2019. *American Journal of Kidney Diseases: The Official Journal of the National Kidney Foundation, 74*(3), 407–416. https://doi.org/10.1053/j.ajkd.2019.01.038

Georgianos, P. I., Vaios, V., Roumeliotis, S., Leivaditis, K., Eleftheriadis, T., & Liakopoulos, V. (2022). Evidence for cardiorenal protection with SGLT-2 inhibitors and GLP-1 receptor agonists in patients with diabetic kidney disease. *Journal of Personalized Medicine, 12*(2), 223. https://doi.org/10.3390/jpm12020223

Inker, L. A., & Titan, S. (2021). Measurement and estimation of GFR for use in clinical practice: Core curriculum 2021. *American Journal of Kidney Diseases: The Official Journal of the National Kidney Foundation, 78*(5), 736–749. https://doi.org/10.1053/j.ajkd.2021.04.016

Kidney Disease: Improving Global Outcomes CKD Work Group. (2013). KDIGO 2012 clinical practice guideline for the evaluation and management of chronic kidney disease. *Kidney International, 3*(1 Suppl. 3), 1–59.

Kidney Disease: Improving Global Outcomes CKD-MBD Work Group. (2017). KDIGO clinical practice guideline update for the diagnosis, evaluation, prevention, and treatment of Chronic Kidney Disease— Mineral and Bone Disorder (CKD-MBD). *Kidney International, 7*(1 Suppl), S1–S130.

Kidney Disease: Improving Global Outcomes (KDIGO) Anemia Work Group. (2012). KDIGO clinical practice guideline for anemia in chronic kidney disease. *Kidney International, 2*(Suppl.), 279–335. https://doi.org/10.1038/ki.2012.270

Kidney Disease: Improving Global Outcomes (KDIGO) Diabetes Work Group. (2020). KDIGO 2020 Clinical practice guideline for diabetes management in chronic kidney disease. *Kidney International, 98*(4S), S1–S115. https://doi.org/10.1016/j.kint.2020.06.019

Kidney Disease: Improving Global Outcomes Lipid Work Group. (2013). KDIGO clinical practice guideline for lipid management in chronic kidney disease. *Kidney International, 3*(Suppl. 3), 1–305.

Kidney Disease: Improving Global Outcomes Work Group. (2021). Clinical practice guideline for the management of blood pressure in chronic kidney disease. *Kidney International, 99*(3S Suppl.), S1–S87.

Kidney Disease: Improving Global Outcomes Work Group. (2022). Clinical practice guideline for diabetes management in chronic kidney disease. *Kidney International, 102*(5S Suppl.), S1–S127.

MacLaughlin, H. L., Friedman, A. N., & Ikizler, T. A. (2022). Nutrition in kidney disease: Core curriculum 2022. *American Journal of Kidney Diseases: The Official Journal of the National Kidney Foundation, 79*(3), 437–449. https://doi.org/10.1053/j.ajkd.2021.05.024

Mendu, M. L., & Weiner, D. E. (2020). Health policy and kidney care in the United States: Core curriculum 2020. *American Journal of Kidney Diseases: The Official Journal of the National Kidney Foundation, 76*(5), 720–730. https://doi.org/10.1053/j.ajkd.2020.03.028

Oliva-Damaso, N., Delanaye, P., Oliva-Damaso, E., Payan, J., & Glassock, R. J. (2022). Risk-based versus GFR threshold criteria for nephrology referral in chronic kidney disease. *Clinical Kidney Journal, 15*(11), 1996–2005. https://doi.org/10.1093/ckj/sfac104

Provenzano, M., Coppolino, G., Faga, T., Garofalo, C., Serra, R., & Andreucci, M. (2019). Epidemiology of cardiovascular risk in chronic kidney disease patients: The real silent killer. *Reviews in Cardiovascular Medicine, 20*(4), 209–220. https://doi.org/10.31083/j.rcm.2019.04.548

Rosenberg, M. (2022). Overview of the management of chronic kidney disease in adults. *UpToDate.*

Schrauben, S. J., Chen, H. Y., Lin, E., Jepson, C., Yang, W., Scialla, J. J., Fischer, M. J., Lash, J. P., Fink, J. C., Hamm, L. L., Kanthety, R., Rahman, M., Feldman, H. I., Anderson, A. H., & the CRIC study investigator. (2020). Hospitalizations among adults with chronic kidney disease in the United States: A cohort study. *PLOS Medicine, 17*(12), e1003470. https://doi.org/10.137/journal.pmed.1003470

Shabaka, A., Cases-Corona, C., & Fernandez-Juarez, G. (2021). Therapeutic insights in chronic kidney disease progression. *Frontiers in Medicine, 8*, 645187. https://doi10.3389/fmed.2021.645187

U.S. Renal Data System. (2020). *USRDS 2020 annual data report: Epidemiology of kidney disease in the United States.* National Institutes of Health, National Institute of Diabetes and Digestive and Kidney Diseases. https://adr.usrds.org/2020/end-stage-renal-disease

Vondracek, S. F., Teitelbaum, I., & Kiser, T. H. (2021). Principles of kidney pharmacotherapy for the nephrologist: Core curriculum 2021. *American Journal of Kidney Diseases: The Official Journal of the National Kidney Foundation, 78*(3), 442–458. https://doi.org/10.1053/j.ajkd.2021.02.342 https://www.cdc.gov/kidneydisease/publications-resources/ckd-national-facts.html

HEMATURIA

Suzanne Barron

DEFINITION

A. Gross hematuria: Visible blood in the urine by the naked eye. Blood can be seen in the urine with only 1 mL of blood in 1 L of urine.

B. Microscopic hematuria: Greater than three red blood cells (RBCs) per high power field (HPF) in a single urinalysis.

INCIDENCE

A. Hematuria is one of the most common urologic diagnoses.

B. Population-based studies have shown prevalence rates of microscopic hematuria ranging from as low as 2% to as high as 31%.

C. Older men have a higher prevalence of hematuria.

D. Incidence rates of associated conditions.

    1. No diagnosis after workup: 60.5%.

    2. Urinary tract infection (UTI): 13%.

    3. Stone disease: 3.6%.

    4. Cancer: 13%.

    5. Glomerular disease: 9.8%.

PATHOGENESIS

A. Glomerular or nephronal hematuria (originates from the nephron).

    1. On microscopic evaluation, RBCs that are dysmorphic (irregular shapes and uneven hemoglobin distribution) often represent glomerular disease. There may be casts.

    2. On urinalysis, the combination of RBCs and significant proteinuria (>1,000 mg/24 hours) most often indicates a glomerular source of hematuria.

    3. Common causes of glomerular hematuria include immunoglobulin A (IgA) nephropathy (Berger disease), thin glomerular basement membrane disease, and hereditary nephritis (Alport syndrome).

B. Extraglomerular hematuria (originates from urologic source): Anything that disrupts the genitourinary (GU) epithelium, which may include irritation, trauma, inflammation, or invasion.

    1. On microscopic evaluation, the RBCs in the urine are isomorphic; have smooth, round membranes; and display even hemoglobin distribution. There may be a small amount of protein in the urine that occurs along with the RBCs.

    2. Associated conditions include tumors, kidney stones, trauma, infection, anatomic abnormalities of the urinary tract such as ureteropelvic junction obstruction, and benign prostatic hypertrophy (BPH).

PREDISPOSING FACTORS

A. Age greater than 35.

B. Smoking history.

C. Recent trauma.

D. Recent urinary tract surgery or instrumentation.

E. BPH.

F. Family history of renal disease.

G. Personal history of nephrolithiasis.

H. Pelvic radiation.

I. Recent febrile illness.

J. Frequent UTIs.

K. Occupational exposure to chemicals and dyes (benzenes or aromatic amines).

L. Medications (abuse of analgesics such as nonsteroidal anti-inflammatory drugs [NSAIDs]).

M. Chronic indwelling catheters (Foley catheters, suprapubic tube catheters).

SUBJECTIVE DATA

A. Common complaints/symptoms.

 1. Flank pain: Possible etiology due to recent trauma, nephrolithiasis, renal cancer, ureteral tumor, or pyelonephritis.

 2. Dysuria/lower urinary tract symptoms (LUTS) such as urgency/frequency and urinary retention: Possible etiology due to UTI, prostatitis, BPH, interstitial cystitis, or bladder stones.

 3. Fever: Etiology due to UTI, prostatitis, or pyelonephritis.

 4. Worm-like (vermiform) clots in the urine: Can occur with bleeding from the upper urinary tract from tumors or masses.

B. Common/typical scenario.

 1. Visual appearance of blood in the urine or presence with microscopic hematuria.

 2. Timing of hematuria during urinary stream: May indicate the site of pathology (i.e., initiation of stream—anterior urethral pathology; termination of stream—bladder neck, prostate, or urethra inflammation/pathology; throughout stream—bladder or upper urinary tract origin).

 3. Aggravating factors.

  a. Pain, recent trauma, or recent vigorous activity/exercise.

  b. Recent upper respiratory infection (associated with glomerulonephritis).

  c. Pseudohematuria from ingestion of certain foods (such as beets) and drugs (Pyridium).

  d. Excessive use of analgesics such as NSAIDs.

C. Family and social history.

 1. Smoking (past or present).

 2. Excessive ingestion of barbecued/smoked foods (associated with link to bladder cancer).

 3. Sexual history (recent sexually transmitted infections [STIs]).

 4. Work history: Exposure to chemicals and dyes in rubber and/or petroleum industries (associated with bladder cancer).

 5. Family history.

  a. GU malignancies.

  b. Primary renal disease.

  c. Polycystic kidney disease.

  d. Nephrolithiasis.

  e. Hypertension.

D. Review of systems.

 1. Constitutional symptoms: Recent weight loss, fevers, or night sweats that may indicate malignancy.

 2. Respiratory: Cough or shortness of breath that may indicate recent upper respiratory infection or tumor invasion.

 3. Musculoskeletal: Generalized pain may indicate excessive NSAID use.

 4. GU: Frequent urination, urinary urgency, flank pain, dysuria, cloudy urine, or foul-smelling urine.

 5. Gynecologic: Menorrhagia.

 6. Gastrointestinal (GI): Nausea, vomiting, or abdominal pain may indicate renal mass or nephrolithiasis.

 7. Neurologic: Confusion, dizziness, or mental status changes may indicate metastatic malignant disease (renal cancer).

 8. Skin: Rashes or pallor that may be associated with systemic lupus erythematosus (SLE).

 9. Hematologic: Excessive bruising or petechiae may indicate blood clotting disorder.

 10. Ear, nose, and throat (ENT): Frequent nosebleeds, rhinorrhea, or sinus congestion.

PHYSICAL EXAMINATION

A. Vital signs.

 1. Temperature: Measurement greater than 101.5°F/ 38.6°C may indicate UTI, pyelonephritis, or prostatitis.

 2. Blood pressure (BP).

  a. Hypertension: Glomerular source or renal failure.

  b. Hypotension: Possible acute blood loss anemia from gross hematuria.

 3. Pulse: Tachycardia, sepsis, or hypovolemia from acute blood loss anemia.

B. Skin: Rashes, pallor, or bruising/lacerations from recent trauma.

C. Edema: Possible nephrotic syndrome (NS); rule out deep vein thrombosis (DVT) from GU malignancy.

D. GU examination.

 1. Costovertebral angle tenderness (CVAT): Nephrolithiasis and pyelonephritis.

 2. Urethral trauma: Urethral caruncle, vaginal prolapse, phimosis, and obvious urethral stricture.

E. Digital rectal examination (DRE).

 1. Boggy, tender warm prostate: Acute prostatitis.

 2. Nodularity: Prostate cancer.

DIAGNOSTIC TESTS

A. Urinalysis.

 1. Color: Red (recent bleeding, most likely urologic source) versus brown or tea color (old blood clots or renal disease).

 2. Proteinuria: Heavy 3 to 4+ (renal disease).

 3. Leukocyte positive and/or nitrite positive: Infection.

 4. Pyuria: Infection.

 5. Red cell casts: Glomerular bleeding.

 6. Crystalluria: Possible nephrolithiasis.

B. Phase contrast microscopy: Helps differentiate renal (presence of distorted RBCs) versus nonglomerular bleeding.

C. Urine culture: Evaluate for infectious sources.
D. Laboratory/bloodwork.
 1. Complete blood count (CBC): Anemia.
 2. Basic metabolic panel: Renal function.
 3. Prothrombin time (PT)/partial thromboplastin time (PTT) and international normalized ratio (INR): Bleeding disorders.
E. Urine cytology.
 1. Recommended for all patients with risk factors for GU malignancy and with LUTS and voiding symptoms.
 2. Not recommended by the American Urological Association as part of routine evaluation of asymptomatic microhematuria.
 3. Negative result does not rule out malignancy.
 4. False-positive results can be seen with calculi or inflammation.
F. Imaging.
 1. CT urogram (CTU) with and without contrast: Gold standard.
  a. Three-phase test.
  b. Used to assess for stones (noncontrast image), tumors of the bladder or kidneys, hydronephrosis, other anatomic abnormalities (contrast image), tumors of the upper tract, and collecting system filling defects (excretory phase).
  c. Contraindicated with a serum creatinine (SCr) greater than 2 mg/dL.
  d. Highest sensitivity and specificity.
 2. MRI/magnetic resonance urography (MRU; MRI urogram): Alternative imaging modality when not able to perform CTU due to renal insufficiency, contrast allergy, or pregnancy.
  a. Less sensitivity at recognizing calculus of the GU tract.
 3. Renal ultrasound: Not as specific or sensitive.
  a. Can be used to grossly rule out clots in bladder or to detect hydronephrosis.
G. Diagnostic procedures/surgery.
 1. Cystoscopy.
  a. Indicated for all patients older than 35 years of age with microscopic hematuria or gross hematuria.
  b. Also indicated for patients younger than 35 years of age with risk factors for GU malignancies and smoking history.
 2. Retrograde pyelogram with or without ureteroscopy (URS): May be performed to evaluate the upper tract in patients who are unable to have intravenous (IV) contrast for the CTU/MRU imaging.
 3. Renal biopsy: Nephrology referral if glomerulonephritis is suspected.

DIFFERENTIAL DIAGNOSIS

A. Pseudohematuria: Certain foods, beets/certain drugs, or phenazopyridine (Pyridium).
B. Hereditary disorders: Polycystic kidney disease, nephropathy, renal tubular acidosis, or cystinuria.
C. Hematologic abnormalities: Bleeding disorders or sickle cell disease.
D. Anatomic abnormalities: Urethral strictures, ureteral strictures, ureteropelvic junction obstruction, urethral caruncle, or phimosis.
E. Vascular malformations (hemangioma).
F. Trauma: Abdominal and pelvic injury (degree of hematuria is a poor indicator of severity of injury).
G. Exercise-induced hematuria.
H. Foreign bodies (catheters, ureteral stents, self-introduced foreign body into the urethra).
I. Infectious (UTI, pyelonephritis, prostatitis, schistosomiasis, tuberculosis).
J. Radiation (radiation cystitis and nephritis).
K. Stones of the GU tract.
L. Malignancy (renal, bladder, ureteral, prostate, penile, urethral, vulvar).
M. Benign tumor.
N. BPH.
O. Endometriosis of urinary tract (cyclic hematuria).
P. Benign essential hematuria (interstitial cystitis, trigonitis).
Q. Glomerulonephritis or renal disorders (IgA nephropathy, drug-induced nephropathy).
R. Overanticoagulation with medications such as warfarin.
 1. Clinical caveat: Patients should still be thoroughly evaluated for other possible causes.

EVALUATION AND MANAGEMENT PLAN

A. General plan.
 1. Urinalysis, urine culture, and laboratory tests (see "Diagnostic Tests").
 2. Urine cytology if indicated.
 3. Imaging (CTU).
 4. Patients with gross hematuria and/or urinary retention.
  a. Place three-way Foley catheter (22–24 Fr most commonly used) and irrigate clots (continuous bladder irrigation with sterile saline solution).
  b. If bleeding is not controlled, propose evaluation with urologic surgery for cystoscopy under anesthesia for clot evacuation/fulguration.
 5. Patients who are voiding without clots or urine retention: Observation, with increase in oral fluid intake.
 6. Patients with gross hematuria or history of trauma for acute blood loss anemia: Monitor with serial hemoglobin and hematocrit and transfuse as indicated.
B. Patient/family teaching points.
 1. Provide patient education and prognosis depending on the cause of the hematuria.
 2. Explain the various tests that are necessary to determine the cause of bleeding and the treatments that may be necessary for control of gross hematuria (e.g., cystoscopy, clot evacuation, Foley catheter placement for bladder irrigation).

▶

3. Help to ease anxiety by providing appropriate analgesics (e.g., lidocaine jelly before placing a three-way catheter or narcotics/anticholinergics for painful bladder spasms due to clot retention/catheter placement).

4. Discuss that benign causes of asymptomatic hematuria are far more common than malignant causes.

C. Pharmacotherapy.

1. No specific medications are primarily indicated to treat hematuria.

2. Appropriate antimicrobials may be used to treat underlying infections.

3. Finasteride may be helpful in controlling bleeding from the prostate.

D. Discharge instructions.

1. Advise patients to refrain from vigorous activity for 1 week after gross hematuria has resolved.

2. Avoid NSAIDs and aspirin (if possible, some patients may need to continue based on history of coronary artery disease) for 3 days.

3. Advise patients that it is normal to have tea-colored urine for a few days as the hematuria is resolving.

4. Recommend that patients drink plenty of fluids.

5. Suggest that patients prevent constipation and straining by taking stool softeners such as docusate sodium.

6. Advise that patients should seek medical attention promptly if they develop bright-red urine, pass clots, are unable to urinate, or have fevers or chills.

FOLLOW-UP

A. Follow-up as indicated for the condition that is causing the hematuria.

B. Once the condition has resolved, reevaluate for microhematuria.

C. In asymptomatic microhematuria with a negative workup, follow up annually for repeat urinalysis/microscopy. If negative for 2 years, release from care. If positive, repeat imaging every 3 years and refer for renal evaluation.

CONSULTATION/REFERRAL

A. Nephrology consult for nephrogenic source of hematuria.

B. Urology consult for stones, tumors of the GU tract, BPH, anatomic evaluation, and control of bleeding.

C. Infectious disease (ID) consult for treatment of infectious sources (pyelonephritis, prostatitis, UTIs, possible tuberculosis workup, or possible schistosomiasis).

D. Rheumatology consult for autoimmune disorders such as SLE.

E. Hematology consult for bleeding disorders.

SPECIAL/GERIATRIC CONSIDERATIONS

A. Screen older adults appropriately for renal function prior to obtaining imaging studies with contrast.

B. The reduced capacity to retain salt and water increases as the kidney ages, predisposing to dehydration.

C. Older individuals are more susceptible to acute kidney injury (AKI) from acute blood loss anemia and certain medications such as NSAIDs.

D. Older adult patients should be monitored closely for hypovolemia that presents with gross hematuria.

CASE SCENARIO: HEMATURIA

A 44-year-old female presents to the ED with a 2-day history of gross hematuria with passage of clots. She is a nonsmoker with no significant past medical history (PMH). She reports normal menses and her last menstrual period was 2 weeks ago. She is an avid runner and often runs 8 to 9 miles about 4 times a week. She reports taking nonsteroidal anti-inflammatory drugs (NSAIDs) routinely to help with muscle and joint aches from running. On exam, the patient appears well-hydrated. Afebrile, vital signs stable. There is no costovertebral angle tenderness (CVAT), with positive mild suprapubic tenderness. There is no edema. Urinalysis is positive for 3+ blood, and negative for nitrites, leukocytes, protein, and glucose. Microscopic urinalysis reveals >182 red blood cells per high power field (RBC/HPF). There are no red cell casts noted. Her serum creatinine (SCr) is 0.8 and her hemoglobin is 10.9. Urine culture is pending. The ED providers consulted with urology and a three-way Foley catheter is inserted for continuous bladder irrigation.

1. What is the next study to order in this patient?
   A. Hepatic function panel
   B. Renal ultrasound
   C. Serial hemoglobin and hematocrit
   D. CT urogram

BIBLIOGRAPHY

American Urologic Association. (2012). Diagnosis, evaluation and follow-up of asymptomatic microhematuria (AMH) in adults. https://www.auanet.org/documents/education/clinical-guidance/Asymptomatic-Microhematuria.pdf

Clifton, M., & Johnston, A. (2020, October). *Medical student curriculum: Hematuria-American Urological Association.* https://www.aua.net.org/education/auauniversity/for-medical-students/medical-students-curriculum/medical-student-curriculum/hematuria

Fatica, R., & Fowler, A. (2009, January). Hematuria. *Cleveland Clinic for Continuing Education.* https://www.auanet.org/guidelines/asymptomatic-microhematuria-(amh)-guideline#x2396

Lambert, M. (2013, May). AUA guideline addresses diagnosis, evaluation and follow-up of asymptomatic microhematuria. *American Family Physician, 87*(9), 649–653.

HYPERCALCEMIA

Divya Monga and Catherine Wells

DEFINITION

A. Serum total calcium greater than 10.2 mg/dL (corrected for low albumin; see Box 5.2).

INCIDENCE

A. Hypercalcemia is a relatively common abnormality that is usually mild in presentation.

B. Approximately 90% of cases of hypercalcemia may be caused by some type of malignancy or hyperparathyroidism.

BOX 5.2   CALCIUM IN HUMANS

Normal total serum calcium is 8.6–10.2 mg/dL.
Normal ionized serum calcium is 1.12–1.3 mmol/L.
Extracellular calcium is found in three forms. 40% of calcium in serum is protein-bound, primarily to albumin. 50% is free (ionized or unbound) calcium. 10% is complexed (i.e., calcium citrate).
Total serum calcium underestimates active calcium. Ionized or unbound calcium is the biologically active form. Correct serum calcium in hypoalbuminemic patients for actual total calcium.   ■ Corrected calcium = serum total calcium + (0.8 × [4 − serum albumin concentration])

99% of total body calcium is found in bones.
PTH and vitamin D regulate serum calcium.
Physiologic functions:
  Bone metabolism
  Electrophysiology of cardiac and smooth muscle
  Coagulation
  Endocrine and exocrine secretory functions

Phosphorus and calcium directly affect each other.
Elevated phosphorus binds to ionized calcium, decreasing unbound, active calcium.
Maintain the optimal relationship between calcium and phosphorous.
  ■ For bone health
  ■ To prevent vascular and soft tissue calcifications

Calcium is an inotrope if given at accelerated doses (due to its effects on cardiac and smooth muscle).
Calcium is critical to the coagulation cascade; thus, low calcium or blocking calcium can lead to bleeding.

PTH, parathyroid hormone.

PATHOGENESIS

A. Calcium is controlled by three major hormones: Parathyroid, calcitriol, and vitamin D.
B. Dysregulation in these hormones can lead to hypercalcemia.
C. Calcium is tightly regulated in the bloodstream; therefore, even mild cases of hypercalcemia are concerning and should be investigated for possible malignancy.

PREDISPOSING FACTORS

A. Women over the age of 50.
B. Patients taking excessive calcium or vitamin D supplements.
C. Cancer.
D. Genetics.
E. Immobility may contribute to release of calcium.
F. Lithium.

SUBJECTIVE DATA

A. Common complaints/symptoms (severity of symptoms depends on the degree and rate of rise in serum calcium).
  1. Gastrointestinal (GI), including nausea, vomiting, and constipation.
  2. Anorexia.
  3. Fatigue and lethargy.
  4. Confusion and impaired concentration.
  5. Severe hypercalcemia.
    a. Cardiac effects, including bradycardia or arrhythmias with EKG changes (shortening of QT interval).
    b. Volume depletion secondary to polyuria and hypercalcemia-induced natriuresis and nephrogenic diabetes insipidus (DI).
    c. Possible acute renal failure if severe and prolonged.
  6. Chronic hypercalcemia.
    a. Possible nephrolithiasis, systemic calcifications (e.g., vascular), and renal failure.

PHYSICAL EXAMINATION

A. Volume status.
B. Cardiac examination.
C. Neurologic examination.
D. Reflexes.
E. Musculoskeletal examination.

DIAGNOSTIC TESTS

A. Serum calcium and phosphorus.
B. 25-hydroxyvitamin D (calcidiol) and 1,25 dihydroyxvitamin D (calcitriol).
C. Intact parathyroid hormone (iPTH).
D. Parathyroid hormone (PTH)-related peptide (PTHrp—secreted by malignant tumor cells).
E. Creatinine and blood urea nitrogen (BUN).
F. Protein electrophoresis and immunofixation (serum and urine), and serum free light chain assay.
G. Alkaline phosphatase for high bone turnover.

▶

H. Thyroid-stimulating hormone (TSH).

I. EKG.

DIFFERENTIAL DIAGNOSIS

A. Malignancy: Likely due to local osteolytic hypercalcemia and/or production of circulating factors that stimulate osteoclastic resorption of the bone. Hematologic malignancies like Hodgkin lymphoma synthesize large amounts of calcitriol.

B. Hyperparathyroidism: Primary, secondary, and tertiary.

C. Paget disease.

D. Milk-alkali syndrome.

E. Thyrotoxicosis.

F. Granulomatous diseases (such as sarcoidosis and tuberculosis).

G. Immobilization.

H. Medication-induced.

1. Vitamin A and D overdose/toxicity.

2. Parenteral nutrition.

3. Thiazide diuretics.

4. Lithium.

5. Estrogens, antiestrogens, and androgens.

6. Calcium supplements and calcium-containing phosphorus binders.

I. Impaired renal function (chronic kidney disease [CKD] or acute kidney injury [AKI]).

EVALUATION AND MANAGEMENT PLAN

A. Goal: To correct the underlying cause of hypercalcemia and prevent complications of hypercalcemia.

B. Step 1: Treat symptoms.

1. Use aggressive volume resuscitation with intravenous (IV) normal saline 0.9% (200–500 mL/hr) in patients with volume depletion and normal heart and kidney function.

2. Manage cardiac effects: EKG changes and hypotension or hypertension.

3. Replace phosphorus if hypophosphatemia is present.

C. Step 2: Treat hypercalcemia and identify the underlying cause.

1. Discontinue all vitamin D and calcium (oral and IV).

2. Acute, severe hypercalcemia.

a. Adequate aggressive volume resuscitation is the first line. In individuals with renal insufficiency and heart failure, judicious and monitored use of loop diuretics may be needed to prevent fluid overload.

b. Possibly arrange for hemodialysis in patients with renal dysfunction.

3. Mild or asymptomatic hypercalcemia. Some therapies may also be, beneficial in combination with severe hypercalcemia management.

a. Calcitonin.

i. Rapid onset of action but with short-term effectiveness (<48 hours) due to tachyphylaxis.

ii. Can be used in initial treatment of severe hypercalcemia along with IV hydration.

iii. Increases renal excretion and decreases osteoclast-mediated bone resorption of calcium.

iv. Dose: 4 to 8 units/kg subcutaneously or intramuscularly (IM) Q12H for a total duration of 24 to 48 hours.

b. Glucocorticoid.

i. Useful in patients with granulomatous disorders or lymphoma.

ii. Decreases calcitriol production, which subsequently lowers intestinal calcium absorption.

iii. Sample regimens: Prednisone 20–60 mg/d PO for 10 days or hydrocortisone 200 mg/d IV for three doses.

c. Bisphosphonate.

i. Examples: Pamidronate and zoledronate.

ii. Potent inhibitors of osteoclast-mediated bone resorption frequently used in hypercalcemia of malignancy.

iii. Due to delayed onset of action, limited role in severe, acute hypercalcemia.

d. Cinacalcet or etelcalcetide.

i. Indication: For outpatient management of primary hyperparathyroidism and secondary hyperparathyroidism of renal origin.

ii. Mimics the effects of calcium (calcimimetic) by binding to the calcium-sensing receptor on the parathyroid gland, thus reducing PTH and serum calcium.

iii. Dosing.

1) Cinacalcet: Initially at 30 mg one to two times daily to max of 180 mg/d. It is given with food to reduce nausea.

2) Etelcalcetide: Initial dosing 5 mg three times weekly IV (after dialysis) to a maximum of 15 mg three times weekly IV (after dialysis).

e. Denosumab.

i. Indicated for hypercalcemia of malignancy.

ii. Delayed onset of action.

iii. Binds to receptor activator of nuclear factor-kappa ligand (RANKL), leading to decreased bone resorption.

iv. Given subcutaneously every 4 weeks with additional doses during the first month of treatment.

D. Step 3: Treat other electrolyte and acid–base disorders.

FOLLOW-UP

A. Hypercalcemia can lead to osteoporosis, kidney stones or failure, nervous system disorders, and arrhythmias.

B. Follow-up of calcium levels is essential to prevent adverse outcomes.

CONSULTATION/REFERRAL

A. Patients should be referred to the appropriate service to treat the underlying disorder.

B. Oncology may be needed for patients with cancer.

C. Endocrine can be consulted for hormonal disorders contributing to hypercalcemia.

D. Nephrology should be consulted if there is renal involvement.

SPECIAL/GERIATRIC CONSIDERATIONS

A. Geriatric patients may be at increased risk due to immobility and dehydration.

B. Sitting or lying for long periods of time can cause calcium to leak into the bloodstream.

C. Severe dehydration can also transiently increase calcium concentration secondary to hypovolemia.

D. Hypercalcemia can contribute to arrhythmias, which further put geriatric patients at risk for adverse events.

CASE SCENARIO: HYPERCALCEMIA

A 30-year-old male with newly diagnosed Hodgkin lymphoma presented with nausea, lethargy, constipation, and abdominal pain for the last 4 days. His blood pressure (BP) was mildly high on presentation. His labs showed slight elevation in blood urea nitrogen (BUN) and creatinine from a normal baseline a month ago. He reports decreased PO intake for the week. His serum calcium was 14 mg/d and serum albumin 3.5 mg/dL.

1. What is the most likely mechanism of the patient's hypercalcemia?

    A. Ectopic synthesis of calcitriol from the lymphoma

    B. Acute kidney injury

    C. Primary hyperparathyroidism

    D. None of the above

BIBLIOGRAPHY

Kraft, M. D., Btaiche, I. F., Sacks, G. S., & Kudsk, K. A. (2005, August). Treatment of electrolyte disorders in adult patients in the intensive care unit. *American Journal of Health System Pharmacy*, 62(16), 1663–1682. https://doi.org/10.2146/ajhp040300

Moe, S. M., & Daoud, J. R. (2004). Disorders of mineral metabolism: Calcium, phosphorous, and magnesium. In D. S. Gipson, M. A. Perazella, & M. Tonelli (Eds.), *National kidney foundation's primer on kidney diseases* (6th ed., pp. 100–112). Elsevier Saunders.

Shane, E. (2018, August 13). Diagnostic approach to hypercalcemia. In J. E. Mulder (Ed.), *UpToDate*. https://www.uptodate.com/contents/diagnostic-approach-to-hypercalcemia

Shane, E., & Berenson, J. R. (2017). Treatment of hypercalcemia. In J. E. Mulder (Ed.), *UpToDate*. https://www.uptodate.com/contents/treatment-of-hypercalcemia

HYPERKALEMIA

Divya Monga and Catherine Wells

DEFINITION

A. Serum potassium concentration of greater than 5.5 mEq/L (Box 5.3).

INCIDENCE

A. Most common in patients with kidney disease (impaired potassium elimination)

PATHOGENESIS

A. Causes.

    1. Redistribution (a net shift of potassium from intracellular to extracellular space).

    2. Total body excess (due to increased potassium ingestion or impaired potassium elimination).

PREDISPOSING FACTORS

A. High-potassium, low-sodium diets.

B. Potassium supplements/certain medications (see below).

C. Renal insufficiency.

SUBJECTIVE DATA

A. Common complaints/symptoms.

    1. General malaise.

    2. Weakness.

    3. Gastrointestinal (GI) complaints.

        a. Nausea and vomiting.

        b. Diarrhea.

    4. Neuromuscular.

        a. Muscle twitching.

        b. Cramping.

        c. Weakness.

        d. Ascending paralysis.

        e. Paresthesia.

        f. Hyperreflexia.

PHYSICAL EXAMINATION

A. Inspect and assess for volume/hydration status: Skin, mucous membranes, and jugular venous distension (JVD).

B. Assess for cardiac and renal comorbidities.

    1. Auscultate and evaluate heart and lung.

    2. Perform neurologic examination.

BOX 5.3 POTASSIUM IN HUMANS

Normal serum potassium concentration is 3.5–5.5 mEq/L.
Serum potassium levels represent extracellular potassium.
The vast majority (98%) of total body potassium is intracellular.

Kidneys excrete 90%–95% of dietary potassium, with the remaining excreted by the gut.
Renal excretion is primarily determined by potassium secretion by the principal cells in the connecting segment and cortical collecting tubule.
Plasma potassium concentration, potassium intake, aldosterone secretion, and sodium and water delivery to the distal potassium secretory sites play a major role in potassium regulation.

Physiologic functions:
    Cellular metabolism
    Glycogen and protein synthesis
    Regulation of the electrical action potential across cell membranes

DIAGNOSTIC TESTS

A. Initial laboratory tests.

1. Serum potassium (preferably plasma).

2. Venous or arterial carbon dioxide (CO_2) or bicarbonate (HCO_3) and/or pH.

B. Other laboratory tests.

1. Comprehensive metabolic panel

2. Complete blood count (CBC).

3. Drug levels (e.g., digoxin).

4. Transtubular potassium gradient (TTKG).

a. (Urine potassium/plasma potassium)/(urine osmolarity/plasma osmolarity).

b. Assessment of the kidney's capability to appropriately conserve potassium.

c. Valid only if the patient is not taking any diuretics or drugs to block the renin–angiotensin–aldosterone system (RAAS), urine osmolarity is greater than 300 mOsm/kg, and urine sodium is greater than 25 mEq/L.

d. Should be greater than 10 during hyperkalemia, indicating that the kidneys are trying to remove potassium.

5. Fractional excretion of potassium (FE_K).

a. Percentage of potassium filtered into the proximal tubule that appears in urine.

b. For normal renal function with average dietary potassium intake, FE_K is approximately 10%.

c. Limited use as above for TTKG and varies with dietary potassium intake and in chronic kidney disease (CKD).

C. Cardiac function tests.

1. EKG changes including:

a. Peaked T-waves, prolonged PR interval, widened QRS complex, and shortened QT interval.

b. Progressive worsening as potassium rises.

c. Bradyarrhythmias.

d. Ventricular fibrillation.

e. Asystole.

DIFFERENTIAL DIAGNOSIS

A. Pseudohyperkalemia: Factitious elevation of the serum potassium caused by in vitro release of potassium from blood cells.

1. Hemolysis during blood draw.

2. Preexisting hemolysis (e.g., sickle cell disease, transfusion reaction, drug-induced).

3. Sampling error (e.g., collected above the level of an infusion).

4. Polycythemia.

5. Thrombocytosis (>500,000–1 million/mm³): Potassium release when clots are formed.

6. Leukocytosis (>100–200,000/mm³): Elevated potassium in serum but not in plasma.

7. Familial pseudohyperkalemia.

B. Redistribution of intracellular potassium (shifts from intracellular to extracellular fluid).

1. Metabolic acidosis or diabetic ketoacidosis: Insulin deficiency.

2. Muscular injury (e.g., trauma and rhabdomyolysis).

3. Succinylcholine.

4. Digoxin overdose.

5. Reduced effective plasma volume/hypertonic state.

a. Severe dehydration.

b. Heart failure.

c. Liver failure.

6. Hyperkalemic periodic paralysis.

7. Medications (toxicity): Beta-blockers, succinylcholine, and digitalis.

8. Prolonged fasting especially in dialysis patients.

C. Impaired elimination.

1. Kidney failure: Acute versus chronic.

2. Medication-induced.

a. Potassium-sparing diuretics.

b. Angiotensin-converting enzyme (ACE) inhibitors.

c. Angiotensin receptor blocker (ARBs).

d. Aldosterone antagonists.

e. Nonsteroidal anti-inflammatory drugs (NSAIDs).

f. Trimethoprim.

g. Heparin.

3. Decreased action of aldosterone/aldosterone deficiency.

a. Medications: ACE inhibitors, ARBs, NSAIDs, potassium-sparing diuretics, antibiotics (trimethoprim, penicillin G potassium), clonidine, cyclosporine, calcineurin inhibitors, heparin, and others.

b. Type IV renal tubular acidosis.

c. Hyporeninemic hypoaldosteronism.

d. Addison disease (primary adrenal insufficiency).

e. Gordon syndrome (type II pseudohypoaldosteronism).

4. Hypocalcemia.

D. Increased ingestion (requires impaired elimination).

EVALUATION AND MANAGEMENT PLAN

A. Step 1: After excluding pseudohyperkalemia, the first step is cardiac stabilization (stabilize the action potential in the myocardium).

1. IV calcium administered as calcium gluconate or calcium chloride transiently stabilizes cardiac muscle but does not decrease serum potassium.

a. Calcium gluconate contains 4.65 mEq Ca++ and calcium chloride contains 13.6 mEq Ca++ in 10 mL of a 10% solution. Adjust doses accordingly.

2. Transient but immediate effect.

3. Usual dose of calcium gluconate is 1,000 mg and calcium chloride is 500 to 1,000 mg infused over 2 to 3 minutes. The dose can be repeated after 5 minutes if EKG changes persist or recur.

4. Central line preferred (especially for calcium or high doses of calcium gluconate).

B. Step 2: Shift potassium to intracellular space. ▶

1. 10 units IV insulin with 50-mL dextrose 50% to prevent hypoglycemia. Repeat as needed. Monitor glucose and potassium closely.
2. High dose beta-agonists such as nebulized albuterol.
3. Sodium bicarbonate in acidotic patients.
   a. NOTE: Correcting acidosis can also lower calcium levels, so monitor levels very closely.
C. Step 3: Remove excess potassium.
   1. Loop diuretics; adequate dosing for renal function.
   2. GI cation exchangers: They bind potassium in the GI tract in exchange for other cations such as sodium or calcium.
   a. Patiromer (Veltassa) as 8.4 g PO once daily.
   b. Sodium zirconium cyclosilicate (SZC): 10 g TID for 48 hours in hyperkalemic emergency.
   c. Sodium polystyrene sulfonate (SPS): Used rarely. Avoid due to complications of bowel necrosis (majority when SPS was administered with sorbitol). If used, given as 15 to 30 g PO every 4 to 6 hours or 30 to 60 g per retention enema.
D. Step 4: Dialysis. Consult a nephrology expert.
   1. Assess all electrolytes and acid–base balance and treat as indicated with nephrology.

FOLLOW-UP

A. Continue to monitor potassium levels for 24 to 48 hours after the last dose of medication to account for the half-life of all medications.
B. Consider chronic treatment, which also includes potassium restriction and increased potassium elimination.
   1. Dietary potassium restriction.
   2. Discontinuation of medications associated with hyperkalemia.
   3. Loop diuretics and GI cation exchangers.
C. Follow up with nephrology and cardiology as needed until potassium is normalized.

CONSULTATION/REFERRAL

A. Consult nephrology for any refractory electrolyte disorder with or without acute kidney injury (AKI) or CKD.
B. Consult endocrinology for any uncontrolled diabetes.

SPECIAL/GERIATRIC CONSIDERATIONS

A. SPS (Kayexalate) is associated with bowel necrosis. Use with caution in all populations, but especially in patients at risk of slow GI motility. Try to avoid use as much as possible.
B. The high doses of beta-agonists required to shift potassium intracellularly can cause tachycardia. Use with caution in patients with preexisting arrhythmias and in other at-risk populations.
C. Patients with CKD and end-stage renal disease (ESRD) as well as high risk of history of cardiac arrhythmias have a higher risk of mortality with hypokalemia than hyperkalemia. Monitor carefully.
D. Patients with chronic hyperkalemia may not require acute lowering of potassium levels for baseline potassium in the absence of EKG changes or other signs/symptoms.

CASE SCENARIO: HYPERKALEMIA

A 30-year-old Black male with end-stage renal disease (ESRD) on hemodialysis (HD) came to the ED with weakness and lethargy after missing HD for the last 1 week. He makes very little urine. His vitals were stable on presentation. His labs showed potassium of 9 mEq/L and bicarbonate of 7mEq/L. EKG showed peaked T-waves.

1. What is the first step in management?
   A. Immediate hemodialysis
   B. Intravenous (IV) calcium gluconate
   C. Furosemide 40 mg IV once
   D. IV isotonic fluids

BIBLIOGRAPHY

Allon, M. (2014). Disorders of potassium metabolism. In D. S. Gipson, M. A. Perazella, & M. Tonelli (Eds.), *National Kidney Foundation's primer on kidney diseases* (6th ed., pp. 90–99). Elsevier Saunders.

Choi, M. J., & Ziyadeh, F. N. (2008, March). The utility of the transtubular potassium gradient in the evaluation of hyperkalemia. *Journal of the American Society of Nephrology*, 19(3), 424–426. https://doi.org/10.1681/ASN.2007091017

Cohnm, J. N., Kowey, P. R., Whelton, P. K., & Prisant, L. M. (2000). New guidelines for potassium replacement in clinical practice. *Archives of Internal Medicine*, 160, 2429–2436. https://doi.org/10.1001/archinte.160.16.2429

Ethier, J. H., Kamel, K. S., Magner, P. O., Lemann, J., & Halperin, M. L. (1990, April). The transtubular potassium concentration in patients with hypokalemia and hyperkalemia. *American Journal of Kidney Diseases*, 15(4), 309–315. https://doi.org/10.1016/s0272-6386(12)80076-x

Kraft, M. D., Btaiche, I. F., Sacks, G. S., & Kudsk, K. A. (2005). Treatment of electrolyte disorders in adult patients in the intensive care unit. *American Journal Health System Pharmacy*, 62(16), 1663–1682. https://doi.org/10.2146/ajhp040300

Pepin, J., & Sheilds, C. (2012). Advances in diagnosis and management of hypokalemic and hyperkalemic emergencies. *Emergency Medical Practice*, 14(2), 1–20.

Sood, M. M., Sood, A. R., & Richardson, R. (2007). Emergency management and commonly encountered outpatient scenarios in patients with hyperkalemia. *Mayo Clinic Proceedings*, 82(12), 1553–1561. https://doi.org/10.1016/S0025-6196(11)61102-6

HYPERMAGNESEMIA

Divya Monga and Catherine Wells

DEFINITION

A. See Box 5.4.
B. Mild hypermagnesemia 2.5 to 4 mg/dL.
C. Moderate hypermagnesemia 4 to 12.5 mg/dL.
D. Severe hypermagnesemia greater than 12.5 mg/dL.

INCIDENCE

A. Hypermagnesemia is rare in patients with normal renal function.

PATHOGENESIS

A. Magnesium is the second most abundant intracellular cation in the body after potassium.
B. It is critical in the functioning of neuromuscular, cardiac, and nervous system functions.
C. Magnesium is vital to vascular tone, heart rhythm, bone formation, and muscle contraction, among many other critical functions.

BOX 5.4 MAGNESIUM IN HUMANS

Normal serum range is 1.5–2.4 mg/dL.
It is found primarily in soft tissue, bone, and muscle.
Approximately 1% of total body magnesium is found in the ECF. 30% of the magnesium found in ECF is protein-bound. The remaining 70% is filterable.
Homeostasis is managed primarily by the kidneys, but the gastrointestinal tract, parathyroid hormone, and serum magnesium concentrations are also involved.
It serves as a cofactor in many enzymatic and biochemical reactions, including reactions involving adenosine triphosphate.

ECF, extracellular fluid.

PREDISPOSING FACTORS
A. Excessive intake of magnesium.
B. Lithium.
C. Hypothyroidism.
D. Decreased glomerular filtration rate (GFR) due to end-stage renal disease (ESRD)/chronic kidney disease (CKD)/acute kidney injury (AKI).

SUBJECTIVE DATA
A. Common complaints/symptoms.
  1. Typically asymptomatic until serum concentrations exceed 4 mg/dL.
  2. Mild/moderate hypermagnesemia.
    a. Nausea, vomiting, flushing, lethargy, and somnolence.
    b. Diminished/absent deep tendon reflexes.
    c. Hypotension.
    d. Bradycardia.
    e. EKG changes such as increased PR interval, increased QRS duration, and increased QT interval.
  3. Severe hypermagnesemia.
    a. Respiratory paralysis and flaccid quadriplegia.
    b. Refractory hypotension.
    c. EKG changes as above and atrioventricular block.
    d. Cardiac arrest.
  4. Hypocalcemia-related symptoms: Moderate hypermagnesemia can inhibit secretion of the parathyroid hormone (PTH), leading to reduction in plasma calcium concentration. Hence, watch for symptoms related to hypocalcemia.

PHYSICAL EXAMINATION
A. Check reflexes.
B. Check blood pressure (BP).
C. Perform cardiac examination.

DIAGNOSTIC TESTS
A. Serum magnesium.
B. Serum creatinine (SCr)/blood urea nitrogen (BUN), intact parathyroid hormone (iPTH), and serum calcium levels.
C. EKG.
D. Evaluation for pregnancy.

DIFFERENTIAL DIAGNOSIS
A. Ingestion.
  1. Magnesium-containing laxatives or antacids.

  2. Accidental ingestion of Epsom salts (magnesium sulfate).
B. Intravenous (IV) magnesium infusion (intentional overdose).
  1. Therapy for preeclampsia and eclampsia.
  2. Parenteral nutrition or magnesium supplementation.
C. Reduced excretion.
  1. Reduced renal function due to CKD or AKI.
D. Theophylline intoxication.
E. Acromegaly.
F. Hypercatabolic state: For example, tumor lysis syndrome.
G. Familial hypocalciuric hypercalcemia.
H. Adrenal insufficiency.

EVALUATION AND MANAGEMENT PLAN
A. Step 1: If severe cardiac symptoms exist, give IV calcium immediately. It can transiently stabilize the neuromuscular and cardiac effects of severe, symptomatic hypermagnesemia.
  1. IV calcium: Usual dose is 100 to 200 mg elemental calcium over 5 to 10 minutes.
B. Step 2: Determine the cause.
  1. Intentional overdose for medical reasons should not be corrected.
  2. If indicated, restrict or discontinue all magnesium-containing agents.
C. Step 3: Treat other electrolyte and acid–base disorders.
D. Step 4: Accelerate renal magnesium clearance.
  1. IV isotonic fluids plus loop diuretics, which can increase urinary excretion of magnesium.
  2. Hemodialysis, which can remove excess magnesium, if all other measures fail, especially in cases of severe neurologic and cardiovascular manifestations.

FOLLOW-UP
A. Hypermagnesemia is a rare occurrence. Follow up with nephrology if persistent.

CONSULTATION/REFFERAL
A. Nephrology should be consulted if hypermagnesemia cannot be explained or requires an intervention such as dialysis.

SPECIAL/GERIATRIC CONSIDERATIONS
A. This is a rare condition that is typically caused by ingestion of excessive magnesium.

CASE SCENARIO: HYPERMAGNESEMIA

A 75-year-old White male with chronic kidney disease (CKD) stage 3 presented to the ED with nausea, vomiting, and lethargy. He has been constipated for the last 1 week and was taking multiple daily doses of magnesium oxide as laxative.

1. What is the most common etiology of the patient's symptoms?
  A. Hyperkalemia
  B. Hypermagnesemia
  C. Inadequate dialysis dose
  D. Hyperphosphatemia

BIBLIOGRAPHY

Kraft, M. D., Btaiche, I. F., Sacks, G. S., & Kudsk, K. A. (2005, August). Treatment of electrolyte disorders in adult patients in the intensive care unit. *American Journal of Health System Pharmacy, 62*(16), 1663–1682. https://doi.org/10.2146/ajhp040300

Moe, S. M., & Daoud, J. R. (2014). Disorders of mineral metabolism: Calcium, phosphorous, and magnesium. In D. S. Gipson, M. A. Perazella, & M. Tonelli (Eds.), *National Kidney Foundation's primer on kidney diseases* (6th ed., pp. 100–112). Elsevier Saunders.

HYPERNATREMIA

Divya Monga and Catherine Wells

DEFINITION

A. Serum sodium greater than 145 mEq/L (Box 5.5).

INCIDENCE

A. Up to 80% of hypernatremia is hospital-acquired. Only 0.1% to 1.4% of hypernatremia is present on admission.
B. Overall inpatient incidence is 1% to 5%, and incidence in critically ill patients is 9% to 26%.
C. Hypernatremia is associated with increased length of stay and is an independent predictor of mortality.
D. Populations at increased risk.
  1. Extremes of age (infants and older adults), especially patients with pulmonary infections or urinary tract infections (UTIs).
  2. Restricted access to water, that is, intubated or debilitated patients.
  3. Altered mental status/neurologic illness.
  4. Chronic debilitating illnesses associated with impaired thirst/dehydration.

PATHOGENESIS

A. Reflects a water deficit relative to total body sodium.
B. Can occur in hypovolemic, euvolemic, and hypervolemic patients.
C. Causes plasma hypertonicity (effect of plasma on cells that causes the cells to shrink).
D. Almost always associated with reduced intake of water with or without loss of the normal thirst response. Otherwise, individuals' normal thirst would encourage them to drink a sufficient amount to correct plasma hypertonicity.
E. Hypovolemic hypernatremia: Represents a pronounced water deficit with a mild sodium deficit and requires impaired thirst or decreased intake of water in addition to losses.
F. Euvolemic hypernatremia: Represents a pure body water deficit.
G. Hypervolemic hypernatremia: Represents minimal decrease or no change in total body water (TBW) with an increase in total body sodium.
H. Acute salt poisoning: Large intake of sodium (whether accidental or intentional), resulting in a rapid rise in sodium and subsequent severe hypertonicity.

PREDISPOSING FACTORS

A. Alterations in thirst.
B. Volume depletion.
C. Hyperglycemia.
D. Certain brain tumors such as pituitary tumors.

SUBJECTIVE DATA

A. Common complaints/symptoms.
  1. Vary depending on the cause, severity, and rate of development of hypernatremia.
    a. Altered skin turgor commonly found in hypovolemic or euvolemic hypernatremia.
    b. Signs of volume overload: Hypervolemic hypernatremia.
  2. Spectrum of neurologic symptoms: Beginning with irritability, dizziness, fatigue, lethargy, and confusion; can progress to seizures and coma.
  3. Other symptoms: Nausea, vomiting, and generalized muscle weakness.
  4. Polyuria.
    a. Definition: 3 L or more per day.
    b. Urine output (UO) exceeding 5 to 10 L per day indicates antidiuretic hormone (ADH) deficiency (as in diabetes insipidus [DI]); these affected patients often crave ice.
  5. Acute salt poisoning: High fever, intracranial hemorrhage, seizures, and coma.

PHYSICAL EXAMINATION

A. Physical examination to assess volume status.
  1. Check skin, mucous membranes, heart, lungs, jugular venous distension (JVD), and edema.
  2. Assess blood pressure (BP) and orthostatic changes.
  3. Determine weight changes.
B. Neurologic assessment (initial and ongoing).

DIAGNOSTIC TESTS

A. Serum sodium.
B. Complete chemistry panel to assess causes.
C. Serum osmolality.
D. Spot urine osmolality (measured).
  1. Greater than 300 mOsm/kg: Urine is concentrated and hypertonic but not necessarily due to sodium. This indicates a relative increase in solute compared with water.
  2. Less than 100 mOsm/kg: Urine is dilute and hypotonic. This indicates a relative increase in water and/or decrease in solute.

▶

BOX 5.5   SODIUM IN HUMANS

Normal serum concentration is 135–145 mEq/L.
It is the most abundant extracellular cation.
The majority of total body sodium is found in cells and plasma water. Additional bound sodium is found (and can accumulate) in bone, cartilage, and connective tissue.
Plasma sodium is approximately the same as interstitial sodium.
Sodium does not cross the blood–brain barrier, but plasma sodium levels and tonicity of plasma affect brain cells.
Changes in serum sodium concentration typically reflect changes in water balance rather than actual changes in total body sodium.

E. Spot urine sodium.

1. Less than 20 mEq/L: Renal sodium retention as in low effective arterial blood volume.

    a. Common with extrarenal volume losses.

2. Greater than 20 to 30 mEq/L: Renal-related losses of electrolytes (sodium).

    a. Common with loop diuretics, osmotic diuresis, or hyperglycemia.

    b. Post-acute kidney injury (AKI) diuresis and postobstructive diuresis.

F. Determination of patient volume status.

1. Consider volume assessment to be unreliable initial diagnostic criteria but is necessary when interpreting hypernatremia-related lab tests.

2. Review and calculate history of fluid intake and output.

DIFFERENTIAL DIAGNOSIS

A. Hypovolemic hypernatremia.

1. Water and salt deficit.

2. Renal losses (urine sodium >20 mEq/L).

    a. Loop diuretics (spot urine osmolality <100 mOsm/kg [hypotonic]).

    b. Postobstructive or post-AKI diuresis.

    c. Osmotic diuresis: Hyperglycemia, mannitol, urea (enteral tube feedings; spot urine osmolality >300 mOsm/kg or 24-hour urine osmolality >1,200 mOsm/kg).

3. Extrarenal losses: Urine sodium less than 20 mEq/L; urine osmolality greater than 300 mOsm/kg (hypertonic).

    a. Gastrointestinal (GI) losses such as vomiting, diarrhea (e.g., acute infectious, osmotic [enteral tube feedings]), nasogastric suctioning, or enterocutaneous fistula.

    b. Skin losses: Perspiration, burns, or severe wounds.

B. Euvolemic hypernatremia.

1. Pure water deficit; body sodium preserved.

2. Renal losses: Hypotonic urine (urine osmolality/plasma osmolality <1).

    a. DI: Inadequate ADH release (spot urine osmolality <100 mOsm/kg).

      i. Central DI: Congenital, head trauma, post neurosurgical surgery, neoplasms, infiltrative disorders (e.g., sarcoidosis), hypoxic encephalopathy, bleeding, infection, aneurysm, and meningitis/encephalitis.

      b. Gestational DI: Peripheral degradation of ADH.

      c. Nephrogenic DI (hereditary): Inadequate renal response to ADH.

        i. X-linked nephrogenic DI.

        ii. Autosomal recessive nephrogenic DI.

      d. Acquired nephrogenic DI: ADH independent urine concentrating defect.

        i. Hypercalcemia or hypokalemia.

        ii. Medication-induced: Lithium, vasopressin V_2 receptor antagonists, demeclocycline, amphotericin B, methoxyflurane, or foscarnet.

        iii. Chronic kidney disease (CKD; e.g., medullary cyst disease, sickle cell disease, amyloidosis, Sjögren syndrome).

        iv. Bartter syndrome.

        v. Malnutrition.

3. Extrarenal losses: Hypertonic urine (urine osmolality/plasma osmolality >1).

    a. Insensible losses.

      i. Cutaneous: Fever, sweating, burns, or increased ambient temperature.

      ii. Respiratory: Tachypnea or mechanical ventilation.

    b. Decreased water intake.

      i. Primary hypodipsia.

      ii. Reset osmostat.

      iii. Decreased access to water (e.g., altered mental status, iatrogenic).

      iv. Water loss intracellular (e.g., seizures, extreme exercise).

C. Hypervolemic hypernatremia.

1. Increased sodium intake (TBW and sodium can be variable).

2. Iatrogenic causes.

    a. Sodium administration (e.g., normal saline, 3% saline, or sodium bicarbonate) via intravenous (IV) or oral routes.

    b. Hyperalimentation.

3. Mineralocorticoid excess.

4. Hypertonic dialysis.

5. Salt ingestion.

EVALUATION AND MANAGEMENT PLAN

A. Initial goal: To replace free water deficit and prevent ongoing water loss. ▶

1. Assess volume status.
2. Calculate water losses and exact replacement necessary to avoid overcorrection.
   a. TBW for lean men is usually 60% of weight in kilogram and for lean women is usually 50% of weight in kilogram. TBW is lower (approximated to 45%) in patients with obesity due to adipose tissue. Older adult patients also have a lower TBW (commonly estimated around 50%).
   b. Free water deficit (L) = current TBW × [plasma Na/140 − 1].
3. Choose appropriate replacement fluid and initial rate of repletion based on acuity and degree of hypovolemia.
4. Estimate ongoing water losses: Renal and extrarenal.
5. Choose an appropriate replacement fluid based on sodium level and underlying cause/diagnosis.
6. Choose replacement rate based on water losses.

B. Hypovolemic hypernatremia.
   1. Step 1: Replace intravascular volume deficit (plasma volume deficit) with isotonic crystalloids within the first several hours. The goal is stable hemodynamics.
   2. Step 2: Replace total free water deficit/loss over 3 to 4 days (include ongoing losses).
      a. Calculate free water deficit (as previously noted).
      b. Choose hypotonic replacement fluid.
         i. 0.45% NaCl IV (½ of the volume given is water).
         ii. Dextrose 5% in water (D5W; oral/gastric tube water, IV).
      c. Replacement rate.
         i. Acute rise in sodium (hypernatremia developed over <48 hours).
            1) Rapid water replacement/correction over 24 hours. Initial fluid regimen: IV D5W at 3 to 6 mL/kg/hr up to a maximum of 666 mL/hr.
         ii. Chronic rise in sodium (hypernatremia developed over >48 hours; NOTE: If unknown whether hypernatremia is acute or chronic, treat as chronic).
            1) Maximum rate for sodium correction = 10 mEq/L per day over 2 to 3 days.
            2) Less than 6 mEq/L per day in older adult patients.
      d. Monitor fluid intake and output closely.
      e. With low sodium intake, do not allow sodium intake to exceed output as this will exacerbate hypernatremia.
      f. Determine and treat the underlying cause.
      g. Perform neurologic checks frequently.
      h. Monitor sodium and blood glucose levels every 4 hours.
      i. Monitor all electrolytes and replace as indicated.
      j. Initially monitor closely in an intensive care setting.

   3. Step 3: Replace ongoing water losses.
      a. Choose fluid with less sodium than current urine concentration.
      b. Monitor sodium at least daily.
      c. Monitor fluid intake and output closely.
      d. Give a low-salt diet.
   4. Step 4: Monitor/replace other electrolyte losses due to polyuria (e.g., hypokalemia, bicarbonate).

C. Euvolemic and hypervolemic hypernatremia.
   1. Step 1: If necessary, correct water deficit (as previously noted).
   2. Step 2: Monitor fluid intake and output closely. Low-salt diet. Do not allow sodium intake to exceed output as this will exacerbate hypernatremia.
   3. Step 3: Define/treat underlying cause.
      a. Review medications.
      b. Consider desmopressin (dDAVP) for central DI (synthetic ADH analog; also increases factor VIII and von Willebrand factor levels—monitor for clotting) at ONE of the following doses:
         i. 0.05 to 0.6 mg daily divided doses PO (needs to be titrated).
         ii. 1mcg Q12h subcutaneously.
         iii. 10 to 20 mcg BID intranasal.
      c. Perform neurologic checks frequently.
      d. Monitor sodium levels every 4 hours, then daily.
      e. Monitor all electrolytes and replace as indicated.
      f. Initially monitor closely in an intensive care setting.
   4. Step 4: Treat other electrolyte and acid–base disorders.

D. Acute salt poisoning: Rapid rise in sodium.
   1. Give a rapid infusion of water to correct at a rate of 1 mEq/L/hr.
   2. Consider hemodialysis for sodium correction.
   3. Closely monitor and avoid overcorrection.

FOLLOW-UP
A. Follow-up depends on the nature of the underlying condition.
B. Hypernatremia needs to be corrected and maintained.

CONSULTATION/REFERRAL
A. Consult nephrology to help regulate hypernatremia.
B. Consult neurosurgery if central DI is responsible for hypernatremia.

SPECIAL/GERIATRIC CONSIDERATIONS
A. Increased age: Decline in TBW, decreased urinary concentrating ability, and impaired thirst; thus, older adult patients lack the same defenses against hypernatremia as younger patients.

CASE SCENARIO: HYPERNATREMIA

A 64-year-old nursing home resident with hemiplegia post cerebrovascular accident (CVA) was brought to the ED for altered mental status and refusal to drink or eat for 4 to 5 days. She has chronic kidney disease stage 3. Her home meds included aspirin, lisinopril, and atorvastatin. She was tachycardic and mildly hypotensive on presentation. Serum sodium on presentation was 181 mEq/L and serum creatinine 3.5 mg/dL (baseline 3).

1. What is the most appropriate intravenous fluid as first-line management of hypernatremia?

  A. Intravenous (IV) normal saline
  B. IV Ringer's lactate
  C. IV dextrose 5% in water
  D. IV albumin

BIBLIOGRAPHY

Kraft, M. D., Btaiche, I. F., Sacks, G. S., & Kudsk, K. A. (2005, August). Treatment of electrolyte disorders in adult patients in the intensive care unit. *American Journal of Health System Pharmacy, 62*(16), 1663–1682. https://doi.org/10.2146/ajhp040300

Lindner, G., Funk, G. C., & Schwarz, C. (2007). Hypernatremia in the critically ill is an independent risk factor for mortality. *American Journal of Kidney Diseases, 50*, 952. https://doi.org/10.1053/j.ajkd.2007.08.016

Sterns, R. H. (2015). Disorders of plasma sodium. *The New England Journal of Medicine, 372*(1), 55–65. https://doi.org/10.1056/NEJMc1501342

HYPERPHOSPHATEMIA

Divya Monga and Catherine Wells

DEFINITION

A. Serum phosphorus greater than 4.5 mg/dL (Box 5.6).

INCIDENCE

A. Hyperphosphatemia is most common in renal impairment (acute or chronic).
B. Sustained hyperphosphatemia is rare in the absence of renal disease.

PATHOGENESIS

A. Homeostasis of phosphate is maintained through gastrointestinal (GI) absorption and renal excretion. Imbalances in either of these mechanisms can result in hyperphosphatemia.

PREDISPOSING FACTORS

A. Acute or chronic kidney disease.
B. Excessive intake is rare, but a potential cause.

SUBJECTIVE DATA

A. Common complaints/symptoms.
  1. Most common and significant manifestations are signs/symptoms of hypocalcemia due to calcium-phosphate precipitation with decrease in ionized calcium.
  2. Can lead to soft tissue calcification due to precipitation of calcium-phosphate crystals in soft tissues, producing symptoms of pruritus, dermatologic changes, and (in severe cases) calciphylaxis.

PHYSICAL EXAMINATION

A. Respiratory examination.
B. Musculoskeletal examination.
C. Dermatologic examination.

DIAGNOSTIC TESTS

A. Serum phosphorus.
B. Serum total calcium, ionized calcium.
C. Venous carbon dioxide (CO_2).
D. Renal function evaluation (blood urea nitrogen [BUN] and serum creatinine [SCr]).

DIFFERENTIAL DIAGNOSIS

A. Renal failure or decreased renal excretion.
  1. In chronic dialysis patients, poor compliance with phosphorus-binding medications.
B. Increased intestinal absorption/exogenous phosphate.
  1. Ingestion of large amounts of phosphate-containing laxatives and enemas like oral sodium phosphate/fleets phospho soda (has been associated with acute phosphate nephropathy if given in patients with chronic kidney disease [CKD]).
  2. Rarely, high-dose fosphenytoin.
  3. Vitamin D overdose.
C. Rapid shifts from intracellular to extracellular.
  1. Acidosis (respiratory or metabolic).
  2. Hemolysis.
  3. Rhabdomyolysis.
  4. Tumor lysis syndrome.
D. Hypoparathyroidism.
E. Hypocalcemia (reciprocal rise).
F. Thyrotoxicosis, acromegaly (rare).
G. Bisphosphonates/fibroblast growth factor receptor (FGFR) inhibitors.
H. Pseudohyperphosphatemia: Due to interference with analytical methods in patients with hyperglobulinemia, hyperlipidemia, hemolysis, and hyperbilirubinemia. Also seen with high-dose liposomal amphotericin use.

EVALUATION AND MANAGEMENT PLAN

A. Step 1: Volume expansion if kidney function intact.
  1. Initial bolus resuscitation.
  2. Continue isotonic intravenous (IV) hydration.
B. Step 2: Emergency treatment for acute and severe hyperphosphatemia due to risk of renal failure.
  1. Calcium replacement (see "Hypocalcemia"). Acute, severe hyperphosphatemia can cause reciprocal hypocalcemia.
  2. Emergency treatment: Renal replacement therapy. Consult nephrology.
  3. Additional management.
    a. Phosphorus binders (as noted in the text that follows) at large doses with meals and snacks, plus a dose at bedtime.
    b. Consultation with a renal dietitian for dietary counseling.
      i. Tightly restrict unnecessary sources of phosphorus in the diet, such as food preservatives and higher phosphorus grains and vegetables.
      ii. Choose an individualized target for protein intake that will not place the patient at risk for ▶

BOX 5.6 PHOSPHORUS IN HUMANS

85% of total body phosphorus is located in bones.
The remaining 14% is intracellular and only 1% is extracellular.
Between 60% and 70% of dietary phosphorus is absorbed by the gastrointestinal tract, in all intestinal segments.
In the kidneys, 70%–80% of filtered phosphorus load is reabsorbed in the proximal tubule.

Two-thirds of ingested phosphorus is excreted in the urine, with the remainder excreted in the stool.
Normal serum phosphorus is 2.5–4.5 mg/dL.
Many physiologic functions:
    Bone and cell membrane composition
    Nerve conduction
    Muscle function
    Cell membrane phospholipid content and function
    Platelet aggregation
    Energy-rich bonds of adenosine triphosphate

nutrition deficiencies or allow excessive phosphorus intake from protein sources.

   c. Continuation of isotonic IV hydration. Consider loop diuretics if needed to increase urine output (UO).

C. Step 3: If nonemergent, assess for cause of hyperphosphatemia.

   1. Hyperphosphatemia management is oral phosphate binders and dietary restriction in patients with chronic renal disease.

     a. Give phosphate binders with food in order to bind dietary phosphorus in the intestinal tract and prevent absorption.

     b. Avoid magnesium- and aluminum-based binders due to risk of accumulation in renal disease.

   2. Phosphorus binders should not be given to patients with acute kidney injury (AKI) due to risk for overcorrection (hypophosphatemia) during recovery.

   3. Current available formulations.

     a. Calcium-based (calcium acetate or calcium carbonate).

     b. Sevelamer.

     c. Lanthanum.

     d. Iron-based (ferric citrate or sucroferric oxyhydroxide).

     e. Dose is specific to formulation used.

D. Step 4: Treat the underlying cause if possible.

E. Step 5: Treat other electrolyte and acid–base disorders.

FOLLOW-UP

A. Calcium levels, phosphate levels, and renal function should be monitored at constant intervals.

CONSULTATION/REFERRAL

A. Nephrology may be consulted if the hyperphosphatemia is associated with renal failure. Endocrinology may be consulted if the patient has hypoparathyroidism.

SPECIAL/GERIATRIC CONSIDERATIONS

A. Older adult patients with CKD are at risk of hyperphosphatemia.

CASE SCENARIO: HYPERPHOSPHATEMIA

A 75-year-old female with history of hypertension on lisinopril and with chronic kidney disease (CKD) stage 4 presented to the hospital with complaints of nausea, vomiting, and muscle cramps. She recently had a colonoscopy for which the bowel preparation used was oral sodium phosphate. Her labs showed marked elevation of creatinine from baseline and severe hyperphosphatemia.

1. What is the most likely diagnosis?
   A. Acute gastroenteritis
   B. Acute appendicitis
   C. Acute phosphate nephropathy
   D. Progression of CKD

BIBLIOGRAPHY

Kraft, M. D., Btaiche, I. F., Sacks, G. S., & Kudsk, K. A. (2005, August). Treatment of electrolyte disorders in adult patients in the intensive care unit. *American Journal of Health System Pharmacy*, 62(16), 1663–1682. https://doi.org/10.2146/ajhp040300

Moe, S. M., & Daoud, J. R. (2014). Disorders of mineral metabolism: Calcium, phosphorous, and magnesium. In D. D. Gipson, M. A. Perazella, & M. Tonelli (Eds.), *National Kidney Foundation's primer on kidney diseases* (6th ed., pp. 100–112). Elsevier Saunders.

Stubbs, J. R., & Yu, A. S. L. (2017). *Overview of the causes and treatment of hyperphosphatemia*. In S. Goldfarb & A. Q. Lam (Eds.), *UpToDate*. https://www.uptodate.com/contents/overview-of-the-causes-andtreatment-of-hyperphosphatemia

HYPOCALCEMIA

Divya Monga and Catherine Wells

DEFINITION

A. Total serum calcium less than 8.6 mg/dL or ionized calcium less than 1.1 mmol/L (see Box 5.2).

INCIDENCE

A. The incidence of hypocalcemia is difficult to quantify.

B. In intensive care patients, hypocalcemia is estimated between 15% and 88% of all patients.

PATHOGENESIS

A. Calcium is necessary for bone mineralization, nerve conduction, muscle relaxation, and cardiac conduction. ▶

B. Calcium is a required element in the clotting cascade.

C. Calcium is available for use in many forms.

    1. Ionized calcium (metabolically active).

    2. Anion bound calcium (bound to phosphate, citrate, etc.)

    3. Protein-bound is the most abundant calcium (primarily albumin-bound).

PREDISPOSING FACTORS

A. Renal failure.

B. Advancing age.

C. Volume depletion.

D. Hepatic insufficiency.

E. Chronic heart failure.

SUBJECTIVE DATA

A. Common complaints/symptoms.

    1. Most specific symptoms are perioral numbness and spasms of the upper and lower extremities.

    2. Severe hypocalcemia can lead to tetany and seizures.

    3. Other neuromuscular, central nervous system (CNS), and cardiovascular symptoms may be present, even with mild to moderate hypocalcemia.

        a. Prolonged QT interval.

        b. Paresthesia.

    4. Chronic hypocalcemia may present with skin manifestations such as brittle and grooved nails, hair loss, dermatitis, and eczema.

PHYSICAL EXAMINATION

A. Cardiac examination.

    1. Assess EKG and rhythm.

    2. Blood pressure (BP).

B. Neurologic examination.

    1. Chvostek sign or Trousseau sign: Increased neuromuscular activity can be demonstrated by tapping over the facial nerve.

    2. Reflexes.

C. Assess for bleeding.

DIAGNOSTIC TESTS

A. Total and ionized serum calcium.

B. Serum phosphorus.

C. Serum magnesium.

D. 25-hydroxyvitamin D.

E. Intact parathyroid hormone (iPTH).

F. Serum albumin.

DIFFERENTIAL DIAGNOSIS

A. Hypoparathyroidism.

B. Pseudohypoparathyroidism (low calcium with low phosphorus also known as iPTH resistance).

C. Hypomagnesemia.

D. Hypoalbuminemia (low total calcium may not reflect actual calcium stores).

E. Vitamin D deficiency.

    1. Poor intestinal absorption (e.g., short bowel, poor nutritional intake).

    2. Lack of sun exposure.

    3. Decreased activation of vitamin D (e.g., cirrhosis, kidney failure).

F. Tissue consumption of calcium.

    1. Acute severe pancreatitis.

    2. Sepsis.

    3. Acute malignancies/blastic bone metastases (excess bone formation).

    4. "Hungry bone syndrome" post parathyroidectomy in chronic kidney disease (CKD) or end-stage renal disease (ESRD) patients with history of hyperparathyroidism.

    5. Acute hyperphosphatemia (e.g., rhabdomyolysis, tumor lysis syndrome).

    6. Citrate infusion (citrate binds to ionized calcium decreasing unbound, active calcium).

        a. Transfusion of blood products preserved with citrate.

        b. Circuit anticoagulation for dialysis/apheresis.

G. Drug-related hypocalcemia.

    1. Calcium chelators.

        a. Citrate (as above).

        b. Lactate.

        c. Foscarnet.

        d. Sodium ethylenediaminetetraacetic acid (EDTA; repeat lab collection).

    2. Bisphosphonates, denosumab, cinacalcet, and foscarnet.

    3. Fluoride poisoning.

    4. Some specific gadolinium-based contrast agents (spurious hypocalcemia).

        a. Gadodiamide and gadoversetamide.

EVALUATION AND MANAGEMENT PLAN

A. Step 1: Replace acute calcium needs.

    1. Intravenous (IV) administration used when rapid correction is required.

    2. Initial dose: 1 g calcium chloride or 3 g calcium gluconate.

        a. Repeat dose as needed.

        b. Calcium chloride contains three times more elemental calcium than calcium gluconate.

    3. Caution: IV calcium can cause vascular and tissue necrosis if extravasation occurs as both calcium chloride and calcium gluconate. A central IV line is recommended for all calcium infusions.

B. Step 2: Assess for ongoing calcium replacement needs and replace as indicated.

    1. Use IV or oral calcium replacement.

    2. Oral calcium supplements used in asymptomatic patients and patients with chronic hypocalcemia.

        a. Calcium carbonate contains maximum elemental calcium compared with other formulations.

        b. Typical dose is calcium carbonate 1,250 mg (equivalent to 500 mg elemental calcium) BID.

        c. Take on empty stomach to maximize absorption of calcium.

    3. Administer vitamin D to increase intestinal absorption of calcium if vitamin is deficient.

        a. NOTE: Patients with renal failure need activated formulas of vitamin D replacement. Consult nephrology for assistance.

C. Step 3: Treat other electrolyte and acid–base disorders (e.g., hypomagnesemia).

FOLLOW-UP

A. Follow-up with an outpatient provider to monitor labs would be advised.

CONSULTATION/REFERRAL

A. Consider consults based on the underlying cause of hypocalcemia and the severity of the condition.

SPECIAL/GERIATRIC CONSIDERATIONS

A. Severe hypocalcemia may result in seizures, tetany, refractory hypotension, or arrhythmias that require a more aggressive approach.

CASE SCENARIO: HYPOCALCEMIA

FS is a 65-year-old with a past medical history (PMH) of chronic kidney disease (CKD) stage 3, heart failure with preserved ejection fraction, and hypertension (HTN). Outpatient labs 2 months ago were checked and all electrolytes were normal. The patient is admitted to the ED due to fever, dyspnea, and shortness of breath, with suspected pneumonia and sepsis with elevated white blood cell (WBC) at 23. On admission, his total calcium is 6.4 mg/dL and albumin is 3.8 mg/dL. Mental status is altered; he cannot answer review of symptoms (ROS).

1. What is the best next step?

A. Check ionized calcium before making any decisions.

B. Order 3 g calcium gluconate intravenous (IV) now, check EKG to assess QT interval, and order ionized calcium level now and to repeat after IV infusion.

C. Order ionized calcium level, order vitamin D and parathyroid hormone (PTH), and order EKG. Once results are received, create a plan.

D. Order 1 g calcium chloride IV now and repeat total calcium level in the morning.

BIBLIOGRAPHY

Goltzman, D. (2000, updated 2016). Approach to hypercalcemia. In K. R. Feingold, B. Anawalt, B. A. Boyce, G. Chrousos, W. W. de Herder, K. Dhatariya, K. Dungan, J. M. Hershman, J. Hofland, S. Kalra, G. Kaltsas, C. Koch, P. Kopp, M. Korbonits, C. S. Kovacs, W. Kuohung, B. Laferrère, M. Levy, E. A. McGee, & D. P. Wilson (Eds.), *Endotext.* MDText.com. https://www.ncbi.nlm.nih.gov/books/NBK279129/

Goltzman, D. (2022). Etiology of hypocalcemia in adults. In C. J. Rossen (Ed.), *Up to Date.* https://www.uptodate.com/contents/etiology-of-hypocalcemia-in-adults?search=hypocalcemia&source=search_result&selectedTitle=1~150&usage_type=default&display_rank=1

Kraft, M. D., Btaiche, I. F., Sacks, G. S., & Kudsk, K. A. (2005, August). Treatment of electrolyte disorders in adult patients in the intensive care unit. *American Journal of Health System Pharmacy, 62*(16), 1663–1682. https://doi.org/10.2146/ajhp040300

Moe, S. M., & Daoud, J. R. (2014). Disorders of mineral metabolism: Calcium, phosphorous, and magnesium. In D. S. Gipson, M. A. Perazella, & M. Tonelli (Eds.), *National Kidney Foundation's primer on kidney diseases* (6th ed., pp. 100–112). Elsevier Saunders.

HYPOKALEMIA

Divya Monga and Catherine Wells

DEFINITION

A. Serum potassium concentration of less than 3.5 mEq/L (see Box 5.3).

INCIDENCE

A. Hypokalemia occurs in 20% of hospitalized patients.

B. Occurs in up to 40% of outpatients treated with thiazide diuretics.

PATHOGENESIS

A. Causes.

1. Total body deficiency (increased losses or decreased intake). This condition may develop as a result of:

a. Gastrointestinal (GI) losses.

b. Renal losses with or without metabolic abnormalities.

c. Decreases in intake that surpass the kidneys' ability to compensate.

2. Redistribution (a net shift of potassium from extracellular to intracellular space).

3. Hypomagnesemia. This causes the kidneys to secrete potassium into the urine at a higher rate than they would with the same potassium levels and higher magnesium levels, leading to hypokalemia or accelerating it.

4. Elevated plasma sodium levels (due to a high-salt diet). These cause the kidneys to lose potassium while making an effort to balance ion neutrality via available ion exchange transporter.

B. If severe and untreated hypokalemia has physiologic consequences.

1. Cardiac arrhythmias.

2. Rhabdomyolysis.

3. Acute renal failure.

4. Kidney fibrosis.

PREDISPOSING FACTORS

A. Nonpotassium-sparing diuretics.

B. Eating disorders.

C. Alcoholism.

SUBJECTIVE DATA

A. Common complaints/symptoms.

1. Palpitations or arrhythmias.

2. GI.

a. Nausea and vomiting.

b. Constipation, ileus.

3. Muscle weakness (severe hypokalemia).

a. Skeletal muscle weakness and paralysis.

b. Respiratory compromise due to diaphragmatic paralysis.

c. Rarely, rhabdomyolysis.

4. Cramping (lower legs).

5. Postural hypotension.

PHYSICAL EXAMINATION

A. Vital signs, including blood pressure (BP).

B. EKG changes.

1. ST-segment depression, T-wave flattening, T-wave inversion, and the presence of U-waves.

2. Can progress to life-threatening and/or fatal arrhythmias and sudden cardiac death.

C. GI system: Abdominal pain and bowel sounds.

D. Musculoskeletal system: Strength.
E. Neurologic examination.

DIAGNOSTIC TESTS
A. Initial lab tests.
  1. Serum potassium (preferably plasma).
  2. Venous or arterial carbon dioxide (CO_2) or HCO_3 and/or pH.
B. Other lab tests.
  1. Complete chemistry panel.
  2. Blood urea nitrogen (BUN) and creatinine to assess kidney function.
C. Estimate of total body extracellular potassium and potassium deficit.
  1. Total body potassium content is about 3,500 mmol or mEq.
    a. 90% is sequestered intracellular.
  2. Total body potassium (mEq/L) = extracellular fluid volume (ECFV) × serum potassium (mEq/L).
    a. ECFV = total body water [0.6 × weight (kg)] × 1/3.
  3. Potassium deficit (mEq/L) =
    a. ECFV × *desired* serum potassium (4.0 or 4.5 mEq/L) − ECFV × serum potassium (mEq/L).
    b. NOTE: This calculation does not account for ongoing losses or intracellular deficits.
D. Assessment for cause of potassium losses.
  1. Trans-tubular potassium gradient (TTKG): Assessment of the kidney's capability to appropriately conserve potassium.
    a. Valid only if the patient is not taking any diuretics or drugs to block the renin–angiotensin–aldosterone system (RAAS).
    b. During hypokalemia, TTKG should be less than 3, indicating the kidneys are conserving potassium.
  2. Urine potassium concentration: 24-hour collection.
E. Cardiac function.
  1. EKG changes including peaked T-waves, prolonged PR interval, widened QRS complex, and shortened QT interval.
  2. Bradyarrhythmias.
  3. Ventricular fibrillation.
  4. Asystole.
F. Severe or prolonged hypokalemia.
  1. Urine myoglobin.
  2. Serum creatinine (SCr) kinase.

DIFFERENTIAL DIAGNOSIS
A. Spurious hypokalemia or pseudohypokalemia.
  1. Leukocytosis greater than 100,000/mm^3.
  2. Insulin dosed immediately prior to lab draw.
B. Redistribution.
  1. Metabolic or respiratory alkalosis.
    a. Increased available insulin.
    b. Insulin overdose.
  2. Catecholamine excess.
    a. Alkalemia.
    b. Familial hypokalemic periodic paralysis.
    c. Thyrotoxicosis.
    d. Factor replacement in megaloblastic anemia.

  e. Medications: Insulin, theophylline toxicity, beta-adrenergic activity/agents (epinephrine), bronchodilators, and caffeine-containing drugs.
C. Increased potassium losses.
  1. GI losses: Prolonged vomiting or diarrhea.
  2. Extrarenal potassium loss (urine potassium <20 mEq/24 hours).
    a. Prolonged diarrhea.
    b. Nasogastric suctioning.
    c. Intestinal potassium binders (e.g., sodium polystyrene sulfonate [SPS] or patiromer).
    d. Poor intake/malnutrition.
    e. Laxative abuse.
    f. Excessive sweating.
    g. Villous adenoma rectosigmoid colon.
  3. Renal potassium loss (urine potassium >20 mEq/24 hours): Non-anion gap (non-AG) metabolic acidosis.
    a. Renal tubular acidosis type I (distal) and type II (proximal).
    b. Liddle syndrome (decreased aldosterone secretion; normal renin level).
    c. Diabetic ketoacidosis and lactic acidosis.
    d. Ureterosigmoidostomy.
    e. Medications: Carbonic anhydrase inhibitors, laxative overuse, and topiramate.
  4. Renal potassium loss (urine potassium >20 mEq/24 hours): Metabolic alkalosis.
    a. Vomiting or nasogastric suction.
    b. Mineralocorticoid excess syndromes (normotensive primary hyperaldosteronism).
    c. Bartter syndrome.
    d. Gitelman syndrome.
    e. Medications: Diuretics (loop, thiazide), especially in the setting of high salt intake.
  5. Renal potassium loss (urine potassium >20 mEq/24 hours): No acid–base disorder.
    a. Elevated renin levels: Malignant hypertension, renovascular disease, and renin-secreting tumor.
    b. Low renin levels: Elevated aldosterone levels (primary hyperaldosteronism, bilateral adrenal hyperplasia, dexamethasone suppression).
    c. Low aldosterone levels.
      i. Mineralocorticoid ingestion.
      ii. Congenital adrenal hyperplasia.
      iii. Cushing syndrome.
      iv. Ectopic adrenocorticotrophic hormone (ACTH).
      v. Tobacco.
      vi. Black licorice.
    d. Excessive sodium intake or retention.
      i. Chronic diuretic therapy.
      ii. Congestive heart failure (CHF).
      iii. Cirrhosis.
    e. Hypomagnesemia.
    f. Enuresis/polyuria: Hypercalcemia, acute kidney injury (AKI) recovery, postobstructive diuresis, and osmotic diuresis (e.g., hyperglycemia).

g. Medications: Aminoglycosides, amphotericin B, high-dose corticosteroids, and mineralocorticoids.
6. Dialysis-associated losses.
7. Other.
   a. Leukemia.
   b. Any disorder causing severe or progressive weakness: Myasthenia gravis and polyneuropathy.

EVALUATION AND MANAGEMENT PLAN

A. Goal: To avoid or resolve the cause of the hypokalemia and treat the condition and its related symptoms.
B. Step 1: Immediate treatment: Potassium supplementation. The total dose is at least equal to the calculated potassium deficit. The calculated dose to replace potassium in extracellular fluid is:
   1. [Ideal plasma potassium mmol/L – actual plasma potassium] × [TBW (L) × extracellular fluid (%)].
     a. Total body water (TBW) = weight (kg) × 0.5 (women), 0.6 (men), 0.45 (older adults).
     b. ECFV is 26% to 30% of TBW.
   2. [4.0 mmol/L–2.5] × [(80 kg × 0.5) × 0.26] = 1.5 × [40 × 0.26] = 1.5 × 10.4 = 15.6 mmol/L or 16.
     a. 16 mmol/L or 16 mEq/L.
     b. Deliver intravenously. Oral doses will be higher due to poor absorption.
     c. This will only replace potassium in the ECFV space. Most potassium losses are in the intracellular space and may be ongoing.
C. Step 2: Repeated calculations and doses for ongoing potassium losses.
   1. Intravenous (IV) supplementation.
     a. Initial dose of 20 to 40 mEq: Common, but in severe hypokalemia will likely need to be repeated.
     b. Dose: 10 to 20 mEq/hr.
     c. Reserved for severe and/or symptomatic hypokalemia or for patients unable to tolerate oral supplementation.
   2. Oral supplementation.
     a. Available in tablet, capsule, or liquid formulations.
     b. Total daily doses: 40 to 100 mEq; sufficient replacement in most cases.
     c. Divided into two to four doses to reduce GI side effects.
     d. Patients with renal dysfunction: Decrease dose by 50% and avoid repeating doses.
D. Step 3: Treatment of underlying disorder.
   1. Correct hypomagnesemia as it can result in refractory hypokalemia.
   2. Decrease or discontinue medications associated with hypokalemia if possible.
   3. Decrease sodium intake (especially with diuretic use).
E. Step 4: Treatment of other electrolyte and acid–base disorders.
F. Step 5: Assessment of need for chronic management.
   1. Some patients will require chronic oral potassium supplements or high-potassium diets.

2. Consider potassium-sparing diuretics (e.g., spironolactone, amiloride, triamterene) in patients on potassium-depleting medications.
3. All patients on potassium-depleting medications need a low-salt diet.

FOLLOW-UP

A. For hypokalemia related to acute episodes, such as severe diarrhea, no follow-up is necessary.
B. Patients on long-term diuretic therapy should have periodic monitoring of serum potassium levels.

CONSULTATION/REFERRAL

A. Consult nephrology for any refractory electrolyte disorder with or without AKI or chronic kidney disease (CKD).
B. Consult endocrinology for any uncontrolled diabetes or other hormone disorders.
C. Consult gastroenterology for refractory symptoms and suspected villous adenoma.

SPECIAL/GERIATRIC CONSIDERATIONS

A. Monitor patients with CKD, CHF, or medications associated with hypokalemia carefully to avoid overcorrecting.

CASE SCENARIO: HYPOKALEMIA

MW is a 65-year-old who weighs 90 kg with a history of severe heart failure with reduced ejection fraction with chronic hypotension and has been taking diuretics for the past 10 years. She presents today with ongoing diarrhea for the past 3 days, weakness, and leg cramps. Today she reports some dizziness and her blood pressure (BP) is slightly lower than normal. She only drinks 32 oz of fluid per day as instructed by her cardiologist. EKG is normal. Admission labs include potassium level of 2.6 mEq/L.

1. How much total potassium should be prescribed?
   A. Potassium chloride 20 mEq intravenous (IV) one-time dose, then repeat the serum potassium level.
   B. Potassium chloride 40 mEq IV one-time dose, then repeat the serum potassium level.
   C. Potassium chloride 40 mEq PO BID.
   D. Potassium chloride 40 mEq IV one-time dose, then repeat the serum potassium level after the infusion is complete and then daily, and start potassium 20 mEq PO once a day.

2. The next morning MW says she feels much better. Her BP is stable and matches her reported outpatient BPs. She is no longer having any muscle cramping. EKG is normal. Diarrhea is improving. Her potassium this morning is 3.1 mg/dL. Other labs are normal. How much potassium should be prescribed today?
   A. Discontinue potassium because she no longer has any symptoms.
   B. Continue potassium chloride 20 mEq PO once a day.
   C. Increase potassium chloride to 20 mEq PO BID.
   D. Continue potassium chloride 20 mEq PO once a day and give an additional dose of potassium chloride 20 mEq intravenously (IV) once now.

BIBLIOGRAPHY

Allon, M. (2014). Disorders of potassium metabolism. In D. S. Gipson, M. A. Perazella, & M. Tonelli (Eds.), *National Kidney Foundation's primer on kidney diseases* (6th ed., pp. 90–99). Elsevier Saunders.

Cohnm, J. N., Kowey, P. R., Whelton, P. K., & Prisant, L. M. (2000). New guidelines for potassium replacement in clinical practice. *Archives of Internal Medicine, 160*, 2429–2436. https://doi.org/10.1001/archinte.160.16.2429

Kraft, M. D., Btaiche, I. F., Sacks, G. S., & Kudsk, K. A. (2005, August). Treatment of electrolyte disorders in adult patients in the intensive care unit. *American Journal of Health System Pharmacy, 62*(16), 1663–1682. https://doi.org/10.2146/ajhp040300

Pepin, J., & Shields, C. (2012). Advances in diagnosis and management of hypokalemic and hyperkalemic emergencies. *Emergency Medical Practice, 14*(2), 1–20.

HYPOMAGNESEMIA

Divya Monga and Catherine Wells

DEFINITION
A. Serum magnesium less than 1.5 mg/dL (see Box 5.4).

INCIDENCE
A. 2% of general population.
B. 10% to 20% hospitalized patients.

PATHOGENESIS
A. Magnesium is the second most abundant intracellular cation in the body after potassium.
B. Most magnesium is stored intracellular (in bone).
C. Magnesium can be ionized, bound to proteins, or bound to anions.
D. It is critical in the functioning of the neuromuscular, cardiac, and nervous systems.
E. Magnesium is vital to vascular tone, heart rhythm, bone formation, and muscle contraction, among many other critical functions.
F. Normomagnesemic cellular depletion of magnesium and total magnesium depletion are associated with refractory hypokalemia and unexplained hypocalcemia.

PREDISPOSING FACTORS
A. Starvation.
B. Alcohol use.
C. Diarrhea.
D. Vomiting.
E. Gastrointestinal (GI) fistulas.

SUBJECTIVE DATA
A. Common complaints/symptoms.
   1. Neuromuscular symptoms similar to or related to hypocalcemia.
      a. Hyperreflexia.
      b. Carpopedal spasm.
      c. Tetany.
      d. Seizures.
      e. Positive Chvostek and Trousseau signs.

2. Severe hypomagnesemia: Possible EKG changes and life-threatening arrhythmias (including torsades de pointes).

PHYSICAL EXAMINATION
A. Neurologic exam including reflexes.
B. Cardiac examination.
   1. EKG.
   2. Vital signs including blood pressure (BP).
C. Musculoskeletal exam.

DIAGNOSTIC TESTS
A. Serum magnesium.
B. Total calcium and ionized calcium (hypomagnesemia is often accompanied by hypokalemia and/or hypocalcemia).
C. Serum Potassium.
D. Serum creatinine (SCr) and blood urea nitrogen (BUN).
E. 24-hour urine collection for magnesium can help differentiate renal versus GI causes.

DIFFERENTIAL DIAGNOSIS
A. Decreased intake.
   1. Chronic alcoholism.
   2. Prolonged fasting.
   3. Protein-calorie malnutrition.
   4. Inadequate supplementation in parenteral nutrition-dependent patients.
B. GI losses.
   1. Inflammatory bowel disease.
   2. Chronic diarrhea.
   3. Laxative abuse.
   4. Malabsorption syndromes.
   5. Surgical bowel resection or small intestinal bypass surgery.
   6. Drug-related poor absorption (proton pump inhibitors).
C. Renal losses.
   1. Drugs.
      a. Diuretics.
      b. Amphotericin B.
      c. Aminoglycosides.
      d. Cyclosporine.
      e. Tacrolimus.
      f. Pentamidine.
      g. Proton pump inhibitors.
      h. Foscarnet.
      i. Cetuximab.
      j. Cisplatin.
   2. High urinary output.
      a. Postobstructive or resolving acute tubular necrosis (ATN) diuresis.
      b. Posttransplant polyuria.
      c. Hypercalcemia.
   3. Inherited hypomagnesemia.
      a. Gitelman syndrome.
      b. Bartter syndrome.
      c. Phosphate depletion.

4. Primary hyperaldosteronism.
5. Chronic metabolic acidosis.
6. Idiopathic renal wasting.

EVALUATION AND MANAGEMENT PLAN

A. Step 1: Initiate intravenous (IV) magnesium replacement 4 g for all patients with severe symptoms or eclampsia/preeclampsia.

   1. Deliver first dose quickly (over 4–5 minutes) if followed by an infusion or repeat slow IV bolus (over 6–12 hours).

   2. Infuse 4 to 6 g over 8 to 12 hours.

     a. Magnesium distributes into tissues slowly, but is rapidly eliminated by the kidney.

     b. Any reduction in kidney function will also reduce ability to eliminate magnesium.

B. Step 2: Replace magnesium.

   1. Available in IV and oral forms.

     a. Use IV replacement for patients with severe depletion, those who cannot tolerate oral replacement, those who have eclampsia/preeclampsia, and those who are symptomatic.

     b. Use oral supplements for chronic hypomagnesemia and asymptomatic states.

       i. Absorption is unpredictable with oral supplements and diarrhea is common.

       ii. Repletion of total body stores takes several days.

   2. Recommended IV doses of magnesium sulfate (dose should be decreased by 50% in patients with renal impairment).

     a. 1 to 4 g if serum magnesium 1 to 1.5 mg/dL.

     b. 4 to 8 g if serum magnesium less than 1 mg/dL.

   3. Oral supplements.

     a. Magnesium oxide 400 mg BID.

C. Step 3: Treat other electrolyte and acid–base disorders.

D. Step 4: Assess cause and initiate a plan for prevention.

   1. Potassium-sparing diuretics can reduce renal magnesium wasting.

FOLLOW-UP

A. Follow-up depends on underlying cause.

B. Patients who have cardiac arrhythmias should be closely followed until magnesium levels are restored.

CONSULTATION/REFFERAL

A. Consult cardiology as needed for cardiac arrhythmias.

B. Consult nephrology for management of renal impairment.

SPECIAL/GERIATRIC CONSIDERATIONS

A. Geriatric patients are at high risk for cardiac arrhythmias and renal impairment.

B. Caution should be used to assure magnesium levels are optimized in this patient population.

CASE SCENARIO: HYPOMAGNESEMIA

JM is a 58-year-old seen in the ED after a syncopal episode. He has no history of medical care and takes no medications. He drinks three to five alcoholic drinks per day. He also complains of foot cramps even after intravenous (IV) hydration and IV potassium replacement. He says this happens at least once every day and nothing helps.

1. What is the most likely cause of the patient's symptoms?
   A. Persistent hypokalemia
   B. Injury as syncope is often associated with falls
   C. Hyponatremia
   D. Hypomagnesemia

2. JM has been admitted for several weeks related to acute decompensated heart failure with reduced ejection fraction for treatments including high-dose IV diuretics. The AGACNP has been replacing potassium with daily doses of IV potassium and struggling to bring the level higher than 3.3 mmol/L. Today the AGACNP additionally ordered a magnesium level, which is 0.6 mg/dL. EKG is normal. What is the best plan of care?
   A. Order IV magnesium 6 g now to infuse over 8 hours.
   B. Start oral magnesium 400 mg once a day.
   C. Order IV magnesium 6 g now to infuse over 30 minutes.
   D. Order IV magnesium 1 g now to infuse over 8 hours.

BIBLIOGRAPHY

Kraft, M. D., Btaiche, I. F., Sacks, G. S., & Kudsk, K. A. (2005, August). Treatment of electrolyte disorders in adult patients in the intensive care unit. *American Journal of Health System Pharmacy, 62*(16), 1663–1682. https://doi.org/10.2146/ajhp040300

Moe, S. M., & Daoud, J. R. (2014). Disorders of mineral metabolism: Calcium, phosphorous, and magnesium. In D. S. Gipson, M. A. Perazella, & M. Tonelli (Eds.), *National Kidney Foundation's primer on kidney diseases* (6th ed., pp. 100–112). Elsevier Saunders.

HYPONATREMIA

Divya Monga and Catherine Wells

DEFINITION

A. See Box 5.5 for further details.

B. Serum sodium less than 135 mEq/L (measured by ion-specific electrode; see Box 5.5).

   1. Mild 130 to 135 mEq/L.

   2. Moderate 125 to 129 mEq/L.

   3. Severe or profound less than 125 mEq/L.

C. Acute hyponatremia: Low serum sodium documented for 48 or fewer hours.

D. Chronic hyponatremia: Low serum sodium that is either documented for greater than 48 hours or onset is unknown.

INCIDENCE

A. The incidence is 15% to 38% in hospitalized patients, with only ~7% incidence in ambulatory settings.

B. In institutionalized geriatric patients, an incidence as high as 53% has been reported.

C. The incidence of moderate and severe hyponatremia (serum sodium <130 mEq/L) is 1%, with a prevalence of 2.5%.

    1. 67% of cases are hospital-acquired and 30% occur in the ICU.

D. Admission of patients with hyponatremia is directly associated with inpatient mortality.

PATHOGENESIS

A. Pseudohyponatremia.

    1. Apparent low sodium with normal plasma and urine osmolality and tonicity.

    2. Often caused by hyperlipidemia or hyperproteinemia.

    3. Normal serum sodium that appears falsely low when using indirect ion-selective electrode (ISE) method to assess plasma for sodium.

      a. The original sample is diluted to 1:10 ratio, measuring whole plasma sodium, assuming the sample contains 93% water and 7% proteins/lipids.

      b. But increased proteins or lipids decrease the ratio of total water, causing a perceived lower than actual sodium level.

    4. Solution: Measurement of sodium via direct ISE and serum sample (undiluted blood).

      a. This is usually a point-of-care test.

B. Dilutional hyponatremia (↑ total body water [TBW] ± ↓ solutes).

    1. Due to transcellular water shifts: Hypertonicity.

      a. Hyperglycemia (>250 mg/dL).

      b. Hypertonic solutions (e.g., mannitol, intravenous immunoglobulin [IVIG]).

C. Solute depletion hyponatremia (↓ solutes + ↑ TBW; requires water intake).

    1. Loss of solute while maintaining water intake.

D. Potassium and sodium.

    1. Potassium is an active cation; sodium is an anion. To maintain electroneutrality, potassium + chloride exchange across cell membranes for sodium.

    2. As a result, when infusing potassium, some potassium ions become intracellular and some sodium ions become extracellular, thus raising sodium levels.

PREDISPOSING FACTORS

A. Older adult patients.

B. Taking psychiatric medications.

C. Cardiac disease.

D. Chronic kidney disease (CKD).

E. Malignancy.

F. Alcoholism.

SUBJECTIVE DATA

A. Common complaints/symptoms.

    1. Neurologic symptoms: Range from mild and nonspecific to severe and potentially fatal.

      a. Severity of symptoms increases with acuity of onset.

        i. Chronic hyponatremia often presents with relatively mild symptoms.

        ii. Acute, severe hyponatremia is associated with marked neurologic deficits.

    2. Neurologic and other symptoms grouped by severity.

      a. Mild symptoms (nonspecific and rarely progress to herniation).

        i. Headache.

        ii. Nausea and vomiting.

        iii. Mild confusion.

      b. Moderate (sometimes known as moderately severe): Most often seen in chronic hyponatremia and thus not associated with impending herniation.

        i. Anorexia.

        ii. Fatigue/malaise.

        iii. Confusion, agitation, disorientation, or forgetfulness.

        iv. Gait disturbance.

        v. Abnormal sensorium (e.g., dizziness).

      c. Severe.

        i. Vomiting.

        ii. Cardiopulmonary distress.

          1) Pulmonary edema.

          2) Acute respiratory failure secondary to tentorial herniation with subsequent brainstem compression.

          3) Cheyne–Stokes respiration.

        iii. Delirium.

        iv. Somnolence/obtundation.

        v. Seizures (10% incidence with severe hyponatremia).

        vi. Pathologic or depressed reflexes.

        vii. Pseudobulbar palsy.

        viii. Coma (Glasgow Coma Scale score ≤ 8).

      d. Other signs (e.g., falls, fractures).

    3. Possible hypovolemia or hypervolemia depending on the etiology of the hyponatremia.

PHYSICAL EXAMINATION

A. Physical examination to assess volume status.

    1. Check skin, mucous membranes, heart, lungs, jugular venous distension (JVD), and edema.

    2. Assess blood pressure (BP) and orthostatic changes.

    3. Determine weight changes.

B. Neurologic assessment (initial and ongoing).

DIAGNOSTIC TESTS

A. Serum sodium.

B. Serum osmolality.

C. Complete chemistry panel including potassium.

D. Spot urine osmolality.

    1. Greater than 300 mOsm/kg: Urine is concentrated/hypertonic but not necessarily due to sodium. This indicates a relative increase in solute compared with water.

    2. Less than 150 mOsm/kg: Urine is dilute/hypotonic. This indicates a relative increase in water and/or decrease in solute.

E. Spot urine sodium.

   1. Less than 20 mEq/L: Renal sodium retention as in low effective arterial blood volume.

   2. 20 mEq/L or more: Diuretics will induce increased urine sodium.

F. Determination of patient volume status.

   1. Volume assessment is known to be unreliable as initial diagnostic criteria in hyponatremia but is necessary when interpreting hyponatremia-related lab tests.

   2. Physical examination to include assessments.

     a. Skin, mucous membranes, heart, lungs, JVD, edema, and weight changes.

     b. BP and orthostatic changes (especially in patients using diuretics).

G. Other lab tests to consider.

   1. Fractional excretion of uric acid (FEUA %) or chloride (FECL %).

     a. These have better specificity and sensitivity than fractional excretion of sodium (FENa %) to help determine volume status and renal clearance of solutes.

   2. Vasopressin levels.

   3. Thyroid-stimulating hormone (TSH).

   4. Glucose and glycosylated hemoglobin.

   5. Cortisol.

DIFFERENTIAL DIAGNOSIS

A. Pseudohyponatremia.

   1. Hypertriglyceridemia greater than 1,000 mg/dL.

   2. Familial hypercholesterolemia.

   3. Proteinemia greater than 10 gm/dL (e.g., multiple myeloma).

B. Dilutional hyponatremia ($\uparrow$ TBW $\pm$ $\downarrow$ solutes).

   1. Impaired free water excretion: Renal tubular water losses.

     a. Endocrine: Hypothyroidism or adrenal/glucocorticoid insufficiency.

     b. Physical/emotional stress.

     c. Syndrome of inappropriate antidiuretic hormone (SIADH).

       i. Central nervous system (CNS) etiologies: Tumor, meningitis, intracranial hemorrhage/hematoma, stroke, or trauma.

       ii. Pulmonary disease: Pneumonia, acute respiratory failure, tuberculosis, or aspergillosis.

       iii. Neoplasm: Small cell carcinoma lung, pancreatic cancer, or duodenal cancer.

       iv. HIV/AIDS.

       v. Postoperative.

     d. Edema syndromes: Nephrotic syndrome (NS), cirrhosis, or heart failure.

     e. Drugs: Amitriptyline, carbamazepine, chlorpropamide, clofibrate, cyclophosphamide, haloperidol, narcotics, nicotine, nonsteroidal anti-inflammatory drugs (NSAIDs), serotonin reuptake inhibitors, thiothixene, thioridazine, vincristine, oxytocin, or 3,4-methylenedioxymethamphetamine (MDMA; also known as ecstasy, E, Molly, X, etc.).

     f. Thiazide diuretics.

     g. Diminished solute intake with ongoing water intake: "Tea and toast" diet or beer potomania.

   2. Excess water intake.

     a. Primary polydipsia.

     b. Dilute infant formula.

     c. Hypotonic intravenous (IV) fluids.

C. Solute depletion hyponatremia ($\downarrow$ solutes + $\uparrow$ TBW; requires water intake).

   1. Renal solute loss.

     a. Diuretic.

     b. Solute diuresis: Bicarbonaturia, ketonuria, glucose, mannitol, or urea diuresis.

     c. Salt wasting nephropathy (e.g., cystic renal diseases, interstitial disease, chronic glomerular disease, partial obstruction).

     d. Mineralocorticoid deficiency.

   2. Nonrenal solute loss.

     a. Gastrointestinal (GI) loss (diarrhea, vomiting, pancreatitis, bowel obstruction).

     b. Cutaneous (sweating, burns).

     c. Blood loss.

     d. Excessive intake of water and sports drinks in athletes, combined with excessive body fluid losses.

EVALUATION AND MANAGEMENT PLAN

A. Step 1: Choose therapy goal and timing of sodium correction based on the following (obtained from history):

   1. Acute hyponatremia with severe symptoms: Emergency treatment (more aggressive treatment).

     a. Sodium 129 mEq/L or less that fell within the past 48 hours, causing severe patient symptoms.

   2. Acute hyponatremia with moderately severe symptoms: Emergency treatment.

     a. Sodium 129 mEq/L or less that fell within the past 48 hours, causing moderate patient symptoms.

   3. Acute hyponatremia with mild symptoms: Nonemergency treatment (most cases).

     a. Sodium 129 mEq/L or less that fell within the past 48 hours, causing mild patient symptoms.

   4. Acute hyponatremia asymptomatic: Nonemergency treatment (most cases).

     a. Sodium 129 mEq/L or less that fell within the past 48 hours, without causing symptoms.

   5. Chronic hyponatremia with any symptoms: Nonemergency treatment.

     a. Sodium 129 mEq/L or less for greater than 48 hours or an unknown period of time, causing any related patient symptoms.

   6. Chronic hyponatremia asymptomatic: Outpatient treatment.

     a. Sodium 129 mEq/L or less for greater than 48 hours, without causing symptoms.

B. Step 2: Set up appropriate monitoring to provide safe care and prevent overcompensation of sodium levels.

   1. Emergency treatment.

     a. Monitor closely in an intensive care setting.

b. Monitor complete fluid intake and output hourly.

i. Do not allow water intake to exceed output as this will exacerbate hyponatremia.

c. Perform neurologic and symptom assessment frequently.

d. Measure sodium levels every 2 to 4 hours until stable and sodium greater than 130 mEq/L, then once daily until sodium is normal and stable.

2. Nonemergency treatment.

a. Monitor in an ED, ICU, or other nursing floor with trained staff.

b. Monitor complete fluid intake and output hourly.

i. Do not allow water intake to exceed output as this will exacerbate hyponatremia.

c. Perform neurologic and symptom assessment frequently.

d. Measure sodium levels every 4 to 6 hours until stable and sodium greater than 130 mEq/L, then once daily until sodium is normal and stable.

3. Outpatient treatment.

a. Only for chronic patients with stable but low sodium.

b. Monitoring and follow-up vary according to cause of hyponatremia.

C. Step 3: Initiate volume correction if hypovolemic.
D. Step 4: Initiate sodium correction therapy according to severity of symptoms.

1. Acute or severe symptomatic hyponatremia.

a. Initial treatment: 3% sodium chloride 100 mL bolus over 10 to 20 minutes.

i. Repeat as needed: Up to three times.

ii. Goal: To raise sodium 5% or 4 to 6 mEq/L and resolve symptoms.

iii. Once goal is met, change to 3% sodium chloride infusion initiated at 0.5 to 2 mL/kg/hr and titrated based on sodium levels until sodium reaches 130 mEq/L.

1) Raise the sodium: 1 mEq/hr.

2) **Maximum** rise in sodium: Up to 10 mEq/L above baseline per 24 hours.

b. Day 1 (first 24 hours): Maximum rise in sodium: 10 mEq/L or 10%.

c. Following days: Raise the sodium up to 8 mEq/L or 10% (maximum).

2. Acute or moderate symptomatic hyponatremia.

a. Initial treatment: 3% sodium chloride infusion given at 0.5 to 2 mL/kg/hr and titrated based on sodium levels until sodium reaches 130 mEq/L.

b. Day 1 (first 24 hours).

i. Goal for day 1: To raise sodium 5% or 4 to 6 mEq/L and resolve symptoms.

ii. Maximum rise in sodium: 10 mEq/L or 10%.

c. Following days.

i. Raise the sodium up to 8 mEq/L or 10% (maximum).

3. Asymptomatic hyponatremia.

a. Water diuresis (unless hypovolemic): Loop diuretics.

b. If not resolved: 3% sodium chloride infusion initiated at 0.5 to 2 mL/kg/hr and titrated based on sodium levels until sodium reaches 130 mEq/L.

c. Day 1 (first 24 hours).

i. Maximum rise in sodium: 10 mEq/L or 10%.

d. Following days.

i. Raise the sodium up to 8 mEq/L or 10% (maximum).

E. Step 5: Other related interventions.

1. Treatment of other electrolyte and acid–base disorders; correct hypokalemia to a potassium of 3.5 to 4.5 mEq/L.

2. Strict fluid intake and output; restrict or supplement intake as needed.

3. Head trauma or hemodynamic instability: Consider consulting nephrology for continuous renal replacement therapy (CRRT) hyponatremia protocols.

a. Slower sodium titration.

b. Controlled management of sodium levels using CRRT.

4. Chronic hyponatremia.

a. Initial therapy.

i. Restrict all water intake (enteral and parenteral) to 1,000 to 2,000 mL/d.

ii. Correct hypokalemia to a potassium of 3.5 to 4.5 mEq/L.

iii. Euvolemic and hypovolemic patients.

1) Administer isotonic saline or balanced crystalloid solution.

2) Discontinue existing/chronic diuretics (assess as possible cause).

iv. Hypervolemic patients.

1) Further restrict all water intake (enteral and parenteral) to 800 to 1,500 mL/d.

2) Give loop diuretics.

v. Replace sodium deficit only if necessary.

1) 3% sodium chloride infusion initiated at 0.5 to 2 mL/kg/hr and titrated based on sodium levels until sodium reaches 130 mEq/L.

2) ± dDAVP 1 to 2 mcg IV or subcutaneously (SC) every 8 hours for 24 to 48 hours.

vi. Only use dDAVP to support a therapy plan that includes sodium replacement and water restriction; dDAVP alone will not correct hyponatremia.

vii. Do not use dDAVP in psychogenic polydipsia or edematous hyponatremia (e.g., congestive heart failure [CHF], cirrhosis).

1) Day 1 (first 24 hours): Maximum rise in sodium: 10 mEq/L or 10%.

2) Following days: Raise the sodium up to 8 mEq/L or 10% (maximum).

b. Patients with high urine cation concentrations.
  i. Give loop diuretics.
  ii. Give vasopressin type 2 (V_2) receptor antagonists, also called vaptans.
  iii. Give salt tablets.
  iv. If resistant to the previously noted therapies, consider demeclocycline, or urea in conjunction with nephrology (demeclocycline is likely to damage kidney function).
5. Overcorrecting hyponatremia.
  a. Risks: Seizures, cerebral edema, osmotic demyelination syndrome (ODS), and death.
  b. If baseline serum sodium is 120 mEq/L or more, no intervention necessary.
  c. If baseline serum sodium is less than 120 mEq/L or if correction exceeds 6 to 8 mEq/L or 10% of the baseline sodium level per day.
  d. Correct sodium level back to the most recent sodium that was within guidelines for correcting at up to 6 to 8 mEq/L or 10% per day.
  E. Give electrolyte free water (D5W) 10 mL/kg and repeat as needed.
  f. Consider also dDAVP 2 mcg IV.
G. Correct sodium quickly, within a few hours of overcorrecting.

FOLLOW-UP

A. Follow-up depends on the underlying cause of hyponatremia.
B. Follow-up should be managed by the primary service that is managing the underlying cause.

CONSULTATION/REFFERAL

A. Consult nephrology if hyponatremia is due to renal disorders.
B. Consult neurology for CNS disorders causing hyponatremia.

SPECIAL/GERIATRIC CONSIDERATIONS

A. A spectrum of diseases and disorders are associated with the geriatric population, predisposing them to hyponatremia, including pulmonary, endocrine, and CNS diseases, as well as cancers.
B. A careful assessment of overall fluid status in older adult patients should be ascertained.
C. Bone stress and fractures.
  1. Sodium is stored in the bone. Hyponatremia induces osteoclasts and thus bone loss.
  2. Chronic hyponatremia is associated with a fourfold increase in osteoporosis (dose- and time-dependent), gait instability, falls in older adults, and increased risk of fractures.
D. Cerebral edema.
  1. Sodium enters the brain only in plasma. Acute changes to plasma tonicity/osmolality cause water to shift in and out of astrocytes. Acute rises in osmolality cause astrocytes to shrink.
  2. Within 48 hours, astrocytes adapt to hyponatremia and intracellular osmolality becomes equal to

plasma osmolality without changing cell volume due to adaptive solutes and osmolytes.
  3. However, this adaptation has consequences such as increased astrocyte susceptibility to injury and poor long-term outcomes.
E. ODS.
  1. Sudden rises in extracellular tonicity/osmolality caused by the treatment/overcorrection of hyponatremia can cause osmotic stress on astrocytes, resulting in demyelination.
  2. ODS initially seems to improve with improvement of hyponatremia.
  3. There is a delayed onset of additional symptoms: Seizures, behavior changes, delusions, swallowing and speech dysfunction, movement disorders, paralysis, and potentially death. Symptoms can be temporary or permanent.
F. Mortality: Mild hyponatremia is associated with increased mortality, but deaths from cerebral edema and ODS are rare.
G. Monitor sodium closely in high-risk populations.
  1. Geriatrics.
  2. Liver disease.
  3. CHF.
  4. CKD.
H. Before treating hyponatremia, rule out and/or treat hypothyroidism, adrenal insufficiency, hyperglycemia, hypertriglyceridemia, and hyperproteinemia.
I. For refractory hyponatremia in patients with CHF, consider adding a low-dose angiotensin-converting enzyme (ACE) inhibitor to the diuretic regimen. Consult nephrology and cardiology experts.
J. For patients with cirrhosis, the primary therapy for hyponatremia is water restriction and a low-salt diet. If diuretics are required, use loop diuretics in combination with potassium-sparing diuretics and monitor potassium carefully.
K. Thiazide diuretics impair urine-diluting capacity, thus exacerbating hyponatremia.

CASE SCENARIO: HYPONATREMIA

RT is a 78-year-old with type 2 diabetes, chronic heart failure with reduced ejection fraction, hyperlipidemia treated with a statin, and mild chronic kidney disease (CKD) on loop diuretics. He presented to the ED with almost 2 days of vomiting and dizziness. His daughter brought him to the ED this morning because he was confused when she checked on him. He has not been able to keep any solid food on his stomach but has been able to drink fluids and has been drinking more water than his cardiologist allows. He has not missed any doses of diuretics for fear of worsening heart failure. His weight was 100 kg on admission. On admission, his creatinine and blood urea nitrogen (BUN) were elevated above his normal baseline, glucose was 103 mg/dL, and sodium was 122 mEq/L. Other labs were normal.

1. What is the first treatment?
  A. 3% sodium 100 mL bolus intravenous (IV) every 20 minutes ×3 to ensure sodium level rises at least 8 mEq/L above baseline

B. 3% sodium 100 mL bolus now over 20 minutes, then reassess both serum sodium and neurologic exam; may repeat ×2 if still symptomatic and if sodium level has not improved by 4 to 6 mEq/L from baseline

C. 3% sodium infusion at 200 mL/hr; repeat sodium level every 6 hours and call if sodium rises more than 4 mEq/L above baseline

D. Normal saline infusion at 200 mL/hr; repeat serum sodium level every 4 hours

BIBLIOGRAPHY

Hoorn, E. J., & Zietse, R. (2017). Diagnosis and treatment of hyponatremia: Compilation of the guidelines. *Journal of American Society Nephrology*, 28, 1–10. https://doi.org/10.1681/ASN.2016101139

Kraft, M. D., Btaiche, I. F., Sacks, G. S., & Kudsk, K. A. (2005, August). Treatment of electrolyte disorders in adult patients in the intensive care unit. *American Journal of Health System Pharmacy*, 62(16), 1663–1682. https://doi.org/10.2146/ajhp040300

Spasovski, G., Vanholder, R., Allolio, B., Annane, D., Ball, S., Bichet, D., Decaux, G., Fenske, W., Hoorn, E. J., Ichai, C., Joannidis, M., Soupart, A., Zietse, R., Haller, M., van der Veer, S., Van Biesen, W., & Nagler, E. (2014, April). Clinical practice guideline on diagnosis and treatment of hyponatremia. *Nephrology, Dialysis, Transplantation*, 29(Suppl. 2), i1–i39. https://doi.org/10.1093/ndt/gfu040

Sterns, R. H. (2015). Disorders of plasma sodium. *The New England Journal of Medicine*, 372(1), 55–65. https://doi.org/10.1056/NEJMra1404489

Sterns, R. H. (2018, September 18). Causes of hypotonic hyponatremia in adults. In J. P. Forman (Ed.), *UpToDate*. https://www.uptodate.com/contents/causes-of-hypotonic-hyponatremia-in-adults

Sterns, R. H. (2018, December 6). *Overview of the treatment of hyponatremia in adults*. In J. P. Forman (Ed.), *UpToDate*. https://www.uptodate.com/contents/overview-of-the-treatment-ofhyponatremia-in-adults

Sterns, R. H., & Silver, M. S. (2016). Complications and management of hyponatremia. *Current Opinion Nephrology Hypertension*, 25(2), 114–119. https://doi.org/10.1097/MNH.0000000000000200

Verbalis, J. G. (2014). Hyponatremia and hypoosmolar disorders. In D. S. Gipson, M. A. Perazella, & M. Tonelli (Eds.), *National Kidney Foundation's primer on kidney diseases* (6th ed., pp. 62–69). Elsevier Saunders.

HYPOPHOSPHATEMIA

Divya Monga and Catherine Wells

DEFINITION
A. See Box 5.6.
B. Serum phosphorus less than 3.5 mg/dL.
C. Moderate hypophosphatemia less than 2.5 mg/dL.
D. Severe hypophosphatemia less than 1 mg/dL.

INCIDENCE
A. Incidence in the general population is typically asymptomatic and estimated to be around 1% to 5%.
B. Incidence is about 3% in all hospitalized patients and up to 70% in ventilated patients.
C. Incidence rises sharply in patients with diabetic ketoacidosis, sepsis, or history of alcoholism.

PATHOGENESIS
A. Homeostasis of phosphate is maintained through gastrointestinal (GI) absorption and renal excretion.
B. Imbalances in either of these mechanisms can result in hypophosphatemia.

C. Severe hypophosphatemia can cause hemolysis, impaired cell function (e.g. platelets, white blood cells [WBCs], and muscle cells), and rhabdomyolysis.

PREDISPOSING FACTORS
A. Eating disorders.
B. Alcoholism.
C. Tumors.
D. Vitamin D deficiency.
E. Refeeding syndrome.
F. Malabsorption.

SUBJECTIVE DATA
A. Common complaints/symptoms.
    1. Depend on magnitude of hypophosphatemia: Moderate and severe before symptomatic.
    2. Muscle weakness.
        a. Diaphragmatic weakness and difficulty with ventilation or weaning mechanical ventilation.
        b. Impaired myocardial contractility.
    3. Neurologic dysfunction.
        a. Irritability ranging to seizures or coma.
        b. Paresthesias.
    4. Hematologic dysfunction, including hemolysis and platelet dysfunction.

PHYSICAL EXAMINATION
A. Vital signs, including blood pressure (BP).
B. Respiratory examination.
C. Musculoskeletal examination.
D. Neurologic examination.
E. GI examination.

DIAGNOSTIC TESTS
A. Serum phosphorus.
B. Total calcium and ionized calcium.
C. 24-hour urine collection for phosphorous to determine if renal excretion is high or low.

DIFFERENTIAL DIAGNOSIS
A. Decreased intestinal absorption.
    1. Malabsorption and chronic diarrhea.
    2. Antacid abuse, excessive calcium supplement use, or overdose of phosphate binders.
    3. Vitamin D deficiency.
    4. Alcoholism.
    5. Malnutrition, starvation, or anorexia.
B. Increased urinary losses.
    1. Primary hyperparathyroidism.
    2. Fanconi syndrome.
    3. Osmotic diuresis.
        a. Postobstructive or resolving acute tubular necrosis (ATN) diuresis.
        b. Glucosuria.
    4. Acetazolamide.
    5. Rickets (X-linked or vitamin D-dependent).
    6. Oncogenic osteomalacia.
    7. Enuresis/polyuria.
        a. Postoperative, especially immediately after kidney transplant.
        b. Extracellular volume expansion.

C. Redistribution (shift to intracellular space).
   1. Alkalosis.
   2. Diabetic ketoacidosis/treatment of hyperglycemia.
   3. Refeeding syndrome (shift of phosphorus intracellularly in response to carbohydrate load).
      a. Malnourished patients are at high risk with total parenteral nutrition.
   4. Alcohol withdrawal.
   5. Severe burns.
   6. Leukemic blast crisis.

EVALUATION AND MANAGEMENT PLAN

A. Step 1: If acute, severe, or symptomatic, replace phosphate intravenously.
   1. Give intravenous (IV) repletion for symptomatic patients with moderate or severe hypophosphatemia or those who cannot tolerate or receive oral supplementation.
      a. Potassium phosphate or sodium phosphate may be given. Sodium phosphate is recommended unless the patient also has hypokalemia.
      b. The initial dose is 0.16 to 0.25 mmol/kg, not to exceed 0.5 mmol/kg.
         i. Give dose over a minimum of 4 to 6 hours.
         ii. Infuse slowly to allow phosphorous to distribute appropriately into the cells before renal excretion of excess extracellular phosphorous.
         iii. Reduce dose by 50% in patients with renal dysfunction.
B. Step 2: Assess for ongoing losses or further phosphorus replacement needs.
   1. Give IV replacement to patients who cannot take or absorb oral phosphorus or patients with ongoing symptoms.
   2. Use oral supplements in patients with asymptomatic mild hypophosphatemia.
      a. May cause or worsen diarrhea.
      b. GI absorption is variable.
      c. Oral formulations contain various amounts of phosphorus, sodium, and potassium.
      d. Common regimen is 250 mg of elemental phosphorus QID.
   3. If oral supplements fail to maintain phosphorous levels, supplement with IV phosphorus.
C. Step 3: Identify and treat cause.
D. Step 4: Treat other electrolyte and acid–base disorders.

FOLLOW-UP

A. Follow-up should occur with the provider who treats the underlying condition causing the electrolyte imbalance.

CONSULTATION/REFFERAL

A. Depends on underlying condition causing hypophosphatemia.
B. Endocrinology should be consulted if the diagnosis is related to hyperparathyroidism.
C. Gastroenterology should be consulted if there is a malabsorption condition.
D. Nephrology should be consulted in renal phosphate wasting.
E. Psychiatry should be consulted for eating disorders.

SPECIAL/GERIATRIC CONSIDERATIONS

A. Older adult patients can develop osteomalacia and be prone to bone pain and fractures.

CASE SCENARIO: HYPOPHOSPHATEMIA

CV is 68 years old and weighs 90 kg. She was admitted to the medical ICU (MICU) for sepsis associated with influenza. She has been mechanically ventilated for 5 days. Her sepsis is recovering but she is still mildly hypotensive, although all vasopressors have been stopped. She failed her initial trial to wean her ventilator yesterday. Her basic metabolic panel labs have been normal. Today the AGACNP additionally collected a phosphorous level, which is 1.2 mg/dL.

1. What is the best next step?
   A. Sodium phosphate 40 mmol intravenous (IV) once over 6 hours. Repeat serum phosphorous level every day with labs.
   B. Potassium phosphate 30 mmol IV now over 2 hours, then repeat phosphorous level. Repeat the dose if the level is <2 mg/dL.
   C. Consult eyes, nose, and throat (ENT) for tracheotomy. Labs are normal and the patient will require prolonged ventilator weaning.
   D. Sodium phosphate 40 mmol IV every day over 4 hours. Add serum phosphorous level every day with labs.

BIBLIOGRAPHY

Kraft, M. D., Btaiche, I. F., Sacks, G. S., & Kudsk, K. A. (2005, August). Treatment of electrolyte disorders in adult patients in the intensive care unit. *American Journal of Health System Pharmacy*, 62(16), 1663–1682. https://doi.org/10.2146/ajhp040300
Moe, S. M., & Daoud, J. R. (2014). Disorders of mineral metabolism: calcium, phosphorous, and magnesium. In D. S. Gipson, M. A. Perazella, & M. Tonelli (Eds.), *National Kidney Foundation's primer on kidney diseases* (6th ed., pp. 100–112). Elsevier Saunders.
Yu, A. S. L., & Stubbs, J. R. (2019, February 12). *Evaluation and treatment of hypophosphatemia*. In A. Q. Lam (Ed.), *UpToDate*. https://www.uptodate.com/contents/evaluation-and-treatment-of-hypophosphatemia

METABOLIC ACIDOSIS

Catherine Harris

DEFINITION

A. Low arterial pH and low HCO_3.
B. Low PCO_2 after respiratory compensation.

INCIDENCE

A. Metabolic acidosis occurs frequently in acute and chronic renal disease and in patients with any type of poisoning from drugs or chemicals. It is a common finding in the hospital setting for a variety of reasons.
B. It is typically classified as having a normal anion gap (non-AG) or a high anion gap (AG).

PATHOGENESIS

A. Metabolic acidosis can be determined by calculating the AG, the first step in distinguishing the type of metabolic acidosis.

  1. The equation to calculate the AG: $AG = Na - (Cl + HCO_3)$.

  2. The normal AG is 12 mEq/L.

B. The causes of metabolic acidosis can be a loss of bicarbonate or the addition of acid.

C. In metabolic acidosis caused by loss of bicarbonate, there is a non-AG.

  1. Gastrointestinal (GI) losses.

   a. Diarrhea.

   b. Ileostomy.

   c. Surgical drains.

  2. Renal losses.

   a. Proximal and distal renal tubular acidosis.

   b. Hypoaldosteronism.

D. In metabolic acidosis caused by addition of acid, the AG is elevated above 12.

  1. Renal failure or uremia.

  2. Lactic acidosis.

  3. Ketoacidosis.

   a. Diabetes.

   b. Ethanol.

   c. Starvation.

  4. Ingestion.

   a. Ethylene glycol.

   b. Methanol.

   c. Paraldehyde.

   d. Salicylate intoxication.

E. In metabolic acidosis, the PCO_2 falls predictably depending on HCO_3 concentration.

  1. To calculate expected change, $PCO_2 = (1.5\ HCO_3^-) + 8 \pm 2$.

  2. If the PCO_2 is not as expected, there is a respiratory acid–base disturbance, too.

F. In AG metabolic acidosis, can be used to discover a second metabolic acid–base disorder.

  1. Gap/HCO_3 – = (measured AG – ideal AG)/(ideal HCO_3 – measured HCO_3^-).

   a. If less than 1, then there is a non-AG metabolic acidosis present.

   b. If greater than 2, then there is a metabolic alkalosis present.

PREDISPOSING FACTORS

A. There are none. Metabolic acidosis is dependent on the cause, which determines the predisposing factors.

SUBJECTIVE DATA

A. Common complaints/symptoms.

  1. Increased respiratory rate.

  2. Drowsiness.

  3. Nonspecific.

B. Family and social history.

  1. Alcohol use or drug abuse.

  2. Occupational history and potential exposure to metals or chemicals.

  3. Genetic disorder associated with a family history of acidosis, typically discovered in childhood.

C. Review of systems.

  1. Neurologic: Blurred vision, vertigo, headache, confusion, and generalized weakness.

  2. Head, ear, eyes, nose, throat: Ringing in the ears, light bothering the eyes, and seeing floaters.

  3. Respiratory: Increased breathing.

  4. Cardiovascular: Chest pain and palpitations.

  5. GI: Diarrhea, vomiting, and pain in the chest that feels like heartburn.

  6. Renal: Increased urination, increased thirst, and urination at night.

  7. Psychiatric: Any history of drug use or depression.

PHYSICAL EXAMINATION

A. Nonspecific physical examination that depends on the underlying cause.

  1. Renal failure: Pallor, drowsiness, asterixis, and pericardial rub.

  2. Diabetic ketoacidosis: Reduced skin turgor, dry mucous membranes, and fruity breath.

  3. Sepsis: Fever, confusion or coma, hypotension, and Kussmaul respirations.

DIAGNOSTIC TESTS

A. Serum electrolytes: Check serum bicarbonate.

B. Arterial blood gas (ABG): pH less than 7.40.

C. AG determination.

D. Base excess/deficit determination to determine the degree of acidosis.

E. Complete blood count (CBC): Look for severe anemia, which can affect oxygen delivery.

F. Urinalysis: Urine pH greater than 5.5 may be associated with certain renal diseases.

  1. Calcium oxalate crystals seen in ethylene glycol toxicity.

G. Beta-hydroxybutyrate.

H. Lactate level.

I. Necessary in certain situations.

  1. Salicylate levels.

  2. Iron levels.

  3. Aldosterone levels.

  4. Ammonium levels.

DIFFERENTIAL DIAGNOSIS

A. For normal AG metabolic acidosis.

  1. Abdomen.

   a. Diarrhea.

   b. Fistulas.

  2. Renal.

   a. Renal tubular acidosis: Addison disease.

   b. Carbonic anhydrase inhibitors.

   c. Post hypocapnia.

   d. Excessive chloride (large volumes of saline).

B. For a high AG metabolic acidosis, use the mnemonic **MUDPILES** to remember the differential diagnosis.

  1. Methanol.

  2. Uremia.

3. Diabetic ketoacidosis.
4. Paraldehyde.
5. Infection, iron, isoniazid, ibuprofen.
6. Lactic acidosis.
7. Ethylene glycol.
8. Salicylates.

EVALUATION AND MANAGEMENT PLAN

A. General plan.
  1. Treat with an alkali therapy to raise plasma pH greater than 7.20.
  2. Calculate the sodium bicarbonate deficit to determine how much must be administered intravenously to raise the serum bicarbonate level to increase the pH greater than 7.20.
  3. Determine the underlying cause of the metabolic acidosis and treat appropriately.
B. Pharmacotherapy.
  1. Metabolic acidosis of any type. Sodium bicarbonate can be used, but treating the underlying issue is critical.
    a. Be cautious of volume overload; loop diuretics can be used to reduce volume as needed.
  2. Methanol or ethylene glycol poisoning. Fomepizole can be used to treat ethylene glycol poisoning.
  3. Uremia. Sodium bicarbonate can be used to keep serum bicarbonate levels above 20 mEq/L.
  4. Diabetic ketoacidosis. Insulin can be used to treat ketoacidosis.
  5. Paraldehyde poisoning. Alkali therapy can be used to correct metabolic acidosis during supportive care; no specific antidote exists.
  6. Infection, iron, isoniazid, or ibuprofen. Antibiotics can be used to treat sepsis and activated charcoal can be used for treatment of poisoning caused by drugs and chemicals.
  7. Lactic acidosis. Alkali therapy such as sodium bicarbonate or tromethamine can be used.
    a. The role of alkali therapy can be controversial.
  8. Ethylene glycol: Fomepizole or ethanol can be used to treat cases of poisoning.
  9. Salicylates: Acetazolamide can treat salicylate poisoning by inducing alkaline diuresis.

FOLLOW-UP

A. The patient needs to follow-up with their primary care provider (PCP) and any appropriate service providers involved in regulating the underlying disease process that causes the metabolic acidosis.

CONSULTATION/REFFERAL

A. Refer to the appropriate service provider related to the cause of the metabolic acidosis.
B. Consult nephrology as quickly as possible in cases that may require hemodialysis.
C. Consult endocrinology for patients who present with diabetic ketoacidosis.

SPECIAL/GERIATRIC CONSIDERATIONS

A. Metabolic complications are common in older adults and can be exacerbated in chronid kidney disease (CKD).
B. Special care to monitor and detect metabolic disturbances should be instituted.

CASE SCENARIO: METABOLIC ACIDOSIS

A 35-year-old female patient with AIDS was brought to the ED with a fever of 102.2°F/39°C and a 3-month history of copious diarrhea. On physical exam, the patient is a well-developed, thin female in moderate distress. Vital signs showed blood pressure (BP) of 100/60, heart rate (HR) 100 beats per minute, and respiratory rate (RR) of 18. Head, ear, eyes, nose, and throat (HEENT) exam was normal. Cardiac exam demonstrated an S1 and S2 without S3, S4, or murmur. Lungs were clear to auscultation and percussion. The abdomen was supple and minimally tender to palpation. Bowel sounds were hyperactive. Stool was guaiac negative. Arterial blood gas (ABG) on admission showed pH of 7.35, PCO_2 of 27 mmHg, PO_2 of 90 mmHg, and bicarbonate of 14 mmol/L. Other labs included sodium (Na) of 136 mmol/L, potassium (K) of 3.4 mmol/L, CL of 112 mmol/L, total carbon dioxide of 14 mmol/L, blood urea nitrogen (BUN) of 30 mg/dL, creatinine of 1.5 mg/dL, and glucose of 105 mg/dL.

1. Which of the following metabolic acidosis states is caused by a loss of bicarbonate resulting in a non-anion gap?
  A. Gastrointestinal (GI) loss such as vomiting
  B. Presence of lactic acidosis
  C. Presence of ketoacidosis from starving
  D. Presence of uremia

2. Which of the following is considered a compensatory mechanism for metabolic acidosis?
  A. Hyperventilation
  B. Hypoventilation
  C. Confusion
  D. Anxiety

BIBLIOGRAPHY

Burger, M., & Schaller, D. (2020). Metabolic acidosis. In *StatPearls [Internet]*. StatPearls Publishing. https://www.ncbi.nlm.nih.gov/books/NBK482146/

Kraut, J. A., & Madias, N. E. (2015, October 15). Metabolic acidosis of CKD: An update. *American Journal of Kidney Diseases*, *67*(2), 307–317. https://doi.org/10.1053/j.ajkd.2015.08.028

Kraut, J. A., & Madias, N. E. (2016, September). Lactic acidosis: Current treatments and future directions. *American Journal of Kidney Diseases*, *68*(3), 473–482. https://doi.org/10.1053/j.ajkd.2016.04.020

Rastegar, M., & Nagami, G. T. (2017, February). Non-anion gap metabolic acidosis: A clinical approach to evaluation. *American Journal of Kidney Diseases*, *69*(2), 296–301. https://doi.org/10.1053/j.ajkd.2016.09.013

Reddy, P., & Mooradian, A. D. (2009, October). Clinical utility of anion gap in deciphering acid-base disorders. *International Journal of Clinical Practice*, *63*(10), 1516–1525. https://doi.org/10.1111/j.1742-1241.2009.02000.x

Thomas, C. P. (2018, October 10). Metabolic acidosis. In V. Batuman (Ed.), *Medscape*. https://emedicine.medscape.com/article/242975-overview

NEPHROLITHIASIS

Timothy Ray

DEFINITION

A. Formation of a kidney stone, an organized mass of crystals that grows on the surface of a renal papilla.

INCIDENCE

A. Renal and ureteral stones are a common problem. In the United States, almost two million outpatient visits with urolithiasis as a primary diagnosis were recorded in 2000.

B. The prevalence has increased from 3.8% (1976–1980) to 8.8% (2007–2010). It coincidentally has increased in concordance with the rising incidence of obesity, higher environmental temperatures, as well as increased use of enhanced diagnostic imaging techniques.

C. Up to the age of 40, the incidence of nephrolithiasis is similar in males and females at approximately 2 per 1,000. However, past age 40, the incidence for males rises to 4 per 1,000 until age 60 and then decreases. After age 40, the incidence for females declines to approximately 1.5 per 1,000. Although rare late in life, even an 80+-year-old male or female may still present with a first stone.

D. The average age of onset is 20s to 30s, with a second peak in the mid-50s. Up to 16% of men and 8% of women will have at least one symptomatic stone by the age of 70 years.

E. It is more common in White people compared with Black, Asian, and Hispanic people.

F. It is more common in southeastern United States, although the reasons are not clear, and is more common in summer due to heat, sunlight exposure, and dehydration, leading to low urine volumes.

G. In stone formers, there are limited data on the rate of recurrence, with some studies showing a recurrence rate of 10% to 30% at 3 to 5 years for idiopathic calcium oxalate stones. Recurrent variability is limited in part due to the many different types of stones and the etiology behind their formation.

PATHOGENESIS

A. Kidney stones occur as a result of an increased burden of a poorly soluble salt excreted into a volume of urine that is insufficient to dissolve it (supersaturation).

  1. In addition to an individual predisposition and/or other factors, there is, especially, lack of inhibitors of crystallization.

  2. Supersaturation of poorly soluble salts (e.g., calcium oxalate) in urine is one factor.

B. However, the main factor, especially in calcium-containing stones, is the accumulation of apatite (calcium phosphate) in the medullary interstitium; this may develop in idiopathic hypercalciuria.

  1. A stone starts to accumulate in the basement membrane of the thin loop of Henle and grows into the medullary interstitium, to finally form the "Randall's plaque," which will erupt, breaking the urothelium of the papilla.

  2. This favors the deposition and aggregation of crystals, resulting in the organized stone.

C. Stone composition breakdown:

  1. Calcium oxalate: 70% to 80%.

  2. Calcium phosphate: 15%.

  3. Uric acid: 8%.

  4. Cystine: 1% to 2%.

  5. Struvite: 1%.

  6. Miscellaneous: Less than 1%.

PREDISPOSING FACTORS

A. Can vary greatly based on the type of kidney stone formation, as well as different populations, environmental circumstances, and clinical situations. Taking a careful patient history and correlating it to the presenting stone event helps not only in treating the acute illness, but also in the preventive care for future stone recurrence.

  1. Idiopathic hypercalciuria.

  2. Obesity, diabetes, and metabolic syndrome: Uric acid stones and calcium oxalate stones.

  3. Dehydration, low fluid intake, and low urine volume (summer months, hot and/or dry weather, athletic, or occupational activities).

  4. High dietary salt.

  5. High oxalate food intake (e.g., spinach, nuts, chocolate, berries, tea, rhubarb, star fruit).

  6. High animal protein diet.

  7. Protein supplements.

  8. Excessive vitamin C supplementation (metabolized to oxalate).

  9. Low calcium diet with main meals of the day.

  10. Bariatric surgery (gastric bypass).

  11. Rapid weight loss/starvation.

  12. Hypocitraturia, metabolic acidosis, hypokalemia, or hypomagnesemia.

  13. Intestinal malabsorption.

  14. Antibiotics (leading to loss of *Oxalobacter formigenes*, a protecting bacteria of the gut microbiota against excess oxalate absorption).

  15. Chronic or recurrent urinary tract infections (UTIs) with urea-splitting organisms such as *Proteus*, *Providencia*, or *Ureaplasma* (struvite stones).

  16. Medications: Topiramate, acetazolamide, atazanavir, indinavir, triamterene, sulfadiazine, sulfasalazine, or felbamate.

  17. Systemic diseases: Primary hyperparathyroidism, distal renal tubular acidosis (type 1), sarcoidosis/tuberculosis, medullary sponge kidney, malignancy, intestinal malabsorption (e.g., Crohn's disease), hyperthyroidism, hypertension, gout, diabetes mellitus, and obesity.

  18. Genetic factors: Mainly related to the development of calcium-based stones, likely due to underlying genetic makeup that predisposes them to abnormal calcium absorption, resorption, and excretion, along with effects on oxalate and citrate pathways.

SUBJECTIVE DATA

A. Asymptomatic stones.

  1. Many times, nephrolithiasis is picked up during an imaging exam of the abdomen that is performed for other purposes.

  2. Asymptomatic phase is most likely to occur in patients who have never had stones previously.

B. Common complaints/symptoms.

1. Flank pain (radiates downward and anteriorly to the abdomen, pelvis, and groin/genitals).
   a. Level of pain can vary greatly and intensity, frequently coming in waves, which often last 20 to 60 minutes.
   b. Site of stone obstruction in the ureter determines the location of pain and can change if the stone migrates down the ureter.
2. Nausea and vomiting.
3. Hematuria (gross or microscopic).
   a. Occurs in the majority of nephrolithiasis patients, although can be undetected in approximately 10% to 30% of episodes.
   b. Tends to occur earlier in acute stone episodes, so by days 3 to 4 the likelihood for hematuria declines greatly.
4. Dysuria and urgency.
5. Complications
   a. Persistent obstruction which can lead to chronic kidney disease (CKD).
   b. Development of infectious condition, which can lead to systemic sepsis rapidly if not caught early.
C. Review of systems.
   1. Establish the onset and characteristics of pain.
   2. Ask about witnessed stone passage.
   3. Ask about stone history.
      a. Age when first stone developed.
      b. Number of stones.
      c. Frequency of stone episodes.
      d. Size of stone (passed or still retained).
      e. Stone composition analysis (if known).
      f. Kidney involved (left, right, or both).
      g. Need of urologic intervention (if yes, response to the intervention).
   4. Previous infection, simple UTI versus systemic urosepsis.
   5. Inquire about diet, at-risk occupations (e.g., pilots, taxi drivers, teachers, athletes), family history, medications, dietary supplements, medical conditions, previous episodes of urolithiasis, and frequency of UTIs.

PHYSICAL EXAMINATION

A. The physical examination is most important for ruling out other conditions. Kidney and ureteral stones have no specific manifestations on physical examination, although need to rule out other etiologies for presentation, that is, flank pain caused by other reasons (see "Differential Diagnosis").
B. Costovertebral angle tenderness (CVAT) can be positive in some cases.

DIAGNOSTIC TESTS

A. Radiologic exams.
   1. *Non*contrast CT scan (stone protocol) is the gold standard.
   2. Renal ultrasound (inexpensive, safe) is a good diagnostic tool to diagnose urolithiasis and rule out

hydronephrosis, especially for frequent stone formers or patients with a contraindication to radiation (e.g., pregnancy).
   3. Plain radiography (kidney–ureter–bladder [KUB]) is used as a serial monitoring device for frequent calcium stone formers to reduce the amount of radiation/cost, as compared with CT, but does not detect hydronephrosis and is less accurate for stone localization than CT or ultrasound. While it can pick up large radiopaque stones, it does not detect noncalcium stones (e.g., uric acid stones), and sensitivity is lowered due to body habitus and bowel contents.
   4. Intravenous pyelography (IVP) can detect hydronephrosis, but is less sensitive and specific than CT for detection of stones. It should not be used in patients with a reduced glomerular filtration rate (GFR) due to risk of contrast-induced acute kidney injury (AKI).
   5. MRI is rarely used as stones are poorly detected, although because it does not involve use of radiation it can be used in pregnancy to localize obstructions. Alternative imaging such as ultrasound is more commonly used in these situations, however.
B. Laboratory analysis.
   1. Serum electrolytes, including calcium and phosphorus.
   2. Blood urea nitrogen (BUN) and creatinine.
   3. Uric acid level.
   4. Urinary labs: pH, uric acid, calcium, oxalate.
   5. In patients with hypercalcemia.
      a. Parathyroid hormone (PTH) level.
      b. 25-OH vitamin D.
      c. 1,25 dihydroxyvitamin D.
   6. A low-serum bicarbonate concentration.
      a. Urine pH.
         i. 6.0 or more: Suggests renal tubular acidosis.
         ii. Greater than 8 urine pH or pyuria: Should lead to urine cultures and consideration of struvite stones.
   7. Ancillary 24-hour urine collection for stone-risk profile is recommended in these situations.
      a. All children with kidney stones.
      b. Metabolically active stones (growing in size or in number within 1 year).
      c. Frequent stone formers (more than two to three episodes).
      d. Noncalcium (e.g., cystine, uric acid) stone formers.
      e. Patients in demographic group not typically prone to stone formation (e.g., African Americans).
C. Radiologic determination of stone composition.
   1. Findings of CT imaging may provide clues as to stone analysis.
   2. Density, location, and appearance can help differentiate types of stones.
      a. Calcium oxalate or calcium phosphate stones tend to be more dense than uric acid, magnesium ammonium phosphate, or cystine stones.

▶

b. Struvite stones are often large and found in the renal pelvis.

c. Patients who have underlying medullary sponge kidney are more predisposed to having bilateral calcium oxalate or calcium phosphate stones, and often found in the corticomedullary junction.

3. Use of dual-energy CT (DECT) can offer better differentiation when it comes to radiologic stone analysis, although cost and radiation exposure make its use less common.

DIFFERENTIAL DIAGNOSIS

A. Pyelonephritis (although in many situations coexist with nephrolithiasis).

B. Peritonitis.

C. In women: Ovarian torsion, ovarian cyst, or ectopic pregnancy.

D. Bleeding within the kidney causing clots, which can occur due to renal cell carcinoma.

E. Gastrointestinal (GI) issues such as acute intestinal obstruction, cholecystitis, diverticulitis, or appendicitis, but would not present with hematuria that is often seen with nephrolithiasis.

F. Acute mesenteric ischemia.

G. Shingles flare on the flank/lateral sides can cause pain similar in location and intensity to acute nephrolithiasis.

EVALUATION AND MANAGEMENT PLAN

A. General plan.

  1. Pain relief.

    a. Patients can be managed at home if they are able to take oral medications and fluids.

    b. Nonsteroidal anti-inflammatory drugs (NSAIDs).

      i. Is the preferred choice for pain control, as long as GFR allows.

      ii. Use of ketorolac for patients in acute care/hospital environment tends to work well, with oral ibuprofen being prescribed for home situations.

      iii. NSAIDs should be stopped 3 days before planned lithotripsy to minimize the risk of bleeding.

    c. Opioids.

      i. Opioids should be reserved for patients with severe pain not controlled by NSAIDs or for patients for which NSAIDs are contraindicated, that is, CKD/AKI, history of GI bleed, or those on anticoagulant therapy.

      ii. Review and documenting patients prior to use of scheduled drugs and limiting narcotic therapy to just during the acute phase of pain is essential and lessens the risk of long-term opioid dependency.

  2. Diet and fluid intake.

    a. Fluid intake.

      i. The mainstay of therapy is to increase the urine volume to more than 2 L/d. Therefore, the patient has to be encouraged to drink around 3 L of fluid per day. Because the risk of stone formation is highest during the nighttime, patients should be encouraged to drink plenty of fluids in the evening.

      ii. Review of patients' overall volume status and underlying cardiac history may impact how aggressive they are hydrated. If the patient has abnormal kidney or cardiac function, for example, low GFR or extraction fraction, then consultation with nephrology or cardiology may be helpful in managing the patient's fluid balance.

    b. Sodium intake.

      i. Urine sodium excretion augments urine calcium excretion.

      ii. Hence, the patient should be instructed to limit dietary sodium to 2 g/d.

    c. Potassium intake.

      i. A higher dietary potassium intake was found to be associated with a substantial reduction in stone formation, possibly due to its impact on reducing urinary calcium excretion.

      ii. Monitoring GFR and serum potassium levels is important before recommending a diet high in potassium.

    d. Dietary calcium.

      i. It has been demonstrated that an adequate calcium intake in the diet decreases kidney stone incidence. This is likely due to intestinal binding of calcium to oxalate, preventing its absorption.

      ii. An age- and gender-appropriate calcium diet is therefore recommended. Calcium supplementation outside of meals should be avoided.

    e. Protein intake.

      i. Increased animal protein intake has been associated with a slightly higher incidence of stone formation.

      ii. Intake of vegetable protein does not seem to have any effect.

B. Specific treatment (for each stone type).

  1. Calcium stones.

    a. Potassium citrate 30 to 60 mEq/d PO.

      i. Would start with 60 mEq/d if 24-hour urinary citrate is less than 150 mg/d.

      ii. Titrate dose to a 24-hour urinary citrate 320 to 640 mg/d and a urinary pH 6.0 to 7.0 to inhibit stone formation.

    b. Thiazide diuretic: Patients with hypercalciuria (24-hour urinary calcium >250 mg/d).

      i. Chlorthalidone 12.5 mg PO daily, or hydrochlorothiazide 12.5 mg PO daily, or indapamide 1.25 mg PO daily.

      ii. If the calcium excretion remains elevated in follow-up 24-hour urinary calcium several months after, the thiazide dose should be increased.

      iii. Monitor labs and volume status for thiazide side effects: Hypovolemia, hyponatremia, hypokalemia, hyperuricemia, and hypercalcemia.

c. Dietary oxalate restriction: Patients with hyperoxaluria (24-hour urinary oxalate >25–30 mg/d). Supplement each meal with calcium carbonate 1 to 1.5 g and snack to bind dietary oxalate in the intestine and prevent absorption.

d. Specific therapy for malabsorptive disorder: First-line treatment for enteric hyperoxaluria.

2. Uric acid stones.

a. Potassium citrate: 30 to 60 mEq/d or BID orally to dissolve retained uric acid stones.

   i. For prevention of new stones: 30 to 60 mEq/d or three times a week titrating urinary pH to greater than 7.0.

   ii. Patient use of colorimetric pH-sensitive urine strips: Check the urinary pH 3 to 4 hours after taking potassium citrate.

b. Low purine and low animal protein diet, if in follow-up the 24-hour urine uric acid is still high (>700 mg/d).

   i. May need to add allopurinol 100 mg/d PO, increasing weekly to 200 to 300 mg/d.

3. Struvite stones (staghorn calculi).

a. Aggressive medical and surgical treatment, since this can lead to renal failure.

   i. Early urologic intervention is advised.

b. Antibiotic therapy to prevent further stone formation due to urease-splitting organisms.

4. Cystine stones.

a. Treatment to decrease cysteine concentration: Water intake as mainstay of therapy.

   i. Trying to achieve 3 to 4 L of urine a day.

   ii. Goal urine cystine concentration less than 243 mg/L.

b. Low-sodium diet 2 g/d.

c. Low-animal protein diet.

d. Potassium citrate: Goal urine pH greater than 7.0 (maintained), which is a difficult task.

   i. Start 20 mEq TID and titrate up to a pH greater than 7.0.

   ii. Monitor labs for serum potassium levels, especially if low GFR.

e. Tiopronin 400 to 1,200 mg/d in three divided doses (comes in 100-mg tablets).

   i. Fewer side effects than D-penicillamine, but still can cause the same side effects (e.g., proteinuria, fever, rash, abnormal taste, arthritis, leukopenia, aplastic anemia, and hepatotoxicity).

C. Additional pharmacologic support.

1. Alpha-blocker: Has been shown to help facilitate spontaneous stone passage after 3 to 4 weeks of therapy.

2. Calcium channel blocker: Can also help with stone passage, however lower stone passage rates than with alpha-blockers.

3. Straining of urine for several days to collect any stone that passes. This will allow more detailed analysis of the type of stone, which will help guide future preventive therapy.

4. Treatment of UTI: Collection of urine culture should be obtained before any antibiotics are started.

5. Antibiotic therapy should be guided by culture results and sensitivity, as well as the minimum inhibitory concentration (MIC).

6. Patients with chronic urinary complications or nephrolithiasis are more prone to having chronic colonization, so empiric use of antibiotics should be avoided unless there is any systemic infectious symptoms.

D. Invasive therapy.

1. Reserved for patients who fail conservative therapy.

2. Need urologic consultation to proceed.

3. Includes:

a. Shock wave lithotripsy (SWL).

b. Ureteroscopy (URS) with laser lithotripsy.

c. Percutaneous nephrolithotomy (PNL).

d. Laparoscopic stone removal.

E. Hospitalization.

1. Stone greater than 5 mm (98% of stones <5 mm will pass spontaneously).

2. Nausea and vomiting; unable to take oral medicine or fluids.

3. Requiring parenteral therapy for pain.

4. Pyelonephritis/UTI or sepsis.

5. Significant stone complications such as hydronephrosis or AKI.

FOLLOW-UP

A. For adult patients with history of only one calcium-containing kidney stone that passed spontaneously, no special follow-up is required.

B. For frequent stone formers (two to three or more episodes), children, or individuals who form noncalcium stones or rare stone types, they need a follow-up in 4 to 6 months with a 24-hour stone risk analysis to monitor the effect of therapy.

C. Follow up for any acute complications, that is, post antibiotic UTI clearance, AKI or fluid/electrolyte abnormality resolving and stabilizing.

D. Initiate preventive therapies.

1. Staying well-hydrated.

2. Avoiding medications that could predispose a patient to further stones.

3. If stone analysis is known, utilize that information to fine-tune and target therapy to lessen further stone growth.

CONSULTATION/REFFERAL

A. Urology.

B. For stones greater than 5 mm as the likelihood of spontaneous passage of stones of this magnitude is low or when complications occur.

C. Radiologic findings indicate any obstructive disease.

D. Multiple or recurrent stones are documented.

1. Nephrology.

a. Presents with AKI, or if CKD shows GFR <60. ▶

b. Electrolyte, acid–base, or fluid abnormalities.

c. Children should be referred to pediatric nephrology.

2. Infectious disease (ID).

3. For complicated UTI or systemic septic conditions.

4. Cardiology.

5. If patient has underlying abnormal cardiac abnormalities that would be impacted by aggressive hydration or if cardiac clearance is needed prior to invasive procedure.

SPECIAL/GERIATRIC CONSIDERATIONS

A. Common in older adults and is associated with multiple comorbidities, including hypertension, coronary artery disease, diabetes mellitus, and CKD.

CASE SCENARIO: NEPHROLITHIASIS

A 47-year-old male presents to his primary care office with a complaint of severe right lateral flank pain. He states that he has had this pain on/off for about a week, with varying levels of intensity. He has intermittent fever, but is afebrile currently, and nonradiating pain, with an intermittent intensity of 2 to 10+. The patient works as a day laborer in a landscaping company. He reports a past medical history (PMH) of seasonal environmental allergies, sciatica, and hyperlipidemia; and a family history of hypertension (HTN) in his father, osteoarthritis in his mother, and a healthy sister. His current medications include seasonal use of over-the-counter (OTC) allergy medicines. He has been taking ibuprofen three to four times a day over the last 4 to 5 days to control the pain. He has no known medication allergies. His vitals showed blood pressure (BP) of 147/76 and heart rate (HR) of 92. Lungs: computed tomography angiography. Heart examination showed RRR, S1, and S2 normal, with no murmurs or rubs. His abdomen was soft, not tender except on the right lateral side and CVA, where there is some generalized nonspecific pain to palpation. He has good bowel sounds. His extremities showed equal/strong distal pulses and no edema. Lab results showed the following: urinalysis, clear yellow and normal except for positive heme/red blood cells (RBC); H/H 16.2/49.3; white blood cell (WBC) 5.8; PLT 225,000; serum creatinine 1.8; sodium 146; potassium 4.8; carbon dioxide (CO_2) 28; glucose 110; chloride 107. After evaluating the patient and reviewing the initial data, the patient's nurse practitioner (NP) is concerned that he may have a kidney stone.

1. What is the best radiologic test that the NP should order to help determine this?

A. Renal ultrasound

B. Kidney–ureter–bladder (KUB) x-ray of the abdomen

C. CT of the abdomen/pelvis, with intravenous (IV) contrast

D. CT of the abdomen/pelvis, without IV contrast

BIBLIOGRAPHY

Assimos, D. G., Krambeck, A., Miller, N. L., Monga, M., Murad, M. H., Nelson, C. P., & Matlaga, B. R. (2016). *Surgical management of stones: American Urological Association/Endourological Society Guideline.* American Urological Association. https://www.auanet.org/education/guidelines/surgical-management-of-stones.cfm

Curhan, G.C. (2021, September). *Up-To-Date.* Kidney stones in adults: Epidemiology and risk factors.

Curhan, G. C., Aronson, M. D., & Preminger, G. M. (2022, May). *Up-To-Date.* Kidney stones in adults: Diagnosis and acute management of suspected nephrolithiasis.

Jindal, G., & Ramchandani, P. (2007, May). Acute flank pain secondary to urolithiasis: Radiologic evaluation and alternate diagnoses. *Radiologic Clinics of North America, 45*(3), 395–410. https://doi.org/10.1016/j.rcl.2007.04.001 vii

Singh, A., Alter, H. J., & Littlepage, A. (2007, November). A systematic review of medical therapy to facilitate passage of ureteral calculi. *Annals of Emergency Medicine, 50*(5), 552–563. https://doi.org/10.1016/j.annemergmed.2007.05.015

Wen, C. C., & Nakada, S. Y. (2007, August). Treatment selection and outcomes: Renal calculi. *The Urologic Clinics of North America, 34*(3), 409–419. https://doi.org/10.1016/j.ucl.2007.04.005

Worcester, E. M., & Coe, F. L. (2008, June). Nephrolithiasis. *Primary Care, 35*(2), 369–391. https://doi.org/10.1016/j.pop.2008.01.005

Ziemba, J. B., & Matlaga, B. R. (2017, September). Epidemiology and economics of nephrolithiasis. *Investigative and Clinical Urology, 58*(5), 299–306. https://doi.org/10.4111/icu.2017.58.5.299

NEPHROTIC SYNDROME

Debra J. Hain

DEFINITION

A. Nephrotic syndrome (NS) is a clinical syndrome with three distinct elements, one physical sign (key feature is edema), and three laboratory test abnormalities of heavy proteinuria, hypoalbuminemia, or hypoproteinemia. Hypercoagulability is an optional feature that some patients will have. NS is a pathognomonic of glomerular disease. Not only is there a risk of acute kidney injury (AKI) but there are also metabolic effects that can impact the health of an individual.

1. Primary or idiopathic.

2. Isolated proteinuria without edema or other features of NS are suggestive of glomerulopathy but may not be associated with the multiple clinical problems that are seen in NS.

B. The National Kidney Foundation defines NS as total urine protein excretion in excess of 3,500 mg/d (equivalent to a total protein to creatinine ratio of >3,000 mg/g), with a decreased serum albumin concentration and edema with or without a decrease in glomerular filtration rate (GFR).

C. The term *nephritic syndrome* is an outdated term characterized by hematuria with red blood cell (RBC) casts, hypertension, and edema with or without decreased GFR. Clinicians may see the term still used.

INCIDENCE

A. Annual incidence in adults is 3 per 100,000 individuals.

B. About 80% to 90% of NS cases are idiopathic.

1. Membranous nephropathy (MN) is the most common primary (idiopathic) disorder in adults and secondary in children.

a. MN is common in White individuals.

b. Focal segmental glomerulosclerosis (FSGS) is the most common lesion for idiopathic NS in adults, particularly Black adults, accounting for about 35% of all cases in the United States, and over 50% of cases are among Black adults.

2. Minimal change disease (MCD) and immuno-globulin A nephropathy (about 90% of cases in children under the age of 10 years and more than 50% are older children) can also be a cause. In adults, it may be an idiopathic condition associated with use of nonsteroidal anti-inflammatory drugs (NSAIDs) or a paraneoplastic effect of malignancy most often associated with Hodgkin lymphoma.

C. About 10% of NS cases are secondary (due to underlying medical conditions).

1. Systemic lupus erythematosus (SLE).
2. Malignancy.
3. Infections (hepatitis B and C, HIV, and malaria).
4. Diabetic nephropathy.

PATHOGENESIS

A. Pathogenesis of NS is related to increased glomerular permeability to albumin and other plasma protein as a consequence of a damaged basement membrane.

B. MN is characterized by immune deposits that form at the base of the foot processes of the glomerular visceral epithelial cell or podocyte.

C. FSGS is multifactorial, but the injury to the foot process on the podocytes seems to be the main cause. Mechanisms include a T-cell-mediated circulating permeability factor, transforming growth factor (TGF), B-cell-mediated matrix synthesis, and genetic podocyte abnormalities.

PREDISPOSING FACTORS

A. Amyloidosis.
B. Diabetes mellitus.
C. Cryoglobulinemia.
D. Sjögren syndrome.
E. SLE.
F. Carcinoma.
G. Leukemia and lymphoma.
H. Melanoma.
I. Multiple myeloma.
J. Infection (bacterial, protozoan, viral); postinfectious glomerulonephritis is a secondary cause.
K. Allergic reaction to insect stings or bites, antitoxins, position ivy, or oak.
L. Malignant hypertension.
M. Sarcoidosis.
N. Genetic syndromes (e.g., familial FSGS, hereditary nephritis [Alport syndrome]).

SUBJECTIVE DATA

A. Common complaints/symptoms.
1. Progressive lower extremity edema.
   a. Marked hypoalbuminemia leads to fluid shifts into the interstitial space by a decrease in plasma oncotic pressure.
   b. Can also be due to the consequence of primary renal sodium retention.
2. Significant fluid weight gain.
3. Fatigue.
4. Exertional dyspnea.
B. Common/typical scenario.
1. Periorbital, genital edema.

2. Ascites.
3. Pleural or pericardial effusion.
4. Adults who present with new onset of edema or ascites and do not have the typical dyspnea seen with heart failure or present with cirrhosis.
C. Review of systems.
1. Determine the onset and duration of symptoms.
2. Determine if weight change has occurred.
   a. If weight gain: How much and over what period of time?
      i. If possible, weigh the patient every day on the same scale and at the same time of day for accurate assessment of weight changes.
3. Ask if any changes in urine output (UO), such as decreased or foamy urine (increased proteinuria).
4. Identify medication or toxin exposure: Risk factors for HIV or hepatitis and symptoms that could be indicative of other causes for edema (e.g., heart failure).
5. Underlying health conditions such as diabetes, SLE, or other systemic disease.
6. History of NS; if yes, when and, if known, what was the cause and treatment?

PHYSICAL EXAMINATION

A. Check vital signs, blood pressure (BP), temperature, heart rate, and respirations; obtain body weight.
1. Evaluate for hypertension, infection, and arrhythmia.
B. Inspect periorbital area, abdomen (ascites), and extremities, assessing for edema.
C. Auscultate heart, lungs, and abdomen.
D. Palpate abdomen, assessing for ascites, and the extremities for edema.

DIAGNOSTIC TESTS

A. The goal of diagnostic testing is to (a) assess for complications, (b) identify the underlying disease, and (c) possibly determine the histologic type of idiopathic NS.
B. Serum and urine tests.
1. Serum chemistry panel to evaluate kidney function (blood urea nitrogen [BUN], creatinine, estimated GFR) and electrolytes.
2. Assess for AKI (see "Acute Kidney Injury" for specific information).
3. Glucose for diabetes mellitus.
4. Blood count and coagulation panel (abnormal suggestive of bleeding disorder).
5. Albumin is the principal urinary protein.
   a. Hypoalbuminemia is found in NS and the mechanism is not totally understood, but it is believed that a substantial fraction of the filtered album is taken up by and catabolized in the proximal tubule, leading to a substantial loss of albumin in the urine.
6. Plasma proteins include clotting inhibitors, transferrin, immunoglobulins, and hormone-carrying proteins such as vitamin D-binding protein.
   a. Anti-streptolysin O.
   b. Antinuclear antibodies (ANA) and double-stranded DNA titers.

c. Assays for C3 nephritic factor with membrano-proliferative glomerulonephritis (MPGN).

d. Antibodies to M-type phospholipase A_2, receptor PLA_2R, are useful in idiopathic MN.

e. Thrombospondin type 1-domain-containing 7A may be useful in idiopathic MN.

7. Lipid panel to assess for hyperlipidemia. The two most common lipid abnormalities in NS are hypercholesterolemia and hypertriglyceridemia. Decreased plasma oncotic pressure appears to stimulate hepatic lipoprotein synthesis.

8. Urine dipstick to confirm proteinuria; protein to creatinine ratio from a random (spot) urine sample to evaluate for nephrotic-range proteinuria (24-hour urine collection is cumbersome for patients and the collection is done incorrectly).

a. Early morning specimen is best.

b. Protein to creatinine ratio greater than 3.0 to 3.5 mg protein/mg creatinine (300–350 mg/mmol).

c. Spot urine may be inaccurate in persons who exercise heavily or in someone who is gaining or losing muscle mass.

d. Hematuria or casts are suggestive of nephritis.

C. Additional tests depending on patient presentation.

1. HIV screening.

2. Liver panel; elevated transaminase may indicate viral hepatitis (if abnormal, obtain viral hepatitis panel). Hepatitis B and C testing.

3. Serum or urine protein electrophoresis (SPEP or UPEP; amyloidosis or multiple myeloma).

4. Rapid plasma regain to determine if syphilis is present.

5. ANA, anti-double-stranded DNA antibody, and complement values (C3 and C4) if connective tissue disorder is suspected.

D. Imaging studies.

1. Chest x-ray: To evaluate for pleural effusion.

2. CT or MRI: Possible to evaluate for neoplastic diseases as secondary cause.

3. Ultrasound (US).

a. Renal US to estimate kidney size, assess echogenicity of kidney, rule out obstruction, and identify kidney calculi.

b. Abdominal to evaluate for ascites.

c. Lower extremity Doppler ultrasound, CT, MRI, or lung ventilation/perfusion scan if thrombosis or pleural effusion is suspected.

4. Echocardiography: For suspected heart failure.

E. Renal biopsy.

1. In children, a kidney biopsy is the standard procedure to determine the cause of proteinuria. In those with NS from a known secondary cause who are responding to treatment, the renal biopsy will not likely add to the treatment. Most nephrologists think biopsy is indicated when the etiology of persistent proteinuria is unknown.

2. It may prove beneficial when trying to determine the best treatment and prognosis in adults with

idiopathic NS of unknown histologic disease type and in those in which the provider is considering underlying SLE as the cause.

3. May be done prior to therapy because you want to make sure what the pathology is and to reduce the chance of reduced tolerance to corticosteriods.

DIFFERENTIAL DIAGNOSIS

A. Liver disease (e.g., cirrhosis).

B. Heart failure.

C. Differential for AKI in NS.

1. Allergic interstitial nephritis.

2. AKI.

a. Acute tubular necrosis (ATN).

b. Prerenal azotemia.

3. Adverse effects from drug therapy.

4. NSAID nephropathy.

5. Renal venous thrombosis.

EVALUATION AND MANAGEMENT PLAN

A. General plan.

1. Confirm NS (evidence of proteinuria and hypoalbuminemia); once confirmed, consult nephrology expert (e.g., physician, nurse practitioner).

2. Assess for common causes (see "Incidence").

3. Assess for complications.

a. Venous thrombosis.

i. Renal veins affected; possible cause of pulmonary embolism.

ii. No evidence for prophylactic anticoagulation: Decision to treat should be considered individually.

b. Infection, especially cellulitis.

i. Maintenance of standard infection control practices.

ii. No strong evidence supporting any specific intervention to prevent infection in adults with NS.

c. AKI.

d. Markedly elevated lipid levels.

B. Patient/family teaching points.

1. Restrict sodium intake to less than 3 g/d (usually 2 g of sodium per day).

2. Restrict fluid to less than 1,500 mL/d; assess fluid volume status on regular basis.

C. Pharmacotherapy.

1. Diuretic therapy to treat edema. There is usually less natriuresis than seen in others due to hypoalbuminemia because of decreased delivery of protein-bound drug to the kidney. In addition, the albuminuria causes binding of the drug within the tubular lumen, so there may be a need for an increased dose to achieve the desired effect.

a. Loop diuretics (act in renal tubule and must be protein-bound to be effective).

i. Oral loop diuretics BID are more effective than once daily.

1) Furosemide 40 mg PO BID or bumetanide 1 mg PO BID is used to start.

2) The dose may be doubled every 1 to 3 days if edema has not improved or the patient is experiencing hypervolemia.

3) Maximum dose of furosemide is 240 mg per dose or 600 mg total per day. If no response to oral drug, consider intravenous (IV) form.

4) IV bolus of 20% human albumin prior to IV diuretic may be considered.

  ii. When edema is severe, it may be necessary to start with IV diuretics.

b. Diuresis should be gradual and guided by daily weights (1–2 kg/d) to prevent hypovolemia.

2. Angiotensin-converting enzyme (ACE) inhibitors or angiotensin receptor blocker (ARBs) are used to reduce proteinuria. However, must evaluate kidney function and potassium, and pay attention to volume status (if hypovolemic, need to replace fluid before initiating therapy).

3. Immunosuppressive therapy: Should be prescribed in collaboration with nephrology expert.

a. Corticosteroids: Used frequently (despite lack of supportive data).

b. Azathioprine (Imuran).

c. Biologics (rituximab, eculizumab).

d. Cyclophosphamide.

e. High-dose immune globulin.

f. Mycophenolate mofetil (CellCept).

4. Nutritional evaluation due to loss in body mas with negative nitrogen balance often occurs in patients with marked proteinuria. Even though the patient may gain weight, it may be due to edema or third spacing. Protein malnutrition may be worse because of the presence of gastrointestinal (GI) symptoms (e.g., anorexia, vomiting).

5. Hypovolemia may occur due to overdiuresis and albumin less than 1.5 g/dL.

6. AKI can occur due to profound proteinuria an hypoabluminemia.

a. Try to avoid NSAIDs and other nephrotic medications/agents.

7. Hypercoagulability: There is an increased risk of arterial and venous thromboemboli (particularly in those with MN).

8. The risk of infection is higher and is one of the leading causes of death in children with NS.

a. Recurrent respiratory tract.

b. Urinary tract infections (UTIs).

c. Peritonitis.

d. Sepsis.

FOLLOW-UP

A. The prognosis is variable depending on the underlying cause, disease histology, and patient clinical factors.

1. Many patients will improve and some will require kidney replacement therapy (KRT).

a. Indications for KRT include severe metabolic acidosis, electrolyte abnormalities (hyperkalemia, hyponatremia, and hyperphosphatemia), and persistent azotemia.

2. Patients with volume overload and cardiopulmonary decompensation for IV diuresis versus ultrafiltration for fluid removal require admission.

3. Follow-up is on an individual basis, but patients should continue with nephrology expert and primary care provider (PCP).

CONSULTATION/REFFERAL

A. Nephrology provider (e.g., nephrologist, nurse practitioner [NP]).

B. Other specialists depending on the underlying cause (e.g., infectious disease [ID], endocrinology, liver specialist).

SPECIAL/GERIATRIC CONSIDERATIONS

A. Consider underlying kidney function when treating with medications.

B. In NS due to AKI requiring dialysis, avoid hypovolemia and hypotension to preserve residual kidney function. Resolution of AKI to baseline kidney function (without requiring dialysis) is possible.

C. Older adults may seem to have a creatinine within normal range due to loss of muscle mass. Use estimated GFR to determine kidney function.

BIBLIOGRAPHY

Beck, L. H., & Salant, D. J. (2010). Membranous nephropathy: Recent travels and new roads ahead. *Kidney International*, 77(9), 765–770. https://doi.org/10.1038/ki.2010.34

Cattran, D. C., & Brenchley, P. E. (2017). Membranous nephropathy: Integrating basic science into improved clinical management. *Kidney International*, 91(3), 566–574. https://doi.org/10.1016/j.kint.2016.09.048

Floege, I. (2015). Introduction to glomerular disease: Clinical presentations. In R. J. Johnson, J. Feehally, & J. Floege (Eds.), *Comprehensive clinical nephrology* (5th ed., pp. 184–197). Elsevier Saunders.

Kerlin, B. A., Ayoob, R., & Smoyer, W. E. (2012). Epidemiology and pathophysiology of nephrotic syndrome—Associated thromboembolic disease. *Clinical Journal of the American Society of Nephrology*, 7(3), 513–520. https://doi.org/ 10.2215/CJN.10131011

Kodner, C. (2009). Nephrotic syndrome in adults: Diagnosis and management. *American Family Physicians*, 80(10), 1129–1134.

Kodner, C. (2016). Diagnosis and management of nephrotic syndrome in adults. *American Family Physician*, 93(6), 479–485.

Korbet, S. M. (2012). Treatment of primary FSGS in adults. *Journal of the American Society of Nephrology*, 23(11), 1769–1776. https://doi.org/10.1681/ASN.2012040389

Lopez, J., & Trachtman, H. (2019). Nephrotic syndrome. In E. V. Lerma, M. A. Sparks, & J. M. Topf (Eds.), *Nephrology secrets* (4th ed., pp. 105–109). Elsevier.

National Kidney Foundation. (2019). Nephrotic syndrome. https://www.kidney.org/atoz/content/nephrotic

Nishi, S., Ubara, Y., Utsunomiya, Y., Okada, K., Obata, Y., Kai, H., & Sato, Y. (2016). Evidence-based clinical practice guidelines for nephrotic syndrome 2014. *Clinical and Experimental Nephrology*, 20(3), 342–370. https://doi.org/10.1007/s10157-015-1216-x

Radhakrishnan, J., & Cattran, D. C. (2012). The KDIGO practice guideline on glomerulonephritis: Reading between the (guide) lines—Application to the individual patient. *Kidney International*, 82(8), 840–856. https://doi.org/10.1038/ki.2012.280

Segal, P. E., & Choi, M. J. (2012). Recent advances and prognosis in idiopathic membranous nephropathy. *Advances in Chronic Kidney Disease*, 19(2), 114–119. https://doi.org/10.1053/j.ackd.2012.01.007

Wu, H. H. L., & Want, A. Y., M. (2022). Kidney replacement therapy in the intensive care unit. *Nephrology Self-Assessment Program*, 21(1), 71–92.

PROSTATITIS

Suzanne Barron

DEFINITION

A. Inflammation of the prostate gland which can be caused by infection or persistent irritation of the gland.
B. The National Institutes of Health divides prostatitis into four groups.
    1. Acute bacterial prostatitis.
    2. Chronic bacterial prostatitis.
    3. Chronic prostatitis/chronic pelvic pain syndrome.
    4. Asymptomatic inflammatory prostatitis.

INCIDENCE

A. Almost 10% of males will have prostatitis over their lifetime.
B. About 90% of these conditions will be related to chronic nonbacterial prostatitis/chronic pelvic pain syndrome.

PATHOGENESIS

A. Acute bacterial prostatitis.
    1. Transmission of bacteria from the urethral meatus, backflow of infected urine into the ejaculatory and prostatic duct after instrumentation with a catheter or cystoscope, implanted bacteria during a prostate biopsy, and hematogenous spread or lymphatic spread of organisms (such as prostatic tuberculosis).
    2. Can be caused by any bacteria, but gram-negative bacteria most likely. The most common organism is *Escherichia coli*.
B. Chronic bacterial prostatitis: Pathophysiology debated but may be related to bacterial biofilms.
C. Chronic nonbacterial prostatitis: Results from chronic inflammation of the prostate gland from persistent irritation that is nonbacterial.
D. Asymptomatic inflammatory prostatitis: Inflammation in the prostate that develops but does not cause symptoms. Usually diagnosed incidentally during imaging.

PREDISPOSING FACTORS

A. Blockage of urine out of the bladder.
B. Phimosis (congenital narrowing of the opening of the foreskin so that it cannot be retracted).
C. Injury to the perineum.
D. Foley catheters.
E. Procedures such as cystoscopy or biopsy of the prostate.
F. Benign prostatic hypertrophy (BPH).

SUBJECTIVE DATA

A. Common complaints/symptoms.
    1. Acute bacterial prostatitis: Fever, chills, malaise, dysuria (painful urination or burning with urination), suprapubic abdominal pain, or urethral discharge. Symptoms occur quickly and patients will appear sick.

    2. Chronic bacterial prostatitis: Intermittent dysuria or recurrent urinary tract infections (UTIs). Symptoms generally occur gradually.
B. Common/typical scenario.
    1. Possible fever, chills, and malaise.
    2. Possible pain with intercourse or defecation.
    3. Arthralgias.
    4. Nocturia.
C. Family and social history.
    1. Ask about number of sexual partners or history of sexually transmitted infections (STIs).
D. Review of systems.
    1. Assess patient for discharge, pain, hematuria, back pain, and weight loss.

PHYSICAL EXAMINATION

A. Check for urethral discharge and inspect the foreskin and penis for any lesions or fluid.
B. Palpate testes and epididymides for inflammation and tenderness.
C. Check for costovertebral angle tenderness (CVAT).
D. Perform rectal examination to evaluate prostate for symmetry, swelling, and tenderness and to determine if the prostate gland is boggy.
E. Avoid massage if acute prostatitis is suspected as this can spread bacteria, increasing the risk of sepsis.

DIAGNOSTIC TESTS

A. Check for infection.
    1. Complete blood count (CBC) with differential.
    2. Urinalysis with urine culture.
    3. Gram stain and culture-expressed prostatic secretions (EPS).
    4. If there is concern for sexually transmitted disease or with urethral discharge, send urine culture for *Chlamydia trachomatis* and *Neisseria gonorrhoeae*.
B. For chronic prostatitis, check:
    1. CBC, serum creatinine (SCr), and blood urea nitrogen (BUN).
    2. Ultrasound, MRI, or biopsy if necessary to rule out other possibilities.

DIFFERENTIAL DIAGNOSIS

A. Anal fistulas.
B. UTI.
C. Epididymitis.
D. Urethritis.
E. Urinary obstruction.
F. Pyelonephritis.

EVALUATION AND MANAGEMENT PLAN

A. General plan.
    1. Acute prostatitis may need intravenous (IV) therapy for severe infection or if patient looks toxic.
    2. Increase fluid intake.
    3. Decrease caffeine and alcohol intake.
B. Patient/family teaching points.
    1. Teach patients how the infection is transmitted.
    2. Suggest that sexual partners may need treatment.
    3. Tell patients to use condoms.
    4. Tell patients to urinate when the urge comes.

C. Pharmacotherapy.
  1. Acute bacterial prostatitis.
    a. Broad-spectrum antibiotics: Treat for 2 weeks' duration.
      1) First-line antibiotics: Trimethoprim/sulfamethoxazole or fluoroquinolone.
      2) Second-line antibiotics: Second-generation cephalosporin.
      3) Third-line antibiotics: Third-generation cephalosporin.
    b. Nonsteroidal anti-inflammatory drugs (NSAIDs) for treating discomfort may be considered.
  2. Chronic bacterial prostatitis.
    a. Traditionally, fluoroquinolone antibiotic treatment for 4 to 6 weeks.
    b. Recent increase in fluoroquinolone resistance. Order culture-specific antibiotics. Consider fosfomycin.
    c. NSAIDs.
    d. Alpha-blockers, which reduce bladder outlet syndrome, may be beneficial.
D. Discharge instructions.
  1. Prevent infection with good hygiene.
  2. Complete the antibiotic treatment as prescribed, which may take up to 1 month.

FOLLOW-UP
A. Evaluate the effectiveness of the treatment plan and resolution of symptoms.
B. Admit patients who appear toxic to the hospital for IV antibiotics.
C. Order imaging with no improvement of symptoms, such as transrectal ultrasound or CT scan pelvis, to rule out prostatic abscess.

CONSULTATION/REFERRAL
A. Consult urology for acute recurrent bacterial infections or persistent infections. Cystoscopy may be required.

SPECIAL/GERIATRIC CONSIDERATIONS
A. Prostatitis may lead to sepsis, particularly in patients with diabetes or chronic renal failure, patients on dialysis, immunocompromised patients, and postsurgical patients with urethral instrumentation. There should be a low threshold to hospitalize these patients if there is a concern.
B. Urinary retention association with acute prostatitis may also require hospitalization.
C. In young men, the most likely cause is a urethral infection from unprotected sexual intercourse. In older men, infection is more likely to be from prolonged catheterization or recent urologic instrumentation.
D. Side effects of long-term antibiotics such as fluoroquinolones especially in the older adult population. Check EKG to assess for prolonged QTc. If prolonged, adjust to alternate antibiotic or monitor frequently.

A 49-year-old male without significant past medical history is currently in the hospital for acute bacterial prostatitis. He is sexually active. He had a transrectal ultrasound-guided prostate biopsy about 1 week ago and received intramuscular gentamicin prior to the procedure. Pathology was negative for prostate cancer. He is currently on day 3 of ciprofloxacin. He initially received a dose of ceftriaxone in the ED. Urine culture is positive for >100,000 colonies of *Escherichia coli*, sensitive to ciprofloxacin. He initially started to improve, but today he has a fever of 103°F/39.4°C with rigors and a heart rate of 120 beats per minute. He reports dysuria and perineal discomfort. He is urinating with low postvoid residual bladder scans.

1. What is the next appropriate step in the management of this patient?
  A. Order a renal/bladder ultrasound.
  B. Order a CT scan of the pelvis.
  C. Add vancomycin to cover possible gram-positive organisms.
  D. Resend urine culture.

BIBLIOGRAPHY
Center for Urology, Rochester, N. Y. (n.d.). Discharge instructions for prostatitis. http://www.cfurochester.com/pdf/discharge-prostatitis.pdf
Davis, N., & Silberman, M. (2021, October). Bacterial prostatitis. In *StatPearls[Internet]*. https://ncbi.nlm.nih.gov/books/NBK459257/
Gupta, N., Mandal, A., & Singh, S. (2008). Tuberculosis of the prostate and urethra. *Indian Journal of Urology*, 24(3), 388–391. https://doi.org/10.4103/0970-1591.42623
Kaplan, D., & Yates, J. (2020, April). *Medical student curriculum: Adult UTI*. American Urological Association. https://www.aua.net/education/auauniversity/for-medical-students/medical-students-curriculum/medical-student-curriculum/adult-uti
Luzzi, G. (2007). Editorial letter. Chronic prostatitis. *New England Journal of Medicine, 356*, 423–424. https://doi.org/10.1056/NEJMc063135
Prostate.net. (n.d.). 5 foods that can cause prostatitis. http://prostate.net/articles/foods-that-cause-prostatitis
Stevermer, J., & Easley, S. (2000, May). Treatment of prostatitis. *American Family Physician, 61*(10), 3015–3022.
Strauss, A., & Dimitrakov, J. (2010, March). New treatments for chronic prostatitis/chronic pelvic pain syndrome. *Nature Reviews Urology, 7*(3), 127–135.
Turek, P. J. (2019, December 6). Prostatitis. In J. P. Taylor 3rd (Ed.), *Medscape*. http://emedicine.medscape.com/article/785418-overviewProstatitis
Xiong, S., Liu, X., Deng, W., Zhou, Z., Li, Y., Tu, Y., Chen, L., Wang, G., & Fu, B. (2020, April). Pharmacological interventions for bacterial prostatitis. *Frontiers in Pharmacology* https://www.frontiersin.org/articles/10.3389/fphar.2020.00504/endNote
Yavasscaoglu, I., Oktay, B., Simpseck, U., & Ozyurt, M. (1999, March). Role of ejaculation in the treatment of chronic non-bacterial prostatitis. *International Journal of Urology, 6*(3), 130–134.

PYELONEPHRITIS

Suzanne Barron

DEFINITION
A. An infection (usually from bacteria) that results in swelling of the kidney. It may affect one or both kidneys.
  1. Uncomplicated.
  2. Complicated: Patients with pregnancy, uncontrolled diabetes, immunocompromise, acute or ▶

chronic kidney disease, kidney transplants, urinary anatomic abnormalities, kidney stones, or urinary obstruction such as hydronephrosis.

INCIDENCE
A. Population-based study of acute pyelonephritis in the United States found overall annual rates of 15 to 17 cases per 10,000 females and 3 to 4 cases per 10,000 males.
B. At least 250,000 cases of pyelonephritis are diagnosed annually in the United States.

PATHOGENESIS
A. Usually results from bacterial invasion from the lower urinary tract (urethra and bladder).
B. Can result from colonization of the vagina with fecal flora.
C. Hematogenous source: From bloodstream infection that reaches renal parenchyma (uncommon). If from a hematogenous source, the offending organism can be gram-positive from bacterial endocarditis.
D. Evidence suggests that bacteria attaches to the urothelium and causes an inflammatory response. Hemolysins allow for bacterial invasion by damaging cells. Infection is most commonly associated with gram-negative bacteria such as *Escherichia coli* and *Klebsiella pneumoniae*. *Other gram-negative bacteria which can cause acute pyelonephritis are Proteus and Enterobacter.*

PREDISPOSING FACTORS
A. Female sex: Shorter urethra, allowing organisms to ascend to the bladder and kidneys.
B. Functional abnormalities: High postvoid residuals or incomplete bladder emptying, and neurogenic bladder.
C. Anatomic conditions: Bladder outlet obstruction/ benign prostatic hypertrophy (BPH) or vesicoureteral reflux.
D. Chronic indwelling catheters.
E. Nephrolithiasis.
F. Diabetes mellitus.
G. Immunosuppression.
H. Alcohol or drug abuse.
I. History of pyelonephritis.
J. Pregnancy.
K. New or multiple sexual partners.
L. History of recent cystitis.

SUBJECTIVE DATA
A. Common complaints/symptoms.
   1. Triad of symptoms: Flank pain, fever, nausea, and vomiting.
   2. Weakness.
   3. Foul-smelling urine.
   4. Hematuria.
   5. Altered mental status.
B. Common/typical scenario.
   1. Onset: Abrupt, usually 1 to 2 days of symptoms.
   2. Location/characteristics.
     a. Sharp and persistent flank pain in one or both kidneys.
     b. Abdominal pain and suprapubic tenderness.
     c. Possible groin pain.

     d. Strong urge to urinate.
     e. Burning on urination.
   3. Fevers/chills: Generally feeling unwell.
   4. Possible past medical history (PMH) of kidney stones, pyelonephritis, or neurogenic bladder with chronic indwelling catheter.
C. Family and social history.
   1. Family history.
     a. Congenital anomalies of the genitourinary (GU) tract.
     b. Nephrolithiasis.
     c. Diabetes mellitus.
     d. History of frequent urinary tract infections (UTIs).
   2. Social history.
     a. Alcohol use.
     b. Drug use (intravenous [IV] drug abuse may be associated with hematogenous spread of staphylococcal infection to the kidney).
     c. Multiple sexual partners.
     d. New sexual partners.
     e. Use of spermicide.
     f. Poor perineal hygiene (fecal incontinence, soiling).
D. Review of systems.
   1. Constitutional: Fevers, chills, or malaise.
   2. Cardiovascular: Palpitations or fast heart rate.
   3. Gastrointestinal (GI): Nausea and vomiting, abdominal pain, and fecal incontinence.
   4. GU: Flank pain, dysuria, foul-smelling urine, hematuria, urgency/frequency, and incontinence.
   5. Neurologic: Confusion and dizziness, especially in older adults.
   6. Gynecologic: Vaginal discharge.
   7. Endocrine: Polyuria, polydipsia, polyphagia (symptoms of diabetes), and night sweats.

PHYSICAL EXAMINATION
A. Vital signs: Evaluate for systemic inflammatory response/sepsis.
   1. Fever.
   2. Tachycardia.
   3. Hypotension.
B. Generalized: Check to see if the patient appears ill; they may have rigors.
C. GU: Evaluate for costovertebral angle tenderness (CVAT; positive in most cases on the side of the infected kidney).
D. Abdominal: Evaluate for suprapubic tenderness (without guarding) and rigidity to rule out other causes of abdominal pain (e.g., acute abdomen, appendicitis).
E. Respiratory: Assess for crackles and decreased breath sounds (signs of pneumonia).
F. Gynecologic examination: Perform if necessary in females to rule out gynecologic disorder or pelvic inflammatory disease.

DIAGNOSTIC TESTS
A. Bloodwork.
   1. Complete blood count (CBC) with differential: Leukocytosis with neutrophil predominance.

2. Basic metabolic panel: Renal failure. Uncommon unless obstruction or sepsis is present.

3. Blood culture: Possible bacteremia.

4. Lactate if there is concern for sepsis.

B. Urinalysis

1. Pyuria greater than 5 to 10 white blood cells per high power field (WBCs/HPF).

2. Positive for leukocytes.

3. WBC casts: Often indicative of pyelonephritis.

4. Nitrites: Positive in most cases if infection is caused by gram-negative bacteria.

5. Red blood cells (RBCs): May or may not be positive.

C. Urine culture.

1. Positive with greater than 100,000 bacteria/mL; 10,000 bacteria/mL in patients with catheterized urine samples.

2. Possibly negative if the patient was on antimicrobials prior to presentation.

D. Imaging: Not necessary in uncomplicated pyelonephritis, but failure to respond to appropriate therapy within 72 hours requires imaging to rule out ureteral obstruction or abscess.

1. Abdominal x-ray (kidney–ureter–bladder [KUB]): Stones may reveal intraparenchymal gas which could be emphysematous pyelonephritis.

2. CT scan of the abdomen and pelvis with and without contrast: Enlarged kidney with perinephric fat stranding. Imaging of choice if there is concern for emphysematous pyelonephritis or renal abscess.

3. Renal ultrasound: Imaging modality of choice for pregnant females (no radiation).

    a. Shows renal enlargement with hypoechoic parenchyma and loss.

DIFFERENTIAL DIAGNOSIS

A. Abdominal disorders.

1. Appendicitis.

2. Cholecystitis.

3. Pancreatitis.

4. Diverticulitis.

5. Peptic ulcer disease.

B. Gynecologic disorders.

1. Ectopic pregnancy.

2. Pelvic inflammatory disease.

3. Ruptured ovarian cyst.

C. Urologic disorders.

1. Nephrolithiasis.

2. Epididymitis.

3. Renal or perinephric abscess.

4. Urethritis.

5. Cystitis.

EVALUATION AND MANAGEMENT PLAN

A. General plan.

1. See Figure 5.1.

2. Obtain urinalysis and urine culture.

3. Obtain bloodwork: CBC, blood cultures, and basic metabolic panel.

4. Start broad-spectrum antibiotics.

    a. Can tolerate oral agents (e.g., ciprofloxacin, trimethoprim, and sulfamethoxazole). Nitrofurantoin should be avoided (does not penetrate kidney well).

    b. Unable to tolerate oral agents (e.g., ampicillin 2 g IV Q6H and gentamicin 1.5 mg/kg Q8H).

5. Use imaging studies for high suspicion of ureteral obstruction and abscess or in cases of complicated pyelonephritis.

6. Hospitalize patients who have systemic inflammatory response syndrome (SIRS), sepsis, dehydration, uncontrollable pain, persistent nausea and vomiting, or complicated cases of acute pyelonephritis.

7. Consult urology if ureteral obstruction is found for stent placement or possible percutaneous nephrostomy drain.

B. Patient/family teaching points.

1. Increase fluids to promote hydration and flushing of the bacteria.

2. Encourage good hygiene and wiping from front to back after urinating to prevent bacteria from colonizing the urethra.

3. Urinate after sexual intercourse to help wash away bacteria.

4. Counsel patient and family that the patient may continue to have fever and flank pain for 2 to 3 days after appropriate treatment has been given. If not clinically improving after 72 hours, patient should be instructed to call and be evaluated with imaging.

5. Reinforce the importance of completing antibiotics for the recommended 14- to 21-day course.

C. Pharmacotherapy.

1. Initiate empiric antibiotics based on local antibiotic resistance. Once urine culture has finalized, switch to an appropriate antimicrobial for 14 to 21 days.

2. Supportive care.

    a. Phenazopyridine as possible help for dysuria.

    b. Antipyretics such as acetaminophen and nonsteroidal anti-inflammatory drugs (NSAIDs) to control fever.

    c. Analgesics for appropriate pain management.

    d. IV fluid hydration to prevent and treat dehydration and sepsis.

D. Discharge instructions.

1. Advise patients to seek medical care for any recurrent symptoms, such as fevers, flank pain, nausea, and vomiting.

2. Advise patients to call if they are unable to tolerate oral antibiotic or develop adverse effects such as rash or diarrhea.

3. Advise patients to drink plenty of fluids.

FOLLOW-UP

A. Instruct patients to follow up within 4 to 6 weeks after completion of antibiotics with a repeat urine culture to verify that infection has cleared.

B. Advise patients to follow up with recurrent symptoms because relapse can occur requiring a second 14-day course of antibiotics.

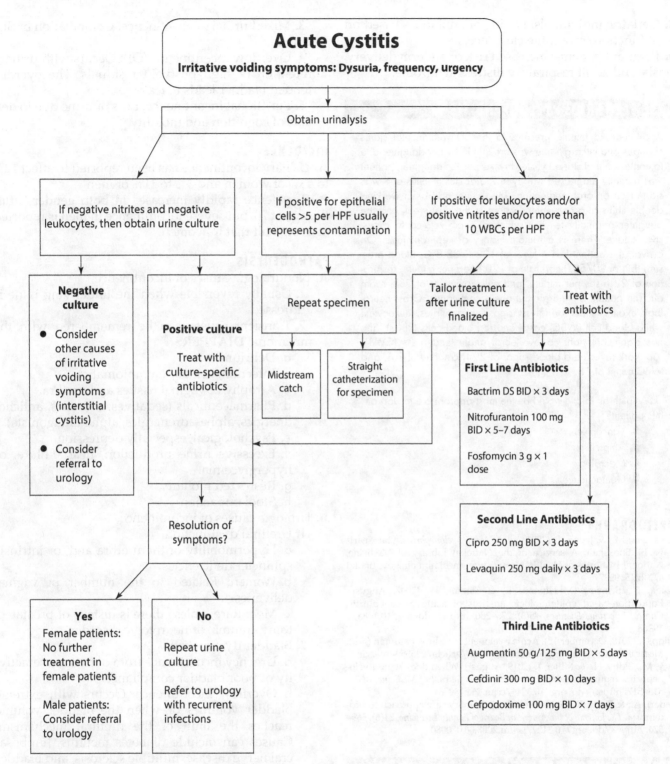

FIGURE 5.1 Acute cystitis algorithm.

HPF, high power field; WBC, white blood cells.

CONSULTATION/REFFERAL

A. Urology consult.

   1. Obstructive ureteral stones.

   2. Nephrolithiasis as a chronic nidus of infection.

   3. Recurrent episodes of pyelonephritis, which warrant evaluation for anatomic anomalies.

B. Infectious disease (ID) consult: Complicated infections and recommendations of duration of treatment.

C. Home infusion consult/home health nursing: If IV antibiotics recommended.

D. Interventional radiology consult: If percutaneous nephrostomy tube is indicated due to ureteral obstruction or for percutaneous drain placement for an abscess.

SPECIAL/GERIATRIC CONSIDERATIONS

A. Diabetic patients: Increased risk of developing emphysematous pyelonephritis.

B. Long-term/recurrent pyelonephritis patients: Development of significant renal scarring.

C. Geriatric individuals: Dosing of antibiotics based on renal function/creatinine clearance.

D. Pregnant patients: Increased risk of preterm delivery, sepsis, and adult respiratory distress syndrome.

CASE SCENARIO: PYELONEPHRITIS

A 64-year-old female presents to the ED with mental status changes and lethargy. She was brought in by her daughter due to confusion that started yesterday. As per the daughter, patient was recently diagnosed with type 2 diabetes mellitus and was started on an oral medication. The patient had been working double shifts at a convenience store in the past week and the daughter originally felt her symptoms were related to excessive fatigue. There is a remote history of nephrolithiasis. On arrival, the patient has a fever of 102°F/38.8°C, blood pressure (BP) of 90/50, heart rate of 120 beats per minute, respiration of 22 resps per minute, and pulse oximeter of 98% room air. The patient is lethargic but obeys commands. Gross neurologic exam is intact. Urinalysis is positive for nitrites, leukocytes, white blood cell (WBC) casts, and red blood cells (RBCs). She has significant right costovertebral angle tenderness (CVAT). Lab work revealed a blood sugar of 294, creatine of 1.4, and WBC count of 18.

1. Which antibiotic would be the most appropriate to start on this patient?

    A. Vancomycin

    B. Ampicillin

    C. Macrobid

    D. Gentamicin

BIBLIOGRAPHY

Belyayeva, M., & Jeong, J. (2021, July). *Acute pyelonephritis*. Stat Pearls NCBI Bookshelf. A service of the National Library of Medicine, National Institutes of Health. https://www.ncbi.nlm.nih.gov/bookds/NBK519537/

Czaga, C., Scholes, D., Hooton, T., & Stamm, W. (2007, August). Population-based epidemiologic analysis of acute pyelonephritis. *Clinical Infectious Diseases, 45*(3), 273–280. https://doi.org/10.1086/519268

Fulop, T. (2018, December 12). Acute pyelonephritis. In V. Batuman (Ed.), *Medscape.* http://emedicine.medscape.com/article/245559-overview

Lacy, M., Sidhy, N., & Miller, J. (2019, August). When does acute pyelonephritis require imaging? *Cleveland Clinic Journal of Medicine, 86*(8), 515–517. https://doi.org/10.3949/ccjm.86a.18096

Naderi, A., & Reilly, R. (2008, December). Primary care approach to proteinuria. *The Journal of the American Board of Family Medicine, 21*(6), 569–574. https://doi.org/10.3122/jabfm.2008.06.070080

URINARY INCONTINENCE

Suzanne Barron

DEFINITION

A. Urinary incontinence is an unintentional loss of urine.

B. Types of incontinence.

    1. Stress urinary incontinence (SUI): Occurs during physical exertion (sneezing, coughing, exercise).

    2. Urgency incontinence (UI): Involuntary loss of urine associated with urgency (bladder spasms).

    3. Mixed urinary incontinence: Combination of SUI and UI.

    4. Overflow incontinence (OI): Occurs with urinary retention or high postvoid residuals. The overdistended bladder leads to leakage.

    5. Functional incontinence: Loss of urine due to deficits of cognition and mobility.

INCIDENCE

A. Urinary incontinence has been reported to affect 12% to 43% of women and 3% to 11% of men.

B. Prevalence rapidly increases in both genders after the age of 70, but severe incontinence in men is reported at about half that in women.

PATHOGENESIS

A. Nonurologic causes of incontinence.

    1. Usually reversible when the underlying issue is addressed.

    2. Transient causes can be remembered with the mnemonic **DIAPPERS**.

        a. Delirium.

        b. Infection, urinary (symptomatic).

        c. Atrophy of vaginal tissues and urethra.

        d. Pharmaceuticals (sedatives, diuretics, anticholinergics, alpha-adrenergics, alpha-antagonists).

        e. Psychological, especially depression.

        f. Excessive urine production, heart failure, or hyperglycemia.

        g. Restricted mobility.

        h. Stool impaction.

B. Urologic causes of incontinence.

    1. Urethral dysfunction.

        a. Hypermobility of the urethra and/or intrinsic sphincter deficiencies.

        b. Women: Related to the number of vaginal deliveries.

        c. Men: Rare, unless there is history of prostatectomy, trauma, or neurologic disorder.

    2. Bladder dysfunction.

        a. Urgency incontinence from detrusor overactivity or poor bladder compliance.

        b. Overflow incontinence: Occurs with extreme bladder volumes or when the bladder volume reaches the limit of the urethral mechanism. Causes can include diabetes mellitus, lumbosacral nerve disease, multiple sclerosis, and bladder outflow obstruction.

PREDISPOSING FACTORS

A. Sex (female > male).

B. Advanced age.

C. Vaginal childbirth.

D. Cognitive impairment.

E. Chronic obstructive pulmonary disease (COPD).

F. Obesity.

G. Pelvic organ prolapse.

H. Smoking.

I. Pregnancy.

J. History of pelvic surgery (hysterectomy, prostatectomy) or pelvic radiation.
K. Poor mobility.
L. Neurologic disorders.
M. Anatomic disorders (e.g., vesicovaginal fistula).
N. Certain medications (diuretics, narcotic pain medication).
O. History of pelvic trauma.

SUBJECTIVE DATA
A. Common complaints/symptoms.
   1. SUI: Leakage of urine involuntarily when laughing, coughing, or sneezing.
   2. UI: Uncontrollable urge to urinate with associated leakage; occurs frequently.
   3. OI: Dribbling of urine, weak stream, and incomplete bladder emptying.
B. Common/typical scenario.
   1. Onset of symptoms: Gradual versus sudden.
   2. Associated pain with incontinence.
   3. Severity: Minimal amount of leakage versus large amount of leakage and soaking through clothes.
   4. Timing and frequency of the incontinence (after sneezing, only occurs at night).
   5. Aggravating factors (e.g., caffeine, citrus).
   6. Alleviating factors (pessary).
   7. Risk factors (vaginal prolapse, recent urinary tract infection [UTI], benign prostatic hypertrophy [BPH], neurologic disorders, trauma).
C. Family and social history.
   1. Smoking.
      a. Tobacco: Irritant to the bladder, causing UI.
      b. Tobacco addiction: Possibly leading to a chronic cough and increased intra-abdominal pressure, damaging the muscles of the pelvic floor and resulting in SUI.
   2. Alcohol: Diuretic effect/central nervous system (CNS) depressant causing OI and UI.
   3. Illicit drugs: Abuse of prescription drugs such as opioids/sedatives causing OI or functional incontinence.
D. Review of systems.
   1. Constitutional: Fevers, chills, and weight gain.
   2. Neurologic: Confusion, altered speech, altered mental status, lower extremity weakness, dizziness, tremors, decreased mobility, and paresthesia (saddle anesthesia).
   3. Respiratory: Chronic cough and chronic bronchitis.
   4. Cardiovascular: Shortness of breath or edema associated with congestive heart failure (CHF).
   5. Abdominal: Constipation, obstipation, or reflux that causes cough.
   6. Genitourinary (GU): Frequency, urgency, hematuria, retention, incomplete bladder emptying, or suprapubic pain.
   7. Gynecologic: Pelvic organ prolapse or leakage of urine from vagina.
   8. Musculoskeletal: Lower back pain.

PHYSICAL EXAMINATION
A. Neurologic.
   1. Assess mental status, motor strength, and sensory status, as well as deep tendon reflexes.
   2. Observe gait.
B. Respiratory: Assess for rhonchi and barrel chest.
C. Cardiovascular: Assess for jugular venous distension (JVD) and edema.
D. Abdomen: Assess for suprapubic tenderness, palpable bladder, and abdominal/pelvic masses.
E. GU.
   1. Perform digital rectal examination (DRE) to evaluate for BPH, prostatitis, and prostate nodules.
   2. Evaluate for rectal fissures and/or fecal impaction.
F. Gynecologic.
   1. Perform Q-tip test: Used to demonstrate urethral hypermobility, which may indicate SUI.
      a. A sterile, well-lubricated Q-tip is placed into the urethra and the patient is then told to cough or strain.
      b. The degree of Q-tip movement is measured. The test is considered positive if the Q-tip moves more than 30 degrees.
   2. Evaluate for vaginal atrophy.
   3. Evaluate for pelvic organ prolapse.
G. Dermatologic: Assess for excoriated skin due to incontinence or presence of fungal infection.

DIAGNOSTIC TESTS
A. Urinalysis and urine culture: Evaluate for infectious source.
B. Postvoid residual: Can be obtained with bladder ultrasound or with a urinary catheter. Volumes greater than 200 mL with associated urinary symptoms should warrant additional testing for possible bladder outlet obstruction or poor bladder contractility.
C. Bloodwork: Basic metabolic panel to evaluate renal function, which may indicate obstructive source.
D. Imaging: Generally not indicated.
E. Urodynamic studies/video-urodynamic studies.
   1. Filling study: Detrusor overactivity and leak point pressure.
   2. Voiding study: Urinary flow rate, postvoid residual, and detrusor sphincter synergy.
F. Cystoscopy: If there is concern for fistula or malignancy.

DIFFERENTIAL DIAGNOSIS
A. UTI (cystitis, prostatitis).
B. Interstitial cystitis.
C. Nocturnal enuresis.
D. Urethral diverticulum.
E. Vesicovaginal fistula.
F. Cauda equina syndrome.
G. Constipation/obstipation.
H. Bladder cancer.
I. Bladder outlet obstruction.

EVALUATION AND MANAGEMENT PLAN
A. General plan.

1. Obtain thorough history to determine the type of urinary incontinence to target treatment.
2. Obtain laboratory studies such as urinalysis, urine culture, and basic metabolic panel.
3. If possible, obtain postvoid residual with bladder scan.
B. Patient/family teaching points.
  1. Encourage smoking cessation and avoidance of alcohol/caffeine.
  2. Encourage keeping a 24-hour voiding diary to help patients understand voiding patterns.
  3. Educate patient about timed voiding, which will help avoid significant bladder distention.
  4. Educate patients with SUI about how to perform Kegel exercises to strengthen pelvic floor muscles. Discuss the role of biofeedback in helping control these muscles.
  5. Educate patients with UI about bladder training (delay voiding for increasing periods of time by inhibiting the desire to void).
  6. Encourage weight loss in obese patients.
  7. Teach patients with OI about how to perform clean intermittent catheterization if necessary.
C. Pharmacotherapy.
  1. SUI.
    a. Currently, no Food and Drug Administration (FDA)-approved medication for SUI.
    b. Topical estrogen in postmenopausal women: Mild benefit.
  2. UI.
    a. First-line therapies: Behavioral therapies such as modification of fluid intake, timed voiding, reduction of bladder irritants, weight loss, and pelvic floor exercises.
    b. Second-line therapies: Medications.
      i. Anticholinergic medications/antimuscarinic medications: Act by binding the muscarinic receptor on the detrusor muscle, decreasing bladder muscle contractility. Medications include oxybutynin, tolterodine, solifenacin, darifenacin, and trospium, with side effects of dry mouth, constipation, and impaired cognitive function.
      ii. Tricyclic antidepressants.
      iii. Direct relaxant effect on bladder muscle.
      iv. Not commonly used due to side effects.
      v. Beta-3-adrenergic receptor agonist (mirabegron): Associated with much less dry mouth and constipation (side effects of anticholinergic medications) but may cause hypertension.
D. Discharge instructions.
  1. Discuss with the patient to call with side effects of medication, such as dry mouth, constipation, confusion, or vision changes.
  2. Instruct the patient to seek medical attention with any fevers, chills, flank pain, or hematuria, which may indicate UTI.
  3. Advise the patient about appropriate care of the skin due to incontinence. Keep the skin clean and dry. Wearing pads may help protect the skin.

  4. Mention that stool softeners or mild laxatives may be needed to prevent constipation.

FOLLOW-UP
A. Follow-up in 3 to 4 weeks for symptom assessment/response to therapy.
B. Biofeedback often requires multiple visits.
C. Instruct the patient to bring their voiding diary to follow-up appointment.
D. For patients on an anticholinergic, check postvoid residual to monitor for urinary retention.

CONSULTATION/REFFERAL
A. Refer to urologist/urogynecologist for persistent symptoms or concern for malignancy or anatomic abnormality.
  1. SUI.
    a. Periurethral bulking agents such as calcium hydroxylapatite.
    b. Pubovaginal sling placement.
    c. Surgical repair of pelvic organ prolapse.
    d. Surgery for BPH (transurethral resection of the prostate [TURP]).
    e. Artificial urinary sphincter for men.
    f. Fit for pessary.
  2. UI.
    a. Percutaneous tibial nerve stimulation.
    b. Intravesical botulinum toxin: High efficacy in patients who have failed other medical treatments.
  3. Cystoscopy to rule out malignancy or anatomic abnormality.
B. Refer to neurology/neurosurgery with any concern for spinal cord injury, compression (cauda equina), or neurologic disorder.

SPECIAL/GERIATRIC CONSIDERATIONS
A. Avoid anticholinergic medication in patients who have a history of acute angle glaucoma.
B. Anticholinergic medication may cause confusion in geriatric individuals.
C. Assess geriatric patients for polypharmacy. Various medications that are commonly given may cause OI (antidepressants, calcium channel blockers, opioid pain medication, sedatives, antihistamines) or UI due to the high volume of urine (diuretics).
D. Consider the cost of pads in geriatric individuals who are on a fixed income. It is estimated that women with severe incontinence pay up to $900 per year for incontinence pads.

CASE SCENARIO: URINARY INCONTINENCE

A 64-year-old male with a past medical history (PMH) significant for hypertension, atrial fibrillation, coronary artery disease, and tobacco abuse presents to the ED with gross hematuria and urinary incontinence for the past 3 days. He denies passage of clots, suprapubic pain, or dysuria. He reports constant dribbling, frequency, and a weak stream. Symptoms started after he was at a wedding 3 days ago where he was drinking alcohol. He is afebrile and afebrile, vital signs stable (AVSS).

1. What would be the best initial study in determining the cause of the patient's incontinence?
  A. Basic metabolic panel
  B. CT scan of the abdomen/pelvis
  C. Bladder ultrasound/postvoid residual
  D. Cystoscopy

BIBLIOGRAPHY

Albala, D., Morey, A., Gomella, L., & Stein, J. (2011). *Oxford American handbook of urology*. Oxford University Press.

Cameron, A., Jimbo, M., & Heidelbaugh, J. (2013). Diagnosis and office-based treatment of urinary incontinence in adults. Part two: Treatment. *Therapeutic Advances in Urology*, 5(4), 189–200. https://doi.org/10.1177/1756287213495100

Cohn, J. A., Brown, E. T., Reynolds, W. S., Kaufman, M. R., Milam, D. F., & Dmochowski, R. R. (2016). An update on the use of transdermal oxybutynin in the management of overactive bladder disorder. *Therapeutic Advances in Urology*, 8(2), 83–90. https://doi.org/10.1177/1756287215626312

Gomella, L., Andriole, G., Burnett, A., Flanigan, R., Keane, T., Koo, H., & Thomas, R. (2015). *The 5-minute urology consult* (3rd ed.). Lippincott Williams & Wilkins.

Gormley, E. A., Kaufman, M., & Takacs, E. (2019, October). *Medical student curriculum: Urinary incontinence-American Urological Association*. https://www.aua.net.org/education/auauniversity/for-medical-students/medical-students-curriculum/medical-student-curriculum/urinary-incontinen

Herbruck, L. (2008). Stress urinary incontinence: An overview of diagnosis and treatment options. *Urology Nursing*, 28(3), 186–198. www.Medscape.com/viewarticle/57833_4

Hesch, K. (2007, July). Agents for treatment of overactive bladder: A therapeutic class review. *Proceedings (Baylor University Medical Center)*, 20(3), 307–314.

Khandelwal, C., & Kistler, C. (2013, April). Diagnosis of urinary incontinence. *American Family Physician*, 87(8), 543–550.

MacDiarmid, S. (2008, Winter). Maximizing the treatment of overactive bladder in the elderly. *Reviews in Urology*, 10(1), 6–13.

Salzman, B., & Hersch, L. (2013, May). Clinical management of urinary incontinence in women. *American Family Physician*, 87(9), 634–640.

Subak, L., Brown, J., Kraus, S., Brubaker, L., Lin, F., Richter, H., Bradley, C. S., & Grady, D. (2006). Diagnostic Aspects of Incontinence Study (DAISy). The "costs" of urinary incontinence for women. *Group, Obstetric Gynecology*, 107(4), 908–916. https://doi.org/10.1097/01.AOG.0000206213.48334.09

Thomas, B. (2015). *The pathophysiology of urinary incontinence: Part 2*. https://www.gmjournal.co.uk/the_pathophysiology_of_urinary_incontinence_part_2_25769830611.aspx

URINARY TRACT INFECTION

Suzanne Barron

DEFINITION
A. Urinary tract infection (UTI): Presence of pathogens in the urinary tract that is causing symptoms in a patient.
B. Asymptomatic bacteriuria: Presence of organisms in the urine but are not causing a patient any illness.

INCIDENCE
A. UTIs account for about seven million office visits annually, affecting men and women.
B. These infections are more common in young, sexually active women than men.
C. 30% to 40% of women will experience one episode per year.
D. Approximately 40% of nosocomial infections are UTIs and most are associated with use of urinary catheters.

PATHOGENESIS
A. UTIs are more common in women because the female urethra:
  1. Is shorter and in closer proximity to the rectum.
  2. Allows bacteria to colonize more easily.
B. UTIs peak in two different age groups in women.
  1. 20 to 40 age group: Predisposed by intercourse.
  2. 55 to 60 age group: Related to declining estrogen levels.

PREDISPOSING FACTORS
A. Conditions that reduce urine flow.
  1. Outflow obstruction: Prostatic hyperplasia, prostatic carcinoma, urethral stricture, or foreign body (calculus).
  2. Neurogenic bladder.
  3. Inadequate fluid uptake.
B. Conditions that promote colonization.
  1. Sexual activity: Increased inoculation.
  2. Spermicide: Increased binding.
  3. Estrogen depletion: Increased binding.
  4. Antimicrobial agents: Decreased indigenous flora.
C. Conditions that facilitate ascent.
  1. Catheterization.
  2. Urinary incontinence.
  3. Fecal incontinence.
D. Conditions in older women, who may be at higher risk for UTIs due to a combination of factors.
  1. Atrophic changes.
  2. Impaired urethral function.
  3. Insufficient fluid intake.
  4. Constipation.
  5. Increased residual urine volume.
E. Genetic predisposition.
  1. Increased colonization ability.
  2. Increased adherence by bacteria to the urinary tract epithelium.

SUBJECTIVE DATA
A. Common complaints/symptoms.
  1. Foul-smelling urine.
  2. Dysuria, increased frequency, or urgency.
  3. Suprapubic pain and discomfort.
  4. Occasional hematuria.
B. Atypical symptoms in older patients.
  1. Confusion.
  2. Delirium.
  3. Falls or adverse behaviors.

PHYSICAL EXAMINATION
A. Possible suprapubic tenderness on palpation.
B. Increasing discharge from vagina.
C. Urinary meatus that may be erythematous or edematous.

D. Negative costovertebral angle tenderness (CVAT).

E. Negative pelvic or prostate examination.

F. Urologic evaluation is required for men with UTI.

DIAGNOSTIC TESTS

A. Urinalysis.

  1. Urine dipstick with clean catch urine necessary.

  2. Positive for blood, leukocyte esterase (detection of white blood cells [WBCs] in the urine), or nitrite positivity.

  3. Leukocyte esterase has a 73% to 84% specificity and 80% to 92% sensitivity for UTI.

B. Urine microscopy.

  1. Pyuria: Finding of WBCs in the urine (>10 WBCs/ high power field [HPF]).

  2. Squamous epithelial cells (more than 15,020 squamous epithelial cells/HPF is suggestive of a contaminated specimen).

  3. Bacteria greater than 15 bacteria/HPF.

  4. Yeast species can sometimes be seen.

C. Urine culture.

  1. >100,000 colonies/mL on a urine culture is considered diagnostic of a UTI.

  2. Lower colony counts obtained by sterile collection or suprapubic aspiration can be indicative of UTI.

DIFFERENTIAL DIAGNOSIS

A. Genital herpes (herpes simplex virus [HSV]).

B. Urethritis.

C. *Chlamydia.*

D. *Trichomonas.*

E. Vaginitis.

F. Prostatitis.

G. Nephrolithiasis.

H. Trauma.

I. Urinary tract tuberculosis.

J. Urinary tract neoplasm.

K. Intra-abdominal abscess.

L. Interstitial cystitis.

N. Overactive bladder.

EVALUATION AND MANAGEMENT PLAN

A. General plan.

  1. See Figure 5.2.

  2. Advise patients on condition, timeline of treatment, and expected course of disease process.

  3. Collect urine culture before starting antibiotics.

  4. Complete all antibiotic regimens.

B. Patient/family teaching points.

  1. Counsel patients about appropriate use of medications (dose, frequency, side effects, need to complete entire course of medications).

  2. Recommend increasing fluid intake to 8 to 10 glasses per day.

  3. Suggest that sitting in a warm tub may relieve symptoms of dysuria.

  4. For women, advise that they wipe front to back after a bowel movement.

  5. For women, advise against using douches.

  6. Tell patients to avoid bubble baths.

  7. Advise that voiding after intercourse may be beneficial.

  8. Use appropriate cleaning for sex toys and advise against sharing sex toys.

C. Pharmacotherapy.

  1. First-line antibiotics.

    a. Bactrim, double strength, orally BID for 3 days.

    b. Nitrofurantoin 100 mg BID for 5 days.

    c. Fosfomycin 3 g as single dose.

  2. Second-line antibiotics.

    a. Ciprofloxacin 250 mg orally BID for 3 days.

    b. Amoxicillin–clavulanate 500/125 mg orally BID for 5 days.

  3. Treatment during pregnancy.

    a. Ampicillin 500 mg orally Q8H for 3 to 7 days.

    b. Amoxicillin–clavulanate 500/125 mg Q8H for 3 to 7 days.

    c. Cephalexin 500 mg Q6H for 3 to 7 days.

    d. Nitrofurantoin 100 mg BID for 5 to 7 days (avoid during first trimester and at term).

    e. Bactrim DS BID for 5 days (avoid during first trimester and at term).

    f. Fosfomycin 3 g orally as single dose.

D. Discharge instructions.

  1. Return to clinic for fever or if symptoms do not improve/progress in 48 to 72 hours.

FOLLOW-UP

A. Follow-up with the primary care provider (PCP).

CONSULTATION/REFFERAL

A. Consult or refer to urology only if complications occur.

SPECIAL/GERIATRIC CONSIDERATIONS

A. Geriatric patients may present with atypical symptoms and require close monitoring of intake versus output during UTI.

B. Patients with chronic kidney disease (CKD) or end-stage renal disease (ESRD) may require antibiotic dose adjustments.

C. Postmenopausal women with recurrent UTIs may benefit from vaginal estrogen

D. Catheter-dependent patients increase in catheter-associated UTI (CAUTI): Develop bacteriuria over time; 10% to 25% of these patients will develop symptoms.

E. Asymptomatic bacteriuria: Does not require treatment unless patient is pregnant or there is a planned urology procedure where mucosal bleeding is expected.

CASE SCENARIO: DYSURIA

A 40-year-old woman presents to the urgent care clinic with reports of foul-smelling urine, urinary frequency, dysuria, and suprapubic discomfort. Symptoms started 3 days ago and have been increasing in severity. She is sexually active. Her last menstrual period was 40 days ago. The patient states she had taken a pregnancy test about 1 week ago and it was negative. She also reports history of irregular menses. She denies

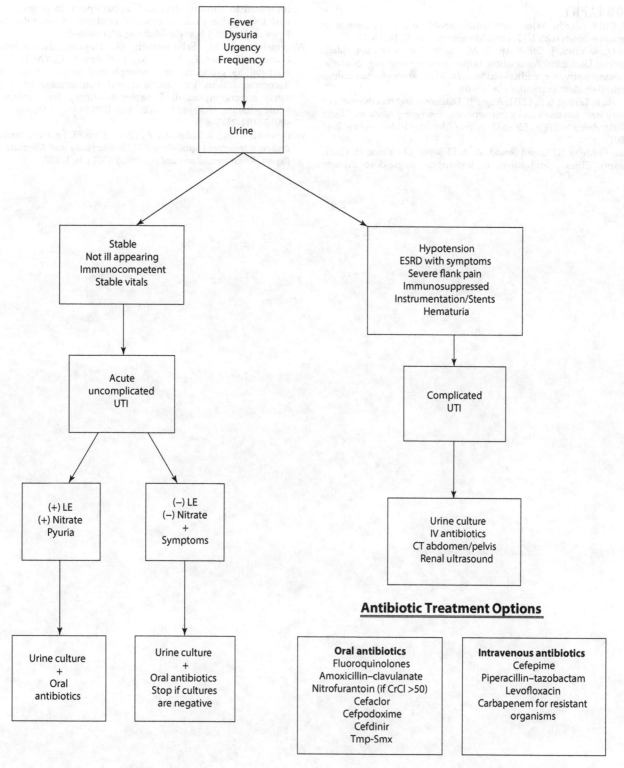

FIGURE 5.2   Urinary tract infection flipped in chronic kidney disease.

CrCl, creatinine clearance; ESRD, end-stage renal disease; IV, intravenous; LE, leukocyte esterase; Tmp-Smx, trimethoprim/sulfamethoxazole; UTI, urinary tract infection.

any significant medical history or frequent urinary tract infections (UTIs). On exam, she is well-appearing, afebrile, vital signs stable (AVSS), no costovertebral angle tenderness (CVAT), with mild suprapubic fullness and tenderness, and no edema. Urine dipstick was positive for leukocyte esterase, and negative for blood, protein, and nitrite. A urine culture is sent and pending. She has no known drug alergies (NKDA).

1. Which antibiotic would be the most appropriate for this patient prior to the results of urine culture?
  A. Ciprofloxacin 250 mg orally BID
  B. Bactrim DS BID for 5 days
  C. Nitrofurantoin 100 mg BID for 7 days
  D. Fosfomycin 3 g orally as a single dose

BIBLIOGRAPHY

Duff, P. (2018, March). Which antibiotics should be used in caution in pregnant women with UTI? *OBG Management, 30*(3), 14, 16–17.

Kaplan, D., & Yates, J. (2020, April). *Medical student curriculum: Adult.* American Urological Association. https://www.auanet.org/education/auauniversity/for-medical-students/medical-students-curriculum/medical-student-curriculum/adult-uti

Lane, D. R., & Takhar, S. S. (2011, August). Diagnosis and management of urinary tract infection and pyelonephritis. *Emergency Medicine Clinics of North America, 29*(3), 539–552. https://doi.org/10.1016/j.emc.2011.04.001

Ramadan El-Mehy, S., Fouad Sanad, Z., & El-Sayed El-Lakwa, H. (2021, January). Efficacy and safety of fosfomycin single-dose therapy compared to nitrofurantoin and cephalosporin in pregnant women with lower urinary tract infection: A randomized controlled trial. *The Egyptian Journal of Hospital Medicine, 82*(4), 626–631.

Wagenlehner, F. M., Schmiemann, G., Hoyme, U., Fünfstück, R., Hummers-Pradier, E., Kaase, M., & Naber, K. G. (2011, February). National S3 guideline on uncomplicated urinary tract infection: Recommendations for treatment and management of uncomplicated community-acquired bacterial urinary tract infections in adult patients. *Urologe A, 50*(2), 153–169. https://doi.org/10.1007/s00120-011-2512-z

Workowski, K. A., & Bolan, G. A. (2015, June 5). Sexually transmitted diseases treatment guidelines, 2015. *Morbidity and Mortality Weekly Report. Recommendations and Reports, 64*(RR-03), 1–137.

KNOWLEDGE CHECK: CHAPTER 5

1. After 2 weeks of treatment with finasteride, a patient calls reporting they have not noted any difference in their lower urinary tract symptoms. The patient previously tried tamsulosin but developed dizziness. What should the clinician advise?

   A. Switch to another 5-alpha-reductase inhibitor such as dutasteride.

   B. Try another alpha-blocker such as terazosin.

   C. Reassure patient that it can take up to 6 months for finasteride to shrink prostatic tissue and to continue therapy.

   D. Discuss nonpharmaceutical treatment such as referral to urology for procedures such as transurethral resection of the prostate (TURP).

2. What is an important fact the practitioner should tell a patient on anticoagulation therapy for atrial fibrillation in the workup of hematuria?

   A. Patients on anticoagulation do not require the same workup as patients who are not on anticoagulation.

   B. The patient should discuss changing to a different anticoagulation medication with their cardiologist.

   C. Most commonly, the cause of the hematuria is benign in nature, but they should still have a thorough workup.

   D. Most cases of hematuria while on anticoagulation are glomerular hematuria and require a nephrology referral.

3. A patient who presented with asymptomatic gross hematuria is stable and ready for discharge from the hospital. During their stay, they have had a urinalysis, urine culture, renal ultrasound, and CT urogram completed without an identifiable cause for the hematuria. What should the practitioner advise the patient to do after discharge?

   A. Follow up with the primary care provider (PCP) for repeat urinalysis in 1 to 2 weeks.

   B. Follow up with urology for a cystoscopy.

   C. Workup is complete and follow up only if blood reappears.

   D. Order an MRI of the abdomen/pelvis for the patient to obtain as an outpatient.

4. While on night call, the nurse practitioner (NP) is called to an ICU patient with a new result for ionized calcium of 0.76 mmol/L. The last result was 1.21 mmol/L 6 hours ago. The patient has been stable on continuous renal replacement therapy (CRRT) using citrate for 2 days, with ionized calcium ranging from 1.07 to 1.34 mmol/L, after a traumatic injury. The patient is bleeding from three chest tubes and returned to the operating room (OR) again today to wash out the abdomen. The patient has received 15 units of packed red blood cell (PRBC) and 10 fresh frozen plasma over the past 2 days. The patient has had a replacement calcium chloride infusing running at a stable rate for the past 2 days. The bedside nurse assured the NP that they have collected this ionized calcium the same as all previous collections and there was no interruption to the calcium infusion. What is the best next step?

   A. Stop the continuous renal replacement therapy (CRRT).

   B. Order an EKG and repeat the ionized calcium before making any changes.

   C. Order 2 g intravenous (IV) calcium chloride IV now, increase the IV calcium replacement infusion, and order a repeat ionized calcium level after the IV calcium bolus.

   D. Call nephrology.

5. A 65-year-old patient with alcoholic cirrhosis still drinks alcohol and is frequently seen in the ED. Today, the emergency medical service (EMS) brings the patient in due to altered mental status and hypotension from outside the nearest liquor store. The patient is still confused and disoriented. On admission, the patient's sodium is 109 mEq/L, potassium is 3.1 mg/dL, magnesium is 1.4 mg/dL, and creatinine is 1.4 mg/dL; other labs are normal. On chart review the nurse practitioner (NP) finds that sodium in the past two admissions was less than 125 mEq/L, and at last discharge sodium was 128 mEq/L. The NP calls the patient's sister who says that the patient is not taking any of the prescribed medications and has been drinking more lately and eating very little. Does the NP need to admit this patient?

   A. No. This is chronic hyponatremia that can be treated as outpatient. Discharge once the patient sleeps off the alcohol intoxication.

   B. Yes. Observation and nonemergent treatment of chronic hyponatremia with new symptoms, including altered mental status.

   C. Yes. Acute kidney injury with severe hypokalemia due to malnutrition and intravenous (IV) hydration.

   D. Cannot answer without more information. Repeat sodium in 6 hours and order a CT of the head.

(*See answers next page.*)

1. C) Reassure patient that it can take up to 6 months for finasteride to shrink prostatic tissue and to continue therapy.

It can take up to 6 months for 5-alpha-reductase inhibitors to shrink prostatic tissue.

2. C) Most commonly, the cause of the hematuria is benign in nature, but they should still have a thorough workup.

Patients on anticoagulation therapy still need a thorough workup. Most commonly, the etiology of gross hematuria is benign in nature.

3. B) Follow up with urology for a cystoscopy.

Patients with gross hematuria need a cystoscopy as part of the workup to rule out any masses in the bladder or changes to the bladder mucosa.

4. C) Order 2 g intravenous (IV) calcium chloride IV now, increase the IV calcium replacement infusion, and order a repeat ionized calcium level after the IV calcium bolus.

While organizational practice may require the NP to call nephrology, the appropriate action is to emergently replace calcium. Citrate binds calcium and requires large replacement doses. In this case, citrate is used both for continuous renal replacement therapy (CRRT) anticoagulant and to anticoagulate blood products so the patient receives a very large dose. Stopping CRRT will not fix the problem. This patient is calcium-deficient. The NP needs to replace the calcium and ensure they are adequately replacing it going forward. Always repeat ionized calcium levels to ensure enough was given. CRRT patients should have ionized calcium check multiple times every day while on therapy.

5. B) Yes. Observation and nonemergent treatment of chronic hyponatremia with new symptoms, including altered mental status.

This is a dilutional hyponatremia common among alcoholics who do not eat or consume solutes, sometimes called beer potomania. Total body water is maintained by drinking fluids, but solutes are lost. Over time, this causes a chronic hyponatremia (lasting more than 48 hours). Chronic symptomatic hyponatremia should be treated slowly and nonemergently to avoid the consequences of overcorrection, but only treat hyponatremia as outpatient if the sodium level is stable; this sodium is not stable. Altered mental status is rarely associated with cerebral pathology, such as bleeding; regardless of decision about CT, there is enough information to admit this patient for observation and treatment of chronic hyponatremia. Restrict water intake, monitor this patient in the hospital due to symptoms, monitor intake and output closely, and slowly replace sodium deficit carefully to avoid raising sodium quickly.

6. What should the practitioner avoid in the physical exam if there is concern for an acute infection of the prostate?

   A. Digital rectal exam
   B. Urethral evaluation and swab
   C. Scrotal/testicular/epididymal exam
   D. Prostate massage

7. How can the practitioner differentiate between acute versus chronic bacterial prostatitis?

   A. Predisposing risk factors
   B. Response to antibiotic therapy
   C. Onset of symptoms
   D. Presence of dysuria

8. When treating pyelonephritis, what is the best imaging study when there is concern for emphysematous pyelonephritis?

   A. Renal ultrasound
   B. Kidney–ureter–bladder (KUB) x-ray
   C. CT scan of the abdomen/pelvis with and without contrast
   D. MRI of the abdomen and pelvis

9. Which antibiotic should be prescribed first line for a suspected case of acute pyelonephritis in an otherwise healthy female while waiting for urine culture and sensitivity to confirm?

   A. Macrobid
   B. Ciprofloxacin
   C. Amoxicillin
   D. Bactrim

10. Stress urinary incontinence in a male with no urologic history would most likely be caused by:

    A. Diabetes mellitus
    B. Neurologic condition such as spinal cord compression
    C. Urinary tract infection
    D. Benign prostatic hypertrophy

(See answers next page.)

6. D) Prostate massage

Prostate massage is contraindicated as it may spread infection causing sepsis.

7. C) Onset of symptoms

Acute prostatitis patients are more likely to have acute illness with fever, and symptoms are more likely to occur suddenly as opposed to gradually with chronic bacterial prostatitis.

8. C) CT scan of the abdomen/pelvis with and without contrast

One of the most serious complications of pyelonephritis is emphysematous pyelonephritis. Emphysematous pyelonephritis is a necrotizing infection of the kidney usually caused by *Escherichia coli* or *Klebsiella pneumoniae*. It occurs more frequently in females and those with a history of diabetes. The diagnosis can be seen on renal ultrasound, but CT scan imaging is typically necessary.

9. D) Bactrim

Most uncomplicated cases of acute pyelonephritis are caused by *Escherichia coli* and patients can be treated effectively with trimethoprim-sulfamethoxazole (TMP-SMX) or a cephalosporin for 14 days.

10. B) Neurologic condition such as spinal cord compression

Stress urinary incontinence in a male with no urologic history would most likely be caused by a neurologic condition such as spinal cord compression.

CHAPTER 6

NEUROLOGY GUIDELINES

Dominick Osipowicz and Jennifer Creed

ANOXIC BRAIN INJURY

DEFINITION

A. Deprivation of oxygen to the brain often due to cardiac arrest, but can occur from any cause, including carbon monoxide poisoning, severe asthma attacks, suffocation, drowning, and strokes.
B. Can be classified into four categories.
   1. Diffuse cerebral hypoxia.
   2. Focal cerebral ischemia.
   3. Global cerebral ischemia.
   4. Cerebral infarction.

INCIDENCE

A. No specific numbers are available to document the incidence or prevalence of anoxic brain injury.
B. The main cause of anoxic brain injury is cardiac arrest (82.4%).
C. Other causes include poisoning, drug overdose, head trauma, stroke, seizures, and severe asthma attacks.

PATHOGENESIS

A. The delivery of oxygen to the brain is highly dependent on its metabolic demand. Overall, this drive is usually higher compared with the rest of the body.
B. Thus, any interruption of blood supply to cerebral vasculature, even in short amounts of time, such as a cardiac arrest, can cause significant brain injury.
   1. Primary brain injury.
      a. Decreased perfusion to the brain: Leads to deprivation of oxygen, glucose, and other nutrients required for brain metabolism.
      b. Release of glutamate, an excitatory neurotransmitter: Along with the release of other excitatory amino acid neurotransmitters, it leads to the formation of free radicals and lipid peroxidation.
      c. Large amounts of sodium and calcium enter the cells: Leads to cytotoxic edema.
      d. Lost regulatory mechanisms of the cell: Leads to cell death.
   2. Secondary brain injury.
      a. Microvascular dysfunction: Occurs from poor perfusion. Small capillaries and arterioles continue to have low perfusion despite restoration of blood flow, resulting in cerebral edema.
      b. Cerebral edema: Can occur from microvascular dysfunction as well as from cell death.
      c. Impaired autoregulation: Increase in intracranial pressure (ICP) leads to a compensatory right shift in pressure regulation resulting in increase in cerebral perfusion pressure (CPP) in order to maintain adequate cerebral blood flow (CBF).
      d. Hyperoxia: Occurs from increased free radicals.
      e. Hyperthermia: Occurs from increased metabolic demand and induction of apoptosis.

PREDISPOSING FACTORS

A. In cardiac arrest, patients may have risk factors associated with cardiac disease.
B. In other causes, patients tend to be younger, especially in respiratory-related anoxic brain injury cases.

SUBJECTIVE DATA

A. Patients with anoxic brain injury will not be able to provide any subjective information so subjective data are not relevant in this situation.
B. However, the interviewer should obtain as much history from others as possible.
   1. Obtain a thorough patient social history through family, friends, or witnesses.
   2. Obtain any information about time, place, and onset.
      a. How long was the person in cardiac arrest or deprived of oxygen? Studies have shown that prolonged CPR (typically >15 minutes) has not led to a good prognosis. These people generally die from this injury within 6 weeks.
   3. Obtain the patient's medical history, medication use, any history of drug or alcohol abuse, or any recent complaints.

PHYSICAL EXAMINATION

A. Thorough neurologic exam: Required.
B. Levels of consciousness.
   1. Coma: State of unresponsiveness. Patients are unaware of their surroundings and are unarousable.
   2. Vegetative state: State of wakefulness without awareness or return of sleep–wake cycles. This results from a severe anoxic injury.
      a. Persistent vegetative state: Vegetative state 1 month after injury.
      b. Permanent vegetative state (PVS): Irreversible. This may occur 3 months after a nontraumatic injury and 1 year following a traumatic brain injury. ▶

3. Minimal consciousness: State that does not fit the definition for PVS. Patients show limited evidence of awareness of themselves or environment that is reproducible. They may have brief periods of meaningful interaction (e.g., simple commands or tracking).

4. Locked-in syndrome: Sustained eye opening, awareness of environment with quadriplegia. Cognition is intact. Vertical eye movements and/or blinking of eyes to communicate.

5. Brain death: Death by irreversible cessation of CBF. Absence of all brainstem functions is characteristic (see "Brain Death" for additional information).

DIAGNOSTIC TESTS

A. Diagnostic tests can be performed but these can be affected by timing and patient temperature. Overall, time is essential to the prognostication process. The longer a clinician waits to prognosticate, the better. In most cases, it is necessary to wait at least 72 hours after rewarming or postarrest without hypothermia to give a prognosis.

B. However, timing should be on a case-by-case basis. Some patients with hypothermia that requires heavy sedation should be given longer than 72 hours because hypothermia can delay drug metabolism.

C. Clinical examination: Traditionally the strongest predictor of outcome. Predictors of poor outcome include:

1. Absent pupillary reflexes.

2. Absent corneal reflexes.

3. Motor response of extensor posturing or no movement.

D. Biochemical markers.

E. Neuroimaging.

1. MRI of the brain: Loss of gray/white matter differentiation. This indicates significant brain injury and is a sign of poor prognosis.

2. CT of the head: Initially, this can be normal, but after about 3 days it shows brain edema and loss of gray/white differentiation.

F. Electrophysiology.

1. Somatosensory evoked potential (SSEP).

2. EEG: Used to determine the presence of underlying brain activity as well as seizures (commonly seen after an anoxic injury).

DIFFERENTIAL DIAGNOSIS

A. Seizure.

B. Hypoglycemia.

EVALUATION AND MANAGEMENT PLAN

A. Hypothermia (see Chapter 7).

B. Supportive care.

1. Ventilatory support.

2. Seizure management: Continuous EEG monitoring for the duration of hypothermia as well as postrewarming period is encouraged.

a. It allows monitoring of not only seizures but the patient's background rhythms.

3. Monitoring of basic labs and evidence of nosocomial infection.

4. Monitoring for evidence of end-organ damage.

C. Family counseling.

1. Inform families of the studies that are performed, including the timeline of these studies; this helps set expectations.

2. Review the results and provide the likelihood of a meaningful recovery versus the possibility of long-term placement.

FOLLOW-UP

A. Case management consultation: Necessary for placement options (long-term facility vs. hospice care).

CONSULTATION/REFERRAL

A. Prompt consultation with a neurologist.

B. Potential consultation with palliative care.

SPECIAL/GERIATRIC CONSIDERATIONS

A. Poor neuroprognostication increases with age of patient and time sustained in a coma.

CASE SCENARIO: UNRESPONSIVENESS AFTER CARDIAC ARREST

A 28-year-old man presents to the ED as an out-of-hospital cardiac arrest. When the emergency medical service (EMS) arrived to the scene, he had pulses but was hypoxic with agonal breathing. Shortly after, he went into pulseless electrical activity (PEA) arrest and required 30 minutes of CPR before return of spontaneous circulation (ROSC) was achieved. He was intubated without need for paralytic. When he arrived to the ED, he was hypotensive to 80/50 and hypothermic to 93.2°F/34°C. He had nonreactive pupils, 4 mm bilaterally, and no corneal, gag, or cough reflex. He extended in the bilateral upper extremities and had triple flexion of the bilateral lower extremities to noxious stimulus. Labs were notable for a lactate of 10.5 and white blood cell (WBC) of 14; his platelets and international normalized ratio (INR) were within normal limits. Urine drug screen was positive for opioids and cocaine. CT of the head was performed and was read as normal. When being transferred back to the room, he developed sudden jerking movements of his arms and legs, which continued until he was given 4 mg of Ativan. He was then transferred to the neurocritical care unit.

1. What would be the next appropriate step?

A. Order continuous EEG.

B. Load with Keppra.

C. Order MRI of the brain with and without contrast.

D. Initiate targeted temperature management.

BIBLIOGRAPHY

Heinz, U., & Rollnik, J. (2015). Outcome and prognosis of hypoxic brain damage patients undergoing neurological early rehabilitation. *BMC Research Notes, 8*, 243. https://doi.org/10.1186/s13104-015-1175-z

Romergyrko, G., Koenig, M., Jia, X., Stevens, R., & Peberdy, M. (2008). Management of brain injury after resuscitation from cardiac arrest. *Neurologic Clinics, 26*(2), 487–506. https://doi.org/10.1016/j.ncl.2008.03.015

Weinhouse, G., & Young, B. (2015). *Hypoxic-ischemic brain injury in adults: Evaluation and prognosis.* In J. L. Wilterdink (Ed.), *UptoDate* https://www.uptodate.com/contents/hypoxic-ischemic-brain-injury-in-adults-evaluation-and-prognosis

BRAIN DEATH

DEFINITION

A. Irreversible loss of all functions of the brain, including loss of brainstem functions.

  1. U.S. law associates brain death with cardiopulmonary death, but specific criteria are not mandatory.

  2. Some states, such as New Jersey, have very specific diagnostic mandates.

    a. Most clinicians rely on guidelines to help guide decision-making.

B. Three key findings that suggest brain death and must be examined.

  1. Coma.

  2. Absence of brainstem reflexes.

  3. Apnea.

C. Once brain death criteria have been established and irreversible loss of brain function is confirmed, patients can be declared brain dead and therefore legally deceased.

INCIDENCE

A. Brain death is declared in approximately 2.3% to 7.5% of all deaths annually.

PATHOGENESIS

A. Causes: Devastating, identifiable, and irreversible neurologic injuries.

B. Main processes resulting in brain death: Mass cerebral edema and downward herniation.

PHYSICAL EXAMINATION (NEUROLOGICAL ASSESSMENT)

A. Prerequisites to clinical examination (note that these could vary by institution; it is important to be familiar with institution guidelines).

  1. Clear clinical or radiographic evidence of widespread brain injury that is compatible with a diagnosis of brain death.

  2. Core body temperature greater than or equal to 36°C or 96.8°F.

  3. Rule out the use of any drug or intoxication that could cause central nervous system (CNS) depression. This must be done through history taking with family and friends, clinical and laboratory testing, and drug screening.

  4. Absence of severe metabolic disturbances as identified by clinical and laboratory data (e.g., severe electrolyte, endocrine, or acid–base abnormalities).

  5. Systolic blood pressure (BP) greater than 100 mmHg.

  6. Identification of an examiner. This can vary according to state and national laws. The examiner should be confident in their understanding of the criteria and comfortable performing all aspects of the examination.

B. Clinical examination. All of the following factors must be checked and confirmed to be absent to determine brain death:

  1. Level of consciousness/mental status.

    a. The patient must be in a nonmedically induced coma.

  2. Motor examination.

    a. The patient must have an absence of brain-originating responses to noxious stimuli.

    b. It is not uncommon to witness spinal-mediated reflexive movements, which are not to be confused with purposeful movements. Examples of spinal-mediated movements include rhythmic facial nerve-innervated muscles, finger flexor movements, "Lazarus sign," triple flexion, positive Babinski sign, or fasciculations of trunk and extremities.

  3. Cranial nerve assessment: Brainstem reflex testing.

    a. Pupillary response: Absent. Pupils are dilated and fixed in a neutral position.

    b. Ocular movement: Absence of vestibulo-ocular reflex bilaterally.

      i. Cold caloric testing: Inject ice cold water into the ear canal and then watch for 2 minutes to ensure there are no eye movements.

    c. Blink response: Absence of corneal reflex bilaterally.

    d. Gag response: Absence of gag reflex bilaterally.

    e. Cough response: Absence of cough reflex with tracheal suctioning.

    f. Respiratory function: Confirmation of apnea.

DIAGNOSTIC TESTS

A. Apnea test.

  1. Prerequisites.

    a. Clinical examination has been performed as described earlier and the findings are consistent with brain death.

    b. Patient has been preoxygenated for 10 minutes and then an arterial blood gas (ABG) is performed.

      i. A partial pressure of oxygen (PaO_2) greater than 200 mmHg and a partial pressure of carbon dioxide ($PaCO_2$) between 35 and 45 mmHg must be present.

    c. Any prior evidence of carbon dioxide (CO_2) retention must be ruled out (e.g., patients with chronic obstructive pulmonary disease [COPD] or severe obesity).

      i. If a patient does have retention, an apnea test cannot be safely and accurately performed and thus a confirmatory ancillary test must be considered.

  2. Actual testing.

    a. Ensure that a physician, respiratory therapist, and nurse are present for the entirety of this test. Testing can range from 8 minutes up to 12 minutes, depending on the stability of the patient during testing. Disconnect the patient from the ventilator ▶

and provide oxygen via a nasal cannula at 6 L/min into the endotracheal tube at the level of the carina.

    i. Alternatively, use a T-piece system with oxygen flow at 12 L/min and use continuous positive airway pressure (CPAP) 10 to 20 cm H_2O, with oxygen flow at 12 L/min.

    ii. Observe respiratory movements.

    iii. Ensure that all clothing is removed and the patient's chest is completely exposed.

    iv. If any respiratory movements are present, place the patient back on the ventilator and abort the test.

b. After the 8- to 12-minute test is performed, draw another ABG sample and result immediately, then place the patient back on the ventilator. Be sure not to place the patient on the ventilator before drawing the ABG.

    i. If the $PaCO_2$ is greater than or equal to 60 mmHg or greater than or equal to 20 mmHg above the baseline, then the test is confirmatory.

3. Complications during apnea testing.

a. Evidence of respiratory insufficiency defined as blood-oxygen saturation (SaO_2)<90% or hemodynamic instability defined as systolic BP <90 mmHg occurs necessitates obtaining an ABG and placing the patient back on the ventilator.

b. If the earlier criteria of $PaCO_2$ >60 mmHg or ≥20 mmHg above baseline are met prior to the 8-minute minimum, the test remains confirmatory.

c. If the patient remains hemodynamically stable and maintains adequate saturations but the test is inconclusive, the test may be repeated for a longer period (10–15 minutes).

d. If the patient does not meet the criteria for confirmatory apnea, ancillary testing may be required.

4. Observation period.

a. Observing for adults is considered optional.

b. Six hours is often recommended, with longer periods, up to 24 hours, recommended in cases of hypoxic ischemic encephalopathy.

c. The 2010 American Academy of Neurology guidelines found insufficient evidence to determine a minimally acceptable observation period.

B. Ancillary testing.

  1. Indications: Limitations to performing the clinical examination or apnea testing. Reasons for considering ancillary testing include:

a. Presence of factors that may affect accurate testing of cranial nerve functions (e.g., preexisting pupillary abnormalities, facial trauma, perforated tympanic membrane, high spinal cord injury).

b. Inability to perform clinical examination or apnea testing.

c. Inability to perform apnea testing due to preexisting CO_2 retention diagnosis.

d. Presence of heavy sedation or neuromuscular paralysis.

2. Specific tests.

a. Cerebral angiography: "Gold Standard" for ancillary testing. A positive study reflects the absence of cerebral perfusion at or beyond the carotid bifurcation or circle of Willis and demonstrates that the external carotid system has blood flow. However, this is invasive, high risk, and requires transportation to the radiology department with an unstable patient. It also carries the risk of false positives when the cranial vault is breached by trauma, surgery, or ventricular drains.

b. Cerebral perfusion study (cerebral scintigraphy or nuclear medicine perfusion test): This method closely resembles cerebral angiography. A positive finding consistent with no cerebral perfusion is the "hollow skull" appearance.

c. Transcranial ultrasound or transcranial Doppler: This method is safe, noninvasive, and inexpensive. However, this method is reliable only if there is a good quality signal and requires expertise in testing both anterior and posterior circulations. Abnormal findings include reverberating flow or small early systolic peaks without diastolic flow.

d. Electroencephalogram: Testing should be performed for at least 30 minutes. This testing must demonstrate no electrical activity and no reactivity to visual, auditory, or sensory stimuli. Testing results can be skewed, especially in the ICU setting; outside activity can be mistaken for cortical activity. Also, the EEG may be flat or isoelectric but cannot evaluate a brainstem that may have viable neurons.

e. Somatosensory evoked potential (SSEPs): In SSEPs, when the median nerve is stimulated and the response is bilateral absence of the parietal sensory cortex, brain death is indicated.

DIFFERENTIAL DIAGNOSIS

A. Various scenarios have been studied and closely resemble brain death. Conditions that therefore must be ruled out include:

  1. Metabolic encephalopathy.

  2. Drug intoxications.

  3. Neuromuscular paralysis.

  4. Guillain–Barré syndrome.

  5. Locked-in syndrome.

  6. Hypothermia.

EVALUATION AND MANAGEMENT PLAN

A. Prognosis and pronouncement of death.

  1. There are no published reports of neurologic recovery after a diagnosis of brain death.

  2. Once brain death criteria are met and brain death has been determined, the person is legally dead and the time of death is given. An attending physician must pronounce a person deceased.

a. Sometimes, there are family objections and delays in discontinuation of life support. These delays can be mitigated through unbiased, ▶

compassionate, family-centered education and engaging the family in medical decisions from admission. As the provider, it is important to show patience, transparency, and consistency in diagnoses and prognoses.

b. Once an unsurvivable prognosis is confirmed, it is an appropriate time to introduce the organ procurement team.

B. Organ procurement.

 1. Each state has an organization that offers its services to hospitals and patients' families to discuss the opportunity for organ donation. This is most often an outlet for families to help cope in a devastating situation.

 2. If a family does decide to donate organs, it may be necessary to treat certain medical problems to preserve the patient's organs. Diabetes insipidus and pulmonary hypertension are two complications that develop early in patients who are diagnosed with brain death and are important to consider.

 3. There are two types of organ donations after death.

   a. Donation after cardiac death.

   i. If the person does not satisfy brain death criteria but does not have a meaningful recovery of life and the family decides to withdraw care but wants to proceed with donation.

   ii. The patient is extubated in the operating room and prepped for surgery, with transplant teams standing by. If the patient dies by cardiac death, they are reintubated and surgery is performed immediately for organ procurement. If the patient does not die within 60 minutes, surgery for donation legally cannot proceed and therefore the patient is made comfortable and allowed to die in a private room.

   b. Donation after brain death.

   i. The patient has already been determined to be brain dead and given a time of death. They can then be taken to the operating room for organ procurement once all arrangements have been made.

CASE SCENARIO: BRAIN DEATH

A 28-year-old man presents to the ED as an out-of-hospital cardiac arrest. When the emergency medical service (EMS) arrived at the scene, he had pulses but was hypoxic with agonal breathing. Shortly after, he went into pulseless electrical activity (PEA) arrest and required 30 minutes of CPR before return of spontaneous circulation (ROSC) was achieved. He was intubated without a need for paralytics. When he arrived at the ED, he was hypotensive to 80/50 and hypothermic to 93.2°F/34°C. He had nonreactive pupils, 4 mm bilaterally, and no corneal, gag, or cough reflex. He extended in the bilateral upper extremities and had triple flexion of the bilateral lower extremities to noxious stimulus. Labs were notable for a lactate of 10.5 and white blood cells (WBC) of 14; his platelets and international normalized ratio (INR) were within normal limits. Urine drug screen was positive for opioids and cocaine. CT of the head was performed and was read as

normal. When being transferred back to the room, he developed sudden jerking movements of his arms and legs, which continued until he was given 4 mg of Ativan. He was then transferred to the neurocritical care unit. The patient was subsequently loaded with levetiracetam 60 mg/kg, which improved but did not completely resolve the clinical seizure activity manifesting as jerking movements in all of his extremities. The patient has been in the neurocritical care unit for 5 days and maximal medical management has been utilized, including a high-dose midazolam and ketamine drip with no improvement in clinical exam. EEG shows that all clinical and electrographic seizures have been suppressed. The neurointensivist covering the unit weaned both midazolam and ketamine drip overnight and attempted a clinical brain death exam in the morning; the result was inconclusive.

 1. What would be the next appropriate step?
   A. Order additional antiepileptics as the patient remains at high risk for status epilepticus.
   B. Order ancillary brain death testing.
   C. Order MRI of the brain without contrast.
   D. Repeat the clinical brain death exam.

BIBLIOGRAPHY

Baker, A., Beed, S., Fenwick, J., Kjerulf, M., Bell, H., Logier, S., & Shepherd, J. (2006). Number of deaths by neurological criteria, and organ and tissue donation rates at three critical care centres in Canada. *Canadian Journal of Anesthesia, 53*(7), 722–726. https://doi.org/10.1007/BF03021632

Burkle, C. M., Schipper, A. M., & Wijdicks, E. F. (2011). Brain death and the courts. *Neurology, 76,* 837–841. https://doi.org/10.1212/WNL.0b013e31820e7bbe

Gardiner, D., Shemie, S., Manara, A., & Opdam, H. (2012). International perspective on the diagnosis of death. *British Journal of Anaesthesia, 108*(Suppl. 1), i14–i28. https://doi.org/10.1093/bja/aer397

Hocker, S., Whalen, F., & Wijdicks, E. F. (2014). Apnea testing for brain death in severe acute respiratory distress syndrome: A possible solution. *Neurocritical Care, 20,* 298–300. https://doi.org/10.1007/s12028-013-9932-0

The Quality Standards Subcommittee of the American Academy of Neurology. (1995). Practice parameters for determining brain death in adults (summary statement). *Neurology, 45,* 1012–1014.

Wijdicks, E. F., Varelas, P. N., Gronseth, G. S., & Greer, D. M. (2010). Evidence-based guideline update: Determining brain death in adults. Report of the Quality Standards Subcommittee of the American Academy of Neurology. *Neurology, 74,* 1911–1918. https://doi.org/10.1212/WNL.0b013e3181e242a8

HEADACHES

DEFINITION

A. Diffuse pain in some part of the head or pain located above the orbitomeatal line of the head.

B. The International Headache Society divides headaches into primary and secondary headaches.

 1. Primary: Benign headaches without any abnormal pathology. More than 90% of headaches are primary. Four types are recognized (for detailed classification, visit ichd-3.org):

   a. Migraine: Characterized by attacks of moderate to severe throbbing headaches that are often unilateral in location, worsened by physical activity, and associated with nausea and/or vomiting, photophobia, and phonophobia. Migraine headaches may last from 4 to 72 hours.

i. Classic migraine: Migraine with aura; the aura usually only lasts up to 60 minutes.

ii. Common migraine: Migraine without aura.

iii. Status migrainosus: Migraine lasting more than 3 days.

b. Tension-type headache (TTH): Most common form of headache that can last from 30 minutes to 7 days. Characterized by bilateral mild to moderate nonthrobbing pressure such as pain, without associated symptoms. Mostly described as a tight band around the head.

c. Trigeminal autonomic cephalalgias (TACs): Less common. Characterized by unilateral headache, and usually prominent cranial parasympathetic autonomic features (such as eyelid edema, nasal congestions, and lacrimation), which are lateralized and unilateral to the headache.

i. Examples include cluster headache, paroxysmal hemicrania, short-lasting unilateral neuralgiform headache attacks with conjunctival injection and tearing (SUNCT) or with cranial autonomic symptoms (SUNA), and hemicrania continua.

d. Other primary headaches.

2. Secondary: Malignant headaches caused by structural lesion or organic pathology. Less than 10% of headaches are secondary.

a. Examples include headaches due to brain tumor, meningitis, substance withdrawal, and intracerebral hemorrhage (ICH).

b. Neuropathies and facial pain.

INCIDENCE

A. Many headache sufferers do not seek medical attention.

B. An estimated 23 million Americans and 240 million people worldwide have migraine headaches each year.

C. Migraine headaches occur in a 3:1 female to male ratio.

D. Episodic TTHs are present in about 46% of the U.S. population.

E. Chronic TTHs are present in approximately 2% of the U.S. population.

PATHOGENESIS

A. The exact mechanism involved in the development of primary headaches is unknown.

B. Headaches usually result from vasodilation/constriction of blood vessels.

C. Migraine headaches are thought to result from activation of meningeal and blood vessel nociceptors, combined with a change in central pain modulation.

D. Activation of the trigeminal system results in release of neuropeptides, which in turn causes neurogenic inflammation and increase in vascular permeability and local dilation of blood vessels, causing pain and associated symptoms via the trigeminal pathway.

E. Decrease in levels of serotonin (5-hydroxytryptamine [5-HT]) has shown to induce migraine.

PREDISPOSING FACTORS

A. Foods containing tyramine (aged cheeses, pickled foods), nitrites (cured meats), monosodium glutamate, or sulfites.

B. Alcoholic beverages, especially red wine and beer.

C. Emotional factors such as stress, anxiety, and depression.

D. Hormonal fluctuations.

E. Decreased sleep or sleep deprivation.

F. Medications: Estrogen, nitroglycerine, or ranitidine.

G. Physical fatigue.

H. Environmental: Weather, odors, sound, bright lights, and barometric changes.

SUBJECTIVE DATA

A. Common complaints/symptoms (red flag symptoms).

1. Every headache evaluation should begin with a search for certain signs and symptoms. The presence of any of these "red flag" symptoms warrants an urgent extensive workup.

2. Systemic symptoms (fever, weight loss) or secondary risk factors (HIV, systemic cancer).

3. Neurologic symptoms or abnormal signs (impaired alertness or consciousness, confusion, weakness, visual loss).

4. Onset: Sudden, abrupt, or split-second.

5. Increased age: New-onset and progressive headache, especially in middle age (>50 years [giant cell arteritis]).

6. Headache history: First headache or different headache (marked change in attack, frequency, severity, or clinical features).

B. Diagnostic criteria.

1. The gold standard for diagnosis of headache is a detailed interview and clinical examination.

2. Headache onset (age, sudden or gradual onset, factors associated with onset such as exercise, sexual activity, Valsalva maneuver, febrile illness).

3. Location of pain: Unilateral, bilateral, or global.

4. Duration (see "Definition" for details).

5. Frequency.

6. Quality: Throbbing, squeezing, band-like, or stabbing.

7. Severity (at onset, at peak, and duration from onset to peak).

8. Associated symptoms such as nausea, vomiting, blurred vision, nasal congestion, mood swings, and so forth.

9. Presence or absence of an aura: Visual scotomas, flashing lights, or facial numbness.

10. Aggravating and relieving factors: Body position or darkness.

C. History.

1. Medication history: Contraceptives, hormonal therapy, vitamins, herbals, and painkillers.

2. General medical history.

3. Family history of headaches.

PHYSICAL EXAMINATION

A. Perform a complete general examination with focus on the head and neck and a full neurologic examination. Generally, these are normal, with no neurologic deficits in primary headaches. A focal neurologic deficit with acute headache predicts central nervous system (CNS) pathology.

B. Observe the body habitus. Patients with pseudo-tumor cerebri tend to be obese.

C. Perform a funduscopic examination to rule out papilledema as in idiopathic intracranial hypertension or diseases with increased intracranial pressure (ICP).

D. Auscultate the skull and orbits for bruits as heard in arteriovenous malformation and fistulas.

E. Palpate and tap the sinus for tenderness in sinus inflammation.

F. Arteries may be tender and harder to palpation in temporal arteritis.

G. Palpate both temporomandibular joints for tenderness and crepitus while the patient opens and closes the jaw.

DIAGNOSTIC TESTS

A. The diagnosis of primary headache is usually made on the basis of headache history, physical examination, and neurologic examination. No specific diagnostic tests are available.

B. The diagnosis of secondary headache involves the following:

1. Complete blood count (CBC), chemistry panel, urinalysis, liver function test, and thyroid profile.

2. Sedimentation rate and C-reactive protein: Elevated in temporal arteritis.

3. Neurologic imaging, which should be considered in patients with any of the following findings:

   a. Thunderclap headache/worst headache of life.
   b. Altered mental status.
   c. Meningismus.
   d. Papilledema.
   e. Acute neurologic deficit.
   f. New-onset headache after age 50.
   g. History of cancer or HIV or immunocompromised state.

4. CT of the head: Best to rule out acute injury and bleed.

5. CT of the paranasal sinuses: To rule out sinusitis.

6. MRI of the brain (more sensitive than CT): Useful to rule out space-occupying lesions, demyelinating lesions, ischemia, and abscess.

7. Magnetic resonance angiography (MRA): Helpful in identifying vascular abnormalities such as aneurysms and arteriovenous malformation.

8. Lumbar puncture: Useful in diagnosing infections, malignancy and subarachnoid hemorrhage, and idiopathic intracranial hypertension.

9. Tonometry: If symptoms suggest acute narrow angle glaucoma (visual halos, corneal edema, shallow anterior chamber).

DIFFERENTIAL DIAGNOSIS

A. Brain tumor.
B. Brain hemorrhage.
C. Seizure.
D. Meningitis.
E. Dissection.
F. Cerebral aneurysm.

EVALUATION AND MANAGEMENT PLAN

A. Migraine headache.

   1. General interventions.
      a. Lifestyle modifications and trigger prevention should be emphasized.
      b. Analgesics such as aspirin, acetaminophen, ibuprofen, and naproxen can be used in mild headaches. Opioids are generally avoided in primary headaches.

   2. Acute migraine: Abortive treatment in inpatient or ED setting.
      a. Nonsteroidal anti-inflammatory drugs (NSAIDs) and corticosteroids: Caution necessary in patients with hepatic or renal impairment, diabetes, or gastritis. One of the following drugs can be used:
         i. Ketorolac 30 mg intravenous (IV).
         ii. Methylprednisolone 100 to 200 mg.
         iii. Dexamethasone 10 to 40 mg.
      b. Neuroleptics: Can be used alone and as pretreatment to ergot derivatives to offset nausea.
         i. Diphenhydramine 25 to 50 mg, lorazepam 0.5 to 1 mg, and/or benztropine 1 mg are often given before neuroleptic to prevent akathisia.
         ii. EKG: Check and avoid neuroleptics if QTc is prolonged.
      c. Antinausea medications can be used to alleviate the sense of nausea, but are also effective in controlling migraines in select patients.
         i. Metoclopramide 10 to 20 mg IV.
         ii. Prochlorperazine 10 to 20 mg IV or intramuscular (IM).
         iii. Droperidol 0.625 to 2.5 mg IV or IM.
         iv. Chlorpromazine 12.5 to 100 mg PO or IV (up to 50 mg only).
      d. Dihydroergotamine 0.5 to 1 mg IV push: Migraine-specific but also helpful in cluster headache. This drug must not be administered if a triptan has been taken in the preceding 24 hours, and it is contraindicated in patients with a history of, or at high risk for, myocardial infarction (MI), or stroke.
      e. Anticonvulsants: Can be useful; given as rapid infusions (over 10–20 minutes).
         i. Valproic acid: 500 to 1,000 mg; can also be useful for cluster headache.
         ii. Levetiracetam: 1,000 to 2,000 mg; maximum recommended dose is 3,000 mg/d.
      f. Magnesium sulfate: 1 to 2 g IV piggyback.
      g. Serotonin (5-HT) receptor agonists: Sumatriptan 6 mg subcutaneous (SC) or 10 mg intranasal.

   3. Migraine prophylaxis: Used when attacks exceed two per month or when acute attacks are refractory. One of the following drugs can be used:

a. Beta-adrenergic blockers: Propranolol is the drug of choice.

b. Tricyclic antidepressants (TCAs): Amitriptyline 25 to 125 mg PO nightly.

c. Serotonin antagonists: Methysergide 1 to 2 mg PO TID.

d. Calcium channel antagonist: Verapamil 40 to 80 mg TID.

e. Anticonvulsant: Valproic acid total 250 mg BID or TID.

B. TTH.

1. Usual abortive treatment can be any simple analgesic.

2. Drug of choice for prophylaxis is amitriptyline 50 to 150 mg/d.

3. Concurrent depression or anxiety disorder needs to be addressed if present.

C. TACs.

1. Abortive treatment.

a. Inhalation of 100% of oxygen for 10 to 15 minutes.

b. Sumatriptan 6 mg SC.

c. Dihydroergotamine IV.

2. Preventive therapy with one of the following:

a. Verapamil is the drug of choice: 80 mg TID; maximum dose is 360 mg/d.

b. Lithium 600 to 1,200 mg/d; monitor lithium levels.

c. Topiramate 100 to 400 mg/d.

d. Gabapentin 1,200 to 3,600 mg/d.

e. Lamotrigine 100 to 300 mg/d (drug of choice for SUNCT).

f. Indomethacin 75 to 150 mg/d (drug of choice for paroxysmal hemicrania).

D. Nonpharmacologic treatment for all types of headaches.

1. Interventions such as acupuncture, biofeedback, nerve block, neurotoxin injections, neurostimulators, and behavioral and psychological therapies are found to be effective in managing headaches.

FOLLOW-UP

A. Patients can follow up with primary providers if headaches are infrequent.

B. Follow up with a headache specialist for more complicated or refractory cases or treatment of persistent headaches.

CONSULTATION/REFERRAL

A. Refer to a headache specialist if there is concern for an underlying pathology of the headaches or if there are any unusual features or symptoms associated with the headaches.

B. Also consider referring patients who are refractory to conventional treatment.

SPECIAL/GERIATRIC CONSIDERATIONS

A. New onset of severe headache in pregnancy or postpartum period should be investigated to rule out cortical sinus thrombosis. MRI is considered safe during pregnancy.

B. Treatment of headache in pregnancy should be coordinated with an obstetrician.

C. Metoclopramide and prochlorperazine are generally considered safe in pregnancy.

D. Ergotamines are absolutely contraindicated in pregnancy.

CASE SCENARIO: FOUR DAYS OF HEADACHE

A 25-year-old woman with a history of migraines presents to the ED with migraine symptoms that have been persistent over the past 4 days. She has one to two migraines monthly, with symptom resolution usually within 2 hours of medication; however, her current headache has failed to respond to sumatriptan which she last took 2 days ago. She takes propranolol as a preventive medication for her migraines but has missed multiple doses due to constant nausea and vomiting. She has been unable to go to work and spends most of her day in bed, in the dark. On exam, the patient's vital signs show heart rate (HR) of 110, blood pressure (BP) of 110/70, and saturation 99% on room air, and she is afebrile. She has sensitivity to light. Her mucous membranes are dry. No papilledema is detected. Neurologic exam is nonfocal. Her labs are notable for a sodium of 132 and creatinine of 1.4. CT of the head is normal.

1. What would be the next appropriate step?

A. Administer single doses of ketorolac and diphenhydramine and discharge to home.

B. Admit to the hospital for intravenous (IV) antiemetics, dihydroergotamine, and steroids.

C. Perform a lumbar puncture.

D. Deliver 100% oxygen for 10 to 15 minutes.

BIBLIOGRAPHY

American Association of Neuroscience Nurses. (2004). Headaches. In M. Bader & L. Littlejohns (Eds.), *AANN core curriculum for neuroscience nursing* (4th ed., Vol. 1, pp. 836–849). Saunders.

Hainer, B., & Matheson, E. (2013). Approach to acute headache in adults. *American Family Physician*, 87(10), 682–687. https://www.aafp.org/afp/2013/0515/p682.html

Hickey, J. (2003). Headaches. In J. Hickey (Ed.), *The clinical practice of neurological and neurosurgical nursing* (5th ed., pp. 603–615). Lippincott Williams.

International Headache Society. (n.d.). IHS headache classification. https://ichd-3.org

Singh, G., Gupta, P., Gupta, A., & Khanal, M. (2011). Clinical approach to a patient with headache. In *Neurology* (Vol. 1, pp. 514–517). Elsevier.

Young, W., Silberstein, S., Nahas, S., & Marmura, M. (2011). *Jefferson headache manual*. Demos Medical.

INTRACEREBRAL HEMORRHAGE

DEFINITION

A. A pathologic accumulation of blood within the parenchyma of the brain.

B. Often confused with intracranial hemorrhage, an umbrella term that encompasses subdural hematoma, epidural hematoma, and subarachnoid hemorrhage, as well as intracerebral hemorrhage (ICH).

INCIDENCE

A. ICH affects 12 to 15 people per 100,000. Incidence increases with age, doubling every 10 years after age 35.

B. Incidence is increased in populations with high prevalence of hypertension, secondary to environmental and genetic factors.

PATHOGENESIS

A. Small vessel vasculopathy, resulting from hypertensive damage to intracranial blood vessels due to chronic or acute hypertension or substance use.

B. Autoregulatory dysfunction, resulting from excessive cerebral blood flow (CBF) after either reperfusion, or hemorrhagic transformation of ischemic strokes.

C. Vascular malformations, resulting from aneurysm rupture or hemorrhage of an arteriovenous malformation.

D. Coagulopathy, resulting from anticoagulation, thrombolysis, and hepatic or bleeding disorder.

E. Hemorrhagic necrosis, of a tumor or infection.

F. Venous outflow obstruction, resulting from cerebral venous thrombosis.

G. Trauma.

H. Cerebral amyloid angiopathy (CAA).

PREDISPOSING FACTORS

A. Modifiable risk factors: Hypertension, cocaine/stimulant use, low cholesterol levels, oral anticoagulants, and excessive alcohol intake.

B. Nonmodifiable risk factors: Age, male sex, African American or Japanese ethnicity, and CAA.

SUBJECTIVE DATA

A. Common complaints/symptoms.
   1. Headache, nausea, vomiting, and seizures.
   2. Decreased score on the Glasgow Coma Scale (GCS).
   3. Focal neurologic signs (such as speech abnormality, facial weakness, cranial nerve palsy, or unilateral limb weakness) can present to varying degrees of severity depending on the location and size of hemorrhage.
   4. Frequency of clinical seizures with ICH is 16%, with the majority occurring at onset.

B. Common/typical scenario.
   1. Severe headache with or without vomiting prompts the patient to go to the hospital, or the patient has a change in mental status and emergency personnel are called to the scene. Typically, bystanders will report nothing unusual has occurred until the moment of the intracranial injury.

C. Family and social history.
   1. Ask about smoking and alcohol use.
   2. Drug use can be associated with ICH in younger patients.
   3. Family history of stroke.

D. Review of systems.
   1. Neurologic: Ask about headache, any weakness, or difficulty speaking.
   2. Cardiac: Ask about history of high blood pressure (BP), irregular heart rate (HR), and if the patient is taking any antiplatelets or anticoagulants.

PHYSICAL EXAMINATION

A. Neurologic: Perform full neurologic examination.
   1. Determine level of consciousness.
   2. Assess language for difficulty understanding speech (receptive) or speaking (expressive).
   3. Assess cranial nerves for deficits, in particular extraocular movements and facial nerves.
   4. Motor assessment: Note any weakness of the limbs.
   5. Sensory assessment: Note any decrease in or lack of sensation on a limb.
   6. Check for symptoms that may provide clue to the location of the hemorrhage.
      a. Basal ganglia/thalamus location: Hemisensory loss, hemiplegia, aphasia, homonymous hemianopsia, eye deviation away from lesion, or upgaze palsy.
      b. Lobar location: Seizures, homonymous hemianopsia, plegia, or paresis of the leg greater than the arm.
      c. Cerebellar location: Ataxia, nystagmus, intractable vomiting, and/or symptoms related to obstructive hydrocephalus (drowsiness, leg weakness, impaired upgaze, blurred, or double vision).
      d. Pons location: Pinpoint pupils, quadriparesis, coma, or locked-in syndrome.

DIAGNOSTIC TESTS

A. Noncontrast head CT: Should be obtained immediately and then 6 hours after admission (Figure 6.1) to assess for hemorrhage expansion.

B. Obtain a stat noncontrast head CT with any neurologic examination change.
   1. Fluid levels seen within hemorrhage on CT scan indicate a coagulopathy (slow oozing of blood over time as seen by different intensities of blood on CT scan).
   2. Hemorrhage volume calculation: ABC/2 (or ABC/3 for hemorrhages secondary to warfarin).
      a. A (diameter in centimeters on CT slice where hemorrhage is largest) ×
      b. B (largest diameter in centimeters 90 degrees to A) ×
      c. C (number of CT slices × slice thickness in centimeters)/2
      d. For example: For a hemorrhage that is 10 mm by 20 mm and extends across 10 slices on a 5-mm thick slice, the volume would be (1 cm × 2 cm × 10 × 0.5)/2 = 5 cm^3.
         i. Most CT images are reconstructed with a 5- or 10-mm thickness.

C. CT angiogram (CTA) of the head and neck: May be helpful to rule out subarachnoid hemorrhage, arteriovenous/cavernous malformation, and brain tumor.

D. MRI of the brain with and without contrast: Should be obtained 4 to 6 weeks post hemorrhage to evaluate for underlying mass if the etiology remains unclear.

DIFFERENTIAL DIAGNOSIS

A. Clinical suspicion is warranted when there is a rapid alteration in neurologic status often in conjunction with signs of an elevation in intracranial pressure (ICP).

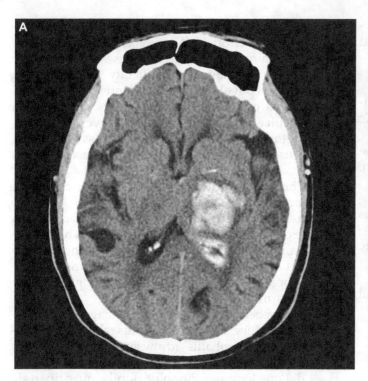
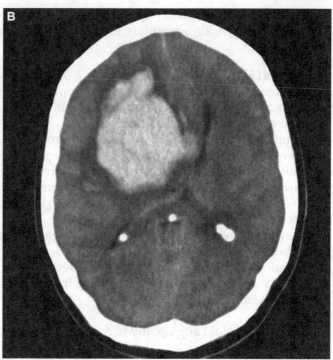

FIGURE 6.1   Head CT scans showing **(A)** basal ganglia hemorrhage due to hypertension and **(B)** right frontal hemorrhage due to amyloid angiopathy.

B. Increased ICP may be evidenced by change in level of consciousness, nausea, vomiting, or headache.

C. The type of neurologic dysfunction brought about by ICH may indicate the location, etiology, and severity of the hemorrhage.

D. Conditions to rule out include arteriovenous malformations, severe hemiplegic migraines, seizures, cerebral aneurysms, and tumors.

EVALUATION AND MANAGEMENT PLAN

A. General plan.

  1. Determine the location of the hemorrhage; this is essential in order to identify risk factors and engage in secondary prevention.

    a. Hypertensive hemorrhages tend to occur most often in the basal ganglia/thalamus, followed by lobar, then cerebellum and then pons.

    b. Amyloid hemorrhages are most common in lobar locations.

    c. Hemorrhages secondary to vascular malformations, tumors, and coagulopathies can occur in any part of the brain.

  2. Medical management.

    a. BP.

      i. Hypertension is associated with hematoma expansion, neurologic deterioration, dependency, and death. Achieving BP control is essential.

        1) Antihypertensive treatment of acute cerebral hemorrhage (ATACH) and intensive BP reduction in acute cerebral hemorrhage (INTERACT) found reduction of systolic BP less than 140 mmHg to be safe and beneficial in improving functional outcomes, if the initial systolic BP is <220 mmHg.

        2) Arterial line and peripheral intravenous (IV) lines should be placed for close monitoring and tight control of BP.

        3) Continuous infusions should be used to maintain BP parameters.

          a) Nicardipine, start 5 mg/hr (max 15 mg/hr).

          b) Clevidipine, start 1 to 2 mg/hr (max 21 mg/hr).

          c) Labetalol, 1 to 2 mg/min (max 2 mg/min).

    b. Coagulopathies.

      i. Any coagulopathies should be addressed and reversed immediately if prudent.

    c. Seizures.

      i. Clinical seizures should be treated with IV antiepileptics.

      ii. Continuous EEG monitoring is necessary for patients with depressed mental status out of proportion to injury.

      iii. Prophylactic antiepileptic medication is not routinely recommended.

    d. ICP.

      i. Monitor ICP with an external ventricular device if the patient has a GCS score of 8 or less and has concomitant hydrocephalus.

    e. Other medical issues.

      i. Hypoglycemia and hyperglycemia should be avoided.

      ii. Normothermia should be maintained; ardently treat fevers.

iii. Deep vein thrombosis (DVT) prophylaxis: After radiographic evidence of hematoma stability is confirmed, SC heparin should be considered in patients with lack of mobility after 1 to 4 days from onset.

3. Surgical management: Surgical management is not warranted in all cases of ICH and is limited in hypertensive hemorrhages to the acutely deteriorating patient as a lifesaving measure. Surgical management is the standard of care in subdural or epidural hematomas, cerebellar ICH, and in patients who have an ICH secondary to a tumor or vascular malformation.

    a. Craniotomy.

      i. This procedure should be considered in patients with a subdural hematoma that is causing midline shift and increased ICP, epidural hematomas, and for removal of tumors associated with ICH.

      ii. Patients with cerebellar ICH who deteriorate neurologically or have brainstem compression and/or hydrocephalus should undergo emergent surgical hematoma evacuation.

    b. Decompressive hemicraniectomy.

      i. This procedure may reduce mortality for comatose patients, those who have large hematomas with significant midline shift, or those with elevated ICP refractory to medical management.

      ii. Decompressive hemicraniectomy is controversial because, although it reduces mortality in comatose patients, morbidity is very profound and outcomes are generally poor, leading to significant impairments of motor, speech, language, and quality of life.

4. Determine prognosis.

    a. Prognosis can be determined using the ICH score.

      i. This simple clinical grading scale (Table 6.1) aids in prognostication at presentation.

      ii. The total score (Table 6.2) represents 30-day mortality risk based on a combination of criteria.

B. Patient/family teaching points.

  1. Depends on the extent of the injury.

    a. If patients are able to participate in their own care, they should be instructed on diet and lifestyle changes, BP control, avoidance of alcohol, and smoking cessation.

    b. If patients are unable to participate in their own care, families need to be given options to care for the patient at home or in a nursing home.

C. Pharmacotherapy.

  1. There are no specific medications for treatment of spontaneous ICH.

    a. Antihypertensive medications to maintain normotension.

    b. Antilipid medications for treatment of atherosclerotic disease.

TABLE 6.1 INTRACEREBRAL HEMORRHAGE SCORE

	Points
Score on Glasgow Coma Scale	
3–4	2
5–12	1
13–15	0
Intracerebral Volume	
≥30 cm^3	1
<30 cm^3	0
Intraventricular Hemorrhage	
Yes	1
No	0
Location	
Infratentorial	1
Supratentorial	0
Age	
≥80 y	1
<80 y	0

Source: From Hemphill, J. C., 3rd, Bonovich, D. C., Besmertis, L., Manley, G. T., & Johnston, S. C. (2001). The ICH score: A simple, reliable grading scale for intracerebral hemorrhage. *Stroke, A Journal of Cerebral Circulation, 32,* 891–897. https://doi.org/10.1161/STR.0000000000000069.

TABLE 6.2 30-DAY MORTALITY RISK FOR SPONTANEOUS INTRACRANIAL HEMORRHAGE

Intracerebral Hemorrhage Score	Mortality (%)
0	0
1	13
2	26
3	72
4	97
5	100
6	100

    c. Patients who need to take antiplatelet medications or need anticoagulation should consult with the neurologist prior to starting.

D. Discharge instructions.

1. If the ICH is small, patients may return home with instructions to slowly return to daily activities.

2. All patients should receive clearance from the neurologist prior to starting antiplatelet or anticoagulation therapy.

FOLLOW-UP

A. Patients should follow up with the neurologist in 6 to 8 weeks from discharge from the hospital or rehabilitation center.

B. Patients who require a nursing home can follow up with specific issues on an as-needed basis.

CONSULTATION/REFERRAL

A. Consult neurology on every ICH patient who comes to the hospital. All patients will require a thorough evaluation of etiology and initiation of secondary prevention.

B. Consult neurosurgery if there is a concern for increased ICP or in patients with a GCS score of less than 13. Patients who have large ICHs should be evaluated for possible surgical intervention.

SPECIAL/GERIATRIC CONSIDERATIONS

A. Older adult patients who present with spontaneous ICH and are diagnosed with amyloid angiopathy are at high risk for hemorrhaging recurrence, up to 30%. There is no known treatment for amyloid angiopathy.

B. Older adult patients with significant volume loss associated with aging or certain disease states, such as dementia or alcoholism, may tolerate larger ICHs with fewer deficits. However, recovery from any lost function in older adults is generally poor.

CASE SCENARIO: INTRAPARENCHYMAL HEMORRHAGE

A 55-year-old man presents to the ED complaining of severe headache, dizziness, and unsteady gait. Upon arrival, his vital signs show a heart rate (HR) of 110, blood pressure (BP) of 167/86, normal respiratory rate, and oxygen saturation (SpO$_2$) of 97%. The patient is afebrile. Exam findings reveal the patient is awake, alert, oriented ×3, follows commands, clear/intact speech, pupils are equal, round and react to light (3 mm, brisk), early-onset malignancies initiative (EOMI), and no facial asymmetry or tongue deviation. Bilateral upper extremity ataxia is present and there is no evidence of weakness or abnormal sensation in all extremities. Labs are within normal limits. Urine drug screen was negative. A noncontrast CT of the head was performed and revealed a moderately sized hyperdensity in the left cerebellar hemisphere.

1. What would be the next appropriate step?

A. Order repeat CT head within 6 hours of admission.

B. Initiate seizure prophylaxis with levetiracetam (Keppra).

C. Initiate strict blood pressure control and start nicardipine drip as needed.

D. Consult neurosurgery for surgical evaluation.

BIBLIOGRAPHY

Anderson, C. S., Heeley, E., Huang, Y., Wang, J., Stapf, C., Delcourt, C., Lindley, R., Robinson, T., Lavados, P., Neal, B., Hata, J., Arima, H., Parsons, M., Li, Y., Wang, J., Heritier, S., Li, Q., Woodward, M., Simes, R. J. … Chalmers, J. (2013). Rapid blood-pressure lowering in patients with acute intracerebral hemorrhage. *The New England Journal of Medicine, 368*, 2355–2365. https://doi.org/10.1056/NEJMoa1214609

Ariesen, M. J., Claus, S. P., Rinkel, G. J., & Algra, A. (2003). Risk factors for intracerebral hemorrhage in the general population: A systematic review. *Stroke, 34*, 2060–2065. https://doi.org/10.1161/01.STR.000008 0678.09344.8D

Arima, H., Huang, Y., Wang, J. G., Heeley, E., Delcourt, C., Parsons, M., & Anderson, C. (2012). Earlier blood pressure-lowering and greater attenuation of hematoma growth in acute intracerebral hemorrhage: INTER ACT pilot phase. *Stroke, 43*, 2236–2238. https://doi.org/10.116 1/STROKEAHA.112.651422

De Herdt, V., Dumont, F., Hénon, H., Derambure, P., Vonck, K., Leys, D., & Cordonnier, C. (2011). Early seizures in intracerebral hemorrhage: Incidence, associated factors, and outcome. *Neurology, 77*, 1794–1800. https://doi.org/10.1212/WNL.0b013e31823648a6

Hemphill, J. C., Bonovich, C. D., 3rd, Besmertis, L., Manley, G. T., & Johnston, S. C. (2001). The ICH score: A simple, reliable grading scale for intracerebral hemorrhage. *Stroke, 32*, 891–897. https://doi.org/10.1161/01.STR.32.4.891

Hemphill, J. C., Greenberg, M. S., 3rd, Anderson, C. S., Becker, K., Bendok, B. R., Cushman, M., & Woo, D. (2015). Guidelines for the management of spontaneous intracerebral hemorrhage: A guideline for healthcare professionals from the American Heart Association/American Stroke Association. *Stroke, 46*, 2032–2060. https://doi.org/10.1161/STR.0000 000000000069

Labovitz, D. L., Halim, A., Boden-Albala, B., Hauser, W. A., & Sacco, R. L. (2005). The incidence of deep and lobar intracerebral hemorrhage in Whites, Blacks, and Hispanics. *Neurology, 65*, 518–522. https://doi.org /10.1212/01.wnl.0000172915.71933.00

Mendelow, A. D., Gregson, B. A., Fernandes, H. M., Murray, G. D., Teasdale, G. M., Hope, D. T., & Barer, D. H. (2005). Early surgery versus initial conservative treatment in patients with spontaneous supratentorial intracerebral haematomas in the International Surgical Trial in Intracerebral Haemorrhage (STICH): A randomised trial. *Lancet, 365*, 387–397. https://doi.org/10.1016/S0140-6736(05)17826-X

Mendelow, A. D., Gregson, B. A., Rowan, E. N., Murray, G. D., Gholkar, A., & Mitchell, P. M. (2013). Early surgery versus initial conservative treatment in patients with spontaneous supratentorial lobar intracerebral haematomas (STICH II): A randomised trial. *Lancet, 382*, 397–408. https://doi.org/10.1016/S0140-6736(13)60986-1

Mould, W. A., Carhuapoma, J. R., Muschelli, J., Lane, K., Morgan, T. C., McBee, N. A., & Hanley, D. F. (2013). Minimally invasive surgery plus recombinant tissue-type plasminogen activator for intracerebral hemorrhage evacuation decreases perihematomal edema. *Stroke, 44*, 627–634. https://doi.org/10.1161/STROKEAHA.111.000411

Naff, N., Williams, M. A., Keyl, P. M., Tuhrim, S., Bullock, M. R., Mayer, S. A., & Hanley, F. D., Jr. (2011). Low-dose recombinant tissue-type plasminogen activator enhances clot resolution in brain hemorrhage: The intraventricular hemorrhage thrombolysis trial. *Stroke, 42*, 3009–3016. https://doi.org/10.1161/STROKEAHA.110.610949

Qureshi, A. I., Palesch, Y. Y., Martin, R., Novitzke, J., Cruz-Flores, S., Ehtisham, A., Ezzeddine, M. A., Goldstein, J. N., Hussein, H. M., Suri, M. F. K., & Tariq, N. (2010). Effect of systolic blood pressure reduction on hematoma expansion, perihematomal edema, and 3-month outcome among patients with intracerebral hemorrhage: Results from the antihypertensive treatment of acute cerebral hemorrhage study. *Archives of Neurology, 67*, 570–576. https://doi.org/10.1001/archneurol.2010.61

Rincon, F., & Mayer, S. A. (2013). The epidemiology of intracerebral hemorrhage in the United States from 1979 to 2008. *Neurocritical Care, 19*, 95–102. https://doi.org/10.1007/s12028-012-9793-y

Stein, M., Misselwitz, B., Hamann, G. F., Scharbrodt, W., Schummer, D. I., & Oertel, M. F. (2012). Intracerebral hemorrhage in the very old: Future demographic trends of an aging population. *Stroke, 43*, 1126–1128. http s://doi.org/10.1161/STROKEAHA.111.644716

van Asch, C. J., Luitse, M. J., Rinkel, G. J., van der Tweel, I., Algra, A., & Klijn, C. J. (2010). Incidence, case fatality, and functional outcome of intracerebral haemorrhage over time, according to age, sex, and ethnic origin: A systematic review and meta-analysis. *The Lancet Neurology, 9*(2), 167–176. https://doi.org/10.1016/S1474-4422(09)70340-0

ISCHEMIC STROKE

DEFINITION
A. A sudden interruption of blood flow to the brain.
B. Classification:
1. Thrombotic strokes: >55%.
2. Embolic strokes: 10% to 30%.
3. Lacunar strokes: 10%.
4. Cryptogenic strokes: 10%.

INCIDENCE
A. Approximately 800,000 strokes occur each year.
1. 610,000 are first-time strokes.
2. 185,000 are recurring strokes.
B. Stroke is the fifth leading cause of death.
C. Stroke is the leading cause of disability. There are approximately seven million stroke survivors in the United States.

PATHOGENESIS
A. Stroke results from decreased cerebral blood flow (CBF) that can be a result of an obstruction (e.g., thrombus or embolus), vasoconstriction, low blood flow states (shock), or anything that deprives oxygen or glucose to the brain.
B. Anaerobic metabolism and lactic acid production compromise the surrounding brain tissue (penumbra), causing ischemia followed by infarction if blood flow is not restored.

PREDISPOSING FACTORS
A. Nonmodifiable.
1. Age greater than 55 years.
2. Sex: Women greater than men.
3. Race: African Americans have a two to three times increased risk compared with White people.
4. Prior stroke or transient ischemic attack (TIA).
5. Family history.
B. Modifiable.
1. Hypertension.
2. Hypercholesterolemia.
3. Diabetes.
4. Atrial fibrillation.
5. Hypercoagulable states.
6. Coronary artery disease.
7. Sleep apnea.
8. Smoking.
9. Alcohol consumption.
10. Use of oral contraceptives.
11. Obesity.
12. Drug use.

SUBJECTIVE DATA
A. Common complaints/symptoms.
1. Depends on the location of the stroke (see discussion in "Transient Ischemic Attack").
B. Common/typical scenario.
1. Sudden, abrupt onset.
2. Typical report from family members: The patient is perfectly fine one moment and then instantly changes.
3. Relationship between typical symptoms and location of stroke (see discussion in "Transient Ischemic Attack").
C. Review of systems.
1. Ask the patient about the following (Table 6.3):
a. Headaches.
b. Speech difficulties.
c. Falls.
d. Dropping objects.
e. Weakness of arms/legs/face.
f. Numbness/tingling.
g. Loss of urine/bowel control.
h. Visual changes: Blurriness, double vision, or loss of vision.

PHYSICAL EXAMINATION
A. Objective data.
1. Level of consciousness.
2. Visual examination.
3. Motor and sensory examination.
4. Speech assessment.
5. Cognitive test.
6. Cranial nerve examination.
B. Use the National Institutes of Health Stroke Scale (NIHSS) to objectively score stroke severity. The tool uses a point range from 0 to 42, with severity increasing with score, and can be accessed through the National Institutes of Health: www.ninds.nih.gov/sites/default/files/NIH_Stroke_Scale.pdf.
1. Used dynamically to assess and then reassess the patient's condition.
2. Scores greater than 13 indicate very severe strokes that may warrant surgical intervention and carry a very high probability of severe disability or death.

DIAGNOSTIC TESTS
A. Initial tests to be done immediately.
1. CT of the head.

TABLE 6.3 TYPICAL FINDINGS OF STROKE SYMPTOMS BASED ON HEMISPHERE

Left hemisphere	Right-sided weakness (face, arm, leg), left gaze preference, dysarthria, aphasia
Right hemisphere	Left-sided weakness (face, arm, leg), right gaze preference, dysarthria, flat affect, may neglect the left side of the body
Brainstem or cerebellum	May have multiple cranial nerve palsies, ataxia, vertigo, dysmetria, visual disturbances especially diplopia, hemiparesis or quadriparesis, locked-in syndrome

a. Should be done immediately if stroke is in the differential diagnosis. From the moment a stroke is suspected, a CT of the head should be completed within 25 minutes.

b. Do NOT delay a CT of the head.

2. Lab tests: Should be done simultaneously with preparing to go to CT of the head.

a. Minimum: Measure glucose prior to CT, but if the patient is a difficult stick obtain the rest of the lab tests after CT of the head.

b. Complete blood count (CBC), basic metabolic panel, prothrombin time (PT)/partial thromboplastin time (PTT)/international normalized ratio (INR).

3. EKG.

B. Other tests to be considered in select patients:

1. CT angiogram (CTA)/CT perfusion (CTP): Shows blood vessels, area of occlusion, and if there is collateral circulation. It can quantify CBF, blood volume, and the presence or absence of penumbra.

2. MRI/magnetic resonance angiography (MRA): To evaluate the extent of stroke.

3. Arterial blood gas (ABG).

4. Cerebral angiography: If a candidate for thrombectomy.

5. Ultrasound of carotids: To evaluate for carotid plaque as the source of stroke.

6. EEG: If seizure is suspected.

DIFFERENTIAL DIAGNOSIS

A. Ischemic stroke.
B. Hemorrhagic stroke.
C. Migraine.
D. Bell's palsy.
E. Seizure.
F. Hypoglycemic/hyperglycemia episode.
G. Sepsis.
H. Benign paroxysmal positional vertigo.
I. Neuromuscular or neurodegenerative disease.
J. Brain tumor.
K. Meningitis.
L. Syncope.
M. Multiple sclerosis.

EVALUATION AND MANAGEMENT PLAN

A. The treatment of stroke should be broken up into three main phases. In the first phase, after the stroke has been identified, the goal of treatment is to minimize the damage as quickly as possible. In the second phase, the goal is to prevent further strokes from occurring. In the third phase, the goal is to return the patient to their functional baseline prior to the stroke occurring.

1. Phase 1 plan.

a. Medical management.

i. Blood pressure (BP) control: The goal of BP management is to avoid complications. BP that is lowered too rapidly can cause increased ischemia, while BP that is too high may cause hemorrhagic conversion.

1) If no thrombolytics are given, treat the following BP:

a) Diastolic BP >140 mmHg: intravenous (IV) infusion.

b) Systolic BP >220 mmHg, diastolic BP 121 to 140 mmHg: IV push medications.

c) Systolic BP <220 mmHg or diastolic BP <120 mmHg: Monitor in the absence of other compelling indications.

2) If thrombolytics are to be given or have been given, treat the following BP:

a) Systolic BP >180 mmHg.

b) Diastolic BP >105 mmHg.

ii. Glucose monitoring.

1) The brain requires glucose for energy. Persistent hyperglycemia is associated with poor neurologic outcomes. Hypoglycemia can cause worsening of ischemia.

2) Goal of glucose monitoring: Maintain euglycemia less than 180 mg/dL.

iii. IV tissue plasminogen activator (tPA) administration.

1) Given to patients with diagnosis of ischemic stroke, once intracranial hemorrhage has been ruled out, who present within a 3-hour time frame for treatment from symptom onset.

2) Some patients may qualify for treatment with IV tPA up to 4.5 hours. However, this is not approved by the Food and Drug Administration (FDA).

b. Surgical management.

i. Endovascular intervention.

ii. Intra-arterial tPA administration.

1) Intra-arterial delivery directly into the clot via endovascular intervention.

2) Given within 6 hours of symptom onset.

3) Delivered directly into the clot.

4) Often used with mechanical clot extraction in large vessel strokes.

iii. Carotid endarterectomy: Rarely done as an emergency.

iv. Hemicraniectomy used for large hemispheric strokes with significant edema.

2. Phase 2 plan: Medical management begins 48 to 72 hours after stroke presentation.

a. Antiplatelet: Low-dose aspirin or clopidogrel should be initiated as soon as intracranial hemorrhage has been ruled out.

i. Aspirin 81 to 325 mg.

ii. Clopidogrel 75 mg.

b. Anticoagulants: Prescribe only if there is an increased cardioembolic risk as determined by the CHA_2DS_2-VAS_c score (Table 6.4 and discussion in "Transient Ischemic Attack").

c. Deep vein thrombosis (DVT) prophylaxis.

d. BP management (see Chapter 3).

3. Phase 3 plan: Rehabilitation.

a. Speech therapy.

b. Physical therapy.

c. Occupational therapy.

B. Patient/family teaching points.

TABLE 6.4 CHA$_2$DS$_2$-VAS$_c$ SCORE CRITERIA

Condition	Points
(C) Congestive heart failure	1
(H) Hypertension	1
(A) Age ≥75 years	2
(D) Diabetes mellitus	1
(C) CVA/TIA/thromboembolic event	2
(V) Vascular disease (prior MI, peripheral artery disease, aortic plaque)	1
(A) Age 65–74 years	1
(F) Female	1

Note: 0 points: No need for antiplatelet or anticoagulants; 1 point: None OR aspirin OR anticoagulant, depending on situation; ≥2 points: Start anticoagulant.
CHA$_2$DS$_2$-VASc, (C) congestive heart failure (H) hypertension (A) age (D) diabetes (S) CVA (V) vascular (A) age (S) sex; CVA, cerebrovascular accident; MI, myocardial infarction; TIA, transient ischemic attack.
Source: From Lip, G. Y., & Halperin, J. L. (2010, June). Improving stroke risk stratification in atrial fibrillation. *American Journal of Medicine, 123*(6), 484–488. https://doi.org/10.1016/j.amjmed.2009.12.013.

1. Note that depression is very common after a stroke.
2. Provide education about the cognitive limitations of the patient.
3. Emphasize that rehabilitation may last as long as 1 year.
4. Encourage lifestyle changes, including smoking cessation, physical activity, and changes in dietary intake.

FOLLOW-UP
A. Patients need to follow up with neurology.
   1. If there has been any intervention, the patient should follow up with a neurosurgeon.

CONSULTATION/REFERRAL
A. Provide referrals to rehabilitation, physical and occupational therapy, nutrition, and speech.

SPECIAL/GERIATRIC CONSIDERATIONS
A. Stroke in adults under 40 is rare.
   1. If it does occur in younger adults, a hypercoagulable workup and transesophageal echocardiogram (TEE) should be initiated in the hospital.
   2. Also consider mechanical causes such as carotid dissection, arteriovenous malformations, or fistulas.
B. Older adults should not be denied treatment due to age alone.
   1. Make sure the patient is assessed for the degree of frailty to help the family make decisions on treatment.
   2. The goal of treatment is to return the patient to baseline. If the baseline for the patient is extremely poor at any age, this should play a stronger role in the decision-making process.

CASE SCENARIO: RIGHT-SIDED HEMIPLEGIA

A 75-year-old man with a history of atrial fibrillation, recently taken off his anticoagulation in preparation for an upcoming surgery, presents to the ED after a fall at home. His wife found him on the floor reaching out to her with his left arm and trying to speak but she could not understand what he was saying. On arrival at the ED, his vital signs showed heart rate (HR) of 101 irregularly irregular, blood pressure (BP) of 230/120, saturating 97% on 2-L nasal cannula, and afebrile. On neurologic exam, he is awake but drowsy, does not follow commands or answer questions (global aphasia), his gaze is to the left, and he has significant right face, arm, and leg weakness with sensory loss. The National Institutes of Health Stroke Scale (NIHSS) score is 21. He is currently protecting his airway.

1. What is the best next immediate step in the management of this patient?
   A. Order complete blood count (CBC) and basic metabolic panel (BMP).
   B. Order CT of the head with CT angiography (CTA) of the head and neck.
   C. Order MRI of the brain.
   D. Order metoprolol 5 mg intravenous (IV) push.

BIBLIOGRAPHY
Adams, H. P., Jr., del Zoppo, G., Alberts, J. M., Bhatt, D. L., Brass, L., Furlan, A., Grubb, R. L., Higashida, R. T., Jauch, E. C., Kidwell, C., Lyden, P. D., Morgenstern, L. B., Qureshi, A. I., Rosenwasser, R. H., Scott, P. A., & Wijdicks, E. F. (2007, May). Guidelines for the early management of adults with ischemic stroke: A guideline from the American Heart Association/American Stroke Association Stroke Council, Clinical Cardiology Council, Cardiovascular Radiology and Intervention Council, and the Atherosclerotic Peripheral Vascular Disease and Quality of Care Outcomes in Research Interdisciplinary Working Groups: The American Academy of Neurology affirms the value of this guideline as an educational tool for neurologists. *Stroke, 38*(5), 1655–1711. https://doi.org/10.1161/STROKEAHA.107.181486

Goldstein, L. B., Bushnell, C. D., Adams, R. J., Appel, L. J., Braun, L. T., Chaturvedi, S., Creager, M. A., Culebras, A., Eckel, R. H., Hart, R. G., Hinchey, J. A., Howard, V. J., Jauch, E. C., Levine, S. R., Meschia, J. F., Moore, W. S., Nixon, J. V., & Pearson, T. A. (2011, February). Guidelines for the primary prevention of stroke: A guideline for healthcare professionals from the American Heart Association/American Stroke Association. *Stroke, 42*(2), 517–584. https://doi.org/10.1161/STR.0b013e3181fcb238

Hughes, S. (2014, May 2). New AHA/ASA stroke secondary prevention guidelines. *Medscape Medical News*, 870–947. https://doi.org/10.1161/STR.0b013e318284056a

Jauch, E. C., Saver, J. L., Adams, Jr., H. P. Bruno, A., Connors, J. J., Demaerschalk, B. M., Khatri, P., McMullan, P. W., & Howard Yonas, H. (2015, June 29). AHA/ASA focused update of the 2013 guidelines for the early management of patients with acute ischemic stroke regarding endovascular treatment: A guideline for healthcare professionals from the American Heart Association/American Stroke Association. *Stroke, 38*(5), 1655–1711.

Mozaffarian, D., Benjamin, E. J., Go, A. S., Arnett, D. K., Blaha, M. J., Cushman, M., de Ferranti, S., Després, J.-P., Fullerton, H. J., Howard, V. J., Huffman, M. D., Judd, S. E., Kissela, B. M., Lackland, D. T., Lichtman, J. H., Lisabeth, L. D., Liu, S., Mackey, R. H., Matchar, D. B. ... Turner, M. B. (2015, January 27). Heart disease and stroke statistics—2015 update: A report from the American Heart Association. *Circulation, 131*(4), e29–e322. https://doi.org/10.1161/CIR.0000000000000152

National Institutes of Health. (2003). *NIH stroke scale*. https://www.ninds.nih.gov/sites/default/files/NIH_Stroke_Scale.pdf

STATUS EPILEPTICUS

DEFINITION

A. Continuous clinical and/or electrographic seizure activity lasting 5 minutes or more, or recurrent seizure activity without return to baseline between seizures.

B. Classification of status epilepticus (SE) is based on semiology, duration, and underlying etiology.

   1. Convulsive SE: Associated with generalized tonic–clonic movements of extremities and mental status impairment; a life-threatening medical emergency.

   2. Nonconvulsive status epilepticus (NCSE): Electrographic seizure activity on EEG without any correlating clinical findings; requires emergent treatment to prevent cortical neuronal damage.

   3. Refractory SE: Clinical or electrographic seizures that do not respond to adequate doses of initial benzodiazepines, followed by a second antiepileptic drug (AED) agent.

   4. Super refractory SE: Clinical or electrographic seizures that continue for ≥24 hours despite anesthetic treatment, or recur on an attempted wean of the anesthetic regimen.

INCIDENCE

A. The annual incidence of SE is 100,000 to 200,000 cases in the United States.

B. Refractory SE occurs in up to 43% of patients with SE.

C. 33% of neuro-ICU patients develop NCSE.

D. 10% of medical ICU patients develop NCSE.

PATHOGENESIS

A. SE results from a neuronal imbalance between excitatory and inhibitory neurotransmitters (gamma-aminobutyric acid [GABA], N-methyl-D-aspartate [NMDA], glutamate) within the central nervous system (CNS).

B. Prolonged epileptic seizures result in lack of oxygen and glucose in brain cells, stimulating the release of excessive amounts of glutamate. Glutamate alters membrane channels, leading to an influx of calcium, which in turn triggers oxygen free radicals and causes cell injury and death.

PREDISPOSING FACTORS

A. Acute processes.

   1. Traumatic brain injury.

   2. Metabolic disturbances: Electrolyte abnormalities, hypoglycemia, and renal failure.

   3. CNS infections.

   4. Cerebrovascular pathology: Ischemic stroke, hemorrhage, cerebral sinus thrombosis, and hypertensive encephalopathy.

   5. Autoimmune encephalitis and paraneoplastic syndromes.

   6. Sepsis.

   7. Drugs: Toxicity, noncompliance with AEDs, and withdrawal from opioids, benzodiazepine, barbiturates, or alcohol.

   8. Anoxic brain injury.

B. Chronic processes.

   1. Preexisting epilepsy.

   2. CNS tumors.

   3. History of CNS pathology (traumatic brain injury, abscess, stroke).

   4. Chronic ethanol abuse.

SUBJECTIVE DATA

A. Common complaints/symptoms.

   1. Generalized convulsive status epilepticus (GCSE): Tonic extension of trunk and extremities, followed by clonic extension. Consciousness is usually lost.

   2. Myoclonic SE: Bursts of brief myoclonic jerks, which increase in intensity until a convulsion occurs. This condition is seen mostly in anoxic encephalopathy or metabolic disturbances, particularly renal failure.

   3. NCSE: Absence of awakening or returning to baseline even after 20 minutes of successful termination of clinical seizures. Symptoms may include coma, confusion, aphasia, staring, automatisms, facial twitching, eye deviation, and agitation.

B. Common/typical scenario.

   1. GCSE usually presents with the classic full-body convulsions and the patient is not aware of the occurrence.

   2. Myoclonic SE typically is seen in what people describe as limb shaking or twitching. Patients are awake and are able to describe the sensation.

   3. In NCSE, patients do not have any signs of twitching or abnormal movements. The only clue to NCSE is the absence of the patient waking up or returning to baseline after an event such as cardiac arrest, intracranial hemorrhage, or any surgery.

C. Family and social history.

   1. The most common cause of SE is a history of epilepsy.

   2. Ask about changes in antiepileptic medications.

   3. Alcohol and drug use can lower the seizure threshold in patients with a history of epilepsy.

D. Review of systems.

   1. In patients with GCSE or NCSE, a review of systems is not obtainable due to the altered level of consciousness.

PHYSICAL EXAMINATION

A. Neurologic examination.

   1. Assess level of consciousness and response to stimuli.

   2. Assess for any speech, memory, or language impairment.

   3. Assess for cranial nerve palsies.

   4. Assess for any sensory or motor deficits in all limbs.

DIAGNOSTIC TESTS

A. Workup should occur simultaneously and in parallel with treatment.

    1. Finger stick blood glucose.

    2. Complete blood count (CBC), comprehensive metabolic panel (CMP), drug screen, AED levels, alcohol levels, arterial blood gas (ABG), serum magnesium, and calcium (total and ionized).

    3. CT of the brain to rule out intracranial pathology.

    4. Continuous EEG monitoring: 24-hour EEG is the gold standard. Most typical pattern in SE is rhythmic high-frequency (>2.5 Hz) activity that increases in amplitude and decreases in frequency, finally terminating abruptly and leaving postictal low-amplitude slowing.

    5. Brain MRI: Seizure focus may show up as a bright signal on diffusion-weighted imaging (DWI) and dark signal on apparent diffusion coefficient (ADC) imaging in a nonvascular territory possibly with leptomeningeal enhancement.

    6. Lumbar puncture and cerebrospinal fluid (CSF) studies.

    7. Toxicology panel: Check for toxins that frequently cause seizures (e.g., isoniazid, tricyclic antidepressants [TCAs], antidepressants, theophylline, cocaine, sympathomimetic, organophosphates, and cyclosporine).

DIFFERENTIAL DIAGNOSIS

A. Movement disorders.

B. Herniation syndromes (decerebrate /decorticate posturing).

C. Psychiatric disorders: Psychogenic nonepileptic seizures, conversion disorder, acute psychosis, or catatonia.

EVALUATION AND MANAGEMENT PLAN

A. General plan.

    1. Treatment of SE should occur quickly and continue sequentially until clinical and electrographic seizures are terminated.

    2. Simultaneous assessment and management of airway, breathing, and circulation should be performed.

    3. Do not withhold seizure medications because of fear of respiratory compromise.

    4. Definitive control of SE should be established within 60 minutes of onset.

    5. Emergent treatment.

        a. Stabilize the patient (airway, breathing, circulation).

        b. Perform cardiac monitoring.

        c. Consider intubation as needed.

        d. Use nutritional resuscitation with 100 mg of thiamine intravenously (IV) followed by 50 mL of 50% dextrose IV push.

        e. Lorazepam (drug of choice for IV administration): 0.1 mg/kg IV at the rate of 2 mg/min (max 4 mg per dose); max total dose 8 mg.

        f. Midazolam is preferred for intramuscular (IM): 0.2 mg/kg IM; max dose 10 mg.

        g. Diazepam (preferred for rectal administration): One-time dose of 10 mg per rectum.

    6. Urgent treatment.

        a. Recommended AEDs include IV fosphenytoin or phenytoin, valproic acid, levetiracetam, and lacosamide. Initial total levels should be drawn after 2 hours of IV loading dose to determine maintenance dose and need to reload.

           i. Load with fosphenytoin 20 mg phenytoin sodium equivalent (PE)/kg at a rate of 150 mg/min. If using phenytoin, the rate should not be more than 50 mg/min. Cardiac monitoring should occur during infusion due to increased risk of QT prolongation and cardiac arrhythmia. An additional 10 mg/kg IV can be given if seizures persist. The maintenance dose is phenytoin 100 mg Q8H. The target free phenytoin level is 2 to 3 mcg/mL. Check serum levels daily.

           ii. Valproic acid: Load with 40 mg/kg (max dose 3,000 mg), infused over 5 to 10 minutes. If seizure persists, additional 20 mg/kg can be given. Maintenance dose is 30 to 60 mg/kg/d in divided doses. Serum valproic goal is 70 to 100 mcg/mL. Check levels daily.

           iii. Levetiracetam: Load with 60 mg/kg (max dose 4,500 mg), infused over 10 minutes. Maintenance dosing is 1,000 to 1,500 mg Q12H. Blood levels are not monitored.

           iv. Lacosamide: Load with 400 mg. Maintenance dosing is 100 to 200 mg BID. Max dose is 400 mg daily. Blood levels are not monitored.

    7. Refractory therapy.

        a. If seizures persist, consider continuous infusion of AEDs. The most commonly recommended are midazolam, propofol, and pentobarbital. Dosing of continuous infusion of AEDs should be titrated to cessation of electrographic seizures or burst suppression.

        b. A period of 24 to 48 hours of electrographic seizure control is recommended prior to slow withdrawal of continuous infusion of AEDs. It is recommended that EEG findings, not serum drug levels, guide therapy.

           i. Midazolam infusion: Load with 0.2 mg/kg, at an infusion rate of 2 mg/min. Begin continuous infusion: 0.05 to 2 mg/kg/hr. For breakthrough seizures, give 0.1 to 0.2 mg/kg bolus and increase infusion by 0.05 to 0.1 mg/kg/hr every 3 to 4 hours.

           ii. Propofol infusion: Load with 1 to 2 mg/kg, infused over 1 minute. Begin continuous infusion at 20 to 200 mcg/kg/min. Use caution when administering high doses (>80 mcg/kg/min) for extended periods of time (>48 hours) to avert risk of propofol infusion syndrome. For breakthrough seizures, increase infusion ▶

rate by 5 to 10 mcg/kg/min every 5 minutes until seizure cessation.

iii. Ketamine infusion: Load with 1.5mg/kg IV. Repeat every 5 minute until seizures stop (max load 4.5mg/kg). Maintain infusion at 1.2 to 7.5mg/kg/hr.

iv. Pentobarbital infusion: Load with 3 to 5 mg/kg IV over 10 to 30 minutes. Begin continuous infusion at 0.5 to 5 mg/kg/hr. For breakthrough seizures, titrate 1 mg/kg/hr every 10 minutes to continuous EEG of 4 to 6 bursts per minute.

FOLLOW-UP

A. Patients will need to follow up with an epileptologist to monitor and control the antiepileptic medications that will be required.

CONSULTATION/REFERRAL

A. A neurologist must be consulted in cases of SE. A neurologist with continuous EEG training and specialty training in epileptology is preferred.
B. Centers without the ability to perform or interpret continuous EEG in patients with SE or NCSE should consider rapid transfer to a higher level of care.

SPECIAL/GERIATRIC CONSIDERATIONS

A. Pregnancy: Lorazepam and fosphenytoin are recommended as initial and urgent therapy. Levetiracetam has shown to be safe in recent studies.

   1. Eclampsia must be considered in patients with SE in pregnancy; delivering the fetus is the best therapy in this situation.

   2. Also, magnesium sulfate is proved to be superior to AEDs in pregnant women with seizures and eclampsia.
B. Anoxic brain injury: Prognosis of SE after hypoxic or anoxic brain injury is poor.
C. Ketamine, an NMDA receptor antagonist, has emerged as a potential treatment for refractory SE associated with autoimmune encephalitis.

CASE SCENARIO: STATUS EPILEPTICUS

A 28-year-old man presents to the ED as an out-of-hospital cardiac arrest. When the emergency medical service (EMS) arrived at the scene, he had pulses but was hypoxic with agonal breathing. Shortly after, he went into pulseless electrical activity (PEA) arrest and required 30 minutes of CPR before return of spontaneous circulation (ROSC) was achieved. He was intubated without a need for paralytics. When he arrived at the ED, he was hypotensive to 80/50 and hypothermic to 93.2°F/34°C. He had nonreactive pupils, 4 mm bilaterally, and no corneal, gag, or cough reflex. He extended in the bilateral upper extremities and had triple flexion of the bilateral lower extremities to noxious stimulus. Labs were notable for a lactate of 10.5 and white blood cell (WBC) of 14; his platelets and international normalized ratio (INR) were within normal limits. Urine drug screen was positive for opioids and cocaine. CT of the head was performed and was read as normal. When being transferred back to the room, he developed sudden jerking movements of his arms and

legs, which continued until he was given 4 mg of Ativan. He was then transferred to the neurocritical care unit. The patient was subsequently loaded with levetiracetam 60 mg/kg, which improved but did not completely resolve clinical seizure activity manifesting as jerking movements in all of his extremities.

1. What would be the next appropriate step?
   A. Order continuous EEG.
   B. Initiate a midazolam drip.
   C. Order MRI of the brain with and without contrast.
   D. Initiate targeted temperature management.

BIBLIOGRAPHY

Bleck, T. (2008). Seizures in the critically ill. In J. E. Parrillo & R. P. Dellinger (Eds.), *Critical care medicine: Principles of diagnosis and management in the adult* (3rd ed., pp. 1367–1383). Mosby. https://doi.org/10.1016/b978-032304841-5.50068-6

Brophy, G. M., Bell, R., Classen, J., Alldredge, B., Bleck, T., Glauser, T., & Vespa, P. (2012). Guidelines for the evaluation and management of status epilepticus. *Neurocritical Care, 17,* 3–23. https://doi.org/10.1007/s12028-012-9695-z

Claassen, J., & Hirsch, L. J. (2009). Status epilepticus. In J. Frontera (Ed.), *Decision making in neurocritical care* (1st ed., Vol. 1, pp. 63–75). Thieme Medical.

Gilmore, R. L., Cibula, J. E., Eisenschenk, S., & Roper, S. N. (2013). Seizures. In J. Layon, A. Gabrielli, & W. Friedman (Eds.), *Textbook of neurointensive care* (2nd ed., Vol. 1, pp. 799–811). Springer Publishing Company.

TRANSIENT ISCHEMIC ATTACK

DEFINITION

A. Temporary blockage of blood flow to the brain (<24 hours) that does not result in permanent damage; often referred to as a "mini-stroke."
B. Majority of transient ischemic attacks (TIAs) demonstrate complete resolution in less than 10 minutes.

INCIDENCE

A. It is estimated that up to 500,000 people a year have a TIA in the United States.
B. Up to 30% of people who report a TIA have a stroke within 5 years.
C. The incidence of a cerebrovascular accident (CVA) has been reported as high as 11% within 7 days.

PATHOGENESIS

A. A TIA occurs when there is blockage of blood to the brain from atherosclerosis, any type of emboli, decreased blood flow/volume to the brain, or constriction of the arteries in the brain.
B. The exact symptoms of a TIA correlate with the particular artery that is affected. The hallmark of a TIA is resolution of symptoms within 24 hours from onset.

PREDISPOSING FACTORS

A. Medical factors.
   1. Hypertension.
   2. Diabetes.
   3. Hyperlipidemia.
   4. Coronary artery disease: Arrhythmias, heart defects, heart infections, or valvular disease.

5. Peripheral artery disease.

6. Obesity.

7. Elevated homocysteine levels.

8. Sickle cell disease.

B. Nonmodifiable risk factors.

1. Family history.

2. Age greater than 55 years.

3. Sex (men more likely than women).

4. Prior TIA.

5. Race, with Hispanics and African Americans at higher risk.

C. Lifestyle factors.

1. Cigarette smoking.

2. Physical inactivity.

3. Poor diet.

4. Excessive alcohol intake.

5. Illicit drug use.

6. Oral contraceptive use.

SUBJECTIVE DATA

A. Common complaints/symptoms.

1. The types of complaints a person would have depend on the area of the brain that is affected. In general, there are three main classifications of TIA/CVA based on circulation patterns.

   a. Anterior circulation symptoms.

     i. Carotid artery: Contralateral motor and sensory loss to arm/leg.

     ii. Anterior cerebral artery: Confusion, personality changes, motor, or sensory loss in leg.

     iii. Middle cerebral artery (majority of TIAs/CVAs): Face asymmetry, motor or sensory loss in arm, slurred speech, or aphasia.

   b. Posterior circulation symptoms.

     i. Contralateral motor or sensory loss.

     ii. Contralateral visual field loss.

     iii. Cortical blindness.

     iv. Dysarthria.

     v. Dysphagia.

     vi. Diplopia.

     vii. Quadriparesis.

   c. Vertebrobasilar circulation symptoms.

     i. Confusion.

     ii. Slurred speech.

     iii. Blurry vision or blindness.

     iv. Weakness of both arms or legs.

     v. Difficulty walking and ataxia.

     vi. Paresthesias.

B. Common/typical scenario.

1. A typical event is described as happening all of the sudden. One moment the person is fine, the next moment the symptoms occur. In the majority of the cases, the symptoms resolve within 10 minutes and the person is back to their previous self.

C. Family and social history.

1. A family history of stroke can raise the risk of stroke, especially if before the age of 65.

2. Smoking, physical inactivity, alcoholism, illicit drug use, and poor diet are all important factors to document.

D. Review of systems.

1. Typically all symptoms will have resolved by the time of the interview, but it is important to document which systems were affected.

   a. Visual fields: Blurry vision, double vision, loss of vision, and/or sense of a curtain being pulled down over one eye (amaurosis fugax).

   b. Language: Slurred speech, difficulty speaking, inability to find words, and/or inability to understand others.

   c. Extremities: Weakness, numbness, tingling, and/or strange sensations.

PHYSICAL EXAMINATION

A. Cranial nerve testing: pupillary reflex, visual fields, extraocular movements, facial sensation, facial movements, hearing, palate elevation, shoulder shrug, tongue extension.

B. Motor strength.

C. Sensory testing.

D. Gait and posture: Walking heel to toe and/or finger to nose test.

DIAGNOSTIC TESTS

A. CT of the head.

B. MRI of the brain within 24 hours.

C. Carotid Doppler: To assess for carotid disease.

D. EKG: To assess for atrial fibrillation.

E. Transthoracic echocardiogram (TTE): To rule out any cardioembolic source.

F. Lab tests: Glucose, chemistry profile, and lipid panel.

1. Consider hypercoagulable workup if younger than 40 years of age or based on history.

2. Consider alcohol levels based on history.

DIFFERENTIAL DIAGNOSIS

A. Ischemic stroke.

B. Hemorrhagic stroke.

C. Migraine.

D. Bell's palsy.

E. Seizure.

F. Hypoglycemic/hyperglycemia episode.

G. Sepsis.

H. Vertigo.

I. Neuromuscular or neurodegenerative disease.

J. Brain tumor.

K. Meningitis.

L. Syncope.

EVALUATION AND MANAGEMENT PLAN

A. General plan.

1. Obtain results from diagnostic tests.

2. Prevent further stroke from modification of risk factors.

3. Manage blood pressure (BP).

4. Initiate lipid control.

5. Maximize blood glucose control.

B. Patient/family teaching points.

1. Assess family baseline understanding of TIAs/CVAs.

2. Educate on risk factor modification.

3. Educate on the role of diet/exercise in preventing future TIAs/CVAs.

4. Educate on the role of pharmacotherapy and adverse effects.

5. Provide pamphlets and educational materials.

6. Introduce smoking cessation plan if indicated.

7. Introduce weight loss program if indicated.

C. Pharmacotherapy.

    1. Antiplatelet drugs: Low-dose aspirin or clopidogrel should be initiated as soon as intracranial hemorrhage has been ruled out.

        a. Aspirin 81 to 325 mg daily.

        b. Clopidogrel 75 mg daily.

    2. Anticoagulants: Prescribed only if there is an increased cardioembolic risk as determined by the $CHA_2DS_2\text{-}VAS_c$ score (see Table 6.4).

    3. Thrombolytics: Not indicated if there is resolution of symptoms.

D. Surgical intervention.

    1. Carotid endarterectomy if a person is symptomatic with severe carotid stenosis (70%–99% blockage).

E. Discharge instructions.

    1. Warning signs of stroke.

    2. What to do if a person suspects a stroke: Call 911.

    3. Possible MedicAlert bracelet if taking a blood thinner.

FOLLOW-UP

A. Follow up with primary care provider (PCP) within 2 weeks.

CONSULTATION/REFERRAL

A. Refer all patients to the neurology team.

SPECIAL/GERIATRIC CONSIDERATIONS

A. Hypercoagulopathy can occur secondary to cancer, pregnancy, and in sickle cell disease. Patients under the age of 40 who present with TIA should undergo a hypercoagulable workup.

CASE SCENARIO: TRANSIENT LEFT FACE AND ARM WEAKNESS

A 60-year-old woman with a medical history of hypertension, hyperlipidemia, diabetes, and tobacco use presents to her primary care provider (PCP) with a 2-hour episode of left face and arm tingling. She notes that she was unable to sign her check very well today. She also reports a mild headache of 2/10. On exam, she has subtle facial weakness with smile, and although her strength is 5/5 in her right arm there is a pronator drift. Her blood pressure (BP) is 185/90. The emergency medical service (EMS) is called and she is transferred to the nearest ED. By the time she arrives and is examined, her symptoms have resolved.

1. What would be the next appropriate step?

    A. Diagnose as complex migraine and discharge home.

    B. Order tissue plasminogen activator (tPA) stat.

    C. Admit to the hospital for further workup for suspected transient ischemic attack (TIA).

    D. Order CT of the head, and if normal then discharge home.

BIBLIOGRAPHY

Easton, J. D., Saver, J. L., Albers, G. W., Alberts, M. J., Chaturvedi, S., Feldmann, E., Hatsukami, T. S., Higashida, R. T., Johnston, S. C., Kidwell, C. S., Lutsep, H. L., Miller, E., & Sacco, R. L. (2009). Definition and evaluation of transient ischemic attack: A scientific statement for healthcare professionals from the American Heart Association/American Stroke, Association Stroke Council, Council on Cardiovascular Surgery and Anesthesia: Council on Cardiovascular Radiology and Intervention; Council on Cardiovascular Nursing; and the Interdisciplinary Council on Peripheral Vascular Disease, The American Academy of Neurology affirms the value of this statement as an educational tool for neurologist. *Stroke, 40*, 2276–2293. https://doi.org/10.1161/STROKEAHA.108.192218

Giles, M. F., & Rothwell, P. M. (2007). Risk of stroke early after transient ischemic attack: A systematic review and meta-analysis. *Lancet Neurology, 6*(12), 1063–1072. https://doi.org/10.1016/S1474-4422(07)70274-0

Johnston, S. C. (2002). Transient ischemic attack. *New England Journal of Medicine, 347*, 1687–1692. https://doi.org/10.1056/NEJMcp020891

Kernan, W. N., Ovbiagele, B., Black, H. R., Bravata, D. M., Chimowitz, M. I., Ezekowitz, M. D., Fang, M. C., Fisher, M., Furie, K. L., Heck, D. V., Johnston, S. C., Kasner, S. E., Kittner, S. J., Mitchell, P. H., Rich, M. W., Richardson, D., Schwamm, L. H., & Wilson, J. A. (2014). Guidelines for the prevention of stroke in patients with stroke and transient ischemic attack: A guideline for healthcare professionals from the American Heart Association/American Stroke Association. *Stroke, 45*, 2160. https://doi.org/10.1161/STR.0000000000000024

Lip, G. Y., & Halperin, J. L. (2010, June). Improving stroke risk stratification in atrial fibrillation. *American Journal of Medicine, 123*(6), 484–488. https://doi.org/10.1016/j.amjmed.2009.12.013

KNOWLEDGE CHECK: CHAPTER 6

1. Which of the following is NOT seen in the pathogenesis of anoxic brain injury?

   A. Influx of sodium and calcium into the cell
   B. Release of the inhibitory neurotransmitter, glutamate
   C. Increased free radicals
   D. Cell death

2. Which of the following describes permanent vegetative state?

   A. Irreversible state of wakefulness without awareness or return of sleep–wake cycle that may occur 3 months after a nontraumatic injury and 1 year following a traumatic brain injury (TBI)
   B. State of unresponsiveness where patients are unaware of their surroundings and are unarousable
   C. Sustained eye opening, awareness of environment with quadriplegia, and intact cognition
   D. Vegetative state after 1 month of injury

3. In most cases, it is necessary to wait at least how many hours before giving a prognosis?

   A. 48 hours
   B. 24 hours
   C. 72 hours
   D. 7 days

4. Which of the following is NOT part of management of a postanoxic brain-injured patient?

   A. Ventilatory support
   B. Continuous EEG monitoring
   C. Monitoring for nosocomial infection
   D. Hyperthermia

5. What are the three types of primary headache?

   A. Migraine, high-altitude headache, trigeminal neuralgia
   B. Migraine, tension-type headache, and trigeminal autonomic cephalalgias
   C. Migraine, tension-type headache, dialysis headache
   D. Medication-overuse headache, migraine, Tolosa–Hunt syndrome

6. When should neurologic imaging be considered for a patient with headache?

   A. Altered mental status
   B. New-onset headache after age 50
   C. Thunderclap headache/worst headache of life
   D. All of the above

7. Which of the following are appropriate abortive treatments for primary headache?

   A. Dihydroergotamine, inhalation of 100% oxygen, Depakote 250 mg PO BID
   B. Amitriptyline, gabapentin, ketorolac, chlorpromazine
   C. Ketorolac, diphenhydramine, sumatriptan, dexamethasone
   D. Ketorolac, diphenhydramine, sumatriptan, verapamil

8. What is the gold standard for diagnosis of headache?

   A. Detailed interview and clinical examination
   B. Complete blood count (CBC), basic metabolic panel (BMP), erythrocyte sedimentation rate (ESR), and C-reactive protein (CRP)
   C. MRI of the brain with and without contrast
   D. Lumbar puncture

9. Which of the following is NOT a modifiable risk factor in stroke?

   A. Hypertension
   B. Hyperlipidemia
   C. Age
   D. Diabetes

10. Which of the following symptoms is most suspicious for a left hemisphere stroke?

    A. Right gaze preference
    B. Vertigo
    C. Aphasia
    D. Double vision

(See answers next page.)

1. **B) Release of the inhibitory neurotransmitter, glutamate**
Glutamate is released, but this is an excitatory neurotransmitter.

2. **A) Irreversible state of wakefulness without awareness or return of sleep–wake cycle that may occur 3 months after a nontraumatic injury and 1 year following a traumatic brain injury (TBI)**
There are different levels of consciousness, ranging from awake and aware to death. State of unresponsiveness where patients are unaware of their surroundings and are unarousable describes coma. Sustained eye opening, awareness of environment with quadriplegia, and intact cognition describe locked-in syndrome. Vegetative state after 1 month of injury describes persistent vegetative state.

3. **C) 72 hours**
In most cases, it is necessary to wait at least 72 hours after rewarming or postarrest without hypothermia to give a prognosis; however, timing should be on a case-by-case basis.

4. **D) Hyperthermia**
Postanoxic brain-injured patients require mechanical ventilation and are at high risk for (a) subclinical seizures, which should be monitored with continuous EEG; and (b) nosocomial infections, which should be monitored with routine cultures. Hyperthermia should be avoided as this can worsen brain injury, and if there are no contraindications anoxic brain-injured patients undergo targeted temperature management between 33°C and 36°C.

5. **B) Migraine, tension-type headache, and trigeminal autonomic cephalalgias**
Headaches are classified into primary and secondary headaches, each with multiple subcategories. Migraine, tension-type headache (TTH), and trigeminal autonomic cephalalgias (TACs) are all classified under primary headaches. Medication-overuse headache, high-altitude headache, and dialysis headache are classified under secondary headaches, while Tolosa–Hunt syndrome and trigeminal neuralgia are classified under neuropathies/facial pains/ and other headaches.

6. **D) All of the above**
Thunderclap headache/worst headache of life, altered mental status, meningismus, papilledema, acute neurologic deficit, new-onset headache after age 50, and history of cancer or HIV or immunocompromised state are all findings that should prompt neurologic imaging. CT of the head is usually a good first choice of imaging as it can rule out life-threatening causes such as subarachnoid hemorrhage and intracerebral hemorrhage, as well as intracranial tumors and abscesses.

7. **C) Ketorolac, diphenhydramine, sumatriptan, dexamethasone**
Abortive treatments include nonsteroidal anti-inflammatory drugs (NSAIDs; ketorolac), corticosteroids (methylprednisolone, dexamethasone), neuroleptics (diphenhydramine), antinausea medications (metoclopramide, prochlorperazine, chlorpromazine), dihydroergotamine, anticonvulsants if given as rapid infusions (Depakote, levetiracetam), magnesium sulfate, serotonin receptor antagonists (sumatriptan), and inhalation of 100% oxygen (for cluster headache). Prophylactic medications include beta-adrenergic blockers (propranolol), tricyclic antidepressants (amitriptyline), calcium channel antagonists (verapamil), and anticonvulsants (Depakote, topiramate, gabapentin).

8. **A) Detailed interview and clinical examination**
A detailed interview and clinical examination are the gold standard for diagnosis of headache and include questions about pain onset, location, duration, frequency, quality, associated symptoms, aura, and aggravating/relieving factors. Basic laboratory testing and imaging can be tailored based on history and exam, while lumbar puncture is usually reserved when there is concern for subarachnoid hemorrhage, infection, or idiopathic intracranial hypertension.

9. **C) Age**
Both nonmodifiable risk factors (age, race, family history) and modifiable risk factors (hypertension, hypercholesterolemia, diabetes, atrial fibrillation, hypercoagulable states, coronary artery disease, sleep apnea, smoking, alcohol consumption, use of oral contraceptives, obesity, and drug use) predispose a person to stroke.

10. **C) Aphasia**
Left hemispheric strokes can cause right-sided hemiparesis, right-sided sensory deficits, left gaze preference, and aphasia (since language center is usually on the left). Right hemispheric strokes cause right gaze preference. Vertigo and double vision are often seen in strokes of the brainstem or cerebellum.

11. What are the blood pressure goals after thrombolytic administration?

  A. Systolic blood pressure (SBP) <220 mmHg, diastolic blood pressure (DBP) <140 mmHg
  B. SBP <140 mmHg, DBP <220 mmHg
  C. SBP <105 mmHg, DBP <180 mmHg
  D. SBP <180 mmHg, DBP <105 mmHg

12. Which imaging should be done immediately if stroke is suspected?

  A. CT of the head
  B. CT angiography (CTA) of the head and neck
  C. Carotid ultrasound
  D. MRI of the brain

13. Which of the following could indicate a transient ischemic attack (TIA)?

  A. A temporary blockage of blood flow to the brain that results in permanent damage
  B. Right arm weakness for 2 days
  C. An area of diffusion restriction on MRI of the brain
  D. An episode of aphasia that lasted 30 minutes

14. Which of the following would NOT be part of the initial transient ischemic attack (TIA) workup?

  A. CT of the head and MRI of the brain
  B. Lower extremity Doppler
  C. Transthoracic echocardiogram (TTE)
  D. Hemoglobin A1C and lipid panel

15. Which of the following is NOT part of the $CHA_2DS_2-VAS_c$ score criteria?

  A. Hypertension
  B. Diabetes
  C. Male sex
  D. Age 64 to 74

16. Which of the following would be part of the management of transient ischemic attack (TIA)?

  A. Starting aspirin 81 mg daily
  B. Follow-up CT scans every 3 months
  C. Avoiding exercise
  D. Switching from cigarettes to chewing tobacco

17. The three key findings suggestive of brain death are:

  A. Coma.
  B. Apnea.
  C. Loss of brainstem reflexes.
  D. Cushing triad.

18. A confirmatory apnea test is characterized by:

  A. Increase of $PaCO_2$ >60 mmHg or increase of 20 mm Hg above baseline.
  B. Decrease of $PaCO_2$ <60 mmHg or decrease of 20 mm Hg below baseline.
  C. No change in $PaCO_2$ over the duration of observation.
  D. Increase of $PaCO_2$ >60 mmHg or decrease of 20 mm Hg below baseline.

19. The following criteria should be met prior to apnea testing for brain death, EXCEPT:

  A. Normothermia
  B. Systolic blood pressure (SBP) >100 mmHg
  C. $PaCO_2$ 35 to 45 mmHg
  D. pH <7.00

20. Ancillary testing of brain death includes all of the following tests, EXCEPT:

  A. Cerebral angiogram
  B. Cerebral scintigraphy
  C. EEG
  D. MRI brain

(See answers next page.)

11. D) SBP <180 mmHg, DBP <105 mmHg
Once a thrombolytic has been administered, strict blood pressure parameters are maintained for the first 24 hours and one should be treated to maintain systolic blood pressure (SBP) <180 mmHg and diastolic blood pressure (DBP) <105 mmHg.

12. A) CT of the head
If stroke is in the differential, a noncontrast CT of the head should be obtained immediately to ensure that no hemorrhage or evolving ischemic stroke is present, and expedite delivery of tissue plasminogen activator (tPA) if indicated. CT angiography (CTA) of the head and neck is often performed right after CT of the head to rule out a large vessel occlusion. Carotid ultrasound and MRI brain can be done at a later time and do not influence the acute stroke care.

13. D) An episode of aphasia that lasted 30 minutes
Transient ischemic attack (TIA) is defined by a temporary blockage of blood flow to the brain that does NOT result in permanent damage and lasts <24 hours. Therefore, a 30-minute episode of aphasia could represent a TIA, whereas 2 days of right arm weakness would represent possible stroke. Diffusion restriction on MRI of the brain indicates an area of ischemia if due to blockage of blood flow; by definition, such changes on MRI represent permanent damage.

14. B) Lower extremity Doppler
In any patient who presents with transient ischemic attack (TIA) symptoms, the standard initial workup will include CT of the head, MRI of the brain, vessel imaging (CT angiography [CTA] of the head and neck and/or carotid Doppler), transthoracic echocardiogram (TTE), and lab work to look for diabetes and elevated low-density lipoprotein (LDL). Lower extremity Doppler would be appropriate if,

for example, TTE demonstrated a patent foramen ovale (PFO).

15. C) Male sex
Male sex is not part of the criteria.

16. A) Starting aspirin 81 mg daily
Initiating antiplatelet drugs, such as aspirin or clopidogrel, would be an appropriate next step in treating transient ischemic attack (TIA). There is no need for serial CT of the head imaging outpatient, especially since TIA would not be detected on CT of the head. Lifestyle changes, including exercise and quitting tobacco, are important steps in lowering stroke risk.

17. A) Coma, B) Apnea, and C) Loss of brainstem reflexes
A diagnosis of brain death is a permanent absence of cerebral and brainstem function, defined as a comatose state, inability to initiate respiratory drive (apnea), and a loss of all brainstem reflexes.

18. A) Increase of $PaCO_2$ >60 mmHg or increase of 20 mmHg above baseline
Inability to initiate respiratory drive in the presence of hypercarbia leads to an increase of $PaCO_2$ above 60 mmHg or an increase in $PaCO_2$ of 20 mmHg above baseline.

19. D) pH <7.00
Prior to apnea testing, all metabolic abnormalities and acid–base imbalances should be corrected to normal ranges to avoid any confounders to completing clinical testing.

20. D) MRI of the brain
MRI of the brain without contrast is not an ideal study to confirm an absence of cerebral perfusion.

21. The most common cause of intracerebral hemorrhage is:

A. Coagulopathy.

B. Hypertension.

C. Cerebral venous thrombosis.

D. Amyloid angiopathy.

22. Initial management of a patient diagnosed with an intraparenchymal hemorrhage should include which of the following?

A. Reversal of coagulopathy

B. Blood pressure management

C. Seizure prophylaxis

D. Emergent ventriculostomy placement

23. For a patient diagnosed with an intracerebral hemorrhage, follow-up imaging to assess for hematoma stability should be performed within:

A. 3 hours from admission.

B. 6 hours from admission.

C. 12 hours from admission.

D. 24 hours from admission.

24. Calculation of intracerebral hemorrhage (ICH) is completed by multiplying A (diameter in centimeters of hemorrhage) × B (diameter in centimeters of hemorrhage 90 degrees from A) × _____, then dividing by 2.

A. Number of CT slices × 0.5 (thickness of slice in centimeters)

B. Number of CT slices × thickness of slice in centimeters

C. Number of CT slices − thickness of slice in centimeters

D. Number of CT slices × 10 (thickness of slice in centimeters)

25. Failure to terminate status epilepticus with appropriate doses of benzodiazepines would prompt the provider to choose one of the following antiepileptics as second-line therapy, EXCEPT:

A. Levetiracetam (Keppra)

B. Fosphenytoin/phenytoin

C. Valproic acid (Depakote)

D. Topiramate (Topamax)

(See answers next page.)

21. B) Hypertension

Chronic uncontrolled hypertension is the most common cause of intracerebral hemorrhage.

22. A) Reversal of coagulopathy and B) Blood pressure management

Reversal of coagulopathy and strict blood pressure (BP) management are essential to achieve hemostasis. Seizure prophylaxis is not indicated in all patients with intraparenchymal hemorrhage. Ventriculostomy should only be inserted if there is concern for elevated intracranial pressure (ICP) and hydrocephalus exists.

23. B) 6 hours from admission

Due to the increased risk of hemorrhagic expansion within the first couple of hours of admission, a repeat CT of the head should be performed within 6 hours.

24. B) Number of CT slices × thickness of slice in centimeters

The correct answer is to multiply A × B × C (calculate the number of CT slices × thickness of slice in centimeters), then divide by 2.

25. D) Topiramate (Topamax)

Topiramate is not a recommended second-line therapy agent; alternatively, phenobarbital can be considered.

CHAPTER 7

TEMPERATURE MANAGEMENT GUIDELINES IN ACUTE BRAIN INJURY

Sarah L. Livesay and Monique Lambert

DEFINITION

A. Elevated body temperature is associated with worse outcomes after acute brain injury. This is seen in a variety of injuries, including traumatic brain injury (TBI), large territory ischemic stroke, hemorrhagic stroke, and hypoxic ischemic encephalopathy (HIE) after cardiac arrest (CA).

  1. Fevers of acute brain injury (either traumatic or vascular in nature) are independently associated with worse outcomes, which are associated with temperatures greater than 99.1°F/37.3°C in a number of studies.

  2. Targeted temperature management (TTM) after CA is associated with improved neurologic recovery in multiple studies.

B. In some instances, lowering the body temperature below normal (induced hypothermia) is associated with either improved control or intracranial pressure (ICP) or improved outcomes.

C. Fever management or TTM to a specific body temperature consists of coordinated interventions, such as the use of antipyretic medications, surface and/or intravascular devices to reduce temperature, and management of shivering and other potential effects of controlling the body temperature.

INCIDENCE

A. Approximately 650,000 adults in the United States experience a CA each year.

B. Fever is common in severe brain injury of multiple etiologies and is associated with secondary brain injury.

PATHOGENESIS

A. Varies according to mechanism of injury.

PREDISPOSING FACTORS

A. Length of hypoperfusion in the case of CA.

B. Severity of neurologic injury.

SUBJECTIVE DATA

A. Events of the CA and resuscitation attempts.

B. Patients with brain injuries may not be alert enough to reliably provide subjective complaints. Patients with spinal cord injury may not be able to describe pain in detail due to sensory or thermoregulatory loss.

C. Review of systems.

  1. Assess patients for fever or symptoms suggesting fever prior to hospital admission.

  2. Inquire about any recent or current known infections, cold/influenza symptoms, or abnormal rashes/skin lesions.

  3. Evaluate for any chills, shivering, or other symptoms suggestive of fever.

  4. In a patient with return of spontaneous circulation (ROSC) post-CA, collect the circumstances of CA, including initial rhythm (if available), length of time to ROSC, and all medications administered.

PHYSICAL EXAMINATION

A. Check blood pressure, pulse, respirations, and temperature.

  1. Temperature monitoring methods are essential in order to obtain accurate and reliable measurements. Continuous monitoring is ideal, but if this is not possible patients' temperatures should be checked on an hourly basis using core methods.

   a. The most accurate source of core temperature monitoring is using a pulmonary artery catheter.

   b. Other core methods of temperature monitoring include intravesicular (bladder), esophageal, and rectal.

   c. Peripheral methods of temperature monitoring include tympanic membrane, axillary, and oral.

B. Look for any lines or drains that may be a nidus for infection.

C. Examine skin thoroughly.

D. Auscultate heart and lungs.

E. Perform a neurologic exam.

DIAGNOSTIC TESTS

A. All tests and imaging should be directed at ruling out infectious causes of fever, as well as venous thromboembolism, transfusion reaction, drug fever, adrenal insufficiency, thyroid storm, and any other noninfectious, noncentral etiologies. Tests should be ordered with discretion and with the individual patient in mind.

B. After CA, testing should be aimed at identifying the cause of CA, early percutaneous reperfusion if indicated, and excluding intracranial causes of CA such as hemorrhagic stroke.

  1. EKG and cardiac enzymes.

EVALUATION AND MANAGEMENT PLAN

A. In patients with acute brain injury other than HIE, an infectious source of fever should be identified and treated. This includes identifying or ruling out infectious and noninfectious sources while actively managing the fever to minimize neurologic injury.

B. In the case of CA, early management should focus on identifying and treating the case of CA if applicable, including early percutaneous coronary intervention (PCI) for myocardial infarction. Instituting TTM can be done concurrently with PCI.

    1. TTM is indicated for any patient after CA who remains unconscious after ROSC. Studies included patients who could receive TTM within 3 to 6 hours of ROSC.

C. TTM goal target temperature and duration differ by etiology of brain injury.

    1. There is mixed literature regarding target temperature after CA. Recent studies suggest no difference in outcomes in decreasing temperature to between 91.4°F/33°C and 96.8°F/36°C. Guidelines in the United States and Europe suggest the provider may choose either target temperature for the first 24 hours. Fever prevention should continue until 72 hours after ROSC.

        a. Certain patient criteria may cause the clinician to choose one temperature over another. For example, a higher temperature may be preferred in patients with bleeding or infection risk, whereas a lower temperature may be helpful in patients with seizures or cerebral edema.

    2. In patients with refractory elevated ICP, inducing hypothermia to a target temperature as low as 91.4°F/33°C may be considered. The target temperature should be individualized to the patient.

        a. Hypothermia in this patient population is effective at controlling ICP but not associated with improved long-term outcomes.

    3. Strategies to prevent and/or manage fever are reasonable in patients with significant brain injury during the acute phase of injury. The exact duration and interventions chosen to control the fever should be individualized to the patient. A randomized clinical trial is currently ongoing and may provide further direction on active fever prevention and management in this patient population.

D. General principles of fever management.

    1. Pharmacologic methods.

        a. Antipyretic agents: Acetaminophen, aspirin, or nonsteroidal anti-inflammatory drugs (NSAIDs).

            i. Acetaminophen is often preferred because aspirin and NSAIDs have undesirable side effects, such as platelet dysfunction and gastrointestinal (GI) upset.

    2. External cooling.

        a. Evaporation such as via water or alcohol sponge baths.

        b. Conduction methods include ice packs or water-circulating cooling blankets or pads. Newer technology in cooling body wraps provides constant monitoring of temperature and adjustment of circulating water to maintain desired body temperature.

        c. Convection (fans and ambient air temperature control) and radiation methods are less effective in these indications.

    3. Invasive cooling methods include cold saline boluses or intravascular catheters that offer constant monitoring of temperature and adjustment of circulating water through catheter balloon to maintain desired body temperature.

    4. Cooling techniques.

        a. TTM is best implemented with advanced temperature technology.

        b. Cooling blankets and intravascular devices are available. There are benefits and drawbacks to each type of technology. Technology should be reviewed for accuracy and degree of temperature control.

            i. Surface cooling is easily applied by the nursing staff, leading to quick induction. Complications may include skin burns if the water temperature is allowed to be very cold for prolonged periods.

            ii. Intravascular cooling may decrease the occurrence of shivering. The intravascular line must be placed by a qualified practitioner, and this must be considered in the induction workflow. Intravascular catheters are associated with higher rates of deep vein thrombosis (DVT).

E. When decreasing body temperature below 96.8°F/36°C, a slow and controlled rewarming period lasting up to 24 hours is necessary to prevent dangerous shifts in electrolytes, such as potassium and rebound cerebral edema.

F. Complications: Many serious complications arise from induction of hypothermia as opposed to normothermia in a patient. Most of these adverse effects are not problematic until core body temperatures are 95°F/35°C or lower. However, a number of complications may occur when attempting maintenance of normal temperatures.

    1. Catheter-related thrombosis and infection, as well as other types of infection.

    2. Skin breakdown; of particular concern when surface cooling devices are used and circulating water temperature is low for prolonged periods of time.

    3. Shivering.

        a. Shivering is an involuntary, rhythmic tremor that consists of oscillatory movements of various skeletal muscle groups. The act of shivering is both an anticipated consequence as well as an adverse effect of therapeutic hypothermia.

        b. Shivering is usually greatest at temperatures between 93.2°F/34°C and 96.8°F/36°C.

    4. Shivering results in increased systemic and cerebral metabolic demand.

        a. The most common and only validated tool for assessment of shivering is the Bedside Shivering Assessment Scale (Table 7.1).

TABLE 7.1 THE BEDSIDE SHIVERING ASSESSMENT SCALE

Score	Definition
0	None: There is no shivering noted on palpation of the masseter, neck, or chest wall.
1	Mild: Shivering is localized to the neck and/or thorax only.
2	Moderate: Shivering involves gross movement of the upper extremities (in addition to the neck and thorax).
3	Severe: Shivering involves gross movements of the trunk and upper and lower extremities.

Source: From Badjatia, N., Strongilis, E., Gordon, E., Prescutti, M., Fernandez, L., Fernandez, A., Buitrago, M., Schmidt, J. M., Ostapkovich, N. D., & Mayer, S. A. (2012). Metabolic impact of shivering during therapeutic temperature modulation: The bedside shivering assessment scale. *Stroke, 39,* 3242–3247. https://doi.org/10.1161/STROKE AHA.108.523654.

i. This scale measures the degree of shivering during induced hypothermia.

ii. It assists in determining the efficacy of non-pharmacologic and pharmacologic interventions.

b. Management of shivering involves using a multimodal approach to counter the effects of shivering, which includes both nonpharmacologic and pharmacologic therapy.

i. Nonpharmacologic agents.

1) Skin counterwarming provided by an air-circulating blanket or focal hand warming.

ii. Pharmacologic agents.

1) Sedatives and hypnotics.
2) Analgesics and opioids.
3) Alpha-agonists.
4) Magnesium supplementation.
5) Neuromuscular blocking agents (NMBAs).

5. Additional systemic complications of induced hypothermia are more likely to occur at lower body temperatures and include the following:

a. Bradycardia is often seen in hypothermia, usually at colder temperatures compared with warmer ones. Cardiac intervals (PR, QRS, QTc) can lengthen. This is generally well-tolerated by the patient and resolves once rewarming has occurred.

b. Central venous pressure (CVP) may increase due to vasoconstriction from cold temperatures.

c. During TTM to lower temperature, there is an increased solubility of oxygen and carbon dioxide, which leads to a decrease in partial pressure of oxygen (PaO_2) and partial pressure of carbon dioxide ($PaCO_2$) and a left shift of the oxygen–hemoglobin dissociation curve. Ventilators may require frequent setting changes during induction of cooling. Arterial blood gas values should be corrected for temperature.

d. At lower body temperature, there is a decreased production of insulin by the pancreas and decreased insulin sensitivity, resulting in higher exogenous insulin needs during hypothermia at lower target temperatures.

e. Increased lactate and ketone levels may be noted in blood or urine samples drawn during TTM to lower target temperatures.

f. As body temperature drops, serum potassium moves intracellularly, resulting in a serum hypokalemia that must be monitored with frequent lab checks and potassium supplementation. However, when the body rewarms, intracellular potassium then shifts extracellularly. Potassium replacement should be less aggressive toward the end of the maintenance period and during rewarming. Rewarming should be slow and controlled to minimize excessive potassium shifts.

g. Fluctuations in additional electrolytes, such as calcium and magnesium, may be seen and should be frequently monitored during TTM.

h. Seizures are estimated to occur in 12% to 22% of patients who are comatose after CA. Clinical signs of seizures may be obscured by coma or sedatives and paralytics administered during TTM. Therefore, seizure activity may be subclinical and the only evidence on EEG monitoring.

i. The available evidence does not support prophylactic treatment, and no specific antiseizure medication is identified as superior in this setting. It is reasonable to undergo frequent or continuous EEG monitoring in patients during TTM to identify subclinical seizures or status epilepticus.

j. During TTM, particularly targeting a lower temperature, patients often experience a *cold diuresis,* or increased urine output during the induction period. This results as hypothermia increases venous return secondary to venous constriction. This, combined with an increase in atrial natriuretic peptide (ANP), decreased antidiuretic hormone (ADH), and tubular dysfunction from the CA, may lead to large-volume diuresis.

k. If uncorrected, this may lead to hypovolemia and hemoconcentration.

l. TTM results in platelet and neutrophil inhibition, particularly at lower target temperatures and longer duration. Patients are at risk for bleeding and infection.

m. In addition to neutrophil dysfunction, patients are at risk for infection as vasoconstriction may lead to decreased white blood cell (WBC) migration to the site of infection and decreased inflammatory response.

FOLLOW-UP

A. Follow-up and postdischarge monitoring are related to the patient's admission diagnosis as well as new issues that may have occurred during hospitalization.

CONSULTATION/REFERRAL

A. Inpatient and outpatient consults are dictated by the diagnosis of each patient.

SPECIAL/GERIATRIC CONSIDERATIONS

A. Geriatric individuals often have unique presentations and require special considerations when gathering a history and physical.

B. Treatment methods may also vary slightly due to multiple comorbidities and less reserve.

1. Skin breakdown is a regular concern in geriatric patients because mobility and skin caliber are lower in these individuals, particularly with external cooling methods.

2. Older patients may not always mount a robust febrile response to infection. They can become hypothermic in an infected state.

3. The effectiveness of different cooling methods increases with advanced age secondary to slower counterregulatory response to small temperature changes, decreased metabolism, decreased vascular response (and as a result, vasoconstriction), and often a lower body mass index (BMI).

4. Medications may need to be adjusted more frequently in older adults, either due to hepatic/renal function or low BMI.

CASE SCENARIO: CARDIAC ARREST

A 68-year-old male with a medical history of coronary artery disease, hyperlipidemia, obesity, and hypertension arrives at the ED after collapsing at the gym. He had a witnessed collapse and received bystander CPR. The gym had an automated external defibrillator (AED) on site, which was applied several minutes prior to arrival of the emergency medical service (EMS). One shock was delivered by the AED and the patient was in sinus tachycardia when EMS arrived. The approximate time of cardiac arrest was estimated at 20 minutes. The patient received intravenous (IV) fluids and norepinephrine for a systolic blood pressure in the 70s when EMS arrived. He was noted to have multiple premature ventricular contractions (PVCs) and ST elevation on EKG and telemetry en route to the hospital. The percutaneous coronary intervention (PCI) team was notified and met him in the ED. In the ED, he was noted to be stuporous, with a Glasgow Coma Scale (GCS) score of 5 (E1, V1, M3), and he was intubated for airway protection. En route to the cardiac catheterization lab, surface cooling gel pads were applied and targeted temperature management (TTM) was started with a goal temperature of 96.8°F/36°C. PCI was initiated and he was noted to have an occluded left anterior descending artery (LAD). The vessel was reperfused and the patient was admitted to the ICU. During the next 12 hours, he was noted to have a Bedside Shivering Assessment Scale (BSAS) of 1 to 2 and the nursing staff instituted surface counterwarming, acetaminophen, buspirone, meperidine, and propofol to successfully control shivering. The patient was noted to have purposeful movements between 18 and 24 hours post-TTM initiation. Fever control was continued for 72 hours postcardiac arrest. His neurologic recovery improved to a GCS score of 15, with some mild confusion persisting on discharge from the ICU. He was discharged from the hospital to home with outpatient speech therapy for cognitive therapy and physical therapy for deconditioning.

1. Which of the following is TRUE regarding the use of intravascular catheters to control temperature in targeted temperature management (TTM)?

A. Catheters are slower than surface pads to reach target temperature.

B. Catheters are associated with less shivering than surface cooling techniques.

C. Catheters are associated with higher rates of deep vein thrombosis (DVT) than surface cooling devices.

D. Catheters are associated with higher rates of skin breakdown than surface cooling devices.

E. Catheters are best reserved for patients at high risk of bleeding during TTM.

BIBLIOGRAPHY

American Geriatrics Society 2019 Beers Criteria Update Expert Panel. (2019). Beers criteria for inappropriate medication use in older patients: An update from the AGS. *Journal of the American Geriatrics Society, 67*(4), 674–694.

Badjatia, N. (2012). *Shivering: Scores and protocols. Critical Care, 16*(Suppl. 2). A9. https://www.ncbi.nlm.nih.gov/pmc/articles/PMC3389469

Badjatia, N., Strongilis, E., Gordon, E., Prescutti, M., Fernandez, L., Fernandez, A., Buitrago, M., Schmidt, J. M., Ostapkovich, N. D., & Mayer, S. A. (2012). Metabolic impact of shivering during therapeutic temperature modulation: The bedside shivering assessment scale. *Stroke, 39*, 3242–3247. https://doi.org/10.1161/STROKEAHA.108.523654

Boggosian, E.G., & Taccone, F.S. (2022). Fever management in acute brain injury. *Current Opinions in Critical Care, 28*(2). https://doi.org/10.1097/MCC.0000000000000918

Callaway, C. W., Donnino, M. W., Fink, E. L., Geocadin, R. G., Golan, E., Kern, K. B., Leary, M., Meurer, W. J., Peberdy, M. A., Thompson, T. M., & Zimmerman, J. Z. (2015). Part 8: Post–cardiac arrest care: 2015 American Heart Association guidelines update for cardiopulmonary resuscitation and emergency cardiovascular care. *Circulation, 132*(18 Suppl. 2). S456–S482. https://doi.org/10.1161/CIR.0000000000000262

Donnino, M. W., Anderen, L. W., Berg, K. M., Reynolds, J. C., Nolan, J. P., Morely, P. T., & Xanthos, T. X. (2015). Temperature management after cardiac arrest, An advisory statement by the Advanced Life Support Task Force of the International Liaison Committee on Resuscitation and the American Association Emergency, Cardiovascular Care Committee and the Council on Cardiopulmonary, Critical Care, Perioperative and Resuscitation. *Circulation, 132*(25). https://doi.org/https://doi.org/10.1161/CIR.0000000000000313

Geri, G., Champigneulle, B., Bougouin, W., Arnaout, M., & Cariou, A. (2015). Common physiological response during TTM. *BMC Emergency Medicine, 15*(Suppl. 1), A14. https://doi.org/10.1186/1471-227X-15-S1-A14

Hocker, S. E., Tian, L., Li, G., Steckelberg, J. M., Mandrekar, J. N., & Rabinstein, A. A. (2013). Indicators of central fever in the neurologic intensive care unit. *JAMA Neurology, 70*(12), 1499–1504. https://doi.org/10.1001/jamaneurol.2013.4354

Nielsen, N., Wetterslev, J., Cronberg, T., Erlinge, D., Gasche, Y., Hassager, C., & Friberg, H. (2013). Targeted temperature management at 33°C versus 36°C after cardiac arrest. *New England Journal of Medicine, 369*(23), 2197–2206. https://doi.org/10.1056/NEJMoa1310519

Rasmussen, T. P., & Girotra, S. (2022, April 10). *A contemporary update on targeted temperature management. American College of Cardiology.* https://www.acc.org/latest-in-cardiology/articles/2021/11/09/13/16/a-contemporary-update-on-targeted-temperature-management

Van Poucke, S., Stevens, K., Marcus, A. E., & Lancé, M. (2014). Hypothermia: Effects on platelet functioning hemostasis. *Thrombosis Journal, 12*, 31. https://doi.org/10.1186/s12959-014-0031-z

Walter, E. J., Hanna-Jumma, S., Carraretto, M., & Forni, L. (2016). The pathophysiological basis and consequences of fever. *Critical Care, 20*(1), 200. https://doi.org/10.1186/s13054-016-1375-5

Weant, K. A., Martin, J. E., Humphries, R. L., & Cook, A. M. (2010). Pharmacologic options for reducing the shivering response to therapeutic hypothermia. *Pharmacotherapy, 30*, 830–841. https://doi.org/10.1592/phco.30.8.830

KNOWLEDGE CHECK: CHAPTER 7

1. Fever of greater than 99.5°F/37.5°C is associated with worse outcomes in which of the following diseases states?

   A. Subarachnoid hemorrhage
   B. Large-volume intracerebral hemorrhage
   C. Hypoxic ischemic encephalopathy
   D. Severe traumatic brain injury
   E. All of the above

2. In a patient who is comatose after return of spontaneous circulation (ROSC), what is the best temperature to choose for targeted temperature management (TTM)?

   A. TTM not indicated in this patient
   B. Target temperature of 91.4°F/33°C
   C. Target temperature of 96.8°F/36°C
   D. Target temperature of either 91.4°F/33°C or 96.8°F/36°C
   E. Target temperature of 99.5°F/37.5°C

3. In a patient with elevated intracranial pressure (ICP) refractory to other medical and surgical treatments, which of the following statements is TRUE regarding the use of induced hypothermia?

   A. Hypothermia is ineffective at controlling elevated ICP.
   B. The body temperature must be decreased to 91.4°F/33°C to be effective.
   C. Hypothermia is not associated with improved long-term outcomes.
   D. Patients are at increased risk of deep vein thrombosis (DVT) during hypothermia.
   E. Informed consent must be obtained to induce hypothermia in this patient population.

(See answers next page.)

1. **E) All of the above**
   In subarachnoid hemorrhage, large-volume intracerebral hemorrhage, hypoxic ischemic encephalopathy, and severe traumatic brain injury, fever of greater than 99.5°F/37.5°C is associated with worse outcomes.

2. **D) Target temperature of either 91.4°F/33°C or 36°C**
   A target temperature of either 91.4°F/33°C or 96.8°F/36°C is appropriate for targeted temperature management (TTM) in a patient who is comatose after return of spontaneous circulation (ROSC).

3. **C) Hypothermia is not associated with improved long-term outcomes.**
   Hypothermia is effective at controlling elevated intracranial pressure (ICP), patient consent is not necessary, and patients are not at increased risk of deep vein thrombosis (DVT) during hypothermia. However, hypothermia is not associated with improved long-term outcomes.

CHAPTER 8

ENDOCRINE GUIDELINES

Kathryn Evans Kreider

DEFINITION

A. Insufficient production of glucocorticoids and/or mineralocorticoids and adrenal androgens as a result of primary adrenal failure or failure of the pituitary or hypothalamus. Cortisol and mineralocorticoids are essential to life due to their role in energy and fluid homeostasis.

  1. Primary adrenal insufficiency (PAI).

    a. Also known as Addison disease.

    b. Deficiency in adrenal hormones as a result of direct injury to the adrenal glands.

    c. Glucocorticoid and mineralocorticoid replacement will be lifelong.

  2. Secondary adrenal insufficiency (SAI).

    a. Insufficient adrenal hormones due to lack of pituitary stimulation.

    b. Adrenal function may recover depending on etiology.

  3. Tertiary adrenal insufficiency (TAI).

    a. Insufficient adrenal hormones due to lack of hypothalamic stimulation on the pituitary.

    b. Adrenal function may recover depending on etiology.

  4. Adrenal crisis (AC).

    a. Potentially fatal condition that occurs when there is heightened need for cortisol in response to stress in the presence of adrenal insufficiency (AI).

    b. May be the initial presentation of AI.

INCIDENCE

A. The prevalence of primary AI is 100 to 140 cases per million.

  1. Women more often affected.

  2. Peak age 30 to 50 years.

B. The prevalence of secondary AI is 150 to 280 cases per million.

  1. Women more often affected.

  2. Peak age around 60 years.

C. The risk of AC in patients with existing AI is 6.3% per patient year.

PATHOGENESIS

A. PAI is caused by destruction of the adrenal cortex, most often by antiadrenal antibodies.

  1. Hormone deficiency occurs when 90% of the cortex is lost.

2. All adrenal hormones may be affected, including mineralocorticoids (aldosterone) and adrenal androgens.

B. Central AI includes SAI and TAI.

  1. SAI is a result of deficient adrenocorticotrophic hormone (ACTH) from the pituitary gland leading to decreased adrenal stimulation.

  2. TAI involves disruption of corticotropin-releasing hormone (CRH), vasopressin, or both, from the hypothalamus, resulting in decreased stimulation of the pituitary gland and reduced ACTH.

  3. The hypothalamic–pituitary axis (HPA) is impaired.

  4. Production of aldosterone and adrenal androgens is unaffected.

PREDISPOSING FACTORS

A. Primary AI.

  1. Presence of other autoimmune conditions (e.g., autoimmune thyroid disease, type 1 diabetes mellitus, autoimmune polyendocrinopathy syndromes).

  2. Disseminated infection (e.g., tuberculosis, HIV, cytomegalovirus, fungal infections).

  3. Adrenal hemorrhage, metastases, or infiltration.

  4. Various genetic disorders (e.g., congenital adrenal hyperplasia, adrenoleukodystrophy).

  5. Use of medications associated with drug-induced AI (e.g., fluconazole, etomidate, phenobarbital, rifampin).

B. Secondary AI.

  1. Pituitary tumor or trauma.

  2. Infections or infiltrative processes (e.g., tuberculosis, meningitis, sarcoidosis).

  3. Pituitary surgery.

C. Tertiary AI.

  1. Most common cause: Long-term use of exogenous glucocorticoids.

  2. Hypothalamic dysfunction secondary to tumors or infiltrative processes.

D. AC.

  1. Abrupt cessation of glucocorticoid use.

  2. Acute physiologic stress in the presence of AI.

  3. Previous AC.

  4. Risk increased if significant comorbidity present.

SUBJECTIVE DATA

A. Common complaints/symptoms.

  1. Tends to be nonspecific with an insidious onset, including:

    a. Weakness and fatigue.

    b. Anorexia and weight loss.

B. Common/typical scenario.
  1. History of the present illness.
    a. Elicit information about onset, duration, and severity of symptoms.
    b. Obtain a detailed medical history.
    c. Inquire about recent illness, injury, trauma, surgery, and procedures.
    d. Evaluate for history of glucocorticoid use.
  2. Other signs and symptoms.
    a. AI.
      i. Abdominal pain.
      ii. Myalgia or arthralgia.
      iii. Depression or anxiety.
      iv. Dizziness or postural hypotension.
      v. Salt craving.
      vi. Skin hyperpigmentation.
      vii. Decreased libido in women (if androgen-deficient).
      viii. Loss of pubic and axillary hair in females (if androgen-deficient).
      ix. Electrolyte imbalances, including hyponatremia and hyperkalemia.
      x. Hypoglycemia.
    b. AC.
      i. Severe weakness.
      ii. Syncope.
      iii. Abdominal pain, nausea, and vomiting.
      iv. Back pain.
      v. Confusion.

PHYSICAL EXAMINATION

A. Vital signs.
  1. Orthostatic hypotension in AI.
  2. Hypotension in AC.
B. Skin.
  1. Hyperpigmentation, particularly sun-exposed areas, skin creases, mucous membranes, scars, and breast areolas.
  2. In females, pubic and/or axillary hair loss.
C. Signs of dehydration.
D. Cardiovascular examination.
E. Mental status examination.
  1. Altered consciousness and delirium in AC.

DIAGNOSTIC TESTS

A. Diagnostic testing for AI should be performed in any hospitalized patient with symptoms suggestive of AI that are otherwise unexplained.
B. AI is usually diagnosed by a low morning (8 a.m.) serum cortisol level and a low stimulated cortisol level.
  1. Cortisol levels are usually at their highest levels in the morning; low levels should raise suspicion of AI.
  2. The diagnosis of AI is likely if the morning cortisol level is less than 5 mcg/dL, and less than 3 mcg/dL is highly suggestive.
  3. A low serum cortisol level (<5 mcg/dL) in addition to a high ACTH level (>66 pmol/L) is highly predictive of AI.

a. ACTH twice the upper limit of normal of the reference range is consistent with PAI.
  4. A high ACTH with a normal cortisol level may be an early indicator of AI.
  5. Do not check "random" cortisols during the day except at 6 to 8 a.m. Normal fluctuations occur later in the day and results cannot be interpreted.
C. The most common stimulation test is the corticotropin stimulation test ("cort-stim"), also known as the ACTH test or cosyntropin test.
  1. This test is the gold standard for diagnosing primary (not secondary) AI.
  2. Cosyntropin is synthetic ACTH given to patients intramuscularly (IM) to stimulate the adrenal glands to produce cortisol.
  3. Cosyntropin testing can be done at any time of day.
    a. Testing is often done early morning (8 a.m.) so morning cortisol levels can be drawn simultaneously.
  4. Steps for performing the cort-stim test include:
    a. Drawing baseline lab tests, including serum cortisol and ACTH.
    b. Administering 250 mcg of cosyntropin IM or intravenously (IV).
    c. Drawing peak serum cortisol level after 30 or 60 minutes.
  5. Peak serum cortisol levels less than 18 mcg/dL indicate AI.
    a. Certain conditions can alter cortisol measurements (alter cortisol-binding globulin [CBG]).
      i. Estrogen-containing contraceptives can falsely increase cortisol.
      ii. Patients with nephrotic syndrome, liver disease, or those with critical illness may have low CBG values and falsely low cortisol levels.
  6. High ACTH levels (often >300 ng/L) are characteristic of PAI.
  7. Renin and aldosterone should be measured to assess mineralocorticoid deficiency if there is a concern for PAI.
    a. PAI is associated with loss of the part of the adrenal gland that produces mineralocorticoid hormones.
      i. Elevated plasma renin and low or inappropriately normal aldosterone is typical.
  8. If SAI or TAI is suspected (pituitary or hypothalamus dysfunction), it is recommended that an endocrinologist be consulted to assist with biochemical testing and confirmatory testing.

DIFFERENTIAL DIAGNOSIS

A. Malnutrition.
B. Gastrointestinal (GI) dysfunction.
C. Malignancy.
D. Failure to thrive.
E. Hyperthyroidism.

EVALUATION AND MANAGEMENT PLAN

A. General plan.

  1. Replacement of glucocorticoid with physiologic dosing; hemodynamic stability.

B. Pharmacotherapy.

  1. If AI is diagnosed in the hospital and the patient is acutely ill/decompensating, stress-dose steroids should be used immediately and continued until the patient show signs of recovery.

  2. If AI or AC is suspected in a hospitalized patient who is acutely ill, start stress-dose steroids prior to receiving the results of diagnostic testing.

    a. Example: Hydrocortisone 50 mg IV Q6H.

    b. Alternative: Hydrocortisone 100 mg IV given immediately, followed by 200 mg hydrocortisone given over 24 hours (continuous IV or intermittent injections).

  3. Stress dosing of steroids should be used for patients with previously diagnosed AI who present to the hospital with acute illness or injury.

  4. Patients should also be given a bolus of IV fluids for acute AC.

    a. 1,000 mL saline or 5% dextrose in saline given within the first hour.

  5. If AI is diagnosed in the hospital and the patient is not acutely ill or demonstrating signs of AC, physiologic dosing may be started with careful consideration to other comorbid conditions and patient acuity.

  6. All patients with confirmed PAI require lifelong glucocorticoid therapy.

    a. Options: May be dosed based on body mass index (BMI) or weight.

      i. Hydrocortisone 15 to 20 mg in the morning and 5 to 10 mg in the afternoon (12–4 p.m.).

      ii. Prednisolone 3 to 5 mg/d total in one to two daily doses.

    b. Patients may occasionally be given glucocorticoid divided into three daily doses.

    c. Dexamethasone should generally be avoided due to potential for Cushing-like features and overreplacement.

  7. Mineralocorticoid replacement should be initiated in all patients who exhibit aldosterone deficiency.

    a. Fludrocortisone should be initiated at doses of 50 to 100 mg/d.

    b. Salt intake should not be restricted.

  8. Response should be measured clinically for both glucocorticoid and mineralocorticoid replacement (blood pressure [BP], weight, energy levels, and signs of glucocorticoid excess; salt craving, postural hypotension, edema).

    a. Electrolytes should be measured to confirm correct mineralocorticoid replacement.

    b. Other biochemical tests are not recommended.

C. Discharge instructions.

  1. Patients should be counseled on signs and symptoms of under- and overreplacement of cortisol.

  2. Patients require a steroid emergency card and a medical alert bracelet.

  3. Patients should be counseled extensively on "sick day rules."

    a. Home management of illness with fever: Patients should double or triple home steroid dose for 2 to 3 days or until recovery; increase electrolyte-containing fluids.

    b. Management of GI-related illness: Patients should inject 100 mg hydrocortisone IM if unable to tolerate oral administration.

    c. Minor to moderate surgical stress: Double or triple home dosing until event is over.

  4. Patients should have a prescription for IM hydrocortisone in case they are unable to take PO steroids.

  5. Patients with mineralocorticoid deficiency should be counseled to increase salt intake on days of excess heat, sweating, or physical activity.

FOLLOW-UP

A. Patients should follow up with an outpatient provider (preferably endocrinologist) every 3 to 6 months until clinically stable, with appointments every 6 to 12 months reasonable thereafter.

B. Patients should be evaluated at each clinical visit for signs and symptoms of over- and underreplacement.

  1. Signs of overreplacement may include insomnia, weight gain, peripheral edema, or hypertension.

  2. Signs of underreplacement are similar to the signs and symptoms of AI.

C. Patients should receive periodic clinical and biochemical evaluation to screen for other autoimmune conditions.

  1. Type 1 diabetes.

  2. Autoimmune thyroid disease.

  3. Pernicious anemia.

  4. Celiac disease.

  5. Premature ovarian failure.

CONSULTATION/REFERRAL

A. Referral to an endocrinologist is recommended to assist with long-term steroid management.

SPECIAL/GERIATRIC CONSIDERATIONS

A. Pregnant patients should be evaluated at least once per trimester; more frequent visits may be required if other complications exist.

  1. A glucocorticoid dose increase may be required in the third trimester.

  2. Stress-dose steroids are required during labor.

CASE SCENARIO: ADRENAL INSUFFICIENCY

Laura is a 42-year-old patient with type 1 diabetes who was brought to the ED by her mother after experiencing an episode of hypoglycemia that caused a fall and loss of consciousness. The patient reports that she has unintentionally lost 10 lb over the last month and has experienced multiple episodes of hypoglycemia, which is not normal for her. She reports significant

(continued)

fatigue. Current medications include insulin glargine 16 units daily and lispro insulin 1:10 carb ratio. Medical history included type 1 diabetes (diagnosed 22 years ago). Upon arrival to the ED, the patient was stable but hypotensive. Her blood pressure (BP) was 85/50, pulse 115, respirations 20, and temperature 98.6°F/37°C. Her physical exam was otherwise normal. Other data included hemoglobin A1C (HbA1C) of 7.1% and point-of-care (POC) blood glucose (BG) of 76 mg/dL; her basic metabolic panel (BMP) revealed sodium of 128 and potassium of 5.4. Her thyroid function was normal and her complete blood count (CBC) was normal. Due to her type 1 diabetes, endocrinology was consulted and requested cortisol/adrenocorticotropic hormone evaluation. The results suggested an adrenocorticotrophic hormone (ACTH) of 265 and a cortisol level of 2.5. Serum aldosterone level was low. The diagnosis of primary adrenal insufficiency (PAI) was confirmed. The patient was started immediately on hydrocortisone 10 mg in the morning and 5 mg in the afternoon, and fludrocortisone 50 mg daily to stabilize her mineralocorticoid levels.

1. What laboratory test differentiates primary adrenal insufficiency (AI) from other types of AI?
   A. Cortisol levels
   B. Cosyntropin stimulation test
   C. Adrenocorticotrophic hormone (ACTH)
   D. Signs and symptoms

2. What treatment is different between primary adrenal insufficiency and other types (secondary or tertiary)?
   A. Dose of steroids
   B. Type of steroids
   C. Use of supplements
   D. Use of fludrocortisone

3. Which of the following conditions puts patients at higher risk for adrenal insufficiency?
   A. High dose of long-term steroids
   B. Type 1 diabetes
   C. Autoimmune thyroid disease
   D. Pituitary surgery
   E. All of the above

4. Which of the following is TRUE regarding the treatment of adrenal insufficiency (AI)?
   A. Hydrocortisone is generally preferred for most patients.
   B. Patients should take the highest dose that is required for maintenance.
   C. Patients will require bone density monitoring annually due to steroid use.
   D. Patients will require annual monitoring for diabetes onset due to steroid use.

BIBLIOGRAPHY

Bornstein, S. R., Allolio, B., Arlt, W., Barthel, A., Don-Wauchope, A., Hammer, G. D., Husebye, E. S., Merke, D. P., Murad, M. H., Stratakis, C. A., & Torpy, D. J. (2016). Diagnosis and treatment of primary adrenal insufficiency: An endocrine society clinical practice guideline. *Journal of Clinical Endocrinology and Metabolism, 101*(2), 364–389. https://doi.org/10.1210/jc.2015-1710

Husebye, E. S., Pearce, S. H., Krone, N. P., & Kämpe, O. (2021). Adrenal insufficiency. *The Lancet, 397*(10274), 613–629. https://doi.org/10.1016/S0140-6736(21)00136-7

Marissa E. Luft

DEFINITION
A. A metabolic disorder due to autoimmune destruction of the pancreatic beta cells.
B. Previously referred to as insulin-dependent diabetes or juvenile-onset diabetes.
C. Further divided into two subgroups based on pathogenesis.
   1. Immune-mediated diabetes.
      a. Autoimmune-mediated destruction of pancreatic beta cells.
      b. Frequently affected with other autoimmune disorders such as Hashimoto thyroiditis, Graves disease, Addison disease, celiac disease, vitiligo, autoimmune hepatitis, myasthenia gravis, and pernicious anemia.
   2. Idiopathic type 1 diabetes.
      a. No known etiologies.
      b. Permanent insulinopenia and prone to ketosis.
      c. No evidence of autoimmunity.
      d. African or Asian ancestry.
      e. Strongly inherited; no human leukocyte antigen association.

INCIDENCE
A. In 2012, approximately 1.25 million American children and adults had type 1 diabetes.
B. Worldwide incidence is increasing by approximately 3% per year.

PATHOGENESIS
A. Autoimmune destruction of pancreatic beta cells; 85% of type 1 diabetes patients have detectable circulating antibodies.
B. Rate of beta cell destruction can vary.
   1. Rapid in infants and children.
   2. Slow in adults.

PREDISPOSING FACTORS
A. Presence of other autoimmune diseases.
B. Family history of diabetes.
C. Viruses.
D. Environmental toxins.

SUBJECTIVE DATA
A. Common complaints/symptoms.
   1. Polyuria (96%).
   2. Polyphagia.
   3. Polydipsia.
   4. Weight loss.
   5. Fatigue.
B. Common/typical scenario.
   1. Patients frequently complain of fatigue and weakness. They may have muscle cramps, blurred vision, and significant polyuria, polydipsia, and polyphagia.
   2. Weight loss occurs over time despite normal or increased appetite.

C. Family and social history.
  1. Ask about family history since there is a strong link to family history.
  2. Ask about type of occupation, that is, shift worker.
  3. Use of alcohol, smoking, or recreational drug use.
  4. Review how much exercise the person gets.
D. Review of systems.
  1. Head, ear, eyes, nose, and throat (HEENT).
    a. Dental issues: Periodontal disease is associated with diabetes.
  2. Psychological.
    a. Depression.
    b. Anxiety.
    c. Disordered eating.
    d. Psychosocial barriers/support.
    e. Barriers to self-management.
  3. Microvascular complications.
    a. Neuropathy.
    b. Nephropathy.
    c. Retinopathy.
  4. Macrovascular complications.
    a. Coronary artery disease (CAD).
    b. Cerebrovascular disease.
    c. Peripheral arterial disease.

PHYSICAL EXAMINATION

A. Height, weight, body mass index (BMI), waist circumference.
B. Vital signs.
C. Funduscopic examination.
D. Thyroid palpation.
E. Skin examination.
  1. Acanthosis nigricans (Figure 8.1).
  2. Lipohypertrophy.
  3. Diabetic dermopathy.
  4. Skin tags.

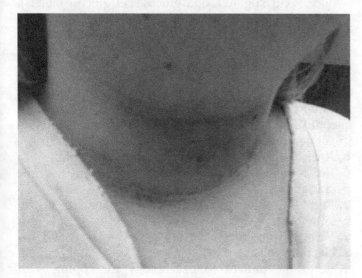

FIGURE 8.1 Acanthosis nigricans is a dark, velvety, hyperpigmentation of the skin, often found at the skin folds.

Source: From Lyons, F., & Ousley, L. (2015). *Dermatology for the advanced practice nurse* (p. 55). Springer Publishing Company.

F. Foot examination.
  1. Inspection, noting mycotic changes to nail or skin.
  2. Vascular examination.
    a. Hair patterns or lack of hair growth.
    b. Pulses (dorsalis pedis and posterior tibial).
    c. Temperature/color.
  3. Reflexes.
    a. Patellar.
    b. Achilles.
  4. Proprioception, vibration, and monofilament sensation.

DIAGNOSTIC TESTS

A. Glycosylated hemoglobin A1C (HgbA1C), fasting glucose, random glucose, or 2-hour glucose tolerance test (GTT) to diagnose.
  1. HgbA1C greater than 6.5%.
  2. Fasting glucose greater than 126 mg/dL.
  3. Random glucose greater than 200 mg/dL with classic symptoms of hyperglycemia.
  4. 2-hour GTT greater than 200 mg/dL.
B. Antibodies to check at the time of diagnosis.
  1. Glutamic acid decarboxylase (GAD).
  2. Islet cell antibodies.
  3. Zinc antibodies.
C. HgbA1C on admission to hospital if no result available for the past 3 months.
D. Annual lab work.
  1. Fasting lipid panel.
  2. Liver function tests.
  3. Urine albumin to creatinine ratio.
  4. Serum creatinine and estimated glomerular filtration rate (GFR).
  5. Thyroid-stimulating hormone (TSH).
E. C-peptide and random glucose to determine insulin production by beta cells.

DIFFERENTIAL DIAGNOSIS

A. Steroid-induced diabetes.
B. Pancreatitis.
C. Cushing disease.
D. Pancreatic endocrine tumor.
E. Gestational diabetes.
F. Maturity-onset diabetes of the young (MODY) type diabetes.
G. Latent autoimmune diabetes in adults (LADA).
H. Type 2 diabetes.
I. Cystic fibrosis-related diabetes.
J. Posttransplant diabetes.
K. Postpancreatectomy diabetes.

EVALUATION AND MANAGEMENT PLAN

A. General plan.
  1. The recommended outpatient comprehensive treatment plan for type 1 diabetes according to the American Association of Diabetes Educators consists of the following seven self-care behaviors:
    a. Healthy eating: The patient should see a registered dietitian for medical nutrition therapy counseling.

b. Being active: At least 150 minutes of moderate-to-vigorous-intensity physical activity spread out over a week is required. This can include resistance exercises and flexibility exercises.

c. Monitoring: It is recommended to test glucose before meals and bedtime (more frequently if needed).

d. Medications (insulin).

   i. Delivery method options: Insulin pen, vial and syringe, and pump.

   ii. Regimen choices (premixed insulin vs. basal and prandial).

   iii. Educate regarding proper storage of insulin.

   iv. Educate regarding different preparation, administration, and site rotation of insulin injection.

   v. Instruct on proper disposal of sharps.

   vi. Educate on symptoms of hypoglycemia.

e. Problem-solving.

f. Healthy coping.

g. Reducing risks.

B. Patient/family teaching points.

  1. Inpatient education focuses on survival skills only.

   a. Checking glucose.

   b. Taking medications.

   c. Diet.

   d. Hypoglycemia treatment.

  2. Outpatient education is more comprehensive and uses the guidelines by the American Association of Diabetes Educators to direct the education. The patient should be referred to outpatient diabetes education at the time of diagnosis, annually thereafter, and as needed or if therapy changes.

C. Pharmacotherapy.

  1. Insulin: Mainstay of therapy.

   a. Initiate therapy using a 0.3 units/kg/d total daily dose.

   b. Follow the 50/50 Rule.

    i. Give one-half of the total daily dose as basal insulin (long-acting insulin).

    ii. Give one-half of the total daily dose as prandial insulin divided evenly between three meals (usually rapid-acting or short-acting insulin).

    iii. Add a gentle correction scale using the same rapid- or short-acting insulin in number 2. Using 1 unit for every 50 points of glucose is above 150 mg/dL.

   c. In the outpatient setting, the patient should learn carbohydrate counting, and then prandial insulin can be dosed as a ratio of 1 unit insulin to the number of grams of carbohydrates.

   d. Consider insulin pump therapy at some point in the future.

  2. Pramlintide.

   a. Delays gastric emptying, blunts secretion of glucagon, and enhances satiety.

   b. Approved by the Food and Drug Administration (FDA) for use in adults with type 1 diabetes; most helpful in treating these patients.

c. Helps with weight loss and reduces insulin dose.

D. Discharge instructions.

  1. Verify the patient's understanding of how to take medications as prescribed.

   a. Dose.

   b. Route.

   c. Frequency.

   d. Relationship to meals.

   e. Proper disposal of sharps.

   f. Rotation of sites for subcutaneous insulin injections.

   g. Need for refrigeration.

  2. Make sure the patient is familiar with dietary restrictions.

   a. The patient should aim for consistent amounts of carbohydrates per meal at first. Then the goal will be to learn to dose insulin to the amount of carbohydrates using carbohydrate counting.

  3. Be sure the patient knows when glucose monitoring is important.

   a. Before meals and bedtime.

   b. Before and after exercise.

   c. Before driving.

   d. More often as needed.

FOLLOW-UP

A. Recommend annual eye examination and podiatry examination.

B. Recommend outpatient education if appropriate.

C. Follow up with an endocrinologist or primary care provider (PCP). Specify how soon the patient should be seen. Specify when to call their provider.

D. Outline hypoglycemia treatment.

  1. Rule of 15:15 g of simple carbohydrates every 15 minutes until glucose is above 70 mg/dL (e.g., ½ cup juice, ½ cup sugared soda, glucose gel, glucose tablets).

  2. Carry glucose tablets or gel at all times.

  3. Instruct the patient to carry a glucagon kit that can be administered by a friend or family member if the patient is unresponsive.

CONSULTATION/REFERRAL

A. Refer the patient to endocrinology for new diagnosis, uncontrolled HgbA1C, multiple complications of diabetes, or comorbid conditions affecting diabetes control.

B. Refer the patient to nephrology for nephropathy.

C. Refer the patient to ophthalmology for yearly eye examination.

D. Refer the patient to podiatry for issues and/or yearly examination.

E. Refer the patient to a dentist (periodontal check, dental cleaning twice a year).

F. Refer the patient to psychology for coping with chronic disease.

SPECIAL/GERIATRIC CONSIDERATIONS

A. Pregnancy.

  1. Retinopathy risk: Counsel the patient on the risk of development or progression of retinopathy. Dilated ▶

eye examination should ideally occur preconception, each trimester, and 1 year postpartum.

2. Potentially teratogenic medications should be stopped.

3. Measurements of fasting and postprandial glucose are recommended.

4. HgbA1C is lower during pregnancy. The target in pregnancy is 6% to 6.5%.

5. Glycemic targets.
   a. Fasting 95 mg/dL or lower.
   b. 1-hour postprandial 140 mg/dL or lower.
   c. 2-hour postprandial 120 mg/dL or lower.

6. Changes in insulin requirements (Table 8.1).
   a. First trimester.
   b. Second trimester.
   c. Third trimester.

7. Labor and delivery: Use regular insulin IV infusion and immediate postpartum until glucose is stable.

8. Postpartum care.
   a. Insulin sensitivity increases with delivery and returns to prepregnancy levels over 1 to 2 weeks.
   b. Prevention of hypoglycemia induced by breastfeeding, erratic sleep, and eating that occurs postpartum.

B. Geriatric.

1. Determine glycemic goals based on expected life span, comorbid conditions, and ability of the patient to self-manage the disease.

2. Use hypoglycemia prevention.

CASE SCENARIO: DIABETES MELLITUS TYPE 1

Steven is a 19-year-old male who presents with recent history of unintentional weight loss, vomiting, diarrhea, abdominal pain, and fatigue. The patient endorsed feeling excessively thirsty and frequent urination. He denied fever, chest pain, shortness of breath, abdominal pain, recent trauma, and recent illness. His physical exam was not significant. The patient's EKG was within normal limits (WNL). Chest x-ray (CXR) was also WNL. Urine analysis was positive for glucose and ketones. Pulmonary hypertension (PH) was noncontributory. His blood pressure (BP) was 122/74, pulse 103, respirations 22, and temperature 97.1°F/36.1°C. Labs included sodium of 138 mEq/L, potassium of 4.9, blood urea nitrogen (BUN) of 32, creatinine (Cr) of 1.3, and hemoglobin of 15 g/dL.

1. What is present on admission that would favor a diagnosis of type 1 diabetes versus type 2 diabetes?
   A. Abdominal pain and fatigue
   B. Polydipsia and polyuria
   C. Weight loss and ketonuria
   D. Tachycardia and afebrile

2. Which hemoglobin A1C (HgbA1C) level is a diagnostic confirmation of diabetes mellitus?
   A. Less than 5.7
   B. 5.7 to 6.4
   C. Greater than or equal to 6.5
   D. Greater than 8

3. Treatment of type 1 diabetes includes healthy eating, increased activity, and tight glucose control with:
   A. Metformin.
   B. Insulin.
   C. Glucose tablets.
   D. Steroids.

4. Insulin administration should follow which rule?
   A. The Golden Rule
   B. The 50/50 Rule
   C. The Dawn Effect Rule
   D. The Rule of 9s.

BIBLIOGRAPHY

Cefalu, W. T. (2017). Standards of medical care in diabetes–2017. *Diabetes Care, 40*(Suppl. 1), s1–s135. https://doi.org/10.2337/dc17-S003

Lyons, F., & Ousley, L. (2015). *Dermatology for the advanced practice nurse* (p. 55). Springer Publishing Company.

Menke, A., Orchard, T., Imperatore, G., Bullard, K., Mayer-Davis, E., & Cowie, C. (2013). The prevalence of type 1 diabetes in the United States. *Epidemiology, 24,* 773–774. https://doi.org/10.1097/EDE.0b013e31829ef01a

Mensing, C. (2011). *The art and science of diabetes self-management education desk reference* (2nd ed.). American Association of Diabetes Educators.

Statistics About Diabetes. (n.d.). http://www.diabetes.org/diabetes-basics/statistics/

DIABETES MELLITUS: TYPE 2

Marissa E. Luft

DEFINITION
A. Relative (rather than absolute) insulin deficiency and peripheral insulin resistance.
B. Previously referred to as noninsulin-dependent diabetes or adult-onset diabetes.

INCIDENCE
A. Accounts for 90% to 95% of all cases of diabetes.
B. According to the 2017 Centers for Disease Control and Prevention's National Diabetes Statistics Report, an estimated 30.3 million Americans or 9.4% of the population had diabetes in 2015 (Table 8.2).

TABLE 8.1   CHANGING INSULIN REQUIREMENTS DURING PREGNANCY

Trimester	First	Second	Third
Insulin requirements	Woman often has decrease in total daily insulin requirements. Woman may experience increased hypoglycemia.	Woman often has rapidly increasing insulin resistance with need for weekly insulin dose adjustments.	Woman often has a leveling off of insulin requirements or a small decrease.

TABLE 8.2   ESTIMATED NUMBER AND PERCENTAGE OF DIAGNOSED AND UNDIAGNOSED DIABETES AMONG ADULTS AGED 18 YEARS AND OLDER, UNITED STATES, 2015

Characteristics	Diagnosed Diabetes Number in Millions (95% CI)[a]	Undiagnosed Diabetes Number in Millions (95% CI)[a]	Total Diabetes Number in Millions (95% CI)[a]
Total	23.0 (21.1–25.1)	7.2 (6.0–8.6)	30.2 (27.9–32.7)
Age in Years			
18–44	3.0 (2.6–3.6)	1.6 (1.1–2.3)	4.6 (3.8–5.5)
45–64	10.7 (9.3–12.2)	3.6 (2.8–4.6)	14.3 (12.7–16.1)
65	9.9 (9.0–11.0)	2.1 (1.4–3.0)	12.0 (10.7–13.4)
Sex			
Female	11.7 (10.5–13.1)	3.1 (2.4–4.1)	14.9 (13.5–16.4)
Male	11.3 (10.2–12.4)	4.0 (3.0–5.5)	15.3 (13.8–17.0)
	Percentage (95% CI)[b]	**Percentage (95% CI)[b]**	**Percentage (95% CI)[b]**
Total	9.3 (8.5–10.1)	2.9 (2.4–3.5)	12.2 (11.3–13.2)
Age in Years			
18–44	2.6 (2.2–3.1)	1.3 (0.9–2.0)	4.0 (3.3–4.8)
45–64	12.7 (11.1–14.5)	4.3 (3.3–5.5)	17.0 (15.1–19.1)
65	20.8 (18.8–23.0)	4.4 (3.1–6.3)	25.2 (22.5–28.1)
Sex			
Female	9.2 (8.2–10.3)	2.5 (1.9–3.2)	11.7 (10.6–12.9)
Male	9.4 (8.5–10.3)	3.4 (2.5–4.6)	12.7 (11.5–14.1)

[a]Numbers for subgroups may not add up to the total due to rounding.
[b]Data are crude, not age-adjusted.
Sources: From 2011–2014 National Health and Nutrition Examination Survey and 2015 U.S. Census Bureau data; National Center for Chronic Disease Prevention and Health Promotion. (2017). *National diabetes statistics report, 2017: Estimates of diabetes and its burden in the United States.* https://www.cdc.gov/diabetes/pdfs/data/statistics/national-diabetes-statistics-report.pdf.

C. In 2015, an estimated 1.5 million new cases of diabetes were diagnosed among U.S. adults older than 18 years.
D. Diabetes was the seventh leading cause of death in 2015.
E. Prevalence varies among different ethnicities (Table 8.3).

PATHOGENESIS
A. Specific etiologies are not known. There is no autoimmune destruction of beta cells.
B. Excess weight causes insulin resistance. Most patients with type 2 diabetes are overweight or obese.
C. Abdominal obesity contributes to increased risk.
D. Ketoacidosis seldom occurs.
E. Hyperglycemia develops gradually; it is often undiagnosed for years before the official diagnosis is made.
F. Insulin secretion is defective and unable to compensate for increased insulin resistance.

PREDISPOSING FACTORS
A. Age; risk is higher as age increases.
B. Obesity, with body mass index (BMI) greater than or equal to 25 kg/m².
C. Lack of physical activity.
D. Women with prior gestational diabetes.
E. History of prediabetes.
F. History of metabolic syndrome.
G. Comorbidities of hypertension and dyslipidemia.
H. Higher rates in certain populations.
  1. African American.
  2. American Indian.
  3. Hispanic or Latino.
  4. Asian American.
I. Strong genetic predisposition.
J. Medications.
  1. Glucocorticoids.
  2. Thiazide diuretics.
  3. Atypical antipsychotics.

TABLE 8.3 PREVALENCE OF DIAGNOSED AND UNDIAGNOSED DIABETES AMONG ADULTS AGED 18 YEARS AND OLDER, UNITED STATES, 2011–2014

Characteristics	Diagnosed Diabetes Percentage (95% CI)	Undiagnosed Diabetes Percentage (95% CI)	Total Percentage (95% CI)
Total	8.7 (8.1–9.4)	2.7 (2.3–3.3)	11.5 (10.7–12.4)
Race/Ethnicity			
Asian, non-Hispanic	10.3 (8.6–12.4)	5.7 (4.0–8.2)	16.0 (13.6–18.9)
Black, non-Hispanic	13.4 (12.2–14.6)	4.4 (3.0–6.2)	17.7 (15.8–19.9)
Hispanic	11.9 (10.3–13.7)	4.5 (3.2–6.2)	16.4 (14.1–18.9)
White, non-Hispanic	7.3 (6.6–8.1)	2.0 (1.5–2.6)	9.3 (8.4–10.2)

Source: From 2011–2014 National Health and Nutrition Examination Survey; National Center for Chronic Disease Prevention and Health Promotion. (2017). *National diabetes statistics report, 2017: Estimates of diabetes and its burden in the United States.* https://www.cdc.gov/diabetes/pdfs/data/statistics/national-diabetes-statistics-report.pdf.

SUBJECTIVE DATA

A. Common complaints/symptoms.
　1. Polyuria.
　2. Blurred vision.
　3. Polydipsia.
　4. Malaise/fatigue.
　5. Frequent urinary tract infections (UTIs) or vaginal candidiasis.
　6. Poor wound healing.
B. Common/typical scenario.
　1. Patients frequently complain of fatigue and weakness. They may have muscle cramps, blurred vision, and significant polyuria, polydipsia, and polyphagia.
　2. Weight loss occurs over time despite normal or increased appetite.
C. Family and social history.
　1. Ask about family history since there is a strong link to family history.
　2. Ask about type of occupation, if the person is a shift worker, use of alcohol, smoking, or recreational drug use.
　3. Review how much exercise the person gets.
D. Review of systems.
　1. Head, ear, eyes, nose, and throat (HEENT).
　　a. Dental issues: Periodontal disease is associated with diabetes.
　2. Psychological.
　　a. Depression.
　　b. Anxiety.
　　c. Disordered eating.
　　d. Psychosocial barriers/support.
　　e. Barriers to self-management.
　3. Microvascular complications.
　　a. Neuropathy.
　　b. Nephropathy.
　　c. Retinopathy.
　4. Macrovascular complications.
　　a. Coronary artery disease (CAD).
　　b. Cerebrovascular disease.
　　c. Peripheral arterial disease.

PHYSICAL EXAMINATION

A. Height, weight, BMI, and waist circumference.
B. Vital signs.
C. Funduscopic examination.
D. Thyroid palpation.
E. Skin examination.
　1. Acanthosis nigricans (see Figure 8.1).
　2. Lipohypertrophy.
　3. Diabetic dermopathy.
　4. Skin tags.
F. Foot examination.
　1. Inspection, noting mycotic changes to nail or skin.
　2. Vascular examination.
　　a. Hair patterns or lack of hair growth.
　　b. Pulses (dorsalis pedis and posterior tibial).
　　c. Temperature/color.
　3. Reflexes.
　　a. Patellar.
　　b. Achilles.
　4. Proprioception, vibration, and monofilament sensation.

DIAGNOSTIC TESTS

A. Hemoglobin A1C (HgbA1C), fasting glucose, random glucose, or 2-hour glucose tolerance test (GTT) to diagnose.
　1. HgbA1C greater than 6.5%.
　2. Fasting glucose greater than 126 mg/dL.
　3. Random glucose greater than 200 mg/dL with classic symptoms of hyperglycemia.
　4. 2-hour GTT greater than 200 mg/dL.
B. HgbA1C on admission to hospital if no result available for the past 3 months.
C. Yearly lab work for patients with diabetes.
　1. Fasting lipid panel.
　2. Liver function tests.
　3. Urine albumin to creatinine ratio.
　4. Serum creatinine and glomerular filtration rate (GFR).

DIFFERENTIAL DIAGNOSIS

A. Prediabetes.

B. Metabolic syndrome.
C. Stress hyperglycemia.
D. Medication-induced hyperglycemia.
E. Posttransplant diabetes.
F. Maturity-onset diabetes of the young (MODY) type diabetes.
G. Latent autoimmune diabetes.
H. Type 1 diabetes.
I. Ketosis-prone diabetes.
J. Pancreatitis.
K. Pancreatic insufficiency.

EVALUATION AND MANAGEMENT PLAN

A. General plan.
  1. The recommended outpatient comprehensive treatment plan most helpful in treating type 2 diabetes according to the American Association of Diabetes Educators consists of the following seven self-care behaviors:
    a. Healthy eating: The patient should see a registered dietitian for medical nutrition therapy counseling.
    b. Being active: At least 150 minutes of moderate-to vigorous-intensity physical activity spread out over a week. This can include resistance exercises and flexibility exercises.
    c. Glucose monitoring.
      i. Oral agents recommended one to two times a day before meals; can vary which meals.
      ii. Insulin recommended before meals and bedtime.
    d. Medications: Oral agents, insulin, and non-insulin (injectable).
      i. Delivery method options: Insulin pen, vial and syringe, and pump.
      ii. Proper storage.
      iii. Preparation, administration, and site rotation.
      iv. Disposal of sharps.
      v. Hypoglycemia symptoms.
    e. Problem-solving.
    f. Healthy coping.
    g. Reducing risks.
B. Patient/family teaching points.
  1. Inpatient education focuses on survival skills only.
    a. Checking glucose.
    b. Taking medications.
    c. Diet.
    d. Hypoglycemia treatment.
  2. Outpatient education is more comprehensive and uses the guidelines by the American Association of Diabetes Educators to direct the education. The patient should be referred to outpatient diabetes education at the time of diagnosis, yearly thereafter, and as needed or if therapy changes.
C. Pharmacotherapy.
  1. Oral agents (Table 8.4).
    a. Metformin: First-line agent.
    b. Sulfonylureas such as glimepiride.
    c. Meglitinides such as repaglinide.
    d. Thiazolidinediones such as pioglitazone.

    e. Alpha glucosidase inhibitors such as acarbose.
    f. Dipeptidyl peptidase-4 (DPP-4) inhibitors such as sitagliptin.
    g. Sodium-glucose cotransporter-2 (SGLT2) inhibitors such as canagliflozin.
    h. Glucagon-like peptide-1 (GLP-1) receptor agonists such as exenatide.
  2. Insulin.
    a. Mainstay of therapy in hospital.
    b. Initiate therapy using one of three different calculations.
      i. For renal patients or those new to insulin, start with 0.3 units/kg/d total daily dose.
      ii. For most patients, start with 0.5 units/kg/d total daily dose.
      iii. For obese patients, insulin-resistant patients, or those on steroids, start with 0.7 units/kg/d total daily dose.
    c. The 50/50 Rule.
      i. Give one-half of the total daily dose as basal insulin (glargine, detemir, degludec).
      ii. Give one-half of the total daily dose as prandial insulin divided evenly between three meals (lispro, aspart, glulisine).
      iii. Add a correction scale using the same rapid-acting insulin used previously.
D. Discharge instructions.
  1. Verify the patient understands how to take the medication as prescribed.
    a. Dose.
    b. Route.
    c. Frequency.
    d. Relationship to meals.
    e. Proper disposal of sharps (for injectables).
    f. Rotation of sites for subcutaneous injections.
    g. Storage.
  2. Make sure the patient is familiar with dietary restrictions.
    a. The patient should aim for consistent amounts of carbohydrates per meal at first. Then the goal will be to learn to dose insulin to the amount of carbohydrates using carbohydrate counting.
  3. Verify the patient is familiar with how to monitor glucose on an ongoing basis.
    a. For oral agents that do not typically cause hypoglycemia.
      i. One to two times a day before meals; can vary which meal.
      ii. Also acceptable: Have HgbA1C checked every 3 to 6 months with their provider as an alternative to checking daily.
    b. For oral agents that can cause hypoglycemia.
      i. Consider initially checking glucose before each meal.
      ii. After a period of time, the patient may go to one to two times a day.
    c. For noninsulin injectable agents such as exenatide.
      i. One to two times a day (hypoglycemia is rare).
    d. For insulin.

TABLE 8.4   ORAL AGENTS USED TO TREAT DIABETES

Oral Agent	Side Effects	Benefits and Considerations
Metformin (first-line agent)	GI side effects; start low and go slow in titrating up dose Extended-release form used to prevent GI side effects	Benefits ■ Inexpensive ■ Does not lead to hypoglycemia Considerations ■ Renally cleared ■ Generally stop when hospitalized ■ Possible vitamin B_{12} deficiency when used long term ■ Lactic acidosis risk (rare: 1/30,000 patients) ■ Contraindications: Estimated GFR <30 mL/min/1.73 m², use with caution if estimated GFR <30 mL/min/1.73 m², acidosis, hypoxemia, and alcohol abuse
Sulfonylureas such as glimepiride	Can cause hypoglycemia Can cause weight gain	Benefits ■ Inexpensive Considerations ■ Hepatically metabolized ■ Renally cleared ■ Caution required in renal and cardiac patients; have active metabolites • Generally stopped while in hospital
Meglitinides such as repaglinide	Short action reduction in postprandial glucose May cause hypoglycemia	Benefits ■ Moderate cost ■ Can use in hospital ■ Effective treatment for steroid-induced hyperglycemia, such as once-a-day prednisone Considerations ■ Hepatically metabolized ■ Renally cleared ■ Frequent dosing
Thiazolidinediones such as pioglitazone	Edema/weight gain/CHF exacerbation Contraindicated in New York Heart Association classes III and IV heart failure Increased risk of MI in rosiglitazone; risk has not been shown in pioglitazone	Benefits ■ Does not cause hypoglycemia ■ Inexpensive Considerations ■ Not used in hospital ■ Delayed onset: Can take up to 12 weeks to achieve peak effect
Alpha glucosidase inhibitors such as acarbose	GI side effects: Gradual dose titration helps prevent	Benefits ■ Minimal systemic absorption ■ Marked reduction in MI rates ■ Moderate cost Considerations ■ Not used in hospital ■ Frequent dosing
DPP-4 inhibitors such as sitagliptin	Minimal side effects Rarely causes hypoglycemia	Benefits ■ Good oral agent for hospital use Considerations ■ Renal dose adjustment (except for linagliptin) ■ Contraindicated in patients with history of pancreatitis ■ High cost

(continued)

TABLE 8.4 ORAL AGENTS USED TO TREAT DIABETES (*CONTINUED*)

Oral Agent	Side Effects	Benefits and Considerations
SGLT2 inhibitors such as canagliflozin	Causes glucosuria Increased risk of genitourinary infections Polyuria, especially when also on diuretics Can cause volume depletion, dehydration, dizziness, and hypotension Cases of DKA	Benefits ■ Shown to improve cardiovascular disease outcomes ■ Empagliflozin (Jardiance) considered best at reducing cardiovascular events Considerations ■ Not for use in hospital ■ High cost
GLP-1 receptor agonists such as exenatide	Once-a-week preparations Prolonged decreased appetite may occur in patients taking these preparations who are admitted to the hospital because medication is likely still having an effect.	Benefits ■ Can aid in weight loss ■ Can improve cardiovascular risk factors ■ Victoza (liraglutide) considered best at reducing cardiovascular events Considerations ■ Should not be used in patients with history of medullary thyroid cancer or history of pancreatitis ■ Use in the hospital is being studied, but not currently recommended ■ Use with narcotic pain medications: Ileus has occurred with GLP-1 receptor agonist use postoperatively in conjunction with narcotic pain medications. Patients should wait until off narcotic pain medications and having no issues with constipation.

CHF, congestive heart failure; DKA, diabetic ketoacidosis; DPP-4, dipeptidyl peptidase-4; GFR, glomerular filtration rate; GI, gastrointestinal; GLP-1, glucagon-like peptide-1; MI, myocardial infarction; SGLT2, sodium glucose cotransporter-2.

    i. Before meals and bedtime.
    ii. Before and after exercise.
    iii. Before driving.
    iv. More often as needed.

FOLLOW-UP

A. Recommend annual eye examination and podiatry examination.
B. Recommend outpatient education if appropriate.
C. Follow up with an endocrinologist or primary care provider (PCP). Specify how soon the patient should be seen. Specify when to call their provider.
D. Outline hypoglycemia treatment.
    1. Rule of 15:15 grams of carbohydrates every 15 minutes until glucose above 70 mg/dL (e.g., ½ cup pop, ½ cup juice, glucose gel, glucose tablets).
    2. Carry glucose tablets or gel at all times.
    3. Instruct the patient (if on insulin) to carry a glucagon kit that can be administered by a friend or family member if the patient is unresponsive.

CONSULTATION/REFERRAL

A. Refer the patient to endocrinology for new diagnosis, uncontrolled HgbA1C, multiple complications of diabetes, and comorbid conditions affecting diabetes control.
B. Refer the patient to nephrology for nephropathy.

C. Refer the patient to ophthalmology every 2 years if negative examinations.
D. Refer the patient to podiatry for issues and/or yearly examination.
E. Refer the patient to a dentist for evaluation of gums and oral health problems associated with diabetes, such as xerostomia, gingivitis, or signs of infection.
F. Refer the patient to psychology for coping with chronic disease.

SPECIAL/GERIATRIC CONSIDERATIONS

A. More than 25% of the U.S. population older than 65 years have diabetes.
B. Diabetes in older adults is associated with higher mortality and reduced functional status.
C. Older adults with diabetes have a higher risk of microvascular and cardiovascular complications of the disease.

CASE SCENARIO: DIABETES MELLITUS TYPE 2

Bette is a 78-year-old female who presents to her primary care provider (PCP) with complaints of increased thirst, frequent non-painful urination, fatigue, intermittent nausea and abdominal pain, nonspecific chest pain, and weight gain. The patient states she has been experiencing these symptoms for a few months. The patient's point-of-care (POC) blood glucose (BG) was 245

(continued)

mg/dL in the PCP office. With the presence of chest pain and elevated BG, the patient's PCP recommends evaluation in the ED. The patient is awake, alert, and oriented on arrival to the ED. EKG, urinalysis (UA), and bloodwork were obtained. EKG was within normal limits, ruling out myocardial infarction (MI). Bloodwork is concerning for hemoglobin A1C (HgbA1C) of 7% and serum glucose of 302 mg/dL. UA was positive for glucose and negative for leukocytes and ketones. PH: Hypertension, obesity, and hypothyroidism. Objective: Blood pressure (BP) 162/74, pulse 98, respirations 26, and temperature 98.1. Lab: Sodium 139 mEq/L, potassium 5, glucose (serum) 302 mg/dL, blood urea nitrogen (BUN) 55 mg/dL, and Cr 1.5 mg/dL.

1. Which piece of data suggests a diagnosis of type 2 diabetes, as opposed to type 1 diabetes?
   A. Serum glucose 302 mg/dL
   B. Absences of ketones in UA
   C. Elevated blood pressure
   D. Elevated Cr

2. Type 2 diabetes accounts for what percentage of diabetes cases in the United States?
   A. Less than 10%
   B. Greater than 50%
   C. Greater than 90%
   D. 1 in every 4

3. Which medication is considered the first-line agent for newly diagnosed type 2 diabetes?
   A. Insulin
   B. Metformin
   C. Sulfonylureas
   D. Thiazolidinediones

4. Patients with diabetes can be prone to hypoglycemic events secondary to medication side effects or alterations in normal state of health. When educating patients about prevention and treatment for hypoglycemic events, include:
   A. The 50/50 Rule.
   B. Rule of 9s.
   C. Rule of 15.
   D. Health Insurance Portability and Accountability Act (HIPAA) rules.

BIBLIOGRAPHY

Cefalu, W. T. (2017). Standards of medical care in diabetes–2017. *Diabetes Care, 40*(Suppl. 1), s1–s135. https://doi.org/10.2337/dc17-S003

Garber, A. J., Abrahamson, M. J., Barzilay, J. I., Blonde, L., Bloomgarden, Z. T., Bush, M. A., Dagogo-Jack, S., DeFronzo, R. A., Einhorn, D., Fonseca, V. A., Garber, J. R., Garvey, W. T., Grunberger, G., Handelsman, Y., Hirsch, I. B., Jellinger, P. S., McGill, J. B., Mechanick, J. I., Rosenblit, P. D., & Umpierrez, G. E. (2017). Consensus statement by the American Association of Clinical Endocrinologists and American College of Endocrinology on the comprehensive type 2 diabetes management algorithm—2017 executive summary. *Endocrine Practice, 23*(2), 207–238. https://doi.org/10.4158/EP161682.CS

Menke, A., Orchard, T., Imperatore, G., Bullard, K., Mayer-Davis, E., & Cowie, C. (2013). The prevalence of type 1 diabetes in the United States. *Epidemiology, 24,* 773–774. https://doi.org/10.1097/EDE.0b013e31829ef01a

Mensing, C. (2011). *The art and science of diabetes self-management education desk reference* (2nd ed.). Publisher American Association of Diabetes Educators.

National Center for Chronic Disease Prevention and Health Promotion. (2017). *National diabetes statistics report, 2017: Estimates of diabetes and its burden in the United States.* https://www.cdc.gov/diabetes/pdfs/data/statistics/national-diabetes-statistics-report.pdf

Statistics About Diabetes. (n.d.). http://www.diabetes.org/diabetes-basics/statistics/

DIABETIC KETOACIDOSIS

Marissa E. Luft

DEFINITION
A. Life-threatening emergency.
B. Absolute insulin deficiency.
C. Severe hyperglycemia.
D. Ketone body production.
E. Systemic acidosis.
F. Develops over 1 to 2 days.

INCIDENCE
A. 18% of cases of diabetic ketoacidosis (DKA) in hospitals are children with type 1 diabetes.
B. 48% of cases of DKA in hospitals are adults with type 1 diabetes.
C. 34% of cases of DKA in hospitals are adults with type 2 diabetes.
D. Higher rate of DKA for persons age less than 45.
E. One to five episodes per 100 people per year.
F. Average mortality is 5% to 10%.

PATHOGENESIS
A. Unchecked gluconeogenesis leads to hyperglycemia.
   1. Increased glucose production.
   2. Decreased glucose uptake.
B. Osmotic diuresis leads to dehydration.
C. Unchecked ketogenesis leads to ketosis.
D. Dissociation of ketone bodies into hydrogen ions and anions leads to anion gap metabolic acidosis; electrolyte abnormalities.

PREDISPOSING FACTORS
A. Illness/infection.
B. Myocardial infarction (MI)/cerebrovascular accident (CVA).
C. Omission of insulin.
D. Minority populations.
E. Newly diagnosed with type 1 diabetes.
F. Poor social support.
G. Mental illness.

SUBJECTIVE DATA
A. Common complaints/symptoms.
   1. Thirst.
   2. Polyuria.
   3. Abdominal pain.
   4. Nausea and vomiting.
   5. Profound weakness.
   6. Fatigue.
   7. Dyspnea.

▶

B. Common/typical scenario.
  1. Patients with any form of diabetes who present with certain symptoms should be evaluated for DKA. These symptoms are abdominal pain, nausea, fatigue, and/or dyspnea.

PHYSICAL EXAMINATION
A. Fruity breath.
B. Vital sign assessment.
  1. Kussmaul respirations.
  2. Supine or orthostatic hypotension.
  3. Diminished peripheral pulses.
  4. Tachycardia.
  5. Hypothermia.
C. Skin examination.
  1. Dry mucous membranes.
  2. Poor skin turgor.

DIAGNOSTIC TESTS
A. Glucose usually greater than 250 mg/dL.
B. Positive blood and urine ketones.
C. Elevated beta hydroxybutyrate.
D. High anion gap (>12 mEq/L).
E. Low arterial pH (<7.3).
F. Low bicarbonate (<15 mEq/L).
G. Serum hyperosmolality greater than 280 mOsm/L.

DIFFERENTIAL DIAGNOSIS
A. Lactic acidosis.
B. Other metabolic acidosis.
C. Starvation ketosis secondary to ketogenic diet.
D. Euglycemic acidosis.
  1. Normal glucose.
  2. Clinical presentation of DKA.
  3. Seen with sodium-glucose cotransporter-2 (SGLT2) inhibitors.
E. Hyperglycemia without ketosis.
F. Hyperosmolar hyperglycemic syndrome.

EVALUATION AND MANAGEMENT PLAN
A. Fluid replacement.
  1. Normal saline (NS) 1 to 2 L over 1 to 2 hours.
  2. Calculation of corrected serum sodium.
   a. High or normal serum sodium: ½ NS at 250 to 500 mL/hr.
   b. Low serum sodium: NS at 250 to 500 mL/hr.
  3. When glucose less than 250 mg/dL: dextrose 5% in normal saline (D5%NS) or ½ NS.
  4. Suggested rate for fluid replacement:
   a. First hour: 1 to 2 L.
   b. Second hour: 1 L.
   c. Third to fifth hours: 500 to 1,000 mL/hr.
   d. Sixth to 12th hours: 250 to 500 mL/hr.
B. Correction of hyperglycemia/metabolic acidosis.
  1. Intravenous (IV) regular insulin infusion.
   a. Bolus: 0.1 to 0.15 units/kg.
   b. Drip rate: 0.1 units/kg/hr.
   c. Check glucose every hour.
    i. If glucose does not decrease by 10% in the first hour, a second loading dose is indicated.

    ii. When glucose is less than 250 mg/dL, slow rate to 0.05 to 1 units/kg/hr until resolution of ketoacidosis.
   d. Continue insulin infusion until anion gap closes (<14 mEq/L).
   e. Initiate subcutaneous basal insulin 2 hours prior to stopping drip.
   f. Refer to hospital DKA protocol.
  2. Acceptable to use subcutaneous insulin to treat DKA as well.
   a. Use insulin analogs: Lispro, aspart, or glulisine.
   b. Check glucose every 2 hours and give a bolus of analog.
    i. Initial dose 0.2 to 0.3 units/kg.
    ii. Then 0.1 to 0.2 units/kg every 2 hours until glucose less than 250 mg/dL.
    iii. When glucose is less than 250 mg/dL, add dextrose to IV fluids as earlier.
    iv. Continue to give 0.05 to 0.1 unit/kg every 2 hours until anion gap closes.
C. Replacement of electrolyte losses.
  1. Watch for life-threatening hypokalemia, which can occur as insulin is infused.
  2. Monitor potassium closely and treat potassium losses aggressively. Anticipatory potassium replacement during treatment of DKA is usually required.
   a. If potassium is greater than 5.5 mEq/L, then no supplementation is immediately required. Reassess within 2 to 4 hours.
   b. If potassium is 4 to 5.4 mEq/L, give 20 mEq of replacement potassium.
   c. If potassium is 3.3 to 4 mEq/L, give 40 mEq of replacement potassium.
   d. If potassium is less than 3.3 mEq/L, hold starting insulin until potassium is replaced. Give potassium 20 to 30 mEq/hr until potassium is greater than 3.3 mEq/L.
  3. A sharp drop in serum phosphorus can also occur with insulin infusion. Treatment is usually not required.
  4. Bicarbonate is not usually given unless pH is less than 7.0 mol/L.
D. Identification and treatment of precipitating causes.
  1. Non-adherence to insulin regimen or psychiatric issues.
  2. Insulin administration error or insulin pump malfunction.
  3. Poor insulin management during illness.
   a. Patients often omit insulin when not eating or having nausea or vomiting.
   b. Patients often forget to check their glucose levels when feeling ill.
  4. Infections.
   a. Intraabdominal.
   b. Pyelonephritis.
   c. Urinary tract infections (UTIs).
   d. Pneumonia.
   e. Influenza.
  5. MI.
  6. Pancreatitis.

7. Steroid therapy prescribed with no instructions about adjusting insulin.

8. CVA.

E. Conversion to a maintenance diabetes regimen; transition to subcutaneous insulin when glucose is less than 200 mg/dL and the anion gap is less than 14 mEq/L.

F. Patient/family teaching points.

1. Sick day management.

2. Survival skills.

3. Glucose monitoring.

4. Insulin administration.

5. Use of ketone strips.

6. Medical alert bracelet.

7. Preventing DKA.

   a. Recognizing signs and symptoms.

   b. Frequency of glucose testing.

   c. Urine ketone testing.

   d. When to call for help.

G. Discharge instructions.

1. Ensure the patient has prescriptions for insulin pen, insulin vial, and needles or syringes.

2. Ensure the patient has prescriptions for glucometer, test strips, and lancets.

3. Ensure the patient has ketone strips.

4. Confirm that a follow-up appointment has been made.

5. Give the patient their physician's contact phone numbers.

FOLLOW-UP

A. Follow-up should occur with the endocrinologist for a management plan to regulate diabetes.

B. Patients may need to follow up with social services for assistance with medications.

CONSULTATION/REFERRAL

A. Refer the patient to psychology/social work for assistance with purchasing medications and equipment and for emotional support.

B. Refer the patient to endocrinology for optimized management of diabetes.

SPECIAL/GERIATRIC CONSIDERATIONS

A. End-stage renal disease patients on dialysis.

1. Absence of osmotic diuresis.

2. Less volume depleted.

3. High serum potassium.

4. Insulin infusion: Only treatment required in a majority of patients.

5. Emergency hemodialysis: Possible treatment in cases where there is pulmonary edema, profound metabolic acidosis, or severe hyperkalemia with EKG changes.

B. DKA in pregnancy.

1. DKA can occur rapidly and at a much lower glucose level in pregnant women with diabetes compared with nonpregnant women with diabetes.

2. All of the effects of DKA on the fetus are not known. Ketoacids and glucose cross the placenta.

3. There is a direct relationship between plasma ketone levels in pregnant diabetic women and lower IQ levels in the child.

4. Presenting symptoms and treatment are the same as in women who are not pregnant.

5. Certain metabolic changes predispose to ketosis.

   a. Increased insulin resistance.

   b. Insulin requirements that rise during pregnancy.

   c. More cases of DKA in second and third trimesters.

6. Accelerated starvation.

   a. Use of large amounts of glucose for energy by the fetus/placenta.

   b. Lower maternal glucose, leading to relative insulin deficiency.

   c. Increase in free fatty acids, which undergo conversion to ketones in liver.

7. Emesis.

8. Stress and fasting state: Can increase insulin antagonistic hormones, which along with dehydration can promote development of ketosis.

9. Lowered buffering capacity.

10. Increased minute alveolar ventilation in pregnancy leading to respiratory alkalosis, which is compensated by increased renal excretion of bicarbonate.

CASE SCENARIO: DIABETIC KETOACIDOSIS

Anna is a 24-year-old female who presents to the ED with altered mental status and hyperglycemia. The patient's point-of-care (POC) blood glucose (BG) was 411 mg/dL. The patient is arousable, but lethargic. Her mother is at bedside. Her mother states that she had been sick with fever and vomiting for a few days prior to admission and that she had been drinking excessive amounts of electrolyte drinks to prevent dehydration. The patient's mother also reports that when she spoke to the patient today she was confused on the phone, so she drove to her home and found her with an altered mental status in bed and looking disheveled, prompting her to call 911. PH: Hypertension, diabetes mellitus type 1, and depression. Objective: Blood pressure 92/54, pulse 123, respirations 28, and temperature 99.1°F/37.3°C. Lab: Sodium 136 mEq/L, potassium 5.4, glucose (serum) 437 mg/dL, blood urea nitrogen (BUN) 35 mg/dL, Cr 1.6 mg/dL, and UA significant for a large amount of ketones.

1. In addition to urine analysis and serum glucose level, what other information helps establish a diagnosis of diabetic ketoacidosis (DKA) in insulin-dependent diabetes mellitus?

   A. Anion gap metabolic acidosis
   B. Anion gap metabolic alkalosis
   C. Anion gap respiratory acidosis
   D. Anion gap respiratory alkalosis

2. What treatment(s) should be started immediately for patients with diabetic ketoacidosis (DKA)?

   A. Bicarbonate infusion
   B. Intravenous (IV) fluids and insulin glucose tolerance test (GTT)
   C. Intubation and mechanical ventilation
   D. IV thiamine

3. Which population is at greatest risk for developing diabetic ketoacidosis (DKA)?

   A. Adults with type 1 diabetes
   B. Children with type 1 diabetes
   C. Adults with type 2 diabetes
   D. Adults >65 years old with type 2 diabetes

4. What is the typical range of blood glucose levels in patients with diabetic ketoacidosis (DKA)?
 A. Greater than 600 mg/dL
 B. Less than 200 mg/dL
 C. Less than 80 mg/dL
 D. Greater than 250 mg/dL

BIBLIOGRAPHY
Cefalu, W. T. (2017). Standards of medical care in diabetes–2017. *Diabetes Care, 40*(Suppl. 1), s1–s135. https://doi.org/10.2337/dc17-S003

Menke, A., Orchard, T., Imperatore, G., Bullard, K., Mayer-Davis, E., & Cowie, C. (2013). The prevalence of type 1 diabetes in the United States. *Epidemiology, 24,* 773–774. https://doi.org/10.1097/EDE.0b013e31829ef01a

Mensing, C. (2011). *The art and science of diabetes self-management education desk reference* (2nd ed.). Publisher American Association of Diabetes Educators.

Statistics About Diabetes. (n.d.). http://www.diabetes.org/diabetes-basics/statistics/

HYPERGLYCEMIC HYPEROSMOLAR STATE

Marissa E. Luft

DEFINITION
A. Severe relative insulin deficiency, resulting in profound hyperglycemia and hyperosmolality.
B. Absence of acidosis.
C. Develops over days to weeks.
D. Typically presents in type 2 diabetes or in patients with no prior diagnosis of diabetes.

INCIDENCE
A. Hyperglycemic hyperosmolar state (HHS) represents less than 1% of hospital admissions of patients with diabetes.
B. Mortality is between 10% and 20%, which is 10 times higher than mortality for diabetic ketoacidosis (DKA).
C. The condition has been reported in children and young adults.

PATHOGENESIS
A. Extreme elevations in glucose.
B. Insulin deficiency.
C. Increased levels of counterregulatory hormones.
 1. Glucagon.
 2. Catecholamines.
 3. Cortisol.
 4. Growth hormone.
D. Increased gluconeogenesis.
E. Decreased use of glucose by peripheral tissues.
F. Higher hepatic and circulating insulin concentrations as well as lower glucagon in HHS compared with DKA.
G. Prevention of ketogenesis.
H. Severe hyperglycemia is associated with a severe inflammatory state.

PREDISPOSING FACTORS
A. Older patients with type 2 diabetes.
B. Patients with more comorbidities.
C. Infection.
 1. Pneumonia.
 2. Urinary tract infection (UTI).
D. No prior diagnosis of diabetes.
E. Stroke.
F. Myocardial infarction (MI).
G. Trauma.
H. Medications.
 1. Glucocorticoids.
 2. Thiazide diuretics.
 3. Phenytoin (inhibits endogenous insulin secretion).
 4. Beta-blockers.
 5. Atypical antipsychotics.

SUBJECTIVE DATA
A. Common complaints/symptoms.
 1. Profound dehydration presenting as a shock-like state.
 2. Mental confusion.
 3. Thirst.
 4. Polyuria.
 5. Nausea and vomiting.
 6. Weakness and fatigue.

PHYSICAL EXAMINATION
A. Ill-appearing, likely with decreased level of consciousness.
B. Vital sign assessment.
 1. Tachycardia.
 2. Hypotension.
 3. Tachypnea.
 4. Decreased core temperature.
C. Neurologic findings. When HHS causes neurologic dysfunction, treatment of HHS results in resolution of neurologic findings. However, when neurologic events cause HHS the neurologic findings remain after resolution of HHS.
 1. Seizures.
 2. Drowsiness and lethargy.
 3. Delirium to coma.
 4. Hemianopsia.
 5. Aphasia.
 6. Paresis.
 7. Positive Babinski sign.
 8. Myoclonic jerks.
 9. Nystagmus.
D. Dermatologic findings.
 1. Acanthosis nigricans (see Figure 8.1).
 2. Diabetic dermopathy.
 3. Dry mucous membranes.
 4. Decreased skin turgor.
 5. Necrobiosis on pretibial surfaces.
E. Funduscopic examination.
 1. Retinopathy.
 2. Premature cataracts.
 3. Xanthelasma.
F. Decreased urine output.

DIAGNOSTIC TESTS
A. Plasma glucose: Greater than 600 mg/dL.
B. Arterial pH: Greater than 7.30 mol/L.

C. Serum bicarbonate: Greater than 18 mEq/L.
D. Urine or serum ketones: Absent or small.
E. Serum beta hydroxybutyrate: Less than 3 mmol/L.
F. Effective serum osmolality: Greater than 320 mOsm/L.
G. Anion gap variable.
H. Hemoglobin and hematocrit elevated due to volume contraction.
I. Leukocytosis usually present.
J. Hemoglobin A1C (HgbA1C).
K. Look for underlying cause using the following:
   1. Chest x-ray (CXR).
   2. Urine analysis.
   3. Blood and urine cultures.
   4. EKG.

DIFFERENTIAL DIAGNOSIS

A. DKA.
B. Hyperglycemia without DKA or HHS.
C. Dehydration.
D. Mental status changes or even coma.
E. Intoxication.
F. Sepsis.
G. Postictal state.
H. Diabetes insipidus.

EVALUATION AND MANAGEMENT PLAN

A. Replacement of fluids.
   1. Treatment of HHS requires more free water and greater volume replacement than in DKA: Can be as much as 10 L fluid deficit.
   2. Rapid and aggressive intravascular volume replacement is necessary.
     a. Use isotonic sodium chloride initially.
     b. Replace one-half of volume in the first 12 hours and then the remainder over the next 12-hour period.
     c. When glucose reaches 250 to 300 mg/dL, switch to D5%NS or ½ normal saline (NS).
   3. Use caution in patients with advanced age, heart failure, and kidney disease.
B. Correction of hyperglycemia.
   1. Use intravenous (IV) insulin or subcutaneous insulin in doses similar to DKA.
   2. Use of insulin without concomitant vigorous fluid replacement increases the risk of shock.
   3. Recheck glucose every 1 to 2 hours.
C. Replacement of electrolytes.
   1. Typically, potassium is not significantly elevated on admission.
   2. Replacement of potassium is required with use of insulin glucose tolerance test (GTT). Add potassium to IV fluids starting at 5 mEq/L or less.
   3. Recheck electrolytes every 2 to 4 hours, as clinically indicated.
   4. Phosphate, magnesium, and calcium are not routinely replaced.
D. Hospitalization.
   1. All patients diagnosed with HHS require hospitalization and virtually all require ICU admission.
   2. Neurologic monitoring, with "neuro" checks every 2 hours, is important.

E. Detection and treatment of underlying pathology.
   1. Some sources advocate prophylactic heparin treatment and broad-spectrum antibiotics until the underlying cause can be established.
F. Conversion to maintenance diabetes regimen prior to discharge.
   1. The patient's extreme hyperglycemia usually indicates extensive beta cell dysfunction.
   2. Initially patients require discharge on full insulin therapy.
   3. Use HgbA1C to help determine glucose control prior to admission.
   4. Make transition to subcutaneous insulin when glucose is less than 200 mg/dL and the anion gap is less than 14 mEq/L.
G. Patient/family teaching points.
   1. Sick day management.
   2. Survival skills.
   3. Glucose monitoring.
   4. Insulin administration.
   5. Medical alert bracelet.
H. Discharge instructions.
   1. Ensure that the patient has prescriptions for insulin pen, insulin vial, and needles or syringes.
   2. Ensure that the patient has prescriptions for glucometer, test strips, and lancets.
   3. Confirm that a follow-up appointment has been made.
   4. Give the patient their physician's contact phone numbers.

FOLLOW-UP

A. Follow-up should occur with the endocrinologist for a management plan to regulate diabetes.
B. Patients may need to follow up with social services for assistance with medications.

CONSULTATION/REFERRAL

A. Refer the patient to psychology for improving adherence to the diabetes regimen.
B. Refer the patient to social work and case management to assist with obtaining medications and resources as needed.

SPECIAL/GERIATRIC CONSIDERATIONS

A. Diabetes in older adults is associated with higher mortality and reduced functional status.
B. Older adults with diabetes have a higher risk of microvascular and cardiovascular complications of the disease.

CASE SCENARIO: HYPERGLYCEMIC HYPEROSMOLAR STATE

Harold is a 62-year-old male who presents to the ED after being found down at home by his wife. The patient's wife states he had complained of feeling "thirsty, foggy, and tired" for a few days prior to admission. The wife also states that the patient thought he was dehydrated from working outside in the garden. The patient is somnolent and unable to participate in the exam.

(continued)

The wife brought his medications from home and shows a bottle of metoprolol, Lipitor, Dilantin, and isosorbide. PH: Coronary artery disease (CAD), seizures, cerebrovascular accident (CVA), and hypertension. Objective: Blood pressure (BP) 92/64, pulse 58, respirations 12, and temperature 97.2°F/36.2°C. Lab: Sodium 152 mEq/L, potassium 3.2, glucose (serum) 957 mg/dL, blood urea nitrogen (BUN) 55 mg/dL, Cr 1.5 mg/dL, urinalysis positive glucose and ketones.

1. Which home medication would increase suspicion for the patient to be presenting with hyperglycemic hyperosmolar state (HHS)?
  A. Metoprolol
  B. Lipitor
  C. Dilantin
  D. Isosorbide

2. What differentiates the diagnosis of hyperglycemic hyperosmolar state (HHS) from diabetic ketoacidosis (DKA) in this patient?
  A. Blood glucose (BG) >800 and no ketones present in UA
  B. No known history of diabetes
  C. Medical history of hypertension
  D. Decreased level of consciousness

3. Which is the treatment for hyperglycemic hyperosmolar state (HHS)?
  A. Large-volume fluid replacement, bicarbonate glucose tolerance test (GTT), intravenous (IV) glucagon
  B. 2 units packed red blood cells (PRBCs), insulin GTT, IV albumin
  C. Large-volume fluid replacement, insulin GTT, electrolyte repletion
  D. Gentle fluid replacement, insulin GTT, IV thyroid hormone

4. Hyperglycemic hyperosmolar state onset:
  A. Is abrupt.
  B. Develops over months to years.
  C. Develops over days to week.
  D. Is a chronic condition.

BIBLIOGRAPHY

Azoulay, E., Chevret, S., Didier, J., Neuville, S., Barboteu, M., Bornstain, C., Darmon, M., Le Gall, J.-R., Vexiau, P., & Schlemmer, B. (2001). Infection as a trigger of diabetic ketoacidosis in intensive care unit patients. *Clinical Infectious Disease, 32*, 30–35. https://doi.org/10.1086/317554

Joint British Diabetes Societies Inpatient Care Group. (2010, March). *The management of diabetic ketoacidosis in adults.* http://www.diabetes.nhs.uk/document.php?o=1336

Kamalakannan, D., Baskar, V., & Barton, D. M. (2003). Diabetic ketoacidosis in pregnancy. *Postgraduate Medical Journal, 79*, 454–457. https://doi.org/10.1136/pmj.79.934.454

Kitabchi, A. E., Umpierrez, G. E., Murphy, M. B., Barrett, E. J., Kreisberg, R. A., Malone, J. I., & Wall, B. M. (2004, January). Hyperglycemic crises in diabetes. *Diabetes Care, 27*(Suppl. 1), S94–S102. https://doi.org/10.2337/diacare.27.2007.S94

Pasuel, F. J., & Umpierrez, G. E. (2014). Hyperosmolar hyperglycemic state: A historic review of the clinical presentation, diagnosis, and treatment. *Diabetes Care, 37*, 3124–3131. https://doi.org/10.2337/dc14-0984

Wordsworth, G., Robinson, A., Ward, A., & Atkin, M. (2014). HHS—Full or prophylactic anticoagulation? *British Journal of Diabetes and Vascular Disease, 14*, 64–66. https://doi.org/10.15277/bjdvd.2014.011

METABOLIC SYNDROME

Marissa E. Luft

DEFINITION
A. Also called insulin resistance syndrome.
B. A group of traits linked to obesity that put people at risk for both cardiovascular disease (CVD) and type 2 diabetes.
C. Must have three of the following:
  1. Waist circumference greater than 40 in. in men and greater than 35 in. in women (varies somewhat by ethnicity depending on which guidelines are used).
  2. Triglyceride level of 150 mg/dL or higher or taking medication for elevated triglyceride levels.
  3. High-density lipoprotein (HDL) below 40 mg/dL for men and below 50 mg/dL for women or taking medication for low HDL.
  4. Blood pressure (BP) above 130/85 mmHg or taking antihypertensives.
  5. Fasting glucose greater than 100 mg/dL or taking medication for elevated blood glucose (BG).
D. Linked to type 2 diabetes, obesity, CVD, polycystic ovarian syndrome, nonalcoholic fatty liver disease, and chronic kidney disease.
E. Patients with metabolic syndrome are at twice the risk of developing CVD over the next 5 to 10 years as individuals without the syndrome. The risk of developing diabetes is five times higher for individuals with metabolic syndrome.

INCIDENCE
A. About 34% of American adults are thought to have metabolic syndrome.
B. Risk increases as people age.
C. Prevalence is higher in non-Hispanic White men than Mexican American and non-Hispanic Black men.
D. The condition is more common in Mexican American women than non-Hispanic Black or non-Hispanic White women.
E. Prevalence is increasing globally due to increased obesity and sedentary lifestyles.

PATHOGENESIS
A. Contributing factors include increased free fatty acid levels, inflammatory cytokines from fat, and oxidative factors.
B. Patients with the characteristics of metabolic syndrome demonstrate a prothrombotic state and a proinflammatory state.
C. Elevated triglycerides and low HDL cholesterol are an atherogenic dyslipidemia condition.
D. The mechanism of how this constellation of risk factors contributes to the development of type 2 diabetes and CVD is not completely understood.

PREDISPOSING FACTORS
A. Sedentary lifestyle.
B. Western diet high in carbohydrates and fats, including saturated fats.
C. Obesity.

D. Family history of diabetes, heart disease, and hyperlipidemia.

SUBJECTIVE DATA

A. Typically, asymptomatic.
B. Patient presentation for a routine physical or a preoperative examination.

PHYSICAL EXAMINATION

A. Look for abdominal obesity: Record height, weight, body mass index (BMI), waist circumference, and waist to hip ratio.
B. Perform a thorough cardiovascular examination.
C. Note skin findings consistent with obesity and insulin resistance.
    1. Skin tags.
    2. Acanthosis nigricans (see Figure 8.1).
D. Note presence of xanthelasma on the medial aspect of eyelids, which is suggestive of hyperlipidemia.

DIAGNOSTIC TESTS

A. Fasting lipid panel.
B. Fasting glucose.

DIFFERENTIAL DIAGNOSIS

A. Type 2 diabetes.
B. Prediabetes.
C. Hyperlipidemia.
D. Hypertension.
E. Obesity.

EVALUATION AND MANAGEMENT PLAN

A. General plan.
    1. Treatment centers on two principles.
      a. Identify individuals with metabolic syndrome.
      b. Use risk factor modification to prevent CVD and type 2 diabetes.
B. Weight loss.
    1. Routinely measure weight and anthropometric measurements.
C. Healthy diet.
    1. Recommend saturated fat less than 7% of total calories.
    2. Reduce trans fats.
    3. Limit dietary cholesterol to less than 2,000 mg/d.
    4. Restrict total fat to 25% to 35% of total calories.
    5. Choose unsaturated fats.
    6. Limit simple sugars.
D. Increased physical activity.
    1. Encourage 30 to 60 minutes of moderate-intensity aerobic activity, preferably daily, supplemented by increase in daily lifestyle activities.
E. Monitoring of BG, lipoproteins, and BP.
F. Treatment of individual risk factors following guidelines for hypertension, hyperlipidemia, and hyperglycemia.
G. Smoking cessation.

FOLLOW-UP

A. Follow-up with primary care provider (PCP) to monitor underlying problems and to treat cardiovascular risk factors.

CONSULTATION/REFERRAL

A. Endocrinology to manage any underlying problems with diabetes.
B. Cardiology to manage cardiovascular risk factors.

SPECIAL/GERIATRIC CONSIDERATIONS

A. The risk of metabolic syndrome increases with age.
B. People with metabolic syndrome are at increased risk of CVDs.

CASE SCENARIO: METABOLIC SYNDROME

Maria is a 55-year-old female who presents to the ED with a chief complaint of palpitations. The patient states she has felt more fatigued and becomes short of breath and has palpitations with minimal activity. EKG and troponins were ordered to rule out myocardial infarction (MI). The patient's serum glucose level was 200. The patient stated she had been taking her insulin regularly and had not had anything to eat yet today. Due to elevated fasting glucose level and elevated blood pressure (BP) at the ED, the patient was admitted for further workup. PH: Hypertension, obesity, type 2 diabetes mellitus (T2DM), and hyperlipidemia. Objective: Blood pressure (BP) 172/86, pulse 110, respirations 22, and temperature 98.7°F/37.1°C. Height: 5 ft 4 in., weight: 138.63 kg, and body mass index (BMI): 52.3. Lab: sodium 136 mEq/L, potassium 5, glucose (serum) 200 mg/dL, blood urea nitrogen (BUN) 42 mg/dL, and Cr 1.3 mg/dL.

1. If the patient is a known type 2 diabetic and has been taking her insulin regularly, why is her fasting glucose elevated?
    A. Insulin resistance syndrome
    B. Myxedema coma
    C. Type 1 diabetes mellitus
    D. Hypertension

2. Which three criteria for diagnosis of metabolic syndrome does this patient present with?
    A. Blood pressure (BP) 172/86, fasting glucose 200, type 2 diabetes mellitus (DM2)
    B. Height <5'5", Cr >0.9, fasting glucose >100
    C. Dyspnea, palpitations, fatigue
    D. Female, elevated blood urea nitrogen (BUN), body mass index (BMI) >50

3. Which is considered the first-line treatment for metabolic syndrome?
    A. Diet and lifestyle modifications
    B. Insulin
    C. Hemodialysis
    D. Aspirin

4. Which age group is at greatest risk for developing metabolic syndrome?
    A. Adolescents
    B. 18 to 24 years old
    C. 45 to 60 years old
    D. >65 years old

BIBLIOGRAPHY

Aguilar, M., Bhuket, T., & Torres, S. (2015). Prevalence of the metabolic syndrome in the United States, 2003–2012. *Journal of the American Medical Association, 313*, 1973–1974. https://doi.org/10.1001/jama.2015.4260

Alberti, K. G., Eckel, R. H., Grundy, S. M., Zimmet, P. Z., Cleeman, J. I., Donato, K. A., Fruchart, J.-C., Philip, W., James, T., Loria, C. M., & Smith, S. C., Jr. (2009). Harmonizing the metabolic syndrome: A joint interim statement of the International Diabetes Federation Task Force on Epidemiology and Prevention; National Heart, Lung, and Blood Institute; American Heart Association; World Heart Federation; International Atherosclerosis Society; and International Association for the Study of Obesity. *Circulation, 120,* 1640–1645. https://doi.org/10.1161/CIRCULATIONAHA.109.192644

American Association of Diabetes Educators. (2008). AADE7 self-care behaviors. *Diabetes Educator, 24,* 445–449.

American Diabetes Association. (2010, January). Diagnosis and classification of diabetes mellitus. *Diabetes Care, 33*(Suppl. 1), S62–S69. https://doi.org/10.2337/dc10-S062

American Diabetes Association. (2012, January). Standards of medical care in diabetes—2012. *Diabetes Care, 35*(Suppl. 1), S11–S63. https://doi.org/10.2337/dc12-s011

American Diabetes Association Professional Practice Committee. (2013, January). American Diabetes Association clinical practice recommendations: 2013. *Diabetes Care, 36*(Suppl. 1), S1–S110.

PHEOCHROMOCYTOMA

Kathryn Evans Kreider

DEFINITION
A. A catecholamine-secreting tumor that typically produces one or more of the following hormones: Epinephrine, norepinephrine, or dopamine.
B. Cardiovascular morbidity and mortality may be high for undiagnosed pheochromocytomas (PCCs) due to catecholamine secretion.
C. PCCs enlarge over time and may cause mass effect if undiagnosed.
D. Paraganglioma is the term used to describe a catecholamine-secreting tumor that exists outside of the adrenal gland, while PCC is a catecholamine-secreting tumor inside the adrenal gland.

INCIDENCE
A. 0.2% to 0.6% of patients in an outpatient setting with hypertension have a PCC.
B. Autopsy studies suggest that 0.05% to 1% of patients have undiagnosed PCCs.
C. Peak incidence is between the fourth and fifth decades of life.
D. Approximately 5% of adrenal incidentalomas are PCCs and 10% to 17% of PCCs may be malignant.
E. PCC should be considered in the workup for malignant hypertension, particularly when the patient reports paroxysmal symptoms, has an adrenal incidentaloma, or has a hereditary predisposition to PCC.

PATHOGENESIS
A. Catecholamine-producing neuroendocrine tumors arising from the adrenomedullary chromaffin cells.
B. Germline mutations: Present in at least one-third of patients presenting with PCC.
C. PCCs may be related to a hereditary condition.

PREDISPOSING FACTORS
A. 30% of patients have a PCC as part of a genetic disorder.
B. Several genetic conditions predispose patients to PCC, including:

1. Multiple endocrine neoplasia (MEN) type 2A.
2. MEN type 2B.
3. Von Hippel–Lindau syndrome.
4. Neurofibromatosis type 1.

SUBJECTIVE DATA
A. Common complaints/symptoms.
　1. Signs and symptoms are present in about 50% of patients.
　2. Symptoms are typically paroxysmal.
　3. Classic triad of symptoms.
　　a. Headache.
　　b. Sweating.
　　c. Tachycardia.
B. Other signs and symptoms.
　1. Cardiovascular (palpitations).
　2. Anxiety/panic attacks.
　3. Nausea.
　4. Abdominal/chest pain.
　5. Flushing.
　6. Weight loss.
　7. Weakness.
　8. Tremor.
　9. Pallor.
　10. Shortness of breath.

PHYSICAL EXAMINATION
A. Vital signs.
　1. Tachycardia.
　2. Hypertension.
　3. Weight loss.
B. Complete cardiovascular examination.
C. Skin examination.
　1. Pallor.
　2. Flushing.

DIAGNOSTIC TESTS
A. Testing for PCC is necessary if there is:
　1. History of PCC.
　2. Symptoms of PCC, especially if they occur in a paroxysmal manner.
　3. Adrenal incidentaloma.
　4. Hereditary predisposition to PCC.
B. Initial testing involves two types of metanephrine tests.
　1. Urinary fractionated metanephrines should be a 24-hour urine collection and include a creatinine level.
　2. Plasma-free metanephrines should be drawn with the patient in the supine position.
　　a. Sympathetic activation occurs in the upright position and can falsely elevate catecholamine levels.
　　b. Ideally, patients should be in the supine position for 30 minutes prior to blood draw.
C. False positive results are common.
　1. Physiologic stress such as hospitalization may elevate hormones and should be considered contributing factors to elevations.
　2. Multiple drugs can cause false positive results, including:

a. Acetaminophen.
b. Beta-blockers: Labetalol and sotalol.
c. Tricyclic antidepressants.
d. Sympathomimetics.
e. Buspirone.
f. Monoamine oxidase (MAO) inhibitors.
g. Cocaine.
3. Confirmatory testing is needed if positive results are believed to be influenced by any of these factors.
4. Mildly elevated levels may suggest false positive results, while true PCC often have clearly elevated levels, two times the normal or more.
D. When biochemical results suggest a PCC, imaging is necessary. A CT scan should be ordered to locate the mass (CT preferred over MRI).
1. CT scan will show Hounsfield units of 10 or greater (<10 is a lipid-rich mass).
E. An MRI should be used in patients when a CT scan cannot be performed (e.g., allergy to CT contrast, or when attempting to limit radiation, such as in pregnant women).
F. All patients with PCCs should consider genetic testing to assess for other related conditions, such as the MEN syndromes.

DIFFERENTIAL DIAGNOSIS
A. Labile essential hypertension.
B. Malignant hypertension.
C. Illegal drug use such as phencyclidine or cocaine.
D. Combining multiple pharmacologic agents such as MAO inhibitors, decongestants, or sympathomimetics.
E. Stroke.
F. Myocardial infarction (MI).
G. Anxiety disorder.
H. Hyperthyroidism.
I. Hypoglycemia (including insulinoma).
J. Alcohol withdrawal.

EVALUATION AND MANAGEMENT PLAN
A. General plan.
1. Treatment involves surgery.
a. Preoperative management.
i. Preoperative medical treatment should occur for 7 to 14 days if possible to stabilize blood pressure (BP) and heart rate.
ii. Patients with hormonally active PCCs should undergo preoperative blockage with an alpha-adrenergic receptor blocker such as phenoxybenzamine or doxazosin. Calcium channel blockers can be used as secondary agents for further BP control.
iii. Beta-blockers can be added after initiation of an alpha-adrenergic receptor blocker to control heart rate. They should not be added before alpha-adrenergic receptor blockers due to the potential for hypertensive crisis if the alpha-adrenergic receptors are unopposed.
iv. Alpha-methyl-para-tyrosine (metyrosine) can be used for a short time preoperatively in combination with an alpha-adrenergic receptor

blocker to further stabilize BP and reduce blood loss and volume depletion during surgery.
v. Initiating a continuous saline infusion the evening before surgery is another helpful approach to minimize volume depletion.
vi. Preoperative diet should include high sodium (>5,000 mg/d) and high fluid intake (>2.5 L/d) to prevent hypotension after tumor removal.
vii. Monitor heart rate, BP, and blood glucose (BG) in the pre- and postoperative periods.
b. Operative procedure.
i. Most PCCs can be removed via minimally invasive adrenalectomy.
ii. Open resection is recommended for large tumors greater than 6 cm or for invasive tumors.
c. Postoperative management.
i. The most common postoperative complications include hypertension, hypotension, and rebound hypoglycemia.
ii. Heart rate, BP, and glucose should be monitored for 24 to 48 hours.
iii. In patients who are at risk for adrenal insufficiency (AI) after surgery, particular attention should be paid to signs and symptoms of AI.
B. Patient/family teaching points.
1. Consider genetic testing, if not already completed, for other potential family members at risk.
2. All first-degree relatives of a mutation carrier should be offered predictive testing.
C. Discharge instructions (if standard accepted guidelines exist, please use discharge template).
1. Monitor BP at home; counseling particularly on the potential for low or labile BP.
2. Monitor postoperative incision for any signs of infection.
3. Discuss the symptoms of PCC and the recommendation for annual biochemical monitoring to ensure long-term disease remission.

FOLLOW-UP
A. Biochemical testing should be repeated 2 to 4 weeks after surgery to ensure complete tumor resection.
B. Annual biochemical monitoring is recommended to assess for recurrent disease.

CONSULTATION/REFERRAL
A. Consultation with an endocrinologist and an endocrine surgeon is preferred for optimal patient outcomes.
B. It is recommended that patients with PCCs be treated by multidisciplinary teams at centers with expertise in this condition. Some studies suggest that there is lower postoperative mortality and shorter hospital stays in high-volume centers, but these data are not conclusive.

SPECIAL/GERIATRIC CONSIDERATIONS
A. Patients with metastatic disease or general complexity should always be referred to high-volume centers with expertise in the management of PCCs.

CASE SCENARIO: PHEOCHROMOCYTOMA

Barbara is a 51-year-old female with no medical history who presents to the ED with dizziness and palpitations. She reports that for the past 3 weeks she has experienced episodes of dizziness, heart racing, and headache. On exam, it is noted that her blood pressure (BP) is 200/105 mmHg and her heart rate is 118 beats per minute (bpm). Cardiac tests including EKG and serial troponins are negative. Her comprehensive metabolic profile, complete blood count (CBC), and thyroid profile are normal. Upon review of her chart, it is noted that the patient had a 1.5-cm adrenal incidentaloma that was noted on an abdominal CT scan 2 years ago but was not evaluated further. The admitting team ordered supine plasma metanephrine levels, which came back elevated at 129 pg/mL (range <62) (metanephrine) with normetanephrines elevated at 275 pg/mL (range <145). A repeat CT scan confirmed a solid adrenal mass that had grown to 2.5 cm and was consistent with pheochromocytoma (PCC). The endocrine surgery team was consulted and the patient was admitted for BP management preoperatively with phenoxybenzamine and metoprolol.

1. Which of the following is commonly reported in patients with PCC?
   A. Paroxysmal symptoms
   B. Weight gain
   C. Hyperthyroidism
   D. Symptoms that improve with rest

2. A patient admitted for trauma related to a motor vehicle accident is showing signs and symptoms of PCC. The patient is currently taking acetaminophen BID (650 mg), labetalol 400 mg daily, and buspirone 15 mg daily for anxiety. What is the next step?
   A. Discuss changing her medications for a time period before hormonal testing is completed.
   B. Order plasma metanephrines.
   C. Order urine metanephrines.
   D. Order abdominal CT scan.

3. What is the purpose of using phenoxybenzamine to control BP in patients with PCC?
   A. Patients require both beta-adrenergic and alpha-adrenergic blockade to prevent severe hypertension or cardiopulmonary crisis perioperatively.
   B. Patients require the use of additional BP meds to lower BP and phenoxybenzamine is the best option.
   C. Beta-adrenergic medications should not be used in patients with PCC.
   D. Alpha-adrenergic medications are the most effective at controlling heart rate.

BIBLIOGRAPHY

Lenders, J. W., Duh, Q.-Y., Eisenhofer, G., Gimenez-Roqueplo, A.-P., Grebe, S. K., Murad, M. H., Naruse, M., Pacak, K., & Young, W. F., Jr. (2014). Pheochromocytoma and paraganglioma: An endocrine society clinical practice guideline. *Journal of Clinical Endocrinology & Metabolism*, 99(6), 1915–1942. https://doi.org/10.1210/jc.2014-1498

Neumann, H. P., Young Jr, W. F., & Eng, C. (2019). Pheochromocytoma and paraganglioma. *New England Journal of Medicine*, 381(6), 552–565. https://doi.org/ 10.1056/NEJMra1806651

PREDIABETES

Marissa E. Luft

DEFINITION
A. Failing pancreatic islet beta cells.
B. State of insulin resistance.
C. Caused by excess body weight, usually abdominal/visceral obesity.
D. Dyslipidemia.
E. Elevated triglycerides.
F. Low high-density lipoprotein (HDL) cholesterol.
G. Hypertension.

INCIDENCE
A. In 2012, 86 million Americans aged 20 and older had prediabetes; this is up from 79 million in 2010.

PATHOGENESIS
A. Insulin resistance: There is a marked decrease in insulin sensitivity 5 years prior to the diagnosis of type 2 diabetes.
B. Relative insulin deficiency; beta cell dysfunction: Beta cell function is increased 3 to 4 years prior to the diagnosis of diabetes and then decreased immediately prior to the diabetes diagnosis.

PREDISPOSING FACTORS
A. Obesity.
   1. Body mass index (BMI) greater than 25 in all, except Asian population.
   2. BMI greater than 23 in Asian Americans.
B. First-degree relative with diabetes.
C. Higher risk in certain populations.
   1. African American.
   2. Latino.
   3. Native American.
   4. Asian American.
   5. Pacific Islander.
D. Women with history of gestational diabetes.
E. History of cardiovascular disease (CVD).
F. Hypertension greater than 140/90 mmHg.
G. HDL less than 35 mg/dL.
H. Triglycerides greater than 250 mg/dL.
I. Women with history of polycystic ovary syndrome.
J. Women who have given birth to a baby weighing over 9 lb.
K. Physically inactive.
L. Physical findings of insulin resistance.
   1. Skin tags.
   2. Acanthosis nigricans (see Figure 8.1).
M. Obstructive sleep apnea.
N. Can have patient take the American Diabetes Association risk test at www.diabetes.org.

SUBJECTIVE DATA
A. Common complaints/symptoms.
   1. Usually asymptomatic.
   2. Patient may present for routine physical or preoperative assessment.

PHYSICAL EXAMINATION

A. Record height, weight, BMI, waist circumference, and waist to hip ratio.
B. Monitor for abdominal obesity.
C. Assess for signs of CVD and peripheral vascular disease.
D. Check for the following signs/symptoms:
  1. Premature arcus cornealis.
  2. Xanthelasma.
  3. Polycystic ovarian syndrome symptoms.
    a. Acne.
    b. Hair loss.
    c. Hirsutism.
  4. Acanthosis nigricans (see Figure 8.1).
  5. Presence of skin tags.

DIAGNOSTIC TESTS

A. Hemoglobin A1C (HgbA1C): 5.7% to 6.4%.
B. Fasting glucose: 100 to 125 mg/dL.
C. Random glucose: 140 to 199 mg/dL.

DIFFERENTIAL DIAGNOSIS

A. Metabolic syndrome.
B. Type 2 diabetes.
C. Obesity.
D. Hypertension.
E. Hyperlipidemia.

EVALUATION AND MANAGEMENT PLAN

A. General plan (lifestyle therapy).
  1. Treat cardiovascular risk factors.
    a. Dyslipidemia.
    b. Hypertension.
  2. Weight loss/management.
    a. This can be achieved through lifestyle, pharmacotherapy, surgery, or a combination of treatments.
    b. Bariatric surgery can be very effective in preventing progression of prediabetes to type 2 diabetes.
  3. Nutrition therapy.
  4. Physical activity.
  5. Sleep.
  6. Community engagement.
  7. Alcohol moderation.
  8. Smoking cessation.
B. Pharmacotherapy.
  1. No medications are approved by the Food and Drug Administration (FDA) solely for management of prediabetes and prevention of type 2 diabetes.
  2. Medications should not be considered the only therapy. All medications should be combined with lifestyle modifications.
  3. Metformin reduces the risk of type 2 diabetes mellitus (T2DM) in prediabetes patients by 25% to 30%.
  4. Acarbose reduces the risk of T2DM in prediabetes patients by 25% to 30%.
  5. Consider with caution use of thiazolidinediones (prevent the development of type 2 diabetes by 60%–75%) or glucagon-like peptide-1 (GLP-1) receptor agonists.

FOLLOW-UP

A. Follow up with primary care provider (PCP) as needed to manage risk factors.

CONSULTATION/REFERRAL

A. Refer the patient to a registered dietitian for diet education/counseling.
B. Refer the patient to a psychologist/counselor for stress reduction and life coaching.
C. An exercise physiologist may help with planning a realistic exercise program.
D. Refer the patient to a lipid clinic for management of hyperlipidemia.

SPECIAL/GERIATRIC CONSIDERATIONS

A. The risk of diabetes increases with age.
B. Microvascular and cardiovascular complications are more common in older adults and should be monitored closely.

CASE SCENARIO: PREDIABETES

James is a 38-year-old male who presents to the preoperative area for elective cardiac catheterization. The patient is assessed by the anesthesiologist, and due to concerns for difficulty with intubation he is admitted to the hospital for further workup prior to the catheterization. The patient's body mass index (BMI) is 37, he endorses signs and symptoms of obstructive sleep apnea, and his blood pressure (BP) is 147/92. On admission, lab results reveal hemoglobin A1C (HgbA1C) of 5.7%, fasting plasma glucose of 124 mg/dL, high-density lipoprotein (HDL) of 42 mg/dL, and triglycerides of 303 mg/dL. PH: Hypertension, obesity, and asthma. Objective: BP 147/92, pulse 102, respirations 28, and temperature 98.9°F/37.2°C.

1. What differential diagnosis is concerning and would require further investigation?
  A. Hypothyroidism
  B. Prediabetes
  C. Polycystic ovarian syndrome
  D. Arcus senilis

2. What is the mainstay of treatment for prediabetes diagnosis?
  A. Diet and lifestyle modifications
  B. Insulin
  C. Thyroidectomy
  D. Continuous positive airway pressure (CPAP) therapy

3. What is the greatest risk factor for being diagnosed with prediabetes?
  A. High-density lipoprotein (HDL) >35
  B. Body mass index (BMI) ≥25 kg/m^2
  C. Sedentary lifestyle
  D. History of schizophrenia

4. Which medication can be used to reduce the likelihood of progression from prediabetes to type 2 diabetes?
  A. Insulin
  B. Metformin
  C. Sulfonylureas
  D. Thiazolidinediones

BIBLIOGRAPHY

Bock, G., Dalla Man, C., Campioni, M., Chittilapilly, E., Basu, R., Toffolo, G., Cobelli, C., & Rizza, R. (2006). Pathogenesis of pre-diabetes: Mechanisms of fasting and postprandial hyperglycemia in people with impaired fasting glucose and/or impaired glucose tolerance. *Diabetes, 55*, 3536–3549. https://doi.org/10.2337/db06-0319

Grundy, S. M. (2012). Pre-diabetes, metabolic syndrome, and cardiovascular risk. *Journal of the American College of Cardiology, 59*(7), 635–643. https://doi.org/10.1016/j.jacc.2011.08.080

THYROID DISORDER: EUTHYROID SICK SYNDROME

Marissa E. Luft

DEFINITION

A. Term designated for patients in which the thyroid organ is normal, but thyroid hormone levels are abnormal. Also referred to as nonthyroidal illness syndrome and can be classified into the following categories:
   1. Low T3 syndrome (most common).
   2. Low T3 and low T4 syndrome.
   3. High T4 syndrome.
   4. Mixed form in which a combination of abnormalities may be found.

INCIDENCE

A. Euthyroid sick syndrome can affect people of all races.
B. It affects male and female patients equally.
C. It occurs in people of any age.

PATHOGENESIS

A. Almost 90% of the hormones secreted by the thyroid gland are T4 and approximately 10% are T3. Most of T4 is converted into T3 in the peripheral tissues, accounting for 90% of the production of T3. The more physiologically active hormone is T3, which is four times more potent than T4.
B. The most common factor in these conditions is reduced extrathyroidal conversion of T4 to T3.
C. With low T3 syndrome, the free triiodothyronine (FT3) is low and the free thyroxine (FT4) is normal.
D. The patient is clinically euthyroid and the leading cause in many circumstances is from systemic illness.
E. The low T3 resolves when the underlying illness clears.
F. The low T3 and low T4 syndrome is usually identified in severely ill patients.
G. The thyroid-stimulating hormone (TSH) early in the illness may be low or normal.
   1. As the illness progresses and recovery ensues, the TSH is often above normal.
   2. Patients with a T4 level below 4 mcg/dL have a mortality rate of 50%. Patients with a T4 level below 2 mcg/dL have a mortality rate of 80%. Mortality rate exceeds 84% in patients who have both severely low T3 and T4 levels.
   3. High T4 syndrome is caused by increased concentrations of thyroid-binding globulin produced in certain liver diseases causing high T4 levels. T4 usually returns to normal within 6 to 8 weeks as the disease stabilizes.

PREDISPOSING FACTORS

A. Acute or chronic illness.
B. Medications.
C. Other endocrine disorders.
D. Burns.
E. Extreme heat or cold.
F. Starvation.

SUBJECTIVE DATA

A. Common complaints/symptoms.
   1. Most often, there are no associated symptoms. Careful history and physical examination will not reveal the typical features of hypothyroidism. Lab values will be abnormal.
   2. If there are symptoms, they are specific to each case.
B. Common/typical scenario.
   1. Patients are usually asymptomatic. The condition is found typically during routine screening for thyroid disease.
C. Family and social history.
   1. No relevant family or social history.
D. Review of systems.
   1. Negative review of systems.

PHYSICAL EXAMINATION

A. There are no particular findings for patients with nonthyroidal illness.
B. The examination findings in each patient reflect the characteristics of the nonthyroidal disease.

DIAGNOSTIC TESTS

A. Total T4.
B. Total T3.
C. TSH.
D. Free T4.
E. Reverse T3.
F. Free T3.

DIFFERENTIAL DIAGNOSIS

A. Hashimoto thyroiditis.
B. Hyperthyroidism.
C. Hypopituitarism.
D. Hypothyroidism.
E. Thyroid dysfunction induced by amiodarone.

EVALUATION AND MANAGEMENT PLAN

A. General plan.
   1. Monitor thyroid levels as needed if the patient becomes symptomatic. Refer to a healthcare provider.
B. Patient/family teaching points.
   1. If symptoms of hypothyroidism or hyperthyroidism occur, call the healthcare provider.
C. Pharmacotherapy.
   1. There is no evidence to date demonstrating the benefit of thyroid replacement in nonthyroidal illness.
D. Discharge instructions.
   1. No clear agreement on treatment exists. Hormone replacement with levothyroxine may not help these patients. Allowing for recovery time of the illness

and checking thyroid function weeks after the illness resolves is the best treatment for euthyroid sick patients.

FOLLOW-UP

A. Follow up with primary care provider (PCP) after release from the hospital.
B. Refer to endocrinology.

CONSULTATION/REFERRAL

A. Referral to an endocrinologist is recommended for monitoring of thyroid function tests both during and after recovery from nonthyroidal illness.

CASE SCENARIO: THYROID DISORDER: EUTHYROID SICK SYNDROME

A 63-year-old male was admitted to the hospital 3 weeks prior for decreased PO intake, increasing confusion, and vomiting. The patient was found to have bowel perforation requiring emergent surgery for resection with colostomy. The patient had difficulty weaning from the ventilator, postoperatively, and has now been incubated for 2 weeks. The patient's hospital course was further complicated by septic shock requiring intravenous (IV) antibiotics, pressors, and insulin glucose tolerance test (GTT). The patient has not shown improvement to date. Consideration of differentials resulted in the ordering of a full panel of bloodwork. PH: Type 2 diabetes mellitus (T2DM), hypertension, hyperlipidemia, schizophrenia, and ETOH (ethyl alcohol) abuse. Objective: Blood pressure (BP) 97/53, pulse 57, respirations 12, and temperature 97.6°F/36.4°C. Lab: Point-of-care (POC) blood glucose (BG) 72 mg/dL, sodium 132 mEq/L, potassium 4.5, white blood cell (WBC) 15,000, hemoglobin 8 g/dL, thyroid-stimulating hormone (TSH) 0.26 mU/L (nl: 0.45–4.5), free T4 0.5 ng/dL (nl: 0.8–1.8), and total T3 31 ng/dL (nl: 80–180).

1. Given the patient's lab results, what would be the immediate next step?
   A. Start IV thyroid hormone replacement.
   B. Consult endocrinology.
   C. Return to the operating room (OR) for emergent thyroidectomy.
   D. Order repeat blood cultures.

2. Given the patient's lab results, what is the working diagnosis?
   A. Hashimoto thyroiditis
   B. Myocardial infarction
   C. Euthyroid sick syndrome
   D. Unknown; repeat blood cultures are needed

3. What is the standard of care for this diagnosis?
   A. Treat and manage the underlying illness.
   B. Order Q8H IV hydrocortisone.
   C. Order 2 units of packed red blood cell (PRBCs).
   D. Serial thyroid CT scans.

4. After a diagnosis of euthyroid sick syndrome, with what frequency should thyroid-stimulating hormone (TSH), T3, and free T4 levels be monitored?
   A. Once a shift
   B. Once a day
   C. Weekly
   D. 2 to 3 months after recovery

BIBLIOGRAPHY

American Association of Clinical Endocrinologists. (2016). *Hyperthyroidism: Information for patients.* http://thyroidawareness.com/sites/all/files/hyperthyroidism.pdf

Brenner, Z., & Porsche, R. (2006). Amiodarone-induced thyroid dysfunction. *Critical Care Nurse, 26*(3), 34–41.

Burch, W. (1994). *Endocrinology* (3rd ed.). Williams & Wilkins.

Burman, K., Ellahham, S., Fadel, B., Lindsay, J., Ringel, M., & Wartofsky, L. (2000). Hyperthyroid heart disease. *Clinical Cardiology, 23*(26), 402–408. https://doi.org/10.1002/clc.4960230605

Carroll, R., & Matfin, G. (2010). Endocrine and metabolic emergencies: Thyroid storm. *Therapeutic Advances in Endocrinology and Metabolism, 1*(3), 139–145. https://doi.org/10.1177/2042018810382481

Dahlen, R., & Kumrow, D. (2002). Thyroidectomy: Understanding the potential for complications. *MEDSURG Nursing, 11*(5), 228–235.

Francis, J., & Jayaprasad, N. (2005). Atrial fibrillation and hyperthyroidism. *Indian Pacing and Electrophysiology Journal, 5*(4), 305–311.

Ganesan, K. (2020, October 30). Euthyroid Sick Syndrome. *StatPearls [Internet].* U.S. National Library of Medicine. https://www.ncbi.nlm.nih.gov/books/NBK482219/

Holcomb, S. (2002). Thyroid diseases: A primer for the critical care nurse. *Dimensions of Critical Care Nursing, 21*(4), 127–133. https://doi.org/10.1097/00003465-200207000-00003

Lee, S. (2018, March 15). Hyperthyroidism and thyrotoxicosis. In R. Khardori (Ed.), *Medscape.* http://emedicine.medscape.com/article/121865-overview

Manzullo, E. F., & Ross, D. S. (2019, February 26). Nonthyroid surgery in the patient with thyroid disease. In J. E. Mulder (Ed.), *UpToDate.* https://www.uptodate.com/contents/nonthyroid-surgery-in-the-patient-with-thyroid-disease

Mathew, V., Misgar, R. A., Ghosh, S., Mukhopadhyay, P., Roychowdhury, P., Pandit, K., Mukhopadhyay, S., & Chowdhury, S. (2011). Myxedema coma: A new look into an old crisis. *Journal of Thyroid Research, 2011,* 1–7. https://doi.org/10.4061/2011/493462

McDermott, M. T. (1970, January 1). Non-Thyroidal Illness Syndrome (Euthyroid Sick Syndrome). *SpringerLink,* Springer. https://link.springer.com/chapter/10.1007/978-3-030-22720-3_26#Sec1

Merrill, E. (2013). A devastating storm. *The Medicine Forum, 14*(12), 24–25. https://doi.org/10.29046/TMF.014.1.012

Roman, S. (2017). *Current best practices in the management of thyroid nodules and cancer.* (PowerPoint slides) https://reachmd.com/programs/cme/current-best-practices-in-the-management-of-thyroid-nodules-and-cancer/8470/transcript/16717/

Ross, D. (2018, September 27). Thyroid function in nonthyroidal illness. In J. E. Mulder (Ed.), *UpToDate.* https://www.uptodate.com/contents/thyroid-function-in-nonthyroidal-illness

Ross, D., & Sugg, S. (2018, September 25). Surgical management of hyperthyroidism. In J. E. Mulder (Ed.), *UpToDate.* https://www.uptodate.com/contents/surgical-management-of-hyperthyroidism

The Nurse Practitioner. (2005). The American Journal of Primary Healthcare. *Thyroid Disorders, 30*(6), 51–52.

Tuttle, R. (2018, January 17). Differentiated thyroid cancer: Clinicopathologic staging. In J. E. Mulder (Ed.), *UpToDate.* https://www.uptodate.com/contents/differentiated-thyroid-cancer-clinicopathologic-staging/print

Umpierrez, G. (2002). Euthyroid sick syndrome. *Southern Medical Journal, 95*(5), 506–513. https://doi.org/10.1097/00007611-200295050-00007

THYROID DISORDER: HYPERTHYROIDISM

Marissa E. Luft

DEFINITION

A. If the thyroid-stimulating hormone (TSH) level is too low, the thyroid is producing too much hormone, specifically T3 and possibly T4. This is called hyperthyroidism.
B. Set of disorders that involve excess synthesis and secretion of thyroid hormones by the thyroid gland, which leads to the hypermetabolic state of thyroid gland-induced thyrotoxicosis.

C. The main autoimmune cause of hyperthyroidism is Graves disease.
D. Three main causes.
   1. Diffuse toxic goiter (Graves disease).
   2. Toxic multinodular goiter.
   3. Toxic adenoma.

INCIDENCE
A. Hyperthyroidism affects approximately three million people.
B. Graves disease.
   1. This is the most common form of hyperthyroidism in the United States, causing approximately 60% to 80% of cases of thyrotoxicosis.
   2. Peak occurrence is between 30 and 60 years of age.
   3. More prevalent in females than in males.
C. Toxic multinodular goiter causes approximately 15% to 20% of thyrotoxicosis, occurring more frequently in regions of iodine deficiency. Toxic adenoma is the cause of approximately 3% to 5% of cases.

PATHOGENESIS
A. Hyperthyroidism results from excess production of thyroid hormone from the thyroid gland.
B. Untreated toxicosis can increase the incidence of cardiovascular and pulmonary complications, skin and bone conditions, and eye disease.

PREDISPOSING FACTORS
A. Genetic factors: Graves disease commonly occurs in multiple members of a family.
B. Autoimmune thyroid disorders.
C. Hashimoto disease.

SUBJECTIVE DATA
A. Common complaints/symptoms.
   1. Palpitations, sweating, extreme fatigue, may have presence of goiter, and weight loss.
B. Common/typical scenario.
   1. Patient presents with extreme fatigue or anxiety and/or significant weight loss over a short period of time and often complains of palpitations.
C. Family and social history.
   1. May have a genetic or familial history.
D. Review of systems.
   1. Cardiovascular: Ask about palpitations or recent increases in BP medications.
   2. Head, ear, eyes, nose, and throat (HEENT): Hair loss.
   3. Psych: Insomnia, anxiety, irritability, nervousness, and increased perspiration.
   4. Endocrine: Menstrual irregularities, weight loss, heat intolerance, and thinning skin.
   5. Musculoskeletal: Muscle weakness, myalgias, and arthralgias.

PHYSICAL EXAMINATION
A. Constitutional: Appears toxic.
B. Cardiovascular: Systolic hypertension with a wide pulse pressure, tachycardia, and atrial fibrillation.
C. HEENT: Palpable diffuse goiter, thyroid bruit, exophthalmos, periorbital edema, proptosis, and lid lag.
D. Neurologic/musculoskeletal: Tremors and hyperreflexia.
E. Dermatologic: Warm moist skin and pretibial myxedema.
F. Psychological: Anorexia and difficulty focusing.

DIAGNOSTIC TESTS
A. TSH level: Most reliable screening measure. It is usually suppressed to an immeasurable level (<0.05 mIU/L) in thyrotoxicosis.
B. Free T4: May or may not be elevated.
C. Free T3: Will be elevated.
D. Thyroid-stimulating immunoglobulin (TSI) or thyrotropin receptor antibodies (G1) to establish Graves disease. Thyroid peroxidase (TPO) level or antimicrosomal antibodies are usually elevated with Graves disease but are usually low or absent in toxic multinodular goiter and toxic adenoma.
E. Thyroid uptake scan to determine the pattern of uptake, which varies with the underlying disorder. Normal radioactive iodine uptake after 6 hours is 2% to 16%; after 24 hours, it is about 8% to 25%. In hyperthyroidism, there will be markedly increased uptake.

DIFFERENTIAL DIAGNOSIS
A. Euthyroid sick syndrome.
B. Thyroiditis.
C. Goiter.
D. Struma ovarii.
E. Graves disease.

EVALUATION AND MANAGEMENT PLAN
A. General plan.
   1. Symptom management helps the patient to establish symptom control with medications.
   2. Further laboratory studies.
     a. Repeat TSH every 6 weeks or as needed until symptoms are controlled.
     b. Check TSI and TPO to rule out Graves disease or Hashimoto thyroiditis, respectively.
   3. Nuclear thyroid scanning to differentiate hyperthyroidism from thyroiditis.
B. Patient/family teaching points.
   1. Definitive treatment plan must be established and coordinated with endocrinology.
   2. Reinforce the need to see endocrinology on a regular basis.
   3. If flu-like symptoms develop while on antithyroid medications, call the provider immediately and stop medications completely.
C. Pharmacotherapy.
   1. Treatment consists of symptom relief with the following drugs:
     a. Beta-blockers: Titrate to heart rate less than 90 beats per minute and to reduce the sympathetic response associated with peripheral conversion of T4 to T3. The effects of beta-blockers are dramatic and rapid (within 10 minutes).

i. Studies have shown that propranolol has the best results in this class of medications.

ii. Other beta-blockers have similar effects and can be used.

b. Antithyroid medications: Prevent thyroid hormone synthesis.

i. Methimazole (Tapazole) is considered the first-line drug therapy.

ii. Propylthiouracil (PTU) is preferred in thyroid storm and in the first trimester of pregnancy.

c. Corticosteroids.

i. Dexamethasone contributes to blocking T4 to T3 conversion, which will control symptoms. Useful in emergencies, but has long-term complications to consider.

2. Radioactive iodine-131 therapy ablates thyroid tissue and is used in cases of:

a. Hyperthyroidism secondary to thyroid cancer.

b. Hyperthyroidism not responsive to medical therapy.

3. Thyroidectomy: May be preferable to radioactive iodine-131 therapy.

a. May be required for large goiters causing airway constriction and severe dysphagia.

b. Thyroid cancers not responsive to radioactive iodine-131 therapy.

D. Imaging studies.

1. Ultrasound, CT scan, and chest x-ray (CXR) are routine. Fine needle aspiration for biopsy, vocal cord evaluation, or esophageal evaluation may be needed depending on the patient's presentation.

2. Monitor for thyroid storm, particularly in the first 18 hours postoperatively.

a. Treat with antithyroid medications until euthyroid.

b. Beta-blockers: Atenolol should be taken 1 hour before surgery to maintain blockade.

E. Discharge instructions.

1. Before discharge, refer the patient to outpatient endocrinology and to ophthalmology, if needed, for eye disease.

FOLLOW-UP

A. Continue to monitor symptoms and thyroid levels.

B. Check TSH 6 weeks after discharge.

CONSULTATION/REFERRAL

A. Refer to endocrinology to manage symptoms and disease progression.

SPECIAL/GERIATRIC CONSIDERATIONS

A. In the acute care setting, the focus should be on the adverse effects of antithyroid medications.

1. Rash.

2. Urticaria.

3. Arthralgia.

4. Hepatotoxicity.

B. Monitoring of results of lab studies is also important.

1. Complete blood count (CBC) for agranulocytosis if the patient develops fever or sore throat, but otherwise not recommend for routine monitoring.

2. Hepatic profile for hepatitis.

C. If fever (>100.5°F/38.1°C) or sore throat develops, the medication will need to be stopped.

CASE SCENARIO: THYROID DISORDER: HYPERTHYROIDISM

Mary is a 35-year-old female who presents with recent history of unintentional weight loss, heat intolerance, diarrhea, and palpitations. The patient denied fever, chest pain, shortness of breath, abdominal pain, nausea, and vomiting. Her physical exam was significant for a moderate, painless goiter. Her EKG revealed sinus tachycardia at 103 beats per minute (bpm) and prolonged QTc of 532 msec. Chest x-ray was within normal limits (WNL). Ultrasound of the thyroid showed an enlarged and hypervascular thyroid gland: Right 7.2 × 2.8 × 3 cm; left 6.6 × 2.6 × 3.2 cm. PH: Seasonal allergies, depression, and anxiety. Objective: Blood pressure (BP) 162/74, pulse 103, respirations 18, and temperature 97.1°F/36.2°C. Lab: Sodium 138 mEq/L, potassium 4.8, white blood cell (WBC) 10,000, hemoglobin 13 g/dL, thyroid-stimulating hormone (TSH) 0.04 mU/L (nl: 0.45–4.5), free T4 75 ng/dL (nl: 0.8–1.8), and free T3 32 ng/dL (nl, 2.0-4.4).

1. Which condition is a rare and life-threatening complication of hyperthyroidism?

A. Myxedema coma

B. Thyroid storm

C. Graves disease

D. Hepatorenal syndrome

2. Which of the following is NOT a treatment option for newly diagnosed hyperthyroidism?

A. Dantrolene

B. Intravenous propylthiouracil (PTU)

C. Thyroidectomy

D. Radioactive iodine

3. What is the predominant cause of hyperthyroidism in the United States?

A. Addison disease

B. Alopecia

C. Graves disease

D. Iodine deficiency

4. It is preferred to delay thyroidectomy until a patient has reached euthyroid state with the treatment of thionamides; however, which finding would require more emergent attention?

A. Tracheal compression by goiter

B. Weight gain

C. Urinary frequency

D. Exophthalmos

BIBLIOGRAPHY

American Association of Clinical Endocrinologists. (2016). *Hyperthyroidism: Information for patients.* http://thyroidawareness.com/sites/all/files/hyperthyroidism.pdf

Brenner, Z., & Porsche, R. (2006). Amiodarone-induced thyroid dysfunction. *Critical Care Nurse, 26*(3), 34–41.

Burch, W. (1994). *Endocrinology* (3rd ed.). Williams & Wilkins.

Burman, K., Ellahham, S., Fadel, B., Lindsay, J., Ringel, M., & Wartofsky, L. (2000). Hyperthyroid heart disease. *Clinical Cardiology, 23*(26), 402–408. https://doi.org/10.1002/clc.4960230605

Carroll, R., & Matfin, G. (2010). Endocrine and metabolic emergencies: Thyroid storm. *Therapeutic Advances in Endocrinology and Metabolism, 1*(3), 139–145. https://doi.org/10.1177/2042018810382481

Dahlen, R., & Kumrow, D. (2002). Thyroidectomy: Understanding the potential for complications. *MEDSURG Nursing, 11*(5), 228–235.

Dillane, D. (2021). Hyperthyroidism. In D. Dillane & B.A. Finegan (Eds.), *Preoperative Assessment*. Springer. https://doi.org/10.1007/978-3-030-58842-7_18

Francis, J., & Jayaprasad, N. (2005). Atrial fibrillation and hyperthyroidism. *Indian Pacing and Electrophysiology Journal, 5*(4), 305–311.

Holcomb, S. (2002). Thyroid diseases: A primer for the critical care nurse. *Dimensions of Critical Care Nursing, 21*(4), 127–133. https://doi.org/10.1097/00003465-200207000-00003

Lee, S. (2018, March 15). Hyperthyroidism and thyrotoxicosis. In R. Khardori (Ed.), *Medscape*. http://emedicine.medscape.com/article/121865-overview

Manzullo, E. F., & Ross, D. S. (2019, February 26). Nonthyroid surgery in the patient with thyroid disease. In J. E. Mulder (Ed.), *UpToDate*. https://www.uptodate.com/contents/nonthyroid-surgery-in-the-patient-with-thyroid-disease

Mathew, V., Misgar, R. A., Ghosh, S., Mukhopadhyay, P., Roychowdhury, P., Pandit, K., Mukhopadhyay, S., & Chowdhury, S. (2011). Myxedema coma: A new look into an old crisis. *Journal of Thyroid Research, 2011*, 1–7. https://doi.org/10.4061/2011/493462

Merrill, E. (2013). A devastating storm. *The Medicine Forum, 14*(12), 24–25. https://doi.org/10.29046/TMF.014.1.012

Roman, S. (2017). *Current best practices in the management of thyroid nodules and cancer*. (PowerPoint slides) https://reachmd.com/programs/cme/current-best-practices-in-the-management-of-thyroid-nodules-and-cancer/8470/transcript/16717/

Ross, D. (2018, September 27). Thyroid function in nonthyroidal illness. In J. E. Mulder (Ed.), *UpToDate*. https://www.uptodate.com/contents/thyroid-function-in-nonthyroidal-illness

Ross, D., & Sugg, S. (2018, September 25). Surgical management of hyperthyroidism. In J. E. Mulder (Ed.), *UpToDate*. https://www.uptodate.com/contents/surgical-management-of-hyperthyroidism

The Nurse Practitioner. (2005). The American Journal of Primary Healthcare. *Thyroid Disorders, 30*(6), 51–52.

Tuttle, R. (2018, January 17). Differentiated thyroid cancer: Clinicopathologic staging. In J. E. Mulder (Ed.), *UpToDate*. https://www.uptodate.com/contents/differentiated-thyroid-cancer-clinicopathologic-staging/print

Umpierrez, G. (2002). Euthyroid sick syndrome. *Southern Medical Journal, 95*(5), 506–513. https://doi.org/10.1097/00007611-200295050-00007

THYROID DISORDER: HYPOTHYROIDISM

Marissa E. Luft

DEFINITION

A. Decreased circulation of free T4/T4, with or without low T3 levels, in the presences of high circulating levels of thyroid-stimulating hormone (TSH).
B. Systemic impacts with varying degree of organ system dysfunction dependent on the level of thyroid deficiency.
C. The predominant cause of hypothyroidism is Hashimoto autoimmune disease.

INCIDENCE

A. Hypothyroidism affects approximately 10 million people.
B. Approximately 10% of women and 3% of men have a diagnosis of hypothyroidism in the outpatient setting.
C. Associated with increased serum cholesterol levels, which may increase the risk of atherosclerosis and heart disease.

PATHOGENESIS

A. Insufficient production of thyroid hormone from the thyroid gland.
B. Categorized into three types based on the origin of dysfunction:
  1. Primary: Originating from the thyroid gland.
  2. Secondary: Originating from the pituitary gland.
  3. Tertiary: Originating from the hypothalamus.

PREDISPOSING FACTORS

A. Age and sex.
B. Family history.
C. Any autoimmune disorder: Autoimmune thyroiditis.
D. Subacute thyroiditis.
E. Radioactive iodine treatment.
F. Thyroid surgery or medications.
G. Postpartum thyroiditis.
H. Congenital condition.

SUBJECTIVE DATA

A. Common complaints/symptoms.
  1. Weight gain, fatigue, forgetfulness, dry hair/nail changes, cold intolerance, and menstrual irregularities.
B. Common/typical scenario.
  1. Patient presents with persistent fatigue and inability to lose weight. The patient will complain that they do not feel right.
C. Family and social history.
  1. May have a familial link.
D. Review of systems.
  1. Constitutional: Inquire about recent viral infections, pervasive fatigue, drowsiness, forgetfulness, and learning difficulties.
  2. Dermatologic: Dry, brittle hair and nails, and itchy skin.
  3. Psychological: Recent depression, feeling sadness, decreased libido, and irritability.
  4. Endocrine: Cold intolerance, menstrual irregularities, and miscarriages.
  5. Musculoskeletal: Muscle cramps and soreness.

PHYSICAL EXAMINATION

A. Cardiovascular: Low blood pressure (BP), bradycardia, and fluid retention.
B. Head, ear, eyes, nose, and throat (HEENT): Periorbital edema, assess for presence of goiter, dysphagia, eyebrow hair loss, and possible scalp hair loss.
C. Neuro/musculoskeletal: Lower extremity fluid retention, myalgia, arthralgia, and hyporeflexia.
D. Dermatologic: Dry, coarse skin and nails.

DIAGNOSTIC TESTS

A. TSH (0.4–5 µIU/mL).
B. Free T4 (0.8–1.8 µg/dL).
C. Thyroid antibodies.
  1. Thyroid peroxidase (TPO) level (<35 IU/mL).

DIFFERENTIAL DIAGNOSIS

A. Anemia.
B. Addison disease.
C. Anovulation.
D. Dysmenorrhea.
E. Cardiac tamponade.
F. Pericardial effusion.
G. Chronic fatigue syndrome.
H. Depression.
I. Thyroiditis.
J. Euthyroid sick syndrome.
K. Goiter.
L. Hypothermia.
M. Constipation.
N. Infertility.
O. Iodine deficiency.
P. Menopause.
Q. Hyperlipidemia.
R. Pituitary disorders.

EVALUATION AND MANAGEMENT PLAN

A. Management.
  1. Normalize thyroid levels by starting thyroid hormone replacement therapy.
  2. Routine laboratory testing every 6 weeks to adjust dose, accordingly, until stabilized.
B. Patient/family teaching points.
  1. Teach patient signs and symptoms of hypothyroidism and when to call provider, including increase in fatigue, unexplained weight gain and fluid retention, increase in hair loss, arthralgias, and myalgias.
  2. Labs must be checked every 6 weeks for a period of time until the medications can be appropriately titrated to patient's tolerance and TSH goal is reached.
C. Pharmacotherapy.
  1. Treatment consists of administering the synthetic thyroid hormone levothyroxine.
    a. Dose is based on weight in kilograms multiplied by 1.6 and can be administered orally or intravenously in the hospital setting at 50% to 80% of the PO dose. It should be taken on an empty stomach first thing in the morning with no food, no other medications or caffeine for at least 1 hour after taking medication, and no supplements for 4 hours after taking medication.

FOLLOW-UP

A. Ensure patient adherence to treatment regimen.
B. Stress the importance of taking medication daily at approximately the same time.
C. Stress the importance of laboratory checks of TSH level every 6 to 8 weeks.
D. Educate regarding the risks of abrupt discontinuation of medication.

CONSULTATION/REFERRAL

A. Once discharged, referral to an outpatient endocrinologist is recommended.

SPECIAL/GERIATRIC CONSIDERATIONS

A. Keep TSH levels for geriatric patients in the midrange to avoid the incidence of cardiac side effects, such as atrial fibrillation or tachycardia.

CASE SCENARIO: THYROID DISORDER: HYPOTHYROIDISM

Bette is 73-year-old female who presents with increasing fatigue and memory impairment for 2 months. The patient also notes constipation and an unintentional weight gain of 10 lb over the past 2 months. The patient denies fever, chest pain, shortness of breath, abdominal pain, nausea, vomiting, or change in appetite. The patient's physical exam is not significant. PH: Hypertension, obesity, congestive heart failure (CHF), and type 2 diabetes (DMII). Objective: Blood pressure (BP) 92/54, pulse 57, respirations 18, and temperature 97.1°F/36.2°C. Lab: Point-of-care (POC) blood glucose (BG) 122 mg/dL, sodium 135 mEq/L, potassium 4.5, white blood cell (WBC) 18,000, hemoglobin 11 g/dL, thyroid-stimulating hormone (TSH) 18 mU/L (nl: 0.45–4.5), free T4 0.7 ng/dL (nl: 0.8–1.8), and free T3 2.3 ng/dL (nl: 2.0–4.4).

1. Which lab value is most concerning?
  A. Point-of-care (POC) blood glucose (BG)
  B. White blood cell (WBC)
  C. Thyroid-stimulating hormone (TSH)
  D. Free T4

2. What is the treatment for newly diagnosed hypothyroidism?
  A. Levophed
  B. Intravenous propylthiouracil (PTU)
  C. Thyroidectomy
  D. Levothyroxine

3. When is the most ideal time to take levothyroxine?
  A. After breakfast
  B. 1 hour after lunch
  C. With dinner
  D. 1 hour before breakfast

4. How often should a patient's thyroid-stimulating hormone (TSH) value be monitored after discharge from hospital?
  A. Weekly
  B. Monthly
  C. Every 6 weeks
  D. Every 3 to 6 months

BIBLIOGRAPHY

American Association of Clinical Endocrinologists. (2016). *Hyperthyroidism: Information for patients.* http://thyroidawareness.com/sites/all/files/hyperthyroidism.pdf

Brenner, Z., & Porsche, R. (2006). Amiodarone-induced thyroid dysfunction. *Critical Care Nurse, 26*(3), 34–41.

Burch, W. (1994). *Endocrinology* (3rd ed.). Williams & Wilkins.

Burman, K., Ellahham, S., Fadel, B., Lindsay, J., Ringel, M., & Wartofsky, L. (2000). Hyperthyroid heart disease. *Clinical Cardiology, 23*(26), 402–408.

Carroll, R., & Matfin, G. (2010). Endocrine and metabolic emergencies: Thyroid storm. *Therapeutic Advances in Endocrinology and Metabolism, 1*(3), 139–145. https://doi.org/10.1177/2042018810382481

Dahlen, R., & Kumrow, D. (2002). Thyroidectomy: Understanding the potential for complications. *MEDSURG Nursing, 11*(5), 228–235.

Francis, J., & Jayaprasad, N. (2005). Atrial fibrillation and hyperthyroidism. *Indian Pacing and Electrophysiology Journal, 5*(4), 305–311.

Holcomb, S. (2002). Thyroid diseases: A primer for the critical care nurse. *Dimensions of Critical Care Nursing*, 21(4), 127–133. https://doi.org/10.1097/00003465-200207000-00003

Lee, S. (2018, March 15). Hyperthyroidism and thyrotoxicosis. In R. Khardori (Ed.), *Medscape*. http://emedicine.medscape.com/article/121865-overview

Manzullo, E. F., & Ross, D. S. (2019, February 26). Nonthyroid surgery in the patient with thyroid disease. In J. E. Mulder (Ed.), *UpToDate*. https://www.uptodate.com/contents/nonthyroid-surgery-in-the-patient-with-thyroid-disease

Mathew, V., Misgar, R. A., Ghosh, S., Mukhopadhyay, P., Roychowdhury, P., Pandit, K., Mukhopadhyay, S., & Chowdhury, S. (2011). Myxedema coma: A new look into an old crisis. *Journal of Thyroid Research*, 2011, 1–7. https://doi.org/10.4061/2011/493462

Merrill, E. (2013). A devastating storm. *The Medicine Forum*, 14(12), 24–25. https://doi.org/10.29046/TMF.014.1.012

Roman, S. (2017). *Current best practices in the management of thyroid nodules and cancer*. (PowerPoint slides) https://reachmd.com/programs/cme/current-best-practices-in-the-management-of-thyroid-nodules-and-cancer/8470/transcript/16717/

Ross, D. (2018, September 27). Thyroid function in nonthyroidal illness. In J. E. Mulder (Ed.), *UpToDate*. https://www.uptodate.com/contents/thyroid-function-in-nonthyroidal-illness

Ross, D., & Sugg, S. (2018, September 25). Surgical management of hyperthyroidism. In J. E. Mulder (Ed.), *UpToDate*. https://www.uptodate.com/contents/surgical-management-of-hyperthyroidism

The Nurse Practitioner. (2005). The American Journal of Primary Healthcare. *Thyroid Disorders*, 30(6), 51–52.

Tuttle, R. (2016). Differentiated thyroid cancer: Clinicopathologic staging. In J. E. Mulder (Ed.), *UpToDate*. https://www.uptodate.com/contents/differentiated-thyroid-cancer-clinicopathologic-staging/print

Umpierrez, G. (2002). Euthyroid sick syndrome. *Southern Medical Journal*, 95(5), 506–513. https://doi.org/10.1097/00007611-200295050-00007

THYROID DISORDER: MYXEDEMA COMA

Marissa E. Luft

DEFINITION
A. A rare (0.22 per 1 million annually) but severe life-threatening form of decompensated hypothyroidism associated with a high mortality rate.
B. Major precipitating factors: Infection and discontinuation of thyroid supplements.

INCIDENCE
A. At present, there are over 300 cases reported in the literature. Myxedema coma is rare and generally unrecognized, with 80% of patients older than 60 years of age.
B. Myxedema coma can occur in younger women, with 36 known cases occurring with pregnant females.
C. A commonly ignored background factor in myxedema coma/crisis is the discontinuation of thyroid supplements in critically ill patients.

PATHOGENESIS
A. Low intracellular T3 secondary to hypothyroidism is the basic underlying pathology.

PREDISPOSING FACTORS
A. Certain medications.
B. Infection and septicemia.
C. Trauma.
D. Withdrawal of thyroid supplements.
E. Underlying cardiovascular disease (CVD).

SUBJECTIVE DATA
A. Complaints/symptoms.
 1. Decreased mentation and extreme lethargy.
B. Common/typical scenario.
 1. Very few cases have occurred in the United States, but usually related to having underlying hypothyroidism. Most likely to be seen in the ICU after hypothyroid medication is discontinued for an extended period of time and a precipitating event occurs, such as sepsis.
C. Family and social history.
 1. Ask about discontinuation of thyroid medications.
D. Review of systems.
 1. Unable to assess due to mental status.

PHYSICAL EXAMINATION
A. Cardiovascular: Hypotension, bradycardia, and EKG changes.
B. Respiratory: Decreased breath sounds and respiratory depression.
C. Neurologic: Poor cognitive function and generalized weakness.

DIAGNOSTIC TESTS
A. Thyroid-stimulating hormone (TSH).
B. Free T4.
C. Nonspecific labs to rule out other disorders, including complete blood count (CBC), urinalysis, blood and urine culture, and serum electrolytes.

DIFFERENTIAL DIAGNOSIS
A. Cerebrovascular accident.
B. Acute psychosis.
C. Hypoglycemia.
D. Hypoxia.
E. Sepsis.
F. Hypothermia.
G. Acute myocardial infarction (MI).
H. Intracranial hemorrhage.
I. Panhypopituitarism.
J. Adrenal insufficiency (AI).
K. Hyponatremia.
L. Gastrointestinal (GI) bleeding.
M. Conversion disorder.

EVALUATION AND MANAGEMENT PLAN
A. General plan.
 1. Consult with an endocrinologist. This is a medical emergency with a high (25%–60%) risk of mortality. If an endocrinologist is not available, confer with a critical care specialist. The advanced practice provider (APP) should not manage this type of patient alone.
 2. Be aware that cardiovascular morbidity occurs, including cardiogenic shock, respiratory depression, hypothermia, and coma.
 3. Achieve normothermia. Warming occurs with administration of thyroid hormone, in most cases both T3 and T4, with gradual slow rewarming via a warming blanket.
 4. Focus on stabilization of cardiac status. Cardiac support is given through administration of thyroid

hormone and IV fluids with stabilization of electrolytes and BG.

5. Achieve optimum ventilation. Ventilation is given through administration of oxygen and, if needed, central or bilevel positive airway pressure or mechanical ventilation.

6. Correct hypoglycemia via dextrose added to maintenance intravenous (IV) infusion.

7. Concomitant AI occurs due to impaired adrenal cellular metabolic functions secondary to lack of thyroid hormone. Administer corticosteroids (hydrocortisone) IV Q8H.

B. Patient/family teaching points.

1. Explain to the patient and family the severity of myxedema crisis and the course of treatment in the intensive care setting.

C. Pharmacotherapy.

1. Give IV triiodothyronine and thyroxine replacement with gradual slow rewarming.

2. Resuscitation and ICU management should be a multidisciplinary team approach.

D. Discharge instructions.

1. Poor outcomes and high mortality rates are associated with myxedema coma; may need nursing home placement, long-term acute care hospital, or hospice care if clinical course is complicated.

FOLLOW-UP

A. Follow-up is dependent on individual outcome.

CONSULTATION/REFERRAL

A. Consultation with an endocrinologist.

B. Consider a palliative care consult due to high mortality rate.

C. Social work consult for placement or family support may be needed.

SPECIAL/GERIATRIC CONSIDERATIONS

A. Poor outcomes are associated with myxedema coma in all age groups.

B. Presentation of advanced hypothyroidism in pregnancy is very unusual and myxedema coma is rare, with fewer than 40 cases reported.

CASE SCENARIO: THYROID DISORDER: MYXEDEMA COMA

Karen is a 69-year-old patient who presents to the ED status post motor vehicle accident. The patient sustained multiple traumatic injuries. She required immediate intubation for airway protection due to decreased level of consciousness. She was transferred to surgical ICU for repair of a femur fracture. Her postoperative chest x-ray (CXR) showed a left lower lobe (LLL) consolidation concerning for aspiration pneumonia and was treated with intravenous (IV) antibiotics. She had difficulty weaning from vent for 1 week postoperatively. RN notified the covering nurse practitioner (NP) that the patient was now hypothermic and not following commands when sedation was titrated down, a change from prior shift. Home medications include levothyroxine 125 mcg PO every day, multivitamin 1 tab PO every day, escitalopram 20 mg every day, and metaxalone 800 mg PO TID. Medical history includes hypothyroidism, depression, and osteoarthritis. Objective: Blood pressure (BP) 85/56, pulse 60, respirations 12, and temperature 96.6. Other data included point-of-care (POC) blood glucose (BG) of 69 mg/dL, sodium of 128 mEq/L, potassium of 4.5, bicarbonate of 29 mEq/L, white blood cell (WBC) of 12,000, hemoglobin of 9 g/dL, thyroid-stimulating hormone (TSH) of 30 mIU/L, free T4 of 10 ng/dL.

1. Given the patient's medical history and acute change in clinical condition, which of the following should be on the list of differential diagnoses?
   A. Prolonged exposure to cold
   B. Hyperglycemia
   C. Myxedema coma
   D. Sepsis

2. What is the gold standard for treatment of myxedema coma?
   A. Intravenous (IV) vancomycin
   B. IV thyroid hormone
   C. IV steroids and pressor support
   D. IV dantrolene

3. Which of the following puts patients at high risk for myxedema coma?
   A. Female and age >65 years old
   B. Prolonged hospitalization
   C. Abrupt withdrawal from levothyroxine
   D. Trauma
   E. All of the above

4. Which of the following is associated with myxedema coma?
   A. Concomitant adrenal insufficiency
   B. Gray hue of skin
   C. Hyperthermia exceeding 104°F/40°C
   D. Lifelong monthly intravenous (IV) thyroid hormone infusions

BIBLIOGRAPHY

American Association of Clinical Endocrinologists. (2016). *Hyperthyroidism: Information for patients.* http://thyroidawareness.com/sites/all/files/hyperthyroidism.pdf

Brenner, Z., & Porsche, R. (2006). Amiodarone-induced thyroid dysfunction. *Critical Care Nurse, 26*(3), 34–41.

Burch, W. (1994). *Endocrinology* (3rd ed.). Williams & Wilkins.

Burman, K., Ellahham, S., Fadel, B., Lindsay, J., Ringel, M., & Wartofsky, L. (2000). Hyperthyroid heart disease. *Clinical Cardiology, 23*(26), 402–408.

Burns, Suzanne M., & Delgado, S. A. (2016). *Cases in Diagnostic Reasoning: Acute & Critical Care Nurse Practitioner.* McGraw-Hill Education.

Carroll, R., & Matfin, G. (2010). Endocrine and metabolic emergencies: Thyroid storm. *Therapeutic Advances in Endocrinology and Metabolism, 1*(3), 139–145.

Dahlen, R., & Kumrow, D. (2002). Thyroidectomy: Understanding the potential for complications. *MEDSURG Nursing, 11*(5), 228–235.

Francis, J., & Jayaprasad, N. (2005). Atrial fibrillation and hyperthyroidism. *Indian Pacing and Electrophysiology Journal, 5*(4), 305–311.

Holcomb, S. (2002). Thyroid diseases: A primer for the critical care nurse. *Dimensions of Critical Care Nursing, 21*(4), 127–133. https://doi.org/10.1097/00003465-200207000-00003

Lee, S. (2018, March 15). Hyperthyroidism and thyrotoxicosis. In R. Khardori (Ed.), *Medscape.* http://emedicine.medscape.com/article/121865-overview

Manzullo, E. F., & Ross, D. S. (2019, February 26). Nonthyroid surgery in the patient with thyroid disease. In J. E. Mulder (Ed.), *UpToDate.* https://www.uptodate.com/contents/nonthyroid-surgery-in-the-patient-with-thyroid-disease

Mathew, V., Misgar, R. A., Ghosh, S., Mukhopadhyay, P., Roychowdhury, P., Pandit, K., Mukhopadhyay, S., & Chowdhury, S. (2011). Myxedema coma: A new look into an old crisis. *Journal of Thyroid Research*, 1–7. https://doi.org/10.4061/2011/493462 2011

Roman, S. (2017). *Current best practices in the management of thyroid nodules and cancer.* (PowerPoint slides) https://reachmd.com/programs/cme/current-best-practices-in-the-management-of-thyroid-nodules-and-cancer/8470/transcript/16717/

Ross, D. (2018, September 27). Thyroid function in nonthyroidal illness. In J. E. Mulder (Ed.), *UpToDate.* https://www.uptodate.com/contents/thyroid-function-in-nonthyroidal-illness

Ross, D., & Sugg, S. (2018, September 25). Surgical management of hyperthyroidism. In J. E. Mulder (Ed.), *UpToDate.* https://www.uptodate.com/contents/surgical-management-of-hyperthyroidism

The Nurse Practitioner. (2005). The American Journal of Primary Healthcare. *Thyroid Disorders, 30*(6), 51–52.

Tuttle, R. (2018, January 17). Differentiated thyroid cancer: Clinicopathologic staging. In J. E. Mulder (Ed.), *UpToDate.* https://www.uptodate.com/contents/differentiated-thyroid-cancer-clinicopathologic-staging/print

Umpierrez, G. (2002). Euthyroid sick syndrome. *Southern Medical Journal, 95*(5), 506–513. https://doi.org/10.1097/00007611-200295050-00007

THYROID DISORDER: THYROID STORM

Marissa E. Luft

DEFINITION
A. State of severe hyperthyroid crisis that causes organ dysfunction.
B. An acute, life-threatening, hypermetabolic state induced by excessive release of thyroid hormones.
C. The severe end of the spectrum of thyrotoxicosis.

INCIDENCE
A. Thyroid storm is most often seen in the context of underlying Graves hyperthyroidism.
B. Although quite rare, it can complicate thyrotoxicosis of any etiology and has a high mortality rate that may approach 10% to 20%.
C. Thyroid marker levels do not adequately address the differences between thyroid storm and hyperthyroidism. To differentiate the severity and potential morbidity of the disease, the Burch–Wartofsky Point Scale (BWPS) can predict the risk of thyroid storm independently from thyroid levels.
D. Thyrotoxicosis is three to five times more common in females, predisposing them to this condition.

PATHOGENESIS
A. Patients with thyroid storm have relatively higher levels of free thyroid hormones.

PREDISPOSING FACTORS
A. Regardless of the underlying etiology, the transition to a state of thyroid storm is usually precipitated by a second superimposed insult. Most often, this is infection.
B. Other associated causes:
  1. Trauma.
  2. Surgery.
  3. Thyroid surgery.
  4. Myocardial infarction (MI).
  5. Diabetic ketoacidosis (DKA).
  6. Pregnancy.
  7. Parturition.
  8. Abrupt cessation of antithyroid medications.
  9. Prescribed or accidental ingestion of excessive amounts of thyroid hormone.

SUBJECTIVE DATA
A. Common complaints/symptoms.
  1. Irritability, emotional lability, and anxiety.
  2. Increased appetite with poor weight gain.
  3. Heat intolerance and excessive sweating.
  4. Fatigue.
  5. Respiratory distress.
  6. Nausea and vomiting, diarrhea, and abdominal pain.
  7. Changes in eyes/visions (proptosis, visual changes), seen only in Graves disease.
B. Common presentation.
  1. Severe florid hyperthyroidism evidenced by extreme irritability, high heart rate, cardiac arrhythmia, nausea, and/or vomiting; in addition, the patient may present with a possible psychosis.
C. Family and social history.
  1. None.
D. Review of systems.
  1. May be difficult to speak to during the acute phase.
  2. Ask about extreme irritability, fatigue, and anxiety.
  3. Ask about palpitations.

PHYSICAL EXAMINATION
A. General: Appears toxic.
B. Cardiovascular: Hypertension with widened pulse pressure, cardiac arrhythmias, and fever.
C. Head, ear, eyes, nose, and throat (HEENT): Goiter and exophthalmos.
D. Neurologic: Tremors, seizure activity, and hyperreflexia.

DIAGNOSTIC TESTS
A. Thyroid-stimulating hormone (TSH).
B. Free T4.
C. Free T3.
D. Liver function tests.
E. Complete blood count (CBC).
F. Comprehensive metabolic panel.
G. Imaging studies, which may include:
  1. Chest x-ray (CXR; rule out congestive heart failure [CHF]).
  2. Head CT (exclude other neurologic conditions).
  3. EKG (identify cardiac arrhythmias).

DIFFERENTIAL DIAGNOSIS
A. Anticholinergic or adrenergic drug intoxication.
B. Anxiety disorders.
C. Central nervous system infections.
D. Heart failure.
E. Hypertension.
F. Hypertensive encephalopathy.
G. Hyperthyroidism.
H. Malignant hyperthermia.

I. Panic disorder.

J. Pheochromocytoma (PCC).

K. Septic shock.

EVALUATION AND MANAGEMENT PLAN

A. General plan.

1. Medical treatment of thyroid storm aims to stop thyroid hormone production within the gland, inhibit the release of thyroid hormone, and inhibit conversion of T4 to T3.

2. An acute care or ICU is most appropriate for management.

3. Antithyroid treatment should be continued until euthyroidism is achieved, at which point a final decision regarding oral medications, surgery, or radioactive iodine therapy can be made.

   a. Occasionally, patients may be severely agitated, limiting further intervention.

   b. Sedatives such as haloperidol or benzodiazepine can be given.

4. Management of Airway, Breathing, Circulation, Disability, and Examination (ABCDE) is crucial.

5. With high fever, acetaminophen is preferable to aspirin, which can increase serum T4 and T3 concentrations by interfering with protein binding.

6. Cooling blankets can also be used, with close attention to slow cooling to decrease metabolic demand.

7. Other elements of supportive care: Intravenous (IV) fluids, electrolyte replacement, and nutritional support.

8. Intubation or noninvasive positive pressure ventilation may also be needed with arterial blood gas (ABG) analysis.

B. Patient/family teaching points.

1. Explanation of what thyroid storm is and the importance of management should be discussed with the patient and family. The ICU is the most appropriate for management to provide careful monitoring.

C. Pharmacotherapy.

1. Beta-blockers.

   a. Propranolol is the first-line choice for beta-blockers providing antiadrenergic effects and inhibiting peripheral conversion of T4 to T3.

2. Propylthiouracil (PTU).

   a. PTU is the thionamide of choice in severe, life-threatening thyroid storm because it blocks conversion of T4 to T3.

   b. PTU should be administered orally or via nasogastric tube in the awake or unresponsive patient with a loading dose of 600 mg followed by a dose of 200 to 250 mg every 4 to 6 hours.

   c. PTU is preferred in the first trimester because it causes less severe birth defects.

3. Methimazole.

   a. Methimazole is recommended for severe nonthreatening thyroid storm because it has a longer half-life than PTU, normalizes T3 more rapidly, and has less hepatotoxicity.

   b. Methimazole is administered in a loading dose of 40 mg PO, with a dose of 20 to 30 mg every 4 to 6 hours (max 120 mg/d).

4. Potassium iodine (SSKI).

   a. 5 drops PO Q6H.

5. Steroids.

   a. 100 mg hydrocortisone IV, then 100 mg Q8H.

D. Definitive therapy.

1. Thyroidectomy.

CONSULTATION/REFERRAL

A. Endocrinology should be consulted in all cases.

FOLLOW-UP

A. Follow-up care with an endocrinologist post hospitalization is recommended.

SPECIAL/GERIATRIC CONSIDERATIONS

A. With pregnancy, lithium carbonate at a dose of 300 mg Q8H can be used when there is contraindication to thionamide therapy. Lithium inhibits thyroid hormone release from the thyroid gland.

CASE SCENARIO: THYROID DISORDER: THYROID STORM

A 43-year-old female presents with increasing anxiety and agitation, in addition to vomiting and diarrhea for 3 days. On the morning of admission, the patient's husband noted the patient to be more lethargic and unable to get out of bed. 911 was called and the patient was brought to the hospital. The patient was found to be tachycardic, tachypneic, and was complaining of visual changes. Chest x-ray (CXR) was obtained and revealed bilateral lower lobe consolidation concerning for pneumonia. Her husband states that she has been under a considerable amount of stress at work and had a productive cough, had been feeling fatigued, and complained of feeling warm for a few days, but did not take her temperature. PH: Hypertension, obesity, depression, and asthma. Objective: Blood pressure (BP) 190/89, pulse 157, respirations 26, and temperature 103.6. Lab: Point-of-care (POC) blood glucose (BG) 122 mg/dL, sodium 135 mEq/L, potassium 4.5, white blood cell (WBC) 18,000, hemoglobin 11 g/dL, and thyroid-stimulating hormone (TSH) 0.17 mU/L (nl: 0.45–4.5), free T4 4.9 ng/dL (nl: 0.8–1.8), and free T3 7.6 ng/dL (nl: 2.0–4.4).

1. Given the patient's lab results, what is the most concerning differential diagnosis?

A. Lung cancer

B. Ectopic pregnancy

C. Thyroid storm

D. Sepsis

2. What tool is used to distinguish thyroid storm from other thyrotoxicosis?

A. FASTS

B. Burch–Wartofsky Point Scale (BWPS)

C. PPS

D. PAINADS

3. What is the first-line treatment for severe life-threatening thyroid storm?

A. Antibiotics

B. Vecuronium bromide

C. Magnesium citrate

D. Propylthiouracil (PTU)

(continued)

4. What is the definitive treatment for thyroid storm?
  A. Thyroidectomy
  B. Radiation
  C. Physical therapy
  D. Transplant

BIBLIOGRAPHY

American Association of Clinical Endocrinologists. (2016). *Hyperthyroidism: Information for patients*. http://thyroidawareness.com/sites/all/files/hyperthyroidism.pdf

Brenner, Z., & Porsche, R. (2006). Amiodarone-induced thyroid dysfunction. *Critical Care Nurse, 26*(3), 34–41.

Burch, W. (1994). *Endocrinology* (3rd ed.). Williams & Wilkins.

Burman, K., Ellahham, S., Fadel, B., Lindsay, J., Ringel, M., & Wartofsky, L. (2000). Hyperthyroid heart disease. *Clinical Cardiology, 23*(26), 402–408.

Carroll, R., & Matfin, G. (2010). Endocrine and metabolic emergencies: Thyroid storm. *Therapeutic Advances in Endocrinology and Metabolism, 1*(3), 139–145. https://doi.org/10.1177/2042018810382481

Dahlen, R., & Kumrow, D. (2002). Thyroidectomy: Understanding the potential for complications. *MEDSURG Nursing, 11*(5), 228–235.

Francis, J., & Jayaprasad, N. (2005). Atrial fibrillation and hyperthyroidism. *Indian Pacing and Electrophysiology Journal, 5*(4), 305–311.

Holcomb, S. (2002). Thyroid diseases: A primer for the critical care nurse. *Dimensions of Critical Care Nursing, 21*(4), 127–133. https://doi.org/10.1097/00003465-200207000-00003

Idrose, A. M. (2015, May 12). Acute and emergency care for thyrotoxicosis and thyroid storm. *Acute Medicine and Surgery, 2*(3), 147–157. https://doi.org/10.1002/ams2.104

Lee, S. (2018, March 15). *Hyperthyroidism and thyrotoxicosis*. In R. Khardori (Ed.), *Medscape*. http://emedicine.medscape.com/article/121865-overview

Manzullo, E. F., & Ross, D. S. (2019, February 26). Nonthyroid surgery in the patient with thyroid disease. In J. E. Mulder (Ed.), *UpToDate*. https://www.uptodate.com/contents/nonthyroid-surgery-in-the-patient-with-thyroid-disease

Mathew, V., Misgar, R. A., Ghosh, S., Mukhopadhyay, P., Roychowdhury, P., Pandit, K., Mukhopadhyay, S., & Chowdhury, S. (2011). Myxedema coma: A new look into an old crisis. *Journal of Thyroid Research, 2011*, 1–7. https://doi.org/10.4061/2011/493462

Merrill, E. (2013). A devastating storm. *The Medicine Forum, 14*(12), 24–25. https://doi.org/10.29046/TMF.014.1.012

Roman, S. (2017). *Current best practices in the management of thyroid nodules and cancer*. (PowerPoint slides) https://reachmd.com/programs/cme/current-best-practices-in-the-management-of-thyroid-nodules-and-cancer/8470/transcript/16717/

Ross, D. (2018, September 27). Thyroid function in nonthyroidal illness. In J. E. Mulder (Ed.), *UpToDate*. https://www.uptodate.com/contents/thyroid-function-in-nonthyroidal-illness

Ross, D., & Sugg, S. (2018, September 25). Surgical management of hyperthyroidism. In J. E. Mulder (Ed.), *UpToDate*. https://www.uptodate.com/contents/surgical-management-of-hyperthyroidism

The Nurse Practitioner. (2005). The American Journal of Primary Healthcare. *Thyroid Disorders, 30*(6), 51–52.

Tuttle, R. (2018, January 17). Differentiated thyroid cancer: Clinicopathologic staging. In J. E. Mulder (Ed.), *UpToDate*. https://www.uptodate.com/contents/differentiated-thyroid-cancer-clinicopathologic-staging/print

Umpierrez, G. (2002). Euthyroid sick syndrome. *Southern Medical Journal, 95*(5), 506–513. https://doi.org/10.1097/00007611-200295050-00007

KNOWLEDGE CHECK: CHAPTER 8

1. What is a primary consideration for checking cortisol levels in hospitalized patients?

   A. Cortisol levels fluctuate throughout the day.
   B. Cortisol levels should ideally be checked between 6 and 8 a.m.
   C. Adrenocorticotrophic hormone (ACTH) should be ordered to differentiate between primary adrenal insufficiency (AI) and other types.
   D. All of the above are primary considerations.

2. A patient arrives to the ED with a suspected adrenal crisis due to report of long-standing glucocorticoids that were abruptly discontinued by accident. The patient is hypotensive and hypoglycemic and has altered mental status. What is the initial recommendation?

   A. Intravenous fluids (IVF)
   B. Intravenous (IV) glucocorticoids
   C. Cortisol testing
   D. Cortisol stimulation test

3. In addition to macrovascular changes responsible for coronary artery disease (CAD), peripheral artery disease (PAD), and cerebrovascular disease, microvascular changes should be monitored as an outpatient. Which of the following specialists should be recommended for follow-up as an outpatient?

   A. Chiropractor and gynecologist
   B. Palliative care and orthodontist
   C. Audiologist and physiatrist
   D. Podiatrist and ophthalmologist

4. Hyperpigmented lesions and dark-brown thickened plaques on the neck, axillae, and abdomen associated with poorly controlled or undiagnosed diabetes are called:

   A. Acanthosis nigricans
   B. Melasma
   C. Vitiligo
   D. Psoriasis

5. What hallmark sign of diabetic ketoacidosis (DKA) is typically present on initial exam and can help establish a differential diagnosis prior to the return of any lab results?

   A. Foul-smelling breath
   B. Deconjugate gaze
   C. Fruity-smelling breath
   D. Cheyne–Stokes breathing

6. Patients with hyperglycemic hyperosmolar state (HHS) are best managed in which setting?

   A. Primary care provider (PCP) office
   B. General medical unit
   C. Telemetry unit
   D. ICU

7. On physical exam, yellowish plaques are noted on the medial aspects of all four eyelids, typically found in patients with a diagnosis of metabolic syndrome. What is this condition called?

   A. Acanthosis nigricans
   B. Melasma
   C. Skin tags
   D. Xanthelasma

8. The primary treatment for pheochromocytoma is surgery. Which of the following is the most important part of surgical referral?

   A. Immediate adrenalectomy
   B. Bilateral adrenalectomy
   C. Blood pressure management prior to surgery
   D. Surgery only if patient is having negative effects from the tumor

9. What major symptom is associated with prediabetes?

   A. Chest pain
   B. Dyspnea
   C. Asymptomatic
   D. Peripheral neuropathy

(See answers next page.)

1. **D) All of the above are primary considerations.**
   It is important to remember that cortisol levels fluctuate throughout the day and should only be interpreted at the early morning time frame. Cortisol levels will be the highest at that time, and if they are low (<5 is suggestive, <3 is diagnostic) it is indicative of adrenal insufficiency.

2. **B) Intravenous (IV) glucocorticoids**
   All patients with suspected adrenal crisis should be treated immediately with IV steroids at stress dosing (three times the normal amount). The patient will also need intravenous fluid (IVF), but this should be a secondary recommendation. Cortisol testing of all kinds can occur later once the patient is stable.

3. **D) Podiatrist and ophthalmologist**
   Microvascular changes associated with diabetes mellitus are neuropathy and retinopathy. Prolonged microvascular damage can cause permanent vision loss as well as numbness in distal extremities, predisposing patients with diabetes to poorly healing wounds and possible need for amputation.

4. **A) Acanthosis nigricans**
   This dermatologic condition is associated with poorly controlled or untreated diabetes. As patients improve health and have improved glucose control, acanthosis nigricans plaques can lighten.

5. **C) Fruity-smelling breath**
   Fruity-smelling breath or breath that smells like nail polish remover/acetone is a signature feature of ketoacidosis. Patients with diabetes are prone to this condition when high levels of ketones accumulate in their blood from the abnormal breakdown of fatty acids secondary to low levels of circulating insulin.

6. **D) ICU**
   Hyperglycemic hyperosmolar state (HHS) is a medical emergency, and all patients with HHS require intensive care level of monitoring and neuro checks every 2 hours.

7. **D) Xanthelasma**
   Yellow plaques on the medial aspect of eyelids, which are suggestive of hyperlipidemia, are known as xanthelasma.

8. **C) Blood pressure management prior to surgery**
   Blood pressure (BP) management is the most important aspect as this can prevent poor outcomes perioperatively and postoperatively. Immediate adrenalectomy is not necessary unless other emergent issues are noted. Bilateral adrenalectomy should never be performed (except in extreme cases with bilateral pheochromocytoma [PCC]) since this will leave the patient with no remaining endogenous cortisol production. Almost all patients with PCC should have surgery (even if no acute or immediate effects are noted) since the long-term prognosis is poor.

9. **C) Asymptomatic**
   Prediabetes is typically diagnosed through routine screening or incidental findings during workup for other conditions. Patients with a diagnosis of prediabetes are typically asymptomatic.

10. Treatment with thyroid hormone is contraindicated in patients who have been diagnosed with euthyroid sick syndrome because it:

A. Interferes with the body's adaptive response.

B. Causes hypotension.

C. Is linked to carbon dioxide retention.

D. Is incompatible with IV dextrose.

11. If a patient with a new diagnosis of hyperthyroidism exhibits symptoms of rash, urticaria, and arthralgias, what is the primary concern?

A. Dangerously elevated FT3 levels

B. Adverse side effects of thionamides

C. Allergy to radioactive iodine

D. Thyroid storm

12. Hypotension may be refractory to vasopressor therapy, until thyroid hormone replacement has reached a significant serum concentration. How should hypotension be treated, in these patients, in the interim?

A. Administration of IV bicarbonate and insulin

B. Trendelenburg position

C. IV fluid boluses

D. IV dextrose

13. What is the most common contributing factor for the development of thyroid storm?

A. Elective surgery

B. Underlying Graves disease

C. Pregnancy

D. Head and neck trauma

(See answers next page.)

10. A) Interferes with the body's adaptive response
Research suggests that the derangement in the body's ability to metabolize free T4 is an adaptive response to conserve energy during critical illness. The iatrogenic administration of thyroid hormone may disrupt this adaptive response and is not recommended, except for special consideration in chronic heart failure patients.

11. B) Adverse side effects of thionamides
Methimazole and propylthiouracil (PTU) are the first- and second-line therapies, respectively, of choice. If patients experience adverse side effects to methimazole, which include rash, urticaria, arthralgias, and hepatoxicity, there is a high likelihood that they will also not tolerate treatment with PTU.

12. C) IV fluid boluses
Treatment of hypotension in patients with myxedema coma can be difficult. There can be a diminished response to IV vasopressors due to the lack of circulating thyroid hormone. Until blood pressure stabilizes as the condition resolves, management of hypotension in these patients requires careful administration of IV fluid boluses while avoiding fluid volume overload.

13. B) Underlying Graves disease
Thyroid storm is most commonly seen in females with a diagnosis of Graves disease.

CHAPTER 9

PSYCHIATRIC GUIDELINES

Aparna Kumar and Elizabeth Jordan

BIPOLAR AND RELATED DISORDERS

DIAGNOSTIC AND STATISTICAL MANUAL OF MENTAL DISORDERS, FIFTH EDITION DEFINITION

Bipolar and related disorders include the diagnoses of bipolar I disorder, bipolar II disorder, cyclothymic disorder, substance- or medication-induced bipolar and related disorder, bipolar disorder related to another medical condition, other specified bipolar and related disorder, and unspecified bipolar and related disorder. In this chapter, bipolar I and II disorders as well as cyclothymic disorder are differentiated.

A. Bipolar I disorder. In order to meet the criteria for bipolar I disorder, mania MUST be present and may follow a depressive or hypomanic episode. The definition of a manic episode is shown in Table 9.1.

1. Distinct period of abnormal and persistent elevated, expansive, or irritable mood, and abnormally and persistent increase in goal-directed activity or energy, lasting at least a week and nearly all day, every day.

2. During the period of mood disturbance and increased energy or activity, *three* (or more) of the following symptoms (four if mood is only irritable) are present to a significant degree and represent a noticeable change from usual behavior.

   a. Inflated self-esteem or grandiosity.

   b. Decreased need for sleep (feeling rested after sleeping very little; e.g., 3 hours for 3 days).

   c. More talkative or feels need to talk.

   d. Flight of ideas or describes racing thoughts.

   e. Distractibility (reported or observed).

   f. Increase in goal-directed activities (may be work, school, sexual, or social) and increase in psychomotor agitation (nongoal directed activity such as pacing).

   g. Excessive involvement in activities that have a high risk for painful consequences (such as spending or buying excessively, engaging in risky behaviors).

3. The mood disturbance is sufficiently severe to cause marked impairment in social and occupational functioning, or to necessitate hospitalization to prevent harm to self or others *OR* there are psychotic features.

4. The episode is not attributable to the physiologic effects of a substance (illicit or prescribed) or to another medical condition.

5. NOTE: All criteria must be fulfilled to be considered a manic episode. A full manic episode that emerges during antidepressant treatment (such as medication) but persists at a fully syndromal level beyond the physiologic effect of treatment is sufficient evidence for a manic episode.

TABLE 9.1 MANIA AND HYPOMANIA COMPARISONS

	Manic Episode	Hypomanic Episode
Duration	1 week or more	4 days or more
Mood	Abnormally and persistently high, irritable, or expansive	
Activity/energy	Abnormally and persistently increased	
Symptoms that are changes from usual behavior	Three or more of inflated self-esteem or grandiosity, ↓ need for sleep, ↑ talkativeness or pressure to talk, flight of ideas or racing thoughts, distractibility (reported or observed), ↑ goal-directed activity or psychomotor agitation, and engagement in activities that have high potential for painful consequences	
Severity	Results in psychotic features, hospitalization, or impairment at work, social, and personal levels	Clear change from usual functioning and others notice this change and NO psychosis, hospitalizations, or impairment
Differential diagnosis	Rule out change from baseline due to substance use, medication use, or underlying medical diagnosis; rule out major depressive disorder, anxiety disorders.	

Source: Adapted with permission from Morrison, J. (2014). DSM-5 made easy: The clinician's guide to diagnosis. Guilford Press.

B. Hypomanic episode (see Table 9.1).

   1. Distinct period of abnormal expansive, elevated, or irritable mood, lasting all day, every day for at least 4 days, that is clearly different from nondepressed mood.

   2. During the same period, three or more (four if mood is only irritable) are present and are a significant change from baseline behavior.

   a. Inflated self-esteem or grandiosity.

   b. Decreased need for sleep (feeling rested after sleeping very little; i.e., 3 hours for 3 days).

   c. More talkative or feels need to talk.

   d. Flight of ideas or describes racing thoughts.

   e. Distractibility (reported or observed).

   f. Increase in goal-directed activities (may be work, school, sexual, or social) and increase in psychomotor agitation (nongoal-directed activity such as pacing).

   g. Excessive involvement in activities that have a high risk for painful consequences (such as spending or buying excessively, engaging in risky behaviors).

   3. Change in behavior is uncharacteristic for the person.

   4. Other people notice the change in mood and functioning.

   5. Episode does not cause marked impairment in social or occupational functioning, does not require hospitalization, and there are no psychotic features. If psychotic features are present, then the episode is considered a manic episode.

   6. The episode is not attributable to the physiologic effects of a substance (illicit or prescribed) or to another medical condition.

   7. NOTE: All criteria must be fulfilled to be considered a hypomanic episode. A hypomanic episode that emerges during antidepressant treatment (such as medication) but persists at a fully syndromal level beyond the physiologic effect of treatment is sufficient evidence for a hypomanic episode. All criteria must be present for a hypomanic episode. Hypomania can exist in bipolar I disorder as well but is not required for diagnosis.

C. Major depressive episode.

   1. Five (or more) of the symptoms listed have been present at the same time in the last 2 weeks and are a change from previous functioning. At least one of the symptoms is (a) depressed mood or (b) loss of interest or pleasure (anhedonia). Symptoms are not related to another medical condition.

   a. Sad mood most of day, every day, either reported by the individual or by observation of others.

   b. Decreased interest in almost all activities most of the day, nearly every day, either reported by the individual or by observation of others.

   c. Changes in appetite and weight loss or weight gain (of 5% or more in a month).

   d. Change in sleep (insomnia or hypersomnia).

   e. Psychomotor agitation or retardation observed by others.

   f. Fatigue or loss of energy.

   g. Feelings of worthlessness or excessive guilt nearly every day.

   h. Decreased ability to think or concentrate or make decisions nearly every day (reported or observed).

   i. Recurring thoughts of death, suicidal ideation without a plan, suicide attempt, or plan for committing suicide.

   2. The mood disturbance is sufficiently severe to cause marked impairment in social, occupational, or important areas of functioning.

   3. The episode is not attributable to the physiologic effects of a substance (illicit or prescribed) or to another medical condition.

   4. Criteria 1 to 3 must be present to be considered a major depressive episode.

   5. NOTE: It is important to understand the context of the episode and whether or not significant loss preceded the change in mood. If so, it is important to distinguish features of major depressive episode (MDE) from those of grief.

D. Bipolar I disorder.

   1. Criteria have been met for manic episode.

   2. Mania and/or depression are not better explained by another diagnosis.

   3. Specifier guidance: The *Diagnostic and Statistical Manual of Mental Disorders*, Fifth Edition (*DSM-5*) describes each diagnosis based on timing (current or most recent), status (severity), presence of psychotic features, and remission status (only applies if does not meet the criteria for mania, hypomania, or major depressive episode). If hypomanic episode, severity and psychotic features specifiers do not apply. If unspecified episode, severity, psychotic features, and remission do not apply.

   a. Timing: Current or most recent episode manic, current or most recent episode hypomanic, current or most recent episode depressed, or current or most recent episode unspecified.

   b. Severity: Mild, moderate, or severe.

   c. Psychotic features: With or without psychotic features.

   d. Remission status: In partial remission or in full remission.

E. Bipolar II disorder.

   1. Must meet the criteria for current or past hypomanic episode and the criteria for current or past major depressive episode.

   2. Specifier guidance: Specifiers are used to indicate the nature of the current episode: Hypomanic or depressed; severity (mild, moderate, severe) and course (partial or full remission).

   3. If depressed, specifiers are mild, moderate, or severe without psychotic features, or severe with mood congruent or incongruent psychotic features, with catatonia, with melancholic features, with mixed features, with anxious distress, or with peripartum onset.

INCIDENCE

A. The 12-month prevalence for bipolar I disorder is 0.6%, with a lifetime male to female ratio of 1:1. The age of onset is about 18 years of age, earlier than in major depressive disorder (MDD).

B. 90% of individuals with a single manic episode have a recurrent mood episode.

C. 60% of manic episodes occur immediately before a major depressive episode.

D. The 12-month prevalence for bipolar II disorder is 0.3%.

PATHOGENESIS

A. The pathogenesis of bipolar disorder is not known. Approximately 60% to 70% heritability has been estimated from twin/pedigree studies, highlighting that heritability is complex and involves genetic changes as well as environmental factors. There is likely genetic overlap with other disorders such as schizophrenia.

B. Brain changes: There are brain changes in bipolar disorder; however it has not been determined if these changes are a result of the disorder or if they precede the disorder.

    1. Decreased connectivity among prefrontal networks and limbic structures.

    2. May be associated with smaller total gray matter volumes, representing a neuroprogressive disorder.

    3. Immune system dysregulations, including elevated cytokines (interleukin-4, tumor necrosis factor-alpha, and C-reactive protein [CRP]) and cytokine receptors, are found in people with bipolar disorder.

PREDISPOSING FACTORS

A. Environmental: Stressful life events appear to play a role in the onset and severity of bipolar disorder.

B. Genetics: Family history is one of the strongest and most consistent predictors of bipolar disorder. Advanced paternal age is also associated with increased risk of bipolar disorder.

C. Sex: Females are more likely to have rapid cycling and mixed states and are more likely to have depressive episodes along with an increased risk of eating disorders and alcohol use disorders.

D. Suicide: Lifetime risk is 15 times greater than that in the general population.

SUBJECTIVE DATA

A. Common complaints/symptoms.

    1. Mania.

        a. Racing thoughts.

        b. Flight of ideas.

        c. Increased focused activity.

        d. Thoughts of grandiosity.

        e. Excessive talking or pressured speech.

    2. Depressive episodes.

        a. Depressed mood.

        b. Loss of energy or fatigue.

        c. Diminished interest in anything.

        d. Weight loss.

        e. Feelings of worthlessness.

B. Common/typical scenario.

    1. A typical scenario starts with an unusual shift in mood, sleep, activity level, and energy. The person may have excessively elevated mood for about a week and then become depressed.

    2. The presence of depression and/or psychosis is not needed for a diagnosis of bipolar and related disorders.

    3. Most people who are diagnosed with bipolar I disorder will have a history of at least one depressive episode.

    4. Cyclothymia is diagnosed when a person has depressive and hypomanic symptoms present at least 50% of the time without meeting the full criteria for depressive or manic episode.

C. Family and social history.

    1. Inquire about family history of mental illness.

    2. Inquire about periods of depression or manic episodes.

    3. Inquire about patterns of sleep and activity level.

    4. Inquire about lifestyle and stressful life events.

D. Review of systems.

    1. Rule out medical causes.

        a. Constitutional: Fever, chills, night sweats, weight loss, fatigue, and loss of appetite.

        b. Endocrine: Excessive thirst or urination, and heat/cold intolerance.

        c. Neurologic: Weakness, headaches, dizziness, tremor, numbness/tingling, seizures/convulsions, fainting, and stroke/transient ischemic attack (TIA).

        d. Cardiovascular: Chest pain, shortness of breath, irregular heartbeat, racing heart, and high blood pressure.

    2. Psychiatric: Irritability, agitation, frustration, sleep disruption, goal-directed activities, and mood fluctuation. Rule out schizoaffective disorder, MDD, cyclothymic disorder, and generalized anxiety disorder; rule out primary insomnia or sleep-related disorder; rule out attention deficit hyperactivity disorder (ADHD).

    3. Substance use: Recent or past alcohol or substance use.

MENTAL STATUS EXAMINATION

A. A mnemonic for elements of the mental status examination (MSE) is: **A**ll **B**orderline **S**ubjects **A**re **T**ough, **T**roubled **C**haracters: **A**ppearance, **B**ehavior, **S**peech, **A**ffect, **T**hought Process, **T**hought Content, **C**ognitive Exam.

    1. Conduct an MSE.

    2. Appearance: Variable. May be overly groomed in mania/hypomania; disheveled if appearing with psychotic features; poor grooming if depressed.

    3. Behavior: Energetic, talkative, excited, funny and/or with psychotic features, disorganized, aggressive, and hostile (mania); can be withdrawn, resistant, or shy (depression). Motor: May see psychomotor retardation in depression; exaggerated movement in ▶

mania; eye contact can be intense (mania); may be easily distractible (mania).

4. Speech: Talkative, fast/pressured, loud, coherent/incoherent, and unable to interrupt (mania); slow, dull, monotonous, slurred, and hesitant (depression).

5. Affect/mood: Affect (perceived by observer) elevated, euphoric, elated, expansive, irritable, anger, hostility, labile mood moving from laughing to crying to irritability, for example (mania). A low frustration tolerance is common; mood (reported by the patient) happy, on top of the world, and intense (mania).

6. Thought process: Flight of ideas (mania), loose associations, disorganization, and incoherence in severe mania.

7. Thought content: Self-confidence and increased self-importance (mania).

8. Perceptual disturbances: Can have delusions (common) or hallucinations; may have paranoia (either depression or mania); mood congruent delusions in mania have themes of wealth and extraordinary abilities or power.

9. Judgment: Usually poor/impaired in mania, variable in depression; may have poor impulse control in mania (up to 75% presenting with aggression).

10. Insight: Poor/impaired in mania, especially if with psychotic features and if delusions/hallucinations present, variable in depression.

11. Cognitive exam: Orientation and memory usually intact in mania and depression, but may be distractible if in manic episode (if grandiose or distracted); may require collateral information from family member or observer for full history.

DIAGNOSTIC TESTS

A. In order to diagnose bipolar disorder, must first rule out potential medical causes of the psychiatric symptoms. This list is not inclusive of all, but provides examples of diagnostic tests that are relevant for particular groups of diagnoses.

   1. Endocrine disorders.
   a. Hyperthyroidism in mania, hypothyroidism in depression: Thyroid function tests.
   b. Diabetes: Fasting blood glucose, hemoglobin A1C, and lipid panel.
   c. Cushing syndrome: Complete blood count (CBC), comprehensive metabolic panel (CMP), 24-hour urinary free cortisol test, late-night salivary cortisol test, low-dose dexamethasone suppression test (LDDST), dexamethasone corticotropin-releasing hormone (CRH) test, and CT/MRI.
   d. Addison disease: CBC, CMP, urinalysis, adrenocorticotrophic hormone (ACTH) stimulation test, thyroid function tests, and CT/MRI.

   2. Neurologic and vascular disorders.
   a. Epilepsy: CBC, CMP, CT/MRI, EEG, and PET scan.
   b. Cerebrovascular disease: CBC, CMP, prothrombin time (PT)/international normalized ratio (INR), CRP, and thyroid function tests.

   c. Tumors: CBC, CMP, ultrasound, x-ray, CT/MRI, and PET scan.
   d. Headaches and head trauma: CBC, CMP, CT/MRI, and EEG.
   e. Lupus: CBC, CMP, liver function tests (LFTs), urinalysis, and antinuclear antibody (ANA).
   f. Multiple sclerosis: CBC, CMP, lumbar puncture, CT/MRI, and electromyography (EMG).

   3. Infectious disease.
   a. HIV/AIDS: HIV testing, tuberculosis (TB) testing, and sexually transmitted disease (STD) testing.
   b. Lyme disease: Two-step Lyme disease testing (enzyme immunoassay (EIA) + EIA or immunofluorescence + western blot or EIA).
   c. Syphilis: Fluorescent treponemal antibody absorption test (FTA-ABS) or rapid plasma reagin (RPR) syphilis.

   4. Vitamin deficiency.
   a. B$_{12}$, folate, niacin, and thiamine.

   5. Medications/substances associated with mania.
   a. Amphetamines: Patient history and urine drug test (UDS).
   b. Corticosteroids: Patient history.
   c. Hallucinogens: Patient history and UDS.
   d. Levodopa: Patient history.
   e. Opiates: Patient history and UDS.
   f. Phencyclidine (PCP): Patient history and UDS.

   6. Screening tools for bipolar and related disorders symptoms: Positive screen DOES NOT indicate a disorder. All screening tools require validation with comprehensive interview/assessment.
   a. Mood Disorder Questionnaire (MDQ).
   b. Young Mania Rating Scale.
   c. Bipolar Depression Rating Scale (BDRS).
   d. Hypomania Checklist (HCL-32): Self-report.

DIFFERENTIAL DIAGNOSIS

A. MDD.
B. Schizophrenia.
C. Generalized anxiety disorder.
D. Posttraumatic stress disorder (PTSD).
E. Substance-induced mood disorder.
F. ADHD.
G. Personality disorders.
H. Cyclothymia.

EVALUATION AND MANAGEMENT PLAN

A. General plan.

   1. Treatment of bipolar disorders is complex: Antidepressants should be avoided unless an individual has refractory depression unresponsive to an atypical antipsychotic (AA), anticonvulsant (such as Lamictal), and/or mood stabilizer. Antidepressant treatment can trigger mania and/or increase the risk of rapid cycling between mania, hypomania, euthymia, and/or depression.

   2. If an antidepressant is used to treat the depressive episode, discontinuation should be considered 6 to 12 months after symptoms have resolved.

B. Patient/family teaching points.

1. Adherence to treatment plan can be challenging due to medication side effects and need for multifactorial and continuous approach to treatment.

2. It is critical to recognize and respond to early warning signs and symptoms of a mood episode (either mania or depression).

3. The patient and family should have resources for coping skills, group support, individual support, and collaboration with clinicians for managing life events and stressors.

4. Encourage patient, family, and support person to learn more about disease course and rationale behind current therapies to increase adherence.

5. Provide management, crisis, and intervention resources in addition to information for local and national support groups, such as the National Alliance on Mental Illness (NAMI).

C. Pharmacotherapy. (This list is not exhaustive but highlights commonly used medications.)

1. *Gold standard* is lithium, which has an indication for acute mania, prophylaxis of depression and suicide, and can be an adjunctive antidepressant treatment in unipolar depression.

a. *Elimination* is almost entirely by the kidneys; therefore, once-a-day dosing is recommended. Lithium 300 mg = 0.3 mEq/L plasma concentration.

b. *Therapeutic range* varies from 0.6 to 1.5 mEq/L (mania: 0.8–1.2 mEq/L, may go as high as 1.5 mEq/L with close monitoring; depression: 0.6–1.0 mEq/L; maintenance 0.7–1.0 mEq/L).

c. *Drug–drug interactions:* Nonsteroidal anti-inflammatory drugs (NSAIDs), including ibuprofen and selective cyclooxygenase-2 (COX-2) inhibitors,diuretics(especiallythiazide)angiotensin-converting enzyme (ACE) inhibitors, and angiotensin II receptor antagonists can increase plasma lithium concentrations. Metronidazole decreases renal clearance and can lead to lithium toxicity. Alkaline agents (such as sodium bicarbonate) can decrease lithium concentrations; use with calcium channel blockers, antipsychotics, selective serotonin reuptake inhibitors (SSRIs) and methyldopa may lead to or worsen neurotoxicity; may prolong the effects of neuromuscular blockade.

d. *Pregnancy:* Must weigh risk–benefit of continued use due to risk of major malformations (slight increase in risk in the general population) and cardiac abnormalities; risk of recurrence of symptoms in pregnancy is high.

e. *Laboratory tests:* Prior to treatment, check human chorionic gonadotropin (HCG) for pregnancy, check weight and height, kidney function tests (with creatinine and urine-specific gravity), thyroid function tests, and CBC (can cause leukocytosis), and repeat every 6 months. Patients over 50 years of age should have an EKG. Initial monitoring for lithium level every 1 to 2 weeks until goal level is reached, then every 2 to 3 months for the next 6 months, then 6 to 12 months once stable. If dose is changed, check level in 1 to 2 weeks.

f. Side effects of lithium at different levels can be seen in Table 9.2.

g. Of note, antipsychotics are also used for monotherapy and combined therapy (such as olanzapine and ziprasidone), but some are indicated for mania, depression, or both. Of note, monitoring for body mass index (BMI), weight, blood pressure, prolactin, lipid profile, and glucose, as well as EKG, is indicated. Side effects such as weight gain and tardive dyskinesia are possible (although to a lesser extent than first-generation antipsychotics).

2. Valproate (Depakote) is indicated for mixed episodes, acute mania, rapid cycling, and maintenance treatment. It is metabolized by the liver.

a. *Drug–drug interactions:* Lamotrigine (Lamictal) should be reduced by 50% if used with valproate. Aspirin and chlorpromazine (and other medications metabolized by CYP2D6 or CYP3A4) can increase the plasma levels of valproate. Valproate can increase the plasma levels of phenytoin and phenobarbital. Caution in patients with alcohol use disorder or regular heavy alcohol use.

b. *Warning:* Do not use if there is history of pancreatitis, serious liver disease, urea cycle disorder, or proven allergy to valproate.

c. *Laboratory tests:* CBC (with platelet count), CMP, LFTs, lipid panel, triglycerides, PT/INR if there is history of bleeding, fasting glucose, and pregnancy test in females. Recheck LFTs, CBC (with platelet count), fasting glucose, and valproic acid (VPA) level every month for the first 3 ▶

TABLE 9.2 LITHIUM TOXICITY AND SIDE EFFECTS

Lithium Level (mEq/L)	Side Effects
1.0–1.5	Tremor
1.5–2.0	Tremor, cog-wheel rigidity, nausea, diarrhea, vomiting, muscle weakness, poor coordination, lethargy, fatigue
2.0–3.0	Blurred vision, dizziness, increased clear urine, tinnitus, ataxia, confusion
>3.0	Delirium, coma, seizures, organ failure, hyperthermia, hypotension, death

months, then every 6 months. Response is based on evaluation of the patient (doses up to trough plasma level of 100 µg/mL generally well tolerated; trough levels up to 125 µg/mL may be needed in some patients with mania. Target dose is usually between 750 and 3,000 mg/d.

d. *Pregnancy:* Consider alternatives to treatment for bipolar disorder and weigh risk–benefit before use. Valproate use during first trimester can increase the risk of neural tube defects (spina bifida) and congenital anomalies. Use of valproate is also associated with developmental delay and lower cognitive test scores after fetal exposure in the absence of other abnormalities.

3. Carbamazepine (Tegretol) can be used for acute mania, mixed episode, and maintenance medication; metabolized in the liver, primarily by CYP4503A4, and is renally excreted; substrate for CYP4503A4 and autoinducer (can induce its own metabolism); also induces CYP4502C9, weakly 1A2, 2C19.

a. *Drug–drug interactions:* Lowers the effectiveness of oral birth control pills. Should not be used concurrently with monoamine oxidase inhibitors (MAOIs) as it has a tricyclic structure. Enzyme-inducing antiepileptics (like phenytoin) can lower levels as can CYP4503A4 inducers. CYP4503A4 inhibitors (like fluoxetine) can increase plasma levels. Can decrease plasma levels of acetaminophen, benzodiazepines, and warfarin, for example. Can cause thyroid dysfunction when used with other anticonvulsants and neurotoxic effects when combined with lithium.

b. *Warning:* Can result in aplastic anemia, agranulocytosis, rare severe dermatologic reactions (such as Stevens–Johnson syndrome), syndrome of inappropriate antidiuretic hormone secretion (SIADH), and can result in cardiac problems. Avoid in patients with bone marrow transplant.

c. *Laboratory tests:* CBC, LFTs, kidney function tests, thyroid function tests, PT/INR, and pregnancy test in female patients. Repeat lab work every 2 to 4 weeks for 2 months, then lab work with carbamazepine level (levels between 4 and 12 µg/mL) every 3 to 6 months throughout treatment. Genetic testing recommended by the Food and Drug Administration (FDA) for people with ancestry across Asia (including South Asian Indians) for the presence of the human leukocyte antigen (HLA) allele (HLA-B*1502). If present, should not use.

d. *Pregnancy:* Use in first trimester is associated with risk of neural tube defects (spina bifida) or other congenital anomalies. Recommend to weigh risk–benefit of discontinuing medication as pregnancy and postpartum are increased periods of symptom relapse. May consider antipsychotics or other medications as alternatives; taper to stop if indicated. Monitor carefully and consume 1 g folate daily if continued.

4. Lamotrigine (Lamictal) is indicated for bipolar maintenance. It has been found effective in bipolar II disorder and bipolar depression as well. Metabolized through the liver through glucuronidation, renally excreted, and can reduce folate concentrations.

a. *Drug–drug interactions:* Valproate increases half-life, needs lower doses of lamotrigine. Can increase risk of rash when used with valproate. Any enzyme-inducing drugs can lower plasma levels; oral contraceptives can decrease plasma levels. Can result in false-positive urine immunoassay for PCP.

b. *Warning:* Risk of serious rash, multiorgan failure associated with Stevens–Johnson syndrome, drug hypersensitivity syndrome; if benign risk with no lab abnormalities and no widespread symptoms, monitor closely; risk of suicidal ideation; risk of Stevens–Johnson syndrome if a patient missed more than 5 days; need to be retitrated; titrate slowly to decrease risk of rash.

c. *Laboratory tests:* Lab testing not required but prudent to check CBC, CMP, thyroid-stimulating hormone (TSH), LFT, and renal function tests; ophthalmologic checks may be done due to the melanin-binding nature of lamotrigine.

d. *Pregnancy:* Risk is not well-studied, but some association with cleft palate or cleft lip; important to weigh risk–benefit for risk of recurrence; may consider alternatives, including antipsychotics; taper to stop if needed.

FOLLOW-UP

A. Patients with bipolar disorder should be followed by a primary care provider (for monitoring of medication side effects and comorbidities), a psychiatric provider (for psychoeducation medication management), a therapist (for increased self-efficacy), and community support (for family support and psychoeducation).

CONSULTATION/REFERRAL

A. Consultation and referral to a specialist are warranted if there are secondary comorbid physical health conditions such as thyroid dysfunction, renal impairment, skin disorders, and/or gastrointestinal side effects.

SPECIAL/GERIATRIC CONSIDERATIONS

A. Support group is critical for long-term support, peer and family support, and education around relapse prevention. Two groups are:

1. Depression and Bipolar Support Alliance.
2. NAMI.

B. Geriatric considerations.

1. If present from a younger age, older adults tend to have fewer episodes of mania.
2. It is important to evaluate for cognitive decline and neurocognitive testing.
3. Mania in older adults can be present in the context of another illness (such as infection). ▶

4. Age-related pharmacodynamic and pharmacokinetic characteristics must be factored into dosing. Reduced enzyme activity (such as CYPA4) necessitates lower dosing in older adults for some antidepressants. The risk of adverse drug reactions is also higher in older adults.

5. Therapy and psychosocial interventions remain relevant in older age adults.

CASE SCENARIO: BIPOLAR DISORDER

A 26-year-old woman with a history of generalized anxiety disorder, diagnosed at 24 years of age, presents to the ED with concerns that "people who work for the government are following her." She reports that she has been awake for the past 3 days and has taken extensive notes about the events over the course of the past 3 days. She also reports that she has spent a great deal of money, and her roommate feels that she is out of control. She reports that she has not eaten for several days nor has she had much to drink because she has been so focused on getting away from the people following her. She has never been on psychiatric medications before this year. To treat her anxiety, she was started on a selective serotonin reuptake inhibitor (SSRI), paroxetine (Paxil) 30 mg daily, approximately 8 weeks ago; the dose was increased last week to 40 mg daily. Her vital signs in the ED showed temperature of 100.4°F/38°C, blood pressure of 90/72, pulse rate of 113, and respiratory rate of 18 breaths per minute. Physical examination findings are unremarkable with the exception of dry oral mucous membranes.

1. What is the most relevant diagnosis to include in the differential diagnosis and the resulting course of action/interventions?

A. Generalized anxiety disorder
B. Major depressive disorder
C. Bipolar disorder
D. Schizophrenia

BIBLIOGRAPHY

American Psychiatric Association. (2013). *Diagnostic and statistical manual of mental disorders* (5th ed.). Author.
Boland, R., Verduin, M., & Ruiz, P (Eds.). (2022). *Kaplan & Sadock's synopsis of psychiatry* (12th ed.). Wolters Kluwer.
BulletPsych. (2020, September 26). *Day #46: Mental status exam in bipolar disorder.* https://www.bulletpsych.com/post/day-46-mental-status-exam-in-bipolar-disorder
Hedya, S., Avula, A., & Swoboda, H. (2021). *Lithium toxicity.* StatPearls [Internet]. https://www.ncbi.nlm.nih.gov/books/NBK499992/
Ljubic, N., Ueberberg, B., Grunze, H., & Assion, H. (2021). Treatment of bipolar disorders in older adults: A review. *Annals of General Psychiatry, 20,* 45.
Morrison, J. (2014). *DSM-5 made easy: The clinician's guide to diagnosis.* Guilford Press.
Pliszka, S. R. (2016). *Neuroscience for the mental health clinician* (2nd ed.). Guilford Press.
Smoller, J., Andreassen, O., Edenberg, H., Faraone, S., Glatt, S., & Kendler, K. (2018). Psychiatric genetics and the structure of psychopathology. *Molecular Psychiatry, 24,* 409–420. https://www.nature.com/articles/s41380-017-0010-4
Stahl, S. M. (2013). *Stahl's essential psychopharmacology: Neuroscientific basis and practical applications* (4th ed.). Cambridge University Press.
Stahl, S. M. (2017). *Stahl's essential psychopharmacology: Prescriber's guide* (6th ed.). Cambridge University Press.

MAJOR DEPRESSIVE DISORDER

DEFINITION

A. Five (or more) of the following symptoms present during the same 2-week period and representing a change from previous functioning. At least one of the symptoms must be either (a) depressed mood or (b) loss of interest or pleasure.

1. Depressed mood most of the day, nearly every day, by subjective report (sad, empty, hopeless) or observed by others (appears tearful).
2. Markedly diminished pleasure in all or most activities.
3. Significant weight loss (more than 5% in a month) or decrease or increase in appetite nearly every day.
4. Insomnia or hypersomnia nearly every day.
5. Psychomotor agitation or retardation nearly every day (observable by others, not merely subjective feelings of restlessness or being slowed down).
6. Fatigue or loss of energy nearly every day.
7. Feelings of worthlessness or excessive or inappropriate guilt (which may be delusional) nearly every day.
8. Diminished ability to think or concentrate, indecisiveness, nearly every day (subjective or observed).
9. Recurrent thoughts of death (not just dying), recurrent suicidal ideation without a specific plan, or a suicide attempt or a specific plan.

B. Symptoms cause clinically significant distress or impairment in social, occupational, or other areas of functioning.
C. The episode is not attributable to the physiologic effects of a substance or to another medical condition.
D. With postpartum onset: If symptoms are within 4 weeks postpartum. Postpartum mental health concerns can often include psychotic symptoms.
E. Mnemonic for evaluation of symptoms: **SIGE CAPS**.

1. Sleep disturbance.
2. Interest and pleasure decrease.
3. Guilt.
4. Energy lower.
5. Concentration decrease.
6. Appetite increase or decrease.
7. Psychomotor agitation or retardation.
8. Suicidal/hopeless.

INCIDENCE

A. The 12-month prevalence is approximately 7%, with increase in 18- to 29-year-olds.
B. Females have 1.5- to 3-fold higher rates than males beginning in early adolescence.
C. Mean age of onset is 40 years of age, with 50% of persons having an onset between the ages of 20 and 50 years.

D. Younger adults have the highest 1-year prevalence of major depressive disorder (MDD), with adolescent females at 20%.

PATHOGENESIS

A. Heritability: 37%.

B. Odds ratio of 2.84 for developing MDD if first-degree relative has diagnosis.

   1. Neurochemical imbalance: The most basic level is the monoamine hypothesis, an imbalance in the following neurotransmitters: norepinephrine, dopamine (DA), and serotonin.

   2. Neurogenesis: This theory posits that neurodevelopment differs in the brain of depressed people. The result is difficulty regulating the hypothalamic–pituitary–adrenal (HPA) axis, which can lead to increased glucocorticoid production and inhibition of neurogenesis.

   3. Neuroplasticity: Atrophy of mature neurons is another theory of depression. This can be due to increased glucocorticoids and decreased brain-derived neurotrophic factor (BDNF), which results in atrophied neurons. This is thought to happen in the hippocampus, of which decreased volumes have also been seen in depression.

PREDISPOSING FACTORS

A. No close interpersonal relationships.

B. Divorced or separated.

C. More common in rural than urban areas.

D. Stressful life events precede the first episode.

E. Depression in older persons is common. Individuals with the following are at higher risk of developing depression: Lower socioeconomic status, loss of spouse, current physical illness, and social isolation.

SUBJECTIVE DATA

A. Common complaints/symptoms.

   1. Agitation or restlessness.

   2. Psychomotor retardation.

   3. Flat affect.

   4. Loss of energy.

   5. Feeling of worthlessness.

   6. Diminished ability to concentrate.

   7. Loss of pleasure in activities.

   8. Recurrent thoughts of death.

B. Common/typical scenario.

   1. Patients may not seek attention for depression but typically complain of other symptoms, such as insomnia, headaches, abdominal upset, and difficulty concentrating.

C. Family and social history.

   1. Depression can be familial.

   2. Social history is noncontributory.

D. Review of systems.

   1. May be useful to rule out medical causes. See "Bipolar and Related Disorders."

MENTAL STATUS EXAMINATION

A. Appearance: Variable. Can be disheveled if depression with psychotic features. Poor grooming if depressed.

B. Behavior: Can be withdrawn, resistant, shy (depression).Motor: May see psychomotor retardation in depression; downcast gaze, hand wringing.

C. Speech: Slow, soft, dull, monotonous, slurred, hesitant (depression), and limited responses to questions.

D. Affect/mood: Affect (perceived by observer) constricted, guarded, and withdrawn; mood (reported by patient) OK, sad, and blue (50% often deny depression).

E. Thought process: Flight of ideas (mania), loose associations, disorganization, and incoherence in severe mania.

F. Thought content: Negative worldviews, rumination, and guilt. Assess for suicidality (10%–15% commit suicide) and homicidal ideation.

   1. Homicidal or assaultive ideation.

     a. Ideation, means, plan, and intent.

     b. Assess for anger, rage, and interpersonal conflict.

     c. If actively homicidal: Inpatient psychiatric hospitalization, notify law enforcement and victim.

   2. Perceptual disturbances/paranoid ideation: Can have hallucinations (auditory common), delusions, paranoia, and mood incongruent delusions.

G. Judgment: Variable in depression.

H. Insight: Variable in depression; if psychotic features may not have insight.

I. Cognitive exam: Orientation and memory usually intact in depression, but up to two-thirds of depressed patients may have cognitive impairment. May require collateral information from family member or observer for full history. Assess orientation to person, place, time, and situation. Assess concentration: Serial 7s, spell "world" backward, or recite the days of the week backward.

J. Suicide risk assessment. NOTE: HIGH RISK for self-harm exists when energy is improving; the individual can carry out the plan.

   1. Ask about ideation: Onset, duration, frequency, active thoughts, lethality, stressors, and use of substances. Ask: "Have you had the thought I wish I were dead or that I wouldn't wake up?" If yes, have you ever had the thought, "I want to kill myself"?

   2. Ask about intent. Ask: "Did you want to harm yourself or end your life?"

   3. Ask about plan: Wish to die, means, and understands consequences. Ask: "Have you ever made a plan to kill yourself? Did you have the intent to do it or was it a thought about doing it?"

   4. Ask about means/access to firearms: Access to carry out plan, taken steps to prepare to end life, lethality. Ask: "Did you ever try to harm or kill yourself? If no, what prevented you, yourself, or someone else?"

   5. Ask about protective (such as family, social connections, faith) or risk factors (such as hopelessness, previous attempt).

   6. Use a validated screening tool to ask the right questions and to understand the next steps. One useful one is the Columbia Suicide Severity Rating Scale ▶

(C-SSRS). Also use a safety planning tool to create a shared framework for referral to services.

K. High-risk populations for suicide. People who are/identify as:

1. Older single White males.
2. Divorced/widowed.
3. Unemployed.
4. Having psychosis.
5. Experiencing homelessness.
6. LGBTQ+.
7. Veterans.
8. Comorbid physical and/or substance use disorder.
9. Previous attempt and/or family history.
10. Access to lethal means.

DIAGNOSTIC TESTS

A. Thyroid function tests.
B. Complete blood count (CBC).
C. Comprehensive metabolic panel (CMP).
D. Based on history: Rapid plasma reagin (RPR), vitamin D level, folate level, B_{12} or thiamine level, and urine drug screen (after discussion with the patient).
E. Differential diagnosis.

1. Endocrine disorders: Hypothyroidism, diabetes, and adrenal dysfunction.
2. Neurologic disorders: Dementia, seizures, tumors, Parkinson disease, sleep apnea, cerebrovascular accident (CVA), and neoplasms.
3. Cardiac disease: Congestive heart failure and hypertension.
4. Infection: Mononucleosis, HIV/AIDS, pneumonia, and tardive dyskinesia (TD).
5. Nutrition deficits: Anemia and low vitamin D/folate/B_{12}/thiamine.
6. Other: Side effects of medications such as cardiac medications, hypnotics, antibacterial medications, antineoplastic medications, analgesics, antiepileptics, or antiparkinsonian drugs.

F. Screening instruments (in public domain): Positive screen DOES NOT indicate a disorder; REQUIRES validation with comprehensive interview/assessment.

1. Patient Health Questionnaire (PHQ)-2.
2. PHQ-9, or PHQ for Adolescents.
3. Mood Disorders Questionnaire (MDQ).
4. Edinburgh Postnatal Depression Scale (EPDS).
5. Geriatric Depression Scale.

DIFFERENTIAL DIAGNOSIS

A. Bipolar disorder, depressed phase.
B. Mood disorder due to general medical condition.
C. Eating disorder.
D. Substance-induced mood disorder.
E. Adjustment disorder with depressed mood.
F. Attention deficit hyperactivity disorder (ADHD).
G. Borderline personality disorder.
H. Complicated grief.
I. Schizophrenia and schizoaffective disorder.

EVALUATION AND MANAGEMENT PLAN

A. General plan.

1. Determine if the patient meets the criteria for MDD, single episode or recurrent, and, if postpartum onset, psychosis or suicidal/homicidal ideation.
2. If the patient is not actively suicidal, homicidal, or has psychosis, discuss treatment options.
3. Recommend psychotherapy for mild to moderate symptoms or if the patient does not wish to start medication.
4. Ensure that bipolar disorder has been ruled out prior to starting antidepressant treatment.

B. Patient/family teaching points.

1. Teach patients about the early signs of relapse and rationale for treatment choices made.
2. Teach family members about depression and how to be supportive.
3. Encourage the patient to learn more about biology behind the disease to increase compliance.
4. Provide information on local support groups and other national resources.

C. Pharmacotherapy.

1. Medication treatment options for depression (Note: Most antidepressants also have indications for anxiety disorders, obsessive-compulsive disorder (OCD), and other diagnoses; important to check Food and Drug Administration (FDA) approvals for each medication).

   a. Selective serotonin reuptake inhibitors (SSRIs).

   i. Black box warning for increase in suicidal thinking up to age 24 (for all antidepressants in *all classes*). Generally considered prudent to continue in pregnancy, with preference toward SSRIs with moderate half-life (not paroxetine [short] nor fluoxetine [long]).

   ii. Risk of serotonin syndrome.

   iii. Discontinuation syndrome: Abrupt discontinuation of medication taken for more than 6 weeks that is more common in medications with short half-lives; usually resolves within 3 weeks. Symptoms can include weakness, nausea, dizziness, headache, increase in anxiety/depression, insomnia, decreased concentration, upper respiratory symptoms, paresthesias, migraine, or headache.

   1) Mnemonic **FINISH** for symptoms related to discontinuation.

   a) Flu-like symptoms.
   b) Insomnia.
   c) Nausea.
   d) Imbalance.
   e) Sensory disturbance.
   f) Hyperarousal.

   2) Treatment of discontinuation syndrome: Place back on medication titrating up slowly; taper slowly if intending to stop medication. May start fluoxetine (Prozac) to help discontinue medications as it has the longest half-life of SSRIs.

iv. Serotonin syndrome (risk with any medication that increases serotonin levels), particularly when multiple agents are used and/or the patient is ill and dehydrated. Serotonin syndrome is a clinical diagnosis with no specific lab tests. Symptoms that present in order of clinical worsening are (a) diarrhea; (b) restlessness; (c) agitation, hyperreflexia, autonomic instability, and fluctuation in vital signs; (d) myoclonus, seizures, hyperthermia, involuntary shivering, and rigidity; and (e) delirium, coma, status epilepticus, cardiovascular collapse, and death. Serotonin syndrome is considered a medical emergency.

    1) Mnemonic **HARMED** for serotonin syndrome symptoms.

        a) Hyperthermia.

        b) Autonomic instability.

        c) Rigidity.

        d) Myoclonus.

        e) Encephalopathy.

        f) Diaphoresis.

    2) Treatment.

        a) Discontinue serotonergic agents.

        b) Sedate using benzodiazepines with goal to eliminate agitation, tremor, clonus, elevated heart rate, and blood pressure.

        c) Initiate supportive therapy including oxygen, intravenous (IV) fluids, and continuous cardiac monitoring.

        d) Other treatments may include nitroglycerine, cyproheptadine (Periactin), methysergide (Sansert), cooling blankets, chlorpromazine (Thorazine), dantrolene (Dantrium), anticonvulsants, mechanical ventilation, and paralyzing agents.

b. Serotonin norepinephrine reuptake inhibitors (SNRIs).

  i. Medications include venlafaxine (Effexor), desvenlafaxine (Pristiq), duloxetine (Cymbalta), and levomilnacipran (Fetzima). Venlafaxine is a weak inhibitor of CYP4502D6 only, while duloxetine is a moderate inhibitor of all CYP450 enzymes.

  ii. May be useful in patients who do not respond to SSRIs.

  iii. Withdrawal effects can be more pronounced for SNRIs.

  iv. Risk of serotonin syndrome is greater with monoamine oxidase inhibitor (MAOI) use within 14 days of initiation or stopping.

  v. Can increase blood pressure; need to monitor; caution in cardiac patients.

  vi. Need to monitor for suicidality, especially in people 24 and under. May be fatal in overdose.

  vii. Little data in pregnancy, but few studies demonstrating adverse effects. Must weigh risk–benefit.

c. Other antidepressants.

  i. Noradrenergic and specific serotonergic antidepressant (NaSSA) more sedating at lower doses; increased appetite; can lower white blood cell (WBC); SolTab.

  ii. Norepinephrine dopamine reuptake inhibitor (NDRI).

    1) Avoid with history of seizure disorder or alcohol use disorder as Wellbutrin can lower the seizure threshold; avoid in history of eating disorder (due to risk of seizure with vomiting/restriction as well as potential weight loss due to Wellbutrin); weight-neutral/some lose weight and little to no sexual dysfunction; can be used to counteract the sexual side effects of SSRIs.

    2) Can be used in ADHD as a second-line treatment, although efficacy to FDA-approved medications has not been compared; may be useful for those with ADHD and comorbidities such as depression or substance use disorder or patients who develop tics on psychostimulants; limited evidence in bipolar disorder, although may be less likely to induce mania or rapid cycling than tricyclic or other antidepressants.

    3) Formulated in immediate-release, sustained-release, and extended-release; dosage should be based on indication and formulation (e.g., smoking cessation = Wellbutrin SR 150 mg BID).

  iii. Serotonin antagonist reuptake inhibitor (SARI) such as trazodone (Desyrel) or nefazodone (Serzone): Can be used for insomnia and is not a controlled substance; should not be given with MAOIs. Nefazodone can slow the metabolism of digoxin. There is a risk of priapism (Trazodone); orthostasis, dizziness, headache, and nausea; hepatotoxicity (Nefazodone); and QTc prolongation.

  iv. Newer antidepressants.

    1) SSRI: 5-hydroxytryptamine agonist such as vortioxetine (Trintellix). Vortioxetine also has action as:

        a) 5HT1B partial agonist.

        b) Antagonist at 5HT3 (may improve nausea, vomiting, and GI symptoms), 5HT1D (may improve cognition), and 5HT7 (may decrease sexual dysfunction).

        c) Side effects include GI upset, hyponatremia, and bleeding.

        d) SSRI-5HT1A receptor agonist: While the effects of the action of this receptor agonist are not known, it appears ▶

to help with quicker onset of action of the medication, such as in vilazodone (Viibryd). Reduce dose to 20 mg when administered with CYP3A4 inducer. Common SSRI side effects persist.

  v. Older antidepressants.

d. Tricyclic antidepressants (TCAs): Block transporter site for norepinephrine and serotonin.

  i. Side effects: Sedation, weight gain, orthostatic hypotension, fine tremor, myoclonic twitches, and antihistaminergic and anticholinergic activity; can result in anticholinergic toxicity (treatment with physostigmine), rash and rare agranulocytosis, leukocytosis, leukopenia, and eosinophilia; and QTc prolongation (EKG over 40 or with history of cardiovascular disease).

  ii. Lethal in overdose; can cause delirium in cognitively impaired and older adults due to their anticholinergic effects. Can exacerbate mania or psychotic features.

  iii. Use caution when given with anticoagulants, which increases the risk of bleeding. Other drug interactions include antiarrhythmics, DA receptor antagonists, central nervous system (CNS) depressants, nicotine, and other sympathomimetics.

  iv. Risk–benefit must be determined in pregnancy and postpartum as some evidence exists that TCAs pass through the placenta and breast milk.

e. MAOIs.

  i. Should not take within 14 days of TCAs. Not used as first- or second-line treatment due to need for dietary changes and drug–drug interactions. Common side effects include orthostatic hypotension, insomnia, weight gain, edema, and sexual dysfunction. Also seen are paresthesias, myoclonus, and muscle pain.

  ii. Risk of hypertensive crisis with tyramine (treatment with alpha-adrenergic agents such as phentolamine).

  iii. Need education on tyramine-free diet, such as to avoid dairy, fish, and processed meats. Even with MAOI patches, dietary changes should be made.

  iv. Many drug–drug interactions: Demerol, over-the-counter (OTC) flu/cold medications, antihypertensives, benzodiazepines, lithium, serotonergic agents, and stimulants.

  v. Caution in older adults as they are more sensitive to side effects. Risk–benefit must be determined in pregnancy and postpartum as some evidence exists that MAOIs pass through the placenta and breast milk.

FOLLOW-UP

A. Weekly follow-up for the first month, then every 2 to 4 weeks as clinically indicated.

B. Provider must watch for high risk of suicide, particularly in the first 2 weeks of antidepressant treatments, when energy and activity improve before mood improves.

CONSULTATION/REFERRAL

A. Consultation with or referral to a psychiatric specialist if the patient fails two full (adequate trial both time and dose) antidepressant trials of at least 8 to 12 weeks at target dose of medication.

B. Referral for psychotherapy as appropriate.

SPECIAL/GERIATRIC CONSIDERATIONS

A. Women of childbearing age: Assess risk and benefit of all medications versus harm of not treating depression in pregnancy and the postpartum. Consult the Pregnancy and Lactation Labelling Rule (PLLR) for latest guidance. Assess risk–benefit of certain medications prior to pregnancy for potential effects on childbearing.

B. Postpartum depression (PPD): Important to assess for PPD with psychosis, as well as anxiety, OCD, and suicidality.

C. Older adults: Assessment of depression in older adults with cognitive problems as pseudodementia may be present. White, widower, older males are at high risk of suicide. Considerations related to aging and drug–drug interactions.

BIBLIOGRAPHY

American Psychiatric Association. (2013). *Diagnostic and statistical manual of mental disorders* (5th ed.). Author.

Boland, R., Verduin, M., & Ruiz, P (Eds.). (2022). *Kaplan & Sadock's synopsis of psychiatry* (12th ed.). Wolters Kluwer.

BulletPsych. (2020, August 16). *Day #25: Mental status exam in depression.* https://www.bulletpsych.com/post/day-25-mental-status-exam-in-depression

Caplan, J. P., & Stern, T. A. (2008). Mnemonics in a nutshell: 32 aids to psychiatric diagnosis. *Current Psychiatry*, 7(10), 27–33.

Pliszka, S. R. (2016). *Neuroscience for the mental health clinician* (2nd ed.). Guilford Press.

Stahl, S. M. (2013). *Stahl's essential psychopharmacology: Neuroscientific basis and practical applications* (4th ed.). Cambridge University Press.

Stahl, S. M. (2017). *Stahl's essential psychopharmacology: Prescriber's guide* (6th ed.). Cambridge University Press.

POSTTRAUMATIC STRESS DISORDER

DEFINITION

A. Exposure to actual or threatened death, serious injury, or sexual violation in one (or more) of the following ways:

1. Directly experiencing the traumatic event(s).

2. Witnessing, in person, the event(s) that occurred to a close family member or close friend, resulting in actual or threatened death.

3. Learning that the traumatic event(s) occurred to a close family member or close friend. In cases of actual or threatened death of a family member or friend, the event(s) must have been violent or accidental.

4. Experiencing repeated or extreme exposure to aversive details of the traumatic event(s) (e.g., first ▶

responders collecting human remains; police officers repeatedly exposed to details of child abuse).

B. Presence of one (or more) of the following intrusive symptoms associated with the traumatic event(s), beginning after the traumatic event(s) occurred:

1. Recurrent, involuntary, and intrusive distressing stories or memories of the traumatic event(s).

2. Recurrent distressing dreams in which the content and/or effect of the dream related to the traumatic event(s) are expressed.

3. Dissociative reactions (flashbacks) in which the individual feels or acts as if the traumatic events were recurring.

4. Intense or prolonged psychological distress at exposure to internal or external cues that symbolize or resemble an aspect of the traumatic event(s).

5. Marked physiologic reactions to internal or external cues that symbolize or resemble an aspect of the traumatic event(s).

C. Persistent avoidance of stimuli associated with the traumatic event(s), beginning after the traumatic event(s) occurred, as evidenced by one or both of the following:

1. Avoidance of or efforts to avoid distressing memories, thoughts, or feelings about or closely associated with the traumatic event(s).

2. Avoidance of or efforts to avoid external reminders (people, places, conversations, activities, objects, situations) that trigger distressing memories, thoughts, or feelings about or closely associated with the traumatic event(s).

D. Negative alterations in cognition and mood associated with the traumatic event(s) beginning or worsening after the traumatic event(s) occurred, as evidenced by two (or more) of the following:

1. Inability to remember an important aspect of the traumatic event(s) (typically due to dissociative amnesia and not the other factors such as head injury, alcohol, or drugs).

2. Persistent and exaggerated negative beliefs or expectations about oneself, others, or the world.

3. Persistent, distorted cognitions about the cause or consequences of the traumatic event(s) that lead the individual to blame themselves or others.

4. Persistent negative emotional state (horror, fear, anger, guilt, shame).

5. Markedly diminished interest or participation in significant activities.

6. Feelings of detachment or estrangement from others.

7. Persistent inability to experience positive emotions.

E. Marked alterations in arousal and reactivity associated with the traumatic event(s) beginning or worsening after the traumatic event(s) occurred, as evidenced by two (or more) of the following:

1. Irritable behavior and angry outbursts typically expressed as verbal or physical aggression toward others/objects.

2. Reckless or self-destructive behavior.

3. Hypervigilance.

4. Exaggerated startle response.

5. Problems with concentration.

6. Sleep disturbances (falling/staying asleep or restless sleep).

F. Duration of the disturbance is more than 1 month.

G. The disturbance causes clinically significant distress or impairment in social, occupational, or other important areas of functioning.

H. The disturbance is not attributed to the physiologic effects of a substance or another medical condition.

I. The diagnosis can be specified as having accompanying depersonalization or derealization. There can also be delayed expression more than 6 months after the event.

INCIDENCE

A. 6.8% lifetime prevalence, with past year prevalence at 3.5%.

B. The lifetime prevalence among women is 9.7% and among men is 3.6%, and is more common in young adults.

C. More common in single, divorced, widowed, and socially withdrawn individuals, especially people from low socioeconomic status backgrounds.

D. The most important risk factor is the severity, duration, and proximity of the person's exposure to the trauma.

E. Symptoms usually develop within the 6 months after the traumatic event, but some people can have delayed onset.

PATHOGENESIS

A. Normal to low levels of cortisol and increased levels of corticotropic releasing factor (CRF), leading to sympathetic activation (increased heart rate, blood pressure, arousal, startle response).

B. Possible alteration in the neurotransmitter system, including serotonin, neuropeptide Y, and decreased gamma-aminobutyric acid (GABA) activity and increased glutamate, leading to dissociation and derealization. Serotonin depletion in the dorsal/medial raphe could contribute to dysregulation between amygdala and hypothalamic–pituitary–adrenal (HPA) axis.

C. Structural changes also contribute: Hippocampus is reduced, amygdala is overly reactive, and the medial prefrontal cortex (which inhibits amygdala) is smaller and less responsive in people with posttraumatic stress disorder (PTSD).

PREDISPOSING FACTORS

A. Childhood trauma.

B. Intimate partner violence.

C. Personality disorder.

D. Female sex.

E. Genetic vulnerability to psychiatric illness.

F. Recent stressful life change.

G. Perception of external locus of control.

H. Co-occurring alcohol and substance use disorder; recent excessive intake.

I. Violence experience in the context of war.
J. Chronic pain and inflammatory bowel diseases.
K. Presence of other psychiatric illness.

SUBJECTIVE DATA

A. Common complaints/symptoms.
  1. Patients who have PTSD have considerable stress that interferes with their ability to interact in the society.
B. Common/typical scenario.
  1. May involve the patient withdrawing from society, job loss, divorce, or even substance abuse.
C. Family and social history.
  1. Ask about family situation, support system, or use of any drugs or alcohol.
D. Review of systems.
  1. Psychiatric: Ask about depression, anxiety, avoidance, withdrawal, constant fear, suicidal thoughts, or complaints of chronic pain.

MENTAL STATUS EXAMINATION

A. Conduct a mental status examination (MSE).
B. Appearance: Variable. May be cooperative or non-cooperative. Can be friendly or hostile. May withhold information. May be well-groomed or poorly groomed.
C. Behavior: Variable. Some patients may present as if they are doing well. Can present consistently with anxiety and/or depression. Can be withdrawn, resistant, and shy (depression). Can be engaged and participative (anxiety). Motor: May see psychomotor retardation (bent over, not moving on own, looking down, poor eye contact) or psychomotor agitation (hand wringing, picking/pulling, pacing, difficulty sitting down).
D. Speech: Variable; normally not as influenced as other diagnoses. May be slowed, soft, minimal initiation of words, monotone if depression present. May be increased rate, tremulous voice if anxiety is present.
E. Affect/mood: Variable. Affect (perceived by the observer): Can be angry, tense, guilty, on edge, fatigued, and may deny problems; can be blunted and can be labile; expansive, euthymic, and constricted. Mood (reported by the patient): Variable. Anxious, sad, and irritable.
F. Thought process: Generally linear and coherent.
G. Thought content: Can have negative world view, guilt, worry, and decreased positive emotion.
H. Suicidal ideation, plan, intentions to act, and access to lethal means: May be present and important to assess.
  1. Assess access to firearms.
I. Homicidal or assaultive ideation.
  1. Ask about specific target and plan.
  2. Perceptual disturbances: Can have flashbacks, intrusive thoughts or sensations, and dissociative experiences.
J. Judgment: Variable and depends on history.
K. Insight: Variable; may include avoidance—patient may or may not have insight into triggers and course of illness.
L. Cognitive exam: Orientation and memory usually intact in PTSD; may impact memory and concentration; may include cognitive exams such as the Mini-Mental State Exam (MMSE) or Montreal Cognitive Assessment (MoCA).

DIAGNOSTIC TESTS

A. Screening instruments.
  1. PTSD Checklist for *Diagnostic and Statistical Manual of Mental Disorders* (Fifth Edition; *DSM-5*; PCL-S).
  2. Clinician-Administered PTSD Scale for PTSD (CAPS-5).
  3. Trauma Screening Questionnaire (TSQ).
  4. Short Screening Scale for PTSD.
  5. Short Form of the PTSD Checklist.

DIFFERENTIAL DIAGNOSIS

A. Adjustment disorder.
B. Acute stress disorder: Distinguished from PTSD based on time frame: Duration is restricted to 3 days to 1 month.
C. Generalized anxiety disorder.
D. Panic disorder.
E. Psychosis.
F. Major depressive disorder (MDD).
G. Borderline personality disorder.
H. Factitious disorders.
I. Dissociative identity disorder.
J. Traumatic brain injury.
K. Epilepsy.
L. Substance use disorders.

EVALUATION AND MANAGEMENT PLAN (ACUTE WITHDRAWAL)

A. General plan.
  1. Psychotherapy.
    a. Trauma-focused cognitive behavioral therapy (TF-CBT).
    b. Present-centered therapy (PCT) or cognitive processing therapy (CPT).
    c. Exposure and response prevention therapy (ExRP).
    d. Eye movement desensitization and reprocessing (EMDR).
B. Pharmacotherapy.
  1. Selective serotonin reuptake inhibitors (SSRIs) are the only Food and Drug Administration (FDA)-approved treatment for PTSD and have the strongest evidence: Paroxetine (Paxil) and sertraline (Zoloft) are the only medications with FDA approval.
  2. Benzodiazepines are not indicated in the treatment of PTSD.
  3. Serotonin norepinephrine reuptake inhibitor (SNRIs) like venlafaxine XR (Effexor SR) and mirtazapine (Remeron) have been shown to be helpful.
  4. Prazosin (Minipress), an alpha1-adrenergic receptor antagonist (AA), has been studied to treat sleep and nightmares: Starting dose 1 mg with therapeutic range usually 6 to 15 mg and limited efficacy above 20 mg. Caution with phosphodiesterase type 5 (PDE-5) inhibitors as they can contribute to symptomatic hypotension. AAs also show evidence for treating nightmares. ▶

5. Trazodone and Suvorexant may be helpful for insomnia.

FOLLOW-UP

A. Coordination with a psychiatric specialist for ongoing treatment and follow-up, as well as therapist, case manager, family, and patient support group. Coordination with primary care provider for any medical issues and rule-outs.
B. Trauma-informed care and interventions have the best outcomes.

CONSULTATION/REFERRAL

A. Consider referral for integrative treatments (complementary and alternative medicine): This may include therapies such as mindfulness, yoga, acupuncture, and massage.

SPECIAL/GERIATRIC CONSIDERATIONS

A. Adaptive coping in older adult patients may be impaired and lead them to engage in substance abuse to manage PTSD symptoms.
B. Older adults may not identify symptoms in the context of a psychological framework, making them less likely to seek treatment.
C. There may be a stigma among older adults about seeking psychological assistance.

BIBLIOGRAPHY

American Psychiatric Association. (2013). *Diagnostic and statistical manual of mental disorders* (5th ed.). Author.
Boland, R., Verduin, M., & Ruiz, P (Eds.). (2022). *Kaplan & Sadock's synopsis of psychiatry* (12th ed.). Wolters Kluwer.
BulletPsych. (2021, May 14). *Day #107: Mental status exam in PTSD.* https://www.bulletpsych.com/post/day-107-mental-status-exam-in-ptsd
Mann, S., & Marwaha, R. (2022). *Posttraumatic stress disorder.* StatPearls [Internet]. https://www.ncbi.nlm.nih.gov/books/NBK559129/
Pliszka, S. R. (2016). *Neuroscience for the mental health clinician* (5th ed.). Guilford Press.
Stahl, S. M. (2013). *Stahl's essential psychopharmacology: Neuroscientific basis and practical applications* (4th ed.). Cambridge University Press.
Stahl, S. M. (2017). *Stahl's essential psychopharmacology: Prescriber's guide* (6th ed.). Cambridge University Press.

SCHIZOPHRENIA

DEFINITION

A. Schizophrenia spectrum and other psychotic disorders include schizophrenia, other psychotic disorders, and schizotypal (personality) disorder. They are defined by abnormalities in one or more of the following five domains: Delusions, hallucinations, disorganized thinking (speech), grossly disorganized or abnormal motor behavior (including catatonia), and negative symptoms.

INCIDENCE

A. 1%, with a lifetime prevalence of 0.6% to 1.9%.
B. Equally prevalent in men and women, but onset differs with more men having onset before the age of 25, with a peak age of 10 to 25 years, and a peak in women at age 25 to 35, with up to 10% of women having onset after the age of 40.

COURSE

A. Onset of psychosis typically occurs between late teens and mid-30s.
B. Onset prior to adolescence is rare.
C. Peak age of first psychotic episode is generally early to mid-20s in males and late-20s in females.
D. Early age of onset was traditionally associated with poorer outcomes, but now thought to be a combination of factors, including male gender, lower educational achievement, prominent negative symptoms, and cognitive impairment.
E. Psychotic symptoms tend to diminish over the lifetime.
F. Negative symptoms are more predictive of prognosis than positive.
G. Cognitive deficits may not improve over the course of the illness.
H. Increased risk of aggression or violence in those with schizophrenia who are not in treatment.
  1. In an acute setting, intramuscular (IM) medication may be needed (benzodiazepine such as lorazepam or antipsychotic medication).
I. There is a higher risk for suicide among those diagnosed with schizophrenia, and it is the leading cause of premature death. 20% to 50% of persons with schizophrenia attempt suicide.
J. Homicide is no more likely than in the general population: Associated with bizarre hallucinations or delusions with predictors of previous violence, dangerous behavior, or hallucinations/delusions with violent content.

PATHOGENESIS

A. The pathogenesis of schizophrenia is unknown.
B. It is a uniquely human condition that appears to be caused by a complex interaction of genes and environment.
C. Studies have shown a strong genetic association, but the understanding of why or how schizophrenia occurs is unknown. Genetic estimates of up to 46% in monozygotic twins.

PREDISPOSING FACTORS

A. Decreased cortical volume in temporal cortex and increased ventral size with decrease in gamma-aminobutyric acid (GABA) interneurons.
B. Born in winter.
C. Raised in urban areas.
D. Early or prenatal infections.
E. Birth complications.
F. Substance use disorders.
G. Advanced paternal age (>50 years).

SUBJECTIVE DATA

A. Diagnostic criteria.
  1. Two or more of the following (at least one of which is from the first three) for at least 1 month:

▶

a. Delusions.

b. Hallucinations (auditory and visual are most common; gustatory, olfactory, and tactile are more common due to an organic etiology).

c. Disorganized speech.

d. Grossly disorganized or catatonic behavior.

e. Negative symptoms (restricted affect, poverty of speech, decreased interests, decreased sense of purpose, decreased social drive).

2. Impairment in functions, such as work, interpersonal relations, self-care, academic, or occupational issues.

3. Continuous symptoms that last for 6 months or longer.

B. Common/typical scenario.

1. Patients commonly present with hallucinations or disorganized speech.

2. Symptoms may be vague in the beginning stages.

3. The first psychotic episode may start in the teen years up to the mid-30s.

C. Family and social history.

1. Risk for schizophrenia is higher in those with first-degree relatives with schizophrenia. This risk is correlated with the closeness of the relation to individual with the diagnosis.

2. Symptoms may affect social and familial relationships.

D. Review of systems.

1. Rule out schizoaffective disorder, other psychotic disorders, major depressive disorder (MDD), and bipolar disorder.

2. Rule out due to substance use or general medical condition.

3. Review of systems in schizophrenia.

a. Positive symptoms.

i. Delusions are fixed beliefs that are not amenable to change in light of conflicting evidence.

1) Persecutory delusions are the most common belief that the individual will be harmed by another individual, organization, or other group.

2) Other forms of delusions: Referential, grandiose, and somatic.

ii. Hallucinations are perception-like experiences that occur without an external stimulus. Auditory hallucinations are the most common in psychotic disorder; however, they can occur with any of the five senses.

iii. Disorganized thinking is typically inferred from the individual's speech.

1) Loose associations (often seen in schizophrenia and mania), derailment, incoherence, tangential, circumstantial, neologisms, echolalia, verbigeration, word salad, and mutism.

iv. Grossly disorganized or abnormal motor behavior may manifest in a variety of ways, ranging from childlike behavior to unpredictable agitation.

b. Negative symptoms account for substantial portion of the morbidity associated with schizophrenia.

i. Diminished emotional expression and avolition are particularly prominent in schizophrenia.

ii. **NEGATIVE TRACK** mnemonic for negative symptoms.

1) **N**egligible response to conventional antipsychotics (first generation).

2) **E**ye contact decreased.

3) **G**rooming and hygiene decline.

4) **A**ffect responses become flat.

5) **T**hought blocking.

6) **I**nattentiveness.

7) **V**olition diminished.

8) **E**xpressive gesture decrease.

9) **T**ime-increases negative symptoms.

10) **R**ecreation/relationship diminish.

11) **A**s: Apathy/alogia/affect flattening/anhedonia/attentional deficits.

MENTAL STATUS EXAMINATION

A. Appearance.

1. Disheveled, obsessively groomed, hygiene, and dress (appropriateness/soiled).

B. Behavior.

1. Can characterize activity by posture, frequency of spontaneous movement, cooperation, or ability to follow directions/commands.

2. Can characterize movement by conscious voluntary movement, unconscious voluntary movement, and involuntary movements.

C. Speech: Assessment of the amount, articulation, modulation, pitch, spontaneity, and cadence of speech.

1. Pressured, verbose, and expansive.

2. Minimally responsive, impoverished, and mutism.

3. Mumbled and garbled.

4. Loud and soft.

5. Spontaneous dialogue versus latency.

6. Stuttering, cluttering, and inflection.

D. Affect/mood.

1. Mood: Patient's subjective report of their emotional state.

2. Affect: Interviewer's observation of patient's emotional state.

3. Reduced emotional responsiveness and/or overly active and inappropriate emotions (extremes of rage, happiness, and anxiety).

E. Thought process/form.

1. Disorders of thought form are observed in the patient's spoken and written language.

a. Loose associations (often seen in schizophrenia and mania), derailment, incoherence, tangential, circumstantial, neologisms, echolalia, verbigeration, word salad, and mutism.

b. Preoccupations.

2. Thought process refers to the way ideas and languages are formed.

▶

a. Flight of ideas, thought blocking, poor abstraction, perseveration, poverty of thought, overinclusion, and circumstantiality.

F. Thought content: Reflect patient's ideas, beliefs, and interpretations of stimuli.

1. Suicidal ideation.
2. Homicidal ideation.
3. Delusions: Persecutory (most common), grandiose, religious, and somatic.
4. Perceptual disturbances.

   a. Auditory hallucinations are most common (voices threatening, accusatory, or insulting).

   b. Command hallucinations put the patient and others at risk of harm.

   c. Visual hallucinations less common in schizophrenia/psychotic disorders.

   d. Tactile, olfactory, and gustatory disturbances are unusual and often associated with an underlying medical/neurologic cause.

G. Cognition.

1. Assess orientation to person, place, and time: Disorientation is not characteristic of schizophrenia.

DIAGNOSTIC TESTS

A. Broad screening: Complete blood count (CBC), blood glucose, comprehensive metabolic panel (CMP), urine drug screen, and liver function tests (LFTs).

B. Exclude specific disorders: Thyroid panel, vitamin B_{12}, folate, HIV, rapid plasma reagin (RPR; with prevalence of syphilis, this should be part of screening), or other infections.

C. Other tests: EEG, chest x-ray, and CT scan/MRI (for first episode, scan is part of the workup).

D. Screening instruments.

1. Brief Psychiatric Rating Scale (BPRS).
2. Scale for Assessment of Negative/Positive Symptoms (SANS/SAPS).
3. Positive and Negative Symptoms Syndrome Scale (PANSS).

DIFFERENTIAL DIAGNOSIS

A. Schizophreniform (less than 6 months of symptoms).
B. Schizoaffective disorder.
C. Brief psychotic disorder.
D. Delusional disorder.
E. Bipolar disorder.
F. MDD.
G. Substance-induced disorder.
H. Psychotic disorder due to general medical condition (as with all psychiatric disorders, onset of symptoms is more commonly insidious: An abrupt change in mental status is likely related to an organic cause).
I. Medical rule-outs.

1. Epilepsy.
2. Neoplasm.
3. AIDS.
4. Vitamin B_{12} deficiency.
5. Heavy metal poisoning.
6. Diabetes mellitus.

7. Cardiovascular disease.
8. Lung disease and cancer (due to high rates of nicotine use in up to 90% of patients, due in part to impairment of nicotine receptors in the brain).

EVALUATION AND MANAGEMENT PLAN

A. General plan.

1. Antipsychotic medications.

   a. First-generation antipsychotics (FGAs) or typical.

      i. Often seen as second line in current practice due to their side effect profile.

      ii. Act on D2 receptors, which result in reduction of positive symptoms as well as unpleasant side effects.

   b. Second-generation antipsychotics (SGAs) or atypical.

      i. Generally regarded as first line, unless clinical history warrants otherwise.

      ii. While each medication has a unique pharmacologic profile, in general SGAs act on both the serotonin 5-HT2A receptors (5HT2A) receptors that have a reciprocal effect on dopamine (DA) release. 5HT2A agonism decreases DA release. 5HT2A antagonism increases DA release (too much DA blockade in the prefrontal cortex is associated with some of the negative symptoms of schizophrenia; Goldberg, et al., 2021).

2. Adverse drug reactions/monitoring considerations.

   a. Medication class box warning: Increased mortality in older adult patients with dementia-related psychosis.

   b. SGAs: Warning for increased risk of metabolic syndrome.

      i. Expert guidelines on screening for all persons treated on SGAs: At baseline, assess family and personal history of cardiovascular disease, weight (body mass index [BMI]), blood pressure, waist circumference, and fasting lipid/glucose; weight is done every 4 weeks; and blood pressure and fasting labs are completed again in 12 weeks. Glucose and lipid changes can occur in the absence of weight gain.

   c. Nearly all antipsychotics carry the risk of QTc prolongation; however, the risk varies by agent.

      i. Those with the least risk include:

         1) SGAs: Aripiprazole.

         2) FGAs: Loxapine.

      ii. Those with the highest risk include:

         1) SGAs: Ziprasidone, quetiapine (moderate risk), and risperidone (moderate risk).

         2) FGAs: Thioridazine and haloperidol (boxed warning for intravenous [IV] dosing).

   d. Risk of tardive dyskinesia on both atypical and typical antipsychotics exists, and assessment of abnormal movements using the Abnormal Involuntary Movement Scale (AIMS) is recommended every 6 months. Risk is higher with typical antipsychotics.

▶

e. Extrapyramidal symptoms.

i. Akathesia: Severe restlessness, inability to remain still.

ii. Parkinsonism-tremor, pill-rolling movements, stiff posture, slow movements.

iii. Dystonia: Involuntary muscle contractions.

1) Can occur in muscles of, extremities, face, neck, abdomen, pelvis, larynx (torticolis, oculogyric crisis, blepharospasms, and laryngospasm).

2) Acute treatment: IM benztropine (Cogentin), IM diphenhydramine (Benadryl), or IV benzodiazapine.

iv. Tardive dyskinesia (TD): nonrhythmic, involuntary movements.

1) Usually develops after long-term treatment.

2) Most often occurs in face and mouth, but can occur in the limbs or trunk.

f. Neuroleptic malignant syndrome (NMS).

1. Risk with new medications, dose increases, or in combination with other dopaminergic medications (including those prescribed for medical reasons).

2. Mnemonic: **FEVER.**

a. Fever.

b. Encephalopathy.

c. Vital sign instability.

d. Enzyme elevation and creatinine phosphokinase (CPK).

e. Rigidity.

3. Cardinal signs/symptoms of NMS: Acute mental status changes with fluctuating consciousness, lead pipe rigidity, and autonomic instability.

4. Labs: Leukocytosis and increased CPK, aspartate aminotransferase (AST), alanine aminotransferase (ALT), and myoglobinuria.

5. Treatment: Stop the offending agent. Supportive care often in ICU setting.

6. Pharmacotherapy treatment of NMS.

a. Bromocriptine: DA agonist used to restore lost dopaminergic tone.

b. Dantrolene: Direct-acting skeletal muscle relaxant.

FOLLOW-UP

A. Follow up with a psychiatric specialist: Should not be treated in primary care setting.

B. Smoking cessation programs.

CONSULTATION/REFERRAL

A. Consultation with primary care providers and referral for ongoing medical follow-up given the high prevalence of medical comorbidities.

B. Referral to psychosocial intervention/training programs and the National Alliance on Mental Illness (NAMI).

C. Referral for co-occurring disorder treatment may be necessary given the high rates of comorbid substance use disorders.

SPECIAL/GERIATRIC CONSIDERATIONS

A. More than two-fifths of older adults with schizophrenia show clinical signs of depression, and the rates of suicide may be higher.

BIBLIOGRAPHY

American Psychiatric Association. (2013). *Diagnostic and statistical manual of mental disorders* (5th ed.). Author.

American Psychiatric Association. (2018). *Resource document on QTc prolongation and psychotropic medications.* https://www.psychiatry.org/File%20Library/Psychiatrists/Directories/Library-and-Archive/resource_documents/Resource-Document-2018-QTc-Prolongation-and-Psychotropic-Med.pdf

Carlat, D. J. (2017). *The psychiatric interview* (4th ed.). Wolters Kluwer.

Farkas, J. (2021, April 17). *Neuroleptic malignant syndrome (NMS). The Internet Book of Critical Care.* https://emcrit.org/ibcc/nms/#:~:text=Neuroleptic%20malignant%20syndrome%20seems%20to,%2C%20lead%2Dpipe%20rigidity

Goldberg, J., Stahl, S., & Schatzberg, A. (2021). *Practical psychopharmacology: Translating findings from evidence-based trials into real-world clinical practice.* Cambridge University Press. https://doi.org/10.1017/9781108553216

Oruch, R., Pryme, I. F., Engelsen, B. A., & Lund, A. (2017). Neuroleptic malignant syndrome: An easily overlooked neurologic emergency. *Neuropsychiatric Disease and Treatment, 13,* 161–175.

Pliszka, S. R. (2016). *Neuroscience for the mental health clinician* (2nd ed.). Guilford Press.

Sadock, B. J., Sadock, V. A., & Ruiz, P. (2015). *Kaplan & Sadock's synopsis of psychiatry: Behavioral sciences/clinical psychiatry* (11th ed.). Wolters Kluwer.

Sadock, B.J., Sadock, V.A., & Ruiz, P. (2018). *Kaplan & Sadock's comprehensive textbook of psychiatry* (10th ed., Vol. 11)). Wolters Kluwer.

Stahl, S. (2020). *Prescriber's guide: Stahl's essential psychopharmacology* (7th ed.). Cambridge University Press. https://doi.org/10.1017/9781108921275

Stahl, S. (2021). *Stahl's essential psychopharmacology: Neuroscientific basis and practical applications* (5th ed.). Cambridge University Press. https://doi.org/10.1017/9781108975292

Stahl, S., Mignon, L., & Muntner, N. (2010). *Stahl's illustrated antipsychotics: Treating psychosis, mania and depression* (2nd ed., Stahl's Illustrated ed.). Cambridge University Press. https://doi.org/10.1017/9780511661136

Stern, T. A., Freudenreich, O., Smith, F. A., Fricchione, G. L., & Rosenbaum, J. F. (2018). *Massachusetts general hospital handbook of general hospital psychiatry* (7th ed.). Elsevier Inc.

Tasman, A., & Mohr, W. (2011). *Fundamentals of psychiatry.* Wiley-Blackwell.

SUBSTANCE USE DISORDERS

DEFINITION

A. Substance-related disorders.

1. A cluster of cognitive, behavioral, and physiologic symptoms indicating that the individual continues using the substance despite significant substance-related problems.

2. An important characteristic of substance use disorders is an underlying change in brain chemistry and persisting beyond detoxification.

3. The diagnosis of a substance use disorder is characterized by a pathologic pattern of behaviors related to use of the substance.

4. All substance use disorders are diagnosed by the following criteria (each substance follows the same diagnostic criterion):

a. A problematic pattern of substance use leading to clinically significant impairment or distress, as ▶

manifested by at least two of the following, occurring within a 12-month period:

    i. The substance is often taken in larger amounts or over a longer period than was intended.

    ii. There is a persistent desire or unsuccessful efforts to cut down or control substance use.

    iii. A great deal of time is spent in activities necessary to obtain the substance, use the substance, or recover from its effects.

    iv. Craving, or a strong desire to urge to use the substance.

    v. Recurrent substance use resulting in a failure to fulfill major role obligations at work, school, or home.

    vi. Continued substance use despite having persistent or recurrent social or interpersonal problems caused or exacerbated by the effects of the substance.

    vii. Important social, occupational, or recreational activities are given up or reduced because of substance use.

    viii. Recurrent substance use in situations in which it is physically hazardous.

    ix. Substance use is continued despite knowledge of having a persistent or recurrent physical or psychological problem that is likely to have been caused or exacerbated by the substance.

    x. Tolerance, as manifested by either of the following:

      1) A need for markedly increased amounts of the substance to achieve intoxication or desired effect.

      2) A markedly diminished effect with continued use of the same amount of the substance.

    xi. Withdrawal, as manifested by either of the following:

      1) The characteristic withdrawal syndrome.

      2) The substance is taken to relieve or avoid withdrawal symptoms.

B. Substance-induced disorders.
  1. Intoxication.
  2. Withdrawal.
  3. Substance/medication-induced mental disorders.

INCIDENCE

A. Alcohol use disorder: Affects approximately 15 % of men and 10% of women.
B. Cannabis 8.5%.
C. Opioids 1.4%.
D. Sedatives 1%.
E. Amphetamines 2%.
F. Cocaine 2.8%.
G. Hallucinogens 1.7%.

PATHOGENESIS

A. Has both a genetic and environmental risk with complex neurobiology.

PREDISPOSING FACTORS

A. Age of first use matters: Odds of alcohol use disorder as an adult go down by 14% for each year a youth does not drink after age 14.
B. Access.
C. Peer groups.
D. Family history.

SUBJECTIVE DATA

A. Common complaints/symptoms.
  1. Craving, irrepressible urge to seek and consume drug substance.
B. Common/typical scenario.
  1. Patients commonly present for either another medical condition or a complication associated with use of the substance.
C. Family and social history.
  1. Behaviors may be learned and there may be a genetic predisposition to addictive substances.
D. Review of systems.
  1. Psychological: Mood symptoms are common in individuals with substance use disorders (SUDs).
  2. Cardiac: Racing heart rate and feeling of palpitations.

MENTAL STATUS EXAMINATION

A. Appearance.
  1. Diaphoretic, lacrimation, piloerection, rhinorrhea, skin assessment (wounds), and scarring at the veins.
  2. Tremor.
  3. Pupils.
    a. Dilated: Opiate withdrawal.
    b. Pinpoint: Opiate intoxication.
    c. Nystagmus: Wernicke.
B. Behavior.
  1. Restless/psychomotor agitation/yawning.
C. Speech.
  1. Quantity, rate, and volume.
  2. Dysarthria.
D. Affect.
  1. Assess for anxiety, agitation, irritability, instability of affect, and dysphoria.
E. Thought content.
  1. Suicidal ideation.
  2. Homicidal ideation.
  3. Delusions: Paranoia may occur in intoxication of multiple substances or substance-induced.
  4. Delirium/withdrawal.
F. Thought process.
G. Perception.
  1. Visual/tactile hallucinations consider intoxication versus substance-induced delirium/withdrawal.
  2. Psychotic symptoms can occur in cocaine, methamphetamine, and hallucinogen intoxication.
H. Cognitive exam.
  1. Disorientation: Consider substance-induced delirium/withdrawal.
  2. Confabulation: Consider Wernicke.

DIAGNOSTIC TESTS

A. Comprehensive metabolic panel (CMP).
B. Liver function tests (LFTs) and kidney function tests.
C. Blood alcohol level.
D. Serum or urine drug screen.
E. Pregnancy test.
F. HIV.
G. EKG.
H. Screening.
   1. Screening, brief intervention, and referral to treatment (SBIRT).
      a. Screening: A healthcare professional assesses for risky substance use behaviors using standardized screening tools such as CAGE.
      b. Brief intervention: A healthcare professional engages a patient showing risky substance use behaviors in a short conversation.
   2. A standard drink.
      a. 12 oz of beer/ale/malt liquor.
      b. 1.5 oz of spirits such as vodka, tequila, gin, whiskey, or rum.
      c. 5 oz of wine.
   3. Positive screen for at-risk drinking.
      a. Men: Greater than 14 drinks a week or greater than four on occasion.
      b. Women: Greater than seven drinks a week or greater than three drinks on occasion.
      c. Elders: Greater than seven drinks a week or greater than one drink on occasion.
   4. CAGE assessment: One yes is a positive screen and needs further assessment.
      a. Have you ever felt the need to Cut down on your substance use?
      b. Have people Annoyed you by criticizing your substance use?
      c. Have you ever felt Guilty about your substance use?
      d. Have you ever felt the need to drink/use first thing in the morning as an Eye opener?

DIFFERENTIAL DIAGNOSIS

A. Attention deficit hyperactivity disorder (ADHD).
B. Bipolar disorder.
C. Trauma-related disorders.
D. Major depression.
E. Anxiety disorders.
F. Other substance use disorders.

EVALUATION AND MANAGEMENT PLAN

A. Motivational interviewing is a patient-centered therapy to help explore and resolve ambivalence.
B. Motivational interviewing also has applications for other chronic health conditions.
C. Management of acute withdrawal.
   1. Alcohol.
      a. High-dose intravenous (IV) thiamine for 3 days (500 mg TID).
      b. Benzodiazepines fixed-tapering-dose regimen (FTDRs) versus symptom-triggered regimen (STR). Caution in liver disease.
      c. Gabapentin taper initiated at 1,200 mg/d dosing and gradually reduced by 300 mg/d. No hepatic metabolism. May reduce cravings.
   2. Opioids.
      a. Symptomatic management.
      b. Methadone taper.
      c. Buprenorphine: Patient must be in moderate withdrawal to prevent precipitated withdrawal.
   3. Cocaine and other stimulants: Benzodiazepines to manage acute intoxication and withdrawal.
   4. Hallucinogens: Benzodiazepines to manage acute intoxication and withdrawal.
D. Hierarchy of detoxification: Sedative/hypnotics and alcohol can be life-threatening. Opioid withdrawal may not be life-threatening; however, medical comorbidities can be life-threatening and/or other substances added to traditional may elevate the risks associated with withdrawal syndromes.
   1. Fentanyl.
   2. Xylazine: A veterinary agent that acts as an alpha-agonist in humans.
E. Assessment of alcohol withdrawal and providing intervention: Risk of seizures after 48 hours of last drink and risk of delirium tremens (DTs) after 72 hours of the last drink.
F. Alcohol withdrawal assessment: Clinical Institute for Withdrawal Assessment for Alcohol (CIWA-AR), and detox is most commonly attempted with a benzodiazepine.
G. Opioid withdrawal assessment: Clinical Opiate Withdrawal Scale (COWS) and detox commonly with buprenorphine or methadone.
H. Alcohol cravings: Naltrexone/Vivitrol, acamprosate, ondansetron, or disulfiram (Antabuse): Need to provide education about products to avoid adverse reactions.
I. Medication-assisted treatment (MAT): Methadone, buprenorphine (can be prescribed by nurse practitioners [NPs] with additional training); suboxone-buprenorphine/naloxone: Naloxone is not absorbed sublingually, added to reduce diversion risk.
J. Nicotine replacement therapy (NRT): NRT options (patch, gum, inhaler), bupropion (Zyban, Wellbutrin), and varenicline (Chantix).

FOLLOW-UP

A. Follow up with a substance use disorder specialist for medications and therapy.

CONSULTATION/REFERRAL

A. Consultation for medical comorbidities.
B. Referral to outpatient support groups such as Alcoholics Anonymous (AA), Narcotics Anonymous (NA), Cocaine Anonymous (CA), and Opioids Anonymous (OA).
C. Referral to treatment: A healthcare professional provides a referral to brief therapy or for additional services.

SPECIAL/GERIATRIC CONSIDERATIONS

A. Substance use in older adults is a rapidly growing problem and may be triggered by retirement; death of a close family member, friend, or even pet; financial strains; or mental or physical decline.

B. Older adult patients may have a decreased ability to metabolize drugs or alcohol.

BIBLIOGRAPHY

American Psychiatric Association. (2013). *Diagnostic and statistical manual of mental disorders* (5th ed.). Author.
Carlat, D. J. (2017). *The psychiatric interview* (4th ed.). Wolters Kluwer.
Drug Enforcement Administration. (2021, February). *Xylazine*. https://www.deadiversion.usdoj.gov/drug_chem_info/Xylazine.pdf
Goldberg, J., Stahl, S., & Schatzberg, A. (2021). *Practical psychopharmacology: Translating findings from evidence-based trials into real-world clinical practice.* Cambridge University Press. https://doi.org/10.1017/9781108553216
Sadock, B. J., Sadock, V. A., & Ruiz, P. (2015). *Kaplan & Sadock's synopsis of psychiatry: Behavioral sciences/clinical psychiatry* (11th ed.). Wolters Kluwer.
Sadock, B. J., Sadock, V. A., & Ruiz, P. (2018). *Kaplan & Sadock's comprehensive textbook of psychiatry* (10th ed., Vol. 11)). Wolters Kluwer.
Stern, T. A., Freudenreich, O., Smith, F. A., Fricchione, G. L., & Rosenbaum, J. F. (2018). *Massachusetts general hospital handbook of general hospital psychiatry* (7th ed.). Elsevier Inc.
Substance Abuse and Mental Health Services Administration. (2019). *Recovery and recovery support.* https://www.samhsa.gov/find-help/recovery

PSYCHIATRIC PATIENT MEDICAL CLEARANCE

DEFINITION

A. Guidelines exist, but no clear definition of what "medical clearance" should include.
B. Review local institutional guidelines.
  1. Purpose: Clearance of a psychiatric patient to transfer to a setting with fewer medical resources.
  2. Guideline: Within reasonable medical certainty, there is no contributing medical condition causing the psychiatric complaints.
C. Assessment for risk of violence: **STAMP**: **S**taring and eye contact, **T**one and volume of voice, **A**nxiety, **M**umbling, and **P**acing.
D. Training in nonviolent crisis intervention and de-escalation.

SUBJECTIVE DATA

A. Common complaints/symptoms.
  1. Delirium.
  2. Confusion.
  3. Agitated behavior.
  4. Suicidal Ideation.
B. Common/typical scenario.
  1. Patients come to the ED or are brought by family or medical services due to an alteration in disposition.
C. Family and social history.
  1. Inquire about substance use, alcohol use, and all medications (prescribed and nonprescribed).
  2. Inquire about falls.
  3. Inquire about family medical and psychiatric history.
  4. Biopsychosocial history.
    a. What led to ED presentation?
    b. Risk to self/others or inability to care for self-due to mental status changes.
    c. Rule out organic or substance-induced causes.
    d. Identify needed medical treatments.
  5. History.
    a. History taking will provide guidance as to what medical testing should occur. Collateral data from a family member, caseworker, group home staff, or someone who knows the patient is critical.
    b. Is this an existing or new psychiatric illness?
    c. Assessment of mental status for acute (more commonly organic in nature) or insidious (more commonly psychiatric in nature) onset, drug interaction, or toxicity (new medication/medication change/overtaking medication).
    d. Relapse of a psychiatric disorder due to nonadherence.
D. Review of systems.
  1. Dermatologic: Ask about bruising or breaks in skin.
  2. Neurologic: Ask about dizziness, confusion, or weakness.
  3. Signs and symptoms of infection.

MENTAL STATUS EXAMINATION

A. Appearance: Hygiene, clothing, body, movements.
B. Behavior and attitude.
  1. Cooperation?
C. Speech: Tone, volume, fluency, spontaneity of responses.
D. Affect: Stabile, labile, appropriate, consistency with self-reported mood.
E. Thought process.
  1. Organized.
  2. Associations: Loose, tangential, circumstantial.
  3. Racing thoughts, flight of ideas.
F. Thought content.
  1. Suicidal ideation, plan, intentions to act, access to lethal means.
    a. Access to firearms.
  2. Homicidal or assaultive ideation.
    a. Specific target?
  3. Perceptual disturbances/paranoid ideations.
    a. Command auditory hallucinations.
G. Cognitive exam.
  1. Assess orientation to person, place, time, and situation.
  2. Assess concentration: Serial 7s, spell "world" backward, and recite the days of the week backward.

DIAGNOSTIC TESTS

A. Laboratory tests will depend on the presenting problem, history, and assessment.
B. Consider:
  1. Drug screen and blood ethanol level.
  2. Any symptoms triggered by return of spontaneous circulation (ROSC) to include assessment of substance use withdrawal and/or intoxication.
  3. Acetaminophen/salicylate level.
  4. Lithium/Depakote levels.

5. Human chorionic gonadotropin (HCG).

6. Basic metabolic panel (BMP).

7. Complete blood count (CBC).

8. Liver function test (LFT).

9. HIV.

10. Rapid plasma reagin (RPR).

11. B$_{12}$/folate levels.

12. EKG/troponins: Unstable angina (UA).

13. Creatine kinase (CK) level.

14. Thyroid stimulating hormone (TSH).

15. Infections workup, blood/urine cultures, chest x-ray.

DIFFERENTIAL DIAGNOSIS

A. Fasting glucose/metabolic disorders.

B. Meningitis (drop coin to see if the patient can look down).

C. Substance use (look up the nose for substance use).

D. Seizure: Postictal (assess tongue for lacerations)

E. Traumatic brain injury.

F. Delirium.

G. Drug overdose.

H. Syphilis.

EVALUATION AND MANAGEMENT PLAN

A. Assess capacity to consent to or refuse treatment. Does this patient have a legal guardian or other surrogate decision-maker? Capacity assessments are based on a patient's understanding, appreciation, reasoning, and expression of choice.

  1. Understanding: Ability to comprehend the information provided about the patient's condition, as well as the risks and benefits of the proposed treatment.

  2. Appreciation: Ability to apply the relevant information to self.

  3. Reasoning: Ability to manipulate the information about their condition rationally.

  4. Choice: The patient can not only express their choice, but it is done so clear and consistently and is consistent with their goals and values.

B. Voluntary versus involuntary commitment: Know your state laws about the process AND transportation.

C. Duty to protect (see earlier) and duty to report (children, older adults, and those without capacity).

D. Inpatient/outpatient or referral to community resource.

CONSULTATION/REFERRAL

A. Psychiatry if available in the hospital, or one can use telemedicine. ED protocols for evaluation of psychiatric cases have been developed by the American College of Emergency Physicians.

B. Consult case management to help the patient find the needed resources for outpatient management.

C. Consult social work for psychosocial needs, such as substance use or transitional housing.

SPECIAL/GERIATRIC CONSIDERATIONS

A. Geriatric patients are more likely to present with delirium to the ED related to medical conditions.

B. Older adult patients who present with a new onset of psychosis should have complete medical workup and assess for substance use disorders (SUDs) and withdrawal.

BIBLIOGRAPHY

American College of Emergency Physicians. (2009). *Massachusetts medical clearance guidelines*. https://www.acep.org/global assets/uploads/uploaded-files/acep/advocacy/state-issues/psychiatric- hold-issues/ma-medical-clearance-guidelines-toxic-screen-ma.pdf

American Psychiatric Association. (2013). *Diagnostic and statistical manual of mental disorders* (5th ed.). Author.

Appelbaum, P. S., & Grisso, T. (1988). Assessing patients' capacities to consent to treatment. *New England Journal of Medicine, 319,* 1635–1638. https://doi.org/10.1056/NEJM198812223192504

Boudreaux, E. D., Niro, K., Sullivan, A., Rosenbaum, C. D., Allen, M., & Camargo, C. A. (2011). Current practices for mental health follow-up after psychiatric emergency department/psychiatric emergency service visits: A national survey of academic emergency departments. *General Hospital Psychiatry, 33*(6), 631–633. https://doi.org/10.1016/j.genhosppsych.2011.05.020

New Jersey Hospital Association. (2011). *Consensus statement: Medical clearance protocols for acute psychiatric patients referred for inpatient admission.* http://www.njha.com/media/33107/ClearanceProtocolsforAcutePsyPatients.pdf

Nordstrom, K., Zun, L. S., Wilson, M. P., Stiebel, V., Ng, A. T., Bregman, B. Anderson, E. L, & Nouri, T. (2012). Medical evaluation and triage of the agitated patient: Consensus statement of the American Association for Emergency Psychiatry project BETA medical evaluation workgroup. *Western Journal of Emergency Medicine, 13*(1), 3–10. https://doi.org/10.5811/westjem.2011.9.6863

Sadock, B.J., Sadock, V.A., & Ruiz, P. (2018). *Kaplan & Sadock's comprehensive textbook of psychiatry* (10th ed., Vol. 11)). Wolters Kluwer.

Stern, T. A., Freudenreich, O., Smith, F. A., Fricchione, G. L., & Rosenbaum, J. F. (2018). *Massachusetts general hospital handbook of general hospital psychiatry* (7th ed.). Elsevier Inc.

Tang, S., Patel, P., Khubchandani, J., & Grossberg, G. (2014). The psychogeriatric patient in the emergency room: Focus on management and disposition. *ISRN Psychiatry, 2014,* 5. https://doi.org/10.1155/2014/413572

KNOWLEDGE CHECK: CHAPTER 9

1. When monitoring a patient on lithium, which of the following should the nurse practitioner remember to teach the patient?

   A. If pregnant, one should immediately stop taking lithium.

   B. Lithium toxicity can happen if someone is sick and dehydrated, or if other medications interact or interfere with lithium levels.

   C. Lithium should not be taken with any other medications.

   D. Baseline lab work is not necessary when someone is on lithium.

2. Which of the following should be the FIRST step if serotonin syndrome is suspected?

   A. Initiate oxygen, intravenous (IV) fluids, and cardiac monitoring.

   B. Apply cooling blankets, give paralytic agents, and initiate ventilation.

   C. Sedate with benzodiazepines to decrease tremor and clonus.

   D. Discontinue the serotonergic agent.

3. A 32-year-old patient with schizophrenia, with previous symptoms of introversion, auditory hallucinations, and cognitive decline, now presents for dysarthria and aggression. Which of the following infectious processes/diseases would be the most important to rule out?

   A. Syphilis

   B. Urinary tract infection

   C. Malaria

   D. Toxoplasmosis

4. A 63-year-old man admitted to the ICU has been determined to have alcohol withdrawal syndrome and has moderate withdrawal symptoms as assessed on the Clinical Institute for Withdrawal Assessment for Alcohol (CIWA-AR). When is the patient most at risk for seizures after drinking cessation?

   A. Within 24 to 48 hours

   B. Only within the first few hours

   C. Within 48 hours

   D. After 72 hours

(See answers next page.)

1. **B) Lithium toxicity can happen if someone is sick and dehydrated, or if other medications interact or interfere with lithium levels.**

   It is critical for the patient to know that it is important to stay hydrated when sick and to not take medication twice if experiencing vomiting/diarrhea. Taking lithium in pregnancy should be determined on a case-by-case basis, and the risks and benefits should be weighed. Ensuring that the patient is stable is critical because pregnancy increases the risk of mood episodes and/or symptom exacerbation. It is important that the patient knows the signs and symptoms of lithium toxicity and knows when to go to the ED if symptoms present. Lithium levels as well as human chorionic gonadotropin (HCG), thyroid function tests, complete blood count (CBC), and kidney function tests are all indicated at baseline. An EKG is also indicated if the patient is 50 years of age or more.

2. **D) Discontinue the serotonergic agent.**

   When serotonin syndrome is a possible diagnosis, the critical step is to stop the offending agent to decrease continued effects. It is also prudent to ensure that all other organic causes have been ruled out. Sedation with benzodiazepines to decrease tremor and clonus would be the second step to decrease tremor, clonus, heart rate, and blood pressure. Initiating oxygen, intravenous (IV) fluids, and cardiac monitoring would likely be the third step once the patient is stable. Applying cooling blankets, giving paralytic agents, and initiating ventilation are additional treatments that may be needed if serotonin syndrome is severe and additional interventions are needed to stabilize the patient.

3. **A) Syphilis**

   Given the rising rates of syphilis, especially as it co-occurs with HIV/AIDs, it is important to rule it out because late-stage syphilis may have long-lasting psychiatric symptoms. While urinary tract infection (UTI) should be ruled out, UTI symptoms tend to occur abruptly and would likely not have a progressively worsening course. While other infectious processes like malaria or toxoplasmosis can also be ruled out, these would be included in the relevant rule-outs if risk factors exist, such as travel to a malaria-prone region or contact with cats for toxoplasmosis. Malaria may have psychiatric symptoms such as delirium, but these are usually seen in the late stage and are not progressive. Toxoplasmosis symptoms may have a presentation in schizophrenia but can be nonspecific in relation to faulty immune activity damaging the neurons.

4. **C) Within 48 hours**

   While withdrawal seizures typically do occur within 12 to 48 hours after cessation of drinking, they *can* appear up to 48 hours after cessation. Some case reports have demonstrated that seizures can occur within a few hours after the last alcoholic drink. Delirium tremens usually occurs around 72 hours in up to 5% of patients after their last drink; however, it can also start between 48 and 96 hours after the last drink and last up to 1 week.

CHAPTER 10

INFECTION GUIDELINES

COLITIS: INFECTIVE

Jennifer W. Parker

DEFINITION

A. Inflammation of the colon caused by an infectious agent (e.g., bacteria, virus, or parasite). Colitis is diagnosed when the patient has diarrhea (passage of three or more unformed stools per day) and has evidence of inflammation in the colon based on at least one of the following:

   1. Positive fecal markers: Elevated leukocytes, positive lactoferrin, or positive calprotectin.

   2. Dysentery: Many small volume stools containing obvious blood or mucus (often associated with fever and abdominal pain).

   3. Mucosal inflammation as identified by colonoscopy or sigmoidoscopy.

B. Duration of symptoms.

   1. Acute: 14 days or fewer (most are infectious and self-limiting).

   2. Persistent: 14 to 30 days.

   3. Chronic: 30 or more days (most are noninfectious).

C. Pseudomembranous colitis caused by the bacteria *Clostridioides difficile* (formerly called *Clostridium difficile)* and often referred to as CDI or *C.Diff* is of special concern and is highlighted in this chapter.

INCIDENCE

A. The vast majority of colitis is viral; only 1.5% to 5.6% of stool cultures produce positive results.

B. Severe diarrhea (four or more liquid stools per day for more than 3 days) is generally bacterial.

C. In the past 30 years, CDI has been increasing in the United States, not only in the healthcare setting but also in the community. There are over half a million infections in the United States per year; one in six cases will get it again within 2 to 8 weeks. The incidence of community-acquired CDI is increasing faster than hospital-acquired, but is typically less severe.

   1. Community-acquired CDI: 51.9 cases per 100,000. The rate of first recurrence is 13.5%, and the death rate within 30 days is 1.3%.

   2. Healthcare-acquired CDI: 95.3 cases per 100,000. The rate of first recurrence is 20.9%, and the death rate within 30 days is 9.3%.

PATHOGENESIS

A. Major causes in the United States.

   1. Viruses: norovirus, rotavirus, adenoviruses, cytomegalovirus (CMV), and astrovirus.

   2. Bacteria: *Salmonella, Campylobacter, Shigella, Escherichia coli* (E. coli), *Yersinia enterocolitica, C. difficile,* and *Mycobacterium tuberculosis.*

   3. Protozoa: *Cryptosporidium, Giardia, Cyclospora,* and *Entamoeba.*

   4. Sexually transmitted infection: *Neisseria gonorrhea, Chlamydia trachomatis,* herpes simplex and *Treponema pallidum.*

B. Diarrhea represents altered changes in the flow of water and electrolytes within an osmotic gradient. Normally the gastrointestinal (GI) tract absorbs about 8 to 9 L of fluid a day, excreting about 200 mL of water in stool.

C. Enteric pathogens, acting primarily on transporter cells or the lateral spaces between cells (which are regulated by tight junctions), alter the balance toward significantly greater excretion and less absorption.

D. Pathogens can alter absorption by either direct or indirect modulation.

   1. Direct modulation involving:

     a. Epithelial ion transport processes.

       i. Evidence from the literature proposes that the rapid onset of diarrhea induced via enteropathogenic *E. coli* (EPEC) may result from direct effects on intestinal epithelial ion transport processes.

     b. Barrier function.

   2. Indirect modulation involving:

     a. Inflammation.

       i. *Shigella* and *Salmonella* species cause an inflammatory diarrhea characterized by fever and polymorphonucleocytes (PMNs) in the stool.

       ii. PMNs regulate absorption through cytokine secretion but also have a more direct role through the secretion of a precursor to adenosine, activating certain transmembrane conductance regulators.

     b. Neuropeptides.

       i. *C. difficile* and rotavirus infection also work indirectly through modulation of ion transport subsequent to cytokine secretion and activation of enteric nerves via neuropeptides.

     c. Loss of absorptive surface.

       i. *Giardia* lead to the loss of brush border absorptive surface and diffuse shortening of villi.

       ii. Similarly, EPEC cause effacement of microvilli, which decreases the surface area for nutrient absorption and causes increased osmolarity of the intestinal contents and malabsorption. ▶

E. CDIs (nosocomial and community-acquired) account for almost all cases of pseudomembranous colitis (acute colitis characterized by formation of an adherent inflammatory membrane that overlays injury site).

1. There is multifactorial activation with enterotoxin A and cytotoxin B. In addition, there is a new strain with increased productions of enterotoxin A and cytotoxin B, as well as binary toxin, with fluoroquinolone resistance.

2. Besides the direct effect of the toxins on tight junctions, and in contrast to other pathogens, *C. difficile* leads to activation of neuropeptides, resulting in inflammation via a necroinflammatory reaction, which activates mast cells, nerves, vascular endothelium, and immune cells.

PREDISPOSING FACTORS

A. Hospitalization, previous CDI, greater than 65 years of age, recent abdominal surgery, use of proton pump inhibitors (PPI), and living conditions (long-term care facilities).

B. International travel: *Shigella, Campylobacter, Salmonella*, enteroinvasive *E. coli* (EIEC), enteroaggregative *E. coli* (EAEC), and others.

C. Foodborne: *Staphylococcus aureus, Bacillus cereus, Clostridioides perfringens*, or *E. coli*.

D. Other risk factors.

1. Antibiotic (Abx) exposure, healthcare exposure (Abx most common to trigger include cephalosporins, clindamycin, carbapenems, trimethoprim, fluoroquinolones, sulfonamides, and penicillin combinations).

2. Exposure to *C. difficile*.

3. HIV or other immune deficiency.

4. Chemotherapy.

5. Enteric tube feeding or other GI tract manipulation.

6. Inflammatory bowel disease (IBD) or other chronic GI disease.

SUBJECTIVE DATA

A. Common complaints/symptoms.

1. Mild: Watery diarrhea three or more times a day and abdominal cramping.

2. Severe: Watery diarrhea 10 or more times a day with abdominal cramping and pain. May also be associated with fever, dehydration, and rapid heart rate.

3. Hematochezia and mucoid discharge.

4. Tenesmus.

5. Urgency.

B. Common/typical scenario.

1. Careful, detailed history of present illness: Important because it can suggest likely cause of the diarrhea.

a. Duration: Acute, persistent, chronic, or change in periodicity.

b. Frequency and characteristics of stool.

   i. Small bowel origin: Watery, large volume, abdominal cramping, bloating, or gas.

   ii. Large bowel origin: Frequent, regular small-volume stools, often tenesmus with bowel movements, and inflammatory signs (e.g., fever and bloody or mucoid stools) are common.

   iii. Inflammatory signs suggest enteric viruses (e.g., CMV, adenovirus), invasive bacteria (e.g., *Salmonella, Shigella, Campylobacter*), or cytotoxic pathogen such as *C. difficile*.

C. Family and social history.

1. Food exposure: Raw or undercooked meat, seafood, unpasteurized dairy products. Timing is important.

a. Less than 6 hours with nausea and vomiting, likely *S. aureus* or *B. cereus*.

b. 8 to 16 hours: Likely *C. perfringens*.

c. Greater than 16 hours: Viral or possibly *E. coli* enterotoxigenic pathogen.

2. Other exposures.

a. Animals (e.g., poultry, petting zoos): *Salmonella*.

b. Travel to resource-limited areas (increased risk of pathogens and certain bacteria).

c. Occupation: Day-care centers likely for *Giardia, Shigella*, or *Cryptosporidium*.

d. Recent hospitalizations: Increased likelihood of CDI.

e. Antibiotic use: Increased likelihood of CDI.

f. Use of PPI: Can increase risk of infectious diarrhea.

g. Anal sexual activity.

D. Review of systems.

1. Neurologic: Lightheadedness and dizziness.

2. Dermatologic: Dry skin.

3. Genitourinary: Frequency of urination and color.

4. Abdominal: Diarrhea, nausea, pain anywhere in the abdomen, bloody stools, loss of appetite, bloating, or distension.

PHYSICAL EXAMINATION

A. Volume status: Hypovolemia.

1. Dry mucous membranes.

2. Tenting of skin or diminished skin turgor.

3. Change in mental status.

4. Dizziness, lightheadedness, and orthostatic blood pressure.

5. Hypotension.

B. Complications: Ileus or peritonitis.

1. Abdominal distention.

2. Abdominal tenderness with percussion or gentle palpitation.

3. Rebound tenderness.

4. Abdominal rigidity.

DIAGNOSTIC TESTS

A. Blood studies: Often not needed for patients with infectious diarrhea but helps determine status of the acutely ill patient. Evaluating for sepsis, dehydration, and electrolyte abnormalities.

1. Serum electrolytes if volume depletion is a concern: Screening for hypokalemia and acute kidney injury (AKI).

2. Complete blood count (CBC): May be of limited help.

    a. Platelet count, partial thromboplastin time (PTT): Concern for hemolytic uremic syndrome.

    b. Leukocytosis: Consistent with CDI.

3. Blood cultures: If high fever is present or sepsis is a concern.

4. Lactate, C-reactive protein (CRP), erythrocyte sedimentation rate (ESR), and procalcitonin (PCT) level if patient has signs and symptoms of sepsis.

B. Stool studies: Generally unnecessary if patients have no comorbidities: Infectious colitis generally resolves on its own, tests should be completed for those with severe illness, high-risk comorbidities, or suggestive history (e.g., travel-related diarrhea), or >7 days of symptoms.

    1. Stool polymerase chain reaction (PCR): Rapid determination of detecting DNA/RNA of 22 pathogens.

    2. Fecal leukocytes: Findings of white blood cell (WBC) count on a test result do *not* differentiate between IBD and infectious colitis; screening test for intestinal inflammation.

    3. Acute bloody diarrhea: Bacterial colitis.

        a. Cultures for enterohemorrhagic *E. coli* (EHEC) and *Entamoeba*.

        b. Shiga toxin direct testing: For many strains of Shiga toxin-producing *E. coli* (STEC).

    4. Stool culture.

        a. *Shigella*, *Salmonella*, and *Campylobacter* are routinely sought.

        b. If STEC, noncholera *Vibrio*, or *Yersinia* is suspected, alert the lab to look for these because specialized techniques are required.

    5. Ova and parasites (O&P): For patients with persistent diarrhea or who are immunocompromised. Unlike bacterial pathogens, which are shed continuously, O&P are shed intermittently.

    6. *C. difficile* toxin: For patients who currently take or have recently taken antibiotics *or* have been hospitalized or recently been in a healthcare facility.

C. Imaging (CT): Not usually warranted unless patient is presenting with acute abdomen.

D. Endoscopy: Not usually warranted.

E. CDI.

    1. Leukocytosis: Can be marked in severe disease (>15,000 cells/mcL).

    2. Volume depletion: Elevated creatinine (Cr), blood urea nitrogen (BUN), and reduced estimated glomerular filtration rate (GFR).

    3. Elevated lactate.

    4. Predictors of mortality.

        a. WBC greater than 35,000 cells/mcL or less than 4,000 cells/mcL.

        b. Significant banding (>10%).

        c. Immunosuppression.

        d. Cardiorespiratory failure.

  5. Need to differentiate *C. difficile* colonization from infection.

    a. Only perform CDI testing on loose stools (unless concern for ileus) when there is a reasonable likelihood of CDI.

    b. Stool studies: If patient used antibiotics within 8 to 12 weeks prior to onset of symptoms.

        i. Culture: Gold standard for identification of *C. difficile*.

            1) Sow times; requires follow-up with toxigenic testing because not all strains produce toxins.

            2) Usually reserved for epidemiologic studies.

        ii. Enzyme immunoassay: Rapid.

            1) Sensitivity of 75% to 94% and specificity of 83% to 98% for identification of toxins A and B.

            2) Low sensitivity may require further diagnostic testing in the face of high clinical suspicion and negative test results.

        iii. PCR: Superior to enzyme immunoassay.

            1) Used by most U.S. hospitals.

            2) High sensitivity and specificity: Single sample is sufficient.

            3) Generally 24 to 48 hours turnaround.

            4) *Does not* differentiate colonization from infection.

DIFFERENTIAL DIAGNOSIS

A. IBD (e.g., ulcerative colitis, Crohn's disease).

B. Ischemic colitis: Vasculitis common in Henoch–Schönlein purpura.

C. Immunodeficiency syndromes (e.g., common variable immunodeficiency, chronic granulomatous disease, Wiskott–Aldrich syndrome, and immunodysregulation, polyendocrinopathy, enteropathy X-linked [IPEX] syndrome).

D. Irritable bowel syndrome.

E. Celiac disease.

COMPLICATIONS

A. Sepsis.

B. Electrolyte imbalance and associated sequela.

C. Toxic megacolon.

D. Aortitis.

E. Infectious aneurysm.

F. Intestinal perforation.

G. Peritonitis.

H. Hemolytic uremic syndrome (HUS).

EVALUATION AND MANAGEMENT PLAN

A. General plan.

    1. Supportive care.

        a. Fluid and electrolyte administration to keep up with losses.

i. Oral is preferred hydration. Severe disease may require oral rehydration solution.

ii. Monitor electrolytes and repletion as necessary.

2. Low-fat, low-dairy (except yogurt or other fermented dairy items) diets: Preferred banana, rice, applesauce, and toast (BRAT) diet.

3. Holding of antimotility therapy (e.g., loperamide, bismuth subsalicylate): Can be harmful with some pathogens; generally alright with inflammatory diarrhea.

B. Pharmacotherapy.

1. Antibiotics.

a. Empiric therapy.

i. Not widely recommended (despite reducing length of illness) due to promotion of antibiotic resistance, likely changes in gut flora, contributing to HUS, and increased risk of CDI.

ii. However, recommended for certain conditions:

1) Severe disease: Greater than six stools per day, fever, hypovolemia requiring hospitalization.

2) Bloody or mucoid stools (likely invasive bacterial infection) unless fever is low or absent.

3) Comorbidities (especially immunocompromising and cardiac diseases), including age greater than 70.

4) *Oral* fluoroquinolones for 3 to 5 days: Preferred treatment for empiric therapy for acute diarrhea of unknown source.

a) Ciprofloxacin: 500 mg BID.

b) Levofloxacin: 500 mg daily.

c) Fluoroquinolone-intolerant patients: Oral azithromycin 500 mg PO daily for 3 days or erythromycin 500 mg PO BID for 5 days.

5) Modify antibiotics as soon as bacteria and antimicrobial susceptibility are identified. Consider infectious diseases consult.

a) Probiotics: Generally not found to improve critical outcomes for patients being treated for CDI.

2. Probiotics: Can be started within 48 hours of initiation of antibiotic treatment on **any patient receiving antibiotics other than for CDI** to lower risk of *C. difficile*, but evidence is low of improved critical outcomes (preventing CDI), but side effects are low as well.

3. Antidiarrheals.

a. Bismuth subsalicylates: Symptomatic improvement in mild or moderate acute diarrhea.

b. Loperamide: May shorten duration of watery diarrhea in otherwise healthy adults and in traveler's diarrhea, but AVOID when there is possibility of toxic megacolon or when fever continues.

4. CDI: History of antibiotic therapy or recent hospitalizations.

a. Discontinuation of offending antibiotic (if possible).

b. *Avoidance* of antimotility medications.

c. Enhanced contact precautions: Handwashing before and after patient contact.

d. Antibiotic therapy: Best to wait for diagnostic confirmation if possible; no treatment if positive toxin assay but asymptomatic.

i. Mild to moderate.

1) Vancomycin 125 mg PO QID × 10 to 14 days.

2) Fidaxomicin 200 mg BID × 10 days.

3) Metronidazole 500 mg PO TID × 10 to 14 days (not first-line treatment; use only if other options not available). Not for use in recurrent CDI infections.

ii. Severe (WBC >15,000 cells/mL × serum albumin <3 g/dL, and/or Cr ≥1.5 baseline).

1) Vancomycin 125 mg PO QID × 10 to 14 days.

iii. Fulminant or complicated.

1) Vancomycin 125 mg PO QID × 10 to 14 days. *Plus*

2) Metronidazole 500 mg IV every 6 to 8 hours. *Plus*

3) Vancomycin via nasogastric tube or rectally.

iv. Recurrent, antibiotic resistant (but recurrent is not equivalent to resistant); after initial treatment, recurrence in 15% to 20% of cases generally 5 to 8 days after treatment. It is important to distinguish a spontaneous recurrence versus antibiotic triggered resistance.

1) Repeat same or alternate antibiotic. Recurrences beyond the second infection should not be treated with metronidazole due to possible neurotoxic effects with prolonged use and decreased effectiveness.

2) Vancomycin pulses and/or tapers for extended duration.

3) Vancomycin for 2 weeks, then rifaximin for 2 weeks (generally not used now that fecal microbiota treatment is available).

4) High-dose vancomycin in combination with *Saccharomyces boulardii* (*not* in immunosuppressed patients).

5) Fecal microbiota treatment: Used in cases of multiple recurrent CDI, moderate CDI with no response to standard antibiotic therapy for 1 week, or severe or fulminate CDI with no response to treatment in 48 hours; relatively high success rate (nearly 90% for recurrent CDI). It involves fecal enemas, colonoscopy with delivery of fecal material, and nasogastric tube delivery of fecal material.

6) Colectomy.

C. Patient/family teaching points.

1. Prevent the spread of *C. difficile* with aggressive handwashing. Do not rely on hand sanitizers because they are ineffective in destroying *C. difficile* spores.

2. Patients need to have a private room.

3. All staff and visitors must wear isolation gowns and gloves while in the room.
D. Discharge instructions.
  1. Avoid unnecessary antibiotics.
  2. Report new or worsening symptoms.
  3. Clean surfaces at home with chlorine-based disinfectants.
  4. Drink fluids to prevent dehydration.

FOLLOW-UP

A. There is generally no role for repeat laboratory testing/testing for a cure with *C. difficile*.
B. Assays may remain positive during recovery.

CONSULTATION/REFERRAL

A. In severe, unresponsive cases, gastroenterology, infectious disease, and/or surgery may need to be consulted.

SPECIAL/GERIATRIC CONSIDERATIONS

A. Older adult patients are generally characterized as having decreased immune function.
B. Short- and long-term hospitalizations have become a critical risk factor in the development of colitis in this population.
C. Mortality rates are also significantly higher in older adult patients.

CASE SCENARIO—COLITIS: INFECTIVE

A 45-year-old woman with no relevant medical history reports to the ED with weakness, dizziness, and diarrhea. She reported that she went to her primary care provider (PCP) 4 days ago with 3 days of watery diarrhea. Her PCP assumed she had viral enteritis and she was sent home to drink lots of fluids. She is found to be tachycardic with heart rate of 123, temperature of 99.8°F/37.7°C, blood pressure of 96/40, respiratory rate of 21, and oxygen saturation of 97% on room air.

1. The nurse practitioner (NP) is admitting the patient and taking her history. She admits to no recent travel, no sick contacts, and no antibiotics in the last 6 months. She does admit going to the dentist 2 weeks ago. What additional tests does the NP request?
  A. Complete blood count (CBC), comprehensive metabolic panel (CMP), stool polymerase chain reaction (PCR)
  B. CT of the abdomen/pelvis
  C. Stool occult blood
  D. Fecal leukocytes

2. Labs come back significant for leukocytosis (white blood cell [WBC] = 15,000, lactate = 3.5, creatinine [Cr] = 2.2, blood urea nitrogen [BUN] = 38, potassium = 2.5) and stool PCR positive for *Clostridioides difficile*. The first line of treatment is:
  A. Start empiric antibiotics.
  B. Bolus patient with intravenous (IV) fluids and trend lactate and vital signs (VS).
  C. Consult gastroenterology.
  D. Make patient nil per os (NPO).

3. Treatment for severe *C. diff* should include all BUT the following:
  A. Loperamide
  B. Oral vancomycin 125 mg QID for 10 days

  C. IV fluid resuscitation
  D. Contact isolation

4. The patient responded well to treatment and was discharged on day 3 of hospitalizations. Discharge teaching included which of the following statements?
  A. You are cured and will likely never get *Clostridioides difficile* infection (CDI) again.
  B. Just take antibiotics until your symptoms have resolved.
  C. You need follow-up testing in 3 days to make sure you no longer have CDI.
  D. Take the entire course of vancomycin and return to PCP if symptoms recur.

BIBLIOGRAPHY

Azer, S. A., & Tuma, F. (2022, January). Infectious colitis. In *StatPearls* [*Internet*]. StatPearls Publishing. https://www.ncbi.nlm.nih.gov/books/NBK544325/

Barkley, T. W., Jr., & Myers, C. M. (2014). *Practice considerations for adult-gerontology acute care nurse practitioners*. Barkley and Associates.

Centers for Disease Control and Prevention. (2021, July 12). *C. diff (Clostridioides difficile)*. https://www.cdc.gov/cdiff/index.html

DuPont, H. L. (2012). Approach to the patient with infectious colitis. *Current Opinion in Gastroenterology, 28*, 39–46. https://doi.org/10.1097/MOG.0b013e32834d3208

Hodges, K., & Ravinder, G. (2010). Infectious diarrhea: Cellular and molecular mechanisms. *Gut Microbes, 1*(1), 4–21. https://doi.org/10.4161/gmic.1.1.11036

Kelly, C. P., Lamont, J. T., & Bakken, J. S. (2019, March 1). *Clostridioides (formerly clostridium) difficile infection in adults: Treatment and prevention*. In E. L. Baron (Ed.), *UpToDate*. https://www.uptodate.com/contents/clostridioides-formerly-clostridium-difficile-infection-in-adults-treatment-and-prevention

Kim, G. K., & Zhu, N. A. (2017). Community-acquired Clostridium difficile infection. *Canadian Family Practice, 63*, 131–132.

Kim, Y. J., Park, K.-H., Park, D.-A., Park, J., Bang, B. W., Lee, S. S., Lee, E. J., Lee, H.-J., Hong, S. K., & Kim, Y. R. (2019). Guideline for the antibiotic use in acute gastroenteritis. *Infection and Chemotherapy, 51*(2), 217. https://doi.org/10.3947/ic.2019.51.2.217

Mayo Clinic. (n.d.). *Laboratory testing for infectious causes of diarrhea*. https://www.mayocliniclabs.com/~/media/it-mmfiles/special-instructions/Laboratory_Testing_For_Infectious_Causes_of_Diarrhea.pdf

Lamont, J. T. (2018, October 25). *Clostridioides (formerly clostridium) difficile infection in adults: Clinical manifestations and diagnosis*. In E. L. Baron (Ed.), *UpToDate*. https://www.uptodate.com/contents/clostridioides-formerly-clostridium-difficile-infection-in-adults-clinical-manifestations-and-diagnosis

Liubakka, A., & Vaughn, B. P. (2016). *Clostridioides difficile* infection and fecal microbiota transplant. *Advanced Critical Care, 27*(3), 324–337. https://doi.org/10.4037/aacnacc2016703

McDonald, L. C., Gerding, D. N., Johnson, S., Bakken, J. S., Carroll, K. C., Coffin, S. E., Dubberke, E. R., Garey, K. W., Gould, C. V., Kelly, C., Loo, V., Sammons, J. S., Sandor, T. J., & Wilcox, M. H. (2018). Clinical practice guidelines for *Clostridioides difficile* in adults and children: 2017 update by the Infectious Disease Society for Healthcare Epidemiology of America (SHEA). *Clinical Infectious Disease, 66*, 987. https://doi.org/10.1093/cid/ciy149

Piccoli, D. A. (2019, January 4). Colitis. In C. Cuffari (Ed.), *Medscape*. http://emedicine.medscape.com/article/927845-overview

Preidis, G. A., Weizman, A. V., Kashyap, P. C., & Morgan, R. L. (2020). AGA technical review on the role of probiotics in the management of gastrointestinal disorders. *Gastroenterology, 159*(2). https://doi.org/10.1053/j.gastro.2020.05.060

Shen, N. T. (2017). Timely use of probiotics in hospitalized adults prevents *Clostridioides difficile* infection: A systematic review with meta-regression analysis. *Gastroenterology, 152*, 1889–1900. https://doi.org/10.1053/j.gastro.2017.02.003

Wedro, B. (2016, June 20). *Colitis*. http://www.emedicinehealth.com/colitis/article_em.htm

COVID-19

Nicole Cavaliere

DEFINITION

A. COVID-19 is an acute respiratory disease caused by the novel coronavirus SARS-CoV-2.
B. Since the first discovery of SARS-CoV-2 infections in December 2019, numerous variants have emerged globally.
C. Initial and early variants included Alpha (2020) and Delta (late 2020–2021).
D. Omicron subvariants have been the predominant strain in the United States beginning in early 2022.

INCIDENCE

A. >97 million cases in the United States from March 2020 to October 2022.
B. Prevalent despite global vaccination efforts and other mitigation strategies (such as facial masks and social distancing).
C. True incidence as of 2022 unknown as many cases are not documented.
D. Severe infections remain more prevalent in the unimmunized population with risk factors.

PATHOGENESIS

A. Single-stranded RNA virus in the genus *Coronavirus* and family Coronaviridae.
B. Structural proteins S (spike), E (envelope), M (membrane), and N (nucleocapsid) are required to make complete virus particle.
C. The S protein on the SARS-CoV-2 virus is responsible for attachment and entry into the target host cell receptor.
D. Transmitted through respiratory droplets. Transmission through fomites is not as prevalent and is consiered low risk. Aerosolization is a possible transmission.
E. Viral shedding by asymptomatic people is a subset of the total infections. Viral titers are in highest concentrations early in the infectious periods, often approximately 1 to 2 days prior to the onset of symptoms.

PREDISPOSING FACTORS

A. Older age, especially >65 years of age.
B. >50 years of age with comorbidities.
C. Comorbidities include cancer, chronic kidney disease, chronic obstructive pulmonary disease (COPD), dementia and other neurologic conditions, diabetes mellitus types 1 and 2, HIV and other immunocompromised individuals, body mass index (BMI) >25, and active tuberculosis.
D. Children and teens <18 years of age at less risk, with exception of those with underlying medical problems.

SUBJECTIVE DATA

A. Common complaints/symptoms.
  1. Common: Fever, cough (dry), and fatigue.
  2. Less common: Pharyngitis, headache, and loss of taste or smell.

3. Serious: Shortness of breath, chest pain, confusion, and cyanosis.
B. Family and social history.
  1. Family history is noncontributory to the acquiescence of this infectious disease.
  2. Patients who are active smokers or with a history of smoking are at higher risk of more severe disease.
  3. Patients living in congregate settings are at higher risk of contracting the disease.
C. Review of systems.
  1. General: Malaise, fever, and shortness of breath.
  2. Head, ear, eyes, nose, and throat (HEENT): Congestion, sore throat, headache, and cough.
  3. Neurologic: Weakness.

PHYSICAL EXAMINATION

A. Many different clinical presentations of COVID-19, particularly based on the variant, are noted. Patients may not exhibit all or any of the following physical examination findings:
  1. Coarse breath sounds, focal wheezing, or rhonchi.
  2. Dyspnea.
  3. Pharyngitis.
  4. Productive and/or nonproductive cough.
  5. Fever, chills, or rigor.
  6. Rhinorrhea.

DIAGNOSTIC TESTS

A. Molecular testing with polymerase chain reaction (PCR) is the gold standard.
  1. High sensitivity but optimal collection techniques via nasal swab are required.
  2. Turnaround time for results is generally 48 to 72 hours.
B. Antigen testing: Detects viral proteins.
  1. Sensitivity not as high as molecular testing (50%–90%).
  2. Quick turnaround time (approximately 15 minutes).
  3. Home antigen testing has increased in popularity and has been accepted by primary care physicians for treatment decisions for those positive for SARS-CoV-2.
C. Serologic testing.
  1. Antibody tests: Assesses N or S protein. Many commercial assays are against the N protein, which will not detect responses to SARS-CoV-2 vaccines.
  2. Overall not recommended due to high rates of false-positives.

DIFFERENTIAL DIAGNOSIS

A. Cannot be distinguished from other causes of viral respiratory infection solely based on clinical presentation.
B. Rule out influenza, respiratory syncytial virus (RSV), and community-acquired pneumonia.
C. For patients who are profoundly hypoxemic, rule out pulmonary embolism, acute myocardial infarction, and chest crisis (such as sickle cell disease).

EVALUATION AND MANAGEMENT PLAN

A. General plan.
   1. Location of care.
      a. Patients with minor symptoms are encouraged to convalesce at home with antiviral and/or supportive over-the-counter (OTC) treatment.
      b. Patients with symptoms that are more severe and life-threatening (such as shortness of breath or hypoxemia) should be treated in the hospital with the appropriate pharmacology treatment and supportive care.
   2. Hospitalization.
      a. Support with non-invasive ventilation (NIV) oxygen, or with intubation and mechanical ventilation if required.
      b. Prone positioning may be employed if there is difficulty with oxygenation despite intubation.
      c. Consider deep vein thrombosis (DVT) prophylaxis for hospitalized patients with increased clotting risk in this subset of patients.
   3. Treat secondary infections.
      a. Evaluate and treat for secondary bacterial or fungal infections.
      b. Evaluate for coinfection with other viral respiratory diseases such as influenza and RSV.
B. Patient/family teaching points.
   1. If not requiring hospitalization, stay home and isolate for a minimum of 5 days.
   2. Mask for 10 to 14 after symptoms appear (longer if patient remains asymptomatic).
   3. Monitor symptoms and seek medical attention if high fever, increasing shortness of breath, or difficulty with oxygenation occurs.
   4. Practice hand hygiene.
C. Pharmacotherapy.
   1. Antivirals (inpatient use only).
      a. Remdesivir.
         i. Intravenous infusion for up to 5 days. U.S. Food and Drug Administration (FDA)-approved for hospitalized patients >12 years of age or 40 kg. Dose: 200 mg IV load on day 1, then 100 mg IV Q24H on days 2 to 5.
         ii. Emergency Use Authorization (EUA) issued for children <12 years of age and weighing 3.5 to 40 kg.
   2. Antivirals (outpatient and inpatient use).
      a. Nirmatrelvir/ritonavir (Paxlovid).
         i. Nirmatrelvir is a SARS-CoV-2 3CLpro protease inhibitor boosted by ritonavir.
         ii. FDA-approved for people >12 years of age with mild to moderate disease outpatient, or inpatients with risk factors for more severe disease.
         iii. Dose: Nirmatrelvir 300 mg (two 150 mg tabs) + ritonavir 100 mg BID PO × 5 days.
         iv. Important to obtain renal and liver serum lab values prior to prescribing and adjust dose as needed.
      b. Molnupiravir.
         i. Ribonucleoside prodrug with activity against coronaviruses.
         ii. FDA-approved for adults (>18 years of age) with mild to moderate COVID-19 with risk factors for severe disease.
         iii. Dose: 800 mg (200 mg caps) PO Q12H × 5 days.
   3. Immunomodulators.
      a. Dexamethasone.
         i. Recommended for patients with severe COVID-19 (requiring oxygen), including those on mechanical ventilation.
         ii. Dosing: Adults and pediatric patient ages 9 and older: 4 mg PO daily × 14 days or until hospital discharge; pediatric patients 2 to 9 years of age: 2 mg PO once daily × 14 days or until hospital discharge.
      b. Tocilizumab.
         i. FDA-approved anti-IL6R (anti-interleukin-6 receptor) monoclonal antibody for CAR-T cell (chimeric antigen receptor T cell) cytokine release syndrome and rheumatoid arthritis.
         ii. National Institutes of Health (NIH) guidelines suggest use in the first 24 hours of ICU care in combination with dexamethasone or with dexamethasone and remdesivir for patients requiring high-flow oxygen.
         iii. Dosing: 8 mg/kg × single dose; can be repeated in 48 hours if no benefit seen.
   4. Antibody-based therapies.
      a. Convalescent plasma.
         i. Serum-containing neutralizing antibodies against SARS-CoV-2.
         ii. Studies with mixed results regarding efficacy. Can be administered inpatient or outpatient.
      b. Monoclonal antibodies (mAb).
         i. Specific to the SARS-CoV-2 spike protein, only offered outpatient in mild to moderate disease.
         ii. After earlier formulations early in the pandemic, the only single mAb on the market approved by FDA is bebtelovimab: Dose 175 mg intravenous (IV) infusion.
   5. Prevention.
      a. Vaccines.
         i. Multiple vaccines worldwide. Three largest distributed in the United States include mRNA vaccines Pfizer/BioNTech (in two doses) and Moderna COVID-19 (in two doses), and adenovirus vaccine JNJ/Janssen (in one dose).
      b. Booster doses have also been approved for waning immunity.

FOLLOW-UP

A. Self-isolation/quarantine for 5 days after the onset of symptoms.
B. Immunity levels vary in individuals based on multiple factors, including severity of disease.
C. Repeated COVID-19 diagnostic tests not warranted after initial positive result, unless for specific purpose (such as travel, procedure, etc.).

▶

CONSULTATION/REFERRAL
A. Primary care provider (PCP) to monitor for long COVID symptoms.
B. May need referral with a pulmonologist following severe disease with postinfection symptoms.

SPECIAL/GERIATRIC CONSIDERATIONS
A. Geriatric population is considered more at risk for more severe disease, particularly those with comorbidities.
B. Masks are recommended in indoor settings for symptomatic or at-risk individuals.

BIBLIOGRAPHY
Auwaerter, P. G. (2022). *Coronavirus COVID-19 (SARS-CoV-2)*. Johns Hopkins Guides. https:hopkinsguides.com/hopkins/view/Johns_Hopkin_HIV_Guide/545303/all/COVID-19

Bhimraj, A., Morgan, R. L., Shumaker, A. H., Lavergne, V., Baden, L., Cheng, V. C.-C., Edwards, K. M., Gandhi, R., Muller, W. J., O'Horo, J. C., Shoham, S., Murad, M. H., Mustafa, R. A., Sultan, S., & Falck-Ytter, Y. (2022). *IDSA guidelines on the treatment and management of patients with COVID-19*. https://www.idsociety.org/practice-guideline/covid-19-guideline-treatment-and-management

NIH. (2022). *COVID-19 treatment guidelines*. https:covid19treatmentguidelines.nih.gov

ENCEPHALITIS

Carey Heck

DEFINITION
A. Inflammation of the brain parenchyma.
B. Viral encephalitis: An acute viral infection of the brain parenchyma characterized by a moderate elevation of white blood cells (WBCs) in the cerebrospinal fluid (CSF) and focal neurologic deficits. These include but are not limited to altered mental status, cognitive impairments, aphasia, hemiparesis, paresthesias, and behavioral changes.
C. Bacterial or fungal encephalitis: Rare.
D. Paraneoplastic and autoimmune encephalitis: Beyond the scope of this text but should be considered in the setting of known history of or concern for cancer and a sterile CSF analysis. Etiology of disease is related to an inflammation of the brain parenchyma secondary to an antibody attack of the neuronal surface cells and/or synaptic proteins.

INCIDENCE
A. Although not as common as bacterial meningitis, encephalitis remains a significant health concern associated with a high rate of morbidity and mortality.
B. Incidence is related to global distribution patterns of viral infections.
C. Global incidence was estimated at 1.4 million cases in 2019, which demonstrated a trend downward over the past 30 years. However, lower socioeconomic regions in South Asia and the Western and eastern sub-Saharan regions of Africa still had the highest rates of encephalitis.

PATHOGENESIS
A. Encephalitis is characterized as an inflammation of the brain parenchyma due to infectious, postinfectious, or noninfectious etiology with symptoms of altered mental status, focal neurologic deficits, and seizures.
B. Viral infection is the most common cause of encephalitis in adults. Herpes simplex virus (HSV) is the leading cause of encephalitis worldwide. HSV is the most common cause of viral encephalitis in the United States accounting for 10% of all cases.
C. In addition to HSV, common causes of infectious encephalitis are varicella herpes zoster virus (VZV), cytomegalovirus (CMV), West Nile virus, influenza, HIV, mumps, rabies, and measles. Also, more than a dozen species of arthropod-borne viruses are known to cause encephalitis.
D. Autoimmune encephalitis.
  1. Anti-N-methyl-D-aspartate receptor (anti-NMDAR), most common form of autoimmune encephalitis.
  2. Anti-NMDAR median age 21 years, with female predominance (4:1).
  3. Associated ovarian teratoma found in up to 58% of younger female patients.
  4. Increasing incidence in younger patients.

PREDISPOSING FACTORS
A. Recent viral illness.
B. Mosquito bites.
C. Tick bites.
D. Exposure to pig, bat, duck, and rodent feces.
E. Rabid animal bites.
F. Travel to areas with known infective vectors.
G. Immunocompromised state.
H. Immunosuppressive therapy.
I. Organ transplantation.

SUBJECTIVE DATA
A. Common complaints/symptoms.
  1. Presentation varies from mild confusion and inappropriate behavior to comatose state.
  2. Affected patients present with cortical findings as viruses gravitate toward the brain parenchyma.
  3. Cortical symptoms include but are not limited to altered mental status, cognitive impairment, aphasias, hemiparesis, paresthesias, and behavioral changes.
  4. Meningeal irritation should not be a symptom. However, it may be seen in patients with meningoencephalitis.
B. Family and social history.
  1. Familial history is often noncontributory.
  2. Social history may reveal recent viral illness and travel abroad, particularly to sub-Saharan Africa, and exposure to rodents, ticks, and mosquitoes.
C. Review of systems.
  1. General: Fatigue, weakness, fever, or chills.
  2. Head, ear, eyes, nose, and throat (HEENT): Headaches.

3. Neurologic: Lethargy, syncope, seizures, muscle weakness, altered sensation, altered speech, or disorientation.

PHYSICAL EXAMINATION

A. Altered mental status: Important distinguishing feature between encephalitis and meningitis. Encephalitis more likely to present with altered mental status.
B. Focal neurologic deficits: Including, but not limited to, cognitive impairments, aphasia, hemiparesis, paresthesias, and behavioral changes.
C. Seizure activity.
D. Nuchal rigidity (unlikely): Including tenderness to palpation and pain with flexion and extension.

DIAGNOSTIC TESTS

A. A noncontrast CT of the head: Required.
  1. Patients will likely have altered mental status, focal neurologic deficits, and new-onset seizures, which raise concern for elevated intracranial pressure; this allows for ruling out a space-occupying lesion.
  2. CT scan of the head with temporal lobe edema that does not follow a vascular pattern is the classic presentation of HSV encephalitis.
B. MRI: Shows demyelination, which may be present in other clinical states with similar presentation.
C. Lumbar puncture: Requisite for all cases of suspected encephalitis unless contraindications are present.
  1. CSF analysis.
    a. Cell count/differential, glucose, protein and Gram stain, and bacterial culture.
    b. Abnormal CSF suggestive of viral encephalitis.
      i. Opening pressure may be elevated.
      ii. CSF WBC count elevated but less than 250 per microliter and lymphocyte dominant.
      iii. CSF red blood cell (RBC) count may be present in HSV encephalitis.
      iv. CSF glucose greater than 60 mg/dL and CSF to serum ratio of greater than 0.6.
      v. CSF protein elevated but less than 150 mg/dL.
      vi. Culture and polymerase chain reaction (PCR) test for virus.
        1) If culture is negative but strong clinical and radiologic suspicion for HSV/VZV encephalitis remains, repeat lumbar puncture in 3 to 5 days and continue treatment.
  2. Contraindications to lumbar puncture.
    a. Systemic anticoagulation.
    b. Thrombocytopenia.
    c. Coagulopathy.
    d. Open sacral wound at L3 to L5 levels.
    e. CT of the head with evidence of increased intracranial pressure and/or mass lesion.
D. EEG: Often abnormal in acute encephalitis.
E. Relevant bloodwork: Complete blood count (CBC), basal metabolic profile (BMP), partial thromboplastin time (PTT)/prothrombin time (PT)/international normalized ratio (INR), lactate, and arterial blood gas.
F. Blood cultures.

DIFFERENTIAL DIAGNOSIS

A. Viral encephalitis.
B. Autoimmune encephalitis
C. Bacterial meningitis.
D. Epidural abscess.
E. Nonconvulsive status epilepticus.
F. Subarachnoid hemorrhage.

EVALUATION AND MANAGEMENT PLAN

A. General plan (viral encephalitis).
  1. Rule out bacterial meningitis due to high risk of morbidity and mortality.
  2. Patient presentation suggestive of central nervous system (CNS) infection.
  3. Follow sepsis guidelines for fluid resuscitation management of septic shock.
  4. Begin broad-spectrum antibiotics as well as antiviral therapy and glucocorticoids if appropriate.
  5. Obtain a "stat" CT of the head without contrast to rule out alternative diagnoses.
  6. Use lumbar puncture with CSF analysis for definitive treatment, and if available meningitis/encephalitis PCR for rapid identification of causative pathogen.
  7. Arrange for hemodynamic management and supportive care.
  8. Admit to ICU for appropriate level of care.
  9. Consider MRI of the brain in patients who fail to improve despite treatment to evaluate alternative diagnoses.
  10. Consider EEG of the brain to evaluate for subclinical seizures in patients with fluctuating neurologic examination or a decreased level of consciousness.
B. Patient/family teaching points.
  1. Worsening neurologic examination may lead to acute respiratory failure requiring intubation and mechanical ventilation.
  2. Seizures may require treatment with antiepileptics. Intubation and mechanical ventilation may be required for patients presenting in status epilepticus.
  3. Evidence of cerebral edema on head CT may prompt aggressive medical management with mannitol and hypertonic saline, including surgical decompression.
  4. Evidence of hydrocephalus on head CT may prompt neurosurgical evaluation and intervention.
  5. Long-term neurologic sequelae are likely with encephalitis.
C. Pharmacotherapy.
  1. Definitive diagnosis of encephalitis: Based on CSF analysis and culture data.
  2. HSV/VZV encephalitis: Acyclovir 10 mg/kg intravenously (IV) Q8H for a duration of 14 to 21 days.
    a. Kidney function should be assessed due to nephrotoxicity of acyclovir.
    b. Poorer patient outcomes associated with a delay of >24 hours in initiation of acyclovir therapy.

3. CMV encephalitis: Ganciclovir 5 mg/kg IV Q12H + foscarnet 60 mg/kg Q8H until symptoms improve.

4. Autoimmune encephalitis.

a. First-line therapy.

i. Methylprednisolone: 1 g daily for 3 to 5 days.

ii. IV immune globulin: 2 g/kg over 5 days (400 mg/kg/d).

iii. Plasma exchange: One session every other day for five to seven cycles.

b. Removal of immunologic trigger (e.g., teratoma).

c. Immunotherapy.

i. Most commonly used with treatment failure with first-line therapy.

ii. Rituximab 375 mg/m² weekly for 4 weeks or 1,000 mg for two doses, 2 weeks apart.

iii. Cyclophosphamide 600 mg/m² to 1,000 mg/m² monthly for 3 to 6 months.

5. HIV encephalitis.

a. Highly active antiretroviral therapy (HAART): Resume or initiate.

b. Patient-specific treatment plan: Refer to infectious disease guidelines for treatment of HIV/AIDS.

6. De-escalation of antimicrobial therapy based on negative cultures or preferably definitive meningitis/encephalitis PCR test.

7. Patients presenting with seizure activity: Prompt initiation of antiepileptics and discontinuation of medications known to reduce seizure potential.

D. Discharge instructions.

1. Patients should be instructed to seek emergency care if they experience signs and symptoms of fever, headache, neck pain, confusion, and muscle weakness.

FOLLOW-UP

A. Patients with neurologic sequelae on discharge are to obtain follow-up with a neurologist.

CONSULTATION/REFERRAL

A. Consider infectious disease consult for atypical pathogens or patients who do not respond to traditional therapy.

B. Consult neurology for patients with neurologic sequelae.

SPECIAL/GERIATRIC CONSIDERATIONS

A. Viral encephalitis in older adult patients may often present with mild confusion, lethargy, and nonspecific neurologic findings. The provider must be vigilant in recognizing patients at high risk for CNS infection and promptly initiate treatment.

B. Prevention strategies (e.g., vaccinations, mosquito control) should be emphasized as treatment options are limited.

CASE SCENARIO: ENCEPHALITIS

A confused, 45-year-old male presents to the ED with his spouse who reports the patient has been increasingly confused over the past 24 hours. Further questioning reveals the patient has had a low-grade fever for 2 days with "flu-like" symptoms. There is no history of recent travel or exposure to other ill individuals. The patient has no significant medical or surgical history. Physical examination reveals no focal neurologic signs or pupillary abnormalities. Laboratory results are within expected values and urine toxicology screen is negative. While at the ED, the patient has a generalized seizure lasting 2 minutes, which resolves spontaneously.

1. Which of the following tests should the advanced practice provider order initially for this patient?
A. Lumbar puncture (LP)
B. Noncontrast head CT
C. MRI
D. PET

2. Based on the suspected diagnosis, the advanced practice provider knows which of the following statements is correct?
A. An emergent consult to neurosurgery for decompressive hemicraniectomy is indicated.
B. Intravenous acyclovir should be initiated only when polymerase chain reaction (PCR) results are available.
C. Broad-spectrum antibiotics plus acyclovir should be started once cerebrospinal fluid (CSF) results are obtained.
D. The patient should be placed in contact isolation to reduce infection risk.

BIBLIOGRAPHY

Abboud, H., Probasco, J. C., Irani, S., ANces, B., Benavides, D. R., Bradshaw, M., Christo, P.C., Dale, C. R., Gernandez-Fournier, M., Flanagan, E. P., Gadoth, A., Geroge, P., Grebenciucova, E., Jammoul, A., Lee, S. T., Li, Y., Matiello, M., Morse, A. M., Rae-Grant, A., . . . Titulaer, M. J. (2021). Autoimmune encephalitis: proposed best practice recommendations for diagnosis and acute management. *Journal of Neurology, Neurosurgery and Psychiatry, 92*(7), 757–768. https://doi.org/10.1136/jnnp-2020-325300

Dalmau, J., & Rosenfeld, M. R. (2018, December 10). *Paraneoplastic and autoimmune encephalitis.* In A. F. Eichler (Ed.), *UpToDate.* https://www.uptodate.com/contents/paraneoplastic-and-autoimmune-encephalitis

Evans, L., Rhodes, A., Alhazzani, W., Antonelli, M., Coopersmith, C. M., French, C., Machado, F.R., Mcintyre, L., Ostermann, M.;., Prescott, H. C., Schorr, C., Simpson, S., Wiersinga, W. J., Alshamsi, F., Angus, D. C., Arabi, Y., Azevedo, L., Beale, R., Beilman, G. … Levy, M. (2021). Surviving sepsis campaign: International guidelines for management of sepsis and septic shock 2021. *Critical Care Medicine, 49*(11), e1063–e1143. https://doi.org/10.1097/CCM.0000000000005337

Shin, Y.-W., Lee, S.-T., Park, K.-I., Jung, K.-H., Jung, K.-Y Sang, S. K, & Chu, K. (2018). Treatment strategies for autoimmune encephalitis. *Therapeutic Advances in Neurological Disorders, 11*, 1–19. https://doi.org/10.1177/1756285617722347

Tyler, K. L. (2018). Acute viral encephalitis. *New England Journal of Medicine, 379*, 557–566. https://doi.org/10.1056/NEJMra1708714

Wang, H., Zhao, S., Wang, S., Zheng, Y., Wang, S., Chen, H., Pang, J., Ma, J., Yang, X., & Chen, Y. (2022). Global magnitude of encephalitis burden and its evolving pattern over the past 30 years. *Journal of Infection, 84*(6), 777–787. https://doi.org/10.1016/j.jinf.2022.04.026

ENDOCARDITIS: INFECTIVE

Nicole Cavaliere

DEFINITION

A. Microbial infection involving the endothelial surface of the heart which may be located in the heart valves (most common), at a ventricular septal defect (VSD) or atrial septal defect (ASD), in the chordae tendineae, or damaged mural endocardium.
B. Characterized by presence of vegetations composed of microorganisms, inflammatory cells, and platelet–fibrin deposits.
C. Classification of infective endocarditis (IE) may be based on the type of presentation, underlying valvular characteristics, and predisposing factors.
D. Acute endocarditis.
  1. Rapid damage to cardiac structures with extracardiac seeding; fulminant illness can develop in days to 2 weeks.
  2. If untreated, can lead to death within weeks.
E. Subacute endocarditis.
  1. Indolent course.
  2. Slow and progressive damage to cardiac structures.
  3. Gradually progressive unless associated with embolic event or ruptured mycotic aneurysm.
F. Short incubation period (<6 weeks) and long incubation period (>6 weeks) are preferred classifications.
G. Heart side used for classification.
  1. Right-sided: Generally from intravenous (IV) drug use.
  2. Left-sided: More common in IV drug use and nondrug users.

INCIDENCE

A. 1.4 to 6.2 cases per 100,000 patients.
B. Life-threatening infection; mortality rates reported anywhere from 14% to 46%.
C. Higher incidence found in the setting of IV drug use, cardiac and vascular prostheses, and nosocomial infections.

PATHOGENESIS

A. Endothelial injury allows either direct infection or the development of a platelet and fibrin thrombus that serves as a site of bacterial attachment.
B. Primary portals of entry include:
  1. Oral cavity.
  2. Skin.
  3. Upper respiratory tract.
  4. Sites of focal infection.
C. Microorganisms adhere to the endothelium, which is often abnormal or damaged. Platelets aggregate at the site.
D. If the organism is resistant to normal bactericidal activity of serum and microbicidal peptides released by platelets, proliferation will occur with formation of microcolonies. Platelet deposition is induced.
E. Tissue factor is elicited from the endothelium and causes a localized procoagulant state.
F. Fibrin deposition occurs. This together with platelet aggregation and microorganism proliferation all generate a vegetation.
  1. Organisms deep within vegetation are metabolically inactive and resistant to antimicrobials.
  2. Surface microorganisms are shed into the bloodstream continuously.
G. Clinical manifestations of IE are a result of cytokine release.
H. Microorganisms associated with IE are dependent on classification (Table 10.1).

PREDISPOSING FACTORS

A. IV drug use predominantly.
B. Advanced age.
C. Degenerative valve disease.
D. Prosthetic valves or other cardiac devices.
E. Chronic rheumatic heart disease (especially in developing countries).
F. Impaired immune system.
G. Hemodialysis.
H. Unrepaired cyanotic congenital heart defect.
I. Poor dental hygiene.
J. Diabetes mellitus.

TABLE 10.1 CLASSIFICATION OF MICROORGANISMS ASSOCIATED WITH INFECTIVE ENDOCARDITIS

	Native Valve Endocarditis		Prosthetic Valve Endocarditis: Time of Onset Related to Valve Surgery in Months			Implantable Cardiac Device	Intravenous Drug Use
	Hospital-acquired	Community-acquired	<2	2–12	>12		
Organism	Staphylococcus aureus, enterococci, streptococci	Streptococci, S. aureus, enterococci	Coagulase-negative staphylococci, S. aureus	Coagulase-negative staphylococci, S. aureus, enterococci	Streptococci, S. aureus, enterococci, coagulase-negative staphylococci	S. aureus, coagulase-negative staphylococci	S. aureus, streptococci

Sources: From Brusch, J. L. (2007). Infective endocarditis and its mimics in the critical care unit. In B. A. Cunha (Ed.), *Infectious diseases in critical care* (2nd ed., pp. 261–262). Informa Healthcare; Thuny, F., Grisoli, D., Collart, F., Habib, G., & Raoult, D. (2012). Management of infective endocarditis: Challenges and perspectives. *Lancet, 379*(9819), 965–975. https://doi.org/10.1016/S0140-6736(11)60755-1.

SUBJECTIVE DATA

A. Common complaints/symptoms.
    1. Flu-like symptoms, including fever and chills.
    2. Night sweats.
    3. Anorexia and weight loss.
    4. Chest pain with breathing.
    5. Shortness of breath.
B. Common/typical scenario.
    1. Depends on the type of IE, location, and patient risk factors.
    2. Fever: Common in most types of IE.
    3. Physical examination findings: Can vary based on location of lesion. New heart murmur often detected.
    4. Need to identify if there has been a recent surgery or illness.
C. Family and social history.
    1. IV drug use.
    2. Predisposing factors (see above).
D. Review of systems.
    1. General: Malaise, chills, or sweats.
    2. Cardiovascular: Recent surgery, dyspnea, or chest pain or pressure.
    3. Respiratory: Dyspnea or cough.
    4. Skin: Discoloration of fingers and toes, pain in fingers and toes, or cutaneous lesions.
    5. Musculoskeletal: Generalized musculoskeletal pain.
    6. Neurologic: Vision changes or headache.
    7. With arterial emboli, review of systems (ROS) can include:
        a. Flank pain.
        b. Hematuria.
        c. Abdominal pain.

PHYSICAL EXAMINATION

A. Cardiac manifestations.
    1. New regurgitant cardiac murmurs (85% of cases): Indicates valve involvement.
    2. S3 heart sound (with heart failure).
B. Noncardiac manifestations.
    1. Janeway lesions: Red spots on the palms of hands or soles of feet.
    2. Osler nodes: Red tender spots under the skin of fingers or toes.
    3. Subungual hemorrhage.
    4. Discoloration of skin, distal phalanges, or extremities (especially with arterial occlusion from emboli).
    5. Roth spots: Conjunctival hemorrhage.
    6. Petechiae.

DIAGNOSTIC TESTS

A. Blood cultures.
    1. Minimum of two sets of blood cultures.
    2. Peripheral venipuncture, different sites.
    3. Drawn at least 1 hour apart. Ideal for 24 hours apart.
B. Other cultures.
    1. Serologic testing for organisms difficult to identify by blood culture alone (e.g., *Bartonella*, *Legionella*).

    2. At time of surgery, detection of pathogens from valve tissue by polymerase chain reaction (PCR) is validated.
C. Other tests.
    1. Complete blood count (CBC) with differential: Evaluate for leukocytosis, thrombocytopenia, and anemia.
    2. Complete metabolic panel: Blood urea nitrogen (BUN) and creatinine to evaluate for immune complex.
    3. Erythrocyte sedimentation rate (ESR), C-reactive protein (CRP), and procalcitonin (PCT): Usually elevated in IE.
    4. Chest radiograph: May demonstrate pulmonary edema (heart failure).
    5. EKG.
        a. With abscess formation, conduction abnormalities such as progressive heart block can occur.
D. Echocardiogram.
    1. Transthoracic echocardiogram (TTE) in all suspected cases less than 12 hours after initial evaluation.
    2. Transesophageal echocardiogram (TEE) in the following circumstances:
        a. Inability to assess valve adequately in TTE.
        b. Suspected IE but negative TTE.
        c. High likelihood for IE: TEE first.
        d. For recurrent IE.
        e. If vegetation is noted.
        f. Clinical suspicion for 3 to 5 days after initial TEE.
E. Other imaging modalities.
    1. Coronary CT angiography (chest CT angiography [CTA] coronary).
        a. In those undergoing surgery for IE.
        b. Preoperative screening: Evaluation for central nervous system (CNS) and intra-abdominal lesions.
        c. Limitations.
            i. Radiation exposure.
            ii. Nephrotoxicity associated with contrast dye.
            iii. Lack of sensitivity to evaluate valve lesions.
    2. MRI.
        a. Tool to detect cerebral embolic events (typically silent) and evaluate for mycotic aneurysms.
        b. Not routinely used.
F. Modified Duke criteria for diagnosis.
    1. Based on clinical, laboratory, and echocardiographic findings.
        a. Definite IE.
            i. Two major criteria. *OR*
            ii. One major criterion and three minor criteria. *OR*
            iii. Five minor criteria.
        b. Possible IE.
            i. One major criterion and one minor criterion. *OR*
            ii. Three minor criteria.
        c. Rejected.
            i. Firm alterative diagnosis.
            ii. Resolution of IE syndrome with antibiotic therapy less than 4 days.
            iii. No pathologic evidence of IE at surgery/autopsy with antibiotics less than 4 days.
            iv. Does not meet the previous criteria.

2. Major criteria.

a. Positive blood culture.

i. Typical microorganisms identified on two separate blood cultures.

1) *Viridans streptococci, Streptococcus bovis,* HACEK group (fastidious gram-negative coccobacillary organisms; HACEK stands for *Haemophilus* species, *Aggregatibacter* species, *Cardiobacterium hominis, Eikenella corrodens,* and *Kingella* species), and *Staphylococcus aureus.*

2) Community-acquired enterococci in the absence of a primary focus.

ii. Persistently positive blood culture, consistent with IE.

1) At least two positive cultures of blood samples drawn greater than 12 hours apart or all of three cultures. *OR*

2) A majority of four or more separate cultures of blood (with first and last sample drawn at least 1 hour apart).

iii. Single positive blood culture for *Coxiella burnetii* or antiphase 1 immunoglobulin G (IgG) antibody titer of 1:800 or more.

iv. Evidence of endocardial involvement: Echocardiogram positive for IE.

1) Oscillating intracardiac mass on valve or supporting structures, in the path of regurgitant jets, or on implanted material in the absence of an alternative anatomic explanation.

2) Abscess.

3) New partial dehiscence of prosthetic valve or new valvular regurgitation (worsening or changing or preexisting murmur not sufficient).

3. Minor criteria.

a. Predisposing factors or IV drug use.

b. Fever: Temperature greater than 100.4°F/38°C.

c. Vascular phenomena: Major arterial emboli, septic pulmonary infarcts, mycotic aneurysm, intracranial hemorrhage, conjunctival hemorrhages, and Janeway lesions.

d. Immunologic phenomena: Glomerulonephritis, Osler nodes, Roth spots, and rheumatoid factor.

e. Microbiologic evidence: Positive blood culture but does not meet a major criterion as previously noted or serologic evidence of active infection with organism consistent with IE.

DIFFERENTIAL DIAGNOSIS

A. Bacteremia from other focal infection.

B. Heart failure.

C. Valve dysfunction not associated with IE (e.g., cord rupture).

D. Peripheral arterial disease.

E. Pulmonary embolism.

F. Heart block related to conduction disease.

G. Mesenteric ischemia.

H. Chronic obstructive pulmonary disease (COPD).

I. Leukemia.

EVALUATION AND MANAGEMENT PLAN

A. General plan.

1. Empiric antimicrobial coverage (see "Pharmacotherapy") is warranted if acute IE is suspected.

2. Blood cultures need to be repeated every 24 to 48 hours until negative.

3. Surgical intervention needs to be considered, especially in the patients indicated here. Definitive treatment may not be possible without valve replacement and/or removal of implantable cardiac devices.

a. Indications for surgical intervention.

i. Moderate to severe refractory heart failure due to valve regurgitation.

ii. Partially dehisced and unstable prosthetic valve.

iii. Persistent bacteremia despite optimal antimicrobial therapy.

iv. *S. aureus* prosthetic valve IE with intracardiac complications.

v. Prosthetic valve endocarditis relapse despite optimal antimicrobial therapy.

vi. Ruptured abscess.

vii. Valve obstruction by vegetation.

b. Considerations for surgical intervention.

i. Perivalvular abscess with or without progressive conduction delays.

ii. Large (>10 mm) hypermobile vegetation noted on TTE (known increased risk of embolic events); recommendation increases strength with associated prior embolic events or valvular regurgitation.

iii. Persistent unexplained fever (>10 days) in culture-negative valve endocarditis.

iv. Poorly responsive or relapsed endocarditis associated with highly resistant microorganisms, such as enterococci or *S. aureus.*

B. Patient/family teaching points.

1. Discussion about potential complications and progression of disease.

2. Early therapy warranted; will need adherence to antimicrobial therapy to prevent resistant organisms.

3. Surgical options need to be discussed, especially as they relate to possible removal of implantable cardiac devices.

4. Education regarding need for central line and long-term IV antibiotics, likely at home; or skilled nursing facility (SNF) if IV drug use is a concern.

5. Education around abstinence from IV drugs, if indicated.

C. Pharmacotherapy.

1. Primary goal: To eradicate infection by sterilizing vegetations.

2. Prolonged IV antimicrobial therapy: Required.

3. Empiric antimicrobial therapy: To be initiated when IE is suspected, after initial blood cultures have been drawn.

▶

4. Typical length of parenteral therapy: 4 to 6 weeks.

5. For patients who undergo surgery, intraoperative tissue cultures should be obtained, with antimicrobial coverage narrowed to identified organisms.

6. For IE associated with implantable cardiac device, antimicrobial therapy is instituted but considered adjunct to device removal (if possible).

7. For common antimicrobial coverage based on the identified microorganism (Table 10.2).

D. Discharge instructions.

1. Instructions about IV antibiotics and central line care, if indicated, should be provided.

FOLLOW-UP

A. Follow-up depends on what therapy is initiated and the needed interventions.

1. A visit with the patient's primary care physician should occur within 3 weeks of discharge.

2. If surgical intervention is required, a visit with the surgical team should occur within 1 to 2 weeks of discharge.

3. Depending on the length of antimicrobial therapy and patient factors, a visit with an infectious disease provider should occur within 1 week of planned antimicrobial discontinuation.

TABLE 10.2. ANTIMICROBIAL COVERAGE IN INFECTIOUS ENDOCARDITIS BASED ON CAUSAL MICROORGANISM

Organism	Antibiotic	Duration	Notes
Streptococcus			
	Penicillin G 12–24 million U/24 hr (continuously or in 4–6 divided doses) IV OR ceftriaxone 2 g/24 hr IV OR vancomycin 30 mg/kg/24 hr IV in 2 divided doses PLUS gentamicin 3 mg/kg/24 hr IV (if prosthetic valve) for the first 2 weeks	4–6 wk	For relative penicillin resistance, use higher dose of penicillin G. Vancomycin should be used in patients who cannot tolerate penicillin. If microorganism is susceptible to ceftriaxone, use as first-line agent.
Staphylococcus (most common is Staphylococcus aureus)			
MSSA of native valve (no foreign devices)	Nafcillin, oxacillin 12 g/24 hr IV in 4–6 equally divided doses OR cefazolin 6 g/24 hr IV in 3 divided doses OR vancomycin 30 mg/kg/24 hr IV in 2 divided doses OR daptomycin >8 mg/kg/dose IV	6 wk	Use penicillin if organism is sensitive; dosing is based on sensitivity and renal function; check creatinine kinase.
MRSA of native valve (no foreign devices)	Vancomycin 30 mg/kg/24 hr IV in 2 divided doses	6 wk	
MSSA of prosthetic valve	Nafcillin, oxacillin 12 g/24 hr IV in 6 equally divided doses PLUS gentamicin 3 mg/kg/24 hr IV in 2–3 divided doses (2 wk) PLUS rifampin 900 mg/24 hr PO in 3 divided doses	6–8 wk	Use gentamicin for a 2-week period to determine susceptibility prior to adding rifampin.
MRSA of prosthetic valve	Vancomycin 30 mg/kg/24 hr IV in 2 divided doses PLUS gentamicin 3 mg/kg/24 hr IV in 2–3 divided doses (2 wk) PLUS rifampin 900 mg/24 hr PO in 3 divided doses	6–8 wk	Use gentamicin for a 2-week period to determine susceptibility prior to adding rifampin.
Enterococcus			
	Penicillin G 18–30 million U/24 hr IV continuously OR in 6 divided doses PLUS gentamicin 3 mg/kg/24 hr (IBW) IV in 2–3 divided doses	4–6 wk	
	Ampicillin 2 g IV every 4 hr PLUS gentamicin 3 mg/kg/24 hr (IBW) IV in 2–3 divided doses	4–6 wk	
	Vancomycin 30 mg/kg/24 hr IV in 2 divided doses PLUS gentamicin 3 mg/kg/24 hr (IBW) IV in 2–3 divided doses	4–6 wk	For penicillin-allergic patients
	Ampicillin 2 g IV every 4 hr PLUS ceftriaxone 2 g IV every 12 hr	6 wk	For Enterococcus faecalis strains with high level of resistance (ampicillin + gentamicin preferable)

IBW, ideal body weight; IV, intravenous; MRSA, methicillin-resistant Staphylococcus aureus; MSSA, methicillin-susceptible Staphylococcus aureus.

CONSULTATION/REFERRAL

A. An infectious disease consult should be obtained to determine appropriate antimicrobial therapy as well as needed duration and follow-up.

B. A cardiac surgery consult may be warranted when surgical indications are present.

C. If indicated, a substance abuse/addiction team consult may be needed.

D. For those with persistent bacteremia without surgical options, it is appropriate to consider a palliative care consultation.

SPECIAL/GERIATRIC CONSIDERATIONS

A. Prophylaxis should be targeted at the *Viridans* group of streptococci.

B. Antibiotic prophylaxis should be considered for patients with the following conditions:

　1. Prosthetic cardiac valve or prosthetic material used for cardiac valve repair.

　2. Previous IE.

　3. Congenital heart disease (CHD).

　4. Unrepaired cyanotic CHD including palliative shunts and conduits.

　5. Repaired congenital heart defect with prosthetic material or device within the past 6 months.

　6. Repaired CHD with residual defects at the site or adjacent to the site of a prosthetic patch or device.

　7. Cardiac transplantation recipients with cardiac valvulopathy.

C. Prophylactic antimicrobials should be considered when patients with the conditions listed in B undergo the following procedures:

　1. Dental procedures that involve manipulation of gingival tissue or the periapical region of the teeth or perforation of the oral mucosa.

　2. Invasive procedures of the respiratory tract that involve incision or biopsy of the respiratory mucosa, such as tonsillectomy and adenoidectomy.

　3. Elective cystoscopy or other urinary tract manipulation in those with an enterococcal urinary tract infection or colonization.

D. General treatment principle: Single dose administered prior to procedure (if not administered before, must be given within 2 hours of procedure).

E. Pharmacotherapy.

　1. Standard oral regimen: Amoxicillin 2 g PO, 30 to 60 minutes prior to procedure.

　2. If unable to take oral therapy: Ampicillin 2 g IV, 30 to 60 minutes prior to procedure.

　3. Penicillin allergy: Cephalexin 2 g PO *OR* clindamycin 600 mg PO *OR* azithromycin 500 mg PO, 30 to 60 minutes prior to procedure.

BIBLIOGRAPHY

Brusch, J. L. (2007). Infective endocarditis and its mimics in the critical care unit. In B. A. Cunha (Ed.), *Infectious diseases in critical care* (2nd ed., pp. 261–262). Informa Healthcare.

Cahill, T. J., Baddour, L. M., Habib, G., Hoen, B., Salaun, E., Pettersson, G. B., Schäfers, H. J., & Prendergast, B. D. (2017, January). Challenges in infective endocarditis. *Journal of the American College of Cardiology, 69*(3), 325–344. https://doi.org/10.1016/j.jacc.2016.10.066

Cuculich, P. S., & Kates, A. M. (2014). *Infective endocarditis. The Washington manual subspecialty consult series, cardiology* (3rd ed., pp. 251–264). Wolters Kluwer Health.

Karchmer, A. W. (2005). Infective endocarditis. In R. O. Bonow, D. L. Mann, D. P. Zipes, & P. Libby (Eds.), *Braunwald's heart disease: A textbook of cardiovascular medicine* (7th ed., pp. 1633–1658). WB Saunders.

Slipczuk, L., Codolosa, J. N., Davila, C. D., Romero-Corral, A., Yun, J., Pressman, G. S., & Figueredo, V. M. (2013). Infective endocarditis epidemiology over five decades: A systematic review. *PLOS ONE, 8*(12), e82665. https://doi.org/10.1371/journal.pone.0082665

Thuny, F., Grisoli, D., Collart, F., Habib, G., & Raoult, D. (2012, March 10). Management of infective endocarditis: Challenges and perspectives. *Lancet, 379*(9819), 965–975. https://doi.org/10.1016/S0140-6736(11)60755-1

INFLUENZA

David J. Bergamo

DEFINITION

A. An acute respiratory illness caused by the orthomyxovirus, influenza.

INCIDENCE

A. 3 to 5 million severe cases and 250,000 to 500,000 deaths annually worldwide.

B. Annually, between 2010 and 2020, in the United States.

　1. Between 9.2 and 41 million related illnesses.

　2. Hospitalization rate between 140,000 and 710,000.

　3. Death rates range between 12,000 and 52,000.

PATHOGENESIS

A. A single-stranded RNA virus attaches to the epithelial cells in the respiratory tract and replicates inside. Ongoing destruction and eradication of these cells occurs.

B. Infectious particles are released through "budding" from the plasma membrane, causing rapid invasion of neighboring cells in a cyclical process.

PREDISPOSING FACTORS

A. All individuals are at risk. Influenza vaccination can decrease risk and severity; however, this efficacy changes annually, pending vaccination and seasonal strain matching.

B. Those at higher risk for complications include children younger than 5 years of age, adults older than 65 years old, pregnant women, long-term care facility residents, Alaskan Natives, and American Indians.

C. Other high-risk groups include patients with underlying neurologic, cardiac, or pulmonary conditions; immunosuppressed individuals (with conditions such as hypogammaglobulinemia, HIV, or cancer); obese patients; and those with other significant comorbid conditions.

SUBJECTIVE DATA

A. Common complaints/symptoms.

　1. Fever.

　2. Diffuse myalgias.

　3. Fatigue.

　4. Cough and respiratory symptoms, including rhinorrhea and sore throat.

5. Headache.

6. Gastroenteritis symptoms (abdominal pain, nausea, vomiting, diarrhea).

B. Common/typical scenario.

1. Symptoms: Abrupt in onset; some patients may remember exact time.

2. Abrupt onset of fever with myalgia and/or headache and respiratory symptoms during influenza season (late fall to early spring): High likelihood for influenza.

C. Family and social history.

1. Positive comorbid conditions or hereditary immunodeficiencies.

2. Recent exposure to individuals with symptoms of influenza: Symptoms generally appear 2 days after exposure (airborne, touching contaminated surfaces).

3. Crowded environments.

D. Review of systems.

1. General: Fever, fatigue, and malaise.

2. Neuro: Headache, anorexia, dizziness, or weakness.

3. Gastrointestinal (GI) symptoms: Uncommon in adults, but are more prominent with certain strains (tends to be seasonal).

4. Respiratory: Nonproductive cough (productive cough is more common in pneumonia).

5. Head, ear, eyes, nose, and throat (HEENT): Runny nose and sore throat.

PHYSICAL EXAMINATION

A. Relatively benign, with nonspecific findings.

B. Constitutional: Ill-appearing and fatigued.

C. Fever: Usually 100°F to 104°F (37.7°C–40°C); rarely much higher other than in complicated cases.

D. Possible hyperemia or cervical lymphadenopathy (more common in younger patients).

E. Mild tachycardia from hypoxia, dehydration, and fever.

F. Pharyngitis.

G. Conjunctivitis.

H. Pulmonary findings: Possibly dry cough, focal wheezing, or rhonchi, but many have normal pulmonary exam.

I. Skin: May appear flushed, warm to hot, with diaphoresis depending on the core body temperature.

DIAGNOSTIC TESTS

A. Clinical diagnosis in patients with influenza symptoms during influenza season or during outbreaks. The combination of fever with cough, sore throat, and myalgia can improve diagnostic accuracy. In periods of outbreak, patients with combinations of any of these symptoms may be reasonably treated with neuraminidase inhibitors without testing.

B. Rapid influenza tests.

1. Polymerase chain reaction (PCR): Most sensitive and specific and can differentiate subtypes.

2. Rapid antigen tests: Result obtained in 15 minutes; less sensitive.

3. Gold standard: Viral culture; may take 72 hours to obtain results.

C. In the acute care setting, consider not testing if it will not change management.

1. Influenza treatment should begin within 48 hours of symptom onset; if symptoms greater than 48 hours, there may not be benefit.

2. If mild symptoms, treatment is generally supportive and may not require targeted treatment.

DIFFERENTIAL DIAGNOSIS

A. HIV.

B. Pneumonia.

C. Cytomegalovirus (CMV).

D. Legionnaires disease.

E. Hantavirus pulmonary disease.

F. Acute respiratory distress syndrome (ARDS).

G. Other viral upper respiratory infections (URIs).

H. Coronavirus (COVID-19).

I. Tick- and mosquito-borne illnesses.

1. However, these tend to present in different seasons or patients have exposure history or travel history.

EVALUATION AND MANAGEMENT PLAN

A. General plan.

1. Usually self-limited; duration can be shortened with use of neuraminidase inhibitors.

a. Therapy has the greatest benefit when given within 30 hours of symptom development, but can typically be started within 48 hours of symptom onset.

2. Airborne isolation.

3. Supportive care.

B. Patient/family teaching points.

1. Handwashing is key to help prevent spread.

2. Annual influenza vaccines for all those who can receive them (most individuals older than 6 months).

a. Consider quadrivalent in those with underlying comorbidities and older adults.

C. Pharmacotherapy.

1. Neuraminidase inhibitors.

a. Oseltamivir (Tamiflu).

i. Most commonly used agent; can cause nausea and vomiting.

ii. Treatment: 75 mg BID for 5 days, starting within 48 hours of symptom onset.

iii. Prophylaxis: 75 mg daily for 10 days within 48 hours of contact with infected person.

b. Zanamivir (Relenza).

i. Inhaled agent that should not be used in patients with pulmonary disease.

ii. Should be avoided in lactose-intolerant patients (powder mixture contains lactose/milk proteins).

c. Peramivir (Rapivab).

i. Intravenous (IV) formulation for those who cannot use oral route.

ii. Treatment: 600 mg IV one dose.

d. Laninamivir.

i. Still under development: Nasal spray.

e. All neuraminidase inhibitors: Can cause neuropsychiatric effects based on their mechanism of action. Less commonly, they may cause skin reactions, including erythema multiforme or Stevens–Johnson syndrome.

f. Adamantane antivirals (amantadine and rimantadine).

i. Target M2 protein of influenza A and therefore not active against influenza B; little to no activity against current influenza A strains.

ii. Amantadine and rimantadine not currently recommended for treatment of influenza A due to high levels of resistance among many circulating strains of influenza.

iii. Amantadine and rimantadine are safe in children older than 1 year of age.

g. Ribavirin.

i. Nucleoside analog active against influenza A and B.

ii. Not Food and Drug Administration (FDA)-approved; rarely used except with consultation of infectious disease specialists via inhaled route.

2. Endonuclease Inhibitors.

a. Baloxavir marboxil (Xofluza).

i. Influenza treatment 40 to <80 kg: 40 mg as a single dose within 48 hours of onset of influenza symptoms.

ii. 80 kg: 80 mg as a single dose within 48 hours of onset of influenza.

3. Tamiflu and Xofluza are the most commonly used therapies, are easy to take, are well-tolerated, and have a generally favorable side effect profile.

FOLLOW-UP

A. Follow-up other than regular visits with primary care physician is usually not required.

CONSULTATION/REFERRAL

A. If hospitalized, consider consultation with infectious disease and pulmonary specialists.

B. If illness is significant, a critical care specialist may be required.

C. In general, influenza tends to be an outpatient illness cared for by primary care and urgent care providers.

SPECIAL/GERIATRIC CONSIDERATIONS

A. Annual influenza vaccination is indicated in all patients who are at least 6 months of age *except*:

1. Patients who have had a severe allergic reaction to prior influenza vaccine (this does not include minor flu-like symptoms).

2. Those with a severe allergic reaction to egg proteins if receiving the live attenuated vaccine (nasal).

B. Immunocompromised patients, pregnant women, and patients 50 years of age or older should *not* receive live attenuated vaccine.

C. Adults under the age of 65 with no significant comorbidities generally have self-limiting disease.

D. Children younger than 5 years of age, but especially under 2 years, are at higher risk of influenza complications.

E. Patients older than 65 years have an increased risk of developing complications.

F. Consider Fluzone (high-dose quadrivalent) vaccine for those in high-risk categories for complications and those over the age of 65.

CASE SCENARIO: INFLUENZA

A 55-year-old female patient presents to the clinic in February complaining of 3 days of rhinorrhea, myalgias, and cough. She states that she had sudden onset of myalgias and a fever of 102.4°F/39.1°C when her symptoms first started but is feeling a little better. She is up-to-date on her vaccinations, but states she had a reaction to the flu shot as a kid, which she describes as muscle aches and fatigue for a couple days. On presentation, she appears nontoxic but tired. Her vitals show heart rate (HR) of 84, respiratory rate (RR) of 14, oxygen saturation of 97%, and blood pressure (BP) of 136/84. Her physical exam is unremarkable with the exception of bilateral expiratory wheezing in the upper lung fields. At the end of the exam, she remarks that she recently broke up with her boyfriend and has been back on the dating scene. She asks if she should tell her last few partners that she has the flu if her rapid test comes back positive.

1. Would you recommend testing the patient for influenza based on your management for the current condition?

A. Yes, I would consider giving her treatment if her rapid flu swab is positive and she is compliant.

B. Yes, I think she is acutely ill and would benefit from therapy that will reduce the duration of her symptoms.

C. No, her symptoms are not consistent with acute influenza and I would not treat her with targeted influenza treatments.

D. No, she is presenting too late to place her on the recommended therapies for influenza and a positive test would not change my targeted therapy.

2. Would you recommend treatment for this patient with Tamiflu or Xofluza?

A. Yes, Tamiflu, because it has been on the market longer and I have seen better results with this drug.

B. Yes, Xofluza, because I am concerned about her compliance and a single dose is always better.

C. Yes, both Tamiflu and Xofluza in combination to help reduce her fever at a rapid rate.

D. No, she is outside of the recommended window to begin antivirals for influenza.

3. Would you recommend she get the flu shot next year?

A. Yes, her reported symptoms of adverse reaction are mild and do not represent a medical contraindication to influenza vaccination.

B. Yes, everyone should get their flu shot no matter their prior reaction.

C. No, her myalgias may represent a precursor to myasthenia gravis and it should be avoided indefinitely.

D. No, the flu shot does not convey any degree of protection to those over the age of 50.

4. Given her current symptoms and past exposures, what other testing considerations should be considered when caring for this patient?

A. Cytomegalovirus (CMV) testing should be considered since she falls into a high-risk category of immunosuppression having been sick for 3 days.

B. She may have acute seroconversion given her recent multiple partners and should be tested for HIV based on her social history inquiry.

C. A stat respiratory panel should be ordered due to her current symptoms and hospital admission should be considered for further workup and intravenous (IV) antibiotics.

D. She should have West Nile testing and follow-up with an infectious disease specialist since she had high fever and myalgias.

BIBLIOGRAPHY

Centers for Disease Control and Prevention. (2022). *National and state healthcare associated infections progress report.* http://www.cdc.gov/HAI/pdfs/progress-report/hai-progress-report.pdf

Centers for Disease Control and Prevention. (2022, February 24). *Disease burden of influenza.* https://www.cdc.gov/flu/about/disease/burden.htm

Colfax, G. N., Buchbinder, S. P., Cornelisse, P. G., Vittinghoff, E., Mayer, K., & Celum, C. (2002, July 26). Conniee sexual risk behaviors and implications for secondary HIV transmission during and after HIV seroconversion. *AIDS, 16*(11), 1529–1535.

Hibberd, P. (n.d.). Seasonal influenza vaccination in adults. *UpToDate.* https://www.uptodate.com/contents/seasonal-influenza-vaccination-in-adults?search=flu+vaccine&source=search_result&selectedTitle=2~142&usage_type=default&display_rank=1

Longo, D., Fauci, A., Kasper, D., Hauser, S., Jameson, J., & Loscalzo, J (Eds.). (2015). *Harrison's principles of internal medicine* (19th ed.). McGraw Hill.

Zachary, K. (n.d.). Seasonal influenza in adults: Treatment. *UpToDate.* https://www.uptodate.com/contents/seasonal-influenza-in-adults-treatment?search=flu+treatment&source=search_result&selectedTitle=1~150&usage_type=default&display_rank=1

MENINGITIS

Carey Heck

DEFINITION

A. Inflammation of the meninges (membranes surrounding the brain and spinal cord).
B. Types of meningitis.
　1. Bacterial meningitis: Acute infection of the meninges and cerebrospinal fluid (CSF) characterized by an elevated number of white blood cells (WBCs) and positive bacterial cultures in the CSF. High rate of morbidity and mortality, especially with delay in treatment.
　2. Viral meningitis: Acute viral infection of the meninges and CSF characterized by a moderate elevation of WBCs in the CSF with negative bacterial cultures. Most common form of meningitis. Course is usually self-limiting and treatment is supportive.
　3. Fungal meningitis: Acute fungal infection of the meninges and CSF characterized by a moderate elevation of WBCs in the CSF, generally with negative bacterial cultures but positive for antibodies of fungal organisms. Like bacterial meningitis, it is associated with significant morbidity and mortality.

4. Aseptic meningitis: Meningeal inflammation not related to an infectious process. Aseptic meningitis is further categorized into three main groups: Systemic diseases including sarcoidosis, Behcet disease, Sjogren syndrome, systemic lupus erythematosus, and granulomatosis with polyangiitis; drug-induced aseptic meningitis, including nonsteroidal anti-inflammatory drugs (NSAIDs), certain antibiotics (sulfamides and penicillins), intravenous (IV) immune globulin, and antiepileptic drugs; and neoplastic meningitis related to solid cancer metastasis or hematologic malignancies.

INCIDENCE
A. Incidence varies by geographic region.
B. Significant reductions in the incidence of meningitis, especially bacterial meningitis, reported in high-income countries with access to vaccinations and healthcare resources. The incidence globally, however, has risen over the past decade, with the highest rates occurring in low-income, densely populated countries without access to healthcare services. Particularly high incidence rates are found in sub-Saharan Africa (often called the "meningitis belt" of Africa).
C. Like bacterial meningitis, fungal meningitis is associated with significant morbidity and mortality.

PATHOGENESIS
A. Pathogens gain entry to the subarachnoid space primarily through the bloodstream, but contiguous entry through paranasal sinuses or neurosurgical sites are also documented. Many pathogens responsible for meningitis, including bacteria, possess surface components that enhance mucosal colonization.
　1. After bacterial colonization, invasion across the epithelium occurs by intra- or intercellular pathways, often mediated by specific adhesions of the bacterial surface.
　2. Following invasion, bacteria survive normal immunologic forces via evasion of the complement system, often due to polysaccharide capsules, and then cross the blood–brain barrier. Complement activation may occur in the CSF, often causing meningeal tissue damage. In the CSF, bacteria can multiply to high concentrations due to the low humoral immunity activity in the CSF. The clinical disease process is due to the interaction of the host inflammatory response and bacterial components once the bacteria enter the CSF.
　3. Once inflammation is present, a series of injuries to the blood–brain barrier epithelium lead to vasogenic brain edema, loss of cerebrovascular regulation, and cerebral hypoperfusion and ischemia, ultimately leading to motor, sensory, or cognitive deficits.
B. Bacterial meningitis: Characterized as a rapidly progressing systemic bacterial illness presenting with fever, headache, and neck stiffness.
C. Cortical brain function: Generally remains intact as brain parenchyma is spared.

D. Types of meningitis and associated causal pathogens.
   1. Bacterial meningitis.
      a. Misdiagnosed, undiagnosed, or untreated bacterial meningitis: Associated with a high rate of morbidity and nearly 100% mortality.
      b. Most common bacterial pathogens: *Streptococcus pneumoniae, Listeria monocytogenes, Neisseria meningitis, Haemophilus influenzae,* and *Staphylococcus aureus.*
         i. Adults: The most common pathogen is *S. pneumoniae.*
         ii. Age older than 60 years and immunocompromised: Highly susceptible to *L. monocytogenes.*
   2. Viral meningitis.
      a. Diagnosis of exclusion given the limited diagnostic tools for isolating individual pathogens.
      b. Most common viral pathogens: Enteroviruses, herpes simplex virus (HSV), varicella herpes zoster virus (VZV), HIV, West Nile virus (WNV).
   3. Fungal meningitis.
      a. Most common fungal pathogens: *Cryptococcus neoformans* and *Coccidioides immitis.*
   4. Aseptic meningitis.
      a. Proposed mechanism of action: Varies depending on the underlying cause.
         i. Systemic diseases: Sarcoidosis and Behcet disease most frequently associated with neurologic manifestations and aseptic meningitis. Treatment generally involves high-dose corticosteroids and immunosuppressive therapy.
         ii. Drug-induced: Difficult to diagnosis; often a delayed diagnosis. CSF: Prognosis is excellent with removal of causative agent.
         iii. Neoplastic meningitis: Incidence increasing due to better control of primary malignancy. Breast, lung, and melanoma are the most common solid tumor cancers associated with neoplastic meningitis. Prognosis is poor.

PREDISPOSING FACTORS

A. Immunocompromised state.
B. Use of immunosuppressive therapy.
C. Organ transplantation.
D. Environmental exposure.
E. Use of intravenous drugs.
F. Lack of immunizations for meningococcus (*Neisseria meningitides*), pneumococcus (*S. pneumoniae*), and *H. influenzae.*
G. Recent brain surgery or trauma (concern for *S. aureus*).
H. Bacterial meningitis is more likely to affect the very young, older adults, and individuals who are immunocompromised.

SUBJECTIVE DATA

A. Common complaints/symptoms.
   1. Severe headache.
   2. Nuchal rigidity: Inability to flex neck forward passively due to increased muscle tone and stiffness; present in 70% of cases of bacterial meningitis.
   3. Hyperthermia/hypothermia.
   4. Altered mental status.
B. Common/typical scenario.
   1. Classic triad of meningitis: Fever, neck stiffness, and headaches.
      a. Found in less than 50% of patients.
      b. However, two out of three symptoms should raise suspicion for meningitis.
   2. Nonspecific symptoms: Altered mental status, lethargy, malaise, nausea, vomiting, diarrhea, photophobia, muscle aches, cough, and sore throat.
C. Family and social history.
   1. Family history: Generally noncontributory.
   2. Social history: Recent illness; travel abroad, particularly sub-Saharan Africa; exposure to rodents, ticks, mosquitos; or individuals residing in close quarters (e.g., students in dormitory housing).
   3. Medication history positive for NSAIDs, certain antibiotics, IV immune globulin, or antiepileptic drugs.
D. Review of systems.
   1. General: Fatigue, weakness, fever, or chills.
   2. Head, ear, eyes, nose, and throat (HEENT): Headaches, neck pain, or neck stiffness.
   3. Neurologic: Lethargy.
   4. Skin: Rash.

PHYSICAL EXAMINATION

A. Nuchal rigidity, including tenderness to palpation and pain with flexion or extension.
B. Kernig test: Pain induced by attempting full extension of the knee while the hip is flexed at 90 degrees. Specificity is high, but sensitivity is limited.
C. Brudzinski test: Passive flexion of the neck induces flexion of the hips. Specificity is high, but sensitivity is limited.
D. Lethargy and suppressed level of consciousness.
E. Focal neurologic deficits, including cranial nerve palsies.
F. Papilledema.
G. Petechial or ecchymotic rash. Petechial rash is relatively specific for meningococcal meningitis, which is caused by *N. meningitides.*

DIAGNOSTIC TESTS

A. Lumbar puncture (LP): Requisite for all cases of suspected meningitis unless contraindications are present. Ideally performed prior to or simultaneously with antibiotic administration. Repeat LP is not necessary unless patient is not responding to therapy.
   1. CSF analysis.
      a. Assessment of cell count/differential, glucose, protein Gram stain, and bacterial culture.
      b. Normal CSF.
         i. Normal opening pressure less than 20 mmHg.
         ii. CSF WBC less than 5 per microliter.
         iii. CSF red blood cells (RBCs; absent).
         iv. CSF glucose greater than 60 mg/dL and CSF to serum ratio of greater than 0.6.

v. CSF protein less than 50 mg/dL.

vi. Sterile culture.

c. Abnormal CSF suggestive of bacterial meningitis.

i. Elevated opening pressure.

ii. CSF WBC greater than 1,000 per microliter and neutrophil dominant.

iii. CSF RBC (absent).

iv. CSF glucose less than 40 mg/dL and CSF to serum ratio of less than 0.4.

v. CSF protein greater than 200 mg/dL.

vi. Culture results in a positive growth for bacterial organism.

d. Abnormal CSF suggestive of viral meningitis.

i. Normal or slightly elevated opening pressure.

ii. CSF WBC less than 250 per microliter and lymphocyte dominant.

iii. CSF RBC (absent).

iv. CSF glucose greater than 60 mg/dL.

v. CSF protein less than 150 mg/dL.

vi. Sterile culture.

e. Abnormal CSF suggestive of fungal meningitis (results may be nonspecific).

i. Elevated opening pressure.

ii. CSF WBC less than 500 per microliter and lymphocyte dominant.

iii. CSF RBC (absent).

iv. CSF glucose less than 40 mg/dL and CSF to serum ratio of less than 0.4.

1) Bacteria ingest glucose, causing a decreased level associated with bacterial meningitis.

v. CSF protein greater than 250 mg/dL.

vi. Sterile culture.

1) Proceed with fungal cultures and fungal antibody testing.

f. Abnormal CSF suggestive of aseptic meningitis.

i. Normal or slightly elevated opening pressure.

ii. CSF WBC less than 250 per microliter and initially neutrophil dominant.

iii. CSF RBC (absent).

iv. CSF glucose greater than 60 mg/dL.

v. CSF protein less than 200 mg/dL.

vi. Sterile culture.

g. WBC/RBC adjustment.

i. A false positive WBC elevation: Often noted in a traumatic LP or a patient with subarachnoid bleed.

ii. Acceptable ratio of WBC to RBC should be approximately 1:700.

2. A noncontrast CT of the head: Required for certain patients prior to LP.

a. Those who present with signs and symptoms concerning for elevated increased intracranial pressure (ICP), altered level of consciousness, new-onset seizures, or focal neurologic deficits.

b. Those with immunocompromised status.

c. Those with a history of central nervous system (CNS) infection, trauma, stroke, cancer, and surgery.

3. Relative contraindications to LP.

a. Systemic anticoagulation.

b. Thrombocytopenia.

c. Coagulopathy.

d. Open sacral wound at the L3 to L5 levels.

e. CT of the head with evidence of increased ICP and/or mass lesion.

B. Laboratory tests.

1. Relevant bloodwork including complete blood count (CBC), basal metabolic profile (BMP), partial thromboplastin time (PTT)/prothrombin time (PT)/international normalized ratio (INR), lactate, and arterial blood gas.

2. Blood cultures.

DIFFERENTIAL DIAGNOSIS

A. Viral encephalitis.

B. Epidural abscess.

C. Nonconvulsive status epilepticus.

D. Subarachnoid hemorrhage.

E. Meningeal tear or CSF leak.

EVALUATION AND MANAGEMENT PLAN

A. General plan.

1. Bacterial meningitis.

a. Blood cultures.

b. Broad-spectrum antibiotic therapy and glucocorticoids

c. Administration of antivirals if there is concern for encephalitis.

d. Obtain "stat" CT of the head if there is altered mental status, focal neurologic deficit, immunocompromised status, or new-onset seizures.

e. LP (ideally performed prior to or simultaneously with antibiotic administration) with CSF fluid analysis for definitive treatment, including meningitis/encephalitis PCR for rapid identification of causative pathogen if available.

f. Continued hemodynamic management and supportive care.

g. MRI of the brain should be considered if the patient fails to improve despite appropriate therapy.

2. Viral meningitis.

a. Spinal fluid suggestive of viral meningitis.

b. De-escalation of antibiotic therapy.

c. Supportive treatment, including but not limited to:

i. Rest.

ii. Fluid resuscitation.

iii. Antipyretics and analgesics as needed.

3. Fungal meningitis.

a. Spinal fluid analysis is likely to be abnormal but may be nonspecific, sending CSF for fungal cultures, and fungal antibody testing.

b. Addition of antifungal medication to antibiotic therapy for bacterial meningitis.

c. Supportive treatment as previously noted.

4. Aseptic meningitis.

a. Treatment as previously noted pending results of LP.

b. De-escalation of antibiotic and antiviral therapy.

c. Treatment of underlying disease (systemic disease with meningeal involvement or neoplastic meningitis) or removal of causative agent (drug-induced meningitis).

d. Supportive treatment.

B. Patient/family teaching points.

1. Worsening neurologic examination may lead to acute respiratory failure requiring intubation and mechanical ventilation.

2. Seizures may require treatment with antiepileptics and, in severe cases, intubation and mechanical ventilation for airway protection.

3. Evidence of cerebral edema on head CT may prompt aggressive medical management with mannitol and hypertonic saline, as well as surgical decompression. Cerebral edema more commonly present in encephalitis rather than meningitis.

4. Evidence of hydrocephalus on head CT may prompt neurosurgical evaluation and intervention.

5. Neurologic sequelae including hearing loss and visual symptoms are very likely post recovery in bacterial meningitis.

6. Public health strategies remain an important element in the prevention and spread of meningitis. Education of parents on the importance of childhood vaccinations is essential. Routine follow-up and review of adult vaccine schedules with patients, especially the pneumococcal vaccine, are recommended.

C. Pharmacotherapy.

1. Treatment is based on specific organism, patient age, and community resistance patterns. Initiation of therapy should begin promptly (within 1 hour of presentation) to avoid associated morbidity and mortality with delay in treatment.

a. Adults: Dexamethasone + ceftriaxone or cefotaxime + vancomycin.

b. Older adults: Dexamethasone + ceftriaxone or cefotaxime + vancomycin + ampicillin.

c. Neurosurgical procedure, shunt infection, head trauma: Vancomycin + antipseudomonal agent.

2. Dexamethasone 10 mg IV Q6H (prior to initiation of antibiotics if able).

a. Evidence is inconclusive, but limited studies demonstrate that the use of dexamethasone correlated with a decrease in mortality and a reduction in hearing loss in adult patients with *S. pneumoniae* meningitis and infants and children with *H. influenzae type B meningitis*.

b. Since the etiology is not known until CSF results are returned, the current recommendation in patients older than 6 weeks with suspected bacterial meningitis is to administer dexamethasone before or with the initial antibiotic dose.

3. Ceftriaxone 2 g IV Q12H (*N. meningitidis, H. influenzae*).

a. Lactam allergy: Substitute with chloramphenicol 50 to 100 mg/kg/d IV divided Q6H.

b. Has good meningeal coverage.

4. Vancomycin 20 mg/kg IV Q12H (*S. pneumoniae*).

5. Ampicillin 2 g IV Q6H (if suspicious for *Listeria monocytogenes*).

a. B-lactam allergy: Substitute with trimethoprim-sulfamethoxazole 5 mg/kg IV Q6H.

6. Acyclovir 10 mg/kg IV Q8H (if suspicious for HSV encephalitis).

7. Imipenem 1 g IV Q6H (if trauma or neurosurgical manipulation).

8. Fluconazole 400 mg IV daily (if suspicious for *C. neoformans* and *C. immitis*). Dosing can be increased to 800 mg to 1,200 mg daily for critically ill patients.

D. Discharge instructions.

1. Instruct patient to seek emergency care if presenting with fever, headache, and stiff neck because this may indicate a worsening infection.

FOLLOW-UP

A. Patients with neurologic sequelae on discharge are encouraged to follow up with a neurologist.

CONSULTATION/REFERRAL

A. Consider an infectious disease consult for patients with atypical pathogens or patients who do not respond to traditional therapy.

SPECIAL/GERIATRIC CONSIDERATIONS

A. Gerontologic patients with a fulminant bacterial meningitis may present with atypical symptoms and deny neck pain or headache. Confusion and lethargy may be the only presenting symptoms.

B. Provider must be vigilant to recognize high-risk patient for CNS infection so that treatment is not delayed.

CASE SCENARIO: MENINGITIS

A previously healthy 70-year-old male patient presents to the ED with complaints of headache, fever, and chills. Physical examination reveals nuchal rigidity, a positive Brudzinski sign, and lethargy. A noncontrast head CT was performed which demonstrated no acute hemorrhage, lesions, or mass effect. A lumbar puncture (LP) was performed. Cerebrospinal fluid (CSF) polymerase chain reaction (PCR) is pending.

1. The advanced practice provider expects which of the following cerebrospinal fluid (CSF) results for the suspected diagnosis?

A. Clear appearance, white blood cell (WBC) <5/mm³ (predominantly lymphocytes), protein 35 mg/dL, glucose 70 mg/dL

B. Clear appearance, WBC 100/mm³ (predominantly lymphocytes), protein 50 mg/dL, glucose 70 mg/dL

C. Turbid appearance, WBC 2,000/mm³ (predominantly neutrophils), protein 250 mg/dL, glucose 20 mg/dL

D. Cloudy appearance, WBC 200/mm³ (predominantly lymphocytes), protein 150 mg/dL, glucose 30 mg/dL

2. Which of the following interventions is indicated initially for this patient?

A. All close contacts should be treated with prophylactic rifampin.

B. Empiric treatment with ceftriaxone and vancomycin should be started.

C. Empiric treatment should include coverage for *Listeria monocytogenes*.

D. Supportive care is the correct treatment for the suspected diagnosis.

BIBLIOGRAPHY

Aksamit, A. J., & Berkowitz, A. L. (2021). Meningitis. *Continuum (Minneap Minn) Neuroinfectious Disease, 27*(4), 836–854. https://oce.ovid.com/9b20ec56-9ae7-4be3-bb60-db4a9349dd30

Mount, H. R., & Boyle, S. D. (2017). Aseptic and bacterial meningitis: Evaluation, Treatment, and Prevention. *American Family Physician, 96*(5), 314–322. https://pubmed.ncbi.nlm.nih.gov/28925647/

Tattevin, P., Tchamgoué, S., Belem, A., Bénézit, F., Pronier, C., & Revest, M. (2019). Aseptic meningitis. *Revue Neurologique, 175*(7–8), 475–480. https://doi.org/10.1016/j.neurol.2019.07.005

Tunkle, A. R. (2018, August 30). *Clinical features and diagnosis of acute bacterial meningitis in adults*. In J. Mitty (Ed.), *UpToDate*. https://www.uptodate.com/contents/clinical-features-and-diagnosis-of-acute-bacterial-meningitis-in-adults

Van de Beek, D., Brouwer, M. C., Koedel, U., & Wall, C. E. (2021). Community-acquired bacterial meningitis. *Lancet, 398*(10306), 1171–1183. https://doi.org/10.1016/S0140-6736(21)00883-7

NECROTIZING FASCIITIS

Catherine Harris

DEFINITION

A. Severe bacterial infection of the fascia (connective tissue that covers and separates the muscles and other internal organs) and overlying subcutaneous fat that causes extensive tissue death.

INCIDENCE

A. Necrotizing fasciitis can occur at any age; however, the mean age is around 50 years.

B. Hospitalizations due to necrotizing fasciitis are gender-neutral.

C. Necrotizing fasciitis occurs randomly and is not linked to similar infections in others.

PATHOGENESIS

A. The most common way of getting necrotizing fasciitis is when the bacteria enter the body through a break in the skin, such as a cut, scrape, burn, insect bite, or puncture wound.

B. The infection spreads along the muscle fascia as a result of its relatively poor blood supply, and muscle tissue may be spared. In addition, overlying tissue can appear unaffected.

C. Necrotizing fasciitis is typically classified based on the microbial source of infection.

  1. Type I: Polymicrobial with aerobic and anaerobic bacteria, such as *Clostridioides, Peptostreptococcus*, and *Bacteroides* species.

  2. Type II: Monomicrobial and generally caused by group A streptococcus (GAS; also known as hemolytic streptococcal gangrene).

PREDISPOSING FACTORS

A. Type I: Certain comorbid conditions.

  1. Diabetes.

  2. Obesity.

  3. Cardiovascular disease.

  4. Peripheral vascular disease.

  5. Liver disease.

  6. Kidney disease.

  7. Cancer.

  8. Other chronic health conditions that weaken the body's immune system.

B. Type II: Risk factors in healthy individuals (no medical history).

  1. Skin injury: Laceration or burn.

  2. Blunt trauma.

  3. Surgery.

  4. Childbirth.

  5. Varicella.

  6. Intravenous (IV) drug use.

SUBJECTIVE DATA

A. Common complaints/symptoms.

  1. Pain: Usually out of proportion to how the area looks; followed by anesthesia (due to thrombosis of small vessels).

  2. Swelling.

  3. Redness.

  4. Fever.

  5. Chills.

  6. Fatigue.

B. Family and social history.

  1. A detailed history is important, as it can suggest the likely cause of the infection.

  2. A careful history, including several factors, should be taken.

   a. Indicate if any trauma occurred at the site.

   b. Onset and duration of symptoms.

   c. Speed at which erythema is spreading.

   d. Existence of any comorbid conditions (medical history).

   e. Any recent swimming in lakes, ponds, or areas of concern.

PHYSICAL EXAMINATION

A. Early on, healthy appearance, but possible rapid progression to ill/septic appearance.

B. Acute tenderness at site of infection.

C. Skin with area of rapidly increasing erythema, bullae, skin necrosis, and/or crepitus; sometimes with dusky or purplish discoloration.

  1. Skin color can change in a few days from red/purple to patchy blue/gray, followed in 3 to 5 days with skin breakdown with bullae with thick pink/purple fluid and frank cutaneous gangrene.

D. Increased warmth and induration at site.

E. Possible crepitus at site.

F. Difficult to palpate muscle groups due to induration, with edema of subcutaneous tissue.

G. If the skin is open, gloved fingers can pass easily between the two layers and may reveal yellowish-green necrotic fascia.

H. If the skin is not open, a scalpel may be needed to open the site.

DIAGNOSTIC TESTS
A. Lab work.
  1. Complete blood count (CBC), basal metabolic profile (BMP), and blood and tissue cultures are necessary.
  2. Lab findings are often nonspecific but may include leukocytosis with a marked left shift; coagulopathy; and elevated creatine kinase (CK), lactate, and creatinine.
B. Imaging: Noncontrast CT and MRI scans (especially in abdominal wall infections).
  1. These can be helpful if gas is identified in the soft tissue and/or fascial planes.
  2. MRI can be overly sensitive.
C. Surgical exploration.
  1. Do *not* delay surgical exploration for results from blood, skin, or wound cultures.
  2. Surgical exploration is the only way to confirm diagnosis. Histopathology of tissue will show extensive tissue damage, including:
    a. Thrombosis of blood vessels.
    b. Abundant bacteria along fascial planes.
    c. Infiltration of acute inflammatory cells.

DIFFERENTIAL DIAGNOSIS
A. Acute epididymitis.
B. Cellulitis.
C. Orchitis.
D. Toxic shock syndrome.
E. Deep vein thrombosis (DVT).
F. Brown recluse spider bite.

EVALUATION AND MANAGEMENT PLAN
A. Surgical emergency. Debridement needs to be done early to minimize tissue loss and possible amputation, and debridement will require review in the operating room every 24 hours.
B. Empiric antibiotics. These should be started immediately. Agents should be broad-based to cover gram-negative and gram-positive organisms and anaerobes. More target-specific antibiotics may be started once tissue cultures and sensitivities are available.
  1. Clindamycin is the antibiotic of choice to cover necrotizing fasciitis for its antitoxin effects.
  2. In addition, the patient requires carbapenems (e.g., imipenem, meropenem, or ertapenem—please note that ertapenem does not cover pseudomonas) or beta-lactamase inhibitor (e.g., piperacillin/tazobactam, ampicillin sodium/sulbactam sodium,

or ticarcillin/clavulanic acid), as well as an agent active against methicillin-resistant *Staphylococcus aureus* (MRSA; e.g., vancomycin, daptomycin, or linezolid).
C. IV fluids: Massive fluids may be necessary due to diffuse capillary leak and hypotension. Also, nutritional support needs to be implemented to help support wound healing.

FOLLOW-UP
A. Repeat imaging of area to make sure there is no lingering infection.
B. Follow up with infectious disease after completion of antibiotics.
C. Follow up with surgery as needed.

CONSULTATION/REFERRAL
A. Consult surgery emergently for surgical intervention.
B. Infectious disease for antibiotic duration.
C. Depending on extent of injury, may need plastic surgery consult for flap.
D. Wound care.

SPECIAL/GERIATRIC CONSIDERATIONS
A. Necrotizing fasciitis is the most frequently overlooked infectious process of the skin in older adults.
B. Skin and soft tissue represent a common site of infection, and it is a recognized focus of sepsis in the older adults.

CASE SCENARIO: NECROTIZING FASCIITIS

A 62-year-old woman presents with a complaint of left hip pain on flexion. She was unable to bear weight on the left leg. The right leg was unaffected. There was no reported trauma or falls and the hip looked unremarkable. Her medical history was also unremarkable aside from seasonal allergies and high cholesterol for which she took no medications. Three weeks ago, the woman had a root canal. Of note, the woman appeared lethargic, pale, and overall not well. Her blood pressure (BP) was 89/50, heart rate (HR) 100 beats per minute, respiratory rate (RR) 20, and temperature 100.4°F/38°C. Within hours, she was found to have a well-demarcated area of redness with palpable subcutaneous crepitus in the surrounding areas. The patient was booked immediately for the operating room.

1. Which of the following is a causal pathogen in necrotizing fasciitis?
  A. *Streptococcus pyogenes* (GAS)
  B. *Ornithodoros moubata*
  C. *Listeria monocytogenes*
  D. *Leishmania infantum*

2. Which of the following is the treatment of choice for necrotizing fasciitis?
  A. No treatment; condition is fatal
  B. 24-hour observation
  C. Immediate surgical debridement
  D. Broad-spectrum antibiotics

BIBLIOGRAPHY

Adachi, S., Takahashi, T., Minami, K., Kurabayashi, H., Inoue, H., Yonekawa, C., Mato, T., Matsumura, T., & Takeshita, K. (2020). Predictors of fatal outcome after severe necrotizing fasciitis; Retrospective analysis in a tertiary hospital for 20 year. *Journal of Orthopaedic Science, 26*(3), 494–499.

Centers for Disease Control and Prevention. (n.d.). *Necrotizing fasciitis: A rare disease, especially for the healthy.* https://www.cdc.gov/features/necrotizingfasciitis

Edlich, R. (2018, October 17). Necrotizing fasciitis workup. In M. S. Bronze (Ed.), *Medscape.* http://emedicine.medscape.com/article/2051157-workup

Ghosh, A., & Johnstone, J. (2013). Necrotizing fasciitis in an immunocompromised elderly woman. *Canadian Journal of Infectious Diseases and Medical Microbiology, 24*(1), 38–39. https://doi.org/10.1155/2013/489587

Goh, T., Goh, L. G., Ang, C. H., & Wong, C. H. (2013). Early diagnosis of necrotizing fasciitis. *British Journal of Surgery, 101*(1), e119–e125. https://doi.org/10.1002/bjs.9371

Lee, C., Kuo, L., Peng, K., Hsu, W., Huang, T., & Chou, Y. (2011). Prognostic factors and monomicrobial necrotizing fasciitis; Gram positive versus gram negative pathogens. *BMC Infectious Diseases, 11*(5). https://doi.org/10.1186/1471-2334-11-5

Misiakos, E. P., Bagias, G., Patapis, P., Sotiropoulos, D., Kanavidis, P., & Machairas, A. (2014). Current concepts in the management of necrotizing fasciitis. *Frontiers in Surgery, 1*, 36. https://doi.org/10.3389/fsurg.2014.00036

Oud, L., & Watkins, P. (2015). Contemporary trends of the epidemiology, clinical characteristics, and resource utilization of necrotizing fasciitis in Texas: A population-based cohort study. *Critical Care Research and Practice, 2015*, 1–9. https://doi.org/10.1155/2015/618067

Southwick, F. S. (2008). *Infectious diseases: A clinical short course* (2nd ed., pp. 268–271). McGraw-Hill Professional Publishing.

OSTEOMYELITIS

Lauren M. Franker

DEFINITION
A. Inflammatory condition of bone secondary to infection; acute or chronic.
B. Classification is based on pathophysiologic mechanism of infection.

INCIDENCE
A. The incidence of osteomyelitis in the United States is largely unknown. The overall incidence rate of occurrence is 21.8 cases per 100,000 person-years. Nonhematogenous osteomyelitis accounts for 80% of infections.

PATHOGENESIS
A. Hematogenous osteomyelitis: Bacteria are seeded into the bone from a bloodstream infection.
 1. In younger adults, often related to trauma or surgery. The most common form is vertebral. May also occur in the sternoclavicular, pelvic, and long bones.
 2. Usually monomicrobial.
B. Nonhematogenous (direct or contiguous) osteomyelitis: Spread from adjacent soft tissues and joints.
 1. Exogenous: Often spread following surgery or trauma with direct inoculation from a contiguous soft tissue infection or chronic open wound.
 2. Most common type of infection in older adults related to joint arthroplasty, lower extremity osteomyelitis related to diabetes mellitus and vascular disease, and osteomyelitis related to decubitus ulceration.
 3. Secondary disease: From diabetes mellitus and vascular insufficiency.
  a. Peripheral vascular disease and poor healing wounds are more likely to lead to bone inflammation.
  b. Patients with diabetic neuropathy are at higher risk of developing osteomyelitis secondary to local spread from diabetic foot infections and unrecognized wounds.
  c. Smoking increases the risk of osteomyelitis from diabetic foot infections and healing fractures.
 4. May be monomicrobial or polymicrobial.
C. Histologic changes.
 1. Infection: Results in bone edema and vascular congestion, leading to small vessel thrombosis.
 2. Medullary and periosteal bloody supply: Compromised. Bone becomes necrotic.
 3. Sequestra: Fragments of dead bone that detach from living bone.
 4. Dead bone: Becomes colonized by a biofilm of bacteria.
D. Microorganisms: Often a function of the location of the osteomyelitis infection.
 1. Most frequent cause of all types of osteomyelitis: *Staphylococcus aureus.*
 2. Hematogenous osteomyelitis: Can occur from aerobic gram-negative rods or from *Pseudomonas aeruginosa* or *Serratia marcescens* in injection drug users.
 3. Nonhematogenous osteomyelitis: *S. aureus* is the most common pathogen in addition to coagulase-negative staphylococci and gram-negative aerobes and anaerobes.
 4. Patients with foreign devices: Coagulase-negative staphylococci.
 5. Polymicrobial diabetic foot infections with decubitus ulcers: May include *Streptococcus* species and *Enterococcus* species.
 6. Less common pathogens associated with clinical conditions: Immunocompromised (*Aspergillus* species, *Mycobacteria tuberculosis, Candida* species), sickle cell disease (*Salmonella* species), HIV infection (*Bartonella henselae*), and tuberculosis (*Mycobacterium tuberculosis*).

SUBJECTIVE DATA
A. Predisposing factors.
 1. Neuropathy.
 2. History of suspicion of intravenous (IV) drug abuse.
 3. Poorly controlled diabetes mellitus.
 4. Peripheral vascular disease.
 5. Chronic or ulcerated wounds.
 6. Sickle cell disease.
 7. History of implanted orthopedic hardware.
 8. History of recent trauma.
B. Common complaints/symptoms.
 1. Hematogenous osteomyelitis.

a. Presents similarly to nonhematogenous disease. Subacute or chronic onset.

b. Patients often have back or neck pain and muscle tenderness, sometimes followed by fever.

2. Nonhematogenous osteomyelitis.

a. Nonspecific symptoms: Pain, edema, erythema, malaise, fever, poor wound healing, drainage from a wound, and tenderness over infected bone.

b. Acute: May present with a more rapid onset of symptoms and more likely to be associated with fever.

c. Chronic: Systemic symptoms not common, presence of fistulous tracts from skin to bone is diagnostics. Long-standing, non-healing ulcers and fractures may also be associated.

C. Family and social history.

1. Medical history: Comorbidities leading to increased risk.

2. Recent surgeries, implants, and so forth.

3. History of diabetes with ulcers.

4. Decubitus ulcers.

5. Peripheral vascular disease.

6. IV drug abuse.

7. Sickle cell disease.

8. Recent trauma.

9. Urinary tract infection (UTI) or pyelonephritis.

D. Review of systems.

1. Constitutional: Possible night sweats, fatigue, malaise, or lethargy.

2. Genitourinary: Signs and symptoms of UTI; loss of bowel or bladder control.

3. Musculoskeletal: Pain, swelling, or redness at site.

4. Skin: Purulent drainage from open wound.

5. Musculoskeletal: Weakness in lower extremities.

PHYSICAL EXAMINATION

A. Erythema, swelling, soft tissue infection, bony tenderness, joint effusion, and decreased range of motion.

B. Chronic wounds/ulcers, tissue necrosis, persistent sinus tract, or exposed bone (ability to probe to bone).

1. Probe to bone test may be useful in lower extremity osteomyelitis owing to vascular insufficiency. Highly suggestive of osteomyelitis.

C. Positive neurologic examination with areas of weakness or sensory loss.

D. Presence of vascular and arterial insufficiency.

DIFFERENTIAL DIAGNOSIS

A. Soft tissue infection.

B. Gout.

C. Charcot arthropathy.

D. Fracture.

E. Malignancy.

F. Bursitis.

G. Osteonecrosis.

H. Sickle cell vaso-occlusive pain crisis.

I. SAPHO syndrome (synovitis, acne, pustulosis, hyperostosis, and osteitis).

DIAGNOSTIC TESTS

A. Laboratory studies.

1. Complete blood cell count.

a. Leukocytosis: Common in acute osteomyelitis but less common in chronic cases.

2. Inflammatory markers: If elevated, can be trended for clinical correlation.

a. Erythrocyte sedimentation rate (ESR).

b. C-reactive protein (CRP): If elevated, often a monitoring parameter of response to antimicrobial therapy.

3. Blood cultures.

B. Imaging studies.

1. Plain film radiography: First-line evaluation for suspected osteomyelitis.

a. Findings can include soft tissue swelling, osteopenia, cortical loss, bony destruction, and periosteal reaction.

b. Used to rule out other bony pathology.

2. Advanced imaging: Often needed to diagnosis following plain film radiography; 50% to 75% of the bone matrix must be destroyed before lytic changes are evident on plain radiographs.

a. Guided by onset of symptoms and patient variables.

3. MRI.

a. High negative predictive value and highly sensitive.

b. Better for early detection when compared with plain radiography.

c. IV contrast media preferred: Useful to distinguish between soft tissue and bone infection and to determine extent of infection. Less useful in areas with surgical hardware due to image distortion.

4. Radionuclide bone skeletal scintigraphy (i.e., three-phase bone scan) combined with CT: May be used if MRI is not possible due to indwelling hardware.

C. Bone biopsy: Diagnostic standard.

1. May be done using open or percutaneous approach, with open being preferable because the sensitivity of percutaneous biopsy is poor.

EVALUATION AND MANAGEMENT PLAN

A. Treatment requires a multifaceted approach that may include antibiotics, surgical intervention, and other modalities.

B. Debridement: Surgical debridement followed by drainage of any associated soft tissue abscess is mainstay of therapy.

1. Surgical debridement: Indicated as part of the initial treatment in the presence of underlying orthopedic hardware and necrotic bone. Removal of hardware may be required.

C. Pharmacotherapy.

1. Antibiotic selection based on cultures identifying causative agent and susceptibilities.

2. In hospitalized patients at risk of methicillin-resistant *Staphylococcus aureus* (MRSA), empiric antibiotic coverage is recommended (nafcillin, oxacillin, or cefazolin).

3. Empiric antimicrobial therapy should target likely pathogens based on acute versus chronic nature of infection, route of infection, and patient risk factors. Most common empiric regimen pending culture data: Vancomycin and a third-generation cephalosporin or beta-lactam/beta-lactamase inhibitor. Combination provides broad gram-positive and gram-negative coverage.

4. When prosthetic joint or spinal implant infections are present, the addition of rifampin to other antibiotics may improve cure rates.

5. Parenteral followed by oral antibiotic therapy is as effective as long-term parenteral therapy. Oral antibiotics have similar cure rates and lower risks and costs compared with parenteral.

6. Parenteral treatment lasts 4 to 6 weeks.

D. Adjunctive therapies: Hyperbaric oxygen therapy.

1. Controversial. Increased oxygen tension has direct antimicrobial effect on anaerobic bacteria. Polymorphonuclear leukocyte killing of organisms is enhanced by increased oxygen tension.

E. Patient/family teaching points.

1. Prolonged duration of antibiotic treatment is necessary.

2. Recurrence is common.

F. Discharge instructions.

1. Complete the course of antibiotics as prescribed.

2. Follow wound care instructions as prescribed.

3. Avoid injury to the area where the infection is located.

4. Report new or worsening symptoms, especially pain, redness, swelling, or drainage in the affected area.

FOLLOW-UP

A. Based on the location of disease and duration of treatment.

CONSULTATION/REFERRAL

A. Orthopedic consult or neurosurgery consult.

B. Interventional radiology consult.

C. Infectious disease consult to determine type and duration of antibiotics.

CASE SCENARIO: OSTEOMYELITIS

A 75-year-old female presents with a 2-day onset of acute low back pain after completing yard work. She denies any radiation to her buttocks. There are no lower extremity paresthesias and no incontinence. She denies any recent fevers, chills, and cough, and no chest pain, palpations, or shortness of breath. Her back pain is worse with range of motion. She has a history of coronary artery disease, diabetes, hypertension, hyperlipidemia, and sleep apnea. Her vital signs include a temperature of 100.9°F/38.2°C, blood pressure (BP) of 110/51, pulse rate of 84 beats per minute, and respiratory rate of 18 breaths per minute. She is awake, alert, and oriented ×3. Her cardiovascular and respiratory examinations are normal. There are no clubbing, cyanosis, or edema in the extremities. Pulses are equal bilaterally and there is no calf tenderness to palpation. The patient does have tenderness to palpation over the mid-lumbar spine. Cranial nerves II to XII are grossly intact. Motor strength is

5/5 in all four extremities. Sensation is intact and she can move all extremities equally. No obvious skin rashes are noted. She has an elevated white blood cell count.

1. The pathogenesis of the patient's osteomyelitis infection can be explained by?

A. Exogenous source

B. Primary source

C. Infectious cause

D. Secondary disease

2. What is the most frequent cause of all types of osteomyelitis?

A. *Candida albicans*

B. *Mycobacteria*

C. *Staphylococcus aureus*

D. *Aspergillus*

3. When accompanied by fever, a diagnosis of osteomyelitis should be considered with the following symptom:

A. Back pain

B. Leg pain

C. Groin pain

D. Chest pain

4. Which laboratory test should be ordered first?

A. Comprehensive metabolic panel (CMP)

B. Erythrocyte sedimentation rate (ESR)

C. Troponin

D. Hemoglobin A1C (HbA1C)

BIBLIOGRAPHY

Bury, D. C., Rogers, T. Y., & Dickman, M. M. (2021). Osteomyelitis: Diagnosis and treatment. *American Family Physician, 104*(4), 395–402. https://www.aafp.org/afp/2021/1000/p395.html

Kremers, H. M., Nwojo, M. E., Ransom, J. E., Wood-Wentz, C. M., Melton, L. J., & Huddleston, P. M. (2015). Trends in the epidemiology of osteomyelitis: A population-based study, 1969 to 2009. *Journal of Bone and Joint Surgery, 97*(10), 837–845. https://doi.org/10.2106/JBJS.N.01350

Schmitt, S. K. (2017). Osteomyelitis. *Infectious Disease Clinics of North America, 32*(2), 325–338. https://doi.org/10/1016.j.idc.2017.01.010

PERITONITIS

Jennifer W. Parker

DEFINITION

A. Inflammation of the peritoneum

B. Considered an acute abdomen.

C. Types.

1. Primary peritonitis: Most often seen as spontaneous bacterial peritonitis (SBP).

a. Considered to be infection of peritoneum/ascitic fluid without a surgically treatable source.

2. Secondary peritonitis: Most common form.

a. Considered to be inflammation of the peritoneum secondary to a surgically treatable source.

3. Tertiary peritonitis: Recurring or chronic peritonitis after adequate treatment of the original disease.

INCIDENCE

A. May be difficult to establish and varies with disease process and type of peritonitis.

   1. Secondary peritonitis is the most common: Accounts for 1% of urgent or emergent hospital admissions and has been estimated to have an overall rate of 9.3/1000.

   2. Patients with ascites from any causes have an incidence rate as high as 18%.

   3. Patients with peritoneal dialysis may have rates as high as 12%.

PATHOGENESIS

A. Peritonitis may be generalized or localized (e.g., abscesses, the leading cause of persistent infection/tertiary peritonitis), and infectious or sterile (e.g., chemical or mechanical).

B. Primary peritonitis (generally SBP) is an acute infection of ascitic fluid, resulting from translocation of bacteria across the gut wall and/or mesenteric lymphatics or, less frequently, due to hematogenous seeding in the presence of bacteremia.

   1. SBP is a complication of any disease that causes ascites, including cirrhosis, heart failure, and Budd–Chiari syndrome. From 10% to 30% of patients with liver cirrhosis develop SBP.

   2. Majority (>90%) of SBP is monomicrobial, with most commonly gram-negative organisms including *Escherichia coli* (40%) and *Klebsiella pneumoniae* (7%); or gram-positive organisms such as *Streptococcus pneumoniae* (15%), other *Streptococcus* strains (15%), and *Staphylococcus* species (3%).

C. Secondary peritonitis is intra-abdominal sepsis generally from a perforated viscus resulting from direct spillage of the luminal organ into the peritoneum.

   1. Causes include perforated peptic ulcer, diverticulitis, appendicitis, necrotizing pancreatitis, perforated bowel, or iatrogenic perforation.

   2. Pathogens differ from the proximal to the distal end of the gastrointestinal (GI) tract (gram-positive is predominant in the upper GI tract, unless the patient is on long-term proton pump inhibitor (PPI) treatment, when gram-negative may become more populous). Contamination from distal small bowel or colon is generally polymicrobial and may include fungi.

   3. Women can experience localized peritonitis from an infected fallopian tube or a ruptured ovarian cyst, as well as pelvic inflammatory disease.

D. Peritoneal dialysis-associated peritonitis.

   1. Causes include and are almost always due to catheter-related infection and are related to touch contamination with pathogenic skin bacteria.

   2. Abdominal pain, cloudy peritoneal effluent due to white cell counts greater than 100 cells/mm^3, purulent drainage at catheter site, or a swollen, tender tunnel site may appear.

E. Secondary peritonitis: Acute or chronic.

   1. Onset can be sudden as when secondary to appendicitis or cholecystitis, or it can be associated with chronic diseases (especially GI) such as Crohn's disease or peptic ulcer disease (PUD), trauma, or recent surgery.

PREDISPOSING FACTORS

A. Primary peritonitis (SBP): Peritonitis without a surgically treatable source.

   1. Decompensated liver failure.

   2. Presence of ascites from any disease process.

   3. Contaminated dialysate.

B. Secondary peritonitis: Peritonitis with surgically treatable source.

   1. Perforation of intestinal tract and abdominal organs.

   2. Trauma.

   3. Peritoneal dialysis.

   4. History of peritonitis.

SUBJECTIVE DATA

A. Common complaints/symptoms.

   1. Primary peritonitis (SBP): Fever and abdominal pain, often accompanied by change in mental status from hepatic encephalopathy and/or sepsis.

   2. Secondary peritonitis: Acute abdominal pain, worse with movement, variable location of pain, high fever, and nausea and vomiting.

      a. Pain can be generalized and dull initially (visceral peritoneum involvement) and then become more localized and severe (parietal layer involvement).

B. Common/typical scenario.

   1. Diagnosis of peritonitis is primarily clinical; thus, history is important.

   2. Specific historical factors include knowledge of previous peritonitis, causes of immunosuppression including the use of immunosuppressive agents, recent abdominal surgery or trauma, presence of diseases (e.g., inflammatory bowel disease, diverticulitis, PUD) that may predispose to intra-abdominal perforations/infections, and travel history.

      a. Primary peritonitis (SBP): Cirrhosis of the liver; hepatitis C, now with ascites.

C. Social history.

   1. Alcohol dependency.

   2. Intravenous (IV) drug use.

   3. Blood transfusion.

D. Review of systems.

   1. Primary peritonitis (SBP).

      a. Constitutional: Feeling poorly, fever, loss of appetite, or generalized weakness.

      b. Neurologic: Change in mental status or dizziness/lightheadedness (secondary to hypotension).

      c. Respiratory shortness of breath, dyspnea on exertion, and inability to take a deep breath.

      d. GI: Diffuse abdominal pain, abdominal tenderness, fever, and often ascites.

   2. Secondary peritonitis.

      a. Constitutional: Fever, chills, diaphoresis, or loss of appetite.

▶

b. Neurologic: Lightheadedness/dizziness (secondary to hypotension).

c. Cardiac: Tachycardia secondary to pain.

d. Respiratory: Shortness of breath and dyspnea (secondary to pain).

e. GI: Acute abdominal pain (worse with movement), nausea and vomiting, and constipation or diarrhea.

PHYSICAL EXAMINATION

A. General appearance: Ill and in severe discomfort.

   1. Peritonitis can often proceed quickly to septic shock and multiple organ dysfunction syndrome (MODS).

B. Vital signs.

   1. Temperature: Often greater than 100.4°F (>38°C), but may be hypothermic (<96.8°F/<36°C).

   2. Tachycardia from presence of inflammatory mediators; fever and hypovolemia from vomiting/shock/third spacing. Patients on beta-blockers may not become truly tachycardic.

   3. Hypotension: Primarily as patients progress with dehydration and shock.

C. Abdomen (patient should be supine, with a pillow underneath their knees; this may allow for improved relaxation of the abdominal wall).

   1. Tenderness to palpitation.

      a. The region of greatest tenderness overlies the site of maximal irritation/pathologic process, even with generalized pain.

   2. Rigidity: Voluntary in anticipation to or response to palpitation or involuntary from peritoneal irritation.

      a. Involuntary rigidity makes peritonitis highly likely.

   3. Increased pain with movement: Possible severe pain caused by coughing or flexing of the hips.

   4. Rebound tenderness (i.e., positive Bloomberg sign): As peritoneum snaps back into place with sudden removal of pressure.

   5. Distension.

   6. Hypoactive to absent bowel sounds: Reflecting generalized ileus (less likely with highly localized infection).

   7. Masses or hernias (occasionally).

   8. Ascites: Especially in SBP.

D. Genitourinary: Oliguria or anuria as patient becomes hypotensive.

E. Integumentary: Presence of signs of liver failure such as jaundice or angiomata if SBP results from cirrhosis.

F. Determine severity of illness with CLIF-SOFA (mortality predictor for acute on chronic liver disease).

DIAGNOSTIC TESTS

A. For all patients.

   1. Paracentesis: For all patients with new ascites and/or hospitalization of cirrhotic patients *prior to* receiving antibiotics.

a. A cell count of >250 or more polymorphonuclear (PMN) leukocytes suggests infection. Patients should be started on broad-spectrum antibiotics immediately, with narrowing of antibiotic treatment following results of culture of ascitic fluid. PMN level is generally available rapidly, whereas cell culture can take 24 to 48 hours.

b. Analysis of ascitic fluid should also include Gram stain; fluid chemistries; serum-ascites albumin gradient; ascitic fluid total protein concentration; and ascitic fluid glucose, lactate dehydrogenase, amylase, and bilirubin concentrations. All of these can help the diagnosis of SBP and/or differentiate SBP from secondary peritonitis.

   2. Plain and upright abdominal films: Evaluation for free air or dilation of large or small bowel.

      a. Free air is present in most cases of anterior gastric and duodenal perforation, less frequent with small bowel and colonic perforations, and rarely present with perforations of the appendix.

      b. Upright films are useful in identifying free air under the diaphragm (usually on the right), which is indicative of viscus perforation.

   3. Chest x-ray (CXR): Elevated diaphragm.

   4. CT of the abdomen with enteral and IV contrast: Evidence of surgically treatable source, ascites, or mass. CT is the optimal diagnostic study for peritoneal abscess and related visceral pathology.

   5. Blood cultures: Often positive.

B. For patients on peritoneal dialysis.

   1. Peritoneal fluid analysis: With white blood cell (WBC) greater than 100 cells/mm³; more than 50% of those are PMN leukocytes.

      a. Low WBC is found even in cases of peritonitis, usually due to the short length of dialysate dwell time or a poor host immune response.

      b. Gram stain of fluid should be completed.

   2. Peritoneal fluid culture: Most commonly gram-positive organisms, such as coagulase-negative *Staphylococcus*.

   3. Peripheral WBC and blood cultures.

   4. Culture of purulent drainage from exit site.

DIFFERENTIAL DIAGNOSIS

A. Primary peritonitis (SBP).

   1. Important to differentiate from secondary peritonitis due to high mortality associated with unnecessary versus postponed surgery.

   2. Other conditions to be considered with ascitic patients: Peritoneal carcinomatosis, tuberculous peritonitis, and alcoholic hepatitis.

B. Secondary peritonitis: Associated with many thoracic and abdominal conditions.

   1. Thoracic conditions leading to diaphragmatic irritation (e.g., empyema).

   2. Retroperitoneal processes: Renal abscess, pyelonephritis, cystitis, and urinary retention.

3. External hernia with intestinal incarceration.
4. Familial Mediterranean fever.
5. Gynecologic disorders: Salpingitis, endometriosis, teratoma, and dermoid cysts.
6. Neoplasms.
7. Vascular conditions: Mesenteric embolus or nonocclusive ischemia, ischemic colitis, and portal or mesenteric vein thrombosis.
8. Splenosis.
9. Vasculitis: Systemic lupus erythematosus and allergic vasculitis.

EVALUATION AND MANAGEMENT PLAN

A. All types of peritonitis: Essential to provide aggressive fluid management to maintain hemodynamic stability.
   1. If at all possible: Avoid vasopressors.
B. Primary peritonitis (SBP).
   1. Empiric antibiotic therapy should be given as soon as possible (but preferably after paracentesis for culture). Antibiotic therapy is indicated in patients with ascites who have temperature >100°F/37.8°C, abdominal pain and/or tenderness, altered mental status, or ascitic fluid polymorphonuclear count >250.
      a. Cefotaxime 2 g Q8H is recognized to produce good results in ascitic fluid (may not need to be renally dosed).
      b. Carbapenems (e.g., meropenem, ertapenem, and imipenem): Generally received for critically ill patients.
      c. Other third-generation cephalosporins and fluoroquinolones may also be appropriate, although resistance to fluoroquinolones is an increasing concern. Fluoroquinolones should also not be used if patient has received them prophylactically
      d. PO therapy requires excellent patient compliance.
      e. Duration of treatment: For standard organisms, a 5-day treatment is generally sufficient. Resistant organisms or *Pseudomonas* or *Enterobacteriaceae* may require 10-day treatments.
   2. Any nonselective beta-blocker (NSBB) should be discontinued (for patients with cirrhosis of the liver, there is a window for NSBB treatment—after diagnosis of variceal hemorrhage and/or ascites but discontinued with diagnosis of SBP).
   3. 25% IV albumin (1.5 g/kg body weight within 6 hours of diagnosis and 1.0 g/kg on day 3) is beneficial with renal dysfunction (creatinine > 1.0 mg/dL, blood urea nitrogen [BUN] >3 0 mg/dL or total bilirubin >4 mg/dL): Should be administered within 6 hours if diagnosis of SBP and on day 3. Octreotide and midodrine may be helpful in addition to albumin once renal failure has developed.
   4. Diuretic therapy concentrates ascitic fluid, thereby raising opsonic activity, which limits recurrence of SBP.
   5. Use of PPIs, which are associated with increased risk of SBP, should be limited.

C. Secondary peritonitis.
   1. Prompt initiation of empiric antibiotic treatment after all cultures have been drawn is necessary to cover gram-negative aerobes, enteric streptococci, and anaerobes (e.g., cefotaxime 2 g IV Q8H with metronidazole 500 mg IV Q8H).
   2. Emergent operative management to eliminate the contamination source is important.
   3. Frequently, patients must be nil per os (NPO) with possible nasogastric tube placement, depending on the source of infection.
   4. Nutritional demands need to be met; many patients develop an ileus after surgery. Consideration of enteral versus parenteral feeding should take place early in the course of treatment. Sepsis will increase nutritional demands.

FOLLOW-UP
A. Primary peritonitis (SBP).
   1. Repeat paracentesis is generally not necessary if patient has cirrhosis and monomicrobial infection.
      a. With an atypical course of SBP, repeat paracentesis in 48 hours.
   2. Prophylaxis is recommended for the many ascitic patients to prevent repeat SBP, including:
      a. Patients with ascites with GI bleed.
      b. Patients with low protein levels in ascitic fluid (<1 g/dL).
      c. Patients with history of SBP.
   3. Prophylactic regimens include:
      a. Ciprofloxacin 750 mg weekly.
      b. Trimethoprim-sulfamethoxazole five doses (Monday to Friday) of double-strength tablets weekly.
      c. Norfloxacin 400 mg daily (NOTE: Long-term prophylaxis with fluoroquinolones is recognized to lead to high-level fluoroquinolone resistance).

CONSULTATION/REFERRAL
A. Peritonitis, with the associated high mortality rates, often requires multiple consults, including:
   1. Surgery (secondary peritonitis).
   2. Infectious disease.
   3. GI.
   4. Nutrition.
   5. Critical care.
   6. Renal (for peritoneal dialysis-associated peritonitis).

SPECIAL/GERIATRIC CONSIDERATIONS
A. Older adult patients may not present with profound guarding and/or abdominal rigidity, which are classic findings of peritonitis.
B. Fever and tachycardia are more common, although these signs are much less specific to peritonitis.
C. Careful history should be taken, and peritonitis cannot be ruled out with just a physical examination in older adult patients.

CASE SCENARIO: PERITONITIS

A 60-year-old male with history of diabetes mellitus type 2 on metformin and Jardiance, hemoglobin A1C [Hgba1C] 6.2%), hypertension (HTN; on Losartan), and obesity (body mass index [BMI] 33) presents to the ED with abdominal pain. The patient was found to be in atrial fibrillation with rapid ventricular response and was started on metoprolol 75 mg daily and returned normal sinus rhythm. Chest x-ray (CXR) showed bilateral mild pleural effusions, with high-sensitivity troponin of 480. CT angiography (CTA) showed mild pulmonary edema and bilateral atelectasis. Echo showed 40% to 45%. The patient was found to have cholecystitis. He underwent cholecystectomy on day 2 of hospitalization. He was treated with intravenous (IV) antibiotics for 2 days and converted to PO oral Augmentin. The patient remained afebrile, but continued to be elevated at 14.

1. The nurse practitioner (NP) up the patient on day 4, and on signout is told the patient should be ready for discharge. Review of systems (ROS) showed dyspnea and malaise. Vital signs are stable except the patient is now requiring 2 to 4 L to keep oxygen saturation (SpO$_2$) >92%, with ambulatory pulse oximeter of 66%. White blood cell (WBC) remains at 13.8 WBC on PO antibiotics. What tests does the NP order?

    A. Blood cultures ×2
    B. Erythrocyte sedimentation rate (ESR), C-reactive protein (CRP), complete blood count (CBC)
    C. CT angiography (CTA)
    D. Chest x-ray (CXR)

2. The next day, the patient is hypothermic with temperature of 97.2°F/36.2°C, heart rate of 85, and white blood cell of 14; CT angiography with no pulmonary embolism, but with bilateral atelectasis, and elevated right hemidiaphragm. The patient's blood glucose on high sliding scale remains in the >300 mg/dL. The patient is flushed appearing on exam, with abdominal firmness and tenderness. Is this patient stable for discharge?

    A. Yes.
    B. No.

3. The NP completes a CT of the abdomen and pelvis, and CT shows stranding and inflammation with fluid accumulation in the gallbladder fossa. What is the first step?

    A. Consult surgery.
    B. Consult gastroenterology.
    C. Attempt paracentesis.
    D. Uptitrate antibiotic therapy.

BIBLIOGRAPHY

Barkley, T. W., Jr., & Myers, C. M. (2014). *Practice considerations for adult-gerontology acute care nurse practitioners.* Barkley and Associates.

Burkart, J. M. (2018, June 1). Clinical manifestations and diagnosis of peritonitis in peritoneal dialysis. In S. Motwani (Ed.), *UpToDate.* www.uptodate.com/contents/clinical-manifestatiosn-and-diagnsosis-of-peritonitis-in-peritoneal-dialysis

Daley, B. J. (2017, January 11). Peritonitis and abdominal sepsis. In P. K. Roy (Ed.), *Medscape.* http://emedicine.medscape.com/article/180234-overview

Daley, B. J. (2021, July 14). Peritonitis and abdominal sepsis. *Background, Anatomy, Pathophysiology.* https://emedicine.medscape.com/article/180234-overview

Ross, J. T., Matthay, M. A., & Harris, H. W. (2018, June 18). Secondary peritonitis: Principles of diagnosis and intervention. *BMJ, 361,* k1407. https://doi.org/ 10.1136/bmj.k1407 PMID: 29914871; PMCID: PMC6889898

Runyon, B. A. (2018, April 11). Spontaneous bacterial peritonitis in adults: Diagnosis. In K. M. Robson (Ed.), *UpToDate.* www.uptodate.com/contents/spontaneous-bacterial-peritontis-in-adults-diagnosis

Runyon, B. A. (2018, September 21). *Spontaneous bacterial peritonitis in adults: Treatment and prophylaxis.* In K. M. Robson (Ed.), *UpToDate.* www.uptodate.com/contents/spontaneous-bacterial-peritontis-in-adults-treatments-and-prophylaxis

Sabatine, M. S (Ed.). (2017). *Pocket medicine: The Massachusetts General Hospital handbook of internal medicine* (6th ed.). Wolters Kluwer.

SYSTEMIC INFLAMMATORY RESPONSE SYNDROME/BACTEREMIA/SEPSIS

Rose Milano

INTRODUCTION

The 2016 Surviving Sepsis Guidelines were reviewed in 2021, resulting in the publication of Surviving Sepsis Campaign: International Guidelines for Management of Sepsis and Septic Shock 2021. The recommendations presented in that document are intended to reflect best practice and provide clinical guidance, but they do not replace a clinician's judgment.

DEFINITION

A. According to the 2016 Surviving Sepsis Campaign, *sepsis* is defined as a medical emergency of life-threatening organ dysfunction caused by a dysregulated host response to infection, requiring immediate treatment and resuscitation.
B. According to the 2016 Surviving Sepsis Campaign, *septic shock* is defined as a subset of sepsis in which underlying circulatory and cellular metabolism abnormalities are profound enough to substantially increase mortality.

RISK IDENTIFICATION

A. Identifying sepsis early allows for early treatment with the intention of improved patient outcomes. Unfortunately, with the plethora of published risk scores and screening tools, the clinician is left to choose which tool they will use. The Surviving Sepsis Campaign does not provide a recommendation of which tool to use, but it does recommend against using the quick Sequential Organ Failure Score (qSOFA) as a single-screening tool when compared with Systemic Inflammatory Response Syndrome (SIRS), National Early Warning Score (NEWS), or Modified Early Warning Score (MEWS) in identifying sepsis or septic shock. Examples of these screening tools available at the time of publication are provided in Table 10.3.

INCIDENCE

A. Sepsis.
    1. According to the Centers for Disease Control and Prevention:
        a. At least 1.7 million adults in the United States develop sepsis annually.
        b. Nearly 270,000 Americans die as a result of sepsis.
        c. One in three patients who die in a hospital had sepsis.
        d. Sepsis starts outside of the hospital in nearly 87% of the cases.
    2. According to the World Health Organization:
        a. In 2017, there were 48.9 million cases and 11 million sepsis-related deaths.

TABLE 10.3 SCREENING TOOLS

Quick Sequential Organ Failure Score

Systolic blood pressure	Less than 100 mmHg
Respiratory rate	Greater than 20 per minute
Altered mental status	Glasgow Coma Scale score less than 15

Systemic Inflammatory Response Syndrome (Criteria)

Body temperature	Greater than 100.4°F/38°C or less than 96.8°F/36°C
Heart rate	Greater than 90 beats per minute
Respiratory rate	Greater than 20 breaths per minute OR Partial pressure of carbon dioxide less than 32 mmHg
Leukocyte count	Greater than 12,000 or less than 4,000 microliters OR Over 10% immature forms or bands

National Early Warning Score

Physiologic parameters	3	2	1	0	1	2	3
Respiratory rate	≤8		9–11	12–20		21–24	25
Oxygen saturation	≤91	92–93	94–95	≥96			
Any supplemental oxygen		Yes		No			
Temperature	≤35.0		35.1–36.0	36.1–38.0	38.1–39.0	≥39.1	
Systolic blood pressure	≤90		101–110	111–219			≥220
Heart rate	≤40		41–50	51–90	91–110	111–130	131
Level of consciousness				A (Alert)			V, P, or U (Voice, Pain, or Unresponsive)

Modified Early Warning Score

Score	3	2	1	0	1	2	3
Respiratory rate		<9		9–14	15–20	21–30	>30
Oxygen saturation (with therapy)	<90						
Heart rate		<40	40–50	51–100	101–110	111–130	>130
Systolic blood pressure	<70	70–80	81–100	101–200			
Temperature		<35.1	35.1–36.5	36.5–37.5	>37.5		
Consciousness				A (Alert)	V (Voice)	P (Pain)	U (Unconscious)

Urine production	<75 mL in the last 4 hours

b. Approximately 85% of sepsis cases worldwide occurred in low- and middle-income countries.

c. Mortality remains high and can exceed 40%.

PATHOGENESIS

A. Systemic effects of sepsis.

1. Immune dysfunction.

a. Dysfunction between the inflammatory and the immunosuppression responses of the immune system.

b. Nonsurvivors of sepsis have been found to have a significant impairment of their B-lymphocytes, which results in decreased production of the antibody immunoglobulin M (IgM). IgM is the largest antibody. It is found in the blood and lymph fluid, and it is the body's immune system's initial response to an infection.

2. Respiratory dysfunction.

a. The lungs are the predominant organ system affected, with the absence of primary pulmonary pathology in many cases.

b. Adult respiratory distress syndrome induced by sepsis in three overlapping phases.

i. Exudative phase where edema and hemorrhage in the alveoli occur within the first few days.

ii. Proliferative phase is characterized by a period of organization and repair.

iii. Fibrotic phase is the final phase, which is characterized by the formation of collagenous fibrosis.

3. Cardiac dysfunction.

a. Septic cardiomyopathy increases mortality up to 50%, has no known specific risk factors, and represents biventricular dysfunction. Three underlying pathologic mechanisms have been identified.

i. Impaired myocardial circulation.

ii. Direct cardiac depression.

iii. Impaired cardiac mitochondrial function.

4. Genitourinary tract.

a. The development of acute kidney injury in sepsis is poorly understood.

b. Current thought is that hypoperfusion causes decreased renal blood flow leading to tubular necrosis.

5. Coagulation dysfunction.

a. Sepsis-induced coagulopathies are important to not miss because they lead to the development of organ dysfunction.

B. Most common bacterial causes of sepsis.

1. *Staphylococcus aureus.*

2. Group A *Streptococcus.*

3. *Escherichia coli.*

4. *Klebsiella* species.

5. *Enterobacter* species.

6. *Pseudomonas aeruginosa.*

C. Fungal and viral sources are also possible causes.

D. Pathophysiology of sepsis is a complex interaction between a host's response to an invading pathogen and the pathogen itself. It starts off as an inflammatory response to an invading organism that is unchecked by a dysfunction of the proinflammatory and anti-inflammatory arms of the immune system, leading to multiple organ dysfunction syndrome (MODS).

1. Most of the time, the response to an invading pathogen is a normal reaction in order to maintain overall integrity of the host. The normal host response may include fever and leukocytosis.

2. Any pathogen that violates at the tissue level is potentially able to evade the host's humeral and cellular immune system, leading to widespread, systemic infection.

3. Although the early phases of sepsis are proinflammatory in nature, if not controlled these may progress to a significant immunosuppressed phase where the host is at an increased risk for secondary infections, along with reactivation of latent viruses.

a. Initially, proinflammatory molecules enter the bloodstream in an effort to ward off the pathogen.

b. With sepsis, an overactive immune response to an infection causes the natural checks and balances to fail. Rather than dissipating, the activated proinflammatory molecules spread beyond the infected area.

c. As these proinflammatory molecules travel, they cause dilation and endothelial damage, leading to leakage of fluid out of the intravascular system and interstitial edema accumulation.

d. This vascular leakage causes disruption of oxygen, nutrients, waste products, and fluids through the capillary walls.

e. If left unchecked, eventually organs become hypoxic and begin to fail.

f. A patient's response to sepsis is highly dependent on a variety of both host variables (e.g., age, comorbidities, genetics) and pathogen factors (e.g., virulence, susceptibility to treatment).

PREDISPOSING FACTORS

A. Sepsis and septic shock

1. Younger than 1 year or over 65 years of age.

2. Immunosuppressed state.

3. Comorbid diseases such as chronic kidney disease, liver disease, and diabetes.

4. Unrecognized, untreated, or undertreated infection.

5. Admission to the ICU or long hospital stays.

6. Invasive devices, such as intravenous (IV) catheters, breathing tubes, and hemodialysis catheters.

7. Previous use of steroids.

8. Malignancy.

9. Burns and other major trauma.

10. Major surgeries.

SUBJECTIVE/OBJECTIVE DATA

A. Sepsis.

1. Fever (temperature greater than 100.4°F/38°C) or hypothermia (temperature less than 96.8°F/36°C).

▶

2. Tachycardia (heart rate greater than 90 beats per minute).

3. Tachypnea (respiratory rate greater than 20 breaths per minute).

4. Leukocytosis (white blood cell [WBC] >12,000/mm³) and leukopenia (WBCs <4,000/mm³) with or without bandemia (more than 10% bands).

5. May progress to altered mental status, oliguria, hypoxia, and ileus.

B. Septic shock is a form of distributive shock with signs of sepsis noted above *PLUS*:

1. Persistent hypotension that is refractory to initial fluid resuscitation.

2. Tissue hypoperfusion resulting in lactic acidosis.

3. Requirement of vasoactive medications.

4. Development of MODS.

C. Family and social history.

1. Use of IV drugs.

2. Family history of diabetes, hepatic disease, cardiovascular disease, or immunosuppression.

3. Medical history: Important because it can suggest a likely source of the infection as the cause of the inflammatory response. It helps to identify the following:

a. Comorbidities.

b. Recent infections.

c. Recent procedures/medical treatments.

d. Implanted devices.

D. Review of systems (highly variable depending on source of infection).

1. Constitutional: Fever, chills, malaise, or fatigue.

2. Respiratory: Dyspnea, cough, or increased oxygen needs.

3. Cardiovascular: Chest pain or palpitations.

4. Gastrointestinal: Localized or diffuse abdominal pain.

5. Genitourinary: Dysuria or decreased urine output.

6. Neurologic: Altered mental status.

7. Integumentary: Cool/cold clammy skin, rash at IV sites, purulent wound, erythema, or warmth.

PHYSICAL EXAMINATION

A. General: Asymptomatic or generally ill-appearing, complaining of fever, chills, or shivering.

B. Neurologic: Altered mental status from baseline, ranging from confusion, malaise, and fatigue to lethargic, to obtunded, to comatose.

C. Respiratory: Tachypnea, dyspnea, cough, respiratory distress, or sputum production.

D. Cardiovascular: Tachycardia with or without murmur; jugular vein distention.

E. Gastrointestinal: Diffuse severe abdominal pain with peritonitis; pain localized depending on source of infection.

1. Right upper quadrant with gallbladder source.

2. Right lower quadrant with appendix source.

3. Left lower quadrant with diverticular disease source.

F. Genitourinary: Costovertebral angle tenderness with acute pyelonephritis or tender prostate on examination, with possible prostatitis.

G. Musculoskeletal: Swelling, joint tenderness, or warmth from septic arthritis.

H. Dermatologic.

1. Cool, clammy, and diaphoretic: Septic shock.

2. Rash, erythema, and induration: Cellulitis.

DIAGNOSTIC TESTS

A. Laboratory.

1. Complete blood count (CBC).

a. Leukocytosis (WBC more than 12,000/mm³) or leukopenia (WBC less than 4,000/mm³) or bandemia (bands more than 10%).

2. Blood cultures, at least two sets, aerobic and anaerobic, prior to antibiotic administration.

3. Urinalysis with culture if indicated.

4. Chemistry panel.

a. Pre-renal azotemia.

b. Hyperbilirubinemia.

c. Elevated liver enzymes.

d. Hyperglycemia.

5. Cardiac enzymes to rule out cardiac cause.

6. Lactate level (marker of tissue perfusion).

7. Procalcitonin level to guide length of antimicrobial therapy.

a. Low levels may indicate reduction of the likelihood of bacterial infection.

b. Not used as a marker for sepsis diagnosis.

8. Coagulation panel (checking for sepsis-induced coagulopathy).

a. Decreased platelets and increased prothrombin time (PT)/international normalized ratio (INR).

9. $PaO_2:FiO_2$ less than 300.

10. Mixed venous saturation of more than 70%.

B. Imaging.

1. Chest x-ray (CXR).

a. May reveal pneumonia or adult respiratory distress syndrome.

2. Plain extremity x-rays.

a. If suspecting necrotizing fasciitis, may reveal presence of gas in the tissues.

3. Abdominal ultrasound.

a. If suspecting biliary tract obstruction.

4. Possible CT scan or MRI: Superior to ultrasound when looking for any potential sources of infection, except those related to the biliary tree.

a. Consider specific CTs if concomitant traumatic injury is suspected; useful in base workup on mechanism of injury.

C. Miscellaneous.

1. EKG if cardiac cause is suspected.

2. Possible lumbar puncture if infection of the neurologic system is suspected.

DIFFERENTIAL DIAGNOSIS

A. Pulmonary embolism.

B. Acute myocardial infarction.

C. Acute pancreatitis.

D. Diabetic ketoacidosis.

E. Massive aspiration.

F. Upper or lower gastrointestinal (GI) hemorrhage.

G. Diuretic-induced hypovolemia.

H. Systemic vasculitis.

I. Cholecystitis.

J. Renal calculi.

K. Adrenal crisis.

L. Toxic shock syndrome.

M. Drug toxicity.

EVALUATION AND MANAGEMENT PLAN

A. Based on updated recommendations from the Surviving Sepsis Campaign: International Guidelines for Management of Sepsis and Septic Shock 2021, the following recommendations listed are only those that are considered either Best-Practice statements or have Strong Recommendations with moderate to high quality of evidence.

1. Recommendation for hospitals and health systems to develop a performance improvement program for sepsis, which should include sepsis screening for acutely ill, high-risk patients, and standard operating procedures for treatment.

2. Recommendation against using qSOFA as a single-screening tool for sepsis or septic shock, when compared with SIRS criteria, NEWS, or MEWS.

3. Recommendation that sepsis and septic shock be considered medical emergencies with resuscitation treatment to begin immediately upon recognition is Best Practice.

4. Recommendation for adults with septic shock on vasopressors that the initial target mean arterial pressure of 65 mmHg be the goal, over higher pressure targets.

5. Recommendation for adults with suspected sepsis/septic shock but yet an unconfirmed infection, continuous re-evaluation, and search for alternative diagnoses and a discontinuation of empiric antibiotics is an alternative illness is either identified or strongly suspected is Best Practice.

6. Recommendation for adults with sepsis without septic shock to initiate rapid assessment of the likelihood of an infectious versus a noninfectious cause of the illness is Best Practice.

7. Recommendation for adults with high risk for methicillin-resistant *Staphylococcus aureus* (MRSA) sepsis septic shock to use of broad-spectrum antimicrobials with MRSA coverage over broad-spectrum antimicrobials without MRSA is Best Practice.

8. Recommendation to optimize antimicrobial dosing strategies based on accepted pharmacokinetic/pharmacodynamic principle and specific drug properties is Best Practice.

    a. Administer one or more broad-spectrum intravenous antimicrobials (to cover all likely bacterial, fungal, and viral pathogens) as soon as possible and within 1 hour after sepsis/septic shock diagnosis.

9. Recommendation for adults with sepsis/septic shock to rapidly identify and treat any anatomic sources of infection with emergent source control is Best Practice.

10. Recommendation for adults with sepsis/septic shock for removal of any intravascular access device

that are possible sources, after alternative vascular access has been established, is Best Practice.

11. Recommendation for adults with sepsis/septic shock to receive crystalloids as first-line fluid replacement and against the use of starches during resuscitation.

12. Recommendation for adults in septic shock which does not respond to fluid resuscitation requiring vasopressors:

    a. Norepinephrine should be first-line agent (strong quality of evidence) and if additional vasopressors are required dopamine and vasopressin have demonstrated a high quality of evidence and moderate quality of evidence, respectively.

13. Recommendation for adults with sepsis-induced adult respiratory distress syndrome (ARDS):

    a. Use low tidal volume ventilation (6 mL/kg) over a high tidal volume (>10 mL/kg).

    b. Use of upper limit goal for plateau pressures of 30 cm H_2O over higher plateau pressures.

    c. Against the use of incremental positive end expiratory pressures (PEEP) titration strategy.

    d. Use of prone positioning during ventilation for greater than 12 hours daily.

14. Recommendation for adults with sepsis/septic shock to use of restrictive (over liberal) transfusion strategy.

15. Recommendation for adults with sepsis/septic shock to use venous thromboembolism (VTE) prophylaxis, unless contraindicated. In addition, use of low molecular weight heparin, over unfractionated heparin, is recommended.

16. Recommendation for adults with sepsis/septic shock to initiate insulin therapy at a glucose level of greater than or equal to 180 mg/dL.

17. Recommendations for long-term outcomes/goals of care are as follows:

    a. Discussing goals of care and prognosis over not having this discussion is Best Practice.

    b. Integrating the principles of palliative care into the treatment plan as soon as appropriate is Best Practice.

    c. Initiating screening for economic and social support and make these referrals as appropriate is Best Practice.

    d. Shared decision-making between intensive care and acute care hospital clinical teams to ensure discharge plans are acceptable and feasible is Best Practice.

    e. Performing medication reconciliation at both intensive care and hospital discharge is Best Practice.

    f. Providing information including intensive care stay, sepsis and related diagnoses, treatments, and common impairments after sepsis to surviving patients and their significant others in written and verbal hospital discharge summary is Best Practice.

    g. Hospital discharge plans should include follow-up with clinicians able to support and manage any new, long-term sequelae as a result of ▶

their illness, as well as follow-up for physical, cognitive, and emotional problems, is Best Practice.

B. The following are still recommended by the Surviving Sepsis Campaign: International Guidelines for Management of Sepsis and Septic Shock 2021. All have Weak Recommendations with low to very low quality of evidence.

1. Surviving sepsis interventions, or "Bundles." "Time of presentation" is defined as the time of the earliest chart annotation consistent with all elements of sepsis or septic shock.

2. Tasks to be accomplished upon the suspicion of adult with sepsis/septic shock.

   a. Measure lactate level and recheck if initial level is elevated.

   b. Obtain blood cultures prior to administering antimicrobials.

   c. Administer broad-spectrum antimicrobials.

   d. Administer 30 mL/kg crystalloids for hypotension.

3. In the event of persistent hypotension after initial fluid administration (mean arterial pressure <65 mmHg), reassess volume status and tissue perfusion and document findings.

4. Assessment of volume status and tissue perfusion indicators.

   a. Focused examination including vital signs, cardiopulmonary status, capillary refill, pulse, and skin findings.

   b. Central venous pressure (CVP).

   c. Dynamic assessment of fluid responsiveness with passive leg raise or fluid challenge.

5. Fluid therapy.

   a. Initial resuscitation fluids with 30 mL/kg of IV crystalloid solution within the first 3 hours of diagnosis of sepsis-induced hypotension.

      i. If additional fluids are required after initial resuscitation, administer IV crystalloid infusion rates based on frequent assessment of hemodynamic status.

6. Antimicrobial therapy.

   a. Narrow empiric antimicrobials as soon as pathogens have been identified by culture/sensitivity results and/or adequate clinical improvements are noted.

   b. Perform daily assessment for de-escalation of antimicrobial therapy over using a fixed duration of therapy.

   c. Suggest against using procalcitonin (PCT) plus clinical evaluation to decide when to start antimicrobials versus clinical evaluation alone.

   d. PCT levels can be used to support shortening the duration of antimicrobial therapy.

7. Corticosteroids.

   a. Not recommended if adequate fluid resuscitation and vasopressor therapy are able to restore hemodynamic stability.

   b. If fluids and vasopressors are not successful, then a daily dose of hydrocortisone 200 mg can be attempted.

8. Nutrition.

   a. Start enteral feeding early (within 72 hours) as soon as patient can tolerate.

   b. Use enteral feeding as opposed to parenteral feeding.

   c. Within the first 7 days of caring for a critically ill adult septic patient, start IV glucose and advance enteral feedings as tolerated over administering parenteral feedings.

9. Renal replacement therapy (RRT).

   a. Use either continuous or intermittent when there are indications for RRT.

SPECIAL/GERIATRIC CONSIDERATIONS

A. Pregnancy.

1. The most common cause of sepsis in pregnant patients is obstruction of the urinary tract.

   a. This may be caused by either hormonal effects of the pregnancy (hydroureters) or the mechanical obstruction of the uterus impinging on the ureters.

B. Geriatrics.

1. Blunted responses: May have insult without meeting the criteria.

2. Medication effects: Blunt heart rate, respiratory rate, and temperature.

3. Possible peritonitis without rebound tenderness.

CASE SCENARIO: SYSTEMIC INFLAMMATORY RESPONSE SYNDROME/BACTEREMIA/SEPSIS

A 57-year-old male professor at the local community college "passed out" during his morning class. Students told the emergency medical service (EMS) they were unable to "wake him up for about 6 minutes." Upon presentation to the ED, he is awake but drowsy, yet able to speak with symmetrical facial expressions. He reports that 3 days prior to admission he had the "flu" and pain in his right buttock, which has felt worse since he woke up this morning. Additional symptoms included general malaise, loss of appetite, and nausea with dry heaves. His initial vital signs showed temperature of 94.7°F/34.8°C, blood pressure (BP) of 90/50 mmHg, supine heart rate (HR) of 110 beats per minute and sitting 125 beats per minute, and respiratory rate (RR) of 28 to 32 per minute. Oxygen saturation was at 90% on 100% nonrebreather mask. Physical exam assessment was unremarkable except for the following: Lethargy, yet responding appropriately; unable to assess lymph nodes due to extreme body habitus. Digital rectal exam showed profuse tenderness and skin showed 5-cm severe erythema with edema/fluctuance and tenderness, with a streak noted extending from his right buttocks to the rectum.

1. Which of the following would be the definitive treatment for this patient diagnosed with septic shock?

   A. Initiate epinephrine intravenously (IV) for hypotension when IV crystalloids have failed to resuscitate.

   B. Administer beta-lactam IV within 1 hour of diagnosis.

   C. Surgical consult for source control.

   D. Initiate parenteral nutritional therapy within 72 hours of diagnosis.

BIBLIOGRAPHY

Abraham, E. (2016). New definitions for sepsis and septic shock: Continuing evolution but with much still to be done. *Journal of American Medical Association, 315*(8), 757–758. https://doi.org/10.1001/jama.2016.0290

Centers for Disease Control and Prevention. (2016). *National and state healthcare associated infections progress report.* http://www.cdc.gov/HAI/pdfs/progress-report/hai-progress-report.pdf

Chakraborty, R. K., & Burns, B. (2021). Systemic inflammatory response syndrome. In *StatPearls.* StatPearls Publishing.

Delinger, R. P., Schorr, C. A., & Levy, M. M. (2017). A user's guide to the 2016 Surviving sepsis campaign. *Intensive Care Medicine, 43*(3), 299–303. https://doi.org/10.1007/s00134-017-4681-8

Evans, L., Rhodes, A., Alhazzine, W., Antonelli, M., Coopersmith, C. M., French, C., Machado, F. R., Mcintyre, L., Ostermann, M., Prescott, H. C., Schorr, C., Simpson, S., Wiersinga, W. J., Alshamsi, F., Angus, D. C., Arabi, Y., Azevedo, L., Beale, R., Beilman, G. ... Dellinger, R. P. Surviving sepsis campaign: International guidelines for management of sepsis and septic shock 2021. *Critical Care Medicine, 49*(11), e1063–e1143. https://doi.org/10.1007/s00134-021-06506-y

Gaieski, D. F., Edwards, J. M., Kallen, M. J., & Carr, B. G. (2013). Benchmarking the incidence and mortality of severe sepsis in the United States. *Critical Care Medicine, 41*(5), 1167–1174. https://doi.org/10.1097/CCM.0b013e31827c09f8

Gupta, S., Sakjuja, A., Kumar, G., McGrath, E., Nanchal, R. S., & Kashani, K. B. (2016). Culture negative severe sepsis: Nationwide trends and outcomes. *Chest, 150*(6), 1251–1259. https://doi.org/10.1016/j.chest.2016.08.1460

Head, L. W., & Coopersmith, C. M. (2016). Evolution of sepsis management: From early goal directed therapy to personalized care. *Advances in Surgery, 50*(1), 221–234. https://doi.org/10.1016/j.yasu.2016.04.002

Longo, D., Fauci, A., Kasper, D., Hauser, S., Jameson, J., & Loscalzo, J (Eds.). (2015). *Harrison's principles of internal medicine* (19th ed.). McGraw Hill.

MacClaren, A., & Spelman, G. (2018, July 6). *Fever in the intensive care unit.* In G. Finlay (Ed.), *UpToDate.* https://www.uptodate.com/contents/fever-in-the-intensive-care-unit

Mahapatra, S., & Heffner, A. C. (2022, January). Septic shock. *StatPearls [Internet].* StatPearls Publishing. https://www.ncbi.nlm.nih.gov/books/NBK430939/

Marino, P. M. (2014). *The ICU book* (4th ed.). Wolters Kluwer/Lippincott Williams & Wilkins.

O'Grady, N. M., Barie, P. S., Bartlett, J. G., Bleck, T., Carroll, K., Kalil, A. C., Linden, P., Maki, D. G., Nierman, D., Pasculle, W., & Masur, H. (2008). & American College of Critical Care Medicine; Infectious Diseases Society of America. Guidelines for evaluation of new fever in critically ill adult patients: 2008 update from the American Association of Critical Care Medicine and the Infectious Diseases Society of America. *Critical Care Medicine, 36*(4), 1330–1349. https://doi.org/10.1097/CCM.0b013e318169eda9

Rhodes, A., Evans, L. E., Alhazzani, L. E., Levy, M. M., Antoneilli, M., Ferrer, R., & Dellinger, P. (2017). Surviving sepsis campaign: International guidelines for management of sepsis and shock: 2016. *Intensive Care Medicine, 43*(3), 304–377. https://doi.org/10.1007/s00134-017-4683-6

Rudd, K. E., Johnson, S. C., Agesa, K. M., Shackelford, K. A., Tsoi, D., Kievlan, D. R., Colombara, D. V., Ikuta, K. S., Kissoon, N., Finfer, S., Fleischmann-Struzek, C., Machado, F. R., Reinhart, K. K., Rowan, K., Seymour, C. W., Watson, R. S., West, T. E., Marinho, F., Hay, S. I. ... Naghavi, M. (2020). Global, regional, and national sepsis incidence and mortality, 1990-2017: Analysis for the Global Burden of Disease Study. *Lancet (London, England), 395*(10219), 200–211.

Singer, M., Deutschman, C. S., Seymour, C. W., Shankar-Hari, M., Annane, D., Bauer, M., & Angus, D. A. (2016). The third international consensus definitions for sepsis and septic shock (Sepsis-3). *Journal of the American Medical Association, 315*(8), 801–810. https://doi.org/10.1001/jama.2016.0287

SEPTIC ARTHRITIS

Yvonne Tumbali

DEFINITION

A. Infection of a joint, generally caused by bacteria, but can be caused by fungi or mycobacteria.

B. Devastating form of acute-onset arthritis; considered an orthopedic emergency, if untreated can result in joint degradation

C. Although all types of septic arthritis are infectious, not all types of infectious arthritis are classified as septic. Systemic diseases that can trigger an inflammatory response in joints include:

1. Lyme disease.
2. Chikungunya: Mosquito-borne illness (in the family of alphaviruses).
3. Rubella.
4. Parvovirus.
5. Hepatitis B and C.

INCIDENCE

A. Incidence is 2 to 10 cases per 100,000 people per year in the general population.

B. The incidence is increased in patients with rheumatoid arthritis or joint prostheses, 30 to 70 per 100,000.

C. The prevalence has been estimated to range from 8% to 27% in adults presenting with one or more acutely painful joints.

D. Mortality has been at the persistent rate of 5% to 15% over the past 25 years.

PATHOGENESIS

A. Hematogenous seeding from bacteremia. Bacteria cause acute synovitis after entering the closed joint space within hours. The synovium is very vascular with no membrane barriers, making it susceptible to seeding by bacteria.

1. Synovial reaction: Results in swift entry of acute and chronic inflammatory cells.
2. Persistent inflammation may lead to joint effusions and elevated pressures, resulting in damage to lymph vessels, lymph node collapse, and joint erosion.
3. Release of cytokines and proteases, which causes cartilage degradation.
4. Bone loss: Evident within a few days.
5. Generally monomicrobial.
6. Most cases (75%): Involvement of only one joint (monoarticular).
   a. Polyarticular infection is commonly seen in rheumatoid arthritis.

B. Joint surgery, joint aspiration, or local steroid injections: Often polymicrobial infections.

C. Puncture wounds or bites: Also possibly inoculant into the joint.

▶

D. Loss of integrity of the gastrointestinal (GI) or urinary tracts may lead to gram-negative bacteremia infections.

E. Bacteria most often involved.

1. *Staphylococcus aureus:* Common cause with increased incidence of methicillin-resistant *Staphylococcus aureus* (MRSA) especially in the United States.

2. Beta-hemolytic streptococci: Next most common.

3. *Neisseria gonorrhoeae:* Most common pathogen among younger, sexually active adults. Was the leading cause in young sexually active adults in the United States, but noted to have decreased since 1980s.

F. Gram-negative bacilli implicated most often in older adult patients and intravenous (IV) drug users.

1. *Klebsiella pneumoniae.*

2. *Escherichia coli.*

3. *Pseudomonas aeruginosa.*

PREDISPOSING FACTORS

A. Age greater than 80 years.

B. Immunocompromised status.

C. Preexisting joint disease (gout, systemic connective tissue disorders).

D. Diabetes mellitus.

E. Rheumatoid arthritis.

F. Disseminated gonococcal infections in young healthy adults. Develops in 1% to 3% of untreated cases of gonorrhea.

G. All substance abuse, particularly IV drug use.

H. Skin infections; cutaneous ulcers.

I. Previous intra-articular corticosteroid injections.

J. Recent joint surgery.

K. Joint prosthesis.

L. Cirrhosis.

M. End-stage renal disease.

N. Penetrating trauma; human or animal bites.

SUBJECTIVE DATA

A. Common complaints/symptoms.

1. Native joints: Acute joint pain, swelling, warmth, erythema, decreased range of motion, fever, chills, or malaise.

2. Prosthetic joints: Possibly minimal symptoms.

B. Common/typical scenario.

1. History of joint swelling, pain, fever, general malaise, or chills of acute onset.

2. Other recent infections (e.g., urinary tract infection [UTI], cellulitis; cutaneous infections from IV drug use; sexually transmitted diseases, particularly gonorrhea; endocarditis).

3. Recent orthopedic surgery or joint replacement: Can be early onset, delayed onset (3–24 months), or late onset (24 months after surgery).

4. History of rheumatoid arthritis; receiving anti-tumor necrosis factor (TNF).

a. Anti-TNF therapy associated with doubling of risk of septic arthritis.

b. Can result in higher mortality because septic arthritis can be mistaken for an acute rheumatoid arthritis flare-up and lead to delay in treatment.

5. History of immunosuppressive diseases, including:

a. Liver disease.

b. Diabetes.

c. Solid tumors.

d. Lymphomas.

e. HIV.

C. Family and social history.

1. History of IV drug use.

2. Smoking history.

3. Sexually active with multiple partners (gonococcal bacterial arthritis).

D. Review of systems.

1. Constitutional: Fatigue, malaise, lethargy, decreased appetite, or recent trauma.

2. GI: Unintentional weight loss, or diarrhea.

3. Genitourinary (GU): Frequent infections.

4. Musculoskeletal: Pain in joint(s), joint swelling, decreased range of motion, or arthritis.

5. Skin: Lesions, erythema, cutaneous wounds, needle marks, or bites.

6. Hematologic/lymphatic: Swollen lymph nodes or exposure to Lyme disease.

PHYSICAL EXAMINATION

A. Low-grade fever.

1. Chills and spiking fever atypical.

2. Fever less likely in older adults.

B. Possible joint swelling, warmth, erythema, and painful joint with limited range of motion.

C. Generally monoarticular. Polyarticular disease is present in about 20% of cases, generally in patients with rheumatoid arthritis or other systemic connective tissue disease.

1. Knee most common (45%–50%).

2. Hip (15%).

3. Shoulder (5%)

4. Ankle (7%–9%).

5. Elbow (8%)

6. Wrists (6–7%).

7. Sacroiliac joints (1%–4%).

8. Axial joint septic arthritis (sternoclavicular, sternomanubrial joints): Most common in IV drug abuse.

D. Joint effusion.

E. Limited active and passive range of motion.

F. Prosthetic joint infections: Later physical findings often minimal.

1. Slight to no swelling.

2. May have draining sinus.

DIAGNOSTIC TESTS

A. Synovial fluid aspiration.

1. Key to identify infectious etiology and considered "gold standard" in diagnosis.

2. Synovial fluid: Check white blood cell (WBC) with differential, crystals, Gram stain, and culture.

3. Leukocyte count and neutrophil percentage: Reliable measure before cultures are available. Synovial fluid leukocyte count greater than 50,000/mm^3 with ▶

polymorphonucleocyte (PMN) leukocyte predominance is usually indicative of septic arthritis but can also be seen in gout. These counts may be lower in patients with prosthetic joints.

4. Cytology: Used to exclude gout or other crystal arthritis types. Mycobacteria and fungi may also be identified by cytology.

5. Cultures.

a. Complete blood count (CBC).

i. Leukocytosis present in most cases but has low sensitivity and specificity.

b. Inflammatory markers.

i. Erythrocyte sedimentation rate (ESR): Useful only in patients with native joint infections without underlying hematologic or rheumatologic conditions.

ii. C-reactive protein (CRP): Typically elevated, but also lacks specificity.

iii. Procalcitonin (PCT): Potential biomarker to distinguish bacterial infections from other inflammatory process; found to be a highly sensitive and specific marker for septic arthritis.

c. Synovial lactate: Suggested to have the best diagnostic accuracy of all markers in septic arthritis. Levels above 10 mmol/L (important laboratory identifies D-lactate produced by bacteria, from L-lactate produced by humans).

d. Radiologic studies.

i. Plain films might show joint space loss but not usually helpful except to rule out an injury that might produce similar symptoms.

ii. CT better than plain films in identifying joint effusion, soft tissue swelling, and abscesses.

iii. MRI sometimes useful in native joint infections to check early cartilage damage. Newer machines may allow for assessment of prosthetics.

iv. Ultrasound useful for inaccessible joints like the hips; guides arthrocentesis in joints not easily accessible.

6. Bone scintigraphy: Sensitive in identifying joint infections but is not specific enough to distinguish infection from other pathologies.

B. Other diagnostics.

1. CT or ultrasound-guided biopsy: Used in axial skeletal joints and sternoclavicular joints.

2. Open biopsy: Highest sensitivity and specificity but is rarely done.

3. Arthroscopy: Useful to evaluate for septic arthritis of the knee.

DIFFERENTIAL DIAGNOSIS

A. Traumatic effusion.

B. Hemarthrosis.

C. Bursitis.

D. Cellulitis.

E. Acute synovitis (inflammation of synovial membrane).

F. Gout or pseudo-gout.

G. Viral arthritis (rubella, hepatitis B and C, HIV).

H. Lyme disease.

I. Reactive arthritis: Seronegative spondyloarthropathies such as Reiter syndrome, psoriatic arthritis, ankylosing spondylitis, and inflammatory bowel disease-related arthritis.

J. Crystal arthritis: Can be present with bacterial arthritis. Diagnosis: microscopic visualization monosodium urate or calcium pyrophosphate crystals.

K. Endocarditis: Can present with sterile synovitis or joint pain similar to septic arthritis. Fifteen percent of patients with infective endocarditis have concomitant septic arthritis or osteomyelitis.

EVALUATION AND MANAGEMENT PLAN

A. General plan.

1. Considered a medical emergency. The mainstay of treatment is timely joint irrigation and treatment with targeted course antibiotics.

2. Early treatment (<7 days from onset): Improved outcome.

3. Antibiotics: First-line treatment.

a. Empiric treatment aimed at most common bacteria of staphylococci and streptococci; with increased MRSA as cause of septic arthritis, include antibiotic active against MRSA, vancomycin.

b. Critically ill patients or higher risk gram-negative infections (older adults, immunocompromised or IV drug users, or concomitant infections such as UTIs, possible use of antibiotics for gram-negative bacteria, such as cefepime or an antipseudomonal beta-lactam).

c. Human or animal bites: Antibiotics active against oral flora, such as ampicillin–sulbactam.

d. Prosthetic joint infections: Vancomycin if methicillin-resistant coagulase-negative staphylococci.

e. Duration of antibiotics.

i. No controlled trials to identify optimal duration; in general, adults are treated for at least 3 to 4 weeks, IV antibiotics for 2 weeks, followed by oral antibiotics for another 1 to 2 weeks.

ii. Gram-negative bacilli including *Pseudomonas aeruginosa* may need 4 to 6 weeks of parenteral therapy.

iii. Gonococcal septic arthritis can be treated with 2 weeks (ceftriaxone).

iv. If associated with osteomyelitis, duration of 6 weeks is recommended.

4. Drainage.

a. Hip, shoulder, and sacroiliac joints: Not easily drained with needle aspiration; may require open arthrotomy with thorough irrigation and debridement of all infected tissues.

b. Sternomanubrial and sternoclavicular joints: Generally managed with open irrigation and debridement.

5. Splinting.

a. Knees splinted in extension.

b. Elbows splinted at 90 degrees.

c. Hips in balanced suspension with no rotation. ▶

d. Joint range of motion to begin when infection improved.

6. Removal of prosthetic joint often necessary.

7. Dental prophylaxis: Should be considered in patients who have prosthetic joints and immunosuppression, diabetes, or rheumatoid arthritis.

B. Pharmacotherapy.

1. Antibiotic therapy: Initiated empirically, then tailored based on Gram stain/cultures after joint aspiration.

a. Most common pathogens: *S. aureus, Staphylococcus epidermidis,* and MRSA, so empiric coverage can be initiated for gram-positive organisms (vancomycin).

b. Ceftriaxone: Empiric coverage for gonococcal infection.

2. Symptom management with acetaminophen and ibuprofen if no contraindications.

C. Patient/family teaching points.

1. Antibiotics are used to treat the infection in septic arthritis.

2. If source control is not achievable with antibiotics alone, the fluid in the joint may be drained.

3. If there is extensive fluid, reaccumulation of fluid, or treatment is ineffective, surgery may be an option.

D. Discharge instructions.

1. Rest painful joints as needed.

2. Elevate joints to reduce swelling and pain.

3. Exercise may help keep joints flexible and reduce pain, but once joints become painful remember to rest them.

4. Nonsteroidal anti-inflammatory drugs (NSAIDs) help reduce swelling, pain, and fever.

FOLLOW-UP

A. Follow up with the orthopedics team.

B. Infectious disease.

C. Physical therapy may be helpful.

CONSULTATION/REFERRAL

A. Consult rheumatology for assistance with diagnosis.

B. Consult orthopedics for anticipated surgical intervention.

C. Infectious disease consult for duration, route, and type of antibiotics.

SPECIAL/GERIATRIC CONSIDERATIONS

A. Immunocompromised patients.

1. Fungal septic arthritis: More common with *Candida* species, *Aspergillus, Histoplasma, Cryptococcus,* and *Sporothrix.*

2. Fungal infections: Challenging to diagnose and treat.

B. Geriatric patients.

1. Comorbid conditions and frailty vulnerable to native and prosthetic joint infections.

2. Inflammatory response: Possibly blunted due to age. Patients may not have overt symptoms such as fever and significant joint swelling, which could delay diagnosis.

3. Advanced age: Significant risk factor for poor outcome.

4. Female predominance after the age of 80.

5. Removal of prosthetics in patients with advanced age: May not be possible.

6. High index of suspicion: Warranted in geriatric patients in any recently symptomatic joint or worsening of preexisting joint disease.

CASE SCENARIO: RIGHT KNEE PAIN

A 55-year-old woman presents to the ED with right knee pain and swelling worsening in the last 24 hours with fever (Tmax 101.5°F/38.6°C) and chills. She works outside as a landscaper and was bending at the knees often while planting flowers and shrubs for the last 2 weeks in a new client's backyard. However, 2 days ago, she noticed some pain, swelling, and redness around the right knee surrounding the joint. She describes the pain as sharp and localized to the right knee, with worsening pain and increased swelling last night and this morning, unable to straighten her right leg fully due to the pain. She took some over-the-counter (OTC) ibuprofen with little relief. Her medical history includes hypertension, childhood asthma, diabetes mellitus, gastroesophageal reflux disease (GERD), and rheumatoid arthritis. She denies chest pain, shortness of breath, back pain, nausea or vomiting, diarrhea, urinary frequency, urgency, and constipation. At the ED, her vital signs include temperature of 101.1°F/38.3°C, pulse rate of 110, with sinus tachycardia on the monitor, respiratory rate of 26 breaths per minute, and blood pressure of 156/78 mmHg. Physical exam reveals alert and oriented to person, place, and time; mild distress; general malaise; normal cardiac and pulmonary exam; and no clubbing, cyanosis, or edema in all extremities, except right knee swelling, erythema, warmth, some fluid medial to the patella as positive bulge sign, pain upon palpation which increased when bending the right knee, and limited active and passive range of motion. Given the symptoms, medical history, recent physical activity, and physical exam, there is an increased suspicion for septic arthritis in the right native knee joint.

1. What medical history places this patient at higher risk for developing septic arthritis?

A. Gastroesophageal reflux disease (GERD)
B. Rheumatoid disease
C. Hypertension
D. Asthma

2. What is the diagnostic test recommended as key or the gold standard to identify and confirm the diagnosis of septic arthritis?

A. Basic metabolic panel with phosphorus and magnesium level
B. Plain knee films
C. Synovial fluid aspiration for white blood cell (WBC), Gram stain, and culture
D. Prothrombin time (PT) and partial thromboplastin time (PTT)

3. The most common bacteria involved in septic arthritis is:

A. *Neisseria gonorrhoeae.*
B. *Pseudomonas aeruginosa.*
C. *Staphylococcus aureus.*
D. *Streptococcus.*

4. Which intravenous (IV) antibiotic is the recommended first line of empiric treatment for the most common bacteria related to septic arthritis in this case?
  A. Vancomycin
  B. Cefepime
  C. Ampicillin
  D. Levofloxacin

BIBLIOGRAPHY

Earwood, J. S., Walker, R. R., & Suge, G. J. C. (2021, December 1). Septic arthritis: Diagnosis and treatment. *American Family Physician, 104*(6), 589–597. https://www.clinicalkey.com/#!/content/playContent/1-s2.0-S0002838X21004196

Elsissy, J. G., Liu, J. N., Wilton, P. J., Nwachuku, I., Gowd, A. K., & Amin, N. H. (2020). Bacterial spetic arthritis of the adult native knee joint. *Journal of Bone and Joint Surgery Reviews, 8*(1). http://dx.doi.org/10.2106/JBJS.RVW.19.00059

Hassan, A. S., Rao, A., Manadan, A. M., & Block, J. A. (2017, December). Peripheral bacterial septic arthritis: Review of diagnosis and management. *Journal of Clinical Rheumatology, 23*(8), 435–444. https://doi.org/10.1097/RHU.0000000000000588

Long, B., Koyfman, A., & Gottlieb, M. (2019, March). Evaluation and management of septic arthritis and its mimics in the ED. *Western Journal of Emergency Medicine, 20*(2), 331–341. https://doi.org/10.5811/westjem.2018.10.40974

McBride, S., Mowbray, J., Caughey, W., Wong, E., Luey, C., Siddiqui, A., Alexander, Z., Playle, V., Askelund, T., Hopkins, C., Quek, N., Ross, K., Orec, R., Mistry, D., Coomarasamy, C., & Holand, D. (2020). Epidemiology, management, and outcomes of large and small native joint septic arthritis in adults. *Clinical Infectious Diseases, 70*(2), 271–279. https://doi.org/10.1093/cid/ciz265

Nair, R., Schweizer, M. L., & Singh, N. (2017, December). Septic arthritis and prosthetic joint infections in older adults. *Infectious Disease Clinics of North America, 31*(4), 715–729. https://doi.org/10.1016/j.idc.2017.07.013

Oliphant, C. M. (2015, November 1). Management of orthopedic infections. *The Journal for Nurse Practitioners, 11*(10), 1036–1042. https://doi.org/https://doi.org/10.1016/j.nurpra.2015.07.015

Osmon, D. R., Berbari, E. F., Berendt, A. R., Lew, D., Zimmerli, W., Steckelberg, J. M., Rao, N., Hanssen, A., & Wilson, W. R. (2013, January). Infectious Diseases Society of America. Executive summary: Diagnosis and management of prosthetic joint infection: Clinical practice guidelines by the Infectious Diseases Society of America. *Clinical Infectious Diseases, 56*(1), 1–10. https://doi.org/10.1093/cid/cis966

Ross, J. J. (2017). Septic arthritis of native joints. *Infections Disease Clinics of North America, 31*(2), 203–218. https://doi.org/10.1016/j.idc.2017.01.001

TUBERCULOSIS

Rose Milano

DEFINITION

A. An infectious, chronic granulomatous disease characterized by the growth of tubercles (nodules).
B. One of the oldest diseases known to affect humans, most frequently affecting the lungs, although up to one-third of cases occur outside of the pulmonary system.

INCIDENCE

A. One of the top 10 leading causes of death worldwide, tuberculosis (TB) ranks higher than malaria and HIV. TB is a leading killer of HIV-positive individuals.
B. One-fourth of the world's population is infected with *Mycobacterium tuberculosis*.
  1. Over 95% of cases and 99% of deaths occur in resource-limited settings.
C. In 2020, there were 2.2 cases per 100,000 persons in the United States.
  1. Cases decreased from 2019, when there were 2.7 cases per 100,000.

PATHOGENESIS

A. General information.
  1. Cause: One of four members of *M. tuberculosis* complex.
    a. *M. tuberculosis, M. africanum, M. orygis, M. bovis.*
  2. Dispersion: Spread by *M. tuberculosis* bacilli-infected airborne droplets, through coughing, sneezing, speaking, and singing.
  3. Lungs are the site of disease in 75% to 80% of cases.
  4. HIV greatly affects spread of TB by promoting and accelerating progression from infection to active state.
    a. Seventy-four percent of HIV-infected TB cases are in sub-Saharan Africa.
B. Primary tuberculosis.
  1. Active disease that develops in previously unexposed patients.
  2. Most cases are not recognized clinically except by a positive TB test.
C. Latent tuberculosis infection (LTBI).
  1. Exposure to *M. tuberculosis* without development of active disease.
    a. *M. tuberculosis* can stay dormant in the exposed host for decades.
  2. Noncontagious: Can turn into active TB disease if left untreated. About 5% to 10% of persons who do not receive treatment for LTBI infection develop active TB disease at some time in their lives.
  3. There is no direct microbiologic tests for diagnosing LTBI.
D. Extrapulmonary TB: Can affect any organ/system in the body. It may occur in 10% to 40% of infected individuals; the most common sites are:
  1. Lymph nodes (tuberculous lymphadenitis).
  2. Pleura.
  3. Upper airways.
  4. Genitourinary tract.
  5. Skeletal.
  6. Central nervous system (CNS)/meninges.
  7. Gastrointestinal (GI).
  8. Pericardium (tuberculous pericarditis).
  9. Miliary/disseminated TB.
E. Drug-resistant TB.
  1. Certain strains of *M. tuberculosis* bacillus are resistant to the drugs normally used to treat the disease.
F. Previous exposure.
  1. Individuals with positive tuberculosis skin test (TST) are less susceptible to a new *M. tuberculosis* infection than individuals with a negative TST.
  2. Previous latent or active TB infections may not confer protective immunity.

PREDISPOSING FACTORS

A. Decreased immune status of the host.
  1. HIV.
  2. Posttransplant patient on immunosuppressive therapy.
  3. Cancer patient on chemotherapy.
  4. Intravenous (IV) drug abuse history.
B. Malnutrition.
C. History of smoking tobacco/alcohol abuse/IV drug use.
D. Chronic renal failure/hemodialysis.
E. Recent infection with pulmonary fibrotic changes.
F. Postjejunoileal bypass/gastrectomy.
G. Older adult individuals with comorbidities and inconsistent immune response.
H. Crowded living conditions.
I. Healthcare workers.
J. Migration from/travel to a country with a high volume of TB cases.
K. Extremes in age: Very young and very old.

SUBJECTIVE DATA

A. Common complaints/symptoms.
  1. Early active TB disease: May be asymptomatic.
  2. Fever.
  3. Unexplained productive cough for more than 2 weeks (cough is seldom a presenting symptom in HIV patients).
  4. Hemoptysis: Sign of advanced infection.
  5. Loss of appetite/weight loss.
  6. Malaise/fatigue.
  7. Night sweats.
B. Common/typical scenario.
  1. Generally, exposure from infected droplets by coughing, sneezing, speaking, or singing.
  2. Slow symptom progression (over months).
    a. Worsening productive cough.
    b. Low-grade fever.
    c. Night sweats.
    d. Fatigue.
    e. Weight loss.
  3. Hemoptysis and/or pleuritic pain, which indicate severe disease.
  4. Detailed medical history: TB.
    a. Presence of TB symptoms: If so, for how long?
    b. Known exposure to individuals with infectious TB disease: When?
    c. Residence in high-risk congregate settings, such as prisons, long-term care facilities, and homeless shelters.
    d. Past medical diagnosis of latent TB or previous known TB disease and previous treatment.
    e. Comorbid diseases, which may increase risk of TB progression, including:
      i. HIV.
      ii. Diabetes mellitus.
C. Family and social history.
  1. TB: An infectious disease with no known genetic predisposition.

  2. Social stigma/poor knowledge about TB: Possibly difficult to obtain accurate history.
  3. Recent travel to areas of known high prevalence of TB, such as Central/South America, Russia, Africa, Eastern Europe, and Asia.
D. Review of systems.
  1. General: Fever, night sweats, weight loss, and fatigue.
  2. Vision: Icteric sclera.
  3. Head/neck: Headache, neck pain, swelling/soreness of lump in throat, and hoarseness.
  4. Respiratory: Shortness of breath, cough, coughing up blood, and pleuritic chest pain.
  5. Neurologic: Change in level of consciousness/mental status and generalized weakness.
  6. Endocrine: Fatigue, polyuria, polydipsia, polyphagia, and weight loss.
  7. Musculoskeletal: Bone/joint pain.
  8. Mental health: Alcohol/drug abuse.
9. Skin/hair: Presence/change in lesions/lumps.

PHYSICAL EXAMINATION

A. General.
  1. Many individuals with primary TB are asymptomatic (about 90% early onset).
  2. Once symptoms present, constitutional symptoms include weakness, fatigue, fever, chills, night sweats, loss of appetite, and jaundice.
B. Head, ear, eyes, nose, and throat (HEENT; TB of eyes, mouth, nose).
  1. Headache (meningeal TB).
  2. Nonhealing oral ulcers/dysphagia (GI tract TB).
  3. Icteric sclera.
  4. Bleeding gums.
  5. Epistaxis.
  6. Hoarseness.
C. Neck (lymphatic TB/pericardial TB).
  1. Lymphadenitis.
  2. Jugular venous distention (late sign of pericardial tamponade).
D. Neurologic (meningeal TB).
  1. Altered mental status and confusion.
  2. Coma.
E. Respiratory (pulmonary TB).
  1. Decreased, absent, and coarse breath sounds.
  2. Dyspnea, tachypnea, sputum production, cough, and hemoptysis (pulmonary TB).
F. Skin.
  1. Jaundice.
  2. Pruritic rash, which may lead to ulcers and abscesses.
  3. Various stages of bruising.

DIAGNOSTIC TESTS

A. Mantoux TST.
  1. Small "wheal" of tuberculin fluid is injected under the skin.
  2. Positive skin test means the individual has been infected with the TB bacteria.

a. Greater than 5 mm induration is positive for:
   i. HIV.
   ii. Recent exposure.
   iii. Fibrotic changes on chest x-ray (CXR).
   iv. Organ transplant.
   v. Patients on immunosuppression medications.
b. Greater than 10 mm induration is positive for:
   i. IV drug users.
   ii. Recent immigrants from high-risk areas.
   iii. Residents/employees of high-risk congregate settings.
   iv. Microbial lab personnel.
c. Greater than 15 mm or more induration is positive for:
   i. Any individual, even with no risk factors.
3. A negative skin test does not exclude a diagnosis of latent TB or active TB disease.
4. Targeted TST programs are recommended for use only in high-risk groups.
B. Approved TB blood tests in the United States: Interferon gamma release assays (IGRAs).
   1. QuantiFERON-TB test.
   2. T-SPOT TB test.
C. Acid-fast bacilli (AFB) testing: Smear and culture.
   1. Culture remains the gold standard for diagnosis and identifying drug susceptibility and genotyping.
   2. Sputum specimens should be obtained from all individuals suspected of having active TB disease, both pulmonary and extrapulmonary, with or without respiratory symptoms.
      a. At least three sputum specimens should be collected at consecutive intervals, 8 to 12 hours apart.
      b. At least one of the specimens should be an early morning specimen.
D. Imaging: Cannot be used alone to distinguish active TB from latent TB.
   1. CXR with a posterior–anterior view is the standard approach.
      a. Although abnormalities may be seen anywhere on a CXR, TB lesions are most often noted in the apical and posterior sections of the upper lobes or superior sections of the lower lobes.
      b. CXRs can be used to rule out active pulmonary TB in an asymptomatic, immunocompetent individual with a positive TST or IGRA.
   2. Chest CT is recommended if any suspicions for TB are noted after CXR.

DIFFERENTIAL DIAGNOSIS

A. Pulmonary TB.
   1. Nontuberculous mycobacterial (NTM) infection.
   2. Fungal infections.
   3. Sarcoidosis.
   4. Lung abscess.
   5. Septic emboli.
   6. Lung cancer.
   7. Lymphoma.
   8. Actinomycosis.

B. Extrapulmonary TB.
   1. Fungal infections.
   2. Non-TB bacterial infections.
   3. Syphilis.
   4. Nodular vasculitis.
   5. Leprosy.
   6. Cat-scratch disease.
   7. Rheumatoid arthritis.
   8. Lupus vulgaris.
   9. Pott disease.
   10. Histoplasmosis.
   11. Constrictive pericarditis.
   12. Bronchiectasis.

EVALUATION AND MANAGEMENT PLAN

A. General plan.
   1. If properly treated, TB caused by drug-susceptible strains is curable in the vast majority of cases. If untreated, the disease may be fatal within 5 years in 50% to 65% of cases.
   2. Medical evaluation for TB disease.
      a. Medical history.
      b. Physical examination.
      c. Test for *M. tuberculosis* infection (IGRA or TST).
      d. CXR.
      e. Bacteriologic examination of clinical specimens.
   3. Goals of treatment if active TB disease has been diagnosed.
      a. Curing the individual.
      b. Preventing morbidity and mortality.
      c. Preventing emergence of multidrug resistant (MDR)-TB.
      d. Interrupting transmission of disease by making patients with active TB disease become patients with latent noninfectious TB.
   4. LTBI: Who should receive treatment?
      a. Individuals with positive IGRA or TST and greater than 5 mm induration.
         i. Those with HIV.
         ii. Those who have had recent contact with person who has active TB disease.
         iii. Those with fibrotic CXR findings and history of prior TB disease.
         iv. Those with organ transplants or other known immunosuppressive conditions, including those who have been receiving the equivalent of 15 mg of prednisone daily for longer than 1 month.
      b. Individuals with positive IGRA or TST and greater than 10 mm induration.
         i. Those who have recently (less than 5 years) arrived in the United States from areas where prevalence of TB is high (Asia, Africa, Eastern Europe, Russia, and Latin America).
         ii. Those who are known IV drug users.
         iii. Those who are residents/employees of high-risk cluster/congregate settings (prisons, nursing homes, homeless shelters, hospitals).
         iv. Those who work in a mycobacteriology lab setting.

v. Those individuals with comorbidities known to increase the risk of infection to active disease (leukemia, diabetes, cancer, renal failure, gastrectomy).

vi. Those with an unaccounted weight loss of 10%.

c. Direct observation therapy (DOT): For individuals who have active TB disease or are at high risk for TB disease *if* they are suspected to be noncompliant with prescribed medications.

B. Patient/family teaching points.

1. Provide information about the disease process.

2. Explain the prescribed medication regimen and the importance of completing the entire treatment, even if the patients are asymptomatic.

3. Give information about possible side effects of the LTBI medications prescribed and when to call the medical provider. Possible side effects include:

a. Fever.

b. Unexplained anorexia.

c. Coffee or cola-colored urine.

d. Icterus.

e. Skin rash.

f. Paresthesias of upper/lower extremities.

g. Fatigue/weakness.

h. Abdominal tenderness, especially right upper quadrant.

i. Easily bruisable.

j. Joint pain.

k. Nausea/vomiting.

C. Pharmacotherapy.

1. Active TB.

a. Two-month intensive phase of isoniazid (INH), rifampin (RIF), pyrazinamide (PZA), and ethambutol (EMB).

i. Intensive phase includes four drugs due to worldwide resistance for INH.

ii. Once drug susceptibility is determined, if isolate is found to be susceptible to both INH and RIF then EMB is not needed and only INH. RIF and PZA are required.

b. Four-month continuation phase of INH and RIF.

2. Latent TB.

a. It is imperative to rule out active TB disease prior to initiating LTBI therapies. If monotherapy with INH is prescribed for active TB disease, drug resistance may develop.

b. Monotherapy with INH: 6-month dosing regimen.

c. Monotherapy with INH: 9-month dosing regimen.

d. INH and rifapentine (RPT) regimen: 12 doses.

e. RIF monotherapy: 4-month regimen.

i. Active TB disease.

ii. Treatment must be for at least 6 months.

iii. Most, but not all, of the *M. tuberculosis* bacilli are killed within the first 8 weeks of treatment.

iv. Undertreatment of the bacilli surviving the initial 8 weeks of treatment can cause the

individual to become ill again, potentially with MDR-TB.

v. Although the Food and Drug Administration (FDA) has approved 10 medications to treat active TB disease, four core medications are used as first-line drugs.

1) INH.

2) RIF.

3) EMB.

4) PZA.

vi. Dosing regimens: Available at the Centers for Disease Control and Prevention website: www.cdc.gov/tb/topic/treatment/tbdisease.htm.

D. Discharge instructions.

1. Provide documentation of the following:

a. TST or IGRA results.

b. Medications to be taken (dose and timing).

c. Possible side effects of medications to watch for.

d. Duration of drug treatment, with date of last dose.

2. Give details of when individual is required to be tested for TB.

3. Name signs and symptoms of active TB disease and stress the importance of seeking medical care if symptoms should arise.

4. Give information about the consequences of noncompliance with the prescribed medication regimen.

5. Describe TB infection control measures and the potential need for isolation.

FOLLOW-UP

A. Assess the state of infection and the infection's response to therapy.

1. Negative culture results are the most important objective measure of response to treatments.

2. Individuals with previously reported positive culture are considered positive until two consecutive negative monthly specimens can be obtained.

B. Check individuals monthly during treatment.

1. Monitor compliance with prescribed medication regimen.

2. Monitor for signs and symptoms of active TB disease.

3. Monitor for signs and symptoms of side effects of medications, especially hepatitis.

a. Jaundice.

b. Loss of appetite.

c. Fatigue.

d. Muscle and/or joint aches.

C. Recognize that active hepatitis and/or end-stage liver disease is a relative contraindication to use of INH or RIF.

1. Individuals with baseline abnormal liver function tests (LFTs) need regular monitoring with physical examination and laboratory evaluation of LFTs.

D. Understand that follow-up recommendations after treatment for active TB disease has been completed include the following:

1. Individuals with a positive response to a 6- to 9-month treatment regimen with both INH and RIF ▶

do not require routine follow-up but should be educated to promptly report a prolonged cough, fever, or weight loss to their medical provider.

2. Individuals with TB bacilli resistant to INH and RIF should be monitored for 2 years after completing the alternative treatment option.

CONSULTATION/REFERRAL

A. TB disease treatment regimens for specific situations require special management and should be administered in consultation with a TB expert.

B. Certain individuals with known or suspected TB should be evaluated by a TB specialist.

1. Pregnant women.
2. Breastfeeding women.
3. Infants and children.
4. HIV-infected individuals.
5. Individuals with known hepatic disease.
6. Individuals with extrapulmonary TB disease.
7. Individuals with drug-resistant TB disease.
8. Individuals with culture-negative TB disease.
9. Individuals with renal insufficiency or end-stage renal disease.

SPECIAL/GERIATRIC CONSIDERATIONS

A. Individuals are no longer considered contagious when they meet *all three* of the following criteria:

1. Three consecutive negative AFB sputum smears collected at 8- to 24-hour intervals with at least one being an early morning specimen.

2. Symptoms have improved clinically.

3. Compliance with prescribed treatment regimen for at least 2 weeks or longer.

B. Special consideration for treatment interruption during initial phase.

1. Interruption is equal to or greater than 14 days: Restarting the treatment from the beginning is recommended.

2. Interruption is less than 14 days: Continuing treatment to complete the total number of doses as originally planned, as long as they are completed within 3 months, is recommended.

C. Special consideration for treatment interruption during the continuation phase.

1. If greater than or equal to 80% of the doses have been given *and* sputum AFB is negative on initial testing, then further dosing may not be needed.

2. If greater than or equal to 80% of the doses have been given *and* sputum AFB is positive on initial testing, then continue and complete therapy as initially prescribed.

3. If less than 80% of the doses have been given *and* the interruption is less than 3 months in duration, then continue and complete therapy as initially prescribed.

4. If less than 80% of the doses have been given *and* the interruption is more than 3 months in duration, then restart therapy from the beginning of the **initial** phase.

D. The rate of TB increases in older adult individuals who live at home.

E. There is a two- to threefold additional increased incidence rate of active TB among nursing home residents.

F. Atypical presentation is not uncommon in older individuals.

1. Approximately 75% present with lung involvement.

2. Miliary TB, meningitis TB, skeletal TB, and genitourinary TB increase with advanced age.

3. Many do not present with cough, hemoptysis, fever, night sweats, or weight loss.

4. Many present with a change in functional capacity, chronic fatigue, cognitive impairment, anorexia, or unexplained low-grade fever.

5. Nonspecific, unexplainable symptoms that persist for weeks to months should alert medical providers to consider the possibility of unrecognized TB.

CASE SCENARIO: TUBERCULOSIS

A 45-year-old male was admitted to the hospital with active tuberculosis and with a history of present illness (HPI) including a worsening dry cough, which did not improve with over-the-counter cough medications, for 6 weeks prior to admission. The day he was admitted, his cough was productive, and purulent, and he admitted to "a couple times I coughed up blood." Upon further questioning, the patient also confirmed he was having night sweats and weight loss. His sputum test results were positive for *Mycobacterium tuberculosis* and he was diagnosed with acute tuberculosis. His medical history was significant for being diagnosed with active tuberculosis 10 years prior, for which he was successfully treated with medications. His significant admitting lab results include negative results for renal and hepatic impairment, along with a negative HIV result, but the susceptibility results for the *M. tuberculosis* organism is pending.

1. Based on the information given and the Infectious Diseases Society of America Guidelines (2016), which of the following medication regimens should be ordered as initial dosing for this patient?

A. Isoniazid (INH) + pyrazinamide (PZA) + ethambutol (EMB) for 2 months

B. Isoniazid (INH) + rifampin (RIF) + pyrazinamide (PZA) + ethambutol (EMB) for 2 months

C. Isoniazid (INH) + rifampin (RIF) + pyrazinamide (PZA) + ethambutol (EMB) for 6 months

D. Isoniazid (INH) + rifampin (RIF) + pyrazinamide (PZA) for 6 months

BIBLIOGRAPHY

Centers for Disease Control and Prevention. (2013). *Core curriculum on tuberculosis: What the clinician should know* (6th ed.). Author https://www.cdc.gov/tb/education/corecurr/pdf/corecurr_all.pdf

Centers for Disease Control and Prevention. (n.d.). *Tuberculosis.* https://www.cdc.gov/tb/default.htm

Deutsch-Feldman, M., Pratt, R. H., Price, S. F., Tsang, A., & Self, J. L. (2021). *Morbidity and mortality weekly report: Tuberculosis – United States,* 70(12), 409–414. 2020

Ehlers, S., & Schaible, U. E. (2013). The granuloma in tuberculosis: Dynamics of a host-pathogen collusion. *Frontiers in Immunology,* 3(411), 1–9. https://doi.org/10.3389/fimmu.2012.00411

Ellner, J. J., & Jacobson, K. R. (2020). Tuberculosis. In L. Goldman & A. L. Schafer (Eds.), *Goldman-Cecil medicine* (25th ed., pp. 2000–2010). Elsevier Saunders.

Lewinsohn, D. M., Leonard, M. K., LoBue, P. A., Cohn, D. L., Daley, C. L., Desmond, E., Keane, J., Lewinsohn, D. A., Loeffler, A. M., Mazurek, G. H., O'Brien, R. J., Pai, M., Richeldi, L., Salfinger, M., Shinnick, T. M., Sterling, T. R., Warshauer, D. M., & Woods, G. L. (2016). Official American Thoracic Society/Infectious Diseases of America/Centers for Disease Control and Prevention clinical practice guidelines: Diagnosis of tuberculosis in adults and children. *Clinical Infectious Diseases, 64*(2), e1–e33. https://doi.org/10.1093/cid/ciw694

Marino, P. M. (2014). *The ICU book* (4th ed.). Wolters Kluwer/Lippincott, Williams & Wilkins.

Mason, P. H., Roy, A., Spillane, J., & Singh, P. (2016). Social, historical and cultural dimensions of tuberculosis. *Journal of Biosocial Science, 48*(2), 206–232. https://doi.org/10.1017/S0021932015000115

Mathew, A. S., & Takalkar, A. M. (2007). Living with tuberculosis: The myths and the stigma from the Indian perspective. *Clinical Infectious Diseases, 45*(9), 1247. https://doi.org/10.1086/522312

Mattu, A., Grossman, S. A., & Rosen, P. L., (Eds.). (2016). *Geriatric emergencies: A discussion-based approach.* John Wiley & Sons.

Menzies, N. A., Swartwood, N., Testa, C., Malyuta, Y., Hill, A. N., Marks, S. M., Cohen, T., & Salomon, J. A. (2021). Time since infection and risks of future disease for individiauls with *Mycobacterium tuberculosis* infection in the United States. *Epidemiology, 32*(1), 70–78. https://doi.org/10.1097/EDE.0000000000001271

Nahid, P., Dorman, S. E., Alipanah, N., Barry, P. M., Brozak, J. L.., Cattamanchi, A., Chaisson, L. H., Chaisson, R. E., Daley, C. L., Grzemska, M., Grzemska, J. M., Ho, C. S., Hopewell, P. C., Keshavjee, S. A., Leinhardt, C., Menzies, R., Merrifield, C., Narita, M., O'Brien, R., . . . Vernon, A (2016). Official American thoracic society/Centers for disease control and prevention/Infectious diseases society of American clinical practice guidelines: Treatment of drug-susceotible tuberculosis. *Clinical Infectious Diseases, 63*(7), e147–e195. https://doi.org/10.1093/cid/ciw376

Rajagopalan, S. (2001). Tuberculosis and aging: A global health problem. *Clinical Infectious Disease, 33*, 1034–1039. https://doi.org/10.1086/322671

Raviglione, M. C. (2015). Mycobacterial diseases: Tuberculosis. In D. L. Kasper, S. L. Hauser, L. J. Jameson, A. S. Fauci, D. L. Longo, & J. Loscalzo (Eds.), *Harrison's principles of internal medicine* (pp. 1102–1122). McGraw-Hill.

Shah, M., & Dorman, S. E. (2021). Latent tuberculosis infection. *The New England Journal of Medicine, 385*(24), 2271–2280.

Weber, C. G. (2014, July 11). *Clinical infectious disease-2017 (The clinical medicine series).* Pacific Primary Care Software PC. *[Kindle]*

World Health Organization. (2018). *Tuberculosis fact sheet.* http://www.who.int/mediacentre/factsheets/fs104/en

KNOWLEDGE CHECK: CHAPTER 10

1. Probiotics should always be started when starting antibiotic therapy in the acute care setting.

   A. True
   B. False

2. Empiric antibiotics that should be started on all patients presenting with acute onset diarrhea include:

   A. Intravenous (IV) levofloxacin.
   B. Oral vancomycin.
   C. Augmentin.
   D. No antibiotic treatment.

3. Within what time frame of symptom onset does influenza treatment need to be started for confirmed influenza?

   A. 24 hours
   B. 30 hours
   C. 48 hours
   D. 72 hours

4. What is always considered an acute abdomen?

   A. Small bowel obstruction (SBO)
   B. Peritonitis
   C. Gastrointestinal (GI) bleed
   D. Cirrhosis of the liver

5. A man with cirrhosis of the liver presents to the ED with acute abdominal pain, bloating, abdominal distension, and ascites. His heart rate is 100, blood pressure is 106/55, temperature is 99.9°F/37.7°C, and oxygen saturation (SpO$_2$) is 90% on room air. What is the first test and urgent consultation to be ordered?

   A. Blood cultures, ID
   B. US of the abdomen, IR
   C. EKG and echo, cardiology
   D. EGD, GI

6. What is the most commonly associated bacteria in a patient with septic arthritis and the antibiotic treatment?

   A. *Staphylococcus aureus* treated with vancomycin
   B. *Neisseria gonorrhoeae* treated with ceftriaxone
   C. *Streptococcus* treated with penicillin
   D. *Pseudomonas aeruginosa* with cefepime

7. Which of the following diagnostic tests has a strong correlation to the diagnosis of septic arthritis?

   A. Synovial white blood cell (WBC) count >50,000 with poly leukocytes
   B. Decreased erythrocyte sedimentation rate (ESR)
   C. Decreased C-reactive protein (CRP)
   D. Leukopenia

(See answers next page.)

1. B) False

Probiotics hold promise to limit antibiotic-associated diarrhea, but studies have shown limited conclusive results. Probiotics have limited side effects, but are rarely covered by insurance and can be costly.

2. D) No antibiotic treatment

Most infectious diarrhea is viral and self-limiting. Oral hydration is the preferred treatment, and intravenous (IV) hydration if patient is not tolerating oral intake. Empiric antibiotics should only be given to the immunocompromised patient, those with certain cardiac diseases, patients older than 70 years, and patients with severe disease. Today, stool polymerase chain reaction (PCR) results are often available within 1 hour.

3. C) 48 hours

Treatment must be started within 48 hours of symptom onset, but maximum efficacy occurs if started within 30 hours.

4. B) Peritonitis

Although small bowel obstruction, gastrointestinal (GI) bleed, and cirrhosis of the liver can all lead to an acute abdomen, peritonitis (which can be caused by the aforementioned) is always considered an acute abdomen.

5. B) US of the abdomen, interventional radiology

Initial concern for spontaneous bacterial peritonitis (SBP) based on history of ascites and abdominal pain requires a paracentesis as soon as possible, prior to starting antibiotics. Bedside ultrasound (US) abdomen will quickly indicate that there is ascitic fluid sufficient to complete the paracentesis. Interventional radiologist should be consulted for an emergency paracentesis. With fever and borderline tachycardia, blood cultures should also be drawn, but consulting Infectious Diseases is not an urgent consult. At this point in the workup, there is no need for endoscopy, and GI does not need to be consulted; there is also no need for an echo and cardiology consult.

6. A) *Staphylococcus aureus* treated with vancomycin

The most common cause of septic arthritis is *Staphylococcus aureus*, which accounts for 52% of cases. Many are a result of staphylococcal infection or transient bacteremia from skin or mucous membrane sources. Vancomycin is the first-line antibiotic especially with the increased occurrence of methicillin-resistant *Staphylococcus aureus* (MRSA).

7. A) Synovial white blood cell (WBC) count >50,000 with poly leukocytes

Synovial WBC >50,000 with increased leukocytes, elevated inflammatory markers (erythrocyte sedimentation rate and C-reactive protein), and increased serum WBC (leukocytosis), along with a strong clinical history, all together can lead to a diagnosis of septic arthritis.

CHAPTER 11

PERIPHERAL VASCULAR GUIDELINES

Cara M. Staley

ACUTE LIMB ISCHEMIA

DEFINITION
A. Acute limb ischemia (ALI) is a sudden decrease in limb perfusion that causes a potential threat to limb viability.

INCIDENCE
A. The incidence of ALI is approximately 1.5 cases per 10,000 persons per year.

PATHOGENESIS
A. Arterial emboli that travel to the extremities predominantly originate from the heart.
B. Paradoxical emboli occur when venous thrombus traverses a cardiac defect and lodges in the arterial circulation.
C. Arterial thrombosis can occur where there is an atherosclerotic plaque or arterial aneurysm at sites of prior revascularization or in patients with thrombophilic conditions.
D. Arterial trauma can occur with interventional catheterization procedures, as well as blunt or penetrating injuries.

PREDISPOSING FACTORS
A. Atrial fibrillation.
B. Recent myocardial infarction.
C. Aortic atherosclerosis.
D. Large vessel aneurysmal disease (e.g., aortic aneurysm, popliteal aneurysm).
E. Prior lower extremity revascularization (angioplasty/stent, bypass graft).
F. Risk factors for aortic dissection.
G. Arterial trauma.
H. Deep vein thrombosis (paradoxical embolism).

SUBJECTIVE DATA
A. Common complaints/symptoms.
  1. The "Six Ps" is the classic presentation of ALI in patients without underlying occlusive vascular disease.
    a. Paresthesia.
    b. Pain.
    c. Pallor.
    d. Pulselessness.
    e. Poikilothermia (cold).
    f. Paralysis.

  2. The sudden and dramatic development of ischemic symptoms in a previously asymptomatic patient is most consistent with an embolus.
B. Common/typical scenario.
  1. Other signs and symptoms.
    a. Patients with known peripheral artery disease (PAD) or those who have undergone prior revascularization may develop symptoms slower (hours to days), depending on whether collateral channels provide flow around the occlusion.
    b. Upper limb ischemia is seldom limb-threatening. Patients often present with a cold feeling and numbness, rather than pain in the arm. Duplex ultrasonography can confirm the diagnosis. The arm often improves with anticoagulation. There should be a low threshold to undertake embolectomy if there is doubt about limb viability.
    c. Blue toe syndrome is typically due to embolic occlusion of digital arteries with atherothrombotic material from proximal arterial sources. There is often a strong pedal pulse and a warm foot. Identification and eradication of the embolic source should be undertaken.
C. Family and social history.
  1. Elicit the onset, duration, and intensity of the "Six Ps" of ALI (paresthesia, pain, pallor, pulselessness, poikilothermia, and paralysis).
  2. Question the patient about previous PAD, prior lower extremity revascularization, and aortic or popliteal aneurysm.
  3. Question the patient about atrial fibrillation, coronary artery disease, recent myocardial infarction, valve disease, and deep vein thrombosis.
  4. Inquire into the patient's history of limb trauma.
  5. Ask the patient about any condition that is a contraindication to administering pharmacologic thrombolytic agents.
D. Review of systems.
  1. Musculoskeletal: Ask about the following:
    a. Temperature and pain of extremity.
    b. Any numbness, tingling, or weakness.

PHYSICAL EXAMINATION
A. Check temperature, pulse, respirations, and oxygen saturation.
B. Take blood pressure on both arms. ▶

C. Inspect: Observe the affected limb and compare with the contralateral limb for mottling, pale, rubra, or necrosis.

D. Auscultate.
   1. Heart and lungs.
   2. Carotid and abdominal aorta pulses.
   3. Pulse of the affected limb with the contralateral limb.
      a. Arm: Brachial.
      b. Leg: Femoral and popliteal.
E. Palpate.
   1. Palpate and compare the pulses of the affected limb with the contralateral limb.
      a. Arm: Brachial, radial, and ulnar pulses.
      b. Leg: Femoral, popliteal, dorsalis pedis, and post tibial pulses.
   2. Check capillary refill of the affected limb and compare with the contralateral limb.
   3. Check limb strength and movement of the affected limb and compare with the contralateral limb.
   4. Check limb sensation of the affected limb and compare with the contralateral limb.
F. Handheld Doppler.
   1. Assess pulses of the affected limb with the contralateral limb and note if the pulse is monophasic, biphasic, or triphasic.
      a. Arm: Brachial, radial, and ulnar pulses.

DIAGNOSTIC TESTS

A. 12-lead EKG to assess for underlying atrial fibrillation or myocardial infarction.
B. If distal leg pulses are detected on handheld Doppler, obtain an ankle brachial index (ABI). An ABI of about 0.3 is diagnostic of subcritical acute ischemia (refer to lower extremity PAD for measuring ABI).
C. Full serum chemistry panel, including urea, creatinine, complete blood count, and baseline coagulation studies.
D. Vascular imaging.
   1. The availability of specific imaging modality and the time required to perform and interpret the study should be weighed against the urgency for revascularization.
   2. Patients should be anticoagulated prior to and during imaging.
   3. CT is the investigation of choice.
   4. Percutaneous angiography is the best choice when an endovascular solution to the arterial occlusion is likely.

DIFFERENTIAL DIAGNOSIS

A. Chronic critical limb ischemia.
B. Acute extremity compartment syndrome.
C. Extensive deep vein thrombosis.
D. Raynaud phenomenon.
E. Nonischemic limb pain from acute gout, neuropathy, spontaneous hemorrhage, or traumatic soft tissue injury.

EVALUATION AND MANAGEMENT PLAN

A. General plan.
   1. Systemic anticoagulation with unfractionated heparin.
      a. Anticoagulation minimizes the risk of further clot propagation and prevents microvascular thrombosis of underperfused distal vessels.
   2. Supportive measures.
      a. Keep nil per os (NPO) by mouth until a definitive treatment plan has been determined.
      b. Intravenous hydration, supplemental oxygen, and analgesia.
      c. Results of vital signs, EKG, and serum panel will guide further therapy.
   3. Treatment selection.
      a. ALI treatment depends on the extent of limb ischemia (Table 11.1).
      b. Class I: ALI may require medical therapy only. Revascularization if contemplated can be performed electively.
      c. Class II: ALI may require revascularization to preserve the affected extremity.

TABLE 11.1 FACTORS AFFECTING RISK OF ABDOMINAL AORTIC ANEURYSM RUPTURE

	Low Risk	Average Risk	High Risk
Diameter	<5 cm	5–6 cm	>6 cm
Expansion	<0.3 cm/y	0.3–0.6 cm/y	>0.6 cm/y
Smoking/COPD	None, mild	Moderate	Severe/steroids
Family history	No relatives	One relative	Numerous relatives
Hypertension	Normal blood pressure	Controlled	Poorly controlled
Shape	Fusiform	Saccular	Very eccentric
Wall stress	Low (35 N/cm^2)	Medium (40 N/cm^2)	High (45 N/cm^2)
Sex		Male	Female

COPD, chronic obstructive pulmonary disease.
Source: From Rahimi, S. A. (2019, January 8). Abdominal aortic aneurysm. In V. L. Rowe (Ed.), *Medscape.* https://emedicine.medscape.com/articl e/1979501-overview.

i. Class IIa: Percutaneous endovascular options are more effective in patients with ischemia of less than 2 weeks in duration. Surgical revascularization is more effective in patients with ischemia of more than 2 weeks.

ii. Class IIb: Requires emergency revascularization. Treatment options will depend on timeliness, personnel, and resource availability.

d. Class III ALI. Revascularization is usually futile and primary amputation should be considered.

4. Endovascular treatment options.
   a. Catheter-directed thrombolysis.
   b. Pharmacomechanical thrombectomy.
   c. Catheter-directed thrombus aspiration.
   d. Percutaneous mechanical thrombectomy.

5. Surgical revascularization options.
   a. Balloon catheter thrombectomy or embolectomy.
   b. Bypass procedures.
   c. Endarterectomy.
   d. Hybrid procedures combining open and endovascular techniques.

B. Pharmacotherapy.
   1. There are no pharmacologic treatment options for ALI.
   2. This is a surgical emergency.
   3. Systemic anticoagulation with a heparin drip may be started to minimize further clot propagation and to prevent microvascular thrombosis.
   4. Administer an initial bolus of 100 mg/kg followed by an intravenous infusion of 1,000 U/hr.
   5. If an urgent operation is not undertaken, heparin should be titrated to maintain an activated partial thromboplastin (aPTT) between 60 and 100 seconds.
   6. Postoperatively, patients will need to be started on long-term oral anticoagulation.

C. Discharge instructions.
   1. Patients will need to be maintained on anticoagulation after surgery and will need to follow up with vascular surgery for the surgical wound. Patients need to be taught about the side effects of anticoagulation therapy and the signs and symptoms of effective wound healing.

FOLLOW-UP
A. Outpatient vascular specialty after 4 to 6 weeks.
B. Outpatient cardiology (if emboli likely to have originated from the heart) after 4 to 6 weeks.

CONSULTATION/REFERRAL
A. ALI is an emergency.
B. Immediate transfer to hospital for urgent vascular consult.

SPECIAL/GERIATRIC CONSIDERATIONS
A. Patients with ALI are usually older adults.

BIBLIOGRAPHY
Cronenwett, J. L., & Johnston, K. W. (2014). *Rutherford's vascular surgery* (8th ed.). Elsevier Saunders.

Gerhard-Herman, M. D., Gornick, H. L., Barrett, C., Barshes, N. R., Corriere, M. A., Drachman, D. E., Fleisher, L. A., Fowkes, F. G. R., Hamburg, N. M., Kinlay, S., Lookstein, R., Misra, S., Mureebe, L., Olin, J. W., Patel, R. A. G., Regensteiner, J. G., Schanzer, A., Shishehbor, M. H., Stewart, K. J., . . . Walsh, M. E. (2016). 2016 AHA/ACC guideline on the management of patients with lower extremity peripheral artery disease: A report of the American College of Cardiology/American Heart Association Task Force on Clinical Practice Guidelines. *Journal of the American College of Cardiology, 69*, 1465–1508. https://doi.org/10.1016/j.jacc.2016.11.008

Mitchell, M. E., & Carpenter, J. P. (2018, March 15). Clinical features and diagnosis of acute lower extremity ischemia. In K. A. Collins (Ed.), *UpToDate*. https://www.uptodate.com/contents/clinical-features-and-diagnosis-of-acute-lower-extremity-ischemia

Rasmussen, T. E., Clouse, W. D., & Tonnessen, B. H. (2011). *Handbook of patient care in vascular diseases* (5th ed.). Wolters Kluwer Health.

AORTIC VESSEL DISEASES: ANEURYSMS OF THE AORTA

DEFINITION
A. An aortic aneurysm is an abnormal enlargement or bulging of the wall of the aorta.
B. An aneurysm can occur anywhere in the vascular tree.
C. The bulge or ballooning may be defined as:
   1. Fusiform: Uniform in shape, appearing equally along an extended section and edges of the aorta.
   2. Saccular aneurysm: Small, lopsided blister on one side of the aorta that forms in a weakened area of the aorta wall.
D. An aneurysm can develop anywhere along the aorta.
   1. Abdominal aortic aneurysms (AAAs) occur in the section of the aorta that runs through the abdomen (abdominal aorta).
   2. Thoracic aortic aneurysms (TAAs) occur in the chest area and can involve the aortic root, ascending aorta, aortic arch, or descending aorta.
   3. Thoracoabdominal aortic aneurysms involve the aorta as it flows through both the abdomen and the chest.

INCIDENCE
A. Approximately 3 to 4 per 100,000 per year.
   1. Intraperitoneal rupture (20%).
   2. Retroperitoneal rupture (80%).
   3. Aortocaval fistula (3%–4%).
   4. Primary aortoduodenal fistula (less than 1%).

PATHOGENESIS
A. Once the aorta reaches a critical diameter (about 6 cm in the ascending aorta and 7 cm in the descending aorta), it loses all distensibility so that a rise in blood pressure to around 200 mmHg (as can occur physiologically during stress or exertion) can exceed the arterial wall strength and may trigger dissection or rupture. This is an emergency that warrants immediate intervention, often surgical.
B. Often occurs as:
   1. Retroperitoneal leak or rupture: If blood leaks into the space around the aorta behind the gut cavity, ▶

then the leak is "contained" by the tissues and the patient is more likely to survive long enough to get to the hospital.

2. Free intraperitoneal rupture: If the rupture is into the gut cavity (the peritoneal cavity), then there are no tissues to "contain" the escape of blood from the aorta and it is much less likely that the patient will survive long enough to be taken to the hospital. Virtually all the blood in the circulation can escape into the peritoneal cavity.

PREDISPOSING FACTORS

A. Genetic: Familial thoracic aortic aneurysm and dissection (TAAD).

B. Connective tissue disorders (Marfan syndrome, Ehlers–Danlos syndrome type IV, and Loeys–Dietz syndrome, which partly resembles Marfan syndrome).

C. Aortitis from giant cell arteritis.

D. Rheumatoid arthritis.

E. Behçet disease.

F. Takayasu arteritis or retroperitoneal fibrosis.

G. Infection, such as syphilis and HIV.

H. Trauma.

I. Weightlifting.

J. Cocaine and amphetamine use.

SUBJECTIVE DATA

A. Common complaints/symptoms.

   1. Most people are unaware that they have an aneurysm because, in most cases, there are no symptoms. However, as aneurysms grow, symptoms may include:

      a. Pulsating enlargement or tender mass felt by a physician when performing a physical examination.

      b. Pain in the back, abdomen, or groin that may be prolonged and not relieved with position change or pain medication.

   2. A ruptured aneurysm usually produces sudden, severe pain and other symptoms such as loss of consciousness or shock, depending on the location of the aneurysm and the amount of bleeding.

B. Common/typical scenario.

   1. Thoracic aneurysm dissection rupture.

      a. TAAs are easily missed or misdiagnosed as cardiac ischemia.

      b. Patients complain of sudden intense and persistent chest or back pain, pain that radiates to the back, trouble breathing, low blood pressure causing feelings of fainting, loss of consciousness, and trouble swallowing.

   2. Abdominal aneurysm dissection or rupture.

      a. With AAA rupture, patients complain of a sudden onset of severe lower back pain that may radiate to the groin, hypotension, or transient lower limb paralysis.

      b. Classic triad of symptoms: Pain, hypotension, and a pulsatile mass.

      c. Most abdominal aneurysms rupture into the retroperitoneal cavity.

      d. Rarely, AAA may rupture into the abdominal veins or the bowel. This may or may not be associated with retroperitoneal rupture.

      e. Emergent surgery is warranted once diagnosis is confirmed with echocardiogram, CT scan, or MRI.

      f. Rupture of an aneurysm is one of the most fatal surgical emergencies, with an overall mortality rate of 90%.

C. Family/social history.

   1. Family history is an independent risk factor for more rapid growth of aortic aneurysms and should be assessed.

   2. First-degree family history of aortic aneurysm or bicuspid aortic valve also elevates risk.

   3. Ask about smoking, which also increases risk of aortic aneurysm.

D. Review of systems.

   1. Head, ear, eyes, nose, and throat (HEENT): Ask about any hoarseness or difficulty swallowing.

   2. Respiratory: Ask if the patient is having any shortness of breath, coughing, difficulty breathing, or chest pain.

   3. Musculoskeletal: Ask about back pain.

PHYSICAL EXAMINATION

A. Transient lower limb paralysis.

B. Right hypochondrial pain.

C. Nephroureterolithiasis.

D. Groin pain.

E. Testicular pain.

F. Testicular ecchymosis (blue scrotum sign of Bryant).

G. Iliofemoral venous thrombosis.

H. Inguinoscrotal mass mimicking a hernia.

I. Patient may show decreased red blood cell (RBC) or hemoglobin due to internal blood loss and increased white blood cell (WBC).

DIAGNOSTIC TESTS

A. An echocardiogram, MRI, or CT scan may help differentiate the diagnosis.

   1. Echocardiogram.

   2. CT and MRI only if the aorta is calcified.

B. Aortic angiogram or arteriogram: An arteriogram or angiogram accurately and directly depicts the vasculature; therefore, it clearly delineates the vessels and any abnormalities.

   1. An abdominal aneurysm would only be visible on an x-ray if it were calcified.

   2. CT scan and ultrasound do not give a direct view of the vessels and do not yield as accurate a diagnosis as the arteriogram.

DIFFERENTIAL DIAGNOSIS

A. Acute gastritis.

B. Appendicitis.

C. Urinary tract infection (UTI).

D. Diverticulitis.
E. Pancreatitis.
F. Cholelithiasis.
G. Small bowel obstruction.
H. Myocardial infarction.

EVALUATION AND MANAGEMENT PLAN

A. General plan.
 1. Uncomplicated aneurysm.
  a. The goals of treatment include:
   i. Preventing the aneurysm from growing.
   ii. Preventing or reversing damage to other body structures.
   iii. Preventing or treating a rupture or dissection.
   iv. Allowing the patient to continue doing normal daily activities.
   v. Following up and screening for risk to prevent occurrence, which is key.
   vi. Evaluating risk factors.
  b. Primary management is rigorous blood pressure control.
  c. Smoking cessation.
  d. Antiplatelet therapy where appropriate.
 2. Dissecting or ruptured aneurysm.
  a. Rupture of aneurysm is an emergency: Patient is often in shock and needs immediate intervention.
   i. Open repair when a rupture occurs as an emergency surgery.
   ii. Emergency endovascular repair for ruptured AAA, thanks to new technology, is now feasible.
   iii. Operative risk is based on patients' comorbidities and hospital factors (Table 11.1).
  b. Type of repair.
   i. Open repair of an AAA involves an incision of the abdomen to directly visualize the aortic aneurysm.
   ii. Endovascular aneurysm repair (EVAR).
B. Patient/family teaching points.
 1. Patients should seek attention if they feel chest pain or they just suddenly "don't feel right."
 2. A strong pulse sensation near the navel or bulge from the abdomen is also a reason to contact a provider right away. Deep constant or severe back or flank pain may be the only symptom a patient has of an expanding aneurysm.
C. Pharmacotherapy.
 1. Uncomplicated aneurysm.
  a. Statins: The role of statin therapy in AAA is unproven, but statins are advised because AAA patients have increased cardiovascular disease (CVD) risk.
  b. Other medical treatment: There is some evidence that the following may reduce the rate of expansion of small aneurysms, but their role is not yet clear:
   i. Doxycycline or roxithromycin.
   ii. Angiotensin-converting enzyme (ACE) inhibitors or losartan.

   iii. Statins.
   iv. Low-dose aspirin.
  c. Evaluate annually for risk of rupture and follow up.
D. Discharge instructions.
 1. Patients with incidentally discovered AAA should be taught to recognize the signs and symptoms of an emergency and be given instructions on what to do next.
 2. Patients who undergo surgery should be taught effective wound care and to assess for signs and symptoms of healing.

FOLLOW-UP

A. Surgical intervention for aneurysm (abdominal or thoracic).
 1. Patients with an incidentally discovered AAA that is less than 3 cm in diameter require no further follow-up.
 2. With AAAs 4 to 5 cm in diameter, elective repair may be of benefit in patients who are young, have a low operative risk, and have a good life expectancy.
 3. If the AAA is 3 to 4 cm in diameter, annual ultrasound imaging should be used to monitor for further dilatation. AAAs 4 to 4.5 cm in diameter should be evaluated with ultrasonography every 6 months, and patients with AAAs greater than 4.5 cm in diameter should be referred to a vascular surgeon.
 4. The decision to treat an unruptured AAA is based on:
  a. Operative risk.
  b. Risk of rupture.
  c. Patient's estimated life expectancy.

CONSULTATION/REFERRAL

A. Consultation should be made immediately to vascular surgery or cardiothoracic surgery for evaluation and general management of patients.

SPECIAL/GERIATRIC CONSIDERATIONS

A. Age is an important predictor of mortality in patients with aortic dissection with or without surgical intervention.
B. Treatment with endovascular aortic aneurysm repair should be strongly considered, particularly in octogenarians.

BIBLIOGRAPHY

Bown, M. J., Fishwick, G., Sayers, R. D., & Bell, P. R. (2007). Repair of ruptured abdominal aortic aneurysm by endovascular technique. *Advances in Surgery, 41,* 63–80. https://doi.org/10.1016/j.yasu.2007.05.005

Hiratzka, L. F., Bakris, G. L., Beckman, J. A., Bersin, R. M., Carr, V. F., Casey, D. E., Jr., Eagle., A, K., Hermann, L. K., Isselbacher, E. M., Kazerooni, E. A., Kouchoukos, N. T., Lytle, B. W., Milewicz, D. M., Reich, D. L., Sen, S., Shinn, J. A., Svensson, L. G., & Williams, D. M. (2010). 2010). ACCF/AHA/AATS/ACR/ASA/SCA/SCAI/SIR/STS/SVM guidelines for the diagnosis and management of patients with thoracic aortic disease. *Circulation, 121*(13), e266–e369. https://doi.org/10.1161/CIR.0b013e3181d4739e

LeFevre, M. L. (2014, August 19). Screening for abdominal aortic aneurysm: U.S. Preventive Services Task Force recommendation statement.

Annals of Internal Medicine, 161(4), 281–290. https://doi.org/10.7326/M14-1204

Moulakakis, K. G., Mylonas, S. N., Dalainas, I., Kakisis, J., Kotsis, T., & Liapis, C. D. (2014, May). Management of complicated and uncomplicated acute type B dissection: A systematic review and meta-analysis. *Annals of Cardiothoracic Surgery, 3*(3), 234–246. https://doi.org/10.3978/j.issn .2225-319X.2014.05.08

Mussa, F. F., Horton, J. D., Moridzadeh, R., Nicholson, J., Trimarchi, S., & Eagle, K. A. (2016). Acute aortic dissection and intramural hematoma: A systematic review. *Journal of the American Medical Association, 316*, 754–763. https://doi.org/10.1001/jama.2016.10026

Rahimi, S. A. (2019, January 8). *Abdominal aortic aneurysm.* In V. L. Rowe (Ed.), *Medscape,* https://emedicine.medscape.com/article/1979501-overview

Svensson, L. G., Kouchoukos, N. T., Miller, D. C., Bavaria, J. E., Coselli, J. S., Curi, M. A., & Sundt, T. M., 3rd. (2008). Expert consensus document on the treatment of descending thoracic aortic disease using endovascular stent-grafts. *The Annals of Thoracic Surgery, 85*(1), S1–S41. https://doi.org/10.1016/j.athoracsur.2007.10.099

Westaby, S., & Bertoni, G. B. (2007, February). Fifty years of thoracic aortic surgery: Lessons learned and future directions. *The Annals of Thoracic Surgery, 83*(2), S832–S834. https://doi.org/10.1016/j.athoracsur.2006.10.098

CAROTID ARTERY DISEASE

DEFINITION
A. Atherosclerosis (waxy substance) plaque builds up inside the carotid arteries and causes carotid artery disease.
B. There are two common carotid arteries, one on each side of the neck. Each divides into internal and external carotid arteries.
   1. The internal carotid arteries supply oxygen-rich blood to the brain.
   2. The external carotid arteries supply oxygen-rich blood to the face, scalp, and neck.

INCIDENCE
A. Carotid artery stenosis is one of the risk factors for stroke. The overall prevalence of asymptomatic carotid artery stenosis in the general population is estimated at ≥50%.
B. The prevalence is higher in patients who harbor additional atherosclerotic lesions, such as coronary artery disease.
C. Patients with severe asymptomatic carotid stenosis have an annual risk of stroke of 2% to 5%.
D. Among those 70 years and older, the prevalence is increased to 12.5%.

PATHOGENESIS
A. Atherosclerosis of the carotid arteries is a diffuse, degenerative disease of the arteries resulting in plaques that consist of necrotic cells, lipids, and cholesterol crystals in the intima of carotid arteries.
B. Arterial narrowing leads to locally increased velocities. A hemodynamic effect is reached when pressure and flow volume are diminished in the poststenotic segment.
C. These plaques can cause stenosis, can crack, or cause injury, allowing platelets to stick to the site to form thrombi and/or rupture, causing embolization, which can cause stroke.

PREDISPOSING FACTORS
A. Smoking.
B. High cholesterol levels in the blood.
C. High blood pressure.
D. Family history of atherosclerosis.
E. Sedentary lifestyle.
F. Diabetes or metabolic syndrome.

SUBJECTIVE DATA
A. Common complaints/symptoms.
   1. Amaurosis fugax (fleeting or transient ipsilateral visual loss).
   2. Transient ischemic attacks (TIAs).
   3. Crescendo TIAs.
   4. Stroke-in-evolution.
   5. Cerebral infarction.
B. Common/typical scenario.
   1. Patients may be asymptomatic with carotid artery disease.
   2. Sometimes it is found on routine surveillance.
   3. Patients oftentimes present with stroke symptoms, which depend on the location of the brain.
   4. Typically patients with a stroke from carotid artery disease present with weakness of extremities and speech difficulties.
C. Family and social history (pertinent findings—positive/negative).
   1. Ask about family history, which has a strong association.
   2. Ask about smoking, dietary habits, and physical activity.
D. Review of systems (pertinent findings—positive/negative).
   1. Neurology: Ask about the following:
      a. Numbness.
      b. Tingling or weakness.
      c. Speech difficulties.
      d. Confusion.
      e. Trouble swallowing.
      f. Visual disturbances.

PHYSICAL EXAMINATION
A. Thorough history.
B. Carotid bruit heard on auscultation.
C. Fundoscopic examination, if the patient presents with amaurosis fugax, hypertensive, or history of TIAs.
D. Cardiac auscultation for murmur.

DIAGNOSTIC TESTS
A. Imaging of the carotid artery is recommended in all patients with symptoms of carotid territory ischemia. This recommendation is based on the significant incidence of clinically relevant carotid stenosis in this patient group and the efficacy of carotid endarterectomy ▶

(CEA) for clinically significant lesions in reducing over-all stroke (grade 1, level of evidence A).

B. Imaging should be strongly considered in patients who present with amaurosis fugax, evidence of retinal artery embolization on fundoscopic examination, or asymptomatic cerebral infarction, and are candidates for CEA. This recommendation is based on the interme-diate stroke risk in this group of patients and the effi-cacy of CEA in reducing the risk of subsequent stroke (grade 1, level of evidence A).

C. Routine screening is *not* recommended to detect clinically asymptomatic carotid stenosis in the general population.

D. Diagnosis.

   1. Carotid duplex ultrasonography, with or without color: Screening test of choice to evaluate for carotid stenosis.

   2. CT angiography (CTA) is preferable to MRI/mag-netic resonance angiography (MRA) for delineating calcium.

   3. Carotid angiography.

   4. Carotid MRA: May be useful in collaborating the finding of an occluded carotid with duplex sonogra-phy; however, this modality tends to overstate the significance of the stenosis.

   5. Aortic arch and carotid arteriography: To evalu-ate the percentage of stenosis.

DIFFERENTIAL DIAGNOSIS

A. Stroke.

B. Intracerebral hemorrhage.

C. Neck trauma.

D. Headache.

E. Vertebral dissection.

F. Vertigo.

EVALUATION AND MANAGEMENT PLAN

A. General plan.

   1. For neurologically symptomatic patients with 50% stenosis or asymptomatic patients with 60% ste-nosis diameter reduction, optimal medical therapy is indicated (grade 1, level of evidence B).

   a. Grading carotid artery stenosis by ultrasound.

      i. Low-degree stenosis: 0% to 40%.

      ii. Moderate stenosis: 50% to 60%.

      iii. Hemodynamically relevant stenosis: Greater than 70%.

      iv. Other simplistic grade is mild stenosis (less than 50%), moderate stenosis (50%–70%), and severe stenosis (70% or greater).

   2. Antiplatelet therapy in asymptomatic patients with carotid atherosclerosis is recommended to reduce overall cardiovascular morbidity, although it has not been shown to be effective in the primary pre-vention of stroke.

   3. Surgical management.

   a. Carotid artery angioplasty and stenting.

      i. Indication for carotid angioplasty and stenting (CAS):

         1) Symptomatic patients with a high-grade stenosis (>70%) who are at high risk for CEA.

         2) Patients who are at high risk for CEA and have asymptomatic carotid stenosis greater than 80%.

         3) CAS is preferred over CEA in *symptom-atic* patients with 50% stenosis and prior ipsilateral operation, tracheal stoma, or external beam irradiation resulting in fibrosis of the tissues of the ipsilateral neck.

   b. CEA.

      i. Indications for CEA:

         1) Symptomatic patients with greater than 70% stenosis: Clear benefit was found in the North American Symptomatic Carotid Endarterectomy Trial (NASCET).

         2) Symptomatic patients with greater than 50% to 69% stenosis: Benefit is marginal; appears to be greater for male patients.

         3) Asymptomatic patients with greater than 60% stenosis: Benefit is significantly less than for symptomatic patients with greater than 70% stenosis.

         4) Generally, symptomatic patients with greater than 50% stenosis and healthy, asymptomatic patients with greater than 60% stenosis warrant consideration for CEA.

         5) Patients who present with repetitive (crescendo) episodes of transient cere-bral ischemia unresponsive to antiplatelet therapy should be considered for urgent CEA.

         6) CEA is preferred over CAS in patients 70 years of age, with long (>15 mm) lesions, preocclusive stenosis, or lipid-rich plaques that can be completely removed safely by a cervical incision in patients who have a vir-gin, nonradiated neck.

         7) Patients with symptomatic carotid ste-nosis will benefit from CEA prior to or con-comitant with coronary artery bypass graft. The timing of the intervention depends on clinical presentation and institutional experience.

         8) Patients with severe bilateral asymp-tomatic carotid stenosis (including steno-sis and contralateral occlusion) should be considered for CEA prior to or concomitant with coronary artery bypass graft.

      ii. Contraindications to CEA.

         1) Patients with severe neurologic deficit following a cerebral infarction.

         2) Patients with an occluded carotid artery.

         3) Concurrent medical illness that would significantly limit the patient's life expectancy.

▶

4) Anatomic issues that would be unfavorable for CEA include the following:
    a) Lesions that extend above C2.
    b) Prior irradiation of the neck.
    c) Prior neck operation.

B. Patient/family teaching points.

  1. Review lifestyle changes.
    a. Smoking cessation.
    b. Weight loss.
    c. Increasing physical activity.
    d. Consuming a healthy diet low in fat and cholesterol.

  2. Remind patients to take medication daily.

  3. Blood pressure management.

  4. Optimum blood sugar control in diabetes.

  5. Manage comorbid conditions.

  6. Educate patients on warning for stroke and regular follow-up.

  7. Patients should be instructed to seek help immediately if they have any worsening symptoms or signs and symptoms of a stroke.

C. Pharmacotherapy.

  1. Perioperative medical management of patients undergoing carotid revascularization should include blood pressure control (<140/80) or beta-blockade (heart rate [HR] 60–80).

  2. Management of cholesterol with statin therapy (low-density lipoprotein [LDL] 100 mg/dL).

  3. Perioperative antithrombotic therapy for CEA should include aspirin (81–325 mg).
    a. Antiplatelet agents (e.g., aspirin, ticlopidine, clopidogrel).
    b. Anticoagulants (e.g., warfarin): Note that use of warfarin in patients with noncardiac emboli is controversial. Anticoagulation is not recommended for treatment of TIA or acute stroke unless there is evidence of a cardioembolic source.

D. Discharge instructions.

  1. Eat a healthy diet.

  2. Limit salt.

  3. Maintain a healthy weight.

  4. Exercise as directed.

  5. Limit alcohol.

  6. Smoking cessation.

FOLLOW-UP

A. Medical therapy recommendation by guideline after intervention.

  1. Aspirin (30–325 mg/d) irreversibly acetylates the cyclooxygenase of platelets, thus inhibiting platelet synthesis of thromboxane.

  2. Ticlopidine (250 mg Q12H) is a thienopyridine that irreversibly alters the platelet membrane and inhibits platelet aggregation. It is approximately 10% more effective than aspirin. Toxicity includes neutropenia and diarrhea.

  3. Clopidogrel (75 mg/d) is used if the risk of neutropenia is low.

  4. Warfarin (titrated international normalized ratio [INR] 2–3) use in patients with noncardiac emboli is controversial.

  5. Antiplatelet therapy with cilostazol may reduce the progression of carotid artery stenosis after stent implantation.

B. Other recommendations for follow-up.

  1. A postoperative duplex ultrasound within 30 days is recommended to assess the status of the endarterectomized vessel.

  2. Imaging after CAS or CEA is indicated to follow contralateral disease progression in patients with 50% contralateral stenosis.

  3. In patients with multiple risk factors for vascular disease, follow-up duplex may be indicated with lesser degrees of stenosis. The likelihood of disease progression is related to the initial severity of stenosis (grade 2, level of evidence C).

  4. Risk factor modification: Lifestyle or medical interventions are implemented in order to address the following risk factors: Hypertension, hypercholesterolemia, and smoking.

CONSULTATION/REFERRAL

A. Referral to a cardiologist.

B. Vascular surgeon is recommended.

C. Intervention cardiologist.

SPECIAL/GERIATRIC CONSIDERATIONS

A. Benefits of CAS versus CEA should be strongly considered in older adults.

B. While older adult patients who had CEA had fewer incidents of stroke than those who had CAS, they had an increased risk of mortality and an increased rate of acute myocardial infarction (AMI).

BIBLIOGRAPHY

Brown, K., Itum, D. S., Preiss, J., Duwayri, Y., Veeraswamy, R. K., Salam, A., & Brewster, L. P. (2015). Carotid artery stenting has increased risk of external carotid artery occlusion compared with carotid endarterectomy. *Journal of Vascular Surgery, 61*(1), 119–124. https://doi.org/10.1016/j.jvs.2014.06.008

Mas, J. L., Trinquart, L., Leys, D., Albucher, J. F., Rousseau, H., Viguier, A., & Chatellier, G. (2008, October). Endarterectomy versus angioplasty in patients with symptomatic severe carotid stenosis (EVA-3S) trial: Results up to 4 years from a randomised, multicentre trial. *Lancet Neurology, 7*(10), 885–892. https://doi.org/10.1016/S1474-4422(08)70195-9

Moore, W. S., Popma, J. J., Roubin, G. S., Voeks, J. H., Cutlip, D. E., Jones, M., & Brott, T. G. (2016, April). Carotid angiographic characteristics in the CREST trial were major contributors to periprocedural stroke and death differences between carotid artery stenting and carotid endarterectomy. *Journal of Vascular Surgery, 63*(4), 851–858. e1. https://doi.org/10.1016/j.jvs.2015.08.119

Ricotta, J. J., Aburahma, A., Ascher, E., Eskandari, M., Faries, P., Lal, B. K., & Moore, W. S. (2011, September). Updated society for vascular surgery guidelines for management of extracranial carotid disease. *Journal of Vascular Surgery, 54*(3), e1–e31. https://doi.org/10.1016/j.jvs.2011.07.031

von Reutern, G. M., Goertler, M. W., Bornstein, N. M., Del Sette, M., Evans, D. H., Goertler, M.-W., Hetzel, A., Kaps, M., Perren, F., Razumovky, A., Shiogai, T., Titianova, E., Traubner, P., Venketasubramanian, N., Wong, L. K. S., & Yasaka, M. (2012). Grading carotid stenosis using ultrasonic methods. *Stroke, 43*, 916–921. https://doi.org/10.1161/STROKEAHA.111.636084

PERIPHERAL ARTERY DISEASE: LOWER EXTREMITY

DEFINITION

A. Lower extremity peripheral artery disease (PAD) is the obstruction of blood flow in the lower extremity arteries.

INCIDENCE

A. The incidence of lower extremity PAD increases with age.
  1. 5% of adults over 50 years of age.
  2. 14.5% of adults over 70 years of age.

PATHOGENESIS

A. Lower extremity PAD is frequently caused by atheroma in the walls of the arteries.
B. PAD, coronary artery disease, and cerebral artery disease are all manifestations of atherosclerosis and commonly occur together.

PREDISPOSING FACTORS

A. Age 70 years and older.
B. Age 50 to 69 years with a history of smoking or diabetes.
C. Age 40 to 49 with diabetes and at least one other risk factor for atherosclerosis.
D. Known atherosclerosis at other sites (e.g., coronary, carotid, renal artery disease).
E. Hypertension.
F. Smoking.
G. Hyperlipidemia.
H. Homocysteinemia.
I. Diabetes.

SUBJECTIVE DATA

A. Common complaints/symptoms.
  1. The PAD Fontaine Classification score lists the common symptoms in accordance with disease progression.
B. Common/typical scenario.
  1. Patient will report painful cramping during walking or exercise.
  2. Elicit the onset, duration, location, and intensity of pain. (Intermittent claudication pain is typically a muscle tightness in the buttock, thigh, or calf that comes on with exercise and is relieved at rest.)
  3. Inquire what aggravates and relieves the pain.
    a. Is the leg pain worse when legs are elevated or down?
    b. Is there resting pain or nocturnal cramping? (With critical limb ischemia [CLI], resting leg pain is aggravated when the legs are elevated.)
  4. Question the patient about cardiovascular-related conditions such as coronary artery disease, myocardial infarction, carotid artery disease, trans-ischemic attack, or strokes.
  5. Question the patient about other medical conditions such as diabetes, chronic kidney disease, heart failure, chronic obstructive pulmonary disease, and hematology conditions.
  6. Inquire about musculoskeletal conditions such as osteoarthritis and spinal degeneration.
C. Review of systems.
  1. Musculoskeletal.
    a. Inquire about aching, tightness, or squeezing pain in the calf, thigh, or buttocks.
    b. Ask about pain before walking versus pain that starts during walking.

PHYSICAL EXAMINATION

A. Atherosclerotic disease is a diffuse process. Therefore, the examination, regardless of the complaint (intermittent claudication, angina, transient ischemic attack [TIA]), should include the entire arterial system.
  1. Check blood pressure in both arms, heart rate (HR), and rhythm.
  2. Inspect full length of the upper and lower extremities: Dry, shiny hairless skin, muscle atrophy, color, necrotic and/or gangrenous ulcers, or evidence of distal embolization in the fingers and/or toes (blue toe syndrome).
  3. Auscultate.
    a. Heart to listen for arrhythmias, gallops, and murmurs.
    b. Carotid, brachial, abdominal aorta, femoral, and popliteal pulses to listen for bruits.
    c. Lung fields.
  4. Palpate.
    a. Abdomen to assess for a pulsatile mass (aortic aneurysm).
    b. Leg: Femoral, popliteal, dorsalis pedis, and post tibial pulses.
    c. Arm: Brachial, radial, and ulnar pulses.
    d. Check capillary refill, strength, and sensation of the upper and lower extremities.
  5. Buerger test to assess for positional rubra (with significant PAD, foot is paler with elevation and then rubrous or cyanotic in the dependent position).
  6. 10-g monofilament foot test to assess for peripheral neuropathy.

DIAGNOSTIC TESTS

A. The ankle brachial index (ABI) has high sensitivity and specificity in identifying PAD. Inclusion of the toe brachial index (TBI) or continuous-wave Doppler (if tissue is intact) assessment increases detection of a serious PAD.
B. Radiologic imaging of arterial leg circulation such as ultrasound, CT, or MRI is best reserved for vascular services as part of treatment decision and workup.
C. Abdominal aorta screening is recommended due to the correlation between peripheral artery disease (PAD) and abdominal aortic aneurysm (AAA). Ultrasound is the modality of choice.
D. Hematologic evaluation: Complete blood count, fasting blood glucose, fasting lipids, serum creatinine, and urinalysis.

DIFFERENTIAL DIAGNOSIS

A. Arterial aneurysm.
B. Arterial dissection.
C. Embolism.
D. Popliteal entrapment syndrome.
E. Adventitial cystic disease.
F. Thromboangiitis obliterans (Buerger disease).
G. Limb trauma.
H. Nonarterial etiologies for limb pain: Neurogenic, musculoskeletal causes, and pathologic.

EVALUATION AND MANAGEMENT PLAN

A. General plan.
  1. PAD management is dependent on symptom severity, comorbid condition, and whether or not the patient will experience a meaningful benefit from a technically successful procedure.
  2. Patients with PAD should have a cardiovascular risk reduction plan.
    a. Smoking cessation is critical.
    b. Treatment of diabetes if applicable to achieve hemoglobin A1C (HbA1C) less than 5.5 mmol/L.
    c. Healthy diet and exercise.
    d. Hematologic evaluation (see "Diagnostics Tests"). Results will guide further therapy.
    e. Additional management plan for patients with intermittent claudication (Fontaine IIa and IIb) includes:
      i. Structured exercise program.
      ii. Referral to vascular service if intermittent claudication is lifestyle-limiting and the patient may benefit from revascularization treatment.
  3. CLI (Fontaine III) and necrosis and gangrene (Fontaine IV) management plan will depend on progression of limb symptoms, comorbid conditions, and conduit availability.
    a. Supportive measures may include:
      i. Wound management.
      ii. Antibiotic therapy if there is underlying cellulitis or wound infection (consider flucloxacillin).
      iii. Pain management.
    b. Vascular treatment may include:
      i. Endovascular revascularization.
      ii. Bypass surgery.
      iii. Digit or limb amputation.
B. Patient/family teaching points.
  1. Patients should seek out a provider if they experience pain, numbness, tingling, weakness, or significant temperature change in their extremities.
  2. Patients should also report open sores that do not heal.
C. Pharmacotherapy.
  1. Antiplatelet therapy with long-term low-dose aspirin.

  2. Treatment of hyperlipidemia with a statin to achieve a low-density lipoprotein (LDL) level less than 100 mg/dL (<70 mg/dL if PAD and a history of coronary or cerebral artery disease).
  3. Treatment of hypertension to achieve a blood pressure less than 140/90 mmHg (<130/80 mmHg for patients with diabetes or renal failure).
  4. Consider pharmacology therapy. In the United States, only pentoxifylline and cilostazol have achieved Food and Drug Administration (FDA) approval for treatment of intermittent claudication.
D. Discharge instructions.
  1. Patients need to be taught to make healthy dietary changes, keep cholesterol levels down, maintain a healthy weight, and stop smoking.

FOLLOW-UP

A. Three-month primary care review of cardiovascular risk management.
B. If treated percutaneously or surgically, outpatient vascular review after 4 to 6 weeks.

CONSULTATION/REFERRAL

A. Consultation and referral are dependent on symptom status. Patients with lower extremity PAD have a wide spectrum of symptoms.
  1. Fontaine classification I, asymptomatic: Conservative management.
  2. Fontaine classification IIa, intermittent claudication greater than 200 m (and nonlifestyle-limiting): Conservative management.
  3. Fontaine classification IIb, intermittent claudication less than 200 m (or lifestyle-limiting): Refer to vascular service.
  4. Fontaine classification III, nocturnal or resting pain: Referral to vascular service.
  5. Fontaine classification IV, necrosis and gangrene: For hospital admission, vascular consult.

SPECIAL/GERIATRIC CONSIDERATIONS

A. Patients with PAD are usually older adults.
B. Younger patients are usually diabetic.

BIBLIOGRAPHY

Cronenwett, J. L., & Johnston, K. W. (2014). *Rutherford's vascular surgery* (8th ed.). Elsevier Saunders.

Mitchell, M. E., & Carpenter, J. P. (2017). *Overview of acute arterial occlusion of the extremities (acute limb ischaemia)*. www.uptodate.com

Neschis, D. G., & Golden, M. A. (2018, June 11). *Clinical features and diagnosis of lower extremity peripheral artery disease*. In K. A. Collins (Ed.), *UpToDate*. https://www.uptodate.com/contents/clinical-features-and-diagnosis-of-lower-extremity-peripheral-artery-disease

Rasmussen, T. E., Clouse, W. D., & Tonnessen, B. H. (2011). *Handbook of patient care in vascular diseases* (5th ed.). Wolters Kluwer Health.

Tehan, P. E., Bray, A., & Chuter, V. H. (2016). Non-invasive vascular assessment in the foot with diabetes: Sensitivity and specificity of the ankle brachial index, toe brachial index and continuous wave Doppler for detecting peripheral arterial disease. *Journal of Diabetes and Its Complications*, 30(1), 155–160. https://doi.org/10.1016/j.jdiacomp.2015.07.019

DEFINITION

A. Upper extremity arterial disease is the obstruction of blood flow in the large and/or small arterial vessels of the upper extremity arteries.

INCIDENCE

A. Upper extremity arterial disease is relatively rare. It accounts for less than 5% of patients presenting with limb ischemia.

PATHOGENESIS

A. Arterial vasospasm: Raynaud phenomenon, ergotism, and vinyl chloride exposure.
B. Arterial obstruction.
   1. Atherosclerosis (main cause of upper extremity arterial disease).
   2. Thoracic outlet compression.
   3. Embolic (e.g., cardiac or thoracic outlet in origin) and aneurysms.
   4. Arteritis (e.g., Takayasu arteritis or giant cell arteritis).
   5. Fibromuscular disease.
   6. Hypersensitivity angiitis.
   7. Iatrogenic, cold, or vibration injury.
   8. Dialysis steal syndrome.
   9. Connective tissue disease (e.g., scleroderma, rheumatoid arthritis, systemic lupus).
   10. Myeloproliferative disorders and hypercoagulable states.
   11. Infection from injection of drugs and arterial procedures.
C. Bilateral symptoms may be from a systemic cause, such as a connective tissue disorder.
D. Unilateral symptoms may be from a discrete occlusive lesion.

PREDISPOSING FACTORS

A. Dependent on pathogenesis.
B. Patients who present with upper extremity ischemia range from young adults with nonatherosclerotic causes to older adult patients with atherosclerosis.
C. Risk factors include smoking, hypercholesterolemia, hypertension, diabetes, and age.

SUBJECTIVE DATA

A. Common complaints/symptoms.
   1. Most patients with upper extremity arterial disease are asymptomatic; the condition is only detected by finding asymmetric arm blood pressures.
B. Common/typical scenario.
   1. Raynaud phenomenon: Predictable sequence of color changes in the finger and/or hand.
      a. Pallor (white), followed by cyanosis (blue), and then rubor (red).
      b. Often associated with finger numbness.

      c. Pain is generally not severe, unless ulceration is present.
      d. Symptoms are activated by exposure to cold and emotional stimuli.
   2. Arm intermittent claudication is an unusual presentation of arm ischemia due to excellent collateral blood flow around the shoulder. However, active adults, particularly manual laborers, may experience arm claudication from subclavian or brachial artery stenosis.
   3. Dizziness, or even syncope, during arm exertion may be from subclavian steal syndrome.
   4. Patients with chronic upper extremity ischemia may complain of change in sensation, hand temperature, and muscle pain with use.
   5. Tissue necrosis includes gangrene and poorly healing ulcerations of the fingers. (Patients may dismiss small ulcers caused by microemboli as inconsequential bruises or sores.)
   6. Acute limb ischemia (ALI) is covered previously.
C. Family and social history.
   1. Elicit the onset, duration, location, and intensity; aggravates and relieves pain.
   2. Inquire about the signs and symptoms of connective tissue disease, such as dry eyes, difficulty swallowing, dry mouth, and arthritis.
   3. Question the patient about any history of trauma, including upper extremity access for peripheral or coronary catheterization.
   4. Inquire about occupational and recreational history regarding exposure to vibrating tools or toxins, as well as repetitive trauma.
   5. Question the patient about cardiovascular-related conditions such as coronary artery disease, myocardial infarction, carotid artery disease, transient ischemic attack (TIA), or strokes.
   6. Question the patient about other medical conditions such as diabetes, chronic kidney disease, heart failure, chronic obstructive pulmonary disease, or hematology conditions.
   7. Inquire about musculoskeletal conditions such as osteoarthritis or rotator cuff injury.
D. Review of systems.
   1. Musculoskeletal: Ask about arm pain with movement and at rest. Ask about any swelling.
   2. Dermatology: Ask about ulceration of fingers or discoloration.

PHYSICAL EXAMINATION

A. Take blood pressure in both arms.
   1. A difference of 10 mmHg or more suggests a hemodynamically significant innominate, subclavian, or axillary artery stenosis.
   2. In cases of suspected claudication, arm blood pressure should be measured at rest and after 2 to 5 minutes of exercise.
B. Inspect.
   1. Hands and fingers; note temperature, color, capillary refill, ulcers, and any other lesions.

2. Fingers for clubbing, which is associated with chronic pulmonary disease. (Patients with clubbing and cold fingers may have low arterial oxygen levels as the basis of their complaint).

3. Fingers for telangiectasia and sclerodactyly, which are commonly seen with advanced scleroderma as well as other connective tissue diseases.

4. Check for splinter hemorrhages in the nail beds, which are seen with emboli.

C. Auscultate.

1. Heart to listen for arrhythmias, gallops, and murmurs.

2. Supraclavicular and infraclavicular fossa to listen for bruits, which may indicate possible subclavian artery stenosis. A supraclavicular pulsatile mass is associated with a subclavian aneurysm or cervical rib.

D. Palpate.

1. Upper extremity pulses.

a. Axillary and proximal brachial artery: The upper medial arm in the groove between the biceps and the triceps muscles.

b. Brachial artery: The antecubital fossa just medial to the biceps tendon.

c. Radial artery: The wrist over the distal radius.

d. Ulnar artery: The wrist over the distal ulna.

2. Carotid, abdominal aorta, femoral, popliteal, dorsalis pedis, and post tibial pulses.

E. Handheld Doppler.

1. Assess upper extremity pulses, including digital pulses, and note if the pulse is monophasic, biphasic, or triphasic.

F. Neurologic examination, including muscle mass, muscle strength, and sensation to assess for compression of the neurovascular bundle (see "Thoracic Outlet Syndrome").

G. Additional bedside examination.

1. Allen test is recommended if there is a difference in arm blood pressure or if there is a reduced radial or ulnar pulse.

a. Allen test should be conducted on both arms.

b. A positive Allen test suggests that there is adequate dual blood supply to the hand.

i. Elevate the hand and ask the patient to clench their fist for 30 seconds.

ii. Pressure is applied over the ulnar and radial arteries to occlude both of them.

iii. The hand is then opened. It should appear blanched.

iv. One artery is tested by releasing the pressure over that artery to see if the hand flushes (color should return within 5–15 seconds).

v. The other artery is then tested in a similar fashion.

2. Adson test and Roos test can assist in assessing for thoracic outlet syndrome (TOS; see "Thoracic Outlet Syndrome").

DIAGNOSTIC TESTS

A. Vascular laboratory: Segmental pressure measurements of the upper extremity and finger pressure measurements and waveforms.

B. Radiologic imaging of arterial arm circulation such as duplex ultrasound, CT, and MRI is best reserved for vascular services as part of treatment decision and workup.

C. Hematologic evaluation.

1. Erythrocyte sedimentation rate, C-reactive protein, antiphospholipid antibodies, antinuclear antibody titer, and rheumatoid factor to screen for underlying autoimmune disease.

2. Platelet count since thrombocytosis can mimic Raynaud phenomenon.

3. Serum protein electrophoresis since serum protein abnormalities may be associated with vasospasms.

4. In patients at risk of or with suspected atherosclerotic disease, fasting lipids, fasting glucose, or serum creatinine.

DIFFERENTIAL DIAGNOSIS

A. Multiple etiologies; see "Pathogenesis."

B. Differential diagnosis includes neurogenic, musculoskeletal, and pathologic causes.

EVALUATION AND MANAGEMENT PLAN

A. General plan.

1. All patients with upper extremity arterial disease should have a cardiovascular risk reduction plan based on their 5-year cardiovascular risk assessment.

2. Treat the underlying cause.

a. Primary Raynaud phenomenon: Conservative management; patients are advised to minimize cold exposure and stress.

b. Emboli: Manage arrhythmia and anticoagulate.

c. Connective tissue diseases: Manage the disease process.

d. Occupational and recreational factors: Advise patients to minimize exposure.

3. Supportive measures.

a. Wound management.

b. Antibiotic if there is underlying cellulitis or wound infection (consider flucloxacillin).

c. Pain management.

4. Vascular treatment may include:

a. Endovascular revascularization.

b. Bypass surgery.

c. Digit or limb amputation.

B. Patient/family teaching points.

1. Patients should seek out a provider if they experience any pain, numbness, tingling, weakness, or significant temperature change in their extremities.

2. Patients should also report open sores that do not heal.

C. Pharmacotherapy.

1. Frequent or severe symptoms.

a. Nifedipine 30 to 180 mg/d or amlodipine 5 to 20 mg/d.

2. Start with lowest dose and gradually increase, if needed, depending on the response.

D. Discharge instructions (if standard accepted guidelines exist, please use discharge template).

1. Make healthy dietary changes.
2. Keep cholesterol levels down.
3. Maintain a healthy weight.
4. Smoking cessation.

FOLLOW-UP

A. Depends on pathogenesis: Outpatient follow-up with vascular, cardiology, or rheumatology service.

B. Three-month primary care review of cardiovascular risk management.

CONSULTATION/REFERRAL

A. Consultation and referral are dependent on the pathogenesis and severity of symptoms.

1. If clinical presentation is suggestive of large vessel disease, refer to vascular service.
2. If hematologic screening is positive for autoimmune disease, refer to rheumatology service.
3. ALI for urgent hospital admission (see "Acute Limb Ischemia").
4. Necrosis and gangrene: For hospital admission, seek a vascular consult.

SPECIAL/GERIATRIC CONSIDERATIONS

A. Older adult patients may not report or experience intermittent claudication.

B. Older adult patients may have decreased blood flow and other circulatory problems that put them at special risk of being unaware of any issues or problems.

BIBLIOGRAPHY

Barshes, N. R. (2017, November 22). *Overview of upper extremity peripheral artery disease*. In K. A. Collins (Ed.), *UpToDate*. https://www.uptodate.com/contents/overview-of-upper-extremity-peripheral-artery-disease

Cronenwett, J. L., & Johnston, K. W. (2014). *Rutherford's vascular surgery* (8th ed.). Elsevier Saunders.

Mitchell, M. E., & Carpenter, J. P. (2017). *Overview of acute arterial occlusion of the extremities (acute limb ischaemia)*. www.uptodate.com

Rasmussen, T. E., Clouse, W. D., & Tonnessen, B. H. (2011). *Handbook of patient care in vascular diseases* (5th ed.). Wolters Kluwer Health.

PERIPHERAL VASCULAR DISEASE

DEFINITION

A. Peripheral vascular disease (PVD) refers to diseases of the blood vessels located outside the heart and brain.

B. Peripheral artery disease (PAD) develops only in the arteries. PAD is the most common form of PVD.

INCIDENCE

A. The Centers for Disease Control and Prevention (CDC) reports approximately 12% to 20% of people over age 60 develop PAD; it affects 15% to 20% of persons older than 70 years of age.

B. PAD affects about 8.5 million Americans.

C. The prevalence of PAD, both symptomatic and asymptomatic, is greater in men than in women, especially in young persons. At very advanced ages, almost no differences exist between sexes. However, age remains the main marker of PAD risk.

D. The estimated prevalence of intermittent claudication in persons aged 60 to 65 years is 35%. However, the prevalence in persons 10 years older (70–75 years) rises to 70%.

PATHOGENESIS

A. PVD is a slow and progressive circulation disorder caused by narrowing, blockage, or spasms in a blood vessel. PAD is considered a set of chronic or acute syndromes, generally derived from the presence of occlusive arterial disease, which causes inadequate blood flow to the limbs.

B. On most occasions, the underlying disease process is arteriosclerotic disease, mainly affecting vascularization to the lower limbs.

C. From the pathophysiologic point of view, ischemia of the lower limbs can be classified as functional or critical due to an imbalance between the needs of the peripheral tissues and the blood supply.

D. Functional ischemia occurs when the blood flow is normal at rest but insufficient during exercise, presenting clinically as intermittent claudication.

E. Critical ischemia is produced when the reduction in blood flow results in a perfusion deficit at rest and is defined by the presence of pain at rest or trophic lesions in the legs.

PREDISPOSING FACTORS

A. Age over 50.
B. Postmenopausal women have a higher risk.
C. Overweight and obesity.
D. Dyslipidemia.
E. Hyperhomocysteinemia.
F. History of cerebrovascular disease or stroke.
G. History of heart disease.
H. History of diabetes.
I. High blood pressure.
J. Family history of high cholesterol, high blood pressure, or PVD.
K. Kidney disease on hemodialysis.
L. Lifestyle choices that can increase risk of developing PVD include:

1. Sedentary lifestyle or not engaging in physical exercise.
2. Unhealthy dietary habits.
3. Smoking increases risk by seven times.
4. Drug use.
5. Excessive alcohol.

SUBJECTIVE DATA

A. Common complaints/symptoms.

1. The first signs of PVD begin slowly and irregularly.
2. Fatigue or cramping in legs and feet that gets worse with physical activity due to the lack of blood flow is the earliest sign patients often report.

3. Leg cramps when lying in bed may occur.

4. Poor hair growth often below the knees.

5. Legs and arms may turn reddish blue or pale.

6. Skin in the extremities may appear pale and thin.

7. Pulses in the extremities may be weak.

8. Ulcers and wounds in legs and toes that will not heal.

9. Toes may appear blue in color and the toenails become thick and opaque.

10. Patients often experience severe burning in toes.

11. In severe cases, pain may occur even at rest, particularly at night when the legs are raised in bed.

12. In a small number of cases (often untreated), tissue death (gangrene) of a foot may result.

13. If an artery higher upstream is narrowed, such as the iliac artery, pain may be experienced in the thighs or buttocks while walking.

B. Common/typical scenario.

1. Patients will typically present with intermittent claudication, which is cramping with exercise that resolves with rest.

2. If the patient has severe disease progression, they may present with pain in the legs that occurs at rest.

C. Family and social history.

1. Ask about family history of any vascular disease or diabetes.

2. Ask about smoking and if the patient has sedentary lifestyle or poor eating habits.

D. Review of systems.

1. Musculoskeletal: Ask about leg cramps, pain at rest, or if patients raise their legs at night.

2. Neurologic: Ask about numbness or severe burning in toes.

3. Dermatologic: Ask about discoloration of extremities, ulcers, or wounds that do not heal, and/or nails that have become thick and opaque.

PHYSICAL EXAMINATION

A. Basic examination of PVD includes assessment for presence of pulses in the lower limbs, including the femoral, popliteal, pedal, and posterior tibial arteries.

B. Auscultation of the abdomen will enable identification of the presence of murmurs, which are indicative of disease in the aorta or the iliac arteries. Auscultation of the inguinal region may reveal the presence of lesions in the external iliac or femoral bifurcation vessels.

C. Check the temperature, color, and capillary refill of the foot. Patients with claudication do not usually show a reduction in temperature or capillary filling.

D. Leg dangling test: A reduction in temperature and paleness, with or without cyanosis or dangling erythrosis, are common in patients with critical ischemia.

E. Patients with PAD have a higher risk of developing critical limb ischemia (CLI).

1. Patients with CLI should undergo expedited evaluation and treatment of factors that are known to increase the risk of amputation.

2. Patients with CLI in whom open surgical repair is anticipated should undergo assessment of cardiovascular risk.

3. Patients with CLI and skin breakdown should be referred to healthcare providers with specialized expertise in wound care.

4. Patients at risk of CLI (those with diabetes, neuropathy, chronic renal failure, or infection) who develop acute limb symptoms represent potential vascular emergencies and should be assessed immediately and treated by a specialist competent in treating vascular disease.

F. Chronic foot and leg ulcers (Table 11.2).

G. Stages of PVD:

1. Stage I is characterized by absence of symptoms. It includes patients who have an extensive occlusive arterial lesion in the legs, or have high risk but present no symptoms of arterial failure. In these situations, patients may present with critical ischemia straight from an asymptomatic stage.

2. Stage II is characterized by presence of intermittent claudication. The intermittent claudication that is typical in patients with PAD is defined as the appearance of pain in muscle masses caused by walking and which ceases immediately after stopping exercise. Of note, a great number of patients report pain in the legs associated with walking, but not with presence of arterial disease. Stage II is itself divided into groups.

a. Stage IIa includes patients with noninvalidating claudication that impedes walking long distances.

b. Stage IIb refers to patients with short claudication or claudication that impedes activities of daily living.

3. Stage III constitutes a more advanced phase of ischemia and is characterized by presence of symptoms at rest. The predominant symptom is usually pain, although patients often report paresthesia and hypoesthesia.

4. Stage IV is characterized by presence of tropical lesions. It is due to the critical reduction of distal perfusion pressure, which is insufficient to maintain tissue tropism. These lesions are situated in the more distal areas of the limb, usually the toes, although on occasions they may present in the malleolus or the heel.

DIAGNOSTIC TESTS

A. The diagnosis is usually made by the typical symptoms, history, and physical examination.

B. Homocysteine level to rule out hyperhomocysteinemia.

C. An ankle brachial index (ABI), toe brachial index (TBI), and/or exercise ABI must be ordered.

D. Pulse volume recording or plethysmography: Recording the pulse wave volumes along the limb by plethysmography is particularly useful in patients in whom arterial calcification prevents a reliable recording ▶

TABLE 11.2 HOW TO DIFFERENTIATE FOOT ULCER AND PAIN

Neuropathic Ulcer	Ischemic Ulcer
Often painless	Extremely painful
Normal pulses	Absent pulses
Typically punched-out appearance	Irregular margins
Often located on the sole or edge of foot or the metatarsal head	Commonly located or starts on the toes
Presence of calluses	Calluses absent or infrequent
Loss of sensation, reflexes, and vibration sense	Variable sensory findings present
Increase in blood flow (arteriovenous shunting)	Decrease in blood flow
Dilated veins	Collapsed veins
Dry, warm foot	Cold foot
Bone deformities	No bony deformities
Red appearance	Pale, cyanotic

Sources: From Armstrong, D. G., & Lavery, L. A. (1998, March 15). Diabetic foot ulcers: Prevention, diagnosis and classification. *American Family Physician, 57*(6), 1325–1332. https://www.aafp.org/afp/1998/0315/p1325.html; Cleveland Clinic. (n.d.). Leg and foot ulcers. http://my.clevelandclinic.org/heart/disorders/vascular/legfootulcer.aspx; Frykberg, R. G. (2002, November 1). Diabetic foot ulcers: Pathogenesis and management. *American Family Physician, 66*(9), 1655–1663. http://www.aafp.org/afp/2002/1101/p1655.html; Jeffcoate, W. J., & Harding, K. G. (2003). Diabetic foot ulcers. *The Lancet, 361*(9368), 1545–1551. https://doi.org/10.1016/S0140-6736(03)13169-8.

of systolic pressures. Transmetatarsal or digital recording provides important information about the state of the vascularization in this zone.

E. Segmental pressure examination or Doppler recording of velocimetric wave can also provide very useful information by means of evaluating changes in the different components of the arterial velocimetric wave.

F. Duplex ultrasound of the extremities is useful in diagnosing the anatomic location and the degree of stenosis of PAD. It may be used in select candidates for endovascular intervention and surgical bypass, and to select the sites of surgical anastomosis. It may also be used for surveillance following femoralpopliteal bypass using venous conduit (but not prosthetic grafts).

G. Imaging techniques are indicated if surgical or endovascular repair is contemplated after identification of a susceptible lesion.

1. CT angiography (CTA) produces an excellent arterial picture; however, it requires iodinated contrast. CTA may be considered to diagnose anatomic location and the presence of significant stenosis in patients with lower extremity PAD and as a substitute for magnetic resonance angiography (MRA) in patients with contraindications to MRA.

2. MRA has virtually replaced contrast arteriography for PAD diagnosis. The advantages of MRA include the following:

a. Excellent arterial picture and no ionizing radiation; noniodine-based intravenous contrast medium rarely causes renal insufficiency or allergic reaction. However, about 10% of patients cannot

utilize MRA due to claustrophobia, having a pacemaker/implantable cardioverter-defibrillator, or because they are obese.

b. The major challenge with MRA is that gadolinium use in individuals with an estimated glomerular filtration rate (eGFR) less than 60 mL/min has been associated with nephrogenic systemic fibrosis (NSF)/nephrogenic fibrosing dermopathy.

c. MRA is useful in diagnosing the anatomic location and the degree of stenosis of PAD, as well as in selecting patients with lower extremity PAD as candidates for endovascular intervention.

DIFFERENTIAL DIAGNOSIS

A. For leg pain or claudication with normal physiologic testing, a provider needs to consider the following (not PAD-related):

1. Symptomatic Baker cyst.

2. Chronic compartment syndrome.

3. Spinal stenosis.

4. Nerve root compression: Arthritis of the hip, ankle, or foot.

EVALUATION AND MANAGEMENT PLAN

A. General plan.

1. The two main goals of PVD treatment are to stop the disease from progressing and to manage pain and symptoms so patients can remain active. The treatments are aimed to lower the risk of serious complications.

2. Antiplatelet therapy.

3. Smoking cessation, as well as avoiding environmental smoking and secondhand smoking.

4. Good glycemic control.

5. Surgical management.

    a. Endovascular revascularization.

        i. Endovascular procedures are effective as a revascularization option in patients with lifestyle-limiting claudication.

        ii. Endovascular procedures are recommended to establish in-line blood flow to the foot in patients with nonhealing wounds or gangrene. A staged approach may be done in patients with ischemic rest pain.

    b. Surgical revascularization: Bypass or graft to restore blood flow. Surgical revascularization is performed; bypass to the popliteal artery with autogenous vein is recommended in preference to prosthetic graft material.

    c. Angioplasty of the blocked peripheral artery is a procedure to open narrowed or blocked blood vessels that supply blood to the legs. Fatty deposits can build up inside the arteries and block blood flow.

B. Patient/family teaching points.

    1. Pain management to enhance activity.

    2. Exercise and physical activity: Structured exercise program and home-based exercise program.

        a. Any exertional limitation of the lower extremity muscles or any history of walking impairment, described as fatigue, aching, numbness, or pain.

        b. The primary site(s) of discomfort in the buttock, thigh, calf, or foot, and the relation of such discomfort to rest or exertion.

    3. Look for any poorly healing or nonhealing wounds of the legs or feet.

    4. Note any pain at rest localized to the lower leg or foot and its association with the upright or recumbent positions.

    5. Watch for postprandial abdominal pain that reproducibly is provoked by eating and is associated with weight loss.

    6. Family history of a first-degree relative with an abdominal aortic aneurysm (AAA).

    7. Pulse intensity should be assessed and should be recorded numerically from 0 to 3 (0 = absent, 1 = diminished, 2 = normal, and 3 = bounding).

C. Pharmacotherapy.

    1. Statin therapy.

    2. Antihypertensive therapy: Angiotensin-converting enzyme (ACE) inhibitors.

    3. Oral anticoagulation (warfarin) in improving lower extremity bypass patency demonstrated improved patency among the subgroup of patients with autogenous vein bypass grafts.

    4. Cilostazol increases blood flow and relieves symptoms of claudication.

D. Discharge instructions.

    1. Patients should be encouraged to maintain a healthy diet, stop smoking, control diabetes, and begin an exercise program.

FOLLOW-UP

A. PVD is a lifelong chronic medical condition. Ongoing care focuses on cardiovascular risk reduction with medical therapy, optimizing functional status with structured exercise, and when indicated revascularization.

B. Patients with PVD who have undergone lower extremity revascularization (surgical and/or endovascular) should be followed up with periodic clinical evaluation and ABI measurement.

C. Duplex ultrasound is recommended for routine surveillance after femoralpopliteal or femoral–tibial–pedal bypass with a venous conduit. Minimum surveillance intervals are approximately 3, 6, and 12 months, and then yearly after graft placement.

CONSULTATION/REFERRAL

A. Interdisciplinary care team members must be included.

B. Care team members may include:

    1. Vascular medical and surgical specialists (e.g., vascular medicine, vascular surgery, interventional radiology, interventional cardiology).

    2. Orthopedic surgeons and podiatrists.

    3. Endocrinologists.

    4. Infectious disease specialists.

    5. Radiology and vascular imaging specialists.

    6. Physical medicine and rehabilitation clinicians.

    7. Orthotics and prosthetics specialists.

    8. Social workers.

    9. Exercise physiologists.

    10. Physical and occupational therapists.

    11. Nutritionists/dietitians.

SPECIAL/GERIATRIC CONSIDERATIONS

A. Older adults may not experience intermittent claudication due to comorbidities that limit walking, such as arthritis, spinal stenosis, heart failure, and pulmonary disease. Hence, management of comorbidities is vital in the management of PAD.

B. Older adults also need a more sensitive diagnostic test for PAD to identify those with asymptomatic PVD.

C. Older adults may also benefit from early diagnosis by screening for asymptomatic PAD.

D. It would be beneficial for older adults to have an established structured or supervised exercise program rather than an unsupervised exercise program.

E. Cilostazol increases maximal walking distance, pain-free walking distance, and the quality of life of the older adult population.

BIBLIOGRAPHY

Alonso-Coello, P., Bellmunt, S., McGorrian, C., Anand, S. S., Guzman, R., Criqui, M. H., Akl, E. A., Vandvik, P. O., Lansberg, M. G., Guyatt, G. H., & Spencer, F. A. (2012, February). Antithrombotic therapy in peripheral artery disease: Antithrombotic therapy and prevention of thrombosis, 9th ed.: American College of chest physicians evidence-based clinical practice guidelines. *Chest, 141*(2 Suppl), e669S–e690S. https://doi.org/10.1378/chest.11-2307

Armstrong, D. G., & Lavery, L. A. (1998, March 15). Diabetic foot ulcers: Prevention, diagnosis and classification. *American Family Physician, 57*(6), 1325–1332. https://www.aafp.org/afp/1998/0315/p1325.html

Cleveland Clinic. (n.d). *Leg and foot ulcers*. http://my.clevelandclinic.org/heart/disorders/vascular/legfootulcer.aspx

Frykberg, R. G. (2002, November 1). Diabetic foot ulcers: Pathogenesis and management. *American Family Physician, 66*(9), 1655–1663. http://www.aafp.org/afp/2002/1101/p1655.html

Gerhard-Herman, M. D., Gornick, H. L., Barrett, C., Barshes, N. R., Corriere, M. A., Drachman, D. E., Fleisher, L. A., Fowkes, F. G. R., Hamburg, N. M., Kinlay, S., Lookstein, R., Misra, S., Mureebe, L., Olin, J. W., Patel, R. A. G., Regensteiner, J. G., Schanzer, A., Shishehbor, M. H., Stewart, K. J. ... Walsh, M. E. (2016). 2016 AHA/ACC Guideline on the management of patients with lower extremity peripheral artery disease: A report of the American College of Cardiology/American Heart Association task force on clinical practice guidelines. *Journal of the American College of Cardiology, 69*, 1465–1508. https://doi.org/10.1016/j.jacc.2016.11.008

Jackson, E. A., Munir, K., Schreiber, T., Rubin, J. R., Cuff, R., Gallagher, K. A., Henke, P. K., Gurm, H. S., & Grossman, P. M. (2014, June 17). Impact of sex on morbidity and mortality rates after lower extremity interventions for peripheral arterial disease: Observations from the blue cross blue shield of Michigan cardiovascular consortium. *Journal of American College of Cardiology, 63*(23), 2525–2530. https://doi.org/10.1016/j.jacc.2014.03.036

Jeffcoate, W. J., & Harding, K. G. (2003). Diabetic foot ulcers. *The Lancet, 361*, 1545–1551. https://doi.org/10.1016/S0140-6736(03)13169-8

Suzuki, J., Shimamura, M., Suda, H., Wakayama, K., Kumagai, H., Ikeda, Y., Akazawa, H., Isobe, M., Komuro, I., & Morishita, R. (2016, April). Current therapies and investigational drugs for peripheral arterial disease. *Hypertension Research, 39*(4), 183–191. https://doi.org/10.1038/hr.2015.134

THORACIC OUTLET SYNDROME

DEFINITION

A. Thoracic outlet syndrome (TOS) is a constellation of signs and symptoms that arise from compression of the neurovascular bundle just above the first rib and behind the clavicle, within the confined space of the thoracic outlet.

INCIDENCE

A. TOS is uncommon and its true incidence is unknown.
B. Most patients are 20 to 50 years old, less than 5% are teenagers, and 10% are older than 50.
C. 70% are female.

PATHOGENESIS

A. Neurogenic thoracic outlet syndrome (nTOS) arises from brachial plexus compression.
  1. It accounts for more than 95% of TOS cases.
  2. It is associated with developmental anomalies of the thoracic outlet and fibrosis of the scalene muscle.
  3. The most common causes are hyperextension neck trauma (motor vehicle accident whiplash) and repetitive stress injuries.
B. Venous thoracic outlet syndrome (vTOS) arises from subclavian vein compression.

  1. It accounts for 3% of TOS cases.
  2. It is often a result of developmental anomalies of the costoclavicular space and repetitive arm activities.
  3. In vTOS, a focal area of scarred subclavian intima narrows the lumen. Thrombus is the final event that occludes the vein.
  4. It is typically asymptomatic until a venous thrombolytic event occurs.
C. Arterial thoracic outlet syndrome (aTOS) arises from subclavian artery compression.
  1. It accounts for 1% of TOS cases.
  2. It is almost always associated with a cervical rib or anomalous rib.
  3. aTOS subclavian artery stenosis is accompanied by poststenotic dilatation that gives the appearance of an aneurysm. Thrombus forms in the dilatation.
  4. It is usually asymptomatic until the arterial emboli dislodges.

PREDISPOSING FACTORS

A. Cervical rib or anomalous rib.
B. Congenital cervical fibrocartilaginous band associated with an incomplete cervical rib.
C. Muscular anomalies.
D. Chronic inflammatory change due to trauma.
E. Fractured first rib or clavicle.
F. Neck mass, for example, goiter, apical lung cancers, thyroid cancers, and lymphoma.
G. Repetitive occupational overhead arm movements (e.g., box stacking) or sporting movements (e.g., pitching, swimming).

SUBJECTIVE DATA

A. Common complaints/symptoms.
  1. nTOS: Pain, dysesthesia, numbness, and weakness, which may not be localized in specific nerve distribution. Symptoms are reproducibly aggravated by elevation or sustained use of the arms or hands.
  2. vTOS: Pain, cyanosis, and edema. Paresthesia in the fingers is typically from swelling in the hand rather than nerve compression. Collateral venous patterning over the ipsilateral shoulder, neck, and chest wall indicates compensatory superficial venous flow from subclavian vein stenosis or occlusion.
  3. aTOS: Pain, pallor, paresthesia, and coldness to hand. Symptoms develop spontaneously unrelated to work or trauma.
B. Common/typical scenario.
  1. Common causes of TOS include physical trauma from car accidents, sports, or repetitive injuries.
  2. Sometimes having an anatomic defect such as an extra rib can cause this.
  3. Patients may complain of numbness or tingling in their arm or fingers and have a weak grip.
C. Family and social history.
  1. Elicit the onset, duration, location, intensity, aggravators, and relievers of symptoms.
  2. Ask about occipital headaches and pain over the trapezius, neck, chest, and shoulder. (Patients with ▶

symptoms confined to the forearm and hand are more likely to have carpal or cubital tunnel syndrome, not nTOS).

3. Enquire about any history of neck trauma (e.g., whiplash, clavicle fracture, fall on slippery surface, tripping downstairs).

4. Enquire about occupational and recreational history of repetitive stress injury (e.g., hours on keyboards, assembly lines).

5. Rule out any secondary causes of upper extremity deep vein thrombosis or arterial thrombosis, such as central venous catheters, pacemakers, or peripheral or coronary catheterization.

D. Review of systems.

1. Musculoskeletal: Ask about arm pain or swelling.

2. Cardiovascular: Ask about cold fingers.

3. Dermatologic: Ask about any changes in skin color, such as lack of color or bluish discoloration.

4. Neurologic: Ask about numbness, tingling, or weakness of extremity.

PHYSICAL EXAMINATION

A. Perform a standard neurologic test.

B. Take blood pressure in both arms. Lower systolic pressure in the affected arm may suggest aTOS.

C. Inspect.

1. Neck and supraclavicular area for pulsatile and nonpulsatile mass.

2. Hands and fingers: Swelling and cyanosis (vTOS), pale, cold, and ischemic changes (aTOS).

3. Skin overlying the ipsilateral shoulder, neck, and chest wall for collateral venous patterning (vTOS).

D. Auscultate.

1. Heart to listen for arrhythmias, gallops, and murmurs.

2. Supraclavicular and infraclavicular fossa to listen for bruits or a thrill (aTOS).

E. Palpate.

1. Carotid and upper extremity pulses: Reduced or absent (aTOS).

2. Palpate scalene muscle to assess for tenderness (nTOS).

F. Perform provocative maneuvers.

1. Adson test.

a. Palpate the radial pulse and then move the patient's upper extremity into an extended, abducted, and externally rotated position.

b. Patient then rotates and laterally flexes the neck to the ipsilateral side while inhaling deeply.

c. A positive test results in reduction or obliteration of the radial pulse.

2. Elevated arm stress test (EAST) or Roos test.

a. Patient seated with arms abducted at 90° in external rotation, elbows flexed to 90°, and head in neutral position.

b. Patient opens and closes hands.

c. The test has a high negative predictive value for nTOS if the patient performs the maneuver for 3 minutes.

DIAGNOSTIC TESTS

A. The predominant clinical signs and symptoms direct the nature of further evaluation depending on the type of TOS.

1. Cervical spine x-ray: Identify bony abnormalities such as cervical ribs, anomalous ribs, or rib/clavicular fracture calluses.

2. Ultrasound: The initial imaging test to evaluate aTOS or vTOS. Provocative shoulder/arm maneuvers are performed under ultrasound.

3. Cross-sectional imaging (CT or MR) and/or electromyography are best reserved for TOS specialists.

4. Hematologic evaluation: There are no specific blood tests for TOS. However, hematologic tests are helpful in ruling out other causes. See "Diagnostic Tests" for "Peripheral Artery Disease: Upper Extremity."

DIFFERENTIAL DIAGNOSIS

A. Neurogenic TOS.

1. Carpal tunnel syndrome.

2. Ulnar nerve compression.

3. Rotator cuff tendinitis.

4. Neck strain/sprain.

5. Fibromyositis.

6. Cervical disc disease.

7. Cervical arthritis.

8. Brachial plexus injury.

B. Arterial TOS.

1. Embolization from other sources.

2. Vasculitis.

3. Radiation arteritis.

4. Connective tissue disorders.

5. Arterial dissection.

6. Atherosclerotic upper extremity disease.

7. Thromboangiitis obliterans.

8. Traumatic.

C. Venous TOS.

1. Acute thrombosis.

2. Lymphedema.

3. Rheumatologic disorders.

4. Cellulitis and allergic reactions.

5. Metabolic or global causes of limb swelling, such as heart failure or myxedema.

EVALUATION AND MANAGEMENT PLAN

A. General plan.

1. Treatment is indicated only for symptomatic patients. Having a cervical rib or other rib anomaly does not indicate a need to intervene.

2. Prevention and rehabilitation: Minimizing work-related overuse syndromes. Input from physical therapists.

3. Thrombolysis.

4. Severe arterial ischemia usually requires surgical embolectomy (with or without intraoperative thrombolysis).

5. Thoracic outlet decompression.

B. Patient/family teaching points.

1. Patients need to avoid repetitive movements and heavy lifting.

2. Diet and exercise can improve symptoms as well.

3. Stretching daily can keep muscles strong and prevent increased pressure on the thoracic outlet.

C. Pharmacotherapy.

1. Medical therapy: Interscalene injection of anesthetic agents, steroids, or botulinum toxin type A.

2. Anticoagulation.

D. Discharge instructions.

1. Patients should follow up with their primary care provider.

2. Surgery may be indicated if medical treatment and physical therapy are not effective.

3. Untreated symptoms can lead to permanent nerve damage so patients should report any worsening symptoms.

FOLLOW-UP

A. As guided by appropriate specialist services (neurology, vascular, or general surgery).

CONSULTATION/REFERRAL

A. Acute ischemia: For hospital admission, seek vascular consult.

B. Nonacute, progressive symptoms, refer to a TOS specialist.

1. Complaints of shoulder, neck, head, chest, and arm problems with activity, elevation, or dangling, with supraclavicular or infraclavicular tenderness, and absence of obvious cervical disc, rotator cuff, or carpal tunnel pathology.

SPECIAL/GERIATRIC CONSIDERATIONS

A. TOS is a complex disease in terms of its etiologies, pathophysiology, diagnosis, and management.

B. TOS is associated with a high incidence of insurance claims and worker compensation issues.

C. Early identification that TOS potentially exists and referral to specialist services are important.

BIBLIOGRAPHY

Goshima, K. G. (2019, January 31). *Overview of thoracic outlet syndromes*. In K. A. Collins (Ed.), *UpToDate*. https://www.uptodate.com/contents/overview-of-thoracic-outlet-syndromes

Illig, K. A., Thompson, R. W., Freischlag, J. A., Donahue, D. M., Jordon, S. E., & Edgelow, P. I. (Eds.). (2013). *Thoracic outlet syndrome*. Springer Publishing Company.

CHAPTER 12

HEMATOLOGY GUIDELINES

Mary L. Wilby

ANEMIA

DEFINITION

A. Anemia is characterized by a lower than normal number of red blood cells (RBCs) and/or level of hemoglobin causing decreased oxygen-carrying capacity.

INCIDENCE

A. Iron deficiency is the most common cause of anemia worldwide, with older adults, women, and children the most often affected.

B. Other causes of anemia vary based on age, gender, and geographic region. Anemias in high-income North American countries, including the United States, are most frequently the result of gastrointestinal (GI) hemorrhage, hemoglobinopathy, and chronic kidney disease.

C. Approximately 240,000 ED visits in the United States result in anemia as the primary hospital discharge diagnosis.

PATHOGENESIS

A. Anemia can be a consequence of bleeding, hemolydeficiency.

B. Blood loss anemia results in a loss of iron-containing RBCs. Hemolysis results in destruction of RBCs, but iron is retained in the body.

C. Microcytic anemia is characterized by RBCs of reduced size. While most commonly associated with iron deficiency, microcytic anemia can be associated with anemia of chronic disease (ACD), thalassemia, and sideroblastic anemia.

D. Macrocytic anemias are characterized by greater than normal mean corpuscular volume. The causes are most often associated with vitamin B_{12} and folate deficiency, antimetabolite drugs including methotrexate, and other causes that interfere with cell metabolism.

E. Pernicious anemia is associated with vitamin B_{12} deficiency caused by the absence of intrinsic factor, a glycoprotein secreted by parietal cells needed for absorption of vitamin B_{12}. Absence of intrinsic factor may be congenital, but is most often caused by an autoimmune-mediated atrophic gastritis.

F. Sideroblastic anemias may be inherited or acquired. Acquired forms may be associated with chronic alcohol abuse, medications including isoniazid, and zinc and lead toxicity.

G. Normocytic anemia, characterized by normal-sized RBCs, may be associated with ACD, hemolysis, acute blood loss, and volume overload. In the acute care setting, hemolysis may be associated with hemolytic uremic syndrome (HUS), thrombotic thrombocytopenic purpura (TTP), disseminated intravascular coagulation (DIC), or heart valve abnormalities.

PREDISPOSING FACTORS

A. Use of nonsteroidal anti-inflammatory drugs (NSAIDs).

B. Peptic ulcer disease.

C. Chronic kidney disease.

D. Uterine fibroids/menorrhagia.

E. Family history of thalassemia, sickle cell disease (SCD), or hereditary spherocytosis.

F. Recent blood transfusion.

G. Nutritional deficiency.

H. Alcohol abuse.

I. Cancer.

J. Connective tissue diseases.

K. Chronic infection such as HIV or tuberculosis (TB).

L. Pregnancy.

M. Intestinal disorders including diverticulosis, inflammatory bowel disease, or celiac disease.

SUBJECTIVE DATA

A. Common complaints/symptoms.

  1. Signs and symptoms of anemia may vary depending on the severity, speed of development, age, and comorbidities of the individual. Tissue hypoxia and the pathologic process contribute to complaints.

  2. Fatigue, weakness, headache, shortness of breath, palpitations, and angina may occur.

  3. Decreased oxygen to the brain often results in confusion, visual changes, and fainting.

  4. Chronic blood loss may not cause symptoms until hemoglobin drops below 8 g/dL.

B. Common/typical scenario.

  1. Other signs and symptoms.

    a. Pale skin, nail beds, conjunctiva, and mucous membranes resulting from shifting of blood away from cutaneous tissues.

    b. Flow-type systolic murmurs may be associated with altered blood viscosity. High output heart failure and ventricular hypertrophy may occur with severe anemia, especially in individuals with established heart disease.

    c. Hemolytic anemia may be associated with increased bilirubin, causing jaundice, splenomegaly, and dark-colored urine.

C. Family and social history.
   1. Onset and duration of symptoms.
   2. Family history of blood disorder.
   3. Associated abdominal pain.
   4. Changes in diet and bowel habits.
   5. Menstrual history, including timing and amount of bleeding.
   6. Medication history.
D. Review of systems.
   1. Head, ear, eyes, nose, and throat (HEENT): Ask about premature graying of hair or burning sensation of tongue.
   2. Neurologic: Ask about numbness or tingling sensations.
   3. Genitourinary: Ask about urine color.
   4. GI: Ask about stool color, any blood in stool, abdominal pain, or cramping.
   5. Ask about dietary habits or unusual habits such as pagophagia.
   6. Dermatologic: Ask about any rashes or redness of skin.
   7. Psychiatric: Ask about fatigue.

PHYSICAL EXAMINATION

A. Check vital signs, including pulse, respirations, and blood pressure.
B. Oral mucosa may be pale, cracked, or dry; tongue may be thickened and smooth with vitamin deficiency.
C. Cardiac examination, noting rate, rhythm, and presence of murmurs.
D. Lung examination, noting rate and adventitious sounds.
E. Abdominal examination, noting evidence of bleeding, distension, peristalsis, abnormal bowel sounds, tenderness, and masses.
F. Rectal examination, noting presence of blood in stool.

G. Skin and mucous membrane examination, noting petechiae, bruising, or pallor of skin, nail beds, and mucous membranes including conjunctiva.
H. Neurologic disturbances may be associated with long-standing vitamin B_{12} deficiency; peripheral neuropathy, alterations in deep tendon reflexes, impaired vibratory sensation, alterations in balance, and impaired mental status may be present.

DIAGNOSTIC TESTS

A. Complete blood count (CBC) including RBC indices.
B. Reticulocyte count.
C. Hemoglobin electrophoresis.
D. Coombs test (antiglobulin test).
E. Serum ferritin.
F. Serum iron.
G. Vitamin B_{12} level.
H. Folate level.
I. Haptoglobin.
J. Lactate dehydrogenase (LDH).
K. Serum creatinine.

DIFFERENTIAL DIAGNOSIS

A. Acute blood loss.
B. Chronic blood loss.
C. Hemolysis.
D. Aplastic anemia.
E. Leukemia.
F. Renal disease.

EVALUATION AND MANAGEMENT PLAN

A. General plan.
   1. See Figure 12.1 for overview of anemia evaluation.
   2. Treatment of anemia is based on identifying and eliminating or ameliorating the cause.

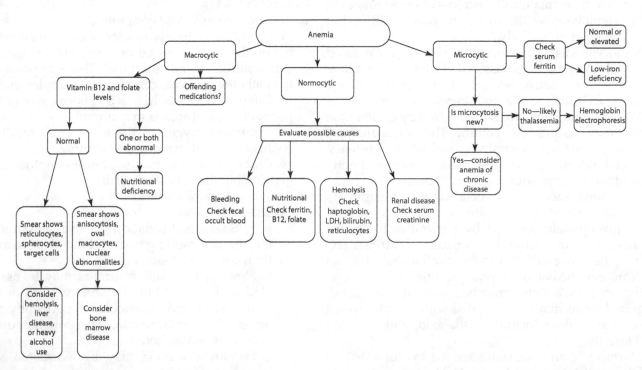

FIGURE 12.1 Overview of anemia evaluation.

LDH, lactate dehydrogenase.

3. The severity of the anemia and its accompanying symptoms determine the treatment.

4. Transfusion is often indicated if/when hematocrit drops to 27% or less.

5. Risks associated with transfusion include fluid overload, transfusion reaction, and iron overload, which must be taken into consideration.

6. Iron deficiency may be treated with increased intake of dietary iron and supplemental iron. Dietary sources are frequently insufficient, and oral and/or intravenous (IV) supplementation are often required.

7. ACD may require treatment when patients become symptomatic with use of medication to stimulate erythropoiesis such as erythropoietin alpha and darbepoetin alfa.

8. Caution should be used when treating with erythropoiesis-stimulating agents as there is an increased risk of stroke, myocardial infarction, and venous thromboembolism (VTE).

B. Patient/family teaching points.

1. Nutritional deficiencies of iron, vitamin B_{12}, and folic acid should be corrected with changes to diet.

2. If taking ferrous sulfate, patients should avoid tea and coffee, which can affect absorption of the drug.

C. Pharmacotherapy.

1. Treatment of anemia is to correct the underlying condition and supplement with ferrous sulfate until anemia is corrected and for several months after it is corrected.

2. Ferrous sulfate 325 mg TID is the standard pharmacologic treatment.

3. Vitamin C 500 units per day can promote absorption of ferrous sulfate.

4. Patients with severe anemia from chronic kidney failure, chemotherapy, or HIV can benefit from epoetin injections.

  a. Dose of epoetin will depend on the severity of anemia, but typically starts at 50 to 100 units per kilogram administered subcutaneously three times per week. Patients will require adequate iron stores prior to starting epoetin injections. The lowest dose possible should be used to reduce the need for transfusion.

D. Discharge instructions (if standard accepted guidelines exist, please use discharge template).

1. Patients are not routinely admitted for anemia unless they are hemodynamically unstable.

2. Discharge planning for a patient who is found to be anemic in the hospital would be to follow up with the primary care provider for further evaluation and workup of anemia in nonacute setting.

FOLLOW-UP

A. Once iron stores have been replenished, there is no need to retest iron studies unless there is evidence of a change in the patient's symptoms or physical examination.

B. Follow-up to identify the cause of the anemia is discussed in the following:

1. Conditions that are unresolved warrant follow-up.

2. ACD often requires ongoing treatment and follow-up under specialist care depending on the cause of the underlying disease.

3. Patients with aggressive forms of thalassemia should be under the care of a hematologist.

4. Patients with vitamin B_{12} deficiency require ongoing care to monitor B_{12} levels and liver function if taking parenteral therapy.

5. Follow-up for patients with folic acid deficiency should consist of periodic monitoring of CBC and serum folate levels.

CONSULTATION/REFERRAL

A. Iron deficiency associated with occult blood loss often requires referral to a gastroenterologist for upper endoscopy and/or colonoscopy, as well as additional testing to identify the source of bleeding.

B. In the case of menorrhagia, referral for follow-up gynecologic care may be needed. Follow-up care of individuals with ACD is dependent on the underlying cause.

C. Referral for care by nephrology, rheumatology, hematology, oncology, gastroenterology, or other specialists may be required.

D. Use of erythrocyte-stimulating factors should be directed by a hematologist or other qualified specialist.

E. Thalassemia may require consultation with hematology for ongoing monitoring.

F. Evidence of sideroblastic anemia should prompt consultation with hematology.

SPECIAL/GERIATRIC CONSIDERATIONS

A. Adults over 50 with occult blood in the stool or iron deficiency anemia should be referred for upper endoscopy and/or colonoscopy given the increased risk of GI malignancy associated with aging.

B. In some cases, the risk associated with the procedure, including perforation, may outweigh the benefits.

CASE SCENARIO: ANEMIA

A 78-year-old man presents to the ED with worsening shortness of breath over the last few days and new onset of chest pain, relieved by rest this morning. He has a history of coronary artery disease, managed with medication. His medical history includes type 2 diabetes that has been well-controlled and osteoarthritis for which he takes 600 mg ibuprofen TID on most days. He walks regularly in his neighborhood but reports that he has had increasing difficulty finishing his usual routine over the last 2 weeks. He denies abdominal pain or change in his stools. A stat complete blood count (CBC) reveals the following: white blood cells 4.6, hemoglobin 9.3, hematocrit 27.5, and platelets 213. The mean corpuscular volume is 80 fL and a test for fecal occult blood is positive. Serum ferritin level is in the low normal range.

1. What is the mostly likely cause of the patient's anemia?
  A. Chronic blood loss associated with nonsteroidal anti-inflammatory drugs (NSAID) use
  B. Acute blood loss associated with peptic ulcer disease

(continued)

C. An undiagnosed gastrointestinal (GI) malignancy
D. Anemia of chronic disease associated with diabetic nephropathy

2. Which of the following should be included in the provider's differential diagnosis? (Select all that apply.)
A. Anemia associated with renal insufficiency
B. An undiagnosed GI malignancy
C. Acute blood loss associated with lower GI bleeding
D. A previously undiagnosed hereditary blood disorder

3. When deciding on a treatment plan, what is the priority?
A. Consult gastroenterology to determine the source of bleeding.
B. Make sure the patient is hemodynamically stable before planning any procedure.
C. Consult hematology to identify the causes of the patient's anemia.
D. Discuss options for addressing the anemia with the patient and their significant other.

4. The provider considers treatment of the patient's anemia with an erythropoietin-stimulating agent. Prior to prescribing this type of agent to treat anemia, what should the provider assess for? (Select all that apply.)
A. Adequate iron stores
B. Renal function
C. Risk factors for venous thrombosis
D. Risk factors for stroke

BIBLIOGRAPHY

Burchum, J. R. (2019). Disorders of red blood cells. In T. L. Norris (Ed.), *Porth's pathophysiology: Concepts of altered health states* (10th ed., pp. 638–662). Wolters Kluwer Health/Lippincott Williams & Wilkins.

Centers for Disease Control and Prevention National Center for Disease Statistics. (2017). *Anemia or iron deficiency.* https://www.cdc.gov/nchs/fastats/anemia.htm

Elder, J. D., Winland-Brown, J. E., & Porter, B. O. (2019). Hematologic disorders. In L. M. Dunphy, J. E. Winland-Brown, B. O. Porter, & D. J. Thomas (Eds.), *Primary care the art and science of advanced practice nursing* (5th ed., pp. 958–991). F. A. Davis.

Kassebaum, N., Jasrasaria, R., Naghavi, M., Wulf, S. K., Johns, N., Lozano, R., Regan, M., Weatherall, D., Chou, D. P., Eisele, T. P., Flaxman, S. R., Pullan, R. L., Brooker, S. J., & Murrayet, C. J. L. (2014). A systematic analysis of global anemia burden from 1990 to 2010. *Blood, 123,* 615–624. https://doi.org/10.1182/blood-2013-06-508325

Palaka, E., Grandy, S., van Haalen, H., McEwan, P., & Darlinton, O. (2020). The impact of CKD anaemia on patients: Incidence, risk factors and clinical outcomes—a systematic literature review. *International Journal of Nephrology, 2020.* https://doi.org/10.1155/2020/7692376 Article ID 7692376

Turner, J., Parisi, M., & Badireddy, M. (2022). Anemia. *StatPearls [Internet]. StatPearls Publishing.* https://www.ncbi.nlm.nih.gov/books/NBK499994/

BLEEDING DIATHESES

DEFINITION

A. Bleeding disorders may occur as a result of abnormalities in platelet number or function, coagulation factors, fibrinolysis, and blood vessel integrity.

B. Deficiencies or inhibitors of clotting factors, whether acquired or inherited, can result in bleeding disorders.

INCIDENCE

A. Bleeding disorders occur frequently in seriously ill patients, and causes may vary from prolonged global clotting tests or isolated thrombocytopenia to composite defects, such as consumption coagulopathies.

B. A prolongation of global clotting times, such as the prothrombin time (PT) or the activated partial thromboplastin time (aPTT), may be apparent in 14% to 28% of critically ill patients.

C. The incidence of a low platelet count (platelet count <150,000 per microliter) in an intensive care population is 35% to 44%. Platelet counts of less than 100,000 per microliter may be seen in another 30% to 50% of patients.

PATHOGENESIS

A. Hemostasis is the process of clot formation at the site of blood vessel injury. Abnormal bleeding is often a result of the absence or dysfunction of one or more of the elements needed in clot formation.

B. Most clotting factors are synthesized by the liver. A final step dependent on vitamin K is required for factors II, VII, IX, and X, and procoagulant proteins C and S. Factor VIII, von Willebrand factor (vWF), and tissue plasminogen activator are produced in the endothelium, including that of the liver. The liver reticuloendothelial system is responsible for metabolizing most clotting factors and fibrin degradation products (FDPs).

C. Coagulation factor inhibitors are antibodies that neutralize a specific clotting factor's function. Alloantibodies occur in patients with inherited factor deficiency. Autoantibodies arise in patients without an inherited factor deficiency. The most commonly inhibited factor is factor VIII.

D. Low platelet counts in critically ill individuals are frequently the result of increased platelet turnover due to thrombin generation, platelet activation, and enhanced platelet–vessel wall interaction. Sepsis is a frequent cause of thrombocytopenia in seriously ill patients. The severity of sepsis may be correlated with the reduction in the platelet count.

E. Drug-induced thrombocytopenia has been associated with a variety of prescription and over-the-counter (OTC) medications, including quinine and some sulfa-containing antibiotics. Antigen–antibody responses lead to the destruction of platelets. Immune thrombocytopenic purpura (ITP) occurs as a result of antibody-induced destruction of platelets or decreased platelet production associated with impaired megakaryocyte function or reduced level of thrombopoietin Primary ITP can occur without any known risk factors, while secondary ITP is a result of an acute or chronic underlying disorder, such as AIDS, systemic lupus erythematosus, lymphoma, or a condition that manifests with a combination of low platelet count, hemolytic anemia, renal failure, neurologic abnormalities, and ▶

fever. This rare disorder stems from introducing certain platelet-aggregating substances into the circulation. In many cases, this is triggered by a lack of an enzyme that breaks down vWF, causing platelet aggregation and adherence to vascular endothelium. While this condition may occur in otherwise healthy people, it is also found in individuals with autoimmune disorders, HIV infection, and pregnancy.

F. Disseminated intravascular coagulation (DIC) is a systemic process that can cause both thrombosis and hemorrhage. The processes associated with coagulation and fibrinolysis become abnormally activated within the vessels and promote ongoing coagulation and fibrinolysis. Consumption of platelets is associated with constant generation of thrombin. Microvascular thrombi, along with inflammation, may cause injury to the microvasculature, resulting in organ dysfunction. Consumption of platelets and low levels of other factors increase the risk of hemorrhagic complications, especially in perioperative patients or those undergoing other invasive procedures. Thrombin generation is triggered and promoted by a lack of thrombin-generating inhibitory mechanisms. Impaired fibrin degradation, due to elevated circulating levels of plasminogen activator inhibitor-type 1 (PAI-1), further promotes intravascular fibrin deposition. Patients with DIC have a low or decreasing platelet count, prolongation of coagulation tests, low plasma levels of coagulation factors and inhibitors, and increased markers of fibrin formation or degradation, including D-dimer or FDPs. No single diagnostic test is used to confirm DIC. The presence of a condition associated with DIC and a combination of laboratory tests are necessary to confirm the diagnosis.

G. von Willebrand disease (vWD) is the most common form of inherited bleeding disorder, resulting from a deficiency or defect of vWF. Individuals with vWD have defects in both platelet function and the coagulation pathway.

H. Hemophilia A is the most common form of hemophilia, accounting for approximately 85% of hemophilia cases. Caused by an X-linked recessive gene, it affects males most often. Although it is a genetic disorder, a number of cases occur without a family history of bleeding. Deficiency or defects of factor VIII are associated with excessive bleeding, most often occurring in soft tissue, joints, and the gastrointestinal (GI) tract. Bleeding may be spontaneous or associated with trauma.

PREDISPOSING FACTORS

A. Thrombotic thrombocytopenic purpura (TTP).
B. Hemolytic uremic syndrome.
C. Chemotherapy-induced microangiopathic.
D. Hemolytic anemia.
E. Severe malignant hypertension.
F. Hemolysis, elevated liver enzymes, and low platelet count (HELLP) syndrome of pregnancy.
G. Preeclampsia.
H. Retained products of conception.
I. Malignancy, especially leukemia.
J. Blood transfusion reaction.
K. Systemic infection.
L. Connective tissue disease.
M. Pancreatitis.
N. Liver disease.
O. Surgery or trauma.
P. Burns.
Q. Snake venom.
R. Chemotherapy-induced bone marrow suppression.

SUBJECTIVE DATA

A. Common complaints/symptoms.
  1. Bruising.
  2. Nose bleeds.
  3. Bleeding gums.
  4. Menorrhagia.
  5. Weakness.
  6. Fatigue.
  7. Abdominal discomfort.
B. Common/typical scenario.
  1. Other signs and symptoms.
    a. Immediate bleeding after vessel injury is frequently associated with platelet disorders.
    b. Large ecchymoses and large, diffusely spreading deep tissue hematomas are common with coagulation disorders.
    c. Bleeding into synovial joints is characteristic of inherited coagulation disorders such as hemophilia.
    d. Petechiae.
    e. Oozing from venipuncture sites.
    f. Uncontrolled postpartum bleeding.
C. Family and social history.
  1. History of HIV infection and malignancy.
  2. History of liver or kidney disease, or malabsorption that is often associated with bleeding.
  3. Medication history, including anticoagulants, nonsteroidal anti-inflammatory drugs (NSAIDs), oral contraceptives, antibiotics, alcohol, and dietary vitamins K and C.
  4. Response to previous hemostatic challenges, including trauma, tooth extraction, pregnancy, surgery, sports, and menstruation.
  5. Family history of bleeding disorders.
D. Review of systems.
  1. Hematologic: Ask about past bleeding problems, any history of anemia, bleeding after any type of surgical procedure or dental procedure, or any transfusions.
  2. GI: Ask about dietary habits or antibiotic use which might contribute to vitamin K deficiency. Ask about liver disease or black tarry stools.
  3. Genitourinary: Ask about any kidney diseases or hematuria.
  4. Endocrine: Ask women about menses. Ask about medications the patient is taking for other conditions.
  5. Dermatologic: Ask about bruising or ecchymosis.

PHYSICAL EXAMINATION
A. Signs of bleeding (e.g., petechiae, mucosal bleeding, soft tissue bleeding, ecchymoses). In hospitalized patients, bleeding from multiple sites can indicate DIC or TTP. Acute extensive mucocutaneous bleeding in a patient previously without symptoms should suggest ITP.
B. Organ enlargement.
C. Joint abnormalities.
D. Signs of systemic disease, including fever and lymphadenopathy.

DIAGNOSTIC TESTS
A. Complete blood count (CBC).
B. Bleeding time.
C. PT.
D. aPTT.
E. Platelet function analysis.
F. Examination of a peripheral blood smear. The following may be required in the presence of abnormalities in screening tests described earlier:
1. Factor deficiencies and inhibitors.
2. Fibrinogen.
3. Fibrin and FDPs.

DIFFERENTIAL DIAGNOSIS
A. Anticoagulant overdose.
B. Acquired factor VIII inhibitors.
C. Local surgical complications.
D. Physical abuse.

EVALUATION AND MANAGEMENT PLAN
A. General plan.
1. Bleeding associated with deficiency of vitamin K can be treated with parenteral vitamin K. Normalization of clotting studies usually follows within several hours. Fresh frozen plasma may be needed in the event of hemorrhage or if emergency surgery is necessary.
2. Individuals with acute or chronic liver disease may require treatment of alterations in clotting functions, fibrinolytic systems, and/or platelet function. When multiple coagulation factors are involved, infusion of fresh frozen plasma is a preferred treatment. Additional treatments may include exchange transfusion and platelet infusion.
3. DIC treatment should be directed at reducing the burden of the underlying disease, controlling thrombosis, and preserving organ function. Controlling the underlying condition is necessary to reduce the stimulus for abnormal clotting and restoring a normal balance of clotting factors. The role of heparin is limited but has been effective when DIC is associated with retained products of conception and when acute promyelocytic leukemia is present. It is contraindicated when there is evidence of central nervous system (CNS), GI, or postoperative bleeding. Interventions for restoring the balance of coagulation factors and platelets include infusion of fresh frozen plasma, cryoprecipitate, and platelets.

4. Individuals with hemophilia should avoid trauma whenever possible. Medications that interfere with platelet function, including NSAIDs, should be avoided.
5. vWD type 1 and some forms of type 2 can be treated with desmopressin to promote hemostasis, treat mucocutaneous bleeding, and prevent bleeding associated with minor procedures. Therapy with antifibrinolytic agents such as tranexamic acid is also beneficial in vWD. Treatment with oral contraceptives or a levonorgestrel-releasing intrauterine device can be very beneficial in women with vWD experiencing menorrhagia. Infusion of von Willebrand concentrate is also an option when desmopressin is not effective.
6. Corticosteroids are often the first line in treatment of ITP. It is cost-effective and easy to administer. Rituximab may be considered as a second-line therapy in patients who do not respond to corticosteroid treatment.
B. Patient/family teaching points.
1. Patients should contact their primary care provider prior to any dental procedures or surgical interventions.
2. Bruising may be spontaneous or recurrent and patients may experience prolonged bleeding after minor cuts or abrasions.
3. Women of childbearing age will need high-risk obstetrics and should carefully plan pregnancies.
C. Pharmacotherapy.
1. Pharmacologic treatment will be based on the underlying cause of bleeding diathesis and is fairly limited.
2. In the acute setting, blood products can be used to control bleeding disorders.
3. Avoidance of medications that interfere with platelet function should be evaluated.
4. Hypoprothrombinemia can be treated acutely with parenteral vitamin K.
5. Minor bleeding or elevated international normalized ratio (INR): 2.5 to 5 mg oral vitamin K one time may be sufficient or can be repeated in 24 hours if needed.
6. Patients who have internal bleeding or who are at high risk for bleeding can be given IV vitamin K 5 to 10 mg diluted in in vitro fertilization (IVF) and infused over 20 minutes. These patients should also receive prothrombin complex concentrate (PCC).
D. Discharge instructions (if standard accepted guidelines exist, please use discharge template).
1. Patients should be instructed on how to recognize signs and symptoms that warrant immediate attention.
2. Patients should also be given instructions on how to control a bleeding source.

FOLLOW-UP
A. In general, medications such as aspirin and NSAIDs should be avoided in patients with abnormal bleeding.
B. Conditions that may pose special risks to individuals with bleeding disorders, including hypertension that ▶

may lead to intracranial bleeding, need close monitoring and treatment.

C. Procedures necessary for preventive care and screening should be planned in cooperation with the patient's hematologist.

D. Dental care such as cleaning and screening colonoscopy can usually be performed with decreased risk of bleeding when supervised carefully and given appropriate hemostatic coverage.

CONSULTATION/REFERRAL

A. Treatment of underlying conditions is important in controlling bleeding in individuals with bleeding diatheses.

B. Consultation with a gastroenterologist/hepatologist is important in the management of advanced liver disease.

C. When thrombocytopenia is present, consultation with a hematologist is warranted.

D. If DIC or thrombocytopenia is associated with sepsis, consultation with an infectious disease specialist is indicated.

E. Bleeding associated with malignancy requires referral to hematology oncology.

F. Bleeding in the setting of pregnancy-related complications requires immediate referral to OB/GYN.

SPECIAL/GERIATRIC CONSIDERATIONS

A. Bleeding disorders in older adults pose special challenges.

B. A number of acquired disorders can present in older adults as a result of alterations in coagulation factors, medications, and comorbid conditions more common with aging.

C. Older adults are more likely to be receiving medications to treat thrombotic disorders, and evidence of bleeding may be dismissed as a side effect of anticoagulants and antiplatelet drugs.

D. Increased risk of bleeding associated with anticoagulants as well as NSAIDs accompanies many physiologic changes of aging.

E. Thrombocytopenia in older adults may be associated with ITP, leukemia, or DIC associated with malignancy or sepsis.

F. Although rare, there is risk of acquired hemophilia and acquired von Willebrand syndrome in older adults.

CASE SCENARIO: BLEEDING DIATHESES

A 35-year-old woman is admitted to the hospital with history of systemic lupus erythematosus and a new onset of easy bruising and recurrent nosebleeds, with a platelet count of 12,000 platelets per microliter or 12×10^9/L. The remainder of her complete blood count (CBC) is normal. She complains of abdominal discomfort and her spleen is moderately enlarged on examination. Serum electrolytes and renal functions are also within normal limits. She denies family history of any type of bleeding disorder. She also denies any previous episodes of irregular bleeding.

1. What is the most likely cause of the patient's condition?
   A. Thrombotic thrombocytopenic purpura

B. Immune thrombocytopenic purpura
C. von Willebrand disease
D. Antiphospholipid syndrome

2. Which features of thrombotic thrombocytopenic purpura (TTP) help differentiate it from immune thrombocytopenic purpura (ITP)?
   A. TTP often presents with fever, renal failure, and hemolytic anemia.
   B. There are few features that differentiate the two conditions.
   C. TTP is not associated with autoimmune diseases.
   D. Platelet count in TTP is normal.

3. Which of the following medications used to treat systemic lupus erythematosus may contribute to risk of bleeding? (Select all that apply.)
   A. Ibuprofen
   B. Hydroxychloroquine
   C. Methotrexate
   D. Aspirin

4. The patient is being discharged from the hospital after bleeding has ceased and platelet count is within a safe range. Discharge instructions should include which of the following? (Select all that apply.)
   A. Monitor for changes in menstrual flow and report them to the patient's healthcare provider.
   B. Notify the patient's dentist about her condition before having any invasive procedures.
   C. Take prophylactic antibiotics prior to any invasive procedures.
   D. Avoid sitting for prolonged periods of time.

BIBLIOGRAPHY

Capriotti, T., & Frizzell, J. P. (2016). *Pathophysiology: Introductory concepts and clinical perspectives* (pp. 285–304). F. A. Davis.

DeSouza, S., & Angelini, D. (2021). Updated guidelines for immune thrombocytopenic purpura: Expanded management options. *Cleveland Clinic Journal of Medicine*, *88*(12), 664–668.

Kahn, A. M. Mydra, H, & Nevarez, A. (2017). Clinical practice updates in the management of immune thrombocytopenia. *Journal of Managed Care and Formulary Management*, *42*(12), 756–763.

Kruse-Jarres, R. (2015). Acquired bleeding disorders in the elderly. *ASH Education Book*, 231–236. 2015(1)

Leung, L. (2021). Overview of hemostasis. P. Mannucci (Ed.), *UpToDate*. https://www.uptodate.com/contents/overview-of-hemostasis?search=overview%20of%20hemostasis&source=search_result&selectedTitle=1~150&usage_type=default&display_rank=1

Levi, M., & Sivapalaratnam, S. (2015). Hemostatic abnormalities in critically ill patients. *Internal and Emergency Medicine*, *10*, 287–296. https://doi.org/10.1007/s11739-014-1176-2

Lillicrap, D. (2013). Von Willebrand disease: Advances in pathogenetic understanding, diagnosis, and therapy. *Blood*, *122*(23), 3735–3740. https://doi.org/10.1182/blood-2013-06-498303

Ma, A. (2022). Approach to the adult with suspected bleeding disorder. In L. L. Leung (Ed.), *UpToDate*. https://www.uptodate.com/contents/approach-to-the-adult-with-a-suspected-bleeding-disorder?search=bleeding%20disorders&source=search_result&selectedTitle=1~150&usage_type=default&display_rank=1

Wimberly, P. (2019). Disorders of hemostasis. In T. L. Norris (Ed.), *Porth's pathophysiology: Concepts of altered health states* (10th ed., pp. 620–636). Wolters Kluwer Health/Lippincott Williams & Wilkins.

COAGULOPATHIES

DEFINITION

A. Strictly speaking, coagulopathy describes a condition that disturbs the blood's ability to clot. For purposes of this text, coagulopathy will refer to hypercoagulability. Bleeding disorders are described elsewhere in this chapter.

B. Hypercoagulability, sometimes referred to as thrombophilia, is an enhanced state of hemostasis that increases the risk of thrombosis and blood vessel occlusion.

C. These conditions are typically created in the presence of increased platelet function or increased activity of the coagulation system. Arterial thrombi are most often associated with turbulent blood flow and are composed of platelets.

D. Hypercoagulability disorders have been characterized as primary (hereditary) or secondary (acquired).

INCIDENCE

A. Approximately 30% of those who present with deep vein thrombosis (DVT) or pulmonary emboli are found to have factor V Leiden. Factor V Leiden is seen primarily in individuals of European descent and in approximately 5% of Whites in the United States.

B. Antiphospholipid antibodies are present in 3% to 5% of the general population and are more prevalent in individuals with systemic lupus erythematosus.

C. Venous thromboembolism (VTE) is not uncommon in the presence of malignancy. Tumor type and stage, location of the tumor, treatment, and comorbid conditions influence risk. It is estimated that as many as 10% of cancer patients develop VTE.

PATHOGENESIS

A. Thrombosis occurs when there is an imbalance in anticoagulation and hemostasis through a variety of mechanisms. Three common factors predispose to thrombosis. These are (a) damage to the lining of the blood vessel wall, (b) a hypercoagulable state, and (c) arterial or venous blood stasis. These three factors are often referred to as the "Virchow's triad." Some patients may have multiple risk factors.

B. Most hereditary thrombophilic disorders are associated with mutations in coagulation proteins, fibrinolytic proteins, platelet receptors, and various other factors. Factor V Leiden, a condition in which a factor V mutation interacts with protein C, leading to increased clot formation, is the most common hereditary condition.

C. Other inherited hypercoagulable states are rarer and include prothrombin gene mutation, hyperhomocysteinemia, antithrombin deficiency, and protein C and protein S deficiency.

D. Antiphospholipid syndrome is the most common acquired hypercoagulable condition. When present, antiphospholipid antibodies are directed against phospholipid–protein complexes, causing risk for both arterial and venous thrombus formation.

E. Protein C and protein S deficiency may also become acquired in some disease states.

F. Increased platelet function may manifest as enhanced platelet adhesion, with clot formation and decreased blood flow. Disturbances in blood flow, as with atherosclerotic plaques, cause endothelial tissue damage. Increased sensitivity of platelets to substances that influence platelet aggregation may increase platelet activity.

G. Elevation in platelet counts above 1,000,000 per microliter, referred to as thrombocytosis, is associated with both thrombosis and bleeding. Primary thrombocytosis is a myeloproliferative disorder associated with a disorder of hematopoietic cells in the bone marrow. Secondary thrombocytosis is often associated with disease states that trigger thrombopoietin production, increasing platelet production. These conditions include surgery, cancer, and chronic inflammatory disorders.

H. Coagulation disorders associated with COVID-19 can present as venous thromboembolic events that may lead to end-organ failure and stroke, and death can occur even when severe respiratory symptoms are absent.

I. Patients with a family history of venous thrombosis in one or more first-degree relatives at a young age (<40 years) are likely to have a hereditary form of thrombophilia.

PREDISPOSING FACTORS

A. Surgery.
B. Cancer.
C. Chronic inflammatory disorders.
D. Atherosclerosis.
E. Diabetes mellitus.
F. Smoking.
G. Pregnancy.
H. Oral contraceptive use.
I. Estrogen replacement therapy.
J. Obesity.
K. Heart failure.
L. Nephrotic syndrome.
M. Polycythemia.
N. Sickle cell disease (SCD).
O. Severe acute respiratory syndrome coronavirus 2 (COVID-19).

SUBJECTIVE DATA

A. Common complaints/symptoms.
 1. Patients with thrombocytosis may experience painful burning and throbbing in the digits associated with arteriole occlusion.
 2. Painful, swollen extremity (usually unilateral).
B. Common/typical scenario.
 1. Other signs and symptoms.
  a. Neurologic impairment consistent with transient ischemic attack or stroke.
  b. Chest pain associated with cardiac ischemia.
  c. Dyspnea associated with pulmonary emboli.
  d. Visual disturbance with retinal ischemia.
C. Family and social history.
 1. History of fetal loss in women with antiphospholipid syndrome.

2. History of unprovoked thrombosis in adults under 45 years of age.
3. Family history of multiple individuals with VTE.
D. Review of systems.
  1. Hematologic: Ask about bruising or previous clotting episodes of the arterial or venous system, such as stroke, myocardial infarction, or small vessel thrombosis.
  2. Rheumatologic: Ask about autoimmune disorders.
  3. Obstetrics: Ask about spontaneous abortions.
  4. Dermatologic: Ask about skin discoloration.

PHYSICAL EXAMINATION
A. Physical examination may yield nonspecific findings.
B. Patients with DVT often present with unilateral swelling, pain, and erythema at the site of venous obstruction.
C. Evidence of arterial thrombosis may manifest in signs of stroke, myocardial infarction, DVT, pulmonary embolism (PE), or digital ischemia.
D. Skin necrosis is associated with warfarin therapy.

DIAGNOSTIC TESTS
A. Complete blood count (CBC).
B. Prothrombin time (PT).
C. Activated partial thromboplastin time (aPTT).
D. Antiphospholipid antibodies.
E. Protein C: May be low in acute thrombosis.
F. Protein S: May be low in acute thrombosis.
G. Factor V Leiden.
H. Antithrombin III: May be low in acute thrombosis.
I. Serum D-dimer concentration: May be elevated in DVT.

DIFFERENTIAL DIAGNOSIS
A. Paroxysmal nocturnal hematuria.
B. Homocysteinemia.
C. Heparin-induced thrombocytopenia.
D. Atherosclerosis.
E. SCD.
F. Myeloproliferative diseases.

EVALUATION AND MANAGEMENT PLAN
A. General plan.
  1. Not all thrombotic episodes are associated with hypercoagulable risk factors and not all individuals with risk factors develop thrombosis.
  2. Workup for coagulopathy is indicated with the presence of idiopathic or recurrent VTE, VTE before the age of 45, VTE with strong family history, VTE in an atypical site, or warfarin-induced skin necrosis.
  3. Patients with arterial thrombosis should be tested for antiphospholipid antibody.
  4. Treatment involves reducing or eliminating factors that lead to thrombosis.
B. Patient/family teaching points.
  1. Women need to avoid oral contraceptives or hormone replacement therapy.

2. Patients may need to be treated with lifelong anticoagulation to prevent further clotting.
3. Patients must be instructed on how to manage bleeding diathesis if on anticoagulation agents.
C. Pharmacotherapy.
  1. Acute events require treatment with anticoagulants, including heparin, warfarin, and other agents.
  2. Immune suppression may be needed in some cases when the condition is refractory to anticoagulants.
D. Discharge instructions.
  1. Patients will need to follow up with hematology.
  2. Any dental procedures or surgical interventions must be done in conjunction with the patient's primary care provider.

FOLLOW-UP
A. Monitoring of anticoagulation therapy posthospitalization is critical to preventing recurrence.
B. Patients should be cautioned to avoid trauma while receiving anticoagulant therapy.
C. Patients with modifiable risk factors, including tobacco use or use of estrogen-containing oral contraceptives, should be counseled about their use.

CONSULTATION/REFERRAL
A. Consultation with a hematologist is critical in the diagnosis and management of patients with hypercoagulable disorders.
B. It is also important that laboratory testing is completed at a facility with experience in utilizing specialized tests.

SPECIAL/GERIATRIC CONSIDERATIONS
A. Aging is accompanied by increased risk of both arterial and venous thromboses.
B. While mechanisms are not entirely clear, a number of coagulation factors, including factors V, VII, VIII, and IX, and von Willebrand factor (vWF), increase with aging. This coupled with other comorbid conditions such as malignancy and structural changes in vascular endothelium contributes to an increased risk of thrombosis in older adults.
C. Special consideration is given for use of anticoagulation in older adults to minimize the risk for bleeding. Careful monitoring of vitamin K antagonists is necessary.
D. Use of direct oral anticoagulants (DOACs) may be an alternative in some cases.
E. Education and monitoring to decrease risk of falls and other forms of trauma are essential in older adults receiving anticoagulation therapy.

CASE SCENARIO: COAGULOPATHIES

A 35-year-old comes to the ED with complaints of pain and swelling of her right arm. The skin is unbroken but there is a small area of ecchymosis at the site of injury and swelling above the site. While there is clearly evidence of injury, posing risk for thrombosis, the patient reports a family history of deep vein

(continued)

thrombosis (DVT) and stroke among several members of her mother's family.

1. Which of the following is a hereditary factor associated with risk of thrombosis?
- **A.** Factor V Leiden
- **B.** Antiphospholipid antibody syndrome
- **C.** Hyperhomocysteinemia
- **D.** Hypercholesterolemia

2. Which of the following should be included in the provider's differential diagnosis?
- **A.** An undiagnosed malignancy
- **B.** Antiphospholipid antibodies
- **C.** Coagulopathy associated with oral contraceptive use
- **D.** Thrombocytosis

3. In addition to deep vein thrombosis, patients with thrombophilic conditions are also at risk of arterial thrombosis. Which of the following may be a manifestation of arterial thrombosis?
- **A.** Superior vena cava (SVC) syndrome
- **B.** Myocardial infarction
- **C.** Unilateral warm, edematous extremity
- **D.** Diffuse erythema of an extremity

4. The patient is being discharged from the hospital on anticoagulants. In addition to education about the safe use of her medication, what other information should be included in her discharge instructions? (Select all that apply.)
- **A.** Avoid prolonged immobility as this can increase risk of vein thrombosis (DVT).
- **B.** Maintain a healthy weight because obesity increases risk of blood clots.
- **C.** Be sure to keep follow-up appointment with the provider for ongoing assessment.
- **D.** Resume all normal activities.

BIBLIOGRAPHY

Ashorobi, D., Ameer, M. A., & Fernandez, R. (2022, January). Thrombosis. In *StatPearls [Internet]*. StatPearls Publishing. https://www.ncbi.nlm.nih.gov/books/NBK538430/

Bauer, K. A. (2021). Risk and prevention of venous thromboembolism in adults with cancer. In L. Leung (Ed.), *UpToDate*. https://www.uptodate.com/contents/risk-and-prevention-of-venous-thromboembolism-in-adults-with-cancer?search=risk%20and%20prevention%20of%20venous&source=search_result&selectedTitle=1~150&usage_type=default&display_rank=1

Bauer, K. A., & Lip, G. Y. (2021). *Evaluating adult patients with established venous thromboembolism for acquired and inherited risk factors*. In L. Leung & J. Mandel (Eds.), *UpToDate*. https://www.uptodate.com/contents/evaluating-adult-patients-with-established-venous-thromboembolism-for-acquired-and-inherited-risk-factors?search=adult%20venous%20thromboembolism&source=search_result&selectedTitle=4~150&usage_type=default&display_rank=4

Hogan, C. (2015). Thrombophilia and hypercoagulable states. In F. J. Domino, R. A. Baldor, J. Golding, & M. B. Stephens (Eds.), *The 5 minute clinical consult premium, 2016* (24th ed., pp. 1092–1093). Wolters Kluwer Health.

Ikewaki, N., Rao, K., Archibold, A. D., Iwasaki, M., Senthilkumar, R., Preethy, S., Kato, S., & Abraham, S. (2020). Coagulopathy associated with COVID-19—Perspectives & preventive strategies using a biological response modifier Glucan. *Thrombosis Journal*, *18*(27). https://doi.org/10.1186/s12959-020-00239-6

Lockwood, C. J., & Bauer, K. A. (2021). *Inherited thrombophilias in pregnancy*. In L. L. Leung & V. Berghella (Eds.), *UpToDate*. https://www.uptodate.com/contents/inherited-thrombophilias-in-pregnancy?search=inherited%20thrombophilias&source=search_result&selectedTitle=3~150&usage_type=default&display_rank=3

Nakashima, M. O., & Rogers, H. J. (2014). Hypercoagulable states: An algorithmic approach to laboratory testing and update on monitoring of direct oral anticoagulants. *Blood Research*, *49*(2), 85–94. https://doi.org/10.5045/br.2014.49.2.85

Schick, P. (2018, January 5). *Hereditary and acquired hypercoagulability*. In S. Nagalla (Ed.), *Medscape*. https://emedicine.medscape.com/article/211039-overview

Wimberly, P. (2019). Disorders of hemostasis. In T. L. Norris (Ed.), *Porth's pathophysiology: Concepts of altered health states* (10th ed., pp. 620–636). Wolters Kluwer Health/Lippincott Williams & Wilkins.

DEEP VEIN THROMBOSIS

DEFINITION
A. Deep vein thrombosis (DVT) describes clot formation in the deep veins, most often in the lower extremities.
B. DVT increases the risk for venous thromboembolism (VTE) to the pulmonary circulation.
C. See Figure 12.2.

INCIDENCE
A. More than 900,000 VTE events occur each year in the United States. Nearly one-third of these result in death.
B. Up to 50% of cases are believed to be idiopathic, with an additional 15% to 25% associated with cancer and 20% associated with surgery.
C. Pulmonary embolism (PE) can occur in up to 50% of patients with untreated DVT.
D. The mortality rate associated with PE is 25% to 30%.

PATHOGENESIS
A. Three factors, often referred to as the Virchow's triad, promote venous thrombosis. These three factors are (a) venous stasis, (b) damage to venous endothelium, and (c) hypercoagulable states. Buildup of clotting factors and platelets promotes thrombus formation in the vessel, often adjacent to a valve. Inflammation associated with the clot promotes additional platelet aggregation, causing the clot to grow proximally.
B. Bedrest and/or immobility are factors often associated with venous stasis.
C. Hypercoagulability may be associated with increased activity of clotting factors or inherited or acquired conditions in which factors that would normally inhibit clotting are deficient.
D. Venous injury can result from surgery, trauma, and venous catheters.
E. Localized symptoms are the result of inflammation and venous obstruction, but symptoms may not be apparent if the vein is deep within the leg due to incomplete occlusion and collateral circulation.

PREDISPOSING FACTORS
A. Immobility.
B. Obesity.

Diagnosis of DVT Algorithm

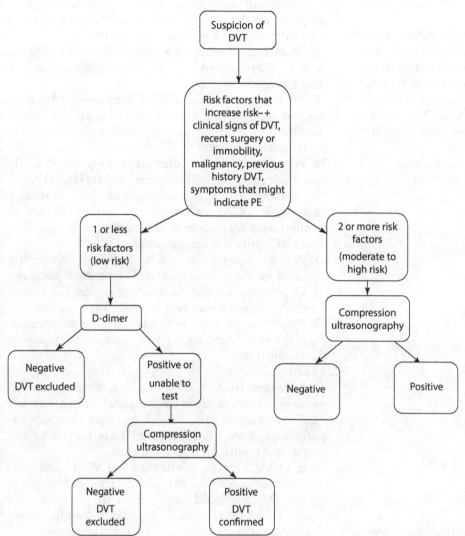

FIGURE 12.2 Diagnosis of DVT.

DVT, deep vein thrombosis; PE, pulmonary embolism.

C. Prolonged dependency (including air travel).
D. Advancing age.
E. Heart failure.
F. Trauma.
G. Medications.
H. Malignancy.
I. Central venous catheters.
J. Pregnancy.
K. Oral contraceptives.
L. Hormone replacement.
M. Nephrotic syndrome.
N. Antiphospholipid antibody syndrome.
O. Hospitalization (especially orthopedic surgery, trauma, spinal cord injury, gynecologic disorders).
P. Inherited clotting disorders, including factor V Leiden mutation, prothrombin mutations, antithrombin deficiency, hyperhomocysteinemia, elevated factor VIII activity, protein C deficiency, and protein S deficiency.

SUBJECTIVE DATA
A. Common complaints/symptoms.
  1. Pain.
  2. Swollen extremity.
  3. Muscle tenderness.
B. Common/typical scenario.
  1. Other signs and symptoms.
    a. Fever.
    b. Increased erythrocyte sedimentation rate.
    c. Increased white blood cell count.
C. Family and social history.
  1. History of recent surgery or trauma.
  2. History of cancer, liver disease, autoimmune disorder, or cardiovascular disease.
  3. History of blood clotting or bleeding problems.
  4. Family history of stroke or other thrombosis.
  5. Immobility.
  6. Recent prolonged travel.
D. Review of systems.
  1. Musculoskeletal: Ask about extremity pain with or without movement, edema, and redness.

PHYSICAL EXAMINATION
A. Physical examination alone is less reliable than when coupled with thorough history.

B. Unexplained extremity swelling, pain, warmth, or erythema may be noted. Pain is frequently described as a cramp or ache in the calf or thigh.

C. The location of the thrombus may influence physical findings. Swelling in the foot and ankle and calf pain are associated with thrombi in the venous sinuses in the soleus muscle and posterior tibial and peroneal veins. Thrombi in the femoral vein are associated with pain in the popliteal area and distal thigh, while those in the iliofemoral veins are manifested by pain and swelling involving the whole leg.

D. Upper extremity swelling along with pain and venous distention may indicate upper extremity DVT.

DIAGNOSTIC TESTS

A. Serum D-dimer concentration.
B. Lower extremity ultrasonography.
C. CT.
D. MRI.
E. Venogram.

DIFFERENTIAL DIAGNOSIS

A. Trauma.
B. Infection.
C. Peripheral artery disease.
D. Chronic venous insufficiency.
E. Postthrombotic syndrome.
F. Lymphedema.
G. Erythema nodosum.
H. Insect bites.
I. Muscle strain.
J. Cellulitis.

EVALUATION AND MANAGEMENT PLAN

A. General plan.
   1. Prompt diagnosis of DVT is facilitated by combining medical history and physical examination, D-dimer testing, and appropriate use of imaging studies.
   2. Hospitalized patients have traditionally been treated with intravenous (IV) heparin followed by warfarin. However, direct oral anticoagulants (DOACs) are also approved for treatment of DVT and PE. All patients receiving anticoagulation must be monitored for signs of bleeding.
   3. Thrombolytic therapy should be reserved for massive PE or extensive DVT.
   4. Contraindications to outpatient management of DVT include surgery within 7 days, cardiopulmonary instability, and severe symptomatic venous obstruction.
   5. Additional contraindications for outpatient treatment include platelet count less than 50,000/microliter, other medical or surgical conditions requiring inpatient management, medical nonadherence, geographic or telephone inaccessibility, impaired hepatic function, impaired renal function (e.g., rising serum creatinine), and inadequate home healthcare support.
   6. The optimal duration of therapy is dictated by the presence of modifiable risk factors for thrombosis.

   7. Long-term anticoagulation is an important consideration for individuals with unprovoked VTE or ongoing prothrombotic risk factors such as cancer and antiphospholipid antibody syndrome.
   8. Short-term therapy is sufficient for most patients with VTE associated with transient triggers such as major surgery.
   9. Inferior vena cava (IVC) filters should be considered for patients with acute VTE and contraindications to anticoagulation. Retrievable filters are preferable.
   10. Warfarin is contraindicated in pregnancy, while low molecular weight heparin (LMWH), dalteparin, enoxaparin, and fondaparinux are pregnancy category B. DOACs are currently contraindicated in women who are pregnant or planning to conceive.
B. Patient/family teaching points.
   1. Patients must be taught to recognize concerning signs for bleeding diathesis while on anticoagulation.
   2. Depending on the medication ordered, patients may need to have routine bloodwork completed.
   3. Patients need to set reminders to take the medications the same time each day to optimize efficacy of the medication.
C. Pharmacotherapy.
   1. Low-dose fractionated or nonfractionated heparin given subcutaneously is the mainstay of treatment.
   2. The availability of LMWH, fondaparinux, enoxaparin, and DOACs has increased the options for acute outpatient treatment of DVT and PE.
      a. DOACs can be as effective as LMWH and vitamin K antagonists such as warfarin.
      b. DOACs should be avoided in patients with advanced renal disease, pregnancy, and lactation.
      c. Warfarin should be avoided in pregnancy.
D. Discharge instructions (if standard accepted guidelines exist, please use discharge template).
   1. Patients will need to follow up with hematology or their primary care provider as an outpatient.
   2. Patients will need instruction on how to monitor for evidence of bleeding.

FOLLOW-UP

A. Patients with DVT should gradually resume activity and avoid immobility.
B. Monitoring of anticoagulation and bleeding risk can be done as an outpatient.
C. Individuals receiving warfarin need regular monitoring of prothrombin time (PT) and international normalized ratio (INR).
D. Platelets should be monitored in patients receiving LMWH and fondaparinux.

CONSULTATION/REFERRAL

A. Consultation with interventional radiology is necessary when considering use of thrombolytics, thrombectomy, stents, or placement of IVC filter.
B. Ongoing follow-up should be provided to patients requiring IVC filter to reduce risks of filter thrombosis.

SPECIAL/GERIATRIC CONSIDERATIONS

A. Increasing age and renal impairment increase risk of VTE in older adults and at the same time increase the risk of bleeding associated with anticoagulant therapy.

B. DOACs may offer an acceptable alternative to warfarin as monitoring is simpler.

C. Alteration in renal function may necessitate dose adjustments or serve as a contraindication to their use.

CASE SCENARIO: DEEP VEIN THROMBOSIS

A 48-year-old man presents to the clinic complaining of lower extremity edema. He denies personal or family history of coronary artery disease or hypercholesterolemia. He denies any recent surgery or trauma. He has a body mass index (BMI) of 30.4. He felt well until this morning and notes that he returned home to the East Coast 2 days ago after a vacation in Hawaii with his family. Physical examination reveals evidence of deep vein thrombosis (DVT).

1. What risk factor for DVT is evident in this case?
  A. Hypercoagulability
  B. Venous stasis
  C. Venous injury
  D. All of the above

2. Which of the following conditions would lead a provider to consider a diagnosis of DVT in a patient who presents with acute onset of lower extremity edema? (Select all that apply.)
  A. Bilateral lower extremity edema
  B. Unilateral lower extremity edema
  C. Recent orthopedic surgery
  D. Recent prolonged travel with dependent lower extremities
  E. History of malignancy

3. Which of the following should be included in the provider's differential diagnosis? (Select all that apply.)
  A. Cellulitis
  B. Lymphedema
  C. Peripheral artery disease
  D. Chronic venous insufficiency

4. Which of the following should the patient report to their provider after discharge? (Select all that apply.)
  A. Bleeding gums
  B. Tarry stool
  C. Sudden onset of lightheadedness
  D. Change in appetite

BIBLIOGRAPHY

Alper, E. C., Ip, I. K., Balthazar, P., Piazza, G., Goldhaber, S. Z., Benson, C. B., Lacson, R., & Khorasani, R. (2018). Risk stratification model: Lower extremity ultrasonography for hospitalized patients with suspected deep vein thrombosis. *Journal of Internal Medicine*, 33(1), 21–25. https://doi.org/10.1007/s11606-17-4170-3

Behravesh, S., Hoang, P., Nanda, A., Wallace, A., Sheth, R. A., Deipolyi, A. R., & Oklu, R. (2017). Pathogenesis of thromboembolism and endovascular management. *Thrombosis*, 2017, 1–14. https://doi.org/10.1155/2017/3039713

Chen, A., Stecker, E., & Warden, B. A. (2020). Direct oral anticoagulation use: A practical guide to common clinical challenges. *Journal of the American Heart Association*, 9(13), e017559. https://doi.org/10.1161/JAHA.120.017559

Desmarais, J., & Dutta, S. (2021). Urgent care diagnosis and management of DVT. *The Journal of Urgent Care Medicine*, 15(2), 13–17.

Kalaizopolulos, D. R., Panagopoulus, A., Samant, S., Galib, N., Kadillari, J., Daniilidis, A., Samartzis, N., Makadia, J., Palaiodimos, L., Kokkinidis, D. G., & Spryrou, N. (2022). Management of venous thromboembolism in pregnancy. *Thrombosis Research*, 211,106–113.

Keller, K., Sabatino, D., Winland-Brown, J. E., Porter, B. O., & Keller, M. B. (2019). Disorders of the vascular system. In L. M. Dunphy, J. E. Winland-Brown, B. O. Porter, & D. J. Thomas (Eds.), *Primary care the art and science of advanced practice nursing* (pp. 520–527). F. A. Davis.

Mefford, L. C. (2019). Disorders of blood flow and blood pressure regulation. In T. L. Norris (Ed.), *Porth's pathophysiology: Concepts of altered health states* (10th ed., pp. 713–752). Wolters Kluwer Health/Lippincott Williams & Wilkins.

Pai, M., & Douketis, J. D. (2022). *Patient education: Deep vein thrombosis (DVT) (Beyond the basics)*. In L. L. Leung (Ed.), *UpToDate*. https://www.uptodate.com/contents/deep-vein-thrombosis-dvt-beyond-the-basics

Streiff, M. B., Agnelli, G., Connors, J. M., Crowther, M., Eichinger, S., Lopes, R., McBane, R. D., Moll, S., & Ansell, J. (2016). Guidance for the treatment of deep vein thrombosis and pulmonary embolism. *Journal of Thrombosis and Thrombolysis*, 41, 32–67. https://doi.org/10.1007/s11239-015-1317-0

Talfur, D. V., & Talfur, A. (2015). Deep vein thrombosis. In F. J. Domino, R. A. Baldor, J. Golding, & M. B. Stephens (Eds.), *The 5 minute clinical consult premium, 2016* (24th ed., pp. 1092–1093). Wolters Kluwer Health.

Wimberley, P. (2019). Disorders of hemostasis. In T. L. Norris (Ed.), *Porth's pathophysiology: Concepts of altered health states* (10th ed., pp. 620–636). Wolters Kluwer Health/Lippincott Williams & Wilkins.

SICKLE CELL CRISIS

DEFINITION

A. Vaso-occlusive crisis (VOC), often referred to as acute painful episode involving the bones, is the most consistent and characteristic feature of sickle cell disease (SCD).

B. Other manifestations of vaso-occlusive disease include stroke, renal infarction, myocardial infarction, infarction, complications of pregnancy, priapism, and venous thromboembolism (VTE).

C. VOCs and their accompanying pain present most frequently in the extremities, chest, and back, although multiple sites may be involved.

INCIDENCE

A. Approximately 5% of the world's population carry an abnormal hemoglobin gene, with SCD being the most predominant form.

B. The greatest burden of the disease lies in sub-Saharan Africa. SCD affects nearly 100,000 individuals in the United States, the majority of whom are African American.

PATHOGENESIS

A. SCD occurs as a result of change in the amino acids of the beta globin chain of the hemoglobin molecule. Under circumstances where deoxygenation occurs, causing a reaction leading to "sickling" of the red blood ▶

cells (RBCs), reoxygenation allows the cell to return to its normal shape; however, repeated sickling damages the cells, leaving them permanently sickled.

B. Chronic hemolysis and high viscosity and vascular occlusion are the two main pathologic processes leading to the symptom most often associated with SCD. Infarction occurs as a result of stasis of the rigid sickle cells in the vascular beds of organs as a result of decreased blood flow. Sickled cells lose their flexibility and are unable to pass through the capillaries. Additionally, sickle cells tend to exhibit more adhesiveness to vascular endothelium and other blood cells, contributing to the obstruction of blood flow.

C. Acute bone pain is one of the most common manifestations of SCD. Pain occurs as a result of activating afferent nerves in bones experiencing ischemia. The long bones, including the femur and humerus, as well as the ribs, vertebrae, pelvis, and sternum, are common sites of pain, often with multiple sites affected at once. Dactylitis, or pain in the hands or feet, is often seen in children. Painful crises may vary in intensity.

D. When arising in other sites, pain can be confused with, or can be an early indication of, another acute complication, such as stroke, liver or splenic sequestration, or constipation associated with opioid use. The etiology of the pain must be identified in order to rule out potential causes of pain other than an uncomplicated VOC, such as cardiac ischemia, pneumonia, or other abdominal complications. VOC can occur in the presence of other complications, making diagnosis more challenging. No diagnostic test is able to rule in or rule out a VOC. Diagnostic tests are most useful in ruling out other causes of pain.

E. Acute abdominal pain may result from vaso-occlusion of mesenteric vasculature, sequestration of blood in the spleen, biliary tract disease, or non-SCD-related conditions. Sequestration most often occurs in the spleen, but the liver and lymph nodes may also be sites of sequestration. If not recognized and treated rapidly, acute sequestration may result in shock and death. Mesenteric syndrome is a rare complication. The patient may present with generalized abdominal pain, localized or rebound tenderness, and rigidity. Paralytic ileus with vomiting, distention, and absence of bowel sounds along with dilated bowel loops and air-fluid levels on abdominal x-ray are hallmarks.

F. Aplastic crisis causing an abrupt drop in circulating hemoglobin can occur as a result of chronic hemolysis and an inability for the bone marrow to recover.

PREDISPOSING FACTORS
A. Exposure to cold.
B. Dehydration.
C. Infection.
D. Physical exertion.
E. Tobacco smoke.
F. Alcohol use.
G. Drug abuse.
H. High altitude.
I. Hypoxic conditions.
J. Physical pain.
K. Pregnancy.
L. Hot weather.
M. Emotional stress.
N. Onset of menses.

SUBJECTIVE DATA
A. Common complaints/symptoms.
  1. Extremity pain.
  2. Chest pain.
  3. Back pain.
B. Common/typical scenario.
  1. Other signs and symptoms.
    a. Abdominal pain.
    b. Tachycardia.
    c. Tachypnea.
    d. Fever.
    e. Pallor.
    f. Jaundice.
C. Family and social history.
  1. Recent history of precipitating factors.
  2. Previous VOC.
  3. Comorbid conditions.
  4. Current treatment regimen, including analgesics and other medications, as well as transfusions.
D. Review of systems.
  1. Ask about pain and where it is located. Pain can affect any part of the body.
  2. Ask about any infections, cough, or fever.
  3. Cardiac: Chest pain and palpitations.
  4. Neurologic: Any weakness or shaking.

PHYSICAL EXAMINATION
A. Vital signs.
B. Oxygen saturation.
C. Skin and mucous membranes, noting pallor or jaundice.
D. Hydration status.
E. Cardiac examination.
F. Lung examination.
G. Abdominal examination.
H. Neurologic examination.

DIAGNOSTIC TESTS
A. Complete blood count (CBC).
B. Blood and urine cultures if febrile.
C. Chest x-ray if pulmonary symptoms.
D. EKG to rule out ischemia.
E. Chemistry panel.
F. Liver function testing.
G. Urinalysis.

DIFFERENTIAL DIAGNOSIS
A. Avascular necrosis.
B. Acute chest syndrome.
C. Gout.
D. Bone infarction.

▶

E. Osteomyelitis.

F. Joint infection.

G. Cerebrovascular accident.

H. Pneumonia.

I. Asthma.

EVALUATION AND MANAGEMENT PLAN

A. General plan.

1. Assessment of pain should occur as quickly as possible and include identification of other serious complications. It is important for providers to realize that most people with SCD have true, severe, life-long pain and do not exhibit drug-seeking behavior or have a substance use disorder.

2. Treatment of acute pain episodes includes providing adequate analgesia, hydration, prophylactic or therapeutic antibiotics after collection of appropriate cultures, and oxygenation if hypoxia is evident.

3. Oral hydration may be inadequate, making intravenous (IV) hydration necessary.

4. Pain management is best directed by the patient's report of pain.

a. Analgesia should be offered within 30 minutes of presentation with an acute painful event.

b. Before prescribing analgesics for an acute painful sickle cell episode, the provider should inquire about and consider any analgesia taken by the patient for this painful episode prior to their arrival at the hospital.

i. The effectiveness of pain relief should be assessed frequently. If the patient with severe pain has not had relief, a second dose of strong opioid should be offered. Continuous infusion of opioids and/or patient-controlled analgesia should be considered if repeated boluses of strong opioid medications are needed within a 2-hour period.

ii. Frequent monitoring for adverse events associated with strong opioids, including respiratory depression and excessive sedation, is advised.

iii. An alternative diagnosis should be considered if the patient does not respond to standard treatment for an acute crisis.

iv. Ketorolac and other nonsteroidal anti-inflammatory drugs (NSAIDs) should be avoided due to risk of renal toxicity. NSAIDs may be appropriate in some selected cases.

v. Patients receiving hydroxyurea should continue their usual dose unless there is evidence of hydroxyurea-related cytopenia.

vi. Prophylaxis for VTE should be considered in all inpatients with acute painful episodes.

vii. Nonpharmacologic measures include:

1) Physical therapy.

2) Relaxation.

3) Distraction techniques.

4) Music therapy.

5) Meditation, which may be beneficial.

6) Prophylactic incentive spirometry, which is recommended to reduce the risk of acute chest syndrome.

7) Heat applications may provide comfort to some patients. Cold applications should be avoided as cold may exacerbate sickling.

B. Patient/family teaching points.

1. Preventing sickle cell crises is the keystone management approach.

2. Patients need to be taught how to recognize their own triggers and to have a self-assessment and treatment plan at home.

3. Prevention of infection is also important.

a. Reinforcing proper hygiene is key.

b. Reinforcing universal precautions is essential.

4. Remind patients that the use of live vaccines is contraindicated in sickle cell due to the immunosuppressive therapy they receive.

C. Pharmacotherapy.

1. A dose of a strong opioid should be offered to all patients with severe pain (7 or greater on a 0–10 scale) and those with moderate pain (4–7 on a 0–10 scale) who have already received some analgesia before their arrival at the hospital.

2. Severe pain episodes require parenteral opioid analgesia and hydration in a hospital setting.

3. The dose of the analgesia should be titrated with the severity of the pain until adequate control is achieved with a scheduled dose regimen, with short-acting agents for breakthrough pain.

4. Meperidine should be avoided due to neurotoxicity associated with high doses.

5. A weak opioid may be considered in those with moderate pain who have not yet received some form of analgesic. Except when contraindicated, acetaminophen should be offered to all patients via a suitable route in addition to opioids.

6. All patients receiving opioids should receive laxatives on a regular basis, as well as antiemetics and antipyretics as needed.

D. Discharge instructions (if standard accepted guidelines exist, please use discharge template).

1. Long-term follow-up is essential.

2. Teach patients to recognize signs of infection and what to do when the signs manifest.

FOLLOW-UP

A. Patients with SCD should have regular follow-up with their hematologist.

B. Those with frequent readmissions for painful crises should be considered for treatment, with hydroxyurea used to increase fetal hemoglobin.

C. Routine laboratory evaluation should include CBC, electrolytes, and renal and liver function tests.

D. Adults should receive all age-appropriate immunizations, including pneumococcal vaccines, influenza, and meningococcal vaccines.

CONSULTATION/REFERRAL

A. Referral for pain management services may be warranted in individuals with chronic pain and when there is concern for opioid abuse.

B. Referral to ophthalmology for annual retinal examination should be considered in all patients.

SPECIAL/GERIATRIC CONSIDERATIONS

A. Improved treatment of patients with SCD has progressively increased their survival over the past 30 years.

B. While the average life expectancy of patients with SCD in the 1970s was less than 20 years, the mean life expectancy in the 1990s among those with the most severe form of the disease increased to 42 years for men and 48 years for women.

C. Cases of individuals living into their 50s and 60s have been well-documented, with additional recent cases indicating some individuals lived into their 80s.

D. Those who survive into later life are more likely to have long-term disease complications, including renal insufficiency.

CASE SCENARIO: SICKLE CELL CRISIS

A 19-year-old male patient presents to the ED complaining of acute chest and back pain. He has a history of sickle cell disease (SCD) that is typically well-managed with an average of one acute crisis annually. He was feeling well until last evening when he began experiencing fever and cough. This morning he had increased shortness of breath, with increased cough with discolored sputum. He rates his pain as 8 on a scale of 0 to 10. He has taken oral oxycodone 5 mg with acetaminophen twice prior to his visit to the ED and reports little relief.

1. Which of the following conditions are known to trigger a painful vaso-occlusive crisis in the presence of SCD? (Select all that apply.)

A. Infection
B. Dehydration
C. Excessive physical exertion
D. Cigarette smoking

2. The patient is admitted to the hospital for treatment of his symptoms. His treatment plan includes parenteral opioids. He is currently requiring IV hydromorphone every 1½ to 2 hours. When prescribing opioids, which option is usually deemed the most effective?

A. Opioids on an as-needed basis every 4 hours
B. Opioids on an as-needed basis every 6 hours
C. Opioids scheduled every 4 hours with additional medication given as needed
D. Patient-controlled analgesics allowing the patient to have control over when he receives the opioid analgesic and provide adequate relief

3. The patient's pain persists and in addition to strong opioids the provider will add nonopioid measures to help reduce pain. Which of the following is an appropriate intervention?

A. Adding intravenous (IV) ketorolac as an adjunctive analgesic
B. Encouraging use of ice packs to the affected painful areas
C. Exchange transfusion
D. Use of distraction techniques

4. The patient's acute pain resolves and he will be discharged home with instructions to taper off of the strong opioid he is taking and resume his previous regimen of oxycodone and acetaminophen. In addition to his prescription for analgesic medications, what other instructions for the patient are needed to reduce risk of complications and readmission after discharge? (Select all that apply.)

A. He should be advised to take a laxative on a regular basis to reduce risk of opioid-induced constipation.
B. He should be advised to continue to drink sufficient amounts of liquids to maintain optimal hydration.
C. He should only take his analgesic medication when pain becomes severe to reduce risk of side effects.
D. He should follow up with his primary care provider to make sure he is kept up to date on immunizations.

BIBLIOGRAPHY

Ballas, S. K., Pullte, D. E., Lobo, C., & Riddick-Burden, G. (2016). Case series of octogenarians with sickle cell disease. *Blood*, 128, 2367–2369. https://doi.org/10.1182/blood-2016-05-715946

DeBaun, M. R. (2022). *Acute vaso-occlusive pain management in sickle cell disease.* In R. A. Larson & L. L. Leung (Eds.), *UpToDate.* https://www.uptodate.com/contents/acute-vaso-occlusive-pain-management-in-sickle-cell-disease?search=sickle%20cell%20crisis&topicRef=110699&source=see_link

Elder, J. D., Winland-Brown, J. E., & Porter, B. O. (2019). Hematological disorders. In L. M. Dunphy, J. E. Winland-Brown, B. O. Porter, & D. J. Thomas (Eds.), *Primary care the art and science of advanced practice nursing* (5th ed., pp. 958–992). F. A. Davis.

Lanzkron, S., Carroll, C. P., & Haywood, C., Jr. (2013). Mortality rates and age at death from sickle cell disease: U.S., 1979–2005. *Public Health Reports*, 128, 110–128. https://doi.org/10.1177/003335491312800206

National Heart, Lung, and Blood Institute. (2014). *Evidence-based management of sickle cell disease: Expert panel report, 2014.* U.S. Department of Health and Human Services.

Vichinsky, E. P. (2020). *Overview of clinical manifestations of sickle cell disease.* In R. A. Larson &. L. L. Leung (Eds.), *UpToDate.* http://www.uptodate.com/contents/overview-of-the-clinical-manifestations-of-sickle-cell disease?search=sickle%20cell%crisis&source=search_result&selectedTitle=1150

KNOWLEDGE CHECK: CHAPTER 12

1. Which of the following conditions are associated with normocytic anemia? (1) Hemolysis, (2) acute blood loss, (3) heart valve abnormalities, (4) iron deficiency.

A. 1 and 2
B. 1 and 3
C. 1, 2, and 3
D. 1 and 4

2. Patients receiving erythropoiesis-stimulating agents require ongoing monitoring for adverse effects. Patients should be cautioned about which of the following?

A. Risk of myocardial infarction and stroke
B. Headache, fever, and myalgia
C. Fatigue, bone pain, and rash
D. Bone pain, flushing, and itching

3. Which of the following is a common form of inherited bleeding disorder?

A. Hemophilia
B. von Willebrand disease
C. Thrombotic thrombocytopenic purpura
D. Immune thrombocytopenic purpura

4. A combination of factors is often associated with bleeding in the setting of chronic liver disease. Which of the following is the most appropriate intervention to treat acute bleeding in a patient with liver disease?

A. Vitamin K injection
B. Fresh frozen plasma infusion
C. Red blood cell transfusion
D. Intravenous corticosteroid

5. Which of the following factors, sometimes referred to as Virchow's triad, are associated with increased risk of clotting?

A. Vessel injury, situations resulting in venous or arterial stasis, and malnutrition
B. Vessel injury, conditions causing hypercoagulability, and thrombocytopenia
C. Vessel injury, conditions causing hypercoagulability, and situations resulting in venous or arterial stasis
D. Cancer, obesity, and prolonged immobility

6. Several factors place older adults at increased risk of coagulopathy. Which of the following are among those factors? (1) Increased amounts of some clotting factors; (2) increased incidence of conditions associated with hypercoagulability, including cancer; (3) structural changes in vascular endothelium; (4) more sedentary lifestyle.

A. 1 and 3
B. 2 and 4
C. 1, 2, and 3
D. 1, 2, 3, and 4

7. Pulmonary embolism (PE) is a serious, life-threatening consequence of deep vein thrombosis (DVT), making prompt diagnosis and treatment critical. Approximately how many people die after diagnosis?

A. 5%
B. 10% to 15%
C. 10% to 30%
D. 30% to 40%

8. Which of the following place otherwise healthy people at risk of DVT?

A. Pregnancy
B. Prolonged time with extremities dependent
C. Use of oral contraceptives
D. All options are correct

9. Which is the most effective means to provide relief of pain in a patient diagnosed with sickle cell disease (SCD) during an acute painful episode?

A. Intravenous (IV) opioids given on an as-needed basis
B. Regularly scheduled IV opioids administered by the nurse
C. Continuous infusion of IV opioids
D. Continuous infusion with patient-delivered as-needed doses given via patient-controlled analgesia (PCA)

10. Providers concerned with potential for opioid abuse may consider reducing the dose of opioids and prescribing ketorolac for patients with sickle cell disease (SCD) and acute pain crisis. Which of the following may be a consequence of this action?

A. Acute kidney injury
B. Fluid retention when given with vigorous intravenous (IV) hydration
C. Constipation
D. Nausea and vomiting

(See answers next page.)

1. C) 1, 2, and 3
Acute blood loss, heart valve abnormalities, and iron deficiency are associated with normocytic anemia.

2. A) Risk of myocardial infarction and stroke
Patients receiving erythropoiesis-stimulating agents should be cautioned for risk of myocardial infarction and stroke.

3. B) von Willebrand disease
von Willebrand disease is a common form of inherited bleeding disorder.

4. B) Fresh frozen plasma infusion
Fresh frozen plasma infusion is the most appropriate intervention to treat acute bleeding in a patient with liver disease.

5. C) Vessel injury, conditions causing hypercoagulability, and situations resulting in venous or arterial stasis
Vessel injury, conditions causing hypercoagulability, and situations resulting in venous or arterial stasis are associated with increased risk of clotting.

6. D) 1, 2, 3, and 4
Increased amounts of some clotting factors; increased incidence of conditions associated hypercoagulability, including cancer; structural changes in vascular endothelium; and more sedentary lifestyle place older adults at increased risk of coagulopathy.

7. C) 10% to 30%
Approximately 10% to 30% of patients die after a diagnosis of pulmonary embolism (PE).

8. D) All options are correct
Pregnancy, prolonged time with extremities dependent, and use of oral contraceptives place otherwise healthy people at risk of deep vein thrombosis (DVT).

9. D) Continuous infusion with patient-delivered as-needed doses given via patient-controlled analgesia (PCA)
Continuous infusion, with the patient given as-needed doses via PCA, is the most effective means to provide relief of pain in a patient diagnosed with sickle cell disease during an acute painful episode.

10. A) Acute kidney injury
Use of ketorolac may cause acute kidney injury.

CHAPTER 13

ONCOLOGY GUIDELINES

BRAIN/CENTRAL NERVOUS SYSTEM MALIGNANCIES

Jennifer Creed

DEFINITION

A. Brain tumors most commonly arise from distant metastasis of other primary malignancies.
B. Primary brain tumors are classified according to the histologic pattern of cell differentiation.
  1. Gliomas.
    a. Most commonly occurring primary brain tumors.
    b. Subtypes include:
      i. Astrocytomas.
        1) Low grade.
          a) Pilocytic astrocytoma (grade I).
          b) Diffuse astrocytoma (grade II).
        2) High grade.
          a) Anaplastic astrocytoma (grade III).
          b) Glioblastoma multiforme (grade IV; most common astrocytoma in adults, 80%).
      ii. Oligodendrogliomas.
      iii. Ependymomas.
  2. Meningiomas.
  3. Nerve sheath tumors.
  4. Pituitary tumors.
  5. Primary central nervous system (CNS) lymphoma (associated with HIV/AIDS and immunosuppression).

INCIDENCE

A. The U.S. incidence rate of primary brain and other CNS tumors in patients 20 years of age and older is 8.5 and 22.38 per 100,000 persons for malignant and non-malignant tumors, respectively.
B. Brain and other CNS tumors are the eighth most common cancer in adults.
C. The 5-year overall survival rate for all malignant brain tumors is ~34%.
D. Survival rates depend on histologic subtype. For example, the 5-year overall survival rates for anaplastic astrocytoma and glioblastoma are 28% and 5%, respectively.

PATHOGENESIS

A. Primary brain tumors proliferate from brain tissue, most commonly from glial tissue.

  1. Tumors that arise from glial tissue include astro-cytomas, oligodendrogliomas, and ependymomas.
  2. Nonglial primary type brain tumors are meningi-omas, schwannomas, craniopharyngiomas, germ cell tumors, and pineal region tumors.
B. Typically, primary brain tumors do not metastasize, although they can.
C. Secondary or metastatic brain tumors originate from another part of the body and spread to the brain.
  1. The most common types include lung, breast, melanoma, colon, and kidney cancer.
  2. Distribution is as follows: Cerebral hemispheres 80%, cerebellum 15%, and brainstem 5%.
  3. Radiographic features can help distinguish meta-static lesions, including presence of multiple lesions, location at the graywhite matter junction, circum-scribed lesions, and vasogenic edema out of propor-tion to lesion size.

PREDISPOSING FACTORS

A. Ionizing radiation.
B. Exposure to cured foods.
C. HIV/AIDS.
D. Immunosuppression.
E. Cytomegalovirus (CMV) infection.
F. Familial predisposition.
  1. Neurofibromatosis type 1 (NF1) and type 2 (NF2).
  2. Li–Fraumeni syndrome.
  3. Turcot syndrome.
  4. Tuberous sclerosis.

SUBJECTIVE DATA

A. Common complaints/symptoms.
  1. Patients with low-grade tumors may initially be asymptomatic.
  2. Neurologic symptoms.
    a. Seizures.
    b. Focal neurologic deficits (weakness, numb-ness, aphasia).
    c. Syncope.
    d. Visual/hearing changes.
    e. Gait instability.
    f. Behavioral/personality changes.
  3. Symptoms related to increased intracranial pres-sure (ICP).
    a. Nausea and/or vomiting.
    b. Headache.
    c. Papilledema.

4. Symptoms/signs associated with pituitary tumors (e.g., prolactinomas).
    a. Bitemporal hemianopsia due to compression of the optic chiasm.
    b. Spontaneous bilateral nipple discharge.
    c. Hypogonadism.

PHYSICAL EXAMINATION

A. Assess for evidence of primary tumors.
B. A full neurologic exam must be performed in all patients with suspected CNS tumors.
    1. Mini-Mental State Examination.
    2. Cranial nerve testing.
    3. Motor strength in all extremities.
    4. Sensory testing.
    5. Reflexes.
    6. Gait and cerebellar assessment.
    7. Rectal tone (if there is concern for spinal pathology).

DIAGNOSTIC TESTS

A. Contrast-enhanced MRI (diagnostic standard).
B. Single-photon emission CT (SPECT) imaging may be used to detect defects in the blood–brain barrier (BBB) and may be considered to distinguish benign from malignant brain lesions.
C. Consider lumbar puncture (LP; contraindicated if there is evidence of elevated ICP).
D. Hormone evaluation for pituitary tumors.
E. If metastatic disease is suspected:
    1. CT of the chest, abdomen, and pelvis with intravenous (IV) contrast.
    2. Biopsy of brain lesion is not necessary if metastatic disease is confirmed.

DIFFERENTIAL DIAGNOSIS

A. Gliomas.
B. Meningiomas.
C. Nerve sheath tumors.
D. Pituitary tumors.
E. Primary CNS lymphomas.
F. Metastatic lesion.

EVALUATION AND MANAGEMENT PLAN

A. General plan.
    1. Management of brain tumors is dependent on definitive pathology for diagnosis.
    2. Biopsy or total resection (if possible) is recommended for all suspected brain malignancies.
    3. The BBB limits CNS penetration of many chemotherapies.
    4. Treatment approach varies depending on grade.
      a. Low-grade glioma (grade I or II).
        i. Maximal safe resection is recommended for all patients.
        ii. Low-risk patients.
          1) Observation postoperatively is reasonable due to slow growth.
          2) MRI should be obtained every 3 to 6 months for the first 5 years, then annually.

        iii. High-risk patients.
          1) Age greater than 40, subtotal resection, or unfavorable molecular features.
          2) Consider radiation and adjuvant chemotherapy.
      b. High-grade glioma (grade III or IV).
        i. Maximal safe resection.
        ii. Combination therapy with adjuvant radiation therapy (RT) and chemotherapy following resection.
        iii. Chemotherapy.
        iv. Targeted therapy.
    5. Seizure prophylaxis.
      a. Patients with no history of seizures generally do not require prophylactic anticonvulsants.
      b. Patients undergoing surgical resection of supratentorial tumors should be placed on prophylactic anticonvulsants for a defined period of time following surgery.
B. Acute care issues in brain/CNS cancers.
    1. Seizures.
    2. Cerebral edema.

FOLLOW-UP

A. Follow-up with the team on a regular basis is important, including medical oncology, radiation oncology, and the neurosurgeon.

CONSULTATION/REFERRAL

A. Referral to a neurosurgeon for biopsy/resection.
    1. Histologic review of the biopsy is the most crucial component of diagnosing brain tumors.
    2. Histologic classification dictates therapeutic approach.
    3. Pathologic review.

SPECIAL/GERIATRIC CONSIDERATIONS

A. Prognosis of patients is highly dependent on tumor location, the ability to resect it, tumor type, and age of the patient.
B. Patients may develop seizures related to the location or aggressiveness of the tumor.

CASE SCENARIO: ALTERED MENTAL STATUS

A 70-year-old woman presents to the ED with a 2-week history of worsening confusion, speech difficulties, and headache. The family notes that over the last day the patient has had right face and arm twitching. They deny any nausea, vomiting, or fever. The patient has a history of breast cancer s/p mastectomy and chemotherapy 15 years prior. On arrival, the patient's vital signs include a temperature of 99.5°F/37.5°C, blood pressure (BP) of 120/70, pulse rate of 68 beats per minute, and respiratory rate of 14 breaths per minute. Her complete blood count (CBC) and basic metabolic panel (BMP) values are all within normal limits. On exam, the patient is awake and attends the examiner. She is oriented to self only. She follows some simple commands but cannot name objects and perseverates. She has paucity of speech and has trouble finding her words. There is no evidence of twitching. Pupils are equally round and reactive to light. Her face is symmetric. Her motor strength is notable for a subtle right arm drift and she appears to have decreased sensation in her right arm and leg. A noncontrast CT of the head shows a large hypodense region in the left temporal lesion causing mass effect on the left midbrain and left thalamus, with a smaller hypodense area in the left thalamus.

1. Which test should be ordered first?
   A. Continuous EEG
   B. MRI of the brain with and without contrast
   C. CT of the chest/abdomen/pelvis
   D. CT angiogram of the head and neck

BIBLIOGRAPHY

Ostrom, Q. T., Patil, N., Cioffi, G., Waite, K., Kruchko, C., & Barnholtz-Sloan, J. S. (2020). CBTRUS statistical report: Primary brain and other central nervous system tumors diagnosed in the United States in 2013–2017. *Neuro-Oncology*, 22(12 Suppl 2), iv1–iv96.

BREAST CANCER

Catherine Harris

DEFINITION

A. Uncontrolled growth of breast cells, usually forming a tumor that can be felt as a lump or seen on x-ray.
B. Malignant tumors invade the surrounding tissues or metastasize to distant body areas.
C. Breast cancer can be curable, and early detection yields a favorable prognosis.

INCIDENCE

A. Breast cancer is the most commonly diagnosed cancer in American women, and approximately 12.4% of women in the United States will develop invasive breast cancer during their lifetime.
B. After increasing for more than 20 years, breast cancer incidence rates in women have stabilized since 2000, possibly related to fewer women using hormone replacement therapy after menopause.
C. Breast cancer is the second leading cause of cancer deaths in women, second only to lung cancer.
D. The chance that a woman will die from breast cancer is about 1 in 36 (~3%).
E. The median age of diagnosis of breast cancer for women in the United States is 68.
F. Fewer than 5% of women diagnosed with breast cancer in the United States are younger than 40.
G. Risk of breast cancer increases with age and is highest in women over the age of 70.
H. Breast cancer is much less common in men than in women, with men in the United States experiencing a 1 in 1,000 lifetime risk of developing breast cancer.

PATHOGENESIS

A. Ductal carcinoma in situ (DCIS).
   1. DCIS is considered noninvasive or preinvasive breast cancer.
   2. The cells that line the ducts of the breast have become dysplastic but remain contained within the walls of the ducts and have not spread into the surrounding breast tissue.
   3. DCIS accounts for approximately 20% of new diagnoses of breast cancer.
B. Lobular carcinoma in situ (LCIS).
   1. LCIS is a collection of abnormal cellular growth inside one or more of the milk-producing glands in the breast (called lobules).
   2. As the abnormal cells have not grown outside of the lobules, it is considered "in situ."
   3. Although it is not considered cancer, it is associated with a higher risk of developing invasive cancer in the future.
   4. LCIS is not very common and usually occurs in premenopausal women.
   5. LCIS is considered higher risk as it typically does not cause symptoms and can be difficult to see on imaging, making it difficult to detect.
   6. It is usually found incidentally when the breast is biopsied for some other reason.
C. Invasive ductal carcinoma (IDC).
   1. This is the most common type of breast cancer and accounts for approximately 80% to 85% of all new breast cancer diagnoses.
   2. IDC (or infiltrating) starts within the duct and grows into the adipose tissue of the breast.
   3. Breaking beyond the ductal wall means it now has the capability to spread to other areas of the body through lymphatic spread.
D. Invasive lobular carcinoma (ILC).
   1. ILC starts in the milk-producing glands (lobules) and invades into the adipose tissue of the breast and therefore can metastasize to other parts of the body.
   2. Accounts for about 10% of breast cancers.
   3. It is considered higher risk as it can be difficult to see on imaging, making detection and monitoring for recurrence difficult.
E. Inflammatory breast cancer (IBC).
   1. IBC is a rare but aggressive form of invasive breast cancer and accounts for about 1% to 3% of all breast cancers.
   2. There may not be a palpable mass or tumor, so it may not be seen on imaging. Sometimes skin thickening can be seen on mammogram.
   3. Often mistaken as cellulitis of the breast, as it presents with redness, warmth, and edema to the skin of the breast, often causing an orange peel appearance.
      a. This is caused not by infection but by cancer cells blocking the lymph vessels in the skin, causing congestion.
      b. If cellulitis is suspected and the patient fails to respond after a course of antibiotics, timely or prompt mammogram and biopsy should be considered.
   4. Time is of the essence with IBC given the strong potential for rapid progression. ▶

5. IBC is considered a more aggressive breast cancer and is associated with poorer prognosis when compared with IDC.

F. Other less common breast cancers and tumors include angiosarcoma, medullary, mucinous, Paget disease, papillary, phyllodes, and tubular.

PREDISPOSING FACTORS
A. Nonmodifiable.
   1. Family history.
   2. Genetic mutation or diagnosis (including BRCA1/2 gene mutations, Cowden syndrome, and Li–Fraumeni syndrome).
   3. Race (White women are more likely to develop breast cancer than other ethnicities).
   4. Sex (women > men).
   5. Personal history of breast cancer.
   6. Breast cellular changes (such as hyperplasia).
B. Modifiable.
   1. Smoking.
   2. Obesity (fat cells produce estrogen).
   3. Increased alcohol consumption (alcohol can limit your liver's ability to control blood levels of the hormone estrogen).
   4. Sedentary lifestyle.
   5. Exposure to estrogen (nulliparity, early onset of menorrhea, delayed onset of menopause, hormone replacement therapy, never breastfeeding).
   6. Use of oral contraceptives (there is an immediate increased risk, but that risk resolves over time after discontinuation).
   7. Prior radiation to the breast or chest wall.

SUBJECTIVE DATA
A. Common complaints/symptoms.
   1. Localized disease.
      a. Pain, swelling, or redness in the breast.
      b. Nipple changes, inversion, or discharge.
      c. Skin changes, thickening, dimpling, or scaling in the breast or nipple.
      d. With lymphatic spread, patients may experience painful or enlarged lymph nodes in the axilla, chest, or neck.
   2. Metastatic disease.
      a. Weight loss and/or change in appetite.
      b. Persistent, nagging, or worsening pain (visceral or bone/joint).
      c. Shortness of breath or cough.
      d. Headache.
      e. Fatigue.
B. Common/typical scenario.
   1. Due to increased awareness and screening, breast cancer can frequently be found on screening mammograms, by self-breast examination, or by providers performing breast surveillance examinations.
   2. When patients present with symptoms outside of the breast, they likely have already developed metastatic disease.

PHYSICAL EXAMINATION
A. In addition to evaluating for disease in the primary site (breast), evaluate for possible metastatic disease.
B. The most common sites of breast cancer metastases are the brain, bone, liver, and lung.
C. Check vital signs, including pulse oximetry.
D. A thorough baseline cardiac examination is important, as some chemotherapies used to treat breast cancer are associated with risk of cardiotoxicity. Many chemotherapies used to treat breast cancer can cause neuropathies, so it is important to assess for any preexisting neuropathies at baseline that may not be related to cancer (such as diabetic neuropathy or prior nerve damage due to injury).
E. Breast examination.
   1. Should be performed in the sitting position with arms at the side and raised above the head, and again while lying supine with the same arm positions. If patient has a self-palpated mass, ask them in which position they were best able to feel the mass. Do not forget to also examine the nipple–areolar complex.
   2. Once the mass is located, measure with a disposable measuring tape by isolating the mass between the thumb and the forefinger and noting the distance between the digits. Note which quadrant of the breast the mass is in.
   3. Assess the skin of the breast, including the skin overlying the mass and the nipple for changes such as redness, peau d'orange appearance, edema, scaliness, or even an open lesion.
   4. If patient notes nipple discharge, the breast can be gently pressed to try and elicit the discharge so the output can be evaluated. If unable to easily express discharge, do not utilize increasing pressure. Sometimes the patient will have discharge that has collected in a bandage or bra which can be evaluated. Note the color, amount, and consistency.
   5. Lymph nodes should also be evaluated in the sitting and supine positions. Include bilateral evaluation of the axilla, supraclavicular, infraclavicular, cervical, and mandibular regions. If lymph nodes are palpated, note the size, consistency, if fixed or mobile, and if the patient reports tenderness with palpation.
F. Evaluate for metastatic disease.
   1. Pulmonary: Observe for signs of dyspnea, increased work of breathing, or retractions; evaluate for pleural effusions (auscultation, percussion, and cacophony).
   2. Musculoskeletal: Bone tenderness or impaired range of motion.
   3. Abdomen: Assess for hepatomegaly, ascites, mass, or tenderness.
   4. Neurologic: Incoordination, focal deficits, visual changes, hearing changes, or decreased strength.

DIAGNOSTIC TESTS
A. History and physical examination.
B. Diagnostic bilateral mammogram with tomosynthesis, which provides higher resolution when evaluating someone who has a known mass or breast abnormality; ▶

ultrasound of the breast as necessary (or as recommended by the radiologist).

C. Breast biopsy and clip placement. Ultrasound of the nodal basin on the ipsilateral side.

D. Pathology review; determination of hormone receptor status (estrogen/progesterone [ER/PR] receptor and human epidermal growth factor receptor 2 [HER2]).

E. Breast MRI when indicated. This is usually recommended by the radiologist if dense breast tissue obscures the mass, there is a question of the size of the mass, or concern is observed for involvement of the chest wall.

F. Breast cancer is predictable. It starts in the breast, moves to the regional lymph nodes, and then metastasizes to distant sites in the body. If nodal ultrasound is negative and there are no findings on physical examination to suggest metastasis, systemic staging is not indicated (per National Comprehensive Cancer Network [NCCN] guidelines). If a suspicious node is noted on imaging or examination, proceed with biopsy of the lymph node. If positive, proceed with metastatic workup.

 1. Complete blood count (CBC) and comprehensive metabolic panel (CMP).

 2. CT of the chest, abdomen, and pelvis with contrast.

 3. Bone scan.

 4. PET scan, if indicated.

G. Diagnosis.

 1. Tissue sample or biopsy is required for diagnosis. Pathology results will help guide the next step of workup, referral/provider evaluation, and recommended interventions.

 2. It is imperative to send biopsy sample(s) for ER/PR and HER-2/neu testing, as these results are required for prognostication and therapy recommendations.

H. Staging: Breast cancer is staged utilizing the American Joint Committee on Cancer (AJCC) tumor, node, metastasis (TNM) system.

DIFFERENTIAL DIAGNOSIS

A. DCIS.
B. LCIS.
C. IDC.
D. ILC.
E. IBC.
F. Paget disease.
G. Abscess.
H. Fibroadenoma.

EVALUATION AND MANAGEMENT PLAN

A. General plan.

 1. Unless there is metastatic disease at the time of presentation, all patients who can tolerate surgery will be offered surgical intervention.

 2. Depending on stage, some patients will also be offered chemo and/or radiation.

 3. If the cancer is estrogen- or progesterone-positive, they may also be offered adjuvant hormone therapy.

 4. Surgery.

 5. Radiation therapy (RT).

 6. Chemotherapy.

 7. Hormone therapy.

 a. About two out of three breast cancers are hormone receptor-positive.

 b. These cells have estrogen (ER-positive) and/or progesterone (PR-positive) receptors on the cell surface that stimulate cell proliferation in the presence of estrogen or progesterone, respectively.

B. Acute care issues in breast cancer.

 1. Breast cancer patients are typically only admitted for surgical resection.

 a. Some procedures, such as segmental mastectomy, are outpatient procedures.

 b. More involved procedures, such as total mastectomy or those receiving immediate breast reconstruction, may require postoperative admission.

 2. Neutropenic fever (also see sections on Leukemias).

 a. Neutropenia may occur as a chemotherapy side effect, and neutropenic patients are highly susceptible to infection.

 b. Neutropenic fever can be life-threatening and can rapidly lead to sepsis.

 c. Diagnostics include CBC with differential, blood cultures, urinalysis with culture, chest x-ray (CXR), sputum culture (if appropriate), intravenous (IV) fluid support (if appropriate), antipyretics, and empiric broad-spectrum antibiotics.

 d. Use of granulocyte colony stimulating factor (G-CSF) may be considered for neutropenia.

 3. Metastatic symptoms.

 a. The most common sites of metastatic spread from breast cancer are the bone, brain, liver, and lung.

 b. Patients with metastatic disease may be admitted for pain management or symptoms resulting from an organ system being affected by disease, such as:

 i. Fluid retention or transaminitis from hepatic metastasis.

 ii. Confusion related to brain metastasis.

 iii. Pain and/or fracture from metastasis to the bone.

FOLLOW-UP

A. See Table 13.1.

CONSULTATION/REFERRAL

A. Medical oncology.

B. Breast surgical oncology.

C. Radiation oncology (can be done prior to or after surgery and/or chemotherapy, or for palliation if metastatic).

D. Fertility specialist, if appropriate.

E. Cardiology referral may be indicated prior to chemotherapy or surgery as chemotherapeutic regimens (e.g., anthracyclines) can cause cardiotoxicity or lead to evaluate for anesthesia clearance.

F. Genetic counseling: If indicated according to the NCCN guidelines.

G. Any patient with suspected breast cancer needs to be seen urgently by a specialist or breast clinic.

TABLE 13.1   BREAST CANCER FOLLOW-UP

	NCCN	ACS/ASCO
History and physical examination	Year 1, every 3–4 months; year 2, every 4 months; years 3–5, every 6 months; year 6+, annually	Years 1–3, every 3–6 months; years 4–5, every 6–12 months; year 6+, annually
Signs of recurrence	No recommendation	Educated and counseled about signs and symptoms
Mammography	6 months after post-BCS radiation therapy annually thereafter	Annually
MRI	No recommendation	Not recommended for routine screening unless patient meets high-risk criteria for increased surveillance
Pelvic examination	Annually, for women on tamoxifen annual exam if uterus present	No recommendation
Routine blood tests	No recommendation	No recommendation
Imaging studies	No recommendation	No recommendation
Tumor marker testing	No recommendation	No recommendation

ACS, American Cancer Society; ASCO, American Society of Clinical Oncology; BCS, Breast Cancer Society; NCCN, National Comprehensive Cancer Network.

H. Consider referrals to support groups and psychiatry for assistance in coping.

SPECIAL/GERIATRIC CONSIDERATIONS
A. Treatment guidelines for older adults patients with breast cancer are limited.
B. Treatment recommendations should be decided in conjunction with the patient and based on life expectancy, as well as the patient's functional status, comorbidities, and social support.

BIBLIOGRAPHY
National Cancer Institute. (n.d.). *Fast stats*. https://seer.cancer.gov/faststats/selections.php?series=cancer
National Comprehensive Cancer Network. (2017, November 10). *Clinical practice guidelines in oncology. Breast cancer (Version 3. 3017)*. National Comprehensive Cancer Network
Runowicz, C. D., Leach, C. R., Henry, N. L., Henry, K. S., Mackey, H. T., Cowens-Alvarado, R. L., & Ganz, P. A. (2016). American Cancer Society/American Society of Clinical Oncology breast cancer survivorship care guideline. *CA: A Cancer Journal for Clinicians, 66*, 43–73. https://doi.org/10.3322/caac.21319

GASTROINTESTINAL CANCERS: COLORECTAL CANCER

Cheryl Pfennig, Rae Brana Reynolds, and Steven H. Wei

DEFINITION
A. Cancer that forms in the tissues of the colon.
B. Most colon cancers are adenocarcinomas and develop from polyps.

INCIDENCE
A. Colorectal cancer is the third most common cancer in both men and women, and is also the third leading cause of cancer deaths.
B. In 2016, there were an estimated 134,490 cases diagnosed in the United States: 39,220 cases of rectal cancer and 95,270 cases of colon cancer.
C. The incidence of colon cancer has continued to decline over the past three decades, likely associated with improved screening and treatment of colorectal polyps. Despite this decline, there were still an estimated 49,140 deaths from colon and rectal cancers in 2016.
D. Greater than 90% of new cases of colorectal cancer occur in patients over the age of 50, with the median onset age at 73.
E. While the risk of colorectal cancer increases with age, in recent years there has been a significant increase in the incidence of colorectal cancer in younger patients.

PATHOGENESIS
A. Colorectal cancer is a complex process that derives from the epithelial cells lining the colon.
B. Genetic mutations, either inherited or acquired, are thought to occur that irritate the lining, causing inflammation and necrosis of the colon.
C. Over time, lesions can develop which can disrupt cellular DNA and cause dysplasia, which can lead to the development of cancer.

PREDISPOSING FACTORS
A. Approximately 2% to 5% of colorectal cancers are hereditary, while the majority of cases are sporadic.
B. Risk factors associated with the development of colorectal cancer include:
   1. Dietary factors, including consumption of red meat, processed meat, and animal fat.
   2. Cigarette smoking.
   3. Inflammatory bowel disease (e.g., ulcerative colitis). ▶

4. History of colorectal cancer or adenomatous polyps.

5. Obesity.

6. Familial syndromes: Familial adenomatous polyposis (FAP) or hereditary nonpolyposis colorectal cancer (HNPCC).

SUBJECTIVE DATA

A. Common complaints/symptoms.

1. Colorectal cancer is often asymptomatic, with symptoms appearing once the disease has become more advanced. Screening colonoscopies often detect early, asymptomatic colorectal cancers.

2. The most common presenting signs and symptoms include:

    a. Abdominal pain.

    b. Anorectal pain.

    c. Iron deficiency anemia.

    d. Weight loss.

    e. Fatigue.

    f. Hematochezia.

    g. Melena.

    h. Bowel changes.

       i. Constipation.

       ii. Diarrhea.

       iii. Urgency.

       iv. Frequency.

       v. Tenesmus.

       vi. Mucous discharge.

    i. Nausea/vomiting.

    j. Urinary dysfunction.

    k. Erectile dysfunction.

PHYSICAL EXAMINATION

A. Gastrointestinal (GI).

1. Percussion.

    a. Dull areas may be present over the tumor site.

    b. A protuberant, tympanic abdomen may be indicative of an obstruction.

2. Auscultate for bowel sounds in all four quadrants.

    a. Absent or decreased bowel sounds are often indicative of obstruction.

3. Palpate for tenderness and/or masses in all four quadrants.

    a. Larger tumors of the colon are often palpable on physical examination in nonobese patients.

    b. Liver is one of the two most common sites for colorectal metastasis, and patients with advanced liver metastasis may have tender hepatomegaly.

4. Digital rectal examination to assess for tumor location, circumferential nature, and sphincter tone.

B. Gynecologic examination in females with rectal cancer is important secondary to the proximity of the rectum to the vagina. Vaginal examination should be performed to evaluate for posterior vaginal wall involvement and to rule out rectovaginal fistula.

C. Evaluate for metastatic disease, primarily liver, lung, and/or lymph nodes.

DIAGNOSTIC TESTS

A. The workup for colorectal cancers includes diagnostic studies to help determine the extent of the disease, as well as the presence of metastatic disease.

1. Colon cancer workup.

    a. Colonoscopy, complete to the cecum with adequately prepped colon.

    b. Pathology review of biopsies.

    c. Laboratory studies: Complete blood count (CBC), comprehensive metabolic panel (CMP), and carcinoembryonic antigen (CEA) level.

    d. CT scan of the chest, abdomen, and pelvis with intravenous (IV) and oral contrast.

2. Rectal cancer workup.

    a. Colonoscopy, complete to the cecum with adequately prepped colon.

    b. Pathology review of biopsies.

    c. Laboratory studies: CBC, CMP, and CEA.

    d. CT scan of the chest, abdomen, and pelvis with IV and oral contrast.

    e. Pelvic MRI is the preferred staging study; however, if not available, perform endorectal ultrasound.

    f. Flexible sigmoidoscopy or rigid proctoscopy is often performed by a surgeon to verify the tumor location for radiation treatment planning and surgery planning.

    g. Enterostomal therapist referral is made for patient education and ostomy site marking.

B. Diagnosis and staging.

1. Colorectal cancer diagnosis is established via tissue biopsy. Colonoscopy is the most common mode to obtain a tissue diagnosis, although an image-guided biopsy of a tumor may confirm the diagnosis.

2. Adenocarcinomas are the most common histologic subtype, accounting for greater than 90% of all cases. Less common histologic subtypes include mucinous carcinoma, signet-ring cell carcinoma, squamous cell carcinoma, and undifferentiated carcinoma.

3. Confirmed tissue diagnosis and a complete workup provide the necessary data to clinically stage colorectal cancer. Proper clinical staging is important as it influences treatment planning and serves as an indicator for prognosis.

4. Staging for colorectal cancer is similar to the staging of many cancers, and utilizes the tumor, node, metastasis (TNM) system.

DIFFERENTIAL DIAGNOSIS

A. Inflammatory bowel disease.

B. Ileus.

C. Ischemic bowel.

D. Diverticulosis.

EVALUATION AND MANAGEMENT PLAN

A. General plan.

1. The primary treatment for colorectal cancer is surgery; however, disease stage and presence of metastatic disease can alter the treatment modalities offered as well as their sequencing.

▶

2. Chemotherapy agents are commonly administered in the adjuvant setting; however, they may be administered in patients with locally advanced disease or with metastatic disease at presentation.
3. Radiation therapy (RT).
4. Surgical management for colorectal cancers.
  a. Should include resection of the primary tumor, as well as the lymphatic, venous, and arterial supply.
  b. Treatment side effects are a potential threat from all three treatment modalities, with the most common including:
    i. Bowel dysfunction.
    ii. Sexual dysfunction.
    iii. Genitourinary dysfunction.
    iv. Neuropathies.
B. Acute care issues in colorectal cancer.
1. Colorectal cancer patients will be admitted to the hospital following surgical resection or for urgent situations including bowel obstructions or perforations.
2. Postoperative hospitalization varies by surgical approach. The average hospital stay is 2 to 7 days, with a shorter average stay for patients who have undergone a minimally invasive surgical approach.
  a. Postoperative management is focused on return of bowel function, ostomy care (if applicable), and pain control.
3. Patients admitted for complications such as bowel obstruction or perforation are managed based on the severity of the complication.
  a. Bowel obstruction.
    i. Nothing by mouth (NPO) and bowel rest.
    ii. Nasogastric tube.
    iii. Surgery: Exploratory laparotomy with possible bowel resection.
  b. Perforation.
    i. NPO and bowel rest.
    ii. Surgery is indicated in the majority of cases to remove the area of perforation and to wash out the abdomen.
    iii. Antibiotics.

FOLLOW-UP

A. Colon cancer recurrence typically occurs within 3 years of resection; therefore, patients should have routine follow-up for at least 5 years after resection.
B. Colonoscopy is necessary after resection for surveillance.

CONSULTATION/REFERRAL

A. Gastroenterology referral for screening is critical in patients who are at high risk for colorectal cancer.
B. Any patient with suspected colon cancer should be referred to surgery immediately. Surgery is the only curative option for localized cancer and should not be delayed.
C. Medical oncology referral for treatment and surveillance.
D. Refer patients to support groups.

SPECIAL/GERIATRIC CONSIDERATIONS

A. Most patients with colorectal cancer are older than 70 years old.
B. Older adult patients may be undertreated and are underrepresented in clinical trials, making treatment guidelines difficult.
C. Life expectancy, quality of life, and patients' functional status should be taken into consideration when determining a plan of action.

BIBLIOGRAPHY

Jasperson, K. W., Tuohy, T. M., Neklason, D. W., & Burt, R. W. (2010). Hereditary and familial colon cancer. *Gastroenterology, 138*(6), 2044–2058.
National Cancer Institute. (2016, September 12). *Surveillance, epidemiology, and end results program.* https://seer.cancer.gov/faststats/selections.php?series=cancer

GASTROINTESTINAL CANCERS: GASTRIC CANCER

Cheryl Pfennig, Rae Brana Reynolds, and Steven H. Wei

DEFINITION

A. A malignant tumor of the stomach.
B. Most cancers of the stomach are adenocarcinomas: Malignant tumors that develop from the cells in the lining of the stomach.

INCIDENCE

A. Gastric cancer is the third most common cause of cancer-related mortality worldwide.
B. In the United States, approximately 22,220 patients are diagnosed annually, 10,990 of whom are expected to die from gastric cancer.
C. The worldwide incidence of gastric cancer has declined over the past few decades, partly due to the recognition of risk factors such as *Helicobacter pylori* and dietary risks.
D. The overall 5-year relative survival rate of all people with stomach cancer in the United States is about 30%.

PATHOGENESIS

A. Gastric cancer is a malignant neoplasm that arises anywhere between the gastroesophageal junction and pylorus.
B. Most tumors are epithelial in origin and classified as adenocarcinomas.
C. *H. pylori* infection is strongly associated with the presence of precancerous lesions that manifest into cancer proliferation. Over 80% of gastric cancers are thought to be attributed to *H. pylori* infection.

PREDISPOSING FACTORS

A. Chronic gastritis caused by:
1. Chronic *H. pylori* infection.
2. Pernicious anemia.
3. Diet.
  a. Diet high in salt and salt-preserved foods, nitrates, nitrites, fried foods, processed meats, and alcohol.

b. Diets low in vegetables (diets high in fruits, vegetables, and fiber are protective against gastric cancer).

B. Obesity.

C. Smoking.

D. Prior gastric surgery.

E. Prior abdominal radiation.

F. Male sex.

G. African American race.

H. Inherited germline mutations in *TP53*, *BRCA2*, and *CDH1*.

SUBJECTIVE DATA

A. Common complaints/symptoms.

1. Unintentional weight loss secondary to insufficient caloric intake caused by tumor-related anorexia, nausea, abdominal pain, early satiety, and/or dysphagia.

2. Bowel changes: Melena or black tarry stools, constipation if treating pain, nausea, anemia, and change in nature or pattern of bowel habits if an obstructing tumor.

3. Persistent vague, epigastric abdominal pain.

4. Dysphagia, especially for tumors in the proximal stomach or gastroesophageal junction.

5. Fatigue secondary to anemia from bleeding tumors.

PHYSICAL EXAMINATION

A. Focused areas of the physical examination for suspected gastric cancer should include:

1. Vital signs.

a. Evaluate weight and recent trends for unintentional weight loss.

b. Heart rate (HR): Tachycardia suggestive of dehydration secondary to poor oral intake.

2. Head, ear, eyes, nose, and throat (HEENT).

a. Evaluate oral mucosa for paleness suggestive of anemia.

b. Evaluate tongue for evidence of thrush.

c. Quality of dentition.

3. Palpate neck and cervical nodal chains for adenopathy suggestive of metastasis.

4. Abdominal examination.

a. Observe for contour of the abdomen and distention, evidence of cachexia.

b. Evaluate the skin, subcutaneous tissue, and umbilicus.

c. Auscultate abdomen noting the frequency and character of bowel sounds, normally 5 to 30 gurgling sounds per minute.

d. Palpation: Prior to palpation, ask about any tender areas and palpate this area last; commonly tender in the epigastric region secondary to reflux.

e. Evaluate for abdominal firmness suggesting carcinomatosis and ascites.

f. Evaluate for nodularity in the umbilical area suggestive of a Sister Mary Joseph nodule demonstrating umbilical metastasis.

g. Palpate for hepatosplenomegaly (HSM) suggestive of metastasis.

DIAGNOSTIC TESTS

A. Complete history and physical examination.

B. Laboratory tests including complete blood count (CBC) with differential and comprehensive metabolic panel (CMP).

C. Upper gastrointestinal (GI) series with barium swallow as initial screening for patients with dysphagia.

D. CT of the chest, abdomen, and pelvis.

E. Esophagogastroduodenoscopy (EGD) for tissue diagnosis and anatomic location.

F. Endoscopic ultrasound (EUS) if no evidence of distant metastatic disease.

G. Diagnostic laparoscopy with biopsy and peritoneal lavage to evaluate for radiographically occult metastatic disease and carcinomatosis.

H. Diagnosis: Tissue diagnosis and anatomic localization of the primary tumor are best obtained by upper GI endoscopy.

I. Staging.

1. Gastric cancers that are 5 cm or more from the gastroesophageal junction are staged using the tumor, node, metastasis (TNM) system as gastric cancers.

2. Gastric cancers that are less than 5 cm from the gastroesophageal junction are staged using the TNM system as esophageal cancers.

DIFFERENTIAL DIAGNOSIS

A. Gastritis.

B. Gastroenteritis.

C. Esophagitis.

D. Esophageal cancer.

E. Peptic ulcer disease.

F. Neoplasm.

EVALUATION AND MANAGEMENT PLAN

A. General plan.

1. Tissue diagnosis and staging evaluation are required for treatment planning.

2. Surgical resection is required for cure of gastric cancer.

3. Surgery followed by chemotherapy ± radiation is the mainstay of treatment.

4. Surgery.

5. Advanced metastatic disease (stage IV) is treated with palliative chemotherapy or on a clinical trial.

B. Acute care issues in gastric cancer.

1. Gastric cancer patients are often only admitted for surgical resection.

2. Postoperative gastric surgery patients without complications will spend 7 to 10 days in the hospital after surgery.

3. The primary focus in the postoperative inpatient setting is nutrition, pain control, monitoring lab work, wound care, and early ambulation.

a. Routine bloodwork including CBC with differential, electrolyte panel, blood urea nitrogen (BUN), and creatinine must be monitored for anemia, infection, electrolyte imbalance/need for replacement, and kidney function.

▶

b. The incision site will be monitored daily for signs of infection and proper healing.

c. The postgastrectomy patient will have a nasogastric tube in place. Once there is no evidence of anastomotic leak, the nasogastric tube may be removed.

d. Supplemental jejunostomy tube feedings will be initiated on postoperative day 1 and will continue until oral intake is adequate.

e. Oral feeding is started 4 to 7 days postoperatively.

f. Upper GI studies are done as indicated (fever, tachycardia, tachypnea, leukocytosis).

g. Early ambulation reduces risk of postoperative pneumonia, ileus, and thrombosis. The goal is to have the patient out of bed the day after the procedure as tolerated.

h. Postoperative cancer patients have a hypercoagulable state; prophylactic enoxaparin is initiated postoperatively and continued for 28 days.

FOLLOW-UP

A. Postgastrectomy complications.

   1. Duodenal stump or anastomotic leak.

     a. Anastomotic leak: Arises from any of the suture/staple lines of the anastomosis.

     b. Duodenal stump leak: Most feared complication of gastrectomy.

     c. Symptoms: Severe abdominal pain, fever, tachycardia, and hypotension.

     d. CT of the abdomen is indicated.

       i. Findings: Pneumoperitoneum, extraluminal contrast, fluid collection, and/or abscess.

     e. Upper GI series (with Gastrografin) may also be performed to assess leak.

     f. Treatment.

       i. Broad-spectrum antibiotics.

       ii. Consider percutaneous drainage of fluid collection/abscess by interventional radiology.

       iii. If leak persists or patient is hemodynamically unstable, they should be taken to the operating room for exploration, drainage, and repair.

   2. Dumping syndrome.

     a. Postgastrectomy patients commonly have rapid transit and report diarrhea.

     b. Dumping syndrome is characterized by diaphoresis, abdominal cramps, and watery diarrhea shortly after intake of concentrated sweets and hyperosmolar liquids.

     c. Diagnosis is based on clinical symptoms.

       i. Gastric emptying studies or upper GI series may be performed.

     d. Treatment.

       i. The primary goal includes dietary changes with frequent small meals that are high in fiber and low in carbohydrates. Avoid food triggers (e.g., simple sugar).

       ii. Octreotide may help but is not typically required.

CONSULTATION/REFERRAL

A. In patients with suspected gastric cancer, consults should be made to gastroenterology, radiation oncology, medical oncology, and surgery.

SPECIAL/GERIATRIC CONSIDERATIONS

A. Most cases of gastric cancer affect older adults.

B. Aggressive treatment and surgery should not be withheld from patients solely due to chronological age.

C. Life expectancy, quality of life, and patients' functional status need to be taken into consideration in conjunction with patients' wishes.

BIBLIOGRAPHY

National Cancer Institute. (2016, September 12). *Surveillance, epidemiology, and end results program.* https://seer.cancer.gov/faststats/selections.php?series=cancer

Siegel, R., Ma, J., Zou, Z., & Jemal, A. (2014). Cancer statistics, 2014. *CA: A Cancer Journal for Clinicians, 64*(1), 9–29.

Zhu, A. L., & Sonnenberg, A. (2012). Is gastric cancer again rising? *Journal of Clinical Gastroenterology, 46*, 804–806.

GASTROINTESTINAL CANCERS: HEPATIC CANCER

Cheryl Pfennig, Rae Brana Reynolds, and Steven H. Wei

DEFINITION

A. Hepatocellular carcinoma (HCC) is the most common form of primary liver cancer in adults.

B. Other cancers that begin in the liver include intrahepatic cholangiocarcinoma (about 10%–20%) and less common tumors such as angiosarcomas, hemangiosarcomas, hepatoblastomas, and malignant epithelioid hemangioendotheliomas.

INCIDENCE

A. Liver cancer occurs primarily in people age 55 to 64, with a median age of 63 at diagnosis.

B. Liver and bile duct cancers are relatively rare in the United States when compared with other cancers.

C. In 2022, an estimated 41,260 cases will be diagnosed in the United States, and about 30,250 people will die of liver and intrahepatic cholangiocarcinoma.

D. Worldwide, liver cancer is the second most common cause of cancer mortality, with the highest incidence rates found in Asia and Africa.

E. The survival rate among individuals with liver cancer varies based on staging at the time of diagnosis.

F. Surveillance, Epidemiology, and End Results (SEER) data estimate that 44% of patients present with localized disease (confined to the primary site), 26% have a disease that has spread to regional lymph nodes, and 19% present with distant metastases.

G. The 5-year relative survival rates for each are 36.1%, 12.8%, and 3.1%, respectively.

H. The incidence and mortality rates of HCC are on the rise in the United States.

PATHOGENESIS

A. There is a strong association with inflammation, necrosis, fibrosis, and cirrhosis in the development of HCC.

B. Some gene mutations have been identified as the cause of uncontrolled division of cells in the liver, leading to development of cancer.

C. HCC has several different subtypes, each with different growth patterns.

PREDISPOSING FACTORS

A. Male sex.

B. Chronic hepatitis B and C virus infections.

C. Alcohol-related cirrhosis.

D. Nonalcoholic fatty liver disease (NAFLD).

E. Exposure to certain chemicals (e.g., nitrites, hydrocarbons, and polychlorinated biphenyls).

F. Dietary intake of aflatoxins (toxic metabolites produced by certain fungi in foods and feeds).

G. Metabolic disorders such as hemochromatosis, Wilson disease, and alpha-1 antitrypsin deficiency.

H. Presence of hepatocellular adenoma (unclear risk of malignant transformation to HCC).

SUBJECTIVE DATA

A. The presentation of liver cancer is dependent on the stage of disease.

B. Common complaints/symptoms.

    1. Fatigue.

    2. Abdominal pain/bloating.

    3. Palpable mass in the right upper quadrant.

    4. Signs and symptoms of liver disease: Ascites, jaundice, splenomegaly, and portal hypertension.

    5. Nausea.

    6. Decreased appetite and early satiety.

    7. Unexplained weight loss.

    8. Fever.

PHYSICAL EXAMINATION

A. Check vital signs.

B. Head and neck.

    1. Evaluate for scleral icterus.

    2. Palpate the neck and supraclavicular area for adenopathy. Look for jugular venous distention.

C. Pulmonary system.

    1. Observe the patient for signs of dyspnea, increased work of breathing, or retractions.

    2. Auscultate all lung fields.

D. Cardiovascular system.

    1. Auscultate heart sounds.

E. Gastrointestinal (GI) system.

    1. Perform a thorough abdominal examination.

    2. Pay close attention to the right upper quadrant.

    3. Assess for a fluid wave/evidence of ascites, hepatomegaly, an umbilical hernia, and caput medusae.

F. Musculoskeletal system.

    1. Observe for signs of muscle wasting and cachexia.

    2. Evaluate lower extremities for pitting edema.

G. Central nervous system (CNS).

    1. Assess cranial nerves II to XII.

H. Skin.

    1. Assess for jaundice, palmar erythema, and spider angiomata.

DIAGNOSTIC TESTS

A. Laboratory evaluation should include complete blood count (CBC), comprehensive metabolic panel (CMP), prothrombin time/partial thromboplastin time/international normalized ratio (PT/PTT/INR), and prealbumin.

B. Tumor markers: Alpha fetoprotein (AFP) and cancer antigen 19–9 (CA 19–9).

C. Multiphasic CT of the chest, abdomen, and pelvis with and without intravenous (IV) contrast.

D. MRI of the abdomen and chest x-ray (CXR) in patients with PO/IV contrast allergy.

E. EKG if considering surgery.

F. Liver tumor biopsy is generally not necessary when considering surgery in the setting of classic imaging findings, elevated tumor markers, and the presence of known risk factors. Patients with fatty liver disease may be referred for biopsy of their underlying (nontumoral) liver to evaluate for percent steatosis and fibrosis, as this impacts their candidacy for surgical resection.

G. Diagnosis.

    1. Diagnosis typically requires a combination of laboratory data, imaging, and biopsy results.

    2. Laboratory data.

        a. Tumor markers are often elevated in patients with liver cancer and can be followed to assess response to therapy or monitored for disease progression.

        b. AFP, while neither specific nor sensitive for HCC, is elevated in 50% to 90% of all patients with HCC.

        c. CA 19–9 is a useful tumor marker and often elevated in cholangiocarcinoma.

    3. Imaging.

        a. Ultrasonography may be used as the initial screening technique in patients being monitored for chronic hepatitis; however, surgical resectability and treatment planning are always based on dedicated, multiphasic imaging of the chest, abdomen, and pelvis.

        b. Triple-phase CT scan with and without IV contrast assesses the blood flow to liver tissue during early arterial, late arterial, and portal venous phases.

        c. CT imaging typically shows arterial phase enhancement in HCC due to increased vascular supply of the tumor from the hepatic artery.

        d. Metastatic adenocarcinomas and cholangiocarcinomas typically enhance during the portal phase on CT.

    4. Biopsy.

        a. Tissue sampling/biopsy is recommended if the patient is not a candidate for surgery and targeted therapy or systemic chemotherapy is being considered.

b. Tissue for pathologic confirmation can be obtained through a percutaneous image-guided biopsy of the liver nodule/mass.

H. Staging.

1. The staging of HCC, like the majority of cancers, follows the American Joint Committee on Cancer (AJCC) tumor, node, metastasis (TNM) system.

2. Higher numbers indicate more advanced disease.

DIFFERENTIAL DIAGNOSIS

A. Cirrhosis.

B. Hepatocellular adenoma.

C. Cholangiocarcinoma.

EVALUATION AND MANAGEMENT PLAN

A. General plan.

1. Patients with HCC may be offered surgery, targeted therapy/chemotherapy, immunotherapy, radiation therapy (RT), liver-directed therapy, or referral for liver transplantation depending on multiple factors present at diagnosis, including:

a. Geographic distribution of disease.

b. Presence of metastatic disease.

c. Age and comorbidities.

d. Cirrhosis.

e. Liver function and reserve volume.

2. Surgery.

3. Targeted therapy/chemotherapy/immunotherapy.

4. RT.

5. Liver-directed therapy includes percutaneous treatments.

a. Radiofrequency microwave ablation.

b. Transarterial chemoembolization (TACE).

c. Radioembolization.

d. Cryotherapy (less common).

e. Ethanol injection (less common).

6. Liver transplantation.

B. Acute care issues in hepatic cancer.

1. Liver cancer patients are often only admitted to the hospital after surgical resection or transplantation.

2. Patients either undergo a partial hepatectomy (removal of a portion of the right or left liver, which may or may not require resection of an entire segment) or a complete right or left hepatectomy. These surgeries can be performed laparoscopically, open, or via a minimally invasive approach. The gallbladder is sometimes removed at the time of liver resection.

3. Liver-directed therapies are generally performed in the outpatient setting but can occasionally require hospital admission.

FOLLOW-UP

A. Postoperative liver surgery patients, without complications, will spend an average of 3 to 7 days in the hospital, depending on the type of surgery performed (laparoscopic vs. open).

B. The primary focus in the postoperative inpatient setting is pain control, early ambulation, monitoring blood counts and liver function tests, wound/drain management, pulmonary toileting to avoid pneumonia, and prevention of blood clots.

C. Patients are evaluated by an inpatient dietitian, who stresses the importance of adequate protein and fluid intake in the perioperative period and after discharge.

CONSULTATION/REFERRAL

A. Most patients are treated by a multidisciplinary team including both surgical and medical oncologists, who formulate a treatment plan based on clinical staging.

B. Hepatobiliary surgeon may be consulted for patients with localized disease and adequate liver function and reserve volume.

C. Medical oncologist may be consulted for patients with metastatic disease (outside of the liver) or if not considered a candidate for surgery.

D. Radiation oncologists may be consulted if RT is being considered in patients with localized disease.

E. A referral to liver transplantation specialist may also be considered in select patients with localized disease but not considered a candidate for liver resection.

F. Prior to surgery, patients are often referred to internal medicine to optimize and manage medical comorbidities in the perioperative period.

G. Patients with active hepatitis virus infections are managed by either infectious disease or hepatology specialists.

SPECIAL/GERIATRIC CONSIDERATIONS

A. Surgical resection and liver transplantation are the only potentially curative treatments for most hepatic cancers.

B. Decisions to aggressively treat or not treat hepatic cancer in the geriatric population should not be based on age alone.

C. Factors such as life expectancy, quality of life, and patients' functional status should be taken into consideration.

BIBLIOGRAPHY

McGlynn, K. G., Petrick, J. L., & El-Serag, H. B. (2021). Epidemiology of hepatocellular carcinoma. *Hepatology*, 73(Suppl 1), 4–13.

National Cancer Institute. (2022, May 5). *Surveillance, epidemiology, and end results program*. https://seer.cancer.gov/faststats/selections.php?series=cancer

GASTROINTESTINAL CANCERS: PANCREATIC CANCER

Cheryl Pfennig, Rae Brana Reynolds, and Steven H. Wei

DEFINITION

A. Adenocarcinoma of the pancreas (referred to as pancreatic cancer) originates from the exocrine cells of the pancreas.

B. Pancreatic cancer comprises more than 95% of pancreatic malignancies.

INCIDENCE

A. Pancreatic cancer is the fourth leading cause of cancer deaths in the United States, with an estimated 53,070 ▶

new cases and 41,780 deaths from pancreatic cancer in 2016.

B. The overall risk of developing pancreatic cancer increases after 50 years of age, and the majority of patients with disease are between the ages of 60 and 80 years.

C. The only potentially curative therapy for pancreatic cancer is surgical resection of the involved portion of the pancreas in patients with localized disease. Unfortunately, 80% of patients have metastatic and locally advanced disease at initial diagnosis, which precludes curative resection for the majority of patients.

D. In patients who have undergone resection with curative intent, only 10% to 27% of patients survive at least 5 years after surgical resection. Meanwhile, the 5-year overall survival rate for all pancreatic cancer stages combined remains low at 8%.

PATHOGENESIS

A. Pancreatic cancer is caused by mutations to DNA.

B. Insults to DNA can be hereditary or environmental, such as alcohol, smoking, drugs, and obesity.

C. Acute pancreatitis and recurrent acute pancreatitis can develop into chronic pancreatitis, which can convert to pancreatic cancer.

D. Most cases of pancreatic cancer are adenocarcinomas.

PREDISPOSING FACTORS

A. Cigarette smoking.
B. Alcoholism.
C. Obesity.
D. Chronic pancreatitis.
E. Diabetes mellitus.
F. Family history.
G. Genetic mutations.

SUBJECTIVE DATA

A. Common complaints/symptoms.
  1. Pain.
  2. Jaundice.
  3. Weight loss.
  4. Steatorrhea.
  5. Nausea.
  6. Hyperglycemia.
  7. Diabetes mellitus.
B. Common/typical scenario.
  1. The pancreas is located proximal to the stomach, small intestine, and bile duct so clinical manifestations of pancreatic cancer usually affect the anatomy and function of these adjacent structures. For example:
    a. A pancreatic tumor obstructing the biliary system could cause jaundice.
    b. Nausea, digestive problems, and weight loss may result from obstruction of the upper digestive tract.
    c. Steatorrhea can result from an obstruction of the pancreatic duct that prevents the passage of digestive enzymes into the intestines.

PHYSICAL EXAMINATION

A. Head and neck: Inspect for scleral icterus and palpate for cervical and supraclavicular lymphadenopathy.
B. Integumentary: Inspect for jaundice.
C. Abdomen: Inspect and palpate for mass effect, ascites, hepatosplenomegaly (HSM), and pain.
D. Weight assessment: Measure weight at each visit especially when nutritionally compromised.
E. Complete a full examination including cardiopulmonary, musculoskeletal, and neurology assessment to evaluate the patient's overall fitness for oncology treatment.

DIAGNOSTIC TESTS

A. Laboratory data.
  1. Complete blood count (CBC).
  2. Comprehensive metabolic panel (CMP).
  3. Prealbumin for nutrition status assessment.
  4. Cancer antigen 19–9 (CA 19–9).
B. Diagnostic imaging.
  1. Multiphase helical CT scan.
    a. A CT scan with contrast can correctly predict resectability in pancreatic cancer with 80% to 90% accuracy.
  2. Endoscopic evaluation.
    a. Esophagogastroduodenoscopy (EGD).
    b. Endoscopic retrograde cholangiopancreatography (ERCP).
C. Staging: The American Joint Committee on Cancer (AJCC) has developed a staging system based on tumor, node, metastasis (TNM) status for pancreatic cancer.

DIFFERENTIAL DIAGNOSIS

A. Acute pancreatitis.
B. Cholangitis.
C. Cholecystitis.
D. Gastric cancer.
E. Peptic ulcer disease.

EVALUATION AND MANAGEMENT PLAN

A. General plan.
  1. Chemotherapy, radiation, and surgery are utilized in the treatment of pancreatic cancer.
  2. The modalities employed and the sequence in which they are administered often depend on the clinical stage of the disease.
  3. Neoadjuvant therapy for pancreatic cancer refers to chemotherapy and/or radiation administered prior to surgery.
  4. Surgery.
    a. The majority of pancreatic cancers arise from the pancreatic head, and these lesions, if resectable, are treated with pancreaticoduodenectomy, commonly known as the Whipple procedure.
    b. Resectable pancreatic tail cancers are treated with a distal pancreatectomy, which can also involve a splenectomy depending on the splenic vessel involvement of the tumor.
  5. Chemotherapy.
  6. Radiation.

FOLLOW-UP
A. Routine follow-up is essential.
B. Patients should have CT imaging at 3- to 6-month intervals for the first 2 years and then annually.

CONSULTATION/REFERRAL
A. Consults should be made to gastroenterology, medical oncology, radiation oncology, and general surgery.

SPECIAL/GERIATRIC CONSIDERATIONS
A. Prognosis for pancreatic cancer is very poor and largely incurable.
B. The 5-year relative survival rate is 7% for all stages of pancreatic cancer.

BIBLIOGRAPHY
Bose, D., Katz, M. H., & Fleming, J. B. (2012). Pancreatic adenocarcinoma. In B. W. Feig & C. D. Ching (Eds.), *The MD Anderson cancer center surgical oncology handbook* (5th ed.). Wolters Kluwer/Lippincott Williams & Wilkins.
Chatterjee, D., Katz, M. H., Rashid, A., Varadhachary, G. R., Wolff, R. A., Wang, H., Lee, J. E., Pisters, P. W. T., Vauthey, J.-N., Crane, C., Gomez, H. F., Abbruzzese, J. L., Fleming, J. B., & Wang, H. (2012). Histologic grading the extent of residual carcinoma following neoadjuvant chemoradiation in pancreatic ductal adenocarcinoma: A predictor for patient outcome. *Cancer, 118*(12), 3182–3190.
Fernandez-del Castillo, C. (2019, January 18). *Clinical manifestations, diagnosis, and staging of exocrine pancreatic cancer.* In D. M. F. Savarese & K. M. Robson (Eds.), *UpToDate.* https://www.uptodate.com/contents/clinical-manifestations-diagnosis-and-staging-of-exocrine-pancreatic-cancer
Karmazanovsky, G., Fedorov, V., Kubyshkin, V., & Kotchatkov, A. (2005). Pancreatic head cancer: Accuracy of CT in determination of resectability. *Abdominal Imaging, 30*(4), 488–500.
Katz, M. H., Wang, H., Fleming, J. B., Sun, C. C., Hwang, R. F., Wolff, R. A., Varadhachary, G., Abbruzzese, J. L., Crane, C. H., Krishnan, S., Vauthey, J.-N., Abdalla, E. K., Lee, J. E., Pisters, P. W. T., & Evans, D. B. (2009). Long-term survival after multidisciplinary management of resected pancreatic adenocarcinoma. *Annals of Surgical Oncology, 16*(4), 836–847.
National Cancer Institute. (2016, September 12). *Surveillance, epidemiology, and end results program.* https://seer.cancer.gov/faststats/selections.php?series=cancer

GYNECOLOGIC CANCERS: CERVICAL CANCER

Diann C. Fernandez

DEFINITION
A. Types of cervical cancer.
  1. The most common type of invasive cervical cancer is squamous cell carcinoma (about 70%–80%).
  2. The second most common subtype is adenocarcinoma (10%–15%).
  3. Other types include adenosquamous carcinoma, adenoid cystic carcinomas, neuroendocrine tumors of the cervix, undifferentiated cervical cancer, and mixed epithelial and mesenchymal tumors.

INCIDENCE
A. Cervical cancer remains the fourth most common cancer of women worldwide with a mortality rate of approximately 52%.
B. About 90% of the new cases and deaths worldwide in 2020 occurred in low- and middle-income countries.
C. Cervical cancer is the third most common gynecologic cancer (after uterine and ovarian cancer) and the 12th most common cancer of women in the United States.
D. An estimated 14,100 new cases of invasive cervical cancer will be diagnosed in 2022, and approximately 4,280 deaths from cervical cancer will occur in the United States in 2022.

PATHOGENESIS
A. Caused by an abnormal growth of cells. Human papillomavirus (HPV) must be present for the majority of cervical cancer to develop.

PREDISPOSING FACTORS
A. Early age of sexual activity: The relative risk of having cervical cancer is 2.5 if the age of first sexual exposure is less than 18 years of age.
B. Multiple sexual partners: Relative risk is 2.8 if the number of partners is five or more.
C. Lower socioeconomic status.
D. A partner with many prior sexual partners or known HPV.
E. Tobacco use.
F. HIV.
G. Long-term immunosuppressive therapy related to solid organ transplant, stem cell transplant (SCT), systemic lupus erythematous, inflammatory bowel disease, or rheumatologic disease.
H. In utero exposure to diethylstilbestrol (DES) increases the risk of clear cell carcinoma of the cervix.
I. HPV infection.
  1. HPV is a double-stranded DNA virus that belongs to the Papillomaviridae family.
  2. There are more than 100 different types of HPV identified, and they are divided into two groups.
    a. Low-risk HPV. Common types: 6, 11, 40, 42, 43, 44, 54, 61, 72, and 81.
    b. High-risk HPV. Most common types: 16, 18, 31, 33, 35, 45, 52, and 58. Subtypes 16 and 18 account for 70% of all cervical cancers.

SUBJECTIVE DATA
A. Common complaints/symptoms.
  1. At early stages, many patients are asymptomatic.
  2. Postcoital bleeding (most common).
  3. Vaginal discharge that can be thin, mucoid, purulent, blood-tinged, and malodorous.
  4. Abnormally heavy or prolonged menses.
  5. Vaginal bleeding becomes heavier, frequent, and may become continuous with progressive disease.
  6. Pelvic or lower back pain, often seen with advanced disease.
B. Common/typical scenario.
  1. The most common cervical lesions are exophytic and friable, arising from the ectocervix.
  2. Endocervical lesions are more commonly adenocarcinomas arising from the mucus-producing glands.
  3. Cervix may be firm with or without mass or ulceration.

4. May find an ulcerated tumor eroding through the cervix.

PHYSICAL EXAMINATION

A. When patients present with symptoms suggestive of cervical cancer, they should undergo complete physical examination including a pelvic examination.

B. It is important to determine if the disease has spread into the parametria or the pelvic sidewalls.

C. Rectovaginal examination is also important to assess for parametrial disease.

D. Examine for distant metastases by palpating the groin and supraclavicular lymph nodes; exam of the right upper quadrant.

DIAGNOSTIC TESTS

A. Pelvic examination, including Pap smear.

B. If no lesions are noted, perform a colposcopy (possible endocervical curettage) to identify any abnormalities.

C. Pathologic confirmation is important for accurate diagnosis. If a visible lesion is noted, obtain a biopsy. The best site to take the biopsy is from the edge of the tumor, where the transition from invasive to noninvasive can be clearly seen.

D. Once diagnosis is confirmed by biopsy, the following tests may be beneficial:

1. Laboratory data: Complete blood count (CBC) and comprehensive metabolic panel (CMP); consider HIV testing.

2. Chest x-ray (CXR).

3. CT imaging to assess extrauterine spread and adenopathy.

4. MRI (best imaging modality to assess extent of disease).

5. PET scan to assess for lymphatic metastasis.

6. Cystoscopy.

7. Proctoscopy.

8. Exam under anesthesia (EUA) may be needed for a thorough examination.

E. Staging.

1. Cervical cancer is staged clinically and with radiologic/surgical evaluation for staging of nodal disease. Clinical staging alone is an option used in low-resource settings.

2. Staging is used to determine the treatment and prognosis.

3. Tumor stage is not changed even after recurrence.

DIFFERENTIAL DIAGNOSIS

A. Cervicitis.

B. Endometrial carcinoma.

C. Vaginitis.

D. Sexually transmitted infections/pelvic inflammatory disease.

EVALUATION AND MANAGEMENT PLAN

A. General plan.

1. Treatments for cervical cancer depend on the age of the patient, type of cervical cancer, stage, and desire for children.

2. Prognostic factors.

    a. Pathologic types.

    b. Tumor size.

    c. Depth of invasion.

    d. Lymphovascular invasion.

    e. Nodal metastases.

3. Surgery is the treatment of choice for stage IA, IB1, and IB2 cervical cancer.

4. Most patients with stage I disease do not require further treatment if they do not have adverse prognostic factors (see the following).

5. Surgical options depend on the stage of cancer and/or are based on their fertility desire.

    a. Simple hysterectomy.

    b. Radical hysterectomy (standard approach for radical hysterectomy is via open abdominal approach).

    c. Fertility-preserving surgeries.

    d. Pelvic exenteration surgery: Type of radical surgery that removes organs from urinary, gastrointestinal (GI), and gynecologic systems.

6. Chemotherapy.

7. Radiation therapy (RT) with or without radiosensitizing chemotherapy.

8. Participation in clinical trial.

B. Acute care issues in cervical cancer.

1. Cervical cancer patients are only admitted for certain types of surgeries.

    a. Radical hysterectomy.

    b. Pelvic exenteration.

    c. Other surgeries, including simple hysterectomy and fertility-preserving surgical procedures, may be outpatient.

2. RT.

3. Other situations where cervical cancer patients may need inpatient admission include postoperative complications, pain control, or due to chemotherapy side effects including nausea, vomiting, and neutropenic fever.

FOLLOW-UP

A. The goals of postoperative management include pain control, fluid and electrolyte balance, early ambulation, and return of bowel and bladder function.

B. Follow-up care should focus on identifying, preventing, and controlling the long-term and late effects of cervical cancer.

C. Coordination of all the patient's providers should be navigated by the primary/leading care provider.

D. Follow-up evaluation every 3 to 6 months for the first 2 years, followed by every 6 months for the next 3 years. Evaluate for signs of recurrence such as abdominal and pelvic pain, leg symptoms such as pain or lymphedema, vaginal bleeding or discharge, urinary symptoms, cough, and weight loss.

E. Annual cervical/vaginal cytology.

CONSULTATION/REFERRAL

A. Gynecologist, gynecologic oncology, radiation oncology, interventional radiologist, and surgery.

SPECIAL/GERIATRIC CONSIDERATIONS

A. Cervical cancer is common in older adult women, and treatment disparities are significantly associated with mortality in this population.

B. Despite evidence that older adult women tolerate treatment well, they are less likely to be offered surgery and adjuvant radiation.

CASE SCENARIO: CERVICAL CANCER

A 64-year-old, G2P2002 woman presents with complaints of postcoital bleeding for 6 to 8 months. The vaginal bleeding lasts for about 1 hour postcoital, then resolves. She denies pelvic/abdominal pain, weight loss, and changes to bowel or bladder function. Her last menstrual period was at age 51. The last well-woman exam was more than 15 years ago. She is referred for gynecologic evaluation. On pelvic exam, she is found to have a normal-sized uterus with a 1 × 3 cm friable exophytic cervical lesion at the 2 o'clock position. Bimanual with rectovaginal exam with free parametria. Cervical biopsy at the 2 o'clock position is done and consistent with squamous cell carcinoma. Lymph node assessment is negative, including inguinal and supraclavicular nodes. The remainder of the physical exam is within normal limits. PET demonstrates no metastatic disease. MRI of the pelvis shows no invasion to adjacent organs nor parametrial involvement. She undergoes total abdominal hysterectomy (TAH)/bilateral salpingo-oophorectomy (BSO). She is diagnosed with stage IB2 cervical cancer, with no adjuvant treatment indicated.

1. Which high-risk human papillomavirus (HPV) types are present in 70% of cervical cancers?

   A. HPV 6 and 11

   B. HPV 31 and 40

   C. HPV 16 and 18

   D. HPV 52 and 58

2. When counseling patients about cervical cancer recurrence, common symptoms to watch for include all of the following EXCEPT?

   A. Cough

   B. Rash

   C. Vaginal bleeding

   D. Abdominal/pelvic pain

BIBLIOGRAPHY

Bruni, L., Albero, G., Serrano, B., Mena, M., Collado, J. J., Gómez, D., Muñoz, J., Bosch, F. X., & de Sanjosé, S. (2021, October 22). ICO/IARC Information Centre on HPV and Cancer (HPV Information Centre). Human papillomavirus and related diseases in the world. Summary Report 22 October 2021.

de Sanjose, S., Quint, W. G., Alemany, L., Geraets, D. T., Klaustermeier, J. E., Lloveras, B., Tous, S., Felix, A., Bravo, L. E., Shin, H. R., Vallejos, C. S., de Ruiz, P. A., Lima, M. A., Guimera, N., Clavero, O., Alejo, M., Llombart-Bosch, A., Cheng-Yang, C., Tatti, S. A., & Retrospective International Survey and HPV Time Trends Study Group. (2011, November). Human papillomavirus genotype attribution in invasive cervical cancer: A retrospective cross-sectional worldwide study. *Lancet Oncology*, 11(11), 1048–1056. https://doi.org/ 10.1016/S1470-2045(10)70230-8. Epub 2010 Oct 15. PMID: 20952254.

Eskander, R. N., & Bristow, R. E. (Eds.). (2014). *Gynecologic oncology: A pocketbook*. Springer Science + Business Media.

Kissel, M., Rambeau, A., Achkar, S., Lecuru, F., & Mathevet, P. (2020). Challenges and advances in cervix cancer treatment in elder women. *Cancer Treatment Reviews*, 84, 101976. https://doi.org/10.1016/j.ctrv.2020.101976 (https://www.sciencedirect.com/science/article/pii/S0305737220300141) ISSN 0305-7372

Noor, R., Tay, E. H., & Low, J. (2014). *Gynaecologic cancer: A handbook for students and practitioners*. Pan Stanford.

Salani, R., Khanna, N., Frimer, M., Bristow, R. E., & Chen, L. M. (2017, July). An update on post-treatment surveillance and diagnosis of recurrence in women with gynecologic malignancies: Society of Gynecologic Oncology (SGO) recommendations. *Gynecologic Oncology*, 146(1), 3–10. https://doi.org/ 10.1016/j.ygyno.2017.03.022 Epub 2017 Mar 31. PMID: 28372871

SEER Cancer Stat Facts: Cervical Cancer. National Cancer Institute. https://seer.cancer.gov/statfacts/html/cervix.html

Sharma, C., Deutsch, I., Horowitz, D., Hershman, D., Lewin, S., Lu, Y.-S., Neugut, A., Herzog, T., Chao, C., & Wright, J. (2012). Patterns of care and treatment outcomes for elderly women with cervical cancer. *Cancer*, 118, 3618–3626. https://doi.org/0.1002/cncr.26589

Siegel, R. L., Miller, K. D., & Jemal, A. (2020). Cancer statistics, 2020. *CA: A Cancer Journal for Clinicians*, 70, 7–30. https://doi.org/10.3322/caac.21590

Sung, H., Ferlay, J., Siegel, R. L., Laversanne, M., Soerjomataram, I., Jemal, A., & Bray, F. (2021). Global cancer statistics 2020: GLOBOCAN estimates of incidence and mortality worldwide for 36 cancers in 185 countries. *CA: A Cancer Journal for Clinicians*, 71, 209–249. https://doi.org/10.3322/caac.21660

GYNECOLOGIC CANCERS: ENDOMETRIAL/UTERINE CANCER

Diann C. Fernandez

DEFINITION

A. Endometrial cancer develops in the lining of the uterus and is the most common type of malignancy of the female reproductive system.

B. More than 90% of all uterine cancers arise from the endometrium (the inner layer) of the uterus. Other uterine cancers develop in the myometrium (the muscle layer) of the uterus, which include uterine leiomyosarcoma, and so forth.

INCIDENCE

A. In 2022, an estimated 65,950 people in the United States will be diagnosed with uterine or endometrial cancer, with 12,550 deaths resulting from the disease.

B. Uterine sarcomas are rare, accounting for <10% of all uterine corpus malignancies, and arise in the myometrium or connective tissue elements of the endometrium.

C. A woman's lifetime risk of developing endometrial cancer is approximately 2.8%.

D. Endometrial cancer represents 3.4% of all new cancer cases in the United States.

E. The majority of women are diagnosed between their 60s and 70s, with a median age of 63.

F. It is the most common gynecologic malignancy.

PATHOGENESIS

A. Endometrial cancer is usually preceded by endometrial hyperplasia, which is an overgrowth of the uterine lining.

B. Adenocarcinomas comprise 80% of endometrial cancers.

   1. Endometrioid carcinoma is the most common subtype and is graded using the International ▶

Federation of Gynecology and Obstetrics (FIGO) classification system.

2. High-risk subtypes include serous endometrial carcinoma (~10%), clear cell carcinoma (<5%), mixed carcinoma, undifferentiated/dedifferentiated carcinoma, and carcinosarcoma.

C. Sarcomas (arising in the myometrium) include leiomyosarcoma, endometrial stromal sarcoma (high grade/low grade), and undifferentiated sarcoma.

PREDISPOSING FACTORS

A. Major risk factors.
   1. Obesity.
   2. Diabetes.

B. Other risk factors.
   1. Increased levels of unopposed estrogen.
   2. Early age at menarche.
   3. Nulliparity.
   4. Late age at menopause.
   5. Older age of 55 or more.
   6. Tamoxifen use for greater than 5 years.
   7. Previous pelvic radiation therapy (RT).
   8. A personal family history of breast or ovarian cancer.
   9. Genetics: Personal or family history of hereditary nonpolyposis colorectal cancer (HNPCC; or Lynch syndrome).

SUBJECTIVE DATA

A. Common complaints/symptoms.
   1. About 90% of women diagnosed with endometrial cancer have abnormal uterine bleeding (i.e., postmenopausal bleeding, recurrent bleeding at irregular intervals, or prolonged or excessive bleeding).
   2. Asymptomatic women can present with an abnormal Pap smear showing atypical or malignant endometrial cells, atypical glandular cells, or adenocarcinoma (which can be endocervical or endometrial).

B. Common/typical scenario.
   1. Endometrial cancer can be discovered incidentally on ultrasonography, CT, or MRI with a thickened endometrial lining.

C. Family and social history.
   1. An accurate history of present illness as well as past medical conditions, family, and social history should be taken.

PHYSICAL EXAMINATION

A. The physical examination should involve a general inspection of the body for abnormalities, palpation of the inguinal and supraclavicular nodes, and inspection of the vulva, anus, vagina, and cervix to evaluate for metastatic lesions.

B. Bimanual and rectovaginal examination should be performed to evaluate the uterus, cervix, adnexa, parametria, and rectum, which may be normal in early-stage endometrial cancer.

C. The size, mobility, and axis of the uterus should be assessed.

D. A biopsy should be performed for any suspicious genital tract lesions detected on examination.

DIAGNOSTIC TESTS

A. Histologic evaluation of endometrial tissue is required for diagnosis.

B. Once endometrial cancer is confirmed, additional studies are needed for treatment planning.
   1. Complete blood count (CBC) with differential.
   2. Serum electrolytes.
   3. Kidney and liver function tests.
   4. EKG.
   5. Transvaginal ultrasound.
   6. CT of the chest, abdomen, and pelvis with intravenous (IV) and oral contrast to rule out extrauterine spread in high-grade malignancies.
   7. MRI of the abdomen and pelvis.
   8. Chest x-ray (CXR; can be used as alternative to CT).
   9. Cancer antigen 125 (CA-125): Can be elevated in some uterine subtypes.
   10. Colonoscopy, sigmoidoscopy, or barium enema.
   11. Mismatch repair protein testing on pathology; if applicable genetic testing.

C. Staging: Endometrial cancer is surgically staged as defined by the 2017 International FIGO criteria.

DIFFERENTIAL DIAGNOSIS

A. Determine source of bleeding.
   1. Cervix.
   2. Vulva.
   3. Vagina.

B. Bleeding can be caused by:
   1. Polyps.
   2. Endometritis.
   3. Neoplasm.
   4. Atrophic changes.

EVALUATION AND MANAGEMENT PLAN

A. General plan.
   1. Treatment is determined based on disease stage and histologic features.
      a. Stage IA and IB.
      b. Stage II.
      c. Stage III and IV.
   2. There are six basic types of treatment for women with endometrial cancer.
      a. Surgery: The standard of care for treatment of endometrial cancer is hysterectomy, bilateral salpingo-oophorectomy (BSO), and surgical staging.
      b. RT: External beam radiation therapy (EBRT) and/or internal radiation/brachytherapy.
      c. Hormone therapy: Progestins, estrogen receptor antagonist, aromatase inhibitors, and gonadotropin-releasing hormone (GNRH) agonists.
      d. Chemotherapy.
      e. Targeted therapy: Lenvatinib, bevacizumab, and mTOR (mammalian target of rapamycin) inhibitors. ▶

f. Immunotherapy: Dostarlimab and pembrolizumab.

g. Participation in clinical trials if available.

3. Fertility-sparing therapy: May be initiated in pre-menopausal patients with grade 1 well-differentiated tumor (recommended by dilation and curettage sampling); stage FIGO IA tumor without involvement of myometrium on MRI, absence of lymphovascular invasion, and without intra-abdominal disease or adnexal mass.

a. Hormone therapy with megestrol and medroxyprogesterone (most common).

b. Levonorgestrel. Progestin intrauterine devices (IUDs) may be used for treatment alone or in combination with oral progestin.

c. Total hysterectomy/BSO/staging after childbearing complete or progression of disease.

B. Acute care issues in endometrial cancer.

1. Endometrial cancer patients are often admitted for surgical management. Surgery can be performed either open laparotomy or minimally invasive via laparoscopic or robotic approach.

2. Postoperative laparotomy patients without complications will spend 3 to 5 days in the hospital after surgery, compared with 1 to 2 days of recovery for patients undergoing minimally invasive surgery (MIS).

FOLLOW-UP

A. Follow-up should occur every 3 to 4 months for the first 2 years, and then every 6 months up to year 5, then annually.

B. Surveillance visit to assess for recurrence should include thorough history and physical exam with pelvic and speculum exam. Most recurrences occur at the vaginal cuff.

C. PET/CT has been shown to be more sensitive or specific than CT alone for recurrence, but further investigation is being evaluated.

D. Pap smears for detection of local recurrence have not been demonstrated.

CONSULTATION/REFERRAL

A. Gynecologic oncology, medical oncology, radiation oncology, and surgery.

SPECIAL/GERIATRIC CONSIDERATIONS

A. Prognosis is favorable for some endometrial cancers.

B. Diagnosis at an early stage of the disease process is a key factor for good prognosis.

C. Surgery is a safe option for older adult women, which significantly extends life with a low rate of complications.

CASE SCENARIO: ENDOMETRIAL CANCER

A 59-year-old, G1P1001 female with menopause at age 52 reports a 2-year history of intermittent vaginal spotting lasting 1 to 2 days. Bleeding has been sporadic and irregular. Her last Pap was 3 years ago, which was negative. Her height is 5'4", weight is 182, and body mass index (BMI) is 31.2. She notes a history of well-controlled hypertension and irregular menstrual cycles most of her adult life. She denies pelvic pain and changes to her bowel or bladder function. There is no family history of cancer. She underwent a transvaginal ultrasound (TVUS) showing 16-mm endometrial stripe, normal-sized uterus with 1-cm fibroid, and normal-sized ovaries. She is referred to gynecology for irregular bleeding and thickened endometrial stripe. Physical exam notes normal-sized cervix without lesions, and uterus with normal shape and size with no palpable adnexal masses. Endometrial biopsy (EMB) performed demonstrates grade 1 endometrioid endometrial cancer. CT imaging is negative. She underwent total laparoscopic hysterectomy (TLH)/bilateral salpingo-oophorectomy (BSO)/staging.

1. Which of the following is NOT generally considered a risk factor for endometrial cancer?

A. Low body mass index (BMI)

B. Personal history of Lynch syndrome

C. Unopposed estrogen therapy

D. Diabetes mellitus

2. What is the most common presenting symptom of endometrial cancer?

A. Abdominal pain

B. Postmenopausal bleeding

C. Fever

D. Constipation

BIBLIOGRAPHY

Chen, L., & Berek, J. (2022). *Endometrial Carcinoma: Clinical features, diagnosis, prognosis, and screening*. In A. Chakrabarti (Ed.), *UpToDate*. https://www.uptodate.com/contents/endometrial-carcinoma-clinical-features-diagnosis-prognosis-and-screening

Leitao, M. M. Jr., Kehoe, S., Barakat, R. R., Alektiar, K., Gattoc, L. P., Rabbitt, C., Chi, D. S., Soslow, R. A., & Abu-Rustum, N. R. (2009, April). Comparison of D&C and office endometrial biopsy accuracy in patients with FIGO grade 1 endometrial adenocarcinoma. *Gynecologic Oncology*, 113(1), 105–108. https://doi.org/10.1016/j.ygyno.2008.12.017 Epub 2009 Jan 23. PMID: 19167049

Nordal, R. R., & Thoresen, S. O. (1997). Uterine sarcomas in Norway 1956–1992: Incidence, survival, and mortality. *European Journal of Cancer*, 33(6), 907–911.

Pecorelli, S. (2009). Revised FIGO staging for carcinoma of the vulva, cervix and endometrium. *International Journal of Gynecology and Obstetrics*, 105(2), 103–104. https://doi.org/10.1016/j.ijgo.2009.02.012

Pecorelli, S. (2010). Corrigendum to "Revised FIGO staging for carcinoma of the vulva, cervix, and endometrium". *International Journal of Gynecology and Obstetrics*, 108(2), 176. https://doi.org/10.1016/j.ijgo.2009.08.009

Plaxe, S., & Mundt, A. (2022). Overview of endometrial carcinoma. In S. Vora & A. Chakrabarti (Eds.), *UpToDate*. https://www.uptodate.com/contents/overview-of-endometrial-carcinoma

Rimel, B. J., Burke, W. M., Higgins, R. V., Lee, P. S., Lutman, C. V., & Parker, L. (2015, May). Improving quality and decreasing cost in gynecologic oncology care. Society of gynecologic oncology recommendations for clinical practice. *Gynecologic Oncology*, 137(2), 280–284. https://doi.org/10.1016/j.ygyno.2015.02.021 Epub 2015 Feb 28. PMID: 25735256

Salani, R., Khanna, N., Frimer, M., Bristow, R. E., & Chen, L. M. (2017, July). An update on post-treatment surveillance and diagnosis of recurrence in women with gynecologic malignancies: Society of Gynecologic Oncology (SGO) recommendations. *Gynecologic Oncology*, 146(1), 3–10. https://doi.org/10.1016/j.ygyno.2017.03.022 Epub 2017 Mar 31. PMID: 28372871

SEER Cancer Stat Facts: Uterine Cancer. National Cancer Institute. https://seer.cancer.gov/statfacts/html/corp.html

GYNECOLOGIC CANCERS: OVARIAN CANCER

Diann C. Fernandez

DEFINITION

A. Ovarian cancers are classified by cells they are derived from.

B. There are three main types of ovarian cancer:

  1. Epithelial tumors (accounting for 95%), that is, serous (high-grade, low-grade), mucinous, endometrioid, and clear cell.

  2. Germ cell tumors, that is, dysgerminoma, yolk sac, embryonal carcinoma, choriocarcinoma, and teratoma.

  3. Sex cord stromal tumors, that is, granulosa cell, thecoma, fibroma, and Sertoli–Leydig.

INCIDENCE

A. It is the second most common cancer among women, with endometrial cancer being first, but it is the most lethal of all gynecologic malignancies.

B. A woman's risk of getting ovarian cancer during their lifetime is about 1 in 78. Their lifetime chance of dying from ovarian cancer is about 1 in 108.

C. Estimated 19,880 new cases in 2022.

PATHOGENESIS

A. The origin and pathogenesis of epithelial ovarian cancer are poorly understood, although dedifferentiation of cells overlying the ovary is thought to be an important source.

B. Ovarian cancer typically spreads by local extension, with significant dissemination within the peritoneal cavity.

C. Ovarian cancer often goes undetected as symptoms are vague and there is no approved screening test. Therefore, patients are typically diagnosed with advanced stages.

PREDISPOSING FACTORS

A. Age.

B. Family history of ovarian, breast, or colon cancer.

C. Genetic predisposition.

D. Reproductive and endocrine abnormalities.

  1. Infertility.

  2. Endometriosis.

  3. Hormonal replacement therapy.

E. Obesity (body mass index [BMI] of ≥30).

SUBJECTIVE DATA

A. Common complaints/symptoms.

  1. Abdominal bloating.

  2. Increase in abdominal girth.

  3. Pelvic/abdominal pain.

  4. Early satiety.

  5. Difficulty eating.

  6. Nausea and vomiting.

  7. Fatigue.

  8. Urinary symptoms (frequency or urgency).

B. Common/typical scenario.

  1. Ovarian cancer is dubbed the "silent killer" due to women presenting with vague symptoms.

  2. Additionally, there are no approved screening methods for ovarian cancer.

  3. Due to the vague symptoms, the majority of women are not diagnosed until they have advanced stage disease.

PHYSICAL EXAMINATION

A. In patients with early disease, physical examination findings are uncommon.

B. Ovarian/pelvic mass, fluid in the abdomen (ascites), pleural effusion, and abdominal mass of a bowel obstruction may be present in advanced disease.

C. Physical examination includes and is not limited to:

  1. General assessment.

  2. Survey of the lymphatic system.

  3. Abdomen: Assess for pain, palpable masses, fluid waves, and bowel sounds.

  4. Pelvic examination: Assess for bleeding, masses, position of cervix if present, and uterine size.

  5. Rectovaginal examination: Assess for bleeding, masses, uterosacral ligaments, and cul-de-sac.

DIAGNOSTIC TESTS

A. Ultrasound, CT, or MRI of the abdomen/pelvis.

B. Tumor markers.

C. Complete blood count (CBC) and comprehensive metabolic panel (CMP).

D. Urinalysis to rule out other causes of pain (urinary tract infection [UTI], kidney stones).

E. Diagnosis.

  1. Final diagnosis is based on the pathologic review of tissue specimen obtained through surgery or biopsy.

  2. Initial surgery (exploratory laparotomy vs. laparoscopic). If there is a strong clinical suggestion for ovarian cancer, laparotomy is preferred for diagnosis and staging.

  3. Fine needle aspiration (FNA) or diagnostic paracentesis should be performed in patients with diffuse carcinomatosis or ascites without an obvious ovarian mass; a thoracentesis if pleural effusion is present.

F. Staging: Ovarian cancer is surgically staged according to the 2017 Eighth Edition American Joint Committee on Cancer (AJCC) and the International Federation of Gynecology and Obstetrics (FIGO) tumor, node, metastasis (TNM) classification system.

DIFFERENTIAL DIAGNOSIS

A. Adnexal tumors.

B. Ectopic pregnancy.

C. Cysts.

D. Endometriosis.

E. Cervicitis.

F. Cancer of surrounding structures.

G. Pelvic inflammatory disease.

H. Uterine leiomyomas.

EVALUATION AND MANAGEMENT PLAN

A. General plan.

  1. All women diagnosed with ovarian, fallopian tube, or peritoneal cancer should have genetic testing and considered for genetic counseling.

2. Surgery.

3. Chemotherapy: Neoadjuvant, adjuvant, intravenous (IV), and IV/intraperitoneal (in optimally debulked patients).

4. Radiation therapy (RT): Not used as first-line treatment; however, it may be used occasionally to treat small, localized recurrent tumors.

5. Hormonal therapy.

6. Targeted therapy.

7. Biotherapy/immunotherapy.

8. Participation in clinical trials, if available.

FOLLOW-UP

A. Follow-up for ovarian cancer is based on the National Comprehensive Cancer Network (NCCN) guidelines for tumor type and stage.

B. Many providers recommend pelvic examination every 2 to 4 months for the first 2 years after completing treatment and every 3 to 6 months for 3 years, then annually after 5 years.

C. Repeat cancer antigen 125 (CA-125) or other tumor markers if initially elevated.

D. Imaging such as CT of the chest/abdomen/pelvis, PET (skull base to thigh), or MRI as clinically indicated based on symptoms.

CONSULTATION/REFERRAL

A. Gynecologic oncologist: Typically will involve surgery, medical oncology, and occasionally radiation oncology.

B. Gastroenterologist: Patients may present primarily with gastrointestinal (GI) complaints.

C. Palliative care: Due to the very poor prognosis, this may be beneficial early on.

SPECIAL/GERIATRIC CONSIDERATIONS

A. Ovarian cancer increases with advancing age, peaking in the seventh decade of life.

B. Discuss aggressive treatment with the patient based on life expectancy, quality of life goals, and functional status.

CASE SCENARIO: OVARIAN CANCER

A 48-year-old G2002 with history of acute pelvic pain and bloating for 3 days is seen by her gynecologist. She underwent a pelvic exam showing palpable left adnexal mass. Last menstrual period (LMP) 4 weeks prior is reported normal. Transvaginal ultrasound (US) shows normal-sized uterus with 6-cm bilateral complex adnexal masses and pelvic ascites. Her CA-125 is 1300. There is no known family history of cancer. Worsening abdominal pain prompted the ED visit. CT imaging shows omental carcinomatosis, bilateral adnexal masses, and abdominal ascites; the lungs are clear. Interventional radiology performed omental biopsy pathology consistent with adenocarcinoma of mullerian origin, consistent with high-grade serous gynecologic malignancy, and suspected ovarian cancer. Paracentesis performed with 3-L ascites is consistent with adenocarcinoma. Initiation of neoadjuvant chemotherapy is planned.

1. What important testing is recommended for this patient with newly diagnosed ovarian cancer?

A. Lipid panel
B. Genetic testing
C. Mammogram
D. Pap smear

2. Following neoadjuvant chemotherapy and imaging showing good response to treatment, what are the typical next steps in the patient's care?

A. Hysterectomy/bilateral salpingo-oophorectomy (BSO)/debulking
B. Surveillance visits every 3 months
C. Omental biopsy
D. Thoracentesis

BIBLIOGRAPHY

American Cancer Society. (2022). *Cancer facts & figures 2022*. Author.

Chen, L., & Berek, J. (2022). Overview of epithelial carcinoma of the ovary, fallopian tube and peritoneum. In A. Chakrabarti (Ed.), *UpToDate*. https://www.uptodate.com/contents/overview-of-epithelial-carcinoma-of-the-ovary-fallopian-tube-and-peritoneum

National Comprehensive Cancer Network Hereditary Cancer Testing Criteria Version 2.2022. https://www.nccn.org/guidelines/guidelines-detail?category=2&id=1503/

Prat, J., Olawaiye, A. B., & Bermudez, A. (2017). Ovary, fallopian tube, and primary peritoneal carcinoma. In M. B. Amin (Ed.), *AJCC Cancer Staging Manual AJCC, Chicago* (8th ed., p. 681). *UpToDate*. https://www.uptodate.com/contents/epithelial-carcinoma-of-the-ovary-fallopian-tube-and-peritoneum-surgical-staging

Salani, R., Khanna, N., Frimer, M., Bristow, R. E., & Chen, L. M. (2017, July). An update on post-treatment surveillance and diagnosis of recurrence in women with gynecologic malignancies: Society of Gynecologic Oncology (SGO) recommendations. *Gynecologic Oncology, 146*(1), 3–10. https://doi.org/10.1016/j.ygyno.2017.03.022, Epub 2017 Mar 31. PMID: 28372871

SEER Cancer Stat Facts: Ovarian Cancer. National Cancer Institute. https://seer.cancer.gov/statfacts/html/ovary.html

HEAD AND NECK CANCERS

Sara Hollstein

DEFINITION

A. Head and neck cancers can arise in the lip, oral cavity, pharynx (nasopharyngeal, oropharyngeal, hypopharyngeal), larynx, nasal cavity, paranasal sinuses, and salivary glands and include a variety of histopathologic tumors.

INCIDENCE

A. In the United States, head and neck cancer accounts for 4% of malignancies, with an estimated 66,470 Americans (48,520 men and 17,950 women) developing head and neck cancer and 15,050 dying (10,940 men and 4,110 women) from the disease in 2022.

B. Head and neck squamous cell carcinoma (HNSCC) comprises more than 90% of head and neck cancers.

PATHOGENESIS

A. Pathophysiology of cancers of the head and neck usually begin in squamous cells of the mucosal lining of the aerodigestive tract.

B. Multiple genetic mutations and changes in protein expressions with the most notable molecular alterations to p53 and estimated glomerular filtration rate ▶

(EGFR) allow for increased tumor proliferation and angiogenesis.

PREDISPOSING FACTORS

A. Tobacco abuse and alcohol account for most cancers of the oral cavity, hypopharynx, larynx, and non-human papillomavirus (HPV) oropharynx carcinomas.

B. Viral infections.

  1. Epstein–Barr virus (EBV; nasopharyngeal cancers).

  2. HPV (oropharyngeal cancers).

  a. HPV 16, 18, 33, and 35 are known for a majority of squamous cell carcinomas of the oropharynx, especially cancers of the lingual, palatine tonsil, and base of the tongue.

  b. HPV vaccine reduces HPV oral infection, but the impact on HNSCC incidence has not been performed in a randomized controlled setting. However, the Food and Drug Administration (FDA) did expand its indication for the HPV vaccination to include oral pharyngeal cancers in 2020 based on current data.

C. Betel nut use: Combination of areca palm nuts, betel leaf, slaked lime, and tobacco commonly used in South Asia.

D. Radiation exposure.

E. Periodontal disease.

F. Immunodeficiency (immunosuppressant use, HIV/AIDS, bone marrow, or organ transplantation).

G. Occupational exposure.

H. Genetic factors (polymorphisms, Fanconi anemia, etc.).

I. Iron deficiency (Plummer–Vinson) associated with elevated risk of squamous cell carcinoma.

J. Gastroesophageal reflux or laryngopharyngeal reflux (laryngeal cancers).

SUBJECTIVE DATA

A. Common complaints/symptoms.

  1. Symptoms and signs vary depending on the subtype and location of the tumor.

  2. Patients may be asymptomatic, but common symptoms include:

  a. Oral or tongue mass, red or white patches, loose teeth, and bleeding gums.

  b. Vision changes and diplopia.

  c. Recurrent sinusitis not improved with antibiotic therapy, epistaxis, and headaches.

  d. Dysphagia.

  e. Pain: Ophthalmalgia, otalgia, odynophagia, sinusitis, and pharyngitis.

  f. Dysarthria, trismus, and hoarseness.

  g. Cervical or supraclavicular adenopathy.

  h. Hearing loss and tinnitus.

  i. Facial numbness, paresthesias, or paralysis.

  j. Dyspnea (metastatic disease involving the lung).

  k. Nausea or vomiting (metastatic disease involving the liver).

  l. Bony pain (metastatic disease involving the bone).

PHYSICAL EXAMINATION

A. Identify the key elements of any mass: Size, size and area of firmness, associated pain, and associated skin changes.

B. Eyes: Tearing, proptosis, and symmetry; grossly assess vision.

C. Ears: Inspect ear canal for drainage and tympanic membrane; grossly assess hearing.

D. Nose and sinus: Sinus pain or tenderness, facial symmetry, nasal patency, nasal septum alignment, and nasal membranes and turbinates.

E. Oral cavity: Assess for dysarthria, tongue mobility, visual examination and palpation of mucous membranes, floor of the mouth, tongue, buccal and gingival mucosa, palates, and posterior pharyngeal wall.

  1. Pharyngeal tumors do require fiberoptic or endoscopic exam for full physical exam evaluation.

F. Neck and lymphatics: Palpate the neck for cervical and supraclavicular lymphadenopathy.

G. Neurologic: Assess cranial nerves II through XII; assess for facial twitching.

H. Common metastatic sites for head and neck cancers are the lung, liver, and bone.

DIAGNOSTIC TESTS

A. History and physical examination.

B. Direct fiberoptic or endoscopic evaluation with biopsy of the primary site.

C. CT or MRI of the head and neck.

D. PET/CT (optional, preferred in lymph node-positive disease).

E. Chest imaging as clinically indicated.

F. Fine needle aspiration (FNA) and/or biopsies of primary tumor and/or nodal disease.

G. Videostroboscopy for patients with dysphonia.

H. EBV quantitative polymerase chain reaction (PCR; for nasopharyngeal cancers).

I. Multidisciplinary team evaluations (dependent on treatment plan and tumor location; see "Consultation/Referral").

J. Staging.

  1. Staging for all oral cancers utilizes the tumor, node, metastasis (TNM) staging outlined by the American Joint Committee on Cancer (AJCC).

  2. TNM staging varies depending on the primary tumor site.

DIFFERENTIAL DIAGNOSIS

A. Infectious, inflammatory, or irritant.

B. Endocrine-associated disease.

C. Neurologically associated processes.

D. Gastroesophageal reflux disease (GERD).

EVALUATION AND MANAGEMENT PLAN

A. General plan (subtypes and treatment).

  1. Treatment for all head and neck cancers depends on TNM stage at diagnosis.

  2. Treatment recommendations vary depending on the primary site and histology of the tumor. Generalized guidelines are outlined here.

▶

a. Early-stage (localized) disease (stage I or II): Definitive radiation therapy (RT) and/or localized resection. RT can be given with systemic therapy dependent on disease type.

b. Advanced disease (stage III or IV) or resections without clear margins. Disease recurrence is high.

   i. Adjuvant or neoadjuvant systemic therapy/radiation with resection as indicated.

   iii. Clinical trial enrollment.

   iv. Palliative care or hospice care.

B. Acute care issues in head and neck cancers.

   1. Patients with HNSCC are rarely admitted except for postoperative management, pain, dehydration, malnutrition, and treatment-related infections.

   2. Acute RT sequelae result in only the area of treated tissue and often start 2 weeks after the start of treatment and can continue to up to 2 to 4 weeks after treatment is completed. Patients with combined systemic and RT may have a higher incidence of side effects. Goals of symptom management are to avoid radiation treatment delays.

   3. Acute radiation-induced dermatitis (dry and moist desquamation).

   a. General care.

      i. Avoid ice packs and heat pads to the area.

      ii. Avoid applying topical applications to the skin prior to treatment.

      iii. Keep the area clean (lukewarm water and synthetic soap), open to air, wear loose-fitting clothing, and avoid the sun.

      iv. Avoid wet shaving the area; electric shaver only.

      v. No powders, perfumes, alcohol-based, and lanolin-free products on the skin. Discuss with

a radiation oncologist their preferred management plan.

      vi. Pain management.

   b. Dry desquamation.

      i. Keep the area moist with prescribed moisturizers following treatment.

   c. Moist desquamation.

      i. May require a treatment break to allow healing.

      ii. Soaks, compresses as prescribed by radiation oncologist.

      iii. Monitor for skin infections (e.g., herpes simplex, *Staphylococcus aureus*).

   4. Sore throat, oral cavity (mucositis).

   a. Avoid acidic or spicy foods, alcohol, and smoking.

   b. Treat dry mouth (xerostomia).

   c. Pain management: Opioids, gabapentin, doxepin, and oral anesthetics (diphenhydramine/lidocaine/antacid mouthwash).

   d. Saline or baking soda rinses.

   e. Keep mouth clean and follow good oral hygiene.

   f. Monitor closely for infections (e.g., oral candidiasis or herpes simplex virus, sepsis).

   g. Palifermin (keratinocyte growth factor).

   5. Weight loss and malnutrition and dehydration.

   a. Due to difficulty eating, mucositis, trismus, difficult mastication, treatment-induced nausea and vomiting.

   b. Management.

      i. Consider parenteral, enteral, or oral nutritional support.

      ii. Refer to nutritionist and record 24-hour recall to document current intake.

      iii. Refer to speech therapy.

      iv. Pain management support if indicated.

TABLE 13.2   HEAD AND NECK CANCER FOLLOW-UP

	H&P	Imaging	Testing	Survivorship Care
Year 1	Every 1–3 months	Based on treatment and concern for residual or recurrence of disease. Standard imaging following treatment is 4–8 weeks if high concern or can be 3–6 if less concern	TSH every 6–12 months if neck RT. Dental evaluation every 6 months if RT affected salivary function/oral area. EBV DNA monitoring if nasal carcinoma	Care plan completion within 1 year. Continue referrals for late and long-term sequelae of treatment
Year 2	Every 2–6 months			
Years 3–5	Every 4–8 months			
Greater than 5 years	Every 12 months			

EBV, Epstein–Barr virus; H&P, history and physical examination; RT, radiation therapy; TSH, thyroid-stimulating hormone.

FOLLOW-UP

A. See Table 13.2.

CONSULTATION/REFERRAL

A. Otolaryngology, medical oncology, radiation oncology, head and neck surgery, and plastic surgery.
B. Nutritionist for weight loss and malnutrition. Gastroenterology for feeding tube placement.
C. Speech, physical, and occupation therapy for pre/posttreatment care. May require specialized lymphedema specialists.
D. Dental evaluation including dental extractions prior to RT.
E. Audiogram depending on tumor location.
F. Social work referral.
G. Counseling, psychologist, and psychiatry as indicated.
H. Tracheostomy care as indicated.
I. Wound management as indicated.
J. Physical and occupational therapy as indicated.
K. Fertility and reproduction counseling as indicated.
L. Tobacco and alcohol session counseling as indicated.

SPECIAL/GERIATRIC CONSIDERATIONS

A. Patients older than 70 years should not be denied systemic therapy based solely on age.
B. Discuss aggressive treatment with the patient. Performance status will be evaluated to determine eligibility for treatments and clinical trial enrollment.
C. Take life expectancy, quality of life, and patients' functional status into consideration.

CASE SCENARIO: HEAD AND NECK CANCER

A 67-year-old male with an oropharynx tumor (stage IVA, T2N2M0), currently in week 5 of concurrent systemic therapy and radiation therapy (RT), is admitted for complaints of dizziness, dysphagia, and oral pain, with worsening fatigue with declining functional impairments. In the outpatient oncology clinic, he receives 1 L of intravenous (IV) fluids following his radiation treatment for orthostatic hypotension with minimal improvement of symptoms. Systemic therapy is held this week due to worsening mucositis, dehydration, and decline. He has had a weight loss of 10% in the last month and previously refused percutaneous endoscopic gastrostomy (PEG) tube placement. He continues to smoke and drink alcohol. He does not have a caregiver at home.

1. What should the initial history include?

2. What other associated symptoms could also be contributing to his symptoms?

3. What treatment options can be offered to treat the oral mucositis?

4. What pain management medications can aid in oral mucositis?

BIBLIOGRAPHY

American Cancer Society. (2022). *Cancer facts & figures 2022.* Author
National Cancer Institute. (2021). *Treatment of head and neck cancer in adults—Health professional version.* https://www.cancer.gov/types/head-and-neck/hp/adult
National Comprehensive Cancer Network. (2021). *Head and neck cancers (Version 1.2022).* https://www.nccn.org/guidelines/guidelines-detail?category=1&id=1437
Poon, C. S., & Stenson, K. M. (2022). *Overview of the diagnosis and staging of head and neck cancer.* https://www.uptodate.com/contents/overview-of-the-diagnosis-and-staging-of-head-and-neck-cancer?search=head%20and%20neck%20cancer&topicRef=3380&source=see_link
Wolf, J. R., & Hong, A. M. (2022). Radiation dermatitis. *UpToDate.* https://www.uptodate.com/contents/radiation-dermatitis?search=radiation%20induced%20dermatitis&source=search_result&selectedTitle=1~150&usage_type=default&display_rank=1

LEUKEMIAS: ACUTE LEUKEMIAS

Alexis C. Geppner

DEFINITION

A. Acute leukemias are a heterogeneous group of rare, clonal hematopoietic/stem cell (HSC) neoplasms exhibiting maturation defects involving myeloid or lymphoid precursor cells.
B. These malignant clones undergo uncontrolled abnormal proliferation and replace the normal bone marrow, causing aberrant differentiation and ineffective hematopoiesis, resulting in granulocytopenia, anemia, and thrombocytopenia.
C. Can originate from HSCs or from committed cells with an inner higher self-renewal potential.
D. Acute leukemia is categorized broadly into acute myeloid/myelogenous leukemia (AML; Tables 13.3, 13.4, 13.5, and 13.6) and acute lymphoblastic leukemia (ALL; Table 13.7 and Figure 13.1).

INCIDENCE

A. AML.
 1. An estimated 20,050 people were diagnosed with AML in the United States in 2022, making up 1% of all new cancer cases.
 2. The incidence of AML is similar to that of solid tumors, with an exponential rise after age 40. The median age of patients at diagnosis is approximately 68 years.
 3. Approximately 85% of patients with newly diagnosed AML are greater than 45 years old.
B. ALL.
 1. An estimated 6,660 people were diagnosed with ALL in the United States in 2022.
 2. Approximately 54% of new cases are diagnosed before age 20, indicating that ALL is primarily a disease of younger patients. The median age of diagnosis is approximately 17 years.

PATHOGENESIS

A. Leukemia develops as a series of genetic changes within a single hematopoietic precursor cell, resulting in alteration/malignant transformation of normal hematopoietic growth and differentiation. This leads to the ▶

TABLE 13.3 FRENCH–AMERICAN–BRITISH CLASSIFICATION OF ACUTE MYELOID LEUKEMIA

Subtype	Description	Details
M0	Minimally differentiated AML	Negative MPO, ≥2 myeloid markers by FC, frequently has complex karyotype associated with poor prognosis
M1	AML without maturation	Less than 10% promyelocytes or more mature myeloid forms
M2	AML with maturation	Subset have t(8;21) associated with favorable prognosis
M3	Acute promyelocytic leukemia	Heavy granulation, bilobed nuclear contour, rarely microgranular variant with inconspicuous granules, often t(15;17) with favorable prognosis
M4	Acute myelomonocytic leukemia	Monocytes and promonocytes >20%; M4Eo contains >5% abnormal eosinophils, associated with inv(16), and favorable prognosis
M5	Acute monocytic leukemia	80% monoblasts, monocytes, or promonocytes; NE stain positive; associated with extramedullary disease and 11q abnormalities
M6	Acute erythroleukemia	>50% erythroid nucleated marrow cells, often severely dyserythropoietic; erythroblasts strongly PAS positive and glycophorin A positive
M7	Acute megakaryocytic leukemia	May have micromegakaryoblasts; diagnosis confirmed by positive CD41 or electron microscopy (platelet peroxidase)

AML, acute myeloid leukemia; CD, cluster of differentiation; FC, flow cytometry; M4Eo, M4 with eosinophilia; MPO, myeloperoxidase; NE, nonspecific esterase; PAS, periodic acid-Schiff.
Source: Adapted from Rodgers, G. P., & Young, N. S. (2013). *The Bethesda handbook of clinical hematology.* Wolters.

accumulation of large numbers of abnormal, immature cells incapable of differentiating into mature hematopoietic cell results.

B. AML.

   1. Thought to be related to the transformation of a single hematopoietic stem cell into a malignant undifferentiated cell with endless proliferation; results in accumulation of abnormal, immature myeloid cells in the bone marrow and peripheral blood (PB).

   2. Can occur de novo or secondary to previous cytotoxic therapy (therapy-related or secondary AML).

   3. Maintained by a pool of leukemia cells with unlimited self-renewal.

C. ALL

   1. Thought to be the result of genetic insults that block lymphoid differentiation and drive aberrant cell proliferation and survival.

   2. Two subtypes depending on lymphocyte lineage affected: T-lymphocytes (T-ALL) or B-lymphocytes (B-ALL).

   3. Risk of central nervous system (CNS) leukemia higher with hyperleukocytosis, T-cell immunophenotype, and mixed-lineage leukemia (MLL) rearrangement. Can enter the CNS via the blood–brain barrier (BBB), the bloodleptomeningeal barrier (BLMB), or the bloodcerebrospinal fluid barrier (BCSFB).

PREDISPOSING FACTORS

A. Sex: Male to female ratio is 4.1 to 1.

B. Age: Median age at diagnosis is approximately 68 years.

C. Race and ethnicity: Slightly higher in European descent; acute promyelocytic leukemia (APL) more common in Hispanic population.

D. Chemical or pesticide exposure: Particularly benzene, petroleum products, and ionizing radiation.

E. Smoking: Most significant controllable risk factor.

F. Prior chemotherapy or high-dose radiation exposure: Alkylating agents, topoisomerase II inhibitors, anthracyclines, and taxanes.

G. Genetic disorders: Down syndrome, Bloom syndrome, Fanconi anemia, Diamond–Blackfan anemia, Shwachman–Diamond syndrome, Li–Fraumeni syndrome, Klinefelter syndrome, neurofibromatosis type 1 (NF1), Kostmann syndrome (severe congenital neutropenia), ataxia–telangiectasia, Wiskott–Aldrich syndrome, and familial mutations of CEBPA, DDX41, and RUNX1.

H. Blood disorders: Myelodysplastic syndrome (MDS), polycythemia vera (PV), paroxysmal nocturnal hemoglobinuria (PNH), myeloproliferative neoplasms (MPNs), and aplastic anemia.

I. Viruses: RNA retroviruses and parvovirus B19 (ALL).

SUBJECTIVE DATA

A. Common complaints/symptoms.

   1. Patients are often symptomatic due to the disease's impact on normal hematopoiesis, causing pancytopenia and/or leukocytosis; however, patients can be initially asymptomatic.

      a. Thrombocytopenia: Easy bruising and bleeding (especially of the mucosal surfaces), epistaxis, and petechiae/purpura.

      b. Anemia: Dyspnea, orthopnea, headaches, and pallor.

      c. Fatigue (most common) often precedes diagnosis for a number of months.

      d. Leukopenia/dysfunctional white blood cells (WBC): Fever and persistent infections not responsive to antibiotics.

TABLE 13.4 WORLD HEALTH ORGANIZATION CLASSIFICATION OF ACUTE MYELOID LEUKEMIA

AML With Recurrent Cytogenetic Translocations
AML with t(8;21)(q22;q22); RUNX1-RUNX1T1
AML with inv(16)(p13.1;q22) or t(16;16)(p13.1;q22); CBFB-MYH11
AML with t(15;17)(q22;q12); PML-RARA
AML with t(9;11)(p22;q23); MLLT3-MLL
AML with t(6;9)(p23;q34); DEK-NUP214
AML with inv(3)(q21;q26.2) or t(3;3)(q21;q26.2); RPN1-EVI1
AML (megakaryoblastic) with t(1;22)(p13;q13); RBM15-MKL1
AML with mutated NPM1
AML with mutated CEBPA

AML With Myelodysplasia-Related Changes

Therapy-Related Myeloid Neoplasms

AML, not otherwise specified
AML with minimal differentiation
AML without maturation
AML with maturation
Acute myelomonocytic leukemia
Acute monoblastic/monocytic leukemia
Acute erythroid leukemia
Acute megakaryoblastic leukemia
Acute basophilic leukemia
Acute panmyelosis with myelofibrosis

Myeloid Sarcoma

Myeloid Proliferations Related to Down syndrome
Transient abnormal myelopoiesis
Myeloid leukemia associated with Down syndrome

Acute Leukemia of Ambiguous Lineage

AML, acute myeloid leukemia.
Sources: Modified from Vardiman, J. W., Thiele, J., Arber, D. A., Borowitz, M. J., Porwit, A., Harris, N. L., Le Beau, M. M., Hellström-Lindberg, E., Tefferi, A., & Bloomfield, C. D. (2009). The 2008 revision of the World Health Organization (WHO) classification of myeloid neoplasms and acute leukemia: rationale and important changes. *Blood, 114,* 937–951. Adapted from Rodgers, G. P., & Young, N. S. (2013). *The Bethesda Handbook of Clinical Hematology.* Wolters.

2. Bone pain/joint pain (due to marrow proliferation).
3. Altered mental status, intermittent/persistent cranial nerve palsies, and priapism (due to leukostasis or leukemia infiltrating the CNS).
4. Ocular, cardiac, pulmonary, or cerebral dysfunction (due to hyperleukocytosis).
5. Palpable lymphadenopathy and/or abdominal distention/bloating.
6. Unexplained weight loss.
7. Loss of appetite.
8. Night sweats (possibly due to cytokine release).

PHYSICAL EXAMINATION
A. Check vital signs, including pulse oximetry, height, and weight.
B. Head and neck.
  1. Evaluate conjunctiva for pallor (anemia) and ocular fundus for hemorrhage or white plaques (related to nerve fiber ischemia).
  2. Evaluate pupils for symmetry and reactivity to light and accommodation (acute intracranial bleed or CNS infiltration).
  3. Carefully examine oropharynx for bleeding, herpetic lesions/aphthous ulcers, oral candidiasis, or gingival hypertrophy (leukemic involvement of the gums; common in monocytic variants of AML).
  4. Evaluate neck/cervical area for lymphadenopathy due to leukemic infiltration (often seen in ALL rather than AML.)
C. Cardiovascular system.
  1. Auscultate heart sounds in all four quadrants. Tachycardia may be present if the patient is profoundly anemic or septic.
  2. Assess for signs of pericardial effusion or cardiac tamponade (hypotension, muffled heart sounds, pericardial friction rub, jugular venous distension [JVD]).
D. Pulmonary system.
  1. Inspect and observe for signs of dyspnea, retractions, and work of breathing.
  2. Auscultate and percuss all lung fields for signs of infection/leukostasis to include pneumonia, pleural effusion, pulmonary embolism, mediastinal mass, or pneumothorax.

TABLE 13.5   RECURRENT GENOMIC REARRANGEMENTS IN ADULT ACUTE MYELOID LEUKEMIA

Rearrangement	Frequency	Concurrent Mutations/Clinical Implications	Prognosis/Outcome
t(15;17)(q22;q21); PML-RARA	5%–13%	*FLT3-ITD*(35%), *FLT3-TKD*(15%), *WT1* (15%); frequency decreases with older age	APL; very good with arsenic trioxide and all-*trans*-retinoic acid therapy
t(8;21)(q22;q22.1); RUNX1-RUNX1T1	1%–6%	*KIT* (25%), *NRAS* (20%), cohesion genes (20%: *RAD21, SMC1A, SMC3*), *ASXL2* (20%), *ASXL1* (10%), *EZH2* (5%); frequency decreases with older age	Favorable risk; inferior with *KIT*
inv(16)(p13.1;q22); CBFB-MYH11	1%–6%	*NRAS* (40%), *KIT*(35%), *FLT3-TKD* (20%), *KRAS*(15%); frequency decreases with older age	Favorable risk
t(9;11)(p21.3;q23.3); MLLT3-KMT2A	1%	*NRAS* (20%), *FLT3-TKD* (10%), *FLT3-ITD* (5%); associated with intermediate-risk deregulated *MECOM* (*EVI1*); associated with therapy-related disease; frequency decreases with older age	Intermediate risk with deregulated *MECOM* (*EVI1*); poor outcomes with t(v;11q23.3)
t(6;9)(p23;q34.1); DEK-NUP214	1%	*FLT3-ITD* (70%), *KRAS* (20%)	Poor outcomes
inv(3)(q21.3;q26.2) or t(3;3)(q21.3;q26.2); GATA2, MECOM (EVI1)	Rare	*NRAS* (30%), *PTPN11* (20%), *SF3B1* (20%), *KRAS* (15%), *GATA2* (15%), *ETV6* (15%), *PHF6* (15%), *RUNX1*(10%), *BCOR* (10%), *ASXL1* (10%_, *NF1* (10%)	Very poor outcomes
t(1;22)(p13.3;q13.3); RBM15-MKL1	Rare	Megakaryoblastic differentiation	Poor outcomes

APL, acute promyelocytic leukemia.
Source: From Bullinger, L., Döhner, K., & Döhner, H. (2017, March 20). Genomics of acute myeloid leukemia diagnosis and pathways. JCO (*Journal of Clinical Oncology*), *35*(9), 934–946. https://doi.org/10.1200/JCO.2016.71.2208.

TABLE 13.6.   RISK STATUS BASED ON CYTOGENETIC AND MOLECULAR ABNORMALITIES

Risk Status	Cytogenetic and Molecular Abnormalities	
Good/better risk	inv(16) or t(16;16) t(8;21) t(15;17) Normal karyotype with NPM1 mutation or isolated CEBPA mutation in the absence of FLT3-ITD	
Intermediate risk	Normal karyotype +8 t(9;11) t(8;21), inv(16), t(16;16) with c-KIT mutation	
Poor risk	Complex karyotype (≥3 clonal chromosomal abnormalities) Monosomal karyotype (at least two monosomies or one monosomy + 1 structural abnormality) −5, 5q-, −7, 7q- 11q23 − non t(9;11) inv(3), t(3;3) t(6;9) t(9;22) Normal karyotype with FLT3-ITD mutation	

CEBPA, CCAAT/enhancer binding protein alpha; c-KIT, CD117 receptor tyrosine kinase; FLT3-ITD, FMS-like tyrosine kinase3-internal tandem duplications; NPM1, nucleophosmin.
Source: Adapted from Rodgers, G. P., & Young, N. S. (2013). *The Bethesda handbook of clinical hematology.* Wolters Kluwer/Lippincott Williams & Wilkins.

TABLE 13.7 FRENCH–AMERICAN–BRITISH CLASSIFICATION OF ACUTE LYMPHOBLASTIC LEUKEMIA

FAB Morphology	Bone Marrow	Cerebrospinal Fluid Cytology
L1: Homogenous blasts, minimal cytoplasm	M1: <5% blasts	CNS-1: No blasts
L2: Increased nuclear heterogeneity, prominent nucleoli	M2: 5%–25% blasts	CNS-2: WBC <5/mcL with blasts
L3: Basophilic cytoplasm with prominent vacuolization	M3: >25% blasts	CNS-3: WBC ≥ 5/mcL with blasts OR symptomatic CNS involvement

CNS, central nervous system; FAB, French–American–British; WBC, white blood cell.
Source: Adapted from Rodgers, G. P., & Young, N. S. (2013). *The Bethesda handbook of clinical hematology*. Wolters Kluwer/Lippincott Williams & Wilkins.

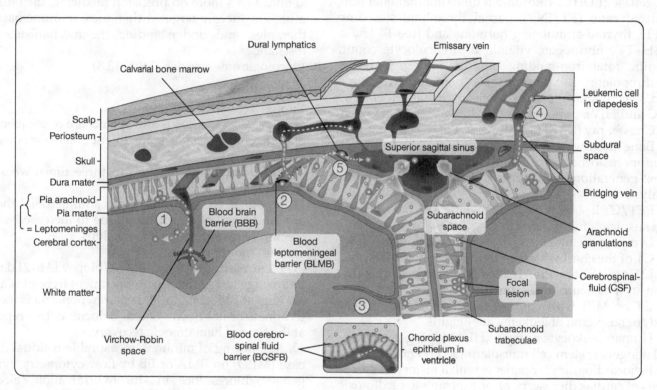

FIGURE 13.1. Potential entry routes for acute lymphoblastic leukemia cells in the central nervous system.

Source: Adapted from Lenk, L., Alsadeq, A., Schewe, D. M. (2020). Involvement of the central nervous system in acute lymphoblastic leukemia: Opinions on molecular mechanisms and clinical implications based on recent data. *Cancer Metastasis Rev, 39,* 173–187.

3. Mediastinal adenopathy is found in 80% of cases of T-cell ALL.

E. Gastrointestinal (GI) system.

  1. Inspect abdomen for distention.

  2. Auscultate for bowel sounds in all four quadrants.

  3. Palpate for hepatosplenomegaly (HSM) due to extramedullary involvement/infiltration of the liver and spleen with leukemia cells. HSM is often found in ALL rather than AML. Massive HSM is rare in de novo acute leukemia and should raise the suspicion of leukemia evolving from a prior hematologic disorder (e.g., chronic myeloid leukemia [CML] or MDS or ALL).

F. Integumentary system.

  1. Inspect skin for pallor (anemia), petechiae and ecchymosis (thrombocytopenia or disseminated intravascular coagulopathy [DIC]), or infiltrative lesions (leukemia cutis/myeloid sarcoma).

  a. Leukemic involvement of the skin occurs in 13% or more of patients and is often found in AML with a monocytic of myelomonocytic component.

  b. Cutis lesions are often nodular and violaceous/blue-gray in color.

  2. Erythematous to violaceous tender nodules and plaques suggest acute neutrophilic dermatosis (Sweet syndrome).

G. CNS.

  1. Perform a full neurologic examination to evaluate for focal neurologic deficits secondary to leukemic involvement.

2. CNS involvement is usually restricted to the leptomeninges.

3. CNS involvement occurs in 3% to 5% of adult ALL at diagnosis and 30% to 40% at relapse.

4. CNS is rare in AML; however, the lack of routine diagnostic lumbar puncture (LP) is the reason this often goes undiagnosed.

DIAGNOSTIC TESTS

A. Complete history, including family history.
B. Physical examination.
C. Laboratory data: Complete blood count (CBC), comprehensive metabolic panel (CMP), lactate dehydrogenase (LDH), prothrombin time/international normalized ratio (PT/INR), partial thromboplastin time (PTT), thyroid-stimulating hormone and free T4 levels (TSH/T4), fibrinogen, vitamin B_{12}, reticulocyte count, ferritin, total iron-binding capacity (TIBC), D-dimer, erythropoietin, B-type natriuretic peptide (BNP), type and screen, and infectious disease screening (hepatitis B/C and HIV).
D. Chest x-ray (CXR) or CT imaging of the chest.
E. Bone marrow aspiration and biopsy: Morphology, immunohistochemistry, flow cytometry, molecular (next-generation sequencing [NGS]), and cytogenetic analysis.
F. PET/CT if staging for ALL, myeloid sarcoma, or clinical suspicion for extramedullary disease.
G. Lymph node biopsy if necessary for staging of ALL.
H. CT of the chest with mediastinal biopsy for T-ALL.
I. LP in patients with ALL or AML with high-risk disease and/or neurologic symptoms.
J. CT or MRI with contrast if neurologic symptoms and/or suspicion of leukemic meningitis.
K. Human leukocyte antigen (HLA) typing if a potential allogeneic stem cell transplant (SCT) candidate.
L. Echocardiogram for patients with a history or symptoms of cardiac disease, or prior exposure to cardiotoxic agents, such as anthracyclines.
M. Central venous access: Peripheral intravenous central catheter (PICC) or central venous catheter (CVC).
N. Diagnosis.

1. Bone marrow aspiration/biopsy required for diagnosis of all types of acute leukemia (documentation of bone marrow infiltration).

2. Lymph node biopsy may be necessary to aid in diagnosis of ALL.

3. Perform LP at diagnosis in all patients with ALL, high-risk disease, and all patients with neurologic symptoms.
O. Classification of acute leukemia.

1. Diagnosis of acute leukemia requires ≥20% blasts (myeloblasts or lymphoblasts) in the bone marrow or PB.

2. Two main classification systems.

a. French–American–British (FAB).
b. World Health Organization (WHO).

DIFFERENTIAL DIAGNOSIS

A. Acute myeloid leukemia.
B. Lymphoma.
C. Aplastic anemia.
D. Idiopathic thrombocytopenic purpura.

EVALUATION AND MANAGEMENT PLAN

A. General plan.

1. The general approach is based on the subtype of leukemia, age, and performance status.

2. Treatment for all patients with acute leukemia (AML and ALL) can be subdivided into two or three phases.

a. Induction chemotherapy.
b. Consolidation chemotherapy.
c. Maintenance chemotherapy.

3. Recent advances in the treatment of the acute leukemias focus more on precision medicine, including mutation-specific targeted therapies, immune-based therapies, and understanding the mechanisms of resistance.
B. Oncologic emergencies (Table 13.8).

FOLLOW-UP

A. Supportive care.

1. Myelosuppression is anticipated as a consequence of both leukemia and the treatment of leukemia with chemotherapy.

2. Bloodwork required two to three times weekly with transfusional support.

3. Broad-spectrum prophylactic antimicrobial therapy during myelosuppression due to increased susceptibility to opportunistic infections.
B. Disease monitoring.

1. Bone marrow aspirate (BMA)/biopsy 14 to 21 days following start of therapy to document hypoplasia.

2. Repeat BMA in 7 to 14 days if hypoplasia is indeterminate or not documented. If documented, repeat at the time of hematologic recovery.

3. Monitoring of minimal/measurable residual disease (MRD) on BMA or PB by flow cytometry, cytogenetic/fluorescence in situ hybridization (FISH) testing, or molecular diagnostics (NGS or polymerase chain reaction [PCR]).

CONSULTATION/REFERRAL

A. Hematology/oncology specialist once leukemia is suspected.

SPECIAL/GERIATRIC CONSIDERATIONS

A. Older adult patients tend to have a poor overall prognosis compared with younger patients, which may be related to some intrinsic poorly understood aspects of the tumor or even host factors.
B. Despite poor prognosis, treatment options should not be based on chronological age alone and should be discussed in detail with the patient.

CASE SCENARIO: ACUTE LEUKEMIAS

A 68-year-old male with a past medical history (PMH) of chronic obstructive pulmonary disease (COPD), diabetes mellitus, hypertension, and diverticulitis presents to the ED with left upper quadrant (LUQ) pain and fatigue. He denies fever, dysuria, hematuria, or recent infections. He is restricted in strenuous activity but still

TABLE 13.8   ONCOLOGIC EMERGENCIES

Oncologic Emergency	Pathophysiology	Signs	Symptoms	Management
TLS	Result of rapid cell turnover Spontaneous or treatment induced	↑ Phosphate, ↓calcium, ↑ potassium, ↑ uric acid, ↑ LDH	Fatigue, weakness, lethargy, edema, syncope, cardiac dysrhythmias	Frequent electrolyte management Corticosteroids IV 0.9% sodium chloride Rasburicase Sodium bicarbonate Allopurinol
Hyperleukocytosis and leukostasis	Leukemic cells poorly deformable and can become lodged in the microvasculature, causing impairment of microvascular perfusion and leading to organ damage	WBC >100 K/mcL with signs/symptoms of tissue hypoxia	Neuro: Confusion, somnolence, CVA Respiratory: Dyspnea, respiratory alkalosis Cardiology: Angina	Cytoreduction (chemotherapy, leukapheresis, hydroxyurea)
Disseminated intravascular coagulation	Excess thrombin generation Consumption of clotting factors and platelets Accelerated fibrinolysis Associated with: APL Gram-negative sepsis L-asparaginase	Positive schistocytes (30%), ↓ platelets, ↓ fibrinogen, ↑ D-dimer, ↑ PT/PTT	Thrombosis and bleeding Dyspnea, hematomas, confusion, headache, memory loss	Treat underlying cause FFP Platelets
Spinal cord compression	Impingement of mass on spinal cord causing increased parenchymal pressure	Abnormalities on MRI	Back pain, motor weakness, urinary retention, urinary and fecal incontinence, gait abnormalities	Corticosteroids (dexamethasone) Radiation therapy Surgical decompression
Hyperviscosity syndrome	High concentrations of serum paraproteins	Retinal hemorrhage, mucosal bleeding	Headache, visual changes, dizziness, altered mental status, CHF, peripheral neuropathy, weakness, fatigue	IV fluids followed by diuresis Plasma exchange

APL, acute promyelocytic leukemia; CHF, congestive heart failure; CVA, cerebrovascular accident; FFP, fresh frozen plasma; IV, intravenous; LDH, lactate dehydrogenase; PT, prothrombin time; PTT, partial thromboplastin time; TLS, tumor lysis syndrome; WBC, white blood cell.

able to do work of light nature. On arrival, vital signs include blood pressure (BP) of 173/84, heart rate (HR) of 98, respiratory rate (RR) of 24, and temperature of 37.7°C (98.8°F). Physical examination is notable for tenderness on palpation of LUQ and left lower quadrant (LLQ). Laboratory results reveal a white blood cell (WBC) count of 208 K/mcL, hemoglobin of 12.1 g/dL, platelet count of 122 K/mcL, and absolute neutrophil count (ANC) of 19.78 K/mcL. Peripheral blood (PB) smear shows 68% immature monocytes and 4% blasts. Chemistry panel is unremarkable except for a creatinine of 1.30 mg/dL, glucose of 279 mg/dL, alkaline phosphatase of 136 IU/L, and lactic acid of 2.5. CT of abdomen and pelvis reveals splenomegaly and numerous mediastinal, right hilar, bilateral axillary, and upper abdominal lymph nodes. Multiple descending colon diverticula are present, with evidence of possible diverticulitis. Bone marrow biopsy reveals 35% monocytoid blasts and immature monocytes (blast equivalents). Next-generation sequencing (NGS) reveals mutations in ASXL1, BCOR, NRAS, and SRSF2. Chromosome analysis testing shows multiple abnormalities including t(3;8)(q26.2;q24.1), der(20), t(3;12), −7, and t(1;3)(q21;p21). Fluorescence in situ hybridization (FISH) is positive for MECOM (EVI1) rearrangement at 86.5% and chromosome 7 rearrangement at 20.5%.

1. What is the diagnosis and French–American–British (FAB) classification of this patient's disease?
   A. M1: Acute myeloid leukemia (AML) without maturation
   B. M2: AML with maturation
   C. M4: Acute myelomonocytic leukemia
   D. M5: Acute monocytic leukemia

2. What is this patient's risk category?
   A. Good risk
   B. Intermediate risk

C. Poor risk

D. Unable to determine at this time

3. What is most concerning about the patient's initial lab values?

A. Lactic acid of 2.5

B. White blood cell (WBC) count of 208 K/mcL

C. Glucose of 279 mg/dL

D. Alkaline phosphatase of 136 IU/L

4. How can/should the patient's response to treatment be monitored?

A. Periodic monitoring of minimal/measurable residual disease (MRD) on bone marrow aspirate (BMA) or peripheral blood (PB) by flow cytometry, cytogenetic/fluorescence in situ hybridization (FISH) testing, or molecular diagnostics (next-generation sequencing [NGS] or polymerase chain reaction [PCR]) depending on treatment

B. Weekly lumbar puncture (LP) with intrathecal chemotherapy

C. Monthly MRI of the brain to check for extramedullary involvement

D. Supportive care

BIBLIOGRAPHY

Birdwell, C., Fiskus, W., Kadia, T. M., DiNardo, C. D., Mill, C. P., & Bhalla, K. N. (2021). EVI1 dysregulation: Impact on biology and therapy of myeloid malignancies. *Blood Cancer Journal, 11*, 64. https://doi.org/10.1038/s41408-021-00457-9

Deak, D., Gorcea-Andronic, N., Sas, V., Teodorescu, P., Constantinescu, C., Iluta, S., Pasca, S., Hotea, I., Turcas, C., Moisoiu, V., Zimta, A. A., Galdean, S., Steinheber, J., Rus, I., Rauch, S., Richlitzki, C., Munteanu, R., Jurj, A., Petrushev, B. … Tomuleasa, C. (2021). A narrative review of central nervous system involvement in acute leukemias. *Annals of Translational Medicine, 9*(1), 68. https://doi.org/10.21037/atm-20-3140

Lenk, L., Alsadeq, A., & Schewe, D. M. (2020). Involvement of the central nervous system in acute lymphoblastic leukemia: Opinions on molecular mechanisms and clinical implications based on recent data. *Cancer Metastasis Reviews, 39*, 173–187. https://doi.org/10.1007/s10555-020-09848-z

Lichtman, M. A. (2017). *Williams manual of hematology*. McGraw-Hill.

National Cancer Institute. (2022, September 12). *Surveillance, epidemiology, and end results program*. https://seer.cancer.gov/statistics/reports.html

Rodgers, G. P., & Young, N. S. (2013). *The Bethesda handbook of clinical hematology*. Wolters Kluwer/Lippincott Williams & Wilkins.

Schiffer, C. A., & Gurbuxani, S. (2022, February 21). Clinical manifestations, pathologic features, and diagnosis of acute myeloid leukemia. In A. G. Rosmarin (Ed.), *UpToDate* https://www.uptodate.com/contents/clinical-manifestations-pathologic-features-and-diagnosis-of-acute-myeloid-leukemia

Singleton, J. M., & Hefner, M. (2022, January). Spinal cord compression. In *StatPearls [Internet]*. StatPearls Publishing. https://www.ncbi.nlm.nih.gov/books/NBK557604/

Stock, W. S., & Thirman, M. J. (2022, March 8). Pathogenesis of acute myeloid leukemia. In A. G. Rosmarin (Ed.), *UpToDate*. https://www.uptodate.com/contents/pathogenesis-of-acute-myeloid-leukemia

Wierzbowska, A., & Czemerska, M. (2021). Clinical manifestation and diagnostic workup. In C. Röllig & G. J. Ossenkoppele (Eds.), *Acute myeloid leukemia. Hematologic Malignancies*. Springer. https://doi.org/10.1007/978-3-030-72676-8_6

Yeung, S., & Manzullo, E. F. (2011). Chapter 46. Oncologic emergencies. In H. M. Kantarjian, R. A. Wolff, & C. A. Koller (Eds.), *The MD Anderson manual of medical oncology*, (2nd ed.). McGraw Hill. https://accessmedicine.mhmedical.com/content.aspx?bookid=379&sectionid=39902077

Zuckerman, T., & Rowe, J. M. (2014). Pathogenesis and prognostication in acute lymphoblastic leukemia. *F1000Prime Reports, 6*, 59.

LEUKEMIAS: CHRONIC LEUKEMIAS

Allison Koblitz

DEFINITION

A. Chronic leukemias are blood cancers that arise from hematopoietic stem cells in the bone marrow.

B. Subtypes:

1. Chronic myeloid leukemia (CML): Myeloproliferative neoplasm (MPN) characterized by Abelson murine leukemia (ABL1) gene fusion on chromosome 9 with chromosome 22 at the breakpoint cluster region (BCR) gene (BCR-ABL1); also known as the Philadelphia chromosome.

2. Chronic lymphocytic leukemia (CLL): Monoclonal disease characterized by accumulation of mature B-cell lymphocytes that progressively accumulate in the blood, bone marrow, and lymphoid tissues.

3. Small lymphocytic leukemia (SLL): Considered the same disease as CLL but is differentiated from CLL based on lymphocyte count ($<5 \times 10^9$/L). Lymphadenopathy and/or organomegaly may or may not be present. Diagnosis should be confirmed with lymph node biopsy if feasible.

INCIDENCE

A. CML.

1. Approximately 15% of newly diagnosed leukemia in the United States, with estimated new cases of 8,860 (0.5% of all new cancer cases) in 2022.

2. The mean age of diagnosis is approximately 67 years old.

3. The estimated deaths from CML in 2022 was 1,220 (0.2% of all cancer deaths). The 5-year survival rate is 70.4% based on 2012 to 2018 data.

B. CLL.

1. Most common type of adult leukemia in the United States, approximately 25% to 30% of newly diagnosed leukemia in the United States, with estimated new cases of 20,160 (1.1% of all new cancer cases) in 2022.

2. The mean age of diagnosis is approximately 70 years old.

3. The estimated deaths from CLL in 2022 was 4,410 (0.7% of all cancer deaths). The 5-year survival rate is 87.9% based on 2012 to 2018 data.

PATHOGENESIS

A. CML.

1. Develops as a result of the BCR-ABL1 fusion on chromosomes 9 and 22 [t(9;22)], which results in expression of the p210 protein (more rarely p190 or p230 is expressed). This protein then allows for unregulated cell division due to deregulated tyrosine kinase activity.

2. Three phases: Chronic (CP), accelerated (AP), and blast (BP). When diagnosed, 90% to 95% are CP-CML. Untreated CP-CML will eventually progress to AP-CML or BP-CML (in an average of 35 years).

B. CLL.

1. Proliferation of B cells that gradually accumulate in the blood, bone marrow, lymph nodes, and spleen.

2. Often an incidental finding on routine bloodwork (complete blood count [CBC]).

3. Can remain indolent, not requiring treatment for years. Aggressive disease requires more upfront treatment.

PREDISPOSING FACTORS

A. Exposure to ionizing radiation.

B. Family history: Estimated six- to ninefold increased risk for direct family members of individuals with CLL.

C. Exposures to certain chemicals: Agent Orange, herbicides, and pesticides.

D. Sex: More common in males.

E. Race/ethnicity: More common in North America and Europe in comparison with Asia.

F. Age: Affects the older adult population (>65 years old).

SUBJECTIVE DATA

A. Common complaints/symptoms.

1. Typically asymptomatic; often an incidental finding (approximately 50% of new CML cases are asymptomatic). Of the presenting symptoms, lymphadenopathy is the most common.

2. Fatigue and malaise.

3. Bleeding or bruising easily.

4. Bone pain and myalgias.

5. B symptoms: Fevers, drenching night sweats, or unintentional weight loss.

6. Organomegaly (splenomegaly and/or hepatomegaly) with associated symptoms (abdominal discomfort/fullness, early satiety).

7. CML transformation to AP or BP more likely to be symptomatic, with the most common symptoms being headaches, bone pain/arthralgias, left upper quadrant (LUQ) abdominal pain (secondary to splenic infarctions), and fever.

PHYSICAL EXAMINATION

A. Vital signs and baseline height and weight.

B. Routine physical examination with focus on:

1. Abdominal assessment: Organomegaly with documentation of baseline spleen and liver size. Splenomegaly is the most common physical finding (40%–50% of cases) with CML.

2. Skin assessment: Bruising.

3. Lymphatics assessment: Cervical, axillary, and inguinal lymph nodes.

C. Assessment of performance status at baseline.

DIAGNOSTIC TESTS

A. CML.

1. CBC with differential: Normal or elevated white blood cell (WBC) count; normal or elevated platelet count; normocytic, normochromic anemia; absolute basophilia or eosinophilia on blood smear.

2. Quantitative polymerase chain reaction (qPCR) for BCR-ABL1 (peripheral blood [PB]).

3. Bone marrow aspiration and biopsy for cytogenetic analysis and morphologic review. Can also use fluorescence in situ hybridization (FISH) on PB if bone marrow biopsy is not appropriate.

4. If AP or BP: Assess cell lineage by flow cytometry, mutational analysis, and human leukocyte antigen (HLA) testing if considering allogeneic stem cell transplant (SCT).

5. Additional lab work: Comprehensive metabolic panel (CMP) and hepatitis B panel.

B. CLL.

1. CBC with differential: ≥5,000 monoclonal B lymphocytes/mcL with clonal confirmation on flow cytometry with immunophenotyping.

2. Additional lab work to consider: CMP, immunoglobulin (Ig) profile, reticulocyte count, haptoglobin, direct antiglobulin, beta-2 microglobulin, lactate dehydrogenase (LDH), uric acid, and infectious disease testing (HIV, hepatitis B and C).

3. PET/CT scan with additional imaging if indicated based on symptoms or if lymph node biopsy is needed.

4. Bone marrow biopsy and aspiration to rule out other diagnoses. Not necessary for diagnosis.

C. CLL staging.

1. Two staging systems.

   a. Rai (Table 13.9).

   b. Binet (Table 13.10).

2. del(11q), del(17p), TP53 mutation associated with poor prognosis for CLL.

DIFFERENTIAL DIAGNOSIS

A. Acute leukemias and myelodysplastic syndrome (MDS).

B. Lymphoma (mantle cell lymphoma [MCL], leukemic marginal zone lymphoma [MZL]).

EVALUATION AND MANAGEMENT PLAN

A. CML treatment.

1. The gold standard treatment of CML are tyrosine kinase inhibitors (TKIs), which include imatinib, dasatinib, nilotinib, and bosutinib.

2. Allogeneic SCT.

B. CML response to therapy.

1. Bone marrow biopsy and aspiration is no longer recommended to monitor for response to therapy as BCR-ABL1 is more sensitive and less invasive.

2. BCR-ABL1 should be monitored every 3 months after initiation of treatment; once BCR-ABL1 is ≤1%, continue to monitor every 3 months for 2 years and then every 3 to 6 months.

3. Complete hematologic response (CHR): Normalization of blood counts (leukocyte count <10,000, platelet count <450,000).

4. Cytogenetic (Ph-positive metaphases) response: Complete cytogenetic response (CCyR) correlates with BCR-ABL1 less than or equal to 1%.

5. Molecular response and treatment milestones.

   a. Early molecular response (EMR): BCR-ABL1 less than or equal to 10%. The goal is to have EMR at 3 and 6 months after initiating treatment.

TABLE 13.9   RAI STAGING FOR CHRONIC LYMPHOCYTIC LEUKEMIA

Stage	Risk	Defining Characteristics
0	Low risk	Lymphocytosis in blood and >40% lymphocytes in the marrow
I	Intermediate risk	Lymphocytosis and presence of lymphadenopathy
II	Intermediate risk	Lymphocytosis and presence of splenomegaly and/or hepatomegaly with or without lymphadenopathy
III	High risk	Lymphocytosis and presence of anemia with or without lymphadenopathy/organomegaly
IV	High risk	Lymphocytosis and presence of thrombocytopenia with or without lymphadenopathy/organomegaly

Note: Anemia is defined as hemoglobin <11 g/dL. Thrombocytopenia is defined as platelets <100,000 mm³. Lymphocytosis is defined as >5 × 10⁹/L.
Source: Adapted from Rai, K. R., Sawitsky, A., Cronkite, E. P., Chanana, A. D., Levy, R. N., & Pasternack, B. S. (1975). Clinical staging of chronic lymphocytic leukemia. *Blood, 46*(2), 219–234.

TABLE 13.10   BINET STAGING FOR CHRONIC LYMPHOCYTIC LEUKEMIA

Stage	Risk/Survival	All Criteria Must Be Met
A	Low risk	Up to two areas of enlarged lymph nodes >1 cm in diameter Platelets >100,000 mm³ Hemoglobin ≥10 g/dL
B	Intermediate risk	Three or more areas of enlarged lymph nodes >1 cm in diameter Platelets >100,000 mm³ Hemoglobin ≥10 g/dL
C	High risk	Three or more areas of enlarged lymph nodes >1 cm in diameter Platelets <100,000 mm³ Hemoglobin <10 g/dL

Source: Adapted from Desai, S., & Pinilla-Ibarz, J. (2012). Front-line therapy for chronic lymphocytic leukemia. *Cancer Control, 19*, 26–36.

b. Major molecular response (MMR): BCR-ABL1 less than or equal to 0.1%. The goal is to have MMR by 12 months after initiating treatment.

c. Deep molecular response (DMR): BCR-ABL1 less than or equal to 0.01%. The goal is to maintain DMR after 12 months of treatment.

d. TKI-resistant disease is defined as a BCR-ABL1 >10% at 6 and 12 months. This would be an indication for BCR-ABL1 kinase domain mutation analysis testing to evaluate for known mutations.

   i. If T315I mutation present, treatment options include ponatinib, asciminib, and omacetaxine.

   ii. If T315I mutation is not present but still concern for TKI resistance, consider second-generation TKI (bosutinib, dasatinib, nilotinib).

   iii. Refer for allogeneic SCT.

c. CLL.

1. Observation is typically recommended as initial treatment.

2. Indications for initiating therapy include:

a. Signs of bone marrow failure: New/worsening cytopenias (hemoglobin <10 g/dL or platelets <100,000 mm³).

b. Massive or enlarging splenomegaly (>6 cm below the left costal margin) or lymphadenopathy (>10 cm in diameter).

c. Worsening lymphocytosis (>50% increase in lymphocyte count over 2 months or doubling of lymphocytes over 6 months).

d. Autoimmune complications (anemia or thrombocytopenia refractory to corticosteroids).

e. New/worsening constitutional symptoms (B symptoms).

3. Prior to initiation of or change to therapy, consider the following:

a. Clinical stage, genetic mutations, and associated prognostic indices.

b. Age/comorbidities/performance status. Age should be considered but should not be a limiting factor when deciding on if/when to treat. Life expectancy and quality of life should also be considered.

c. Toxicity profile of treatment options.

4. Frontline therapy: Ibrutinib, acalabrutinib ± obinutuzumab, or venetoclax + obinutuzumab.

a. Ibrutinib and acalabrutinib may initially cause an increase in WBC count and is not a sign of treatment failure.

b. Venetoclax is associated with an increased risk of tumor lysis syndrome (TLS) with initiation of treatment. TLS labs (CMP, magnesium level, phosphorus level, uric acid, and LDH) should be monitored closely. Consider allopurinol for TLS prophylaxis.

5. Future considerations for treatment: CD19 chimeric antigen receptor therapy (CAR-T).

6. Richter's transformation: Histologic transformation of CLL to diffuse large B-cell lymphoma (DLBCL) or Hodgkin lymphoma (HL).

a. Occurs in 2% to 10% of patients; pathogenesis is not well-understood.

b. Associated with poor prognosis; typically not chemosensitive. Occurs more frequently in patients who have received multiple previous chemoimmunotherapy regimens.

c. Median survival of 5 to 12 months after transformation if previously received chemoimmunotherapy; if no previous treatment, median survival is approximately 46 months.

d. Diagnosis should be confirmed by excisional lymph node biopsy.

e. Treatment per guidelines for DLBCL or HL.

D. Associated considerations.

1. Autoimmune cytopenias.

a. Autoimmune hemolytic anemia (AIHA): Positive Coombs test, decreased hemoglobin, increased reticulocyte count, elevated LDH, elevated indirect bilirubinemia, and low haptoglobin levels.

i. First-line treatment is steroids.

ii. Consider intravenous immunoglobulin (IVIG), Rituxan, or splenectomy in steroid-refractory patients.

iii. Occurs in approximately 15% of patients diagnosed with CLL.

b. Immune thrombocytopenia (ITP): Decreased platelet count, hemoglobin/WBC normal, and normal coagulation studies.

i. Diagnosis of exclusion. Must rule out other causes of thrombocytopenia (e.g., medications, microangiopathy, infections).

ii. Treatment.

1) Frontline treatment is intravenous (IV) steroids tapered to PO steroids.

2) IVIG raises platelet count more rapidly than steroids, but the duration of response is shorter than with steroids.

3) Rituxan and/or splenectomy can be considered in steroid-refractory patients.

2. Central nervous system (CNS) disease.

a. Documented mostly in association with AP or BP-CML. Patients present with mental status changes and/or new neurologic symptoms or deficits.

b. Imaging including CT of the head/brain or MRI of the brain to rule out other etiologies.

c. LP with cerebrospinal fluid (CSF) sampling to assess cell count and differential, flow cytometry, and cytology.

d. For negative CSF testing, prophylactic intrathecal (IT) chemotherapy should be given. If CSF testing is positive, refer for IT chemotherapy treatment. Dasatinib has been reported to cross the blood–brain barrier (BBB) and therefore would be the TKI of choice in the setting of CNS involvement.

3. Hypogammaglobulinemia.

a. A decrease in Ig levels that is associated with recurrent or a predisposition to infections (most commonly sinopulmonary infections).

b. Common complication of B-cell malignancies (CLL). Can also occur with the use of ibrutinib, anti-CD20 antibodies (rituximab), and Bruton's tyrosine kinase (BTK) inhibitors (venetoclax).

c. In the setting of hypogammaglobulinemia (IgG level <400–500 mg/dL) and recurrent infections, consider IVIG therapy.

FOLLOW-UP

A. Routine follow-up for all patients should occur once every 6 to 12 months and include a physical examination and CBC.

B. CLL patients are at a higher risk for other types of cancer, particularly nonmelanomatous skin cancers. Routine monitoring for cancer with yearly skin checks should occur, as well as additional workup if patient reports new or worsening symptoms.

CONSULTATION/REFERRAL

A. Hematology oncology.

B. Additional referrals (dermatology, interventional radiology for port placement, etc.) should be considered on an individualized basis.

SPECIAL/GERIATRIC CONSIDERATIONS

A. CLL is the most common type of leukemia and typically affects the older adult population (with the median age at diagnosis being 70 years old). With the aging population and longer life expectancy, CLL will likely become more prevalent with increased morbidity and mortality in older adults.

B. TKIs are typically well-tolerated; however, the more severe/acute symptoms reported are as follows:

1. Dasatinib: Pleural effusions, pulmonary artery hypertension, hemorrhage (especially if on other anticoagulation), and cytopenias.

2. Nilotinib: Hyperglycemia, QTc prolongation (check EKG at baseline, 7 days after starting nilotinib, and then periodically), occlusive vascular events, and pancreatitis.

3. Imatinib: Weight gain, fatigue, edema, myalgias, nausea, and cytopenias.

4. Bosutinib: Gastrointestinal (GI) disturbances and elevated transaminases.

CASE SCENARIO: CHRONIC LEUKEMIA

A 67-year-old female with chronic myeloid leukemia (CP-CML) diagnosed 3 years ago started on dasatinib 100 mg daily following diagnosis. She has been followed every 3 months with ongoing good response as evidenced by undetectable BCR-ABL1 p210 levels. She presents to the hospital with shortness of breath. Chest x-ray (CXR) shows pneumonia and a moderate-large right-sided pleural effusion. She is prescribed a course of azithromycin. She presents 3 months later with ongoing shortness of breath; repeat CXR shows a persistent pleural effusion.

1. What is the next course of action?
   A. Prescribe another and/or different course of antibiotics.
   B. Order thoracentesis for diagnostic and/or therapeutic purposes.
   C. Switch to a different tyrosine kinase inhibitor (TKI) therapy.
   D. Monitor symptoms and repeat imaging in 3 months.

2. The nurse practitioner (NP) has found that the pleural effusions are related to dasatinib. The patient is switched to nilotinib. What is the recommended EKG monitoring for a patient starting on nilotinib?
   A. At baseline, 7 days after initiation of therapy, and then periodically
   B. Every 30 days
   C. Every week ×4 and then as needed
   D. EKG monitoring is not necessary

3. After switching to nilotinib, what will the plan be for monitoring/evaluation?
   A. Bone marrow aspiration and biopsy every 3 months until BCR-ABL1 is negative.
   B. No change in the monitoring plan is indicated as the patient has been on a tyrosine kinase inhibitor (TKI) for multiple years.
   C. Refer for allogeneic stem cell transplant.
   D. Check BCR-ABL1 every 3 months; once BCR-ABL1 is ≤1%, continue to monitor every 3 months for 2 years and then every 3 to 6 months.

4. The patient has had ongoing major molecular response (MMR) after switching to nilotinib. The NP continues to monitor as recommended, and 2 years into treatment BCR-ABL1 turns positive again. The NP has confirmed medication compliance. What is the next course of action?
   A. Continue to monitor but check the BCR-ABL1 more frequently.
   B. Stop nilotinib and consider an alternative tyrosine kinase inhibitor (TKI) or treatment plan.
   C. Check a BCR-ABL1 kinase domain mutation analysis.
   D. Refer for allogeneic stem cell transplant (SCT).

BIBLIOGRAPHY

Celik, S., Kaynar, L., Guven, Z. T., Baydar, M., Keklik, M., Çetin, M., Ünal, A., & Demirkan, F. (2021). Secondary hypogammaglobulinemia in patients with chronic lymphocytic leukemia receiving ibrutinib therapy. *Indian Journal of Hematology and Blood Transfusion, 38,* 282–289.
Eichhorst, B., Robak, T., & Montserrat, E. (2020). Chronic lymphocytic leukaemia: ESMO Clinical Practice Guidelines for diagnosis, treatment, and follow-up. *Annals of Oncology, 32*(1), 23–33.
Hallek, M., Cheson, B. D., Catovsky, D., Caligaris-Cappio, F., Dighiero, G., Döhner, H., Hillmen, P., Keating, M., Montserrat, E., Chiorazzi, N., Stilgenbauer, S., Rai, K. R., Byrd, J. C., Eichhorst, B., O'Brien, S., Robak,

T., Seymour, J. F., & Kipps, T. J. (2018). iwCLL guidelines for diagnosis, indications for treatment, response assessment and supportive management of CLL. *Blood, 131*(25), 2745–2760.
Hallek, M., & Othman, A. (2021). Chronic lymphocytic leukemia: 2022 update on diagnostic and therapeutic procedures. *American Journal of Hematology, 96*(12), 1679–1705.
Jabbour, E., & Kantarjian, H. (2018). Chronic myeloid leukemia: 2018 update on diagnosis, therapy, and monitoring. *American Journal of Hematology, 93*(3), 442–459.
Medeiros, B. C., Possick, J., & Fradley, M. (2018). Cardiovascular, pulmonary, and metabolic toxicities complicating tyrosine kinase inhibitor therapy in chronic myeloid leukemia: Strategies for monitoring, detecting, and managing. *Blood Reviews, 32*(4), 289–299.
National Cancer Institute. (2022, May 09). *Cancer stat facts: Leukemia – Chronic Myeloid Leukemia (CML).* https://seer.cancer.gov/statfacts/html/cmyl.html
National Cancer Institute. (2022, May 09). *Cancer stat facts: Leukemia – Chronic Lymphocytic Leukemia (CLL).* https://seer.cancer.gov/statfacts/html/clyl.html
Shallis, R. M., & Podoltsev, N. (2019). What is the best pharmacotherapeutic strategy for treating chronic myeloid leukemia in the elderly? *Expert Opinion on Pharmacotherapy, 20*(10), 1169–1173.

LEUKEMIAS: MYELODYSPLASTIC SYNDROMES

Lori Sheneman

DEFINITION
A. Myelodysplastic syndrome (MDS) consists of a group of heterogeneous myeloid neoplasms associated with ineffective hematopoiesis.
B. They are characterized by the morbidities of their cytopenias and the potential to evolve into acute myeloid leukemia (AML).

INCIDENCE
A. The incidence rate of MDS is approximately 4.5 per 100,000 people per year (Platzbecker, 2021).
B. MDS is a disease of older individuals (median age at diagnosis: 70–75 years of age), with incidence peaking at 55.4 per 100,000 people among those who are 80 years of age and older (Platzbecker, 2021).

PATHOGENESIS
A. MDS develops when a clonal population of dysplastic hematopoietic stem cells are present among precursor and mature bone marrow blood cells.
B. MDS can be characterized as primary (de novo) or therapy-related (t-MDS) due to previous exposure to cytotoxic chemotherapy or radiation therapy (RT).

PREDISPOSING FACTORS
A. More common in males.
B. Increases with age.
C. Exposure to chemotherapy or RT.
D. Environmental exposure such as long-term work exposure to benzene and other chemicals.

SUBJECTIVE DATA
A. Common complaints/symptoms: Patient presentation is typically related to cytopenias and may include:
   1. Fever.
   2. Dyspnea.
   3. Fatigue.
   4. Ecchymoses.

5. Bleeding.

6. Recurrent infections.

B. Medical history.

   1. Timing, severity, and pace of abnormal cytopenias.

   2. Transfusion history.

   3. Pneumonias, urinary tract, and other recurrent/frequent infections.

PHYSICAL EXAMINATION

A. Vital signs: Assess for tachycardia due to anemia or weight.

B. General: Assess for pallor or weakness.

C. Head, ear, eyes, nose, and throat (HEENT): Assess oral cavity for hemorrhagic bullae, gingival bleeding, and mucosal ulcerations. Evaluate eyes for hemorrhagic conjunctiva.

D. Cardiopulmonary: Assess for signs of heart failure and adventitious breath sounds consistent with infection.

E. Gastrointestinal (GI): Assess for hepatosplenomegaly (HSM) and hematochezia.

F. Skin: Assess for petechiae and ecchymoses.

DIAGNOSTIC TESTS

A. Laboratory.

   1. Complete blood count (CBC) with differential.

   2. Peripheral blood (PB) smear.

   3. Comprehensive metabolic panel (CMP) with serum uric acid and lactate dehydrogenase (LDH).

   4. Thyroid function tests.

   5. Serum erythropoietin, vitamin B_{12}, folate, and iron studies.

B. Bone marrow aspirate (BMA) and biopsy, including cytogenetics, next-generation sequencing (NGS), and flow cytometry.

C. Diagnostic criteria.

   1. MDS diagnostic criteria are primarily based on the World Health Organization (WHO) guidelines correlated with the clinical presentation (Table 13.11).

   2. Risk stratification and prognostic scoring system.

DIFFERENTIAL DIAGNOSIS

A. Other causes of dysplasia.

   1. Nonmalignant: Nutritional deficiencies, toxic exposures, drugs and biologic exposures, infection, congenital disorders, autoimmune disorders, and sideroblastic anemia.

   2. Malignant: Hairy cell leukemia and large granular lymphocytic leukemia.

EVALUATION AND MANAGEMENT PLAN

A. General plan.

   1. Treatment of MDS is based on risk stratification of the disease and comorbidities of the patient.

   2. Treatment is focused on supportive management of cytopenias (e.g., blood and platelet transfusions, ▸

TABLE 13.11 2008 AND 2016 WHO CLASSIFICATIONS OF MYELODYSPLASTIC SYNDROME

2008 WHO Classification	2016 WHO Classification
RCUD encompassing RA, RN, and RT	MDS-SLD
RCMD	MDS-MLD
RARS	MDS-RS (SF3B1 mutation)
	MDS-RS-SLD
	MDS-RS-MLD
MDS associated with isolated del(5q)	MDS with isolated del(5q)
	MDS-EB
RAEB-1	MDS-EB-1
RAEB-2	MDS-EB-2
MDS, unclassified	MDS, unclassifiable
	With 1% blood blasts
	With single lineage dysplasia and pancytopenia
	Based on defining cytogenetic abnormality
Refractory cytopenia of childhood	Refractory cytopenia of childhood

MDS, myelodysplastic syndrome; MDS-EB, MDS with excess blasts; MDS-MLD, MDS with multilineage dysplasia; MDS-RS, MDS with ringed sideroblasts; MDS-RS-MLD, MDS-RS with multilineage dysplasia; MDS-RS-SLD, MDS-RS with single lineage dysplasia; RA, refractory anemia; RAEB-1, refractory anemia with excess blasts-1; RAEB-2, refractory anemia with excess blasts-2; RARS, refractory anemia with ringed sideroblasts; RCMD, refractory cytopenia with multilineage dysplasia; RCUD, refractory cytopenia with unilineage dysplasia; RN, refractory neutropenia; RT, refractory thrombocytopenia; WHO, World Health Organization.

growth factors) and prolonging the time to disease progression (i.e., transformation to AML).

B. Supportive care pharmacotherapy.

1. Anemia: Darbepoetin (Aranesp) or erythropoietin (Procrit).

2. Iron overload from repeated transfusions: Iron chelation therapy.

C. Pharmacotherapy.

1. Hypomethylating agents (HMA): Azacitidine (Vidaza, Onureg) or decitabine (Dacogen, Inqovi).

2. Lenalidomide (Revlimid) for MDS with del(5q).

3. Luspatercept (Reblozyl) for MDS with ringed sideroblasts (MDS-RS).

4. Intensive chemotherapy can be considered after failure of HMA, as a bridge for patients going for allogeneic stem cell transplant (SCT).

D. Other treatment and only chance of a cure: Allogeneic hematopoietic SCT.

E. Disease progression to AML is defined by the presence of 20% or more myeloid blasts in bone marrow or PB. This is associated with poor prognosis and response to standard treatment options.

FOLLOW-UP

A. Focus on response to therapy and monitor for signs or symptoms of disease progression.

B. Frequency of visits determined by the oncologist; will include CBCs to monitor hematologic response and transfusion needs.

C. A bone marrow biopsy and aspirate may be warranted if there is concern for disease progression.

CONSULTATION/REFERRAL

A. Patients with MDS need to be referred to hematology-oncology.

SPECIAL/GERIATRIC CONSIDERATIONS

A. Management of the disease in the older adult population presents a challenge due to concomitant morbidities, which preclude toleration of intensive chemotherapy regimens.

B. Patients with MDS have high utilization rates of EDs and require frequent transfusions.

CASE SCENARIO: MYELODYSPLASTIC SYNDROMES

Mr. Jones is a 72-year-old male with a past medical history of hypertension and hyperlipidemia and who is seeing his primary care provider (PCP) for a 6-month checkup. He notes increased bruising over the past month. On review of his complete blood count (CBC) over the past 2 year, there was progressive pancytopenia. His current labs are as follows: white blood cell 3.3 with an absolute neutrophil count (ANC) of 1,200, hemoglobin (Hgb) of 8.2, mean corpuscular volume of 108, and platelet count of 82. After further investigation, the patient notes increased fatigue and dyspnea on exertion.

1. What would be the first step of working Mr. Jones up?

A. Bone marrow biopsy

B. Treating with darbepoetin

C. Further labs studies: Peripheral smear, iron studies, ferritin, B_{12}, folate, serum erythropoietin, thyroid studies

D. Monitor patient; no further intervention at this time

2. Mr. Jones' workup showed no evidence of nutritional or metabolic causes. What would be the next step in his workup?

A. Refer to a hematologist/oncologist for bone marrow biopsy/aspirate and further follow-up.

B. Start supportive transfusion support.

C. Monitor the patient; no further intervention at this time.

D. Advise to limit exposure to toxic chemicals.

3. Mr. Jones's bone marrow results are consistent with myelodysplastic syndrome (MDS). Cytogenetics were normal. Next-generation sequencing (NGS) revealed a single mutation, RUNX1. How should Mr. Jones's MDS be classified?

A. MDS, unclassified (MDS-U)

B. MDS with multilineage dysplasia (MDS-MLD)

C MDS with single-lineage dysplasia (MDS-SLD)

D. MDS with isolated del(5q) (MDS del(5q))

4. How is it best to support Mr. Jones and help maintain quality of life?

A. Darbepoetin with transfusion support as needed

B. Hospice care

C. A routine to improve diet and exercise

D. Monitor labs for evidence of transformation to acute myeloid leukemia (AML)

BIBLIOGRAPHY

Aster, J., & Stone, R. (2022). Clinical manifestations and diagnosis of myelodysplastic syndromes (MDS). *UpToDate.*

Garcia-Manero, G., Chein, K. S., & Montalban-Bravo, G. (2020). Myelodysplastic syndromes: 2021 update on diagnosis, risk stratification and management. *American Journal of Hematology, 95*, 1399–1420.

Hasserjian, R. (2019). Myelodysplastic syndrome update. *Pathobiology, 86*, 7–13.

Hellstrom-Lindberg, E., Tobiasson, M., & Greenberg, P. (2020). Myelodysplastic syndromes: Moving towards personalized management. *Haematologica, 105*, 1765–1779.

Platzbecker, U., Kubasch, A. S., Homer-Bouthiette, C., & Prebet, A. (2021). Current challenges and unmet medical needs in myelodysplastic syndromes. *Leukemia, 35*, 2182–2198.

LEUKEMIAS: MYELOPROLIFERATIVE NEOPLASMS

Shannon B. Holloway

DEFINITION

A. Myeloproliferative neoplasms (MPNs) are characterized by clonal myeloproliferation without dysplastic features, thus differing from myelodysplastic syndrome (MDS).

B. Myelofibrosis (MF), polycythemia vera (PV), and essential thrombocythemia (ET) comprise a heterogeneous group of neoplasms characterized by overproliferation of immature and mature cells of the myeloid lineage, often associated with bone marrow hypercellularity and fibrosis, and splenomegaly.

INCIDENCE

A. The prevalence of MF, PV, and ET in the United States is 13,000, 148,000, and 134,000, respectively.

B. The reported worldwide annual incidence rates of MPNs range from 1.15 to 4.99 per 100,000.

PATHOGENESIS

A. Molecular pathogenesis is linked to activation of the JAK/STAT (Janus kinase/signal transducer and activator of transcription) signaling pathway in MPNs with resultant gene mutations in *JAK2*, *CALR*, and *MPL* identified.

B. Typically predominate in one lineage depending on the disease.

PREDISPOSING FACTORS AND COMPLICATIONS

A. Age greater than 65.

B. History of thrombosis.

C. Major complications of MPNs include thrombosis, bleeding, or evolution to acute myeloid leukemia (AML) or a fibrotic phase of the disease.

SUBJECTIVE DATA

A. Common complaints/symptoms.

  1. Most patients with MPNs are typically asymptomatic, with abnormal blood counts often prompting further evaluation.

  2. Fatigue, pruritus, night sweats, bone pain, fever, and weight loss are common complaints.

  3. The Myeloproliferative Neoplasm Symptom Assessment Form (MPN-SAF) is a validated tool used to assess clinically relevant MPN symptoms such as abdominal pain, early satiety, abdominal discomfort, inactivity, vasomotor symptoms, difficulty concentrating/sleeping, night sweats, fever, pruritus, bone pain, weight loss, and depressed mood.

B. Common/typical scenario.

  1. Some patients present with bleeding or sequelae of thrombosis (transient ischemic attack, myocardial infarction, stroke, deep vein thrombosis, pulmonary embolism, headaches, migraines, dizziness, lightheadedness, coldness of the fingers and toes).

  2. PV is diagnosed when an otherwise unexplained increased hemoglobin/hematocrit/red blood cell mass is accompanied by the presence of a *JAK2* mutation along with a decreased erythropoietin level.

  3. MF is characterized by a leukoerythroblastic blood picture, splenomegaly, and bone marrow fibrosis that cannot be attributed to another myeloid disorder.

  4. ET is a diagnosis of exclusion, representing clonal or autonomous thrombocytosis not classifiable as PV, primary myelofibrosis, chronic myeloid leukemia (CML), or MDS.

PHYSICAL EXAMINATION

A. Skin: Facial plethora (flushed face), excoriations from scratching secondary to pruritus, and petechiae.

B. Abdomen: Splenomegaly, hepatomegaly, abdominal distention, and tenderness to palpation typically in the left upper quadrant (LUQ).

C. Head and neck: Epistaxis, hemorrhagic bullae, or gingival bleeding in oral cavity.

DIAGNOSTIC TESTS.

A. Complete blood count (CBC) with differential.

B. Comprehensive metabolic panel (CMP) with serum uric acid and lactate dehydrogenase (LDH).

C. Erythropoietin level and iron studies.

D. Vitamin B_{12} level.

E. Evaluate for acquired von Willebrand disease.

  1. Prothrombin time/international normalized ratio (PT/INR) and partial thromboplastin time (PTT).

  2. Factor VIII.

  3. Gold standard: Ristocetin activity test.

F. Peripheral blood (PB) smear.

G. Bone marrow aspiration and biopsy.

H. Abdominal ultrasound to assess splenomegaly/hepatomegaly.

I. CT scan of the abdomen and pelvis with contrast to assess splenomegaly/hepatomegaly and for obscure venous thrombosis.

J. Diagnosis: According to the World Health Organization (WHO) diagnostic criteria, laboratory findings and a bone marrow aspiration and biopsy are necessary to confirm a diagnosis of ET, PV, and MF.

K. Human leukocyte antigen (HLA) testing typing for stem cell transplant (SCT).

DIFFERENTIAL DIAGNOSIS

A. Acute lymphoblastic leukemia (ALL).

B. AML.

C. Chronic lymphocytic leukemia (CLL).

D. Chronic myelogenous leukemia.

E. Non-Hodgkin lymphoma (NHL).

F. MDS.

EVALUATION AND MANAGEMENT PLAN

A. General plan.

  1. The overall goal of treatment for patients with ET and PV is to prevent thrombosis and bleeding.

  2. The most frequent complication of ET/PV is thrombosis, which can include myocardial infarction, pulmonary embolism, deep vein thrombosis, or cerebrovascular accident.

  3. There is a risk stratification process that assesses a patient's risk for thrombohemorrhagic complications.

B. Treatment of ET.

  1. Low-risk patients.

    a. Managed with observation.

    b. Low-dose aspirin can be added to a low-risk patient's regimen on a case-by-case basis.

  2. High-risk patients.

    a. Treated with a cytoreductive agent.

    b. In addition, all high-risk patients must be on low-dose aspirin.

    c. Patients with a history of thrombosis should be treated with anticoagulant therapy.

C. Treatment of PV.

  1. Risk stratification based on thrombosis history, leukocyte count, age, and mutations using their Mutation-Enhanced International Prognostic Scoring System (MIPSS).

  2. Low-risk patients: Therapeutic phlebotomy and daily low-dose aspirin are indicated in low-risk patients.

  3. High-risk patients: Initially treated with phlebotomy to attain hematocrit goal of less than 45% and are then placed on ruxolitinib or a cytoreductive agent such as hydroxyurea.

▶

4. Daily-low dose aspirin recommended, and patients with preexisting thrombus must be treated with anticoagulation.

D. Staging of MF.

   1. Risk stratification.

      a. Three main prognostic scoring systems are used for MF risk stratification.

         i. The International Prognostic Scoring System (IPSS) is used at initial diagnosis and scores are based on age, hemoglobin level, leukocyte count, and circulating peripheral blasts.

         ii. The Diagnostic International Prognostic Scoring System (DIPSS) is used if karyotyping is not available during the course of treatment.

         iii. The Diagnostic International Prognostic Scoring System-Plus (DIPSS-Plus) is used if karyotyping is available during the course of treatment and includes platelet count and transfusion needs, as well as unfavorable karyotype.

   2. MF grading based on bone marrow biopsy.

E. Treatment of MF.

   1. The treatment approach for PMF, post-PV, or post-ET MF is the same.

   2. Referral to specialized centers with experts in MF and SCT is recommended.

   3. Watch and wait approach is appropriate for low-risk patients.

   4. Ruxolitinib or fedratinib (*JAK2* inhibitors) and pacritinib (kinase inhibitor).

   5. Allogeneic hematopoietic SCT is the only curative option.

   6. Disease progression to AML is defined by the presence of 20% or more myeloid blasts in bone marrow or PB. This is associated with poor prognosis and response to standard treatment options.

FOLLOW-UP

A. Changes in symptom status should be reported immediately to providers; prompt evaluation should include a CBC at a minimum.

B. Follow-up to monitor response to treatment should occur every 3 to 6 months, or more frequently if there is a change in symptoms.

CONSULTATION/REFERRAL

A. Refer to an oncologist specializing in MPNs.

B. MPNs are relatively rare, and smaller community-type oncologists may not have extensive experience in treatment options or access to major clinical trials that could benefit patients.

SPECIAL/GERIATRIC CONSIDERATIONS

A. Supportive care should be an integral part of treatment.

B. MPNs are more prevalent in older adults, who are at increased risk of cardiovascular and other comorbidities, such as congestive heart failure, peripheral vascular disease, stroke, thromboembolism, renal disease, liver disease, and infections.

CASE SCENARIO: MYELOPROLIFERATIVE NEOPLASMS

A 70-year-old man presents to his primary care physician with complaints of fatigue, worsening night sweats and abdominal fullness, and facial itching for 3 weeks. He also reports unintentional weight loss of 15 lb in the past 3 months and recent upper respiratory tract infection (URI), treated with antibiotics. His past medical history (PMH) is notable for hypertension and diabetes mellitus and left hip replacements surgery. His vital signs are within normal limits. His physical exam is remarkable for a flushed face, marked splenomegaly, lower extremity edema, and a fine resting tremor. His last visit to a provider was over 2 years ago prior to his recent treatment for URI.

1. Which presenting symptoms are worrisome for myeloproliferative neoplasm (MPN)?

  A. Fatigue

  B. Abdominal fullness

  C. Weight loss

  D. All of the above

2. Which physical findings is common with myeloproliferative neoplasm (MPN)?

  A. Flushed face

  B. Lower extremity edema

  C. Fine resting tremor

  D. All of the above

3. What additional workup would be helpful?

  A. Complete blood count

  B. Bone marrow biopsy

  C. Abdominal ultrasound

  D. All of the above

4. What would be some treatment options if this patient has myelofibrosis (MF)?

  A. Watch and wait

  B. *JAK2* inhibitors

  C. Stem cell transplant

  D. All of the above

BIBLIOGRAPHY

Arber, D. A., Orazi, A., Hasserjian, R., Thiele, J., Borowitz, M. J., Le Beau, M. M., Bloomfield, C. D., Cazzola, M., & Vardiman, J. W. (2016). Revision to the World Health Organization classification of myeloid neoplasms and acute leukemia. *Blood*, *127*, 2391.

Barbui, T., Thiele, J., Gisslinger, H., Finazzi, G., Vannucchi, A. M., & Tefferi, A. (2016). The 2016 revision of WHO classification of myeloproliferative neoplasms: Clinical and molecular advances. *Blood Review*, *30*(6), 453–459.

Cervantes, F., Dupriez, B., Pereira, A., Passamonti, F., Reilly, J. T., Morra, E., & Tefferi, A. (2009). New prognostic scoring system for based on a study of the International Working group for myelofibrosis research and treatment. *Blood*, *113*(13), 2895–2901.

Choi, C. W., Bang, S., Jang, S., Jung, C. W., Kim, H. J., Kim, H. Y., Kim, S.- J., Kim, Y.-K., Park, J., & Won, J. H. (2015). Guidelines for the management of myeloproliferative neoplasms. *Korean Journal of Internal Medicine*, *30*(6), 771–788.

Greenfield, G., McMullin, M. F., & Mills, K. (2021). Molecular pathogenesis of the myeloproliferative neoplasms. *Journal of Hematology & Oncology*, *14*, 103. https://www.fda.gov/drugs/new-drugs-fda-cders-new-molecular-entities-and-new-therapeutic-biological-products/novel-drug-approvals-2022

Mehta, J., Wang, H., Idbal, S. U., & Mesa, R. (2014). Epidemiology of myeloproliferative neoplasms in the United States. *Leuk Lymphoma*, 55, 595–600.

Mesa, R. A., Niblack, J., Wadleigh, M., Verstovsek, S., Camoriano, J., Barnes, S., Tan, A. D., Atherton, P. J., Sloan, J. A., & Tefferi, A. (2007). The burden of fatigue and quality of life in myeloproliferative disorders (MPDs): An international Internet-based survey of 1179 MPD patients. *Cancer*, 109(1), 68.

Mesa, R., Jamieson, C., Bhatia, R., Deininger, M. W., Gerds, A. T., Gojo, I., Gotlib, J., Gundabolu, K., Hobbs, G., Klisovic, R. B., Kropf, P., Mohan, S. R., Oh, S., Padron, E., Podoltsev, N., Pollyea, D. A., Rampal, R., Rein, L. A. M., Scott, B ... Sundar, H. (2016). Myeloproliferative neoplasms. *Journal of the National Comprehensive Cancer Network*, 14(2), 1572–1611.

National Comprehensive Cancer Network. Myeloproliferative Neoplasms Guidelines (Version. (2/2022-April 13, 2022). https://www.nccn.org/professionals/physician_gls/pdf/mpn.pdf

Passamonti, F., Cervantes, F., Vannucchi, A. M., Morra, E., Rumi, E., Pereira, A., Guglielmelli, P., Pungolino, E., Caramella, M., Maffioli, M., Pascutto, C., Lazzarino, M., Cazzola, M., & Tefferi, A. (2010). A dynamic prognostic model to predict survival in primary myelofibrosis: A study by the IWG-MRT. *Blood*, 115, 1703–1708.

Shallis, R. M., Wang, R., Davidoff, A., Ma, X., Podoltsev, N. A., & Zeidan, A. M. (2020). Epidemiology of the classical myeloproliferative neoplasms: The four corners of an expansive and complex map. *Blood Reviews*, 42, 100706.

Skoda, R., Duek, A., & Grisouard, J. (2015). Pathogenesis of myeloproliferative neoplasms. *Experimental Hematology*, 43(8), 599–608.

Tefferi, A., Guglielmelli, P., Lasho, T. L., ColtroG, Finke., M, C., Loscocco, G. G., Sordi, B., Szuber, N., Rotunno, G., Pacilli, A., Hanson, C. A., Ketterling, R. P., Pardanani, A., Gangat, N., & Vannucchi, A. M. (2020). Mutation-enhanced international prognostic systems for essential thrombocythemia and polycythemia vera. *British Journal of Haematology*, 189, 291–302.

Thiele, J., Kvasnicka, H. M., Facchetti, F., Franco, V., van der Walt, J., & Orazi, A. (2005). European consensus on grading bone marrow fibrosis and assessment of cellularity. *Haematologica*, 90(8), 1128–1132.

Vainchenker, W., & Constantinescu, S. N. (2013). JAK/STAT signaling in hematologic malignancies. *Oncogene*, 32, 2601–2613.

Vannucchi, A. M., Barbui, T., Cervantes, F., Harrison, C., Kiladjian, J. J., Kröger, N., Thiele, J., Buske, C., &ESMO Guidelines Committee. (2015). Philadelphia chromosome-negative chronic myeloproliferative neoplasms: ESMO clinical practice guidelines for diagnosis, treatment and follow-up. *Annals of Oncology*, 26(5), 85–99.

LUNG CANCER

Courtney Robb

DEFINITION

A. Lung cancer is the uncontrolled growth of abnormal cells that form in the tissues of one or both lungs, usually in the cells lining air passages. These abnormal cells divide rapidly to form tumors.

B. The two main types are nonsmall cell lung cancer (NSCLC) and small cell lung cancer (SCLC).

  1. NSCLC.

    a. NSCLC is the most common type of lung cancer, comprising 85% of the lung cancer diagnoses.

    b. There are three histologic subtypes of NSCLC arising from different lung cells, which have similar prognosis and treatment.

      i. Adenocarcinoma.

        1) Most common subtype of NSCLC, making up roughly 40% of lung cancers, and it is the most common type of lung cancer found in nonsmokers.

        2) Originates in glandular cells that typically secrete mucus.

      ii. Squamous cell carcinoma.

        1) Typically linked to a history of smoking.

        2) Tumors are often located in the central area of the lungs near the main bronchus.

        3) Comprises 25% to 30% of lung cancer diagnoses.

        4) Originates in the flat cells that coat the inside of the airways called squamous cells.

      iii. Large cell (undifferentiated) carcinoma.

        1) Accounts for 10% to 15% of lung cancers. Also, linked to history of smoking.

        2) Can occur anywhere in the lung but often appears as a large peripheral mass on chest radiograph.

        3) Tends to grow and spread quickly.

        4) Due to its tendency for rapid growth and metastasis, it is more difficult to treat.

  2. SCLC.

    a. SCLC, previously known as oat cell lung cancer, accounts for 15% to 20% of all lung cancers.

    b. Associated with a poor prognosis due to the advanced stage (usually metastatic) at the time of diagnosis.

INCIDENCE

A. Lung cancer is the second most common cancer in both women and men, accounting for approximately 14% of all new cancer diagnoses. However, it is the number one cause of cancer deaths in both women and men each year.

B. More individuals die annually from lung cancer than of breast, prostate, and colon cancer combined.

C. Lung cancer primarily occurs in people over the age of 65, with less than 2% being younger than age 45.

D. The average age at diagnosis is 70 years old.

E. The 5-year survival rate among individuals with lung cancer varies based on staging at the time of diagnosis. However, if diagnosed and treated early, it can be cured.

F. There is up to a 92% 5-year survival with stage IA. This number declines with advancing stage to 68% with stage IB, 60% with stage IIA, 53% with stage IIB, 36% with stage IIIA, and less than 30% with stage IIIB and below.

PATHOGENESIS

A. Lung cancer can be divided into two broad categories: Small cell and nonsmall cell carcinoma.

  1. Small cell carcinoma is almost exclusively caused by exposure to cigarette smoking.

  2. Nonsmall cell carcinoma (adenocarcinoma, squamous cell and large cell carcinoma) can be caused by other environmental factors, such as:

    a. Smoking.

    b. Radon gas.

    c. Pollution.

    d. Asbestos.

    e. Radiation.

    f. Toxic dust.

    g. Coal.

    h. Diesel.

    i. Arsenic.

PREDISPOSING FACTORS

A. History of smoking (cigarette/cigar/pipe/marijuana). This is dose-dependent, meaning increased quantity and duration of smoking increases the risk of lung cancer.

B. Exposure to radon or asbestos.

C. History of lung cancer in the immediate family.

D. Exposure to Agent Orange or other carcinogens.

E. Diagnosis of another respiratory disease such as chronic obstructive pulmonary disease (COPD), emphysema, chronic bronchitis, or pneumonia.

F. Contact with secondhand smoke.

SUBJECTIVE DATA

A. Common complaints/symptoms.

1. Cough, especially if persistent (the most common).
2. Shortness of breath.
3. Hemoptysis.
4. Pain in the chest, back, or shoulder unrelated to cough.
5. Changes in voice or becoming hoarse.
6. Recurrent lung problems, like bronchitis or pneumonia.
7. Wheezing.
8. Bone pain (with bone metastasis).
9. Headaches (with intracranial metastasis).
10. Unexplained weight loss.
11. Fatigue.

B. Common/typical scenario.

1. Patients are frequently asymptomatic, with symptoms only developing once the disease is well-advanced.
2. Often, lung cancer is discovered incidentally on chest imaging.

PHYSICAL EXAMINATION

A. Check vital signs, including pulse oximetry.

B. Head and neck.

1. Evaluate pupils for symmetry and reaction to light. Tumor in the lung apex can cause compression of the cervical sympathetic plexus, which can cause Horner syndrome (ptosis, miosis, and anhidrosis).
2. Palpate the neck and supraclavicular area for adenopathy.
3. Evaluate the neck for facial edema, facial cyanosis, or jugular vein distention (JVD), which could indicate superior vena cava (SVC) syndrome if the tumor is obstructing the SVC.

C. Pulmonary system.

1. Observe for signs of dyspnea, increased work of breathing, or retractions.
2. Auscultate lung sounds in all lung fields. Lung tumor can lead to obstruction and collapse of a lobe or entire lung or postobstructive pneumonia. Pleural effusions may develop as well. All of these scenarios would lead to decreased breath sounds in those areas of the lung affected.
3. Percussion of the lung will be dull with collapsed lobes of the lung or pleural effusion.

D. Cardiovascular system.

1. Auscultate heart sounds, which should be normal. If the tumor has direct cardiac involvement, or pericardial effusion has developed, the heart sounds may be affected.
2. Assess for signs of cardiac tamponade, such as hypotension, distant/muffled heart sounds, pericardial rub, or JVD.

E. Gastrointestinal (GI) tract.

1. Auscultate for bowel sounds in all four quadrants.
2. Palpate for hepatomegaly. One of the most common sites of lung metastasis is the liver, which can manifest as tender hepatomegaly.

F. Musculoskeletal system.

1. Bone is another area of common metastasis.
2. Patients may report bone pain or tender spots on examination, including the spine.
3. Lung cancers that arise in the lung apex, called Pancoast tumors, can cause shoulder or scapula pain that radiates down the arm.

G. Central nervous system (CNS).

1. A neurologic examination should be performed to evaluate for any focal neurologic deficits that may be produced by intracranial metastases or spinal cord compression.
2. Evaluation for neuropathy, decreased sensation, or decreased strength should be performed.

DIAGNOSTIC TESTS

A. Laboratory data.

1. Complete blood count (CBC).
2. Comprehensive metabolic panel (CMP).
3. Prothrombin time/international normalized ratio (PT/INR) and partial thromboplastin time (PTT).

B. Imaging and procedures.

1. Chest x-ray (CXR).
2. CT of the chest with contrast for evaluation of size of mass, any other nodules/masses, enlarged lymph nodes, and/or involvement of adjacent structures.
3. PET/CT scan to assess for metastatic disease.
4. Endobronchial ultrasound (EBUS) to evaluate mediastinal lymph nodes.
5. Brain MRI to evaluate for metastatic disease.

C. Biopsy: Interventional radiology (IR) CT-guided biopsy.

D. Ancillary tests prior to surgery.

1. EKG.
2. Pulmonary function test (PFT).

E. Diagnosis: Tissue sample or biopsy is required for diagnosis; these are typically obtained through a CT-guided biopsy of the lung nodule/mass.

F. Staging is one of the most important elements in determining therapeutic options and prognosis. The staging for NSCLC and SCLC differs as noted in the following:

1. NSCLC.

a. Like the majority of cancers, NSCLC is staged by the tumor, node, metastasis (TNM) system.

b. Higher numbers indicate more advanced lung cancer.

c. Staging determines the approach to treatment (e.g., surgery, chemotherapy, radiation, or combination of treatment modalities).

2. SCLC.

a. SCLC has a two-stage system: Limited versus extensive stage.

i. Limited stage: Localized to one hemithorax. Lymph nodes may be involved but they too must be located in the ipsilateral hemithorax in relation to the primary tumor.

ii. Extensive stage: Involves lung cancer in both hemithoraces and/or metastasis to other organs and/or contralateral nodal metastasis. Staging determines the approach to treatment (chemoradiation vs. chemotherapy alone).

DIFFERENTIAL DIAGNOSIS

A. Adenocarcinoma.
B. Squamous cell carcinoma.
C. Large cell carcinoma.
D. Small cell carcinoma.
E. Pulmonary nodule.
F. Hamartoma.
G. Neuroendocrine tumor.
H. Metastasis from other primary cancer.
I. Granulomatous disease.

EVALUATION AND MANAGEMENT PLAN

A. General plan.

1. Based on staging, patients will be offered chemotherapy, radiation, and/or surgery either alone or in combination with one another.

2. Targeted therapies.

3. Immunotherapy.

B. Acute care issues in lung cancer.

1. Lung cancer patients are often admitted for surgical resection.

a. Pneumonectomy: Removal of the entire lung.

b. Lobectomy: The most common surgical procedure in lung cancer patients, with removal of a single lobe of the lung.

c. Segmental resection: Removal of a segment/portion of the involved lobe.

d. Sleeve resection: Consider when the cancer is confined to the bronchus or pulmonary artery and requires bronchoplastic reconstruction.

e. Wedge resection: Removal of a small peripheral nodule; performed only on lung cancer patients with limited pulmonary reserve.

2. Postoperative lung surgery patients, without complications, will spend 3 to 5 days in the hospital after surgery.

3. The primary focus in the postoperative inpatient setting includes the following: Pain control, monitoring lab work, wound care, chest tube management, pulmonary toileting to avoid pneumonia, and early ambulation.

a. Pain control.

i. May be managed by epidural, intercostal nerve block, and/or PO/intravenous (IV) pain medications.

ii. Optimizing pain control leads to faster recovery as pain control allows the patient to deep-breathe, deep-cough, and ambulate, thereby reducing the risk of pneumonia.

b. Monitoring laboratory data: Routine bloodwork including CBC with differential, electrolyte panel, blood urea nitrogen (BUN), and creatinine must be monitored for anemia, infection, electrolyte imbalance/need for replacement, and kidney function.

c. Infection.

i. The incision site will be monitored daily for signs of infection and proper healing.

ii. Pulmonary toileting with the incentive spirometer and acapella apparatuses is crucial to prevent pneumonia in the postoperative lung resection patient.

iii. Early ambulation is also crucial to reducing the risk of postoperative pneumonia.

d. Pneumothorax prevention/monitoring.

i. The postlung surgery patient will have anywhere from one to two chest tubes placed in the operating room and managed in the recovery unit.

ii. Chest tubes are placed on wall suction to help reinflate the lung and allow for fluid drainage.

iii. The chest tube is a closed system that will need to be monitored for air leak and fluid drainage daily.

iv. Daily CXRs should also be performed.

v. Once there is evidence of no air leak and the CXR shows an inflated lung, the chest tube may be removed.

FOLLOW-UP

A. Frequency of follow-up visit depends on cancer stage and is most frequent during the first 2 years post treatment, when the risk of recurrence is highest.

B. Perform physical exam and CT imaging for cancer surveillance and to manage any posttreatment complications.

C. Assess for health-related quality of life at baseline and during follow-up visits.

CONSULTATION/REFERRAL

A. Most lung cancer patients are seen by:

1. Medical oncologist, who orders chemotherapy, targeted therapy, or immunotherapy.

2. Radiation oncologist, who offers radiation therapy (RT).

3. Cardiothoracic surgeon to formulate a treatment plan based on clinical staging.

SPECIAL/GERIATRIC CONSIDERATIONS

A. Much evidence exists to suggest that older adults with good functional status can tolerate combination chemotherapy in the treatment of lung cancer.

B. Chronological age alone should not dictate treatment options.

C. Providers should work with patients to decide on the best alternatives of management.

CASE SCENARIO: LUNG CANCER

A 73-year-old patient with a 30 pack-year history of smoking and emphysema comes to the clinic complaining of new cough and worsening shortness of breath. A chest x-ray (CXR) is performed for further evaluation and a 2-cm nodule is noted on the x-ray. A CT of the chest with contrast is ordered and shows a spiculated 2-cm lesion in the left upper lobe concerning for malignancy.

1. What is the next order that should be placed to obtain a diagnosis?

    A. Complete blood count (CBC) with differential
    B. PET/CT
    C. EKG
    D. Interventional radiology biopsy

2. Once lung cancer diagnosis is confirmed, what other exams are needed to help stage this patient and rule out metastatic disease?

    A. Angiogram and brain MRI
    B. Brain MRI and PET/CT
    C. Pulmonary function test and stress test
    D. Echocardiogram and PET/CT

3. The patient's biopsy shows squamous cell carcinoma. What part of the patient's history involves the leading risk factor for this type of cancer?

    A. Age
    B. Sex
    C. Smoking history
    D. Emphysema

4. Based on this patient's age, a consult with medical oncology would not be recommended as the patient is too old to receive any systemic treatment.

    A. True
    B. False

BIBLIOGRAPHY

National Cancer Institute. (2016, September 12). *Surveillance, epidemiology, and end results program.* https://seer.cancer.gov/faststats/selections.php?series=cancer

National Cancer Institute. (2022, March 16). *Non small cell lung cancer.* https://www.nccn.org/professionals/physician_gls/pdf/nscl.pdf

Weerakkody, Y., & Worsley, C. (2021, December 7). *Lung cancer (staging-IASLC).* 8th edition). https://radiopaeidia.org/articles/lung-cancer-staging-iaslc-8th-edition?lang=us

LYMPHOMAS: HODGKIN LYMPHOMA

Melissa Barnett

DEFINITION

A. Malignancies that develop from lymph nodes and lymphoid tissues are broadly classified into Hodgkin lymphoma (HL) and non-Hodgkin lymphoma (NHL).

B. HL, which originates in germinal center or postgerminal center B-lymphocytes, is characterized by the presence of a distinctive type of giant cell called a Reed–Sternberg cell in the background of reactive cells.

INCIDENCE

A. HL accounts for approximately 10% of all lymphomas and approximately 0.4% of all cancers diagnosed annually in the developed world.

B. The median age at diagnosis is 39 years.

C. In 2020, an estimated 8,480 patients were diagnosed with HL and an estimated 970 patients died of HL.

D. In the United States, the most common subtype of HL is classic HL, followed by mixed cellularity, lymphocyte-rich, and lymphocyte-depleted.

PATHOGENESIS

A. HL occurs due to the clonal proliferation of malignant Hodgkin/Reed–Sternberg cells in the background of reactive cells.

B. The proliferation of these malignant cells causes lymphadenopathy and enlargement of lymphoid tissue/organs (e.g., spleen).

C. Lymphoma generally spreads to contiguous lymph nodes following lymph vessels.

PREDISPOSING FACTORS

A. Epstein–Barr virus (EBV) infection.

B. Immunosuppression (e.g., patients with HIV infection or long-term immunosuppressant use).

C. Family history of HL.

D. Most patients who develop HL have no identifiable risk factors.

SUBJECTIVE DATA

A. Common complaints/symptoms.

  1. Painless lymphadenopathy, frequently in the neck, axilla, or groin, is the most common presenting complaint. Occasionally, lymph nodes can become painful after consuming alcohol.

  2. B symptoms: Unintentional weight loss, fever, and night sweats.

B. Common/typical scenario.

  1. Other signs and symptoms.

    a. Generalized pruritus.
    b. Fatigue.
    c. Lack of appetite.
    d. Cough, difficulty breathing, or chest pain secondary to large mediastinal mass or lymphadenopathy. Often a mediastinal mass will be discovered incidentally on a routine chest radiograph.

C. Family and social history.

  1. Ask about previous malignancy, prior treatment with chemotherapy or radiation therapy (RT), history of immunosuppressive illnesses such as HIV, and family history of malignancy.

D. Review of systems.

  1. Elicit the presence or absence and the duration of symptoms.

  2. Determine the patient's performance status as this can impact future treatment options.

PHYSICAL EXAMINATION

A. A complete physical examination, including vital signs, should be performed.

B. Special attention should be paid to the size and number of palpable peripheral lymph nodes and the presence or absence of hepatosplenomegaly (HSM).

C. Comprehensive neurologic examination should be performed to assess for central nervous system (CNS) involvement.

DIAGNOSTIC TESTS

A. Definitive diagnosis is made by lymph node biopsy. An excisional biopsy is preferred for diagnosis, but often core biopsy of an involved node is sufficient.

B. Complete workup should include complete blood count (CBC), erythrocyte sedimentation rate (ESR), comprehensive metabolic panel (CMP), lactate dehydrogenase (LDH), pregnancy test in women with childbearing potential, and HIV serology.

C. Clinical staging, including the following evaluations, should also be completed:

   1. Full-body PET/CT scan.

   2. Bilateral bone marrow biopsy/aspiration should be considered if the patient has pancytopenia or if there is suspicion of marrow involvement based on imaging.

   3. Lumbar puncture (LP) and/or dedicated brain imaging, only if CNS involvement is suspected.

D. HL is staged per the Ann Arbor staging.

E. Other important tests to consider include pulmonary function tests and echocardiogram, as they will likely be needed for assessment prior to chemotherapy or RT.

DIFFERENTIAL DIAGNOSIS

A. Reactive processes such as infectious or autoimmune conditions.

B. HIV.

C. NHL.

D. Other solid tumors.

E. Any disease with lymphadenopathy needs to be considered.

EVALUATION AND MANAGEMENT PLAN

A. General plan.

   1. Treatment based on the stage of the disease at diagnosis, but can involve chemotherapy, RT, and immunotherapy, either alone or in combination.

   2. The most common frontline chemotherapy regimens used are ABVD (doxorubicin, bleomycin, vinblastine, and dacarbazine) or BV + AVD (brentuximab vedotin, doxorubicin, vinblastine, and dacarbazine).

   3. RT is generally reserved for patients with bulky disease at diagnosis.

   4. High-dose chemotherapy followed by autologous or allogeneic stem cell transplant (SCT) may be indicated for refractory or recurrent disease.

FOLLOW-UP

A. Based on individual needs and individual oncologists.

B. Basic schedule includes:

   1. Visits every 3 to 6 months for first 2 years, every 6 to 12 months in years 3 to 5, and annually after year 5.

   2. Usual tests are physical examination, bloodwork, imaging as indicated, and surveillance of symptom changes.

CONSULTATION/REFERRAL

A. Immediate referral to an oncologist should be made when HL is suspected or diagnosed.

SPECIAL/GERIATRIC CONSIDERATIONS

A. HL is one of the most curable malignancies in adults; however, survival rates in older adult patients are significantly lower than in younger patients.

BIBLIOGRAPHY

Hoppe, R. T., Advani, R. H., Ai, W. Z., Ambinder, R. F., Armand, P., Bello, C. M., Benitez, C. M., Bierman, P. J., Boughan, K. M., Dabaja, B., Gordon, L. I., Hernandez-Ilizaliturri, F. J., Herrera, A. F., Hochberg, E. P., Huang, J., Johnston, P. B., Kaminski, M. S., Kenkre, V. P., Khan, N. … Ogba, N. (2020). Hodgkin Lymphoma, Version 2.2020. NCCN Clinical Practice Guidelines in Oncology. *Journal of the National Comprehensive Cancer Network*, 18(6), 755–781. https://doi.org/10.6004/jnccn.2020.0026

National Cancer Institute. (2022, April 27). *Surveillance, epidemiology, and end results program*. https://seer.cancer.gov/statfacts/html/hodg.html

LYMPHOMAS: NON-HODGKIN LYMPHOMA

Alycia Rosendale

DEFINITION

A. Malignancies that develop from lymph nodes and lymphoid tissues are broadly classified into Hodgkin lymphoma (HL) and non-Hodgkin lymphoma (NHL).

B. NHL encompasses a diverse group of diseases with more than 50 distinct subtypes, which are further classified by histology and clinical presentation. These various subtypes are determined based on the cells from which they arise (B-cells, T-cells, natural killer cells) or by their degree of indolence versus aggressiveness.

C. Patients with indolent lymphomas typically survive for several years even without therapy. However, patients with aggressive lymphomas may only have months to live.

INCIDENCE

A. NHL is relatively common in the United States, with over 80,000 estimated cases in 2022 (accounting for 4.2% of all cancer diagnoses), as compared with approximately 8,000 cases of HL in 2022.

B. The majority of NHL cases are B-cell neoplasms (85%), whereas T-cell/natural killer (NK)-cell neoplasms account for only 15% of NHLs.

C. Most often NHL is diagnosed between the ages of 65 and 74, although it is seen in all age groups.

D. Rates of new cases have remained relatively stable, although the rate of mortality has slowly decreased over the last decade. The 5-year relative survival was 73.8% in 2012 to 2018.

PATHOGENESIS

A. Tumors associated with NHL originate from lymphoid tissues.
B. Most NHLs come from B-cell expansion.

PREDISPOSING FACTORS

A. Immunodeficiency states.
B. Epstein–Barr virus (EBV) infection.
C. HIV infection.
D. Human T-lymphotropic virus type 1 (HTLV-1) infection.
E. Autoimmune rheumatoid diseases (lupus, Sjögren, rheumatoid arthritis).
F. Herbicide/pesticide exposure.

SUBJECTIVE DATA

A. Common complaints/symptoms.
   1. Rapidly enlarging lymph nodes (most commonly in the neck or abdomen).
   2. B symptoms: Fever greater than 100.4°F/38°C, drenching night sweats, and unintentional weight loss of greater than 10% body weight.
B. Common/typical scenario.
   1. Other nonspecific symptoms: Malaise, fatigue, chronic pain, early satiety, and cough/chest discomfort (seen with mediastinal involvement).
   2. Approximately 34% of all patients present with primary extranodal lymphoma at the time of diagnosis; the gastrointestinal (GI) tract is the most common site, followed by the skin.

PHYSICAL EXAMINATION

A. Vital signs.
B. Head and neck: Facial edema/jugular venous distension (JVD) can indicate superior vena cava (SVC) syndrome (most commonly seen in primary mediastinal lymphoma).
C. Lymphatics: Cervical, axillary, inguinal, and Waldeyer ring (tonsils, base of tongue, nasopharynx).
D. Cardiopulmonary: Evaluate for signs of dyspnea/airway obstruction, evidence of malignant pleural effusion (decreased breath sounds/crackles), and signs of pericardial effusion/tamponade.
E. Abdomen: Evaluate for hepatomegaly/splenomegaly and ascites.
F. Neurologic: Evaluate for signs of spinal cord compression, altered mental status, memory impairment, or cranial nerve dysfunction.

DIAGNOSTIC TESTS

A. Laboratory data.
   1. Complete blood count (CBC) with differential.
   2. Comprehensive metabolic panel (CMP).
   3. Magnesium.
   4. Phosphorus.
   5. Lactate dehydrogenase (LDH).
   6. Uric acid.
   7. Coagulation studies: Prothrombin time/international normalized ratio (PT/INR) and partial thromboplastin time (PTT).
B. Lymph node biopsy (excisional or core biopsy).
C. PET/CT scan.
D. Bone marrow biopsy.

E. Lumbar puncture (LP) and brain/spine MRI if at risk for central nervous system (CNS) involvement.
F. Formal ophthalmologic examination if at risk for/confirmed CNS involvement (can also rarely be seen in mantle cell lymphoma [MCL] and marginal zone lymphoma [MZL]).
G. Hepatitis B and C serologies (risk of reactivation due to Rituxan).
H. HIV screen.
I. ±Serum protein electrophoresis (SPEP).
J. ±Echocardiogram (for patients who will receive an anthracycline).
K. Diagnosis/staging.
   1. Definitive diagnosis is confirmed with excisional or core needle biopsy (not fine needle aspiration [FNA]).
   2. The Lugano classification system, based on Ann Arbor staging, is the most widely used classification system employed in NHL.

DIFFERENTIAL DIAGNOSIS

A. Solid tumors.
B. Hematologic malignancies.
C. Hodgkin lymphoma.

EVALUATION AND MANAGEMENT PLAN

A. General plan.
   1. The indicated treatment varies greatly depending on the type of NHL, staging, and age/performance status/comorbidities.
   2. A majority of NHL is treated with chemotherapy alone, although there are variants of indolent lymphoma in which watchful waiting is appropriate.
   3. For some subtypes, radiation therapy (RT) is indicated as monotherapy.
   4. Infrequently, surgery is employed for excision of lymphoid tumors.
   5. Stem cell transplant (SCT; autologous or allogenic) is typically reserved for aggressive/late-stage disease or for relapsed/refractory NHLs.
B. Acute care issues in lymphomas.
   1. Neutropenic fever (see sections on Leukemias).
   2. Tumor lysis syndrome (TLS; see sections on Leukemias).
   3. Superior vena cava (SVC) syndrome.
      a. Obstruction of blood flow through the SVC caused by external lymph node compression or by thrombus within the vena cava and is most commonly seen associated with cases of primary mediastinal B-cell lymphoma.
      b. Clinical presentation most commonly reveals dyspnea, cough, facial swelling, upper extremity edema, or chest pain.
      c. Treatment should be initiated after the cause of the obstruction is clarified so as not to confound accurate diagnosis, and is focused on treating the underlying cause with chemotherapy and/or radiation. A short course of high-dose steroids can also be considered with radiation. Stent placement or surgical bypass is reserved for severe cases and rarely utilized.
   4. Spinal cord compression.

a. Involvement of the spinal cord is not an unusual finding in patients with NHLs, and spinal cord compression typically manifests as severe back pain at the level of involvement, weakness (typically involving lower extremities), or paresthesia below the level of spinal involvement, and bladder/bowel dysfunction (late finding).

b. Diagnosis is confirmed with MRI.

c. High-dose steroids and RT are the mainstays of treatment.

FOLLOW-UP

A. Based on individual needs and individual oncologists.

B. Basic schedule includes:

1. Visits every 3 to 6 months for the first 2 years, every 6 to 12 months in years 3 to 5, and annually after year 5.

2. Usual tests are physical examination, bloodwork, imaging as indicated, and surveillance of symptom changes.

CONSULTATION/REFERRAL

A. Hematologic oncology to manage patients with NHL.

B. Radiation oncology and surgery for placement of ports should be initiated.

C. Infectious disease is often consulted to manage neutropenic fevers.

SPECIAL/GERIATRIC CONSIDERATIONS

A. Older adult patients with NHL show similar features and prognostic factors as younger patients, suggesting similar treatment strategies should be offered to both groups.

B. Chronological age should not be the main determinant in treatment options, even in older adult patients older than 80 years.

CASE SCENARIO: NON-HODGKIN LYMPHOMA

A 68-year-old male with past medical history (PMH) of hypertension and a remote history of intravenous (IV) drug use several years ago presents to the ED complaining of chest pain and difficulty breathing. He was given nitroglycerin in the ambulance which did not improve his pain. While taking his history, he also admits to complaints of drenching night sweats, fatigue, and unintentional weight loss over the last few weeks. He also describes "swelling like a golf ball" on the left side of his neck that has grown over the last week but has not caused him any pain. His vital signs on arrival include temperature of 98.9°F/37.2°C, blood pressure (BP) of 134/85, heart rate (HR) of 72, and respiratory rate of 17 breaths per minute. On exam, the patient appears in mild distress and has facial swelling. The nurse practitioner (NP) notes left-sided, nontender, firm cervical lymphadenopathy and distension of the veins in his neck. His heart has regular rate and rhythm with no murmurs present. Lungs reveal crackles in bilateral bases. Abdominal exam is benign. EKG shows normal sinus rhythm and no ST elevations or abnormalities. First troponin is negative. A chest x-ray reveals mediastinal widening and pleural effusion.

1. Which of the exam findings or complaints are most concerning for B symptoms?

A. Chest pain not improved with nitroglycerin

B. Night sweats, fatigue, unintentional weight loss

C. Nontender, firm cervical lymphadenopathy

D. Facial swelling

2. Based on the patient's presentation, the NP is concerned for superior vena cava (SVC) syndrome. What treatment options will the NP discuss with the patient?

A. Thoracentesis

B. Nebulizers and supplemental oxygen

C. Chemotherapy or radiation

D. Surgery

3. The NP is suspicious for lymphoma as the cause of the patient's superior vena cava (SVC) syndrome. The patient is currently stable and the NP would like to have a definitive diagnosis prior to initiating treatment for SVC syndrome. Which study will help make a definitive diagnosis?

A. Fine needle aspiration (FNA)

B. MRI

C. PET scan

D. Core biopsy

4. Biopsy results returned confirming diffuse large B-cell lymphoma and the patient has been consented to begin chemotherapy. Prior to initiating, which additional lab studies will the NP order?

A. HIV and hepatitis panel

B. Blood cultures

C. Thyroid function tests

D. Lipid panel

BIBLIOGRAPHY

Krol, A. D. G., le Cessie, S., Snijder, S., Kluin-Nelemans, J. C., Kluin, P. M., & Noordijk, E. M. (2003). Primary extranodal non-Hodgkin's lymphoma (NHL): The impact of alternative definitions tested in the Comprehensive Cancer Centre West population-based NHL registry. *Annals of Oncology, 14*(1), 131–139. https://doi.org/10.1093/annonc/mdg004

National Cancer Institute. (n.d.). *Surveillance, epidemiology, and end results program*. https://seer.cancer.gov/statfacts/html/nhl.html

MULTIPLE MYELOMA

Jo Ann M. Davidson

DEFINITION

A. Plasma cell dyscrasias are a group of heterogeneous disorders that stem from the malignant proliferation of monoclonal plasma cells.

INCIDENCE

A. Multiple myeloma (MM) is primarily a disease of older adults, and the median age at diagnosis is 65.

B. MM represents approximately 1% of all cancers and approximately 10% of all hematologic malignancies.

C. It is the second most common hematologic cancer. ▶

D. Almost all cases evolve from an asymptomatic, premalignant stage called monoclonal gammopathy of undetermined significance (MGUS).

PATHOGENESIS
A. Plasma cell dyscrasias arise from the monoclonal proliferation of plasma cells.

PREDISPOSING FACTORS
A. Familial cases are rare. Only about 2.4% of all multiple myeloma cases are familial.
B. Twice as common in Black persons.
C. More common in males than in females.
D. Occupational exposures may contribute, such as:
  1. Pesticides/herbicides such as Agent Orange.
  2. Petroleum workers.
  3. Woodworkers.
  4. Leather workers.
  5. Ionizing radiation.

SUBJECTIVE DATA
A. Common complaints/symptoms.
  1. The clinical presentation of plasma cell dyscrasias is quite variable. Bone pain is the most common presenting symptom.
  2. Patients with MM often present with signs/symptoms related to plasma cell proliferation in the bone marrow and/or renal dysfunction.
    a. Elevated total protein: Due to hypersecretion of monoclonal immunoglobulin (Ig) and light chains; often associated with decreased albumin.
    b. Bone involvement: Osteolytic lesions and pathologic fractures.
    c. Normocytic, normochromic anemia with complaints of weakness and fatigue.
    d. Renal failure (acute or chronic) due to cast nephropathy or hypercalcemia.
    e. Recurrent infections due to impaired antibody response, neutropenia, and increase in monoclonal Ig levels.
    f. Hypercalcemia.
B. Common/typical scenario.
  1. Patients may also present with an extramedullary plasmacytoma (soft tissue mass comprised of clonal plasma cells) that can cause spinal cord compression, cauda equina syndrome, severe back pain, paresthesia, and/or radiculopathy.
  2. AL amyloidosis can lead to amyloid deposition in any organ, and patients can present with congestive heart failure, renal failure, hepatomegaly, skin changes, neuropathy, gastroparesis, or diarrhea depending on the organ system(s) involved.

PHYSICAL EXAMINATION
A. Head and neck: Conjunctival pallor due to anemia; macroglossia.
B. Musculoskeletal: Localized bone tenderness.
C. Lymphatics: Assess for lymphadenopathy.

D. Neurologic: Vertebral compression fractures and/or plasmacytomas can cause neurologic deficits if there is spinal cord or nerve compression.
E. Integumentary: Petechiae and purpura due to thrombocytopenia.

DIAGNOSTIC TESTS
A. Laboratory data.
  1. Complete blood count (CBC) with differential.
  2. Comprehensive metabolic panel (CMP) and calcium level.
  3. Serum protein electrophoresis with immunofixation electrophoresis (SPEP/IFE).
  4. 24-hour urine protein electrophoresis with immunofixation electrophoresis (UPEP/IFE): Bence Jones proteinuria.
  5. Serum free light chain assay (kappa and lambda).
  6. Serum Ig levels (IgA, IgG, IgM, IgD, IgE).
  7. Beta-2 microglobulin for staging and prognostication.
  8. Lactate dehydrogenase (LDH) for staging and prognostication.
B. Imaging.
  1. Bone survey with plain films to assess for axial and appendicular lytic bone lesions (less sensitive, used only if other screening modalities are not available).
  2. Low-dose, whole-body CT scan to assess for lytic lesions: Study of choice to detect osteolytic disease per the International Myeloma Working Group (IMWG).
  3. PET/CT to assess for subtle bone lesions and/or plasmacytomas.
  4. Consider MRI to rule out osteolytic lesions that cannot be seen on bone survey or CT, assessing extramedullary disease, or concern for cord compression.
C. Bone marrow aspiration and biopsy.
  1. Evaluation includes fluorescence in situ hybridization (FISH).
D. Diagnosis.
  1. **CRAB** criteria for symptomatic myeloma.
    a. **C**alcium (hypercalcemia): Serum calcium greater than 11 mg/dL.
    b. **R**enal insufficiency: Serum creatinine greater than 2 mg/dL or CrCl (creatinine clearance) less than 40 mL/min.
    c. **A**nemia: Hemoglobin less than 10 g/dL.
    d. **B**one lesions: One or more osteolytic lesions on bone survey, MRI, CT, or PET/CT.
  2. Diagnosis includes one or more CRAB criteria *PLUS* clonal plasma cells less than or equal to 60%, involved to uninvolved serum free light chain (FLC) ratio less than or equal to 100 mg/L, and more than one focal lesion (5 mm or more) on MRI.
E. Staging and risk stratification.
  1. Staging systems for newly diagnosed myeloma patients.
    a. Revised International Staging System (R-ISS): More commonly used.
    b. DurieSalmon staging.
    c. Mayo Clinic Risk Stratification for Multiple Myeloma (mSMART).

DIFFERENTIAL DIAGNOSIS
A. Non-Hodgkin lymphoma (NHL).
B. Amyloidosis.
C. Solitary plasmacytoma.
D. Waldenstrom macroglobulinemia.

EVALUATION AND MANAGEMENT PLAN
A. General plan.
　1. Treatment depends on the plasma cell dyscrasia.
　2. Therapy options for MM and amyloidosis.
　　a. Patients typically receive two to six cycles of systemic induction chemotherapy followed by autologous stem cell transplant (SCT; if eligible) or maintenance chemotherapy (if ineligible for transplant or after transplant).
　　b. Systemic chemotherapy (induction and maintenance). Drug classes include:
　　　i. Proteosome inhibitors such as bortezomib, carfilzomib and ixazomib.
　　　ii. Immunomodulating drugs (IMiDs) such as lenalidomide, thalidomide, and pomalidomide.
　　　iii. Histone deacetylase (HDAC) inhibitors such as vorinostat and panobinostat.
　　　iv. Steroids such as dexamethasone.
　　　v. Monoclonal antibodies such as daratumumab and elotuzumab.
　　c. Autologous SCT.
　　d. Allogeneic SCT.
　　　i. Not commonly utilized for MM as upfront therapy.
　　　ii. Can be considered in patients with plasma cell leukemia, refractory myeloma, relapsed myeloma, or young patients with high-risk disease (based on FISH data).
　　e. Chimeric antigen receptor therapy (CAR-T): Immune therapy targeting T-cells.
　　f. Radiation therapy (RT) for treatment of solitary plasmacytomas, pathologic or impending pathologic fracture, and palliative pain control.
　　g. Surgical intervention.
　　　i. Vertebroplasty or kyphoplasty may be indicated in patients with vertebral compression fractures.
　　　ii. Excisional biopsy may be performed to confirm plasmacytomas.
B. Supportive care.
　1. Bone disease.
　　a. All patients with osteolytic lesions and/or pathologic fractures should be initiated on bisphosphonates and calcium/vitamin D supplements.
　　b. Prior to initiation of bisphosphonate, patients must be evaluated by a dentist to assess for periodontal disease and risk of jaw osteonecrosis.
　2. Infectious prophylaxis (viral, bacterial).
　3. Thromboembolic prophylaxis (e.g., low-dose aspirin).
　4. Pain management if indicated.

C. Emergencies and inpatient management.
　1. Pain management.
　　a. Pain is primarily due to skeletal fractures and bone pain from lytic lesions.
　　b. Pharmacologic therapy.
　　　i. Avoid nonsteroidal anti-inflammatory drugs (NSAIDs) due to nephrotoxicity.
　　　ii. Oral or intravenous (IV) analgesics.
　　c. Surgical intervention for collapsed vertebral body.
　　　i. Vertebroplasty: Injection of bone cement (methyl methacrylate) under fluoroscopy.
　　　ii. Kyphoplasty: Placement of inflatable bone tamp prior to injection of bone cement.
　2. Hypercalcemia.
　　a. Due to osteolysis and/or renal failure.
　　b. Check ionized calcium and corrected calcium = serum calcium + 0.8 (normal albumin − serum albumin).
　　c. Rule out other causes (e.g., hyperparathyroidism, thyrotoxicosis, medications, hypervitaminosis D).
　　d. If asymptomatic and corrected calcium less than 12 mg/dL, patient may not require immediate treatment.
　　e. Therapeutic intervention.
　　　i. Simultaneous administration of:
　　　　1) Hydration: Isotonic saline for volume expansion.
　　　　2) Calcitonin: Dose of 4 IU/kg.
　　　　3) Bisphosphonates (e.g., zoledronic acid, pamidronate).
　　　ii. Consider dialysis for patients with severe hypercalcemia.
　　　iii. Repeat serum calcium.
　3. Renal failure.
　　a. Due to light chain deposition in renal tubules (light chain cast nephropathy).
　　b. Correct electrolyte abnormalities.
　　c. Careful review of medications and discontinue or dose-adjust nephrotoxic agents.
　　d. Consider kidney biopsy: Stain for Congo red to rule out amyloidosis.
　　e. IV hydration.
　　f. Consider dialysis.
　4. Tumor lysis syndrome (TLS: See sections on Leukemias.
　5. Spinal cord compression.
　　a. Due to vertebral compression fracture and/or plasmacytoma.
　　b. Symptoms vary depending on the location of compression and may include:
　　　i. Back pain.
　　　ii. Motor deficits.
　　　iii. Paresthesia.
　　　iv. Bowel/bladder incontinence or dysfunction.
　　　v. Gait ataxia.
　　c. Emergent evaluation with MRI of cervical, thoracic, and/or lumbar spine.

d. If a mass is present, arrange biopsy of lesion for diagnosis.

e. Requires emergent steroids, RT, and/or neuro-surgical decompression.

6. Hyperviscosity syndrome.
    a. Symptoms and signs include:
        i. Blurred vision.
        ii. Papilledema.
        iii. Headache.
        iv. Neurologic symptoms.
        v. Oral/nasal bleeding.
        vi. Stupor/coma.
    b. Obtain IgM and serum viscosity levels.
    c. Requires emergent plasmapheresis if symptomatic (not based on serum viscosity level).

FOLLOW-UP

A. Typically includes blood/urine tests, radiologic testing, and bone marrow evaluation. Frequency determined by disease status and risk stratification.

B. Long-term surveillance varies on a case-by-case basis.

CONSULTATION/REFERRAL

A. Consult medical oncologists, radiation oncologists, and surgical oncologists specializing in MM.

SPECIAL/GERIATRIC CONSIDERATIONS

A. Long-term and late effects of treatment can develop in survivors months or even years after treatment.
    1. These effects can be physical and/or emotional.
    2. Teach patients to identify and report them to their providers.

B. Patients older than 70 years should not be denied chemotherapy based solely on age.
    1. Aggressive treatment should be discussed with the patient.
    2. Autologous SCT can be safely done in older adults depending on functional status and comorbid conditions.
    3. Life expectancy, quality of life, and functional status should be taken into consideration.

CASE SCENARIO: MULTIPLE MYELOMA

Mr. J.D. is a 67-year-old African American male who presents to his primary care provider (PCP) with complaint of low back pain for the past 2 weeks which is now increasing in intensity. He denies any injuries but does report that the pain radiates to the back of his legs. He is also experiencing subjective complaint of fatigue. His past medical history (PMH) includes gastroesophageal reflux disease (GERD), diabetes mellitus (DM) type 2 (diet-controlled), depression, hypertension, and osteoporosis. His family history includes esophageal cancer in his father, who is deceased, and colon cancer in his younger brother, who is still living. His physical exam is benign, including neurologic assessment, except for tenderness with palpation over the spinous processes of the lumbar spine.

1. What imaging studies, if any, would be ordered to evaluate his low back pain?
    A. MRI of the lumbar spine
    B. X-rays of the lumbar spine
    C. No imaging studies warranted at this time; conservative management only
    D. CT scan of the lumbar spine

2. Mr. J.D. returns to his primary care provider's (PCP) office for follow-up. His x-rays showed compression fractures and possible lytic lesions in his lumbar spine. What is the next step for this patient?
    A. MRI of the cervical, thoracic, and lumbar spine if there is concern for spinal cord compression
    B. Low-dose, whole-body CT scan if no concern for spinal cord compression
    C. Whole-body PET-CT
    D. Referral to orthopedics

3. On low-dose, whole-body CT scan, Mr. J.D. was found to have new compression fractures at L1 to L4, 50% height loss at L3, and scattered lytic lesions throughout his axial skeleton. Due to the concern for multiple myeloma, the patient should have:
    A. A referral to orthopedics
    B. A bone marrow biopsy
    C. Lab work for multiple myeloma workup: Complete blood count (CBC) with differential, comprehensive metabolic panel (CMP), serum protein electrophoresis with immunofixation electrophoresis (SPEP/IFE), 24-hour urine protein electrophoresis with immunofixation electrophoresis (UPEP/IFE), serum free light chain assay (kappa and lambda), serum immunoglobulin levels (IgA, IgG, IgM, IgD, IgE), beta-2 microglobulin, and lactate dehydrogenase (LDH)
    D. A referral to hematology

4. Mr. J.D.'s pertinent lab results showed a hemoglobin of 8.2 g/dL, creatinine of 2.10 mg/dL, calcium of 11.1 mg/dL, beta-2 microglobulin of 2.96 mg/L, monoclonal protein of 3,300 mg/dL, serum free kappa of 88.1 mg/dL, and serum immunofixation showed immunoglobulin G (IgG)-kappa monoclonal protein. What is the next step?
    A. Refer to hematology for bone marrow biopsy.
    B. Follow lab results every 3 to 6 months.
    C. Refer to allergy/immunology for hypergammaglobulinemia.
    D. Refer to nephrology for acute kidney injury.

BIBLIOGRAPHY

Bird, S., Cairns, D., Menzies, T., Boyd, K., Davies, F., Cook, G., Drayson, M., Gregory, W., Jenner, M., Jones, J., Kaiser, M., Owen, R., Jackson, G., Morgan, G., & Pawlyn, C. (2021). Sex differences in multiple myeloma biology but not clinical outcomes: Results from 3894 patients in the myeloma XI trial. *Clinical Lymphoma, Myeloma, & Leukemia, 21*(10), 667–675.

Blocka, J., Durie, B. G. M., Huhn, S., Mueller-Tidow, C., Försti, A., Hemminki, K., & Goldschmidt, H. (2019). Familial cancer: How to successfully recruit families for germline mutation studies? Multiple myeloma as an example. *Clinical Lymphoma, Myeloma, & Leukemia, 19*(10), 635–644.

Rajkumar, S. V. (2020). Multiple myeloma: 2020 update on diagnosis, risk stratification and management. *American Journal of Hematology, 95*(5), 548–567.

SARCOMA

Morgan Mount

DEFINITION

A. Sarcomas are divided into two broad categories.
1. Soft tissue sarcoma.
2. Bone sarcoma.

B. Soft tissues include adipose, muscle, tendinous, fibrous, and vascular tissues, and there are at least 60 subtypes of soft tissue sarcoma. Examples include:
1. Gastrointestinal (GI) stromal sarcoma.
2. Angiosarcoma.
3. Liposarcoma.
4. Rhabdomyosarcoma.
5. Leiomyosarcoma.

INCIDENCE

A. In 2016, there was an estimated 12,310 new cases of soft tissue sarcomas and 4,990 patients died of the disease.

B. In 2016, there was an estimated 3,260 new cases of bone sarcomas and 1,550 patients died of the disease.

C. Although very rare in adults (about 1%), sarcomas comprise ~15% of all pediatric cancers.

D. Males are affected more frequently than females.

PATHOGENESIS

A. Sarcomas, as with many cancers, are often associated with cytogenetic abnormalities or molecular mutations.

B. Sarcomas have a wide range of clinical behaviors and outcomes depending on the subtype and extent of disease.

C. Expert pathologic review is necessary to determine the specific subtype. Differentiation patterns can be difficult to ascertain as there are at least 60 different histologic subtypes.

D. Classification of sarcomas depends on tissue appearance, histologic grade, and cell of origin.

PREDISPOSING FACTORS

A. Genetic factors.

B. Exposure to radiation.

C. Exposure to chemical carcinogens (e.g., Agent Orange, polyvinyl chloride).

SUBJECTIVE DATA

A. Common complaints/symptoms.
1. Sarcomas can occur in any anatomic area: About 46% occur in lower extremities, 18% occur in the torso, 13% occur in the upper extremities, 13% occur in the retroperitoneum, and 9% occur in the head and neck.
2. The clinical presentation depends on the tumor's location.
3. Patients often present with:
   a. Swelling.
   b. Palpable soft tissue or bone mass.
   c. Pain.

4. Patients may present with:
   a. Constitutional symptoms such as fever, weight loss, and night sweats.
   b. Neurologic symptoms if there is involved nerve compression.
5. Patients with a mass increasing in size or a mass greater than 5 cm should undergo evaluation for possible sarcoma with imaging (x-rays, CT, and/or MRI).

PHYSICAL EXAMINATION

A. Vital signs.

B. Musculoskeletal: Evaluate location, size, and mobility of palpable mass.

C. Neurologic: Assess for any sensory/motor deficits, gait abnormality, and strength.

D. Evaluate for metastatic disease.
1. Lymphatics: Assess for adenopathy.
2. Cough: Assess for metastatic spread to the lung.
3. Ascites: Retroperitoneal sarcomas can metastasize to the liver producing fluid wave.

DIAGNOSTIC TESTS

A. General plan.
1. Imaging.
   a. CT or MRI for suspected soft tissue sarcoma. MRI typically preferred in extremities.
   b. Conventional x-ray imaging should be performed for suspected bone sarcoma followed by MRI.
   c. Consider PET scan.
2. Biopsy.
   a. Definitive diagnosis is based on biopsy of the mass. Core needle biopsy is typically sufficient to make an accurate diagnosis.
   b. Fine needle aspiration (FNA) is not recommended.
3. Molecular/cytogenetic markers.
4. Metastatic evaluation.
   a. May include MRI with gadolinium to evaluate for bone metastasis.
   b. CT of the chest and/or abdomen to assess for lung or liver metastasis.
   c. Consider whole-body PET.

B. Staging.
1. Complete staging includes CT scan of the chest, abdomen, and pelvis and bone scan to assess for metastatic disease.
2. For Ewing sarcoma, an MRI of the spine should be performed to assess for bone marrow metastases.
3. Soft tissue sarcomas (except retroperitoneal sarcomas): The tumor, node, metastasis (TNM) staging system is used.
4. Bone sarcomas: The Musculoskeletal Tumor Society (MSTS) staging system is used.

DIFFERENTIAL DIAGNOSIS

A. Lipoma.

B. Carcinoma.

C. Neuroma.

EVALUATION AND MANAGEMENT PLAN

A. General plan.

1. Treatment and prognosis vary depending on the subtype, location, and extent of disease.

2. Therapy includes a combination of systemic therapy, radiation, surgery, and in some cases targeted therapy.

3. For localized sarcomas, surgical excision is the mainstay of treatment.

4. For metastatic disease, unresectable disease, large tumors (>5 cm), and tumors that are located in deeper tissues or have visceral involvement, systemic chemotherapy ± radiation is often given followed by surgery if indicated.

5. Chemosensitivity and choice of treatment differ based on histologic subtype.

B. Acute care issues in sarcoma.

1. Local surgical resections can be attempted as outpatient for very small superficial tumors.

2. Patients are usually admitted for extensive surgery or toxic chemotherapy.

3. Postoperative management usually focuses on pain control, wound care, pulmonary toileting, and early ambulation.

4. Complex aggressive chemotherapy usually requires inpatient admission.

　　a. High-dose chemotherapeutic combinations are employed depending on the type of sarcoma.

　　b. Two-dimensional echocardiography as excellent left ventricular function is needed for use of doxorubicin-containing chemotherapy, which is usually incorporated into first-line chemotherapy for most soft tissue sarcomas.

　　c. Routine bloodwork including electrolyte panel, blood urea nitrogen (BUN), and creatinine must be monitored for electrolyte imbalance/need for replacement and kidney function.

FOLLOW-UP

A. Complete within first 3 weeks. If assessing response to chemotherapy, reimage every two cycles.

B. Surveillance is every 3 months for the first 2 years, every 4 to 6 months for 2 years, and then annually.

C. An MRI or CT of the primary site may be indicated along with a chest x-ray (CXR) or CT of the chest to assess for lung metastasis.

CONSULTATION/REFERRAL

A. Referrals for patients with suspected sarcoma should be referred to a multidisciplinary sarcoma center so they can be followed by a surgical oncologist, medical oncologist, and radiation oncologist.

B. Orthopedic oncology should be consulted if the primary site is in an extremity or the spine.

SPECIAL/GERIATRIC CONSIDERATIONS

A. Sarcomas are rare but malignant tumors. Older adult patients are more often diagnosed with high-stage sarcomas and have a higher mortality rate.

CASE SCENARIO: SARCOMA

The patient is a 57-year-old male firefighter in excellent shape who was lifting a heavy object at work and felt a "pull" in his right upper extremity. Occupational health told him it was a biceps tear. A general surgeon in the community attempted to drain the "hematoma" but his needle penetrated a solid mass. The patient went on to have MRI of the right humerus which revealed a large 10-cm, enhancing soft tissue mass. Biopsy reveals a myxofibrosarcoma. The patient is told he would need an amputation of his right upper extremity.

1. Which of the following types of biopsy is most appropriate?

　　A. Fine needle aspiration in two different locations of the tumor

　　B. Excisional biopsy

　　C. Core needle biopsy

　　D. No biopsy indicated

2. What would be the most appropriate scan to assess for lung metastasis?

　　A. Lung metastasis unlikely so no lung imaging is ordered

　　B. CT of the chest with intravenous (IV) contrast

　　C. MRI of the chest with and without IV contrast

　　D. Chest x-ray posteroanterior and lateral

3. The patient has no distant metastasis and core needle biopsy revealed myxofibrosarcoma, high grade 3/3. What is the next step?

　　A. Present the case at the multidisciplinary sarcoma tumor board

　　B. Proceed with radiation

　　C. Proceed with surgery

　　D. Proceed with proton therapy

4. The patient's two-dimensional (2D) echocardiogram showed an ejection fraction of 65%. His health history and lab work are unremarkable. He has excellent family support. What chemotherapy regimen should be recommended?

　　A. Paclitaxel (Taxol)

　　B. Pembrolizumab (Keytruda)

　　C. Imatinib (Gleevec).

　　D. Doxorubicin (Adriamycin)/ifosfamide (Ifex)

BIBLIOGRAPHY

Lawrence, W., Jr., Donegan, L. W., Natarajan, N., Mettlin, C., Beart, R., & Winchester, D. (1987). Adult soft tissue sarcomas. A pattern of care survey of the American College of Surgeons. *Annals of Surgery, 205*(4), 349–359.

National Cancer Institute. (2016, September 12). *Surveillance, epidemiology, and end results program.* https://seer.cancer.gov/faststats/selections.php?series=cancer

SKIN CANCER

Krista M. Rubin

DEFINITION

A. Two main types.

　　1. Melanoma (most aggressive).

2. Nonmelanoma (NMSC; also known as keratinocyte carcinoma, which is becoming the preferred term to differentiate from other skin cancers more accurately).

    a. Basal cell carcinoma (BCC; most common).

    b. Squamous cell carcinoma (SCC; second most common).

3. Other types of skin cancer include Merkel cell carcinoma, Kaposi sarcoma (associated with HIV), cutaneous lymphoma, and skin adnexal tumors. Together these comprise <1% of all skin cancers.

INCIDENCE

A. Skin cancer is the most common type of cancer worldwide.

B. An estimated 5.4 million keratinocyte carcinomas are diagnosed in the United States each year.

    1. 8 out of 10 of those are BCCs.

    2. Excellent prognosis when detected and managed early, but if left untreated can result in significant morbidity and cosmetic disfigurement.

    3. Deaths are uncommon; approximately 2,000 per year.

C. An estimated 99,780 cases of invasive melanoma will be diagnosed in the United States in 2022 with 7,650 deaths.

D. The incidence of melanoma is increasing at a greater rate than any other type of cancer.

E. The majority of people who develop melanoma are White men over age 55.

F. The overall lifetime risk of developing melanoma is 1 in 38 for Whites, 1 in 167 for Hispanics, and 1 in 1,000 for Blacks.

G. Melanoma survival for all stages at diagnosis is 93%; decreases with more advanced disease.

    1. Localized disease 99%.

    2. Regional disease 68%.

    3. Distant disease 30%, but significant clinical advances in the past decade have dramatically improved outcomes for patients with advanced melanoma.

PATHOGENESIS

A. The primary cause of most skin cancer is exposure to UV radiation, both solar and artificial.

B. UV radiation induces both direct and indirect DNA damage that ultimately leads to mutations in key cancer genes responsible for cell survival proliferation and differentiation.

C. Mutations in p53 (tumor suppressor gene) are highly associated with NMSCs.

D. Most melanomas arise from healthy skin, with only about 25% arising from a preexisting mole.

PREDISPOSING FACTORS

A. Light or fair skin that freckles or burns easily and those with red or blond hair, and blue or green eyes.

B. Male with age greater than 50 years.

C. Excess sun exposure and UV-based artificial tanning.

D. Family history of skin cancer.

E. Personal history of skin cancer.

F. History of sunburns, especially early in life.

G. History of indoor tanning.

H. Chronic immunosuppression, particularly solid organ transplant recipients.

I. Individuals with dysplastic or atypical nevi, with several large nondysplastic nevi, with many small nevi, or with moderate freckles.

J. Chemical exposure to arsenic, chromium, polycyclic aromatic hydrocarbons, or benzene.

K. Chronic skin ulcers, nonhealing wounds, or burn scars.

L. Associated genetic syndromes; basal cell nevus syndrome, xeroderma pigmentosum, oculocutaneous albinism, familial atypical multiple mole and melanoma syndrome, epidermolysis bullosa, and Fanconi anemia are associated with an increased risk of skin cancer.

SUBJECTIVE DATA

A. Common complaints/symptoms.

    1. There are some general physical characteristics of malignant skin lesions but the appearance may vary with each skin cancer.

    2. The most common sign of skin cancer is a change in the skin, including:

        a. A new growth.

        b. BCCs commonly present as "nonhealing sores," often ulcerated, sometimes eczematous in appearance.

        c. A change in appearance of a mole.

        d. Scar elevation (thickening or rising of a previously flat mole).

        e. Surface changes (scaling, erosion, oozing, bleeding, or crusting).

        f. Surrounding skin changes (redness, swelling, or small new patches of color around a larger lesion [satellite pigmentations]).

        g. Sensory changes (itching, tingling, or burning).

        h. Changes in consistency (friability).

    3. Metastatic melanoma signs and symptoms include:

        a. Unexplained weight loss or fatigue.

        b. Enlarged or tender lymph nodes: Regional lymph nodes are the most common site of initial metastasis in patients with melanoma and may be the first presenting sign in metastatic melanoma of unknown primary.

        c. Shortness of breath, persistent cough, and hemoptysis.

        d. Bone pain.

        e. Headaches, numbness, weakness, or decreased sensation.

        f. Seizures.

        g. Anorexia, abdominal pain, dysphagia, small bowel obstruction, hematemesis, and melena.

PHYSICAL EXAMINATION

A. Integumentary system.

1. Total body skin should be examined, including the scalp, dorsal feet, soles, toe webs, nails, and genitals.

2. Assess the total number of nevi present on patient's skin and differentiate between typical and atypical lesions using the ABCDE (asymmetry, border, color, diameter and evolving) criteria.

3. Melanoma lesions are more likely to be asymmetrical, have irregular borders, appear very dark black or blue, or have more variation in color than a benign mole and may be greater than 6 mm in diameter.

4. Visualize and palpate skin cancer excision scars and the surrounding skin (assessing recurrence or for in-transit/satellite metastasis) and evaluate regional lymph node basin(s).

B. Lymphatic system.

1. Melanoma may disseminate through the lymphatics.

2. Palpate for enlarged or hard lymph nodes.

C. Pulmonary system.

1. Observe for tachypnea, dyspnea, or labored breathing.

2. Auscultate all lung fields for lung sounds.

3. Melanoma metastasis to the lungs may cause persistent cough, shortness of breath, pain in the chest, or pleural effusion.

D. Cardiovascular system.

1. Auscultate heart sounds for abnormal findings to evaluate the presence of a tumor that has direct cardiac involvement.

2. Assess for signs of hypotension, jugular venous distension (JVD), or pericardial rub.

3. Cardiac symptoms, pericardial effusion, and cardiac tamponade are associated with cardiac metastasis of melanoma.

E. Gastrointestinal (GI) tract.

1. Auscultate bowel sounds in four quadrants.

2. Palpate for hepatomegaly or tenderness to palpation.

3. Liver metastases may also cause ascites.

F. Musculoskeletal system.

1. Bone metastasis of melanoma can cause bone pain and discomfort.

2. Examine for any tender area including spine.

G. Central nervous system (CNS).

1. A neurologic examination is essential to evaluate for any intracranial metastases.

2. Evaluate for decreased strength, altered sensation, and/or neuropathy.

DIAGNOSTIC TESTS

A. Biopsy.

1. For primary skin lesions, choice of biopsy technique depends on lesion size, location, and shape, but should provide enough tissue to assess the full thickness of the lesion.

B. Nodal basin ultrasound and/or lymphoscintigraphy.

C. Imaging.

1. CT of the chest/abdomen/pelvis with intravenous (IV) contrast.

2. Consider whole-body PET/CT.

3. Consider brain MRI with IV contrast.

4. If clinically indicated, perform a neck CT with IV contrast.

D. Laboratory studies.

1. Complete blood count (CBC), chemistry panel including liver function tests, and serum lactate dehydrogenase (LDH) level for patients with advanced melanoma. Elevated LDH levels are associated with worse survival and may predict survival for patients with stage IV melanoma and are incorporated into melanoma staging.

E. Staging.

1. Accurate staging for any cancer is essential for defining prognosis and subsequent recommendations for treatment and follow-up care.

2. The American Joint Committee on Cancer (AJCC) is the most commonly used in the United States and employs the TNM (tumor, node, metastasis) classification.

DIFFERENTIAL DIAGNOSIS

A. BCC.

B. SCC.

C. Malignant melanoma.

D. Benign lesions.

EVALUATION AND MANAGEMENT PLAN

A. General plan.

1. Based on staging, the treatment options include surgery, topical therapy, immunotherapy, targeted therapy, radiation therapy (RT; e.g., stereotactic radiosurgery or whole brain radiation). Chemotherapy is rarely used.

2. Surgery is the treatment of choice for resectable primary tumors.

3. For metastatic and unresectable disease, systemic therapy is generally recommended.

4. Immunotherapy (specifically immune checkpoint inhibitors [ICIs]) is now considered standard first-line therapy in advanced SCC and advanced melanoma.

5. Targeted therapy: For advanced melanoma in tumors found to harbor a BRAF mutation.

6. RT: For high-risk primary or recurrent tumors, as palliative therapy (for painful or bleeding metastatic tumors), or for melanoma brain metastases.

7. Topical for low-risk BCC and SCC.

B. Acute care issues in skin cancers.

1. Most of the surgical procedures are done on an outpatient basis; however, hospitalization is indicated for complex surgeries and depends on reconstructive techniques.

2. Wound care, Jackson-Pratt (JP) drain management and pain management, and monitoring for infection are the main areas of focus during postoperative management.

3. Management of acute cancer or cancer treatment-related complications.

FOLLOW-UP

A. Determined by cancer stage, risk of developing additional skin cancers, and other factors such as the patient's awareness and ability to detect early signs and symptoms of the disease.
B. Generally includes performing physical and skin examinations, review of systems, and may include laboratory tests and scans.

CONSULTATION/REFERRAL

A. Patients with suspected skin cancer should be referred to dermatology, medical oncology, radiation oncology, and surgical oncology.

SPECIAL/GERIATRIC CONSIDERATIONS

A. The white-skinned older adult population represents the largest patient group at risk of developing skin cancer.
B. Treatment of skin cancer in the older adult population should be based on life expectancy, quality of life, and the patient's functional status, and not solely on chronological age.

CASE SCENARIO: SKIN CANCER

The nurse practitioner (NP) is seeing Sally, a 49-year-old female with red hair and blue eyes, for her annual wellness physical examination. The NP notices a 3-mm ulcerated lesion on the side of her left temple. Sally says she thought it was a pimple and she must have picked at it. She thinks it has been there for a couple of months. It is not itchy, nor has it bled.

1. The likely diagnosis is:
  A. Acne
  B. Squamous cell carcinoma
  C. Melanoma
  D. Basal cell carcinoma

2. Sally becomes very anxious at the possibility of having cancer. The NP says:
  A. Most basal cell carcinomas (BCCs) have an excellent prognosis.
  B. BCC is an aggressive skin cancer associated with poor prognosis.
  C. BCC is a rare form of skin cancer seen primarily in individuals with dark skin.
  D. BCC is not considered malignant as it is so common.

BIBLIOGRAPHY

American Cancer Society. (2022a). *Key statistics for basal and squamous cell skin cancers.* https://www.cancer.org/cancer/melanoma-skin-cancer.html

American Cancer Society. (2022b). *Cancer facts and figures.* https://www.cancer.org/content/dam/cancer-org/cancer-facts-and-statistics/annual-cancer-facts-and-figures/2022/2022-cancer-facts-and-figures.pdf

Babadzhanov, M., Doudican, N., Wilken, R., Stevenson, M., Pavlick, A., & Carucci, J. (2020). Current concepts and approaches to Merkel cell carcinoma. *Archives of Dermatological Research, 313*(3), 129–138. https://doi.org/10.1007/s00403-020-02107-9

Conforti, C., & Zalaudek, I. (2021). Epidemiology and risk factors of melanoma: A review. *Dermatology Practical & Conceptual, 11*(Suppl 1), e2021161S. https://doi.org/10.5826/dpc.11s1a161s

Khandelwal, A. R., Echanique, K. A., St. John, M., & Nathan, C. A. (2021). Cutaneous cancer biology. *Otolaryngologic Clinics of North America, 54*(2), 259–269. https://doi.org/10.1016/j.otc.2020.11.002

Parker, E. R. (2021). The influence of climate change on skin cancer incidence – A review of the evidence. *International Journal of Women's Dermatology, 7*(1), 17–27. https://doi.org/10.1016/j.ijwd.2020.07.003

Skin Cancer Foundation. (2022). *Skin cancer facts and statistics.* https://www.skincancer.org/skin-cancer-information/skin-cancer-facts/

Swetter, S. M., Tsao, H., Bichakjian, C. K., Curiel-Lewandrowski, C., Elder, D. E., Gershenwald, J. E., Guild, V., Grant-Kels, J. M., Halpern, A. C., Johnson, T. M., Sober, A. J., Thompson, J. A., Wisco, O. J., Wyatt, S., Hu, S., & Lamina, T. (2019). Guidelines of care for the management of primary cutaneous melanoma. *Journal of the American Academy of Dermatology, 80*(1), 208–250. https://doi.org/10.1016/j.jaad.2018.08.055

Walker, H. S., & Hardwicke, J. (2021). Non-melanoma skin cancer. *Surgery (Oxford), 40*(1), 39–45. https://doi.org/10.1016/j.mpsur.2021.11.004

KNOWLEDGE CHECK: CHAPTER 13

1. MRI of the brain shows necrotic irregular mass crossing the corpus callosum, with vasogenic edema. What is the most likely diagnosis?

   A. Cerebral abscess
   B. Metastatic lesion
   C. Meningioma
   D. High-grade astrocytoma

2. What are the three subtypes of gliomas?

   A. Astroglioma, oligodendroglioma, meningioma
   B. Astroglioma, oligodendroglioma, ependymoma
   C. Meningioma, oligodendroglioma, pituitary tumor
   D. Central nervous system (CNS) lymphoma, oligodendroglioma, ependymoma

3. When examining a patient, which symptom would be most concerning for elevated intracranial pressure?

   A. Arm numbness
   B. Decreased hearing
   C. Vomiting
   D. Speech difficulty

4. What would be a reasonable treatment plan for a low-grade glioma in a low-risk patient?

   A. Maximal safe resection only
   B. Maximal safe resection with surveillance MRIs every 3 to 6 months
   C. Maximal safe resection plus chemotherapy
   D. Maximal safe resection radiation and chemotherapy

5. Which of the following symptoms is associated with cervical cancer?

   A. Postcoital bleeding
   B. Copious vaginal discharge
   C. Pain in the back, buttocks, or legs
   D. All of the above

6. What is the most common subtype of cervical cancer?

   A. Adenosquamous
   B. Squamous cell
   C. Neuroendocrine tumors
   D. Adenocarcinoma

7. What is the most common gynecologic malignancy in the United States?

   A. Cervical cancer
   B. Ovarian cancer
   C. Endometrial cancer
   D. Vulvar cancer

8. Fertility-sparing treatment options for premenopausal patients with IA grade 1 endometrioid endometrial cancer include all of the following EXCEPT:

   A. Megestrol
   B. Whole pelvic radiation
   C. Levonorgestrel intrauterine device (IUD)
   D. Medroxyprogesterone

9. Which of the following symptoms can be present in a patient with newly diagnosed ovarian cancer?

   A. Bloating and abdominal distention
   B. Unexpected weight loss
   C. Urinary frequency or urgency
   D. All of the above

10. The subtypes of ovarian cancer include all of the following EXCEPT:

    A. Sex cord stromal tumors
    B. Germ cell tumors
    C. Epithelial tumors
    D. Sarcomatous tumors

11. When treating acute moist radiation desquamation, the following should be recommended EXCEPT:

    A. Apply hot or cold packs to the affected area for comfort.
    B. Apply compresses and soaks as prescribed by the radiation oncologist.
    C. Keep the area clean (lukewarm water and synthetic soap) and open to air, wear loose-fitting clothing, and avoid the sun.
    D. Monitor for concomitant skin infections (e.g., herpes simplex, *Staphylococcus aureus*).

(See answers next page.)

1. **D) High-grade astrocytoma**
High-grade astrocytomas appear as a mass with heterogeneous intensity as a result of central necrosis, hemorrhage, hypervascularity, and edema, and disseminate along the white matter tracts and may cross the corpus callosum to involve the contralateral hemisphere, generating the classically described butterfly lesion. Cerebral abscess has true restricted diffusion, metastatic lesions are often multifocal, and meningiomas are extra-axial masses with a broad dural base.

2. **B) Astroglioma, oligodendroglioma, ependymoma**
Astrogliomas, oligodendrogliomas, and ependymomas develop when the glial cells of the brain parenchyma divide abnormally. Meningiomas grow from the meninges, namely the dura mater, while pituitary tumors are restricted to the pituitary gland and primary central nervous system (CNS) lymphomas originate from lymphocytes.

3. **C) Vomiting**
Any focal neurologic deficit on exam can be concerning for a brain malignancy, but when a tumor grows too large with increasing surrounding vasogenic edema, it can cause increased intracranial pressure (ICP) that causes nausea, vomiting, headache, blurry vision, and lethargy. This can become a neurologic emergency leading to decreased level of consciousness and respiratory depression, and even cause brain herniation and death if not treated quickly.

4. **B) Maximal safe resection with surveillance MRIs every 3 to 6 months**
Both low- and high-grade gliomas warrant maximal safe resection. If they are low grade *without* risk features, such as older age (>40), subtotal resection, or unfavorable molecular features, then observation with surveillance MRIs is reasonable.

5. **D) All of the above**
For patients with symptoms, the most common is irregular bleeding or postcoital bleeding. Some nonspecific complaints include vaginal discharge, which can include foul odor. More advance disease may include pain in the back, buttocks, and legs, with unilateral leg swelling and changes to bowel/bladder habits.

6. **B) Squamous cell**
Squamous cell carcinoma accounts for 70% to 80% of invasive cervical cancer. Adenocarcinoma accounts for 10% to 15%. Adenosquamous and neuroendocrine are rare.

7. **C) Endometrial cancer**
In the United States, the most common gynecologic cancer is endometrial cancer, followed by ovarian cancer and cervical cancer.

8. **B) Whole pelvic radiation**
Premenopausal women with grade 1 well-differentiated tumor without myometrial involvement on MRI, without lymphovascular invasion, and without intra-abdominal disease/adnexal mass can be offered fertility-sparing treatment with close follow-up. These include options A, C, and D. However, treatment with whole pelvic radiation would lead to infertility.

9. **D) All of the above**
In general, symptoms related to ovarian cancer are vague and nonspecific. They can include all of these symptoms, which can oftentimes lead patients to see gastroenterologist and urologist prior to seeking gynecologic care.

10. **D) Sarcomatous tumors**
The subtypes of ovarian cancer include sex cord stromal tumors, germ cell, and epithelial tumors.

11. **A) Apply hot or cold packs to the affected area for comfort.**
Extreme temperature changes such as hot and cold packs can further damage the dermal layers and result in further injury worsening the desquamation. This can result in treatment delays. Only apply products discussed and approved by the radiation oncologist and at the timing recommended around the scheduled treatments.

12. What is thought to be the pathogenesis of acute lymphoblastic leukemia (ALL)?

A. A result of genetic insults that block lymphoid differentiation and drive aberrant cell proliferation and survival

B. Always arises secondary to Epstein–Barr virus (EBV)

C. Most often occurs secondary to previous cytotoxic chemotherapy

D. Related to the transformation of a single hematopoietic stem cell into a malignant undifferentiated cell with endless proliferation; results in accumulation of abnormal, immature myeloid cells in the bone marrow and peripheral blood

13. Which of the following biochemical features is NOT seen in tumor lysis syndrome (TLS)?

A. Hyperuricemia
B. Hyperkalemia
C. Hypercalcemia
D. Hyperphosphatemia

14. What is the only chance of a cure for myelodysplastic syndrome?

A. Transfusion support
B. Darbepoetin
C. Hypomethylating agents
D. Allogeneic stem cell transplant

15. What are the risk factors for developing myelodysplastic syndrome (MDS)?

A. Eating red meat
B. Drinking alcohol
C. Exposure to chemotherapy and radiation, or environmental exposure to benzenes and other chemicals
D. Excessive exercising

16. Which is the most prevalent myeloproliferative neoplasm (MPN) in the United States?

A. Essential thrombocythemia (ET)
B. Polycythemia vera (PV)
C. Myelofibrosis (MF)
D. They all occur in equal frequency

17. Gene mutations commonly seen in MPNs include:

A. JAK2
B. CALR
C. HAL6
D. Both JAK2 and CALR

18. From which cell type are most non-Hodgkin lymphomas derived?

A. T-cells
B. Natural killer cells
C. B-cells
D. Myeloid cells

19. A patient with known non-Hodgkin lymphoma who has not yet started treatment presents with severe lower back pain and inability to walk. What study should be ordered to evaluate for spinal cord compression?

A. X-ray of the lumbar spine
B. MRI of the spine
C. PET scan
D. CT of the abdomen/pelvis

20. Who is most likely to develop melanoma?

A. A 49-year-old female with red hair and blue eyes
B. A 38-year-old Hispanic male with a family history of squamous cell carcinoma in his 50-year-old brother
C. A 72-year-old non-Hispanic White male with blue eyes
D. A 25-year-old female with a history of multiple sunburns as a child

(See answers next page.)

12. **A) A result of genetic insults that block lymphoid differentiation and drive aberrant cell proliferation and survival**

All other answers are related to acute myeloid leukemia (AML).

13. **C) Hypercalcemia**

Hypocalcemia, not hypercalcemia, is seen in tumor lysis syndrome (TLS).

14. **D) Allogeneic stem cell transplant**

Myelodysplastic syndrome (MDS) is a disease involving pluripotent hematopoietic stem cells; therefore, the only possible cure is replacing them with healthy cells (Hellstrom-Lindberg et al., 2020).

15. **C) Exposure to chemotherapy, radiation, or environmental exposure to benzenes and other chemicals**

Exposure to chemotherapy, radiation, and other environmental exposures can cause clonal mutations in the bone marrow leading to MDS.

16. **B) Polycythemia vera (PV)**

The prevalence of myelofibrosis (MF), PV, and essential thrombocythemia (ET) in the United States is 13,000, 148,000, and 134,000, respectively.

17. **D) Both *JAK2* and *CALR***

Molecular pathogenesis in myeloproliferative neoplasms (MPNs) is linked gene mutations in *JAK2*, *CALR*, and *MPL*.

18. **C) B-cells**

Non-Hodgkin lymphomas (NHLs) originate from the lymphoid tissues, and most NHLs are derived from B-cells.

19. **B) MRI of the spine**

An urgent MRI should be ordered to evaluate for spinal cord compression followed by prompt treatment with steroids ± radiation therapy.

20. **C) A 72-year-old non-Hispanic White male with blue eyes**

Each of these individuals has an increased risk of developing melanoma, but an individual is at highest risk based on age, race, and sex. From age 50 on, significantly more men develop melanoma than women, and the majority of individuals who develop melanoma are White men over the age of 55. Adding to the risk is having blue eyes.

CHAPTER 14

IMMUNE SYSTEM, CONNECTIVE TISSUE, AND JOINTS GUIDELINES

BACK PAIN

Joanne Elaine Pechar

DEFINITION

A. Pain in the lower back region, which may or may not have a radicular component.

B. Low back pain (LBP) is categorized into three groups, based on the duration of symptoms.

   1. Acute LBP: Pain that is 6 weeks or less in duration.

   2. Subacute LBP: Pain that continues between 6 and 12 weeks.

   3. Chronic LBP: Pain that is more than 3 months in duration.

C. Types of LBP.

   1. Benign back pain is a dull, aching pain that generally worsens with movement but improves with rest and lying.

   2. Tumor- or infection-related back pain typically presents with constant and dull pain. This pain is unrelieved by rest and is worse at night, therefore often awakening the patient.

   3. Disc herniation is worsened by coughing, Valsalva maneuver, and sitting, and is relieved by lying in the supine position.

   4. Spinal stenosis is associated with bilateral (and occasionally unilateral) sciatic pain that is worsened by activities such as walking, prolonged standing, and back extension. Pain is relieved by rest and forward flexion.

   5. Pain referred to the back is usually unaffected by posture and the common origin is the abdomen and pelvis.

   6. Radicular or "root" pain is greater in intensity and radiates from the spine to the leg in a specific nerve root distribution. Sneezing, coughing, lifting heavy objects, or straining may elicit an intense or sharp pain. Any maneuver that leads to nerve root stretching evokes radicular pain such as straight leg raise (SLR) or bending at the waist.

INCIDENCE

A. The lifetime incidence of LBP is 70% and has an incidence of 5% per year.

B. The peak incidence of LBP is in the age range of 40s to 50s.

C. LBP is the second most common reason for physician visits in the United States.

D. For approximately 90% of the patients, the most common cause of LBP is related to disc degeneration.

E. Back symptoms are the most common cause of disability in those under 45 years old.

PATHOGENESIS

A. LBP presents suddenly from an accident, fall, whiplash injury, or heavy lifting.

B. LBP develops gradually as a result of age-related changes to the spine.

C. Bony overgrowth (osteophytes) or disc herniation may directly impinge on spinal nerve roots or the spinal cord itself and can lead to instability and misalignment of the spine, which produces pain and neurologic deficits.

D. Radiculopathy is caused by compression, inflammation, or injury to a spinal nerve root.

E. Sciatica is a form of radiculopathy caused by compression of the sciatic nerve, the large nerve that travels through the buttocks and extends down the back of the leg.

F. Spondylolisthesis is a condition in which a vertebra of the lower spine slips out of place, pinching the nerves exiting the spinal column.

   1. Slippage of the anterior spine forward leaving posterior elements behind.

G. Spinal stenosis is the narrowing of the spinal column, which then leads to pressure on the spinal cord and nerves.

   1. The spinal cord pressure can cause pain or numbness with walking or standing and may, over time, lead to leg weakness and sensory loss. Symptoms typically are relieved by sitting.

   2. This is also known as neurogenic claudication.

   3. Symptoms are usually bilateral.

   4. Patients treated with surgery experience relief of back and leg pain. Within 7 to 10 years, 25% develop recurrent stenosis.

H. Spondylosis or osteoarthritis (OA) is back pain-induced movement of the spine associated with stiffness and older age.

   1. Osteophytes may contribute to spinal canal stenosis, lateral recess stenosis, or neural foraminal narrowing.

▶

I. Vertebral metastases.

   1. Systemic cancer patients typically present with back pain not relieved by rest. Early diagnosis is crucial.

   2. Multiple myeloma, lymphoma, and metastatic carcinoma of the breast, bronchus, prostate, thyroid, kidney, stomach, and uterus are the common malignant tumors that involve the spine.

   3. Primary lesion may be small and asymptomatic.

   4. Pain is constant and dull and often unrelieved by rest and is generally worse at night, interrupting sleep.

   5. Vertebral body fracture in the setting of a healthy young or middle-aged patient should alert provider the possibility of underlying metastasis.

J. Vertebral osteomyelitis.

   1. Presents as back pain unrelieved by rest with focal spine tenderness and with elevated erythrocyte sedimentation rate (ESR), C-reactive protein (CRP), and white blood cell (WBC).

   2. Motion becomes limited and there is percussion-induced tenderness over the spine and pain with jarring of the spine.

   3. Primary sources of infection are skin, lungs, and urinary tract.

   4. Intravenous (IV) drug abuse is a significant risk factor.

   5. Most often caused by staphylococci infection.

   6. A common finding is the destruction of the vertebral bodies and disc space.

   7. MRI with and without contrast is the gold standard for diagnosis.

K. Spinal epidural abscess.

   1. Necessitates urgent surgical treatment.

   2. Failure to diagnose and treat has led to cases of paraplegia or death from sepsis.

   3. Most often caused by staphylococci infection carried in the bloodstream or is introduced into the epidural space from an osteomyelitic lesion. Another avenue of infection is the IV self-administration of drugs and contaminated needles.

   4. Main symptoms are low-grade fever, leukocytosis, and persistent and severe localized pain that is intensified by pressure and percussion over the vertebral spine.

L. Lumbar adhesive arachnoiditis.

   1. A result of inflammation within the arachnoid space.

   2. Fibrosis can cause clumping of nerve roots.

M. Intraspinal hemorrhage.

   1. Occurs during subarachnoid, subdural, and epidural bleeding.

   2. Sudden, excruciating midline back pain ("strike of a dagger") often with rapidly evolving paraparesis, urinary retention, and leg numbness.

   3. Common causes are coagulopathy (mainly on blood thinners) and spinal arteriovenous malformation (AVM).

PREDISPOSING FACTORS

A. The first attack typically occurs between ages 30 and 40.

B. African American female patient.

C. Diet high in calories and fat.

D. Inactive lifestyle.

E. Obesity.

F. Cigarette smoking.

G. Occupation: Job that requires heavy lifting, pushing, pulling, or twisting.

SUBJECTIVE DATA

A. History.

   1. Pain worse at night.

   2. Cancer history.

   3. History of chronic infection (especially lung, skin, and genitourinary).

   4. History of trauma.

   5. Bowel and bladder incontinence.

   6. Glucocorticoid use.

   7. IV drug use.

   8. History of rapidly progressive neurologic deficit.

B. Common complaints/symptoms.

   1. LBP with radiation to buttocks, legs, or feet.

   2. Paraspinal muscle spasms.

   3. Muscle stiffness.

   4. Paresthesias.

   5. Gait disturbances.

   6. Numbness.

C. Common/typical scenario.

   1. Neurogenic claudication (low back, buttock, or leg pain, which may be relieved by sitting or with rest, induced by walking or standing).

   2. Fecal or urinary incontinence.

   3. Large postvoid residual greater than 100 mL and overflow incontinence.

   4. Perianal or perineal sensory loss.

   5. Dermatomal sensory loss.

   6. Focal leg weakness, paralysis, and hyporeflexia in the legs.

   7. Elevated ESR, CRP, and human leukocyte antigen (HLA), if an infection is present.

   8. Fever.

D. Family and social history.

   1. Family history is typically noncontributory.

   2. Social history.

     a. Smoking, which is associated with LBP.

     b. Dietary and eating habits.

     c. Obesity is a major cause of LBP.

     d. Elicit drug use.

E. Review of systems.

   1. Elicit the onset, frequency, duration, and location of symptoms.

   2. Inquire if the pain is worse during activity, at rest, or at night.

   3. Inquire about exacerbating factors.

   4. Inquire if the pain radiates to the lower extremities.

   5. Inquire about associated symptoms, such as numbness, tingling, weakness, and sensory deficits.

   6. Determine if there is any recent loss or change in bowel or bladder function.

7. Check if there is symptom improvement after taking pain medications.

8. Determine whether the patient has a history of trauma and chronic infection.

9. Check for signs of systemic disease, which include history of cancer, age greater than 50 years, unexplained weight loss, duration of pain greater than 1 month, nighttime pain, and unresponsiveness to previous therapies.

PHYSICAL EXAMINATION

A. Check vital signs: Blood pressure, heart rate, respiration, and temperature; check weight.
  1. Unexplained fever.
  2. Unexplained weight loss.
B. Inspect.
  1. Examine the back for any warmth, erythema, swelling, purulent drainage, or abscess.
  2. Inspect the curvature of the spine.
  3. Observe for signs of previous surgery.
C. Check for tenderness or pain using palpation along the spine.
  1. Percussion tenderness over the spine.
  2. Presence of abdominal, rectal, or pelvic mass.
  3. Tenderness over spinous process or jarring by gentle percussion may indicate the presence of local inflammation, infection, pathologic or traumatic compression fracture, metastasis, epidural abscess, or disc lesion.
D. Check for radicular pain associated with straight leg test.
  1. SLR test is positive if the test causes radicular pain of the affected leg radiating below the knee.
  2. SLR sign is elicited by passive flexion of the leg at the hip while the patient is in a supine position. The maneuver stretches the L5 to S1 nerve roots and sciatic nerve passing through the hip.
  3. Lasegue sign is when the compression of the L5 or S1 root is detected.
E. Complete neurologic examination including:
  1. Motor strength.
  2. Sensation.
  3. Deep tendon reflexes.
F. Check back range of motion (ROM): Flexion, extension, side bending, and rotation.
  1. Determine when and under what conditions the pain worsens or begins.
G. Check hip ROM: Possible referred pain from hip pathology.
  1. Internal or external rotation of the leg at the hip.
H. Assess gait.
  1. Observation of the gait may reveal a subtle limp, a pelvic tilt, or stiffness of bearing, which is indicative of a disinclination to bear weight on a painful leg.
I. Perform digital rectal examination to assess rectal sphincter tone or anal sphincter laxity.

DIAGNOSTIC TESTS

A. Spine x-ray or film.
  1. Anteroposterior, lateral, and oblique views.
  2. Demonstrates fractures, disc space narrowing, osteophyte formation, tumor, instability, displacement of vertebral bodies, and most importantly bone infiltration by cancer or myeloma.
B. MRI scan.
  1. Provides axial and sagittal views, which demonstrate normal and pathologic discs, ligaments, nerve roots, epidural fat, and shape and size of the spinal canal.
  2. Gold standard study in cases of suspected spinal infection, neoplasm, and epidural compression syndromes.
  3. Administration of gadolinium enhances regions of inflammation and tumor but not particularly helpful in degenerative disc diseases of the spine. The decision to administer an IV contrast agent depends on the degree of suspicion of infiltration of the bones or spinal canal by cancer or the need to detect spine nerve root tumors.
C. CT scan.
  1. Useful in evaluating vertebral fractures, facet joints, and posterior elements of the spine.
  2. CT myelography is the best substitute imaging to diagnose an epidural abscess or cord compression when metallic devices, such as pacemaker, preclude MRI use.
D. Nuclear medicine bone scan.
  1. Can also be used if infection and tumor are suspected.
E. Electromyography (EMG) and nerve conduction studies are also helpful in suspected root and nerve diseases.
F. Laboratory tests.
  1. Routine laboratory studies such as ESR, CRP, complete blood count (CBC), blood cultures, and urinalysis are rarely needed for nonspecific acute LBP if the duration is under 3 months.
  2. Acute phase reactants such as ESR and CRP are helpful in screening spinal osteomyelitis, epidural abscess, or myeloma.
  3. HLA if ankylosing spondylitis (AS) is suspected.
  4. Serum protein electrophoresis if myeloma is suspected.
G. All the aforementioned tests must be interpreted in the context of history and clinical examination; otherwise they are subject to overuse and overinterpretation.

DIFFERENTIAL DIAGNOSIS

A. Degenerative disc disease.
B. Spinal stenosis.
C. Spondylosis and spondylolisthesis.
D. Discitis.
E. Vertebral osteomyelitis.
F. Spinal cord or cauda equina compression.
G. Herniated intervertebral disc.

▶

H. Spinal epidural abscess.

I. AS.

J. Spine-related bone tumors.

K. Metastatic cancer.

L. Scoliosis and hyperkyphosis.

M. Vertebral compression fracture.

N. Myofascial pain syndrome.

O. Fibromyalgia pain syndrome.

P. Lumbosacral strain and sprain.

EVALUATION AND MANAGEMENT PLAN

A. General plan.

  1. General intervention.

    a. Bedrest for a few days. Limit bending, lifting, and twisting.

    b. Physical therapy and aerobic exercise.

    c. Local application of ice in the acute phase followed by heat and massage.

    d. Brace is indicated for adolescents with spine curvature between 20 and 40 degrees.

    e. Lying on the side with knees and hips flexed or supine with a pillow under the knees can relieve the pain.

  2. Adjunct therapy.

    a. Transcutaneous electrical nerve stimulation (TENS).

    b. Biofeedback.

    c. Acupuncture.

  3. Red flags: Indications for imaging.

    a. Concern for malignancy: Age 50 years or older, history of cancer, unexplained weight loss, pain unrelieved by bedrest, pain lasting more than a month, or LBP failure to improve in 1 month.

    b. Concern for infection: Elevated ESR greater than 20, IV drug abuse, urinary tract infection, skin infection, or fever.

    c. Concern for compression fracture: Corticosteroid use and/or age 50 or older.

    d. Concern for neurologic problem: Sciatica.

    e. New fecal or urinary incontinence.

  4. Surgical intervention.

    a. Indications for surgery when *all three* criteria are met:

      i. Evidence of disc herniation as demonstrated by an imaging study.

      ii. Worsening clinical picture with neurologic deficit.

      iii. Failed improvement after 4 to 6 weeks of conservative treatment.

      iv. NOTE: Cauda equina and spinal cord compression syndromes need urgent surgical decompression in 24 to 48 hours of symptom onset.

      v. Imaging demonstrates compressive abscess or epidural collection.

    b. Types of spine surgery.

      i. Vertebroplasty and kyphoplasty are minimally invasive treatments to repair compression fractures of the vertebrae.

      ii. Spinal laminectomy or spinal decompression is used to treat spinal stenosis.

        1) The lamina or bony walls of the vertebrae and bone spurs are removed. The goal of the procedure is to open up the spinal column to remove pressure on the nerves.

      iii. Discectomy or microdiscectomy is recommended to remove herniated discs from pressing on the nerve roots or the spinal cord.

      iv. Foraminotomy is an operation that enlarges the foramen, which is where a nerve root exits the spinal canal. The enlargement removes the blockage and relieves pressure, caused by bulging discs, on the nerve.

      v. Spinal fusion is used to treat degenerative disc disease and spondylolisthesis.

        1) The disc between two or more vertebrae is removed and the adjacent vertebrae are fused together by bone grafts or metal devices secured by screws.

        2) Spinal fusion can be performed through the abdomen with a procedure known as an anterior lumbar interbody fusion, or it may be performed through the back in a procedure called posterior lumbar fusion.

      vi. Irrigation and debridement with or without removal of instrumentation and delayed primary wound closure is the process of removing infection and infected tissues from the spinal canal.

        1) Two-step process with plastic surgery where spine drains and wound vacuum-assisted closure (VAC) therapy is used to assist in wound closure, promote healing, and prevent reinfection, especially in deep wound infections.

        2) Acute infected cases are managed with IV antibiotic therapy in combination with surgery.

B. Patient/family teaching points.

  1. Counsel in regard to exercise therapy.

  2. Counsel about smoking cessation and weight loss.

  3. Counsel about ergonomic interventions for prevention of occupational LBP.

C. Pharmacotherapy.

  1. First-line agents: Nonsteroidal anti-inflammatory drugs (NSAIDs) and Tylenol. Avoid NSAIDs after fusion.

  2. Muscle relaxants: Cyclobenzaprine, diazepam, carisoprodol, metaxalone, Robaxin, or tizanidine.

  3. Opioids or narcotics.

  4. Antidepressants and anticonvulsants.

  5. Transforaminal or epidural steroid injections. ▶

D. Discharge instructions.

  1. Patients should participate in physical therapy and start with first-line pharmacologic agents for pain management.

  2. If pain does not get better with treatment or it worsens, the patient should call the healthcare provider.

  3. Patients should also call if they suddenly feel something pop or snap in the back or if they have questions or concerns about their condition or care.

  4. Patients should seek urgent attention if a change in bowel or bladder habits is observed.

FOLLOW-UP

A. Patients who have not improved after 4 to 6 weeks of conservative therapy and who did not receive imaging during initial evaluations require follow-up.

B. Patients presenting with persistent and worsening symptoms should have an MRI for further evaluation.

CONSULTATION/REFERRAL

A. Patients without concerns for a particular etiology who have not improved after 12 weeks need imaging and referral to orthopedic spine surgery or neurosurgery specialists for further evaluation and treatment.

B. Patients with symptoms of spinal cord compression or severe neurologic deficits should have immediate MRI for further evaluation and also receive urgent specialist referrals.

SPECIAL/GERIATRIC CONSIDERATIONS

A. When performing pain assessment in a cognitively impaired older adult, the American Geriatrics Society encourages the integration of the following six behavioral domains:

  1. Facial expressions.

  2. Verbalizations or vocalizations.

  3. Body movements.

  4. Changes in interpersonal interactions.

  5. Changes in activity patterns or routines.

  6. Mental status changes.

B. Clinicians should be mindful of older patients with dementia and chronic LBP and should accordingly adjust pain management.

  1. Dementia can alter pain reporting, pain behaviors, and pain coping.

  2. Older patients may not reliably communicate the need for analgesic medications.

C. Due to harmful side effects in older patients with noncancer pain, nonopioid medications are preferred to opioids.

D. Doses of opioid medications should be reduced in older adults and also titrated slowly.

  1. Decrease initial dose by 25% for a 60-year-old patient and by 50% for an 80-year-old patient.

CASE SCENARIO: BACK PAIN

A 55-year-old patient with a medical history of ventricular tachycardia presents with chronic low back pain (LBP) for more than 6 months. She reports a constant and dull mid-LBP worse at night and unrelieved by rest, interrupting her sleep, with intermittent radiculopathy down to her left knee. She denies any recent fall, trauma, or motor vehicle collision, but reports a 20-lb weight loss in the last 2 months. On arrival, her vital signs include blood pressure of 132/65, pulse rate of 82 beats per minute, respiratory rate of 18 breaths per minute, and temperature of 97.5°F/36.3°C. The provider performs a detailed neurologic exam and notes tenderness to palpation to the lumbar spine with no focal neurologic deficits. The patient denies leg weakness, paresthesias, numbness, and bowel or bladder dysfunction.

1. Which spine exam should be performed next?
  A. Log roll test
  B. Straight leg raise test
  C. Spurling maneuver test
  D. Hoffman sign or reflex test

2. What is the patient's indication for imaging?
  A. Concern for malignancy
  B. Concern for infection
  C. Concern for compression fracture
  D. Concern for neurologic problem

3. The patient reports that she has a pacemaker in place. What would be the most appropriate test to define her lumbar spine pathology?
  A. CT myelogram
  B. MRI scan
  C. Bone scan
  D. Plain lumbar x-ray films

4. What is the common malignant tumor that involves the spine?
  A. Metastatic carcinoma of the brain
  B. Metastatic carcinoma of the pancreas
  C. Metastatic carcinoma of the breast
  D. Metastatic carcinoma of the liver

BIBLIOGRAPHY

Deyo, R. A., & Tsui-Wu, Y. (1987). Descriptive epidemiology of low-back pain and its related medical care in the United States. *Spine*, 12(3), 264–268. https://doi.org/10.1097/00007632-198704000-00013

Jameson, J., Fauci, A. S., Kasper, D. L., Hauser, S. L., Longo, D. L., & Loscalzo, J. (Eds.). (2020). *Back and neck pain*. In A. Fauci (Eds.), *Harrison's manual of medicine* (20th ed.). https://accessmedicine.mhmedical.com/content.aspx?bookid=2738&sectionid=227556477

Ju, D. G., Yurter, A., Gokaslan, Z. L., & Sciubba, D. M. (2014). Diagnosis and surgical management of breast cancer metastatic to the spine. *World Journal of Clinical Oncology*, 5(3), 263–271. https://doi.org/10.5306/wjco.v5.i3.263

Knight, C., Deyo, R., Staiger, T., & Wipf, J. (2017, December 6). Treatment of acute low back pain. In L. Kunins (Ed.), *UpToDate*. https://www.uptodate.com/contents/?source=search_result&search=acute%20low%20back%20pain&selectedTitle=1

Parvizi, J. (2010). *High yield orthopaedics*. Saunders/Elsevier.

Ropper, A. H., Samuels, M. A., Klein, J. P., & Prasad, S. (Eds.). (2019). Pain in the back, neck, and extremities. In A. Ropper, & R. H. Brown (Eds.),

Adams and Victor's principles of neurology (11th ed.). McGraw Hill http s://accessmedicine.mhmedical.com/content.aspx?bookid=1477&sec tionid=117185855

Swiontkowski, M. F., & Stovitz, S. D. (2006). *Manual of orthopaedics* (6th ed.). Lippincott Williams & Wilkins.

Wheeler, S. G., Wipf, J. E., Staiger, T. O., Deyo, R. A., & Jarvik, J. G. (2018, July 12). Evaluation of low back pain in adults. In L. Kunins, & S. I. Lee (Eds.) *UpToDate*. https://www.uptodate.com/contents/evaluation-of -low-back-pain-in-?source=search_result &search=acute%20low%20 back%20pain&selectedTitle=226

Wright, R., Malec, M., Shega, J. W., Rodriguez, E., Kulas, J., Morrow, L., Rodakowski, J., Semla, T., & Weiner, D. K. (2016). Deconstructing chronic low back pain in the older adult—Step by step evidence and expert-based recommendations for evaluation and treatment: Part XI: Dementia. *Pain Medicine, 17*(11), 1993–2002. https://doi.org/10.1093/ pm/pnw247

COMPARTMENT SYNDROME OF THE LOWER LEG

Joanne Elaine Pechar

DEFINITION

A. A surgical limb-threatening emergency which refers to a buildup of pressure within a muscle compartment (surrounded by a closed fascia) leading to a decline in tissue perfusion in the injured extremity and causing permanent damage and irreversible ischemic necrosis of the muscles and nerves.

B. A serious complication typically results from a crush injury to a large bone. There is an increase in closed compartmental pressure causing ischemic changes and diminished microcirculation within the soft tissues.

INCIDENCE

A. The average annual overall incidence of acute compartment syndrome (ACS) is 3.1 cases per 100,000 people.

B. Due to relatively larger muscle mass in men, ACS is 10 times more prevalent particularly in young men compared with women.

C. Tibial fractures caused by trauma account for approximately 75% of ACS cases; blunt soft tissue injury is the second leading cause.

D. Mechanisms of injury associated with a high risk of ACS include automobile versus pedestrian injuries, proximal tibia and fibula ballistic injuries, and tibia fractures during soccer or football injuries.

E. The most common sites of ACS are (in descending order of prevalence) the calf, forearm, thigh, upper arm, hand, and foot.

F. ACS is most common among younger patients under 35 years old due to a greater incidence of high-impact injuries, stronger fascial structures, and increased muscle bulk.

G. ACS is not always associated with trauma or injury.

PATHOGENESIS

A. ACS develops when the intracompartmental pressure (ICP) exceeds venous capillary pressure.

B. Arteriovenous pressure gradient theory.

  1. Ischemia begins when local blood flow cannot meet the metabolic demands of the surrounding affected tissue.

  2. As compartment pressure rises, venous outflow is reduced and venous pressure rises, leading to a decrease in the arteriovenous pressure gradient.

  3. Without intervention, due to arteriolar compression, microcirculation is compromised and blood is shunted away from intracompartmental tissues, which ultimately reduces tissue perfusion. Inadequate tissue perfusion and oxygenation results in soft tissue ischemia, cellular necrosis, anoxia, and irreversible death of the cells if not treated rapidly.

  4. In patients with ACS, myonecrosis may occur within 2 hours of injury.

  5. Irreversible ischemic injury to myoneural issues within the compartment occurs after 6 to 8 hours of circulatory failure.

    a. Reperfusion following prolonged ischemia leads to viable muscle and nerve salvage, which can induce systemic inflammatory response syndrome (SIRS), acute respiratory distress syndrome (ARDS), metabolic acidosis, hypotension, cardiac arrhythmias, myoglobinemia, renal failure, and death.

C. Anatomy of the lower leg.

  1. There are four compartments in the lower leg: Anterior, lateral, superficial posterior, and deep posterior.

  2. Each individual compartment encloses specific muscles, nerves, arteries, veins, and bones.

  3. The most common location of ACS is the anterior compartment or anterior tibial compartment of the lower extremity.

PREDISPOSING FACTORS

A. Trauma-related closed tibial shaft fracture is the major contributing factor to ACS and accounts for one-third of all ACS cases.

B. List of traumatic and nontraumatic ACS etiologies.

  1. Vascular: Reperfusion therapy, arterial puncture or injury, hemorrhage, deep vein thrombosis (DVT), intravenous (IV) infusions, and intraosseous infusions.

  2. Soft tissue: Crush injury, contusion, fall, direct blow, burn skin and skeletal traction, insect bite, and snake bite.

  3. Iatrogenic: Drugs such as anticoagulants; bleeding disorders; circumferential wraps, casts or splints, constrictive dressings, tourniquets, and long leg brace; extravasations of drugs, contrast media, and fluids; prolonged lithotomy positioning; prolonged immobilization; viral myositis; and diabetic muscle infarction.

SUBJECTIVE DATA

A. Common complaints/symptoms.

  1. The cardinal and earliest symptom of ACS is pain out of proportion.

  2. Persistent burning pain at rest.

  3. Pain reproduced with passive stretch of the affected muscle compartment.

B. Common/typical scenario.

1. Massive swelling of the limb with firm and tense feeling on deep palpation.

2. Reduced two-point discrimination or vibration sense.

3. Loss of light touch sensation.

C. Family and social history.

1. Family and social history are noncontributory as the cause of ACS is typically related to injury or surgery.

D. Review of systems.

1. Severe pain out of proportion to injury and what is otherwise expected is often an early and sensitive sign of ACS.

a. Pain described as severe, burning, deep, and worse with passive stretch of the involved muscle.

b. Most patients at risk of ACS have sustained trauma, fracture, or injury to the nerve or soft tissue, which may be the source of pain.

c. The injured extremity becomes swollen and tense as ACS develops. Increasing ICP builds up on nerve fibers and injured components within the compartment.

d. Obtunded patients, patients emerging from anesthesia, or patients receiving nerve blocks may not accurately report pain.

e. In the late stages of ACS, pain may not be a subjective clinical finding as pain receptors and nerve fibers are at high risk of ischemic necrosis and death.

2. Paresthesia in the distribution of any sensory nerves within the compartment.

a. Onset, which suggests the first signs of ischemic nerve dysfunction, is within approximately 30 minutes to 2 hours following injury.

PHYSICAL EXAMINATION

A. Paralysis is found in the late stages of ACS.

1. A higher ICP leads to ischemic neuronal tissues and nerve dysfunction and subsequent paresthesia, paresis, and ultimately complete paralysis.

2. Motor function may deteriorate within 4 hours of muscle tissue ischemia.

3. At 8 to 24 hours of ischemia, motor and sensory loss is irreversible.

B. Pulselessness is a late finding, which is a poor indicator of ACS.

1. As ICP rises, a loss of limb pulses indicates a decline in arterial perfusion.

C. Pallor.

1. Presence of pallor and longer capillary time in the injured limb indicate direct arterial injury.

D. Poikilothermia.

1. Presence of coolness or a change in the temperature of the affected extremity.

DIAGNOSTIC TESTS

A. High index of clinical suspicion and the "6 Ps" cardinal symptoms: Pain, pallor, poikilothermia, paresthesia, paralysis, and pulselessness.

B. Measuring limb ICP.

1. Stryker pressure monitoring device: A handheld digital monitor for single tissue fluid pressure readings. To measure, the clinician injects 0.3 mL of saline solution into each of the four leg compartments (Figure 14.1). This device has been shown to be very accurate, with a sensitivity of 94% and a specificity of 98%.

2. An ICP of 30 mmHg or above is considered a critical threshold for diagnosis of ACS, and if ICP is elevated emergent decompression should be considered.

3. Normal pressure of a tissue compartment falls between 0 and 8 mmHg in resting stage.

4. ICP should be measured in each compartment of interest but within 5 cm from the injured or fractured site.

C. Delta pressure.

1. Delta pressure is the difference between the diastolic pressure and the measured ICP.

2. Delta pressure of less than or equal to 30 mmHg is diagnostic of ACS.

D. Laboratory assessments.

1. Creatinine kinase (CK), renal function, basic metabolic panel (BMP), urinalysis, and urine myoglobin are recommended.

2. Rising CK levels >1,000 U/mL or presence of myoglobinuria is indicative of ACS given rhabdomyolysis is present in 40% of ACS with traumatic injuries.

3. BMP may show elevated creatinine and hyperkalemia, which are most often due to associated rhabdomyolysis.

E. Cases of missed ACS diagnosis are accounted for a decrease in or loss of consciousness, spinal or epidural anesthesia, poor clinical judgment, and presence of prior or inadequate fasciotomies.

F. ACS carries a significant legal risk in medical practice. Legal claims for ACS found that 32% of the cases were due to delay in treatment and 23% due to misdiagnosis.

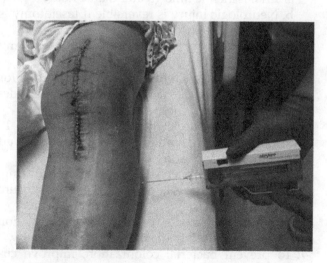

FIGURE 14.1   An advanced practice provider monitoring for compartment syndrome.

G. Delay in diagnosis can result in poor patient outcomes, including chronic pain, infection, muscle necrosis, rhabdomyolysis, renal failure, muscle contractions, amputation, and even death.

H. Missed diagnosis is associated with clinician inexperience, patient sedation, polytrauma, soft tissue, and overreliance on clinical signs and symptoms.

DIFFERENTIAL DIAGNOSIS

A. DVT.
B. Thrombophlebitis.
C. Cellulitis.
D. Necrotizing fasciitis.
E. Peripheral vascular injury.
F. Rhabdomyolysis.
G. Shin splints.
H. Stress fractures.

EVALUATION AND MANAGEMENT PLAN

A. General plan.
   1. Restore blood flow, minimize tissue damage, decrease tissue pressure, and restore functional loss.
   2. Standard treatment: Emergent fasciotomy is a surgical limb-saving procedure to decompress the affected compartments and prevent critical limb ischemia.
      a. Two types of surgical technique: Single or double incision.
         i. Single-incision technique involves a single long incision made from the head of the fibula to the lateral malleolus.
         ii. Double-incision technique is the most common fasciotomy method: The four-compartment technique incorporates two longitudinal anterolateral and posteromedial incisions. Posterior compartments are opened medially and lateral compartments from the lateral side.
   3. The preferred time interval to restore perfusion is 4 to 6 hours.
      a. An absolute indication for fasciotomy is an arterial ischemic time greater than 4 hours.
      b. Neurologic injury is reversible if fasciotomy is performed within 4 hours.
      c. Neurologic injury is irreversible if fasciotomy is further delayed until 12 hours.
   4. In 48 to 72 hours, a return to surgery is needed for reevaluation of muscle viability and wound debridement of nonviable tissues.
   5. Once ACS is completely resolved within 7 to 10 days, the fasciotomy wound is left open for delayed complete primary closure or skin grafting.
      a. Wound closure techniques: Shoelace suturing, elastic band closure, and vacuum-assisted closure (VAC).
   6. Prophylactic fasciotomy had a higher amputation rate than those undergoing therapeutic fasciotomy.
   7. To prevent bacterial colonization, improve circulation, and approximate wound edges, a negative

pressure wound therapy is used for assisted closure of fasciotomy wounds.
   8. Fasciotomy complications include further surgery for delayed wound closure or skin grafting, pain and nerve injury, permanent muscle weakness or paralysis, and chronic venous insufficiency.
   9. Nonoperative treatment measures.
      a. Loosening compression dressings, "bivalving" casts, and complete removal of splints and casts.
      b. Elevation of the affected extremity to facilitate venous drainage, reduce edema, and maximize tissue perfusion.

B. Patient/family teaching points.
   1. ACS is a surgical emergency that can develop quickly and is a medical condition requiring rapid diagnosis and management.
   2. Early diagnosis of ACS is critical to avoiding morbidity.
   3. Permanent damage to muscles and nerves can occur within hours, which can necessitate amputation if not addressed immediately and not appropriately diagnosed and treated.
   4. Keep the affected limb propped up on pillows so the limb is level with the heart.
   5. Do not put any compressive bandages over the site.

C. Pharmacotherapy.
   1. There is no pharmacologic treatment for ACS; only surgery will reduce the pressure in the compartment.

D. Discharge instructions.
   1. Seek care immediately if the pain or swelling does not improve, fever or rash develops, or the injured limb becomes cold or numb.
   2. Contact the provider with questions or concerns.

FOLLOW-UP

A. Follow-up is needed in 1 to 2 weeks for neurovascular examination, control of swelling, and wound check to ensure complete wound healing.

CONSULTATION/REFERRAL

A. Early consultation and collaboration with orthopedic or vascular surgery is critical for limb salvage and to prevent possible devastating complications, such as the following.
   1. Wound infection.
   2. Paralysis.
   3. Permanent nerve damage.
   4. Contractures.
   5. Amputation.
   6. Rhabdomyolysis.
   7. Multiorgan failure.
   8. Sepsis.
   9. Death.

SPECIAL/GERIATRIC CONSIDERATIONS

A. Diagnosis of ACS may be delayed with older patients who received epidural anesthesia and who sustained neurovascular injuries following total knee arthroplasty (TKA).

1. Continuous epidural analgesia can mask pain associated with passive stretching, therefore delaying diagnosis.

2. Older patients may develop foot drop or peroneal nerve injury following TKA.

B. ACS remains difficult to diagnose, with clinical high index of suspicion remaining as the cornerstone of decision-making.

CASE SCENARIO: COMPARTMENT SYNDROME OF THE LOWER LEG

A 70-year-old patient presents to a local hospital, status post day 3 from a right knee arthroplasty, with a medical history of atrial fibrillation, cardiomyopathy, deep vein thrombosis (DVT), and hypertension. Three years ago, he was placed on warfarin (Coumadin) due to provoked DVT and pulmonary embolism (PE) after his hip replacement surgery. He was started on a heparin drip immediately after his knee surgery to prevent venous thromboembolism (VTE) as recommended by his hematologist. His vital signs include a temperature of 98°F/36.6°C, blood pressure of 150/75, pulse rate of 85 beats per minute, and respiratory rate of 22 breaths per minute. During rounds, the advanced practice provider found his right knee and leg extremely swollen. The patient's main complaint was severe pain, especially during passive flexion of his right toes; he reports some feeling of tingling to his right foot. On assessment, he can barely move his right big toe and ankle, with a muscle strength grade of 2/5 plantar flexion and 2/5 dorsiflexion. On palpation, he has +2 dorsalis pedis pulse. He receives general anesthesia with no regional block.

1. What is the next best course of action?
   A. Turn off heparin drip.
   B. Take off Ace wrap dressing.
   C. Elevate the legs.
   D. Apply ice therapy.

2. What is a late finding and poor indicator of acute compartment syndrome (ACS)?
   A. Poikilothermia
   B. Pain out of proportion
   C. Pallor
   D. Pulselessness

3. Which test would best measure limb intracompartmental pressure?
   A. Stryker pressure monitoring device
   B. Delta pressure
   C. Alpha pressure
   D. Creatinine kinase (CK)

4. What is the critical threshold of intracranial pressure (ICP) indicative of acute coronary syndrome (ACS) diagnosis?
   A. 5 mmHg or above
   B. 10 mmHg or above
   C. 30 mmHg or above
   D. 15 mmHg or above

BIBLIOGRAPHY

Asprey, D. P., & Dehn, R. W. (2013). *Essential clinical procedures*. Elsevier Health Sciences.

Azar, F. M., Canale, S. T., & Beaty, J. H. (2017). *Campbell's operative orthopaedics*. Elsevier.

Donaldson, J., Haddad, B., & Khan, W. S. (2014). The pathophysiology, diagnosis and current management of acute compartment syndrome. *The Open Orthopaedics Journal, 8*(1), 185–193. https://doi.org/10.2174/1874325001408010185

Gahtan, V., & Costanza, M. J. (Eds.). (2015). *Essentials of vascular surgery for the general surgeon*. Springer.

Glass, G. E., Staruch, R. M., Simmons, J., Lawton, G., Nanchahal, J., Jain, A., & Hettiaratchy, S. P. (2016). Managing missed lower extremity compartment syndrome in the physiologically stable patient: A systematic review and lessons from a Level I trauma center. *The Journal of Trauma and Acute Care Surgery, 81*(2), 380–387. https://doi.org/10.1097/TA.0000000000001107

Long, B., Koyfman, A., & Gottlieb, M. (2019). Evaluation and management of acute compartment syndrome in the emergency department. *The Journal of Emergency Medicine, 56*(4), 386–397. https://doi.org/10.1016/j.jemermed.2018.12.021

Murdock, M., & Murdoch, M. M. (2012). Compartment syndrome: A review of the literature. *Clinics in Podiatric Medicine and Surgery, 29*(2), 301–310. https://doi.org/10.1016/j.cpm.2012.02.001

Pechar, J., & Lyons, M. M. (2016). Acute compartment syndrome of the lower leg: A review. *The Journal for Nurse Practitioners, 12*(4), 265–270. https://doi.org/10.1016/j.nurpra.2015.10.013

Raza, H., & Mahapatra, A. (2015). Acute compartment syndrome in orthopedics: Causes, diagnosis, and management. *Advances in Orthopedics, 2005*, 1–8. https://doi.org/10.1155/2015/543412

Schmidt, A. H. (2017). Acute compartment syndrome. *Injury, 48*(Suppl. 1), S22–S25. https://doi.org/10.1016/j.injury.2017.04.024

Stahel, P. F., Mauser, N., Gissel, H., Henderson, C., Hao, J., & Mauffrey, C. (2013). Acute lower-leg compartment syndrome. *Orthopedics, 36*(8), 619–624. https://doi.org/10.3928/01477447-20130724-07

Vegari, D. N., Rangavajjula, A. V., Dilorio, T. M., & Parvizi, J. (2014). Fasciotomy following total knee arthroplasty: Beware of terrible outcome. *The Journal of Arthroplasty, 29*(2), 355–359. https://doi.org/10.1016/j.arth.2013.05.013

Wesslén, C., & Wahlgren, C. M. (2018). Contemporary management and outcome after lower extremity fasciotomy in non-trauma-related vascular surgery. *Vascular and Endovascular Surgery, 52*(7), 493–497. https://doi.org/10.1177/1538574418773503

JOINT PAIN

Dolores Diana Zollo

DEFINITION

A. Discomfort, pain, or inflammation usually felt in the hands, feet, hips, knees, or spine. It can affect any part of the joint extending from the bone, cartilage, ligaments, tendons, or muscles.

   1. Arthralgia: True joint pain within the joint capsule.
   2. Arthritis: Joint inflammation that causes pain.
   3. Tendonitis: Inflammation of the tendons or flexible bands that connect the muscle to the bone. Typically more prevalent in the elbow, heel, or shoulder, and is caused by overuse activities.
   4. Bursitis: Inflammation of the bursa sac (a flat, fluid-filled sac that provides cushioning where skin, muscles, tendons, and ligaments rub over the bones) caused by overuse and is mostly found in areas around the hip, knee, elbow, or shoulder.

▶

B. Usually categorized into *two groups* based on duration of symptoms:

1. Acute joint pain: Pain resolving after 6 weeks or less after onset of symptoms (e.g., viral, bacterial infection, gout, pseudogout, reactive arthritis [ReA], or joint disorder flare-up).

2. Chronic joint pain: Pain that extends past 6 weeks in duration after onset of symptoms (e.g., inflammatory disorders such as rheumatoid arthritis [RA], psoriatic arthritis [PsA] and systemic lupus erythematosus [SLE], or osteoarthritis [OA]).

C. The causes include various self-limiting illnesses and others that can be debilitating and life-threatening.

D. The most common form of joint pain is OA or degenerative joint disease (DJD), which presents over time when the cartilage, the protective cushion in between the bones, wears away. The joints become painful and stiff, resulting in decreased joint mobility on both active and passive range of motion (ROM).

E. Joint pain limits the function of the joint and can decrease a person's ability to do simple tasks. Severe joint pain can affect the quality of life.

F. Of note, nonarticular disorders very rarely demonstrate crepitus, swelling, instability, and/or actual joint deformity.

INCIDENCE

A. It is estimated that approximately 5% of primary care office visits are for joint pain, with OA being the most common disease.

PATHOGENESIS

A. Sources of pain within the joint include the joint capsule, periosteum, ligaments, subchondral bone, and synovium, but not the articular cartilage, which lacks nerve endings.

B. The basic pathophysiologic types of joint disease and pain stem from synovitis, enthesopathy, crystal deposition, infection, and structural or mechanical derangements.

PREDISPOSING FACTORS

A. A combination of clinical, laboratory, and imaging data can help differentiate patients likely to have self-limited disease from those likely to have persistent arthritis.

B. Prediction models based on patients with early arthritis have identified a number of features associated with persistent and/or erosive disease, including:

1. Duration of symptoms prior to presentation.
2. Older age.
3. Male sex assigned at birth.
4. High body mass index (BMI).
5. Duration of morning stiffness.
6. Number of tender or swollen joints.
7. Involvement of lower extremities.
8. Elevated acute phase reactants.
9. Rheumatoid factor (RF).
10. Anticyclic citrullinated peptide (anti-CCP) antibody.
11. Erosive change on baseline radiograph.
12. HLA-DRB1 shared epitope alleles.

SUBJECTIVE DATA

A. Common complaints/symptoms.

1. Pain may be constant or intermittent (e.g., hip, knee, ankle, shoulder, or hand pain).
2. Complaints of the joint feeling stiff, achy, or sore.
3. Complaints of a burning, throbbing, or "grating" sensation in the joint.
4. Soft tissue swelling or effusions.
5. Joint erythema or warmth.
6. Joint contractures or deformity.
7. Myalgias and muscle spasms.
8. Muscle weakness.

B. Common/typical scenario.

1. Rash.
2. Fever.
3. Crepitus.

C. Family and social history.

1. Family history may have a role in joint pain. Specific questions inquiring about autoimmune diseases in the family should be addressed.
2. Patient's daily routine may provide insight into causes of repetitive injuries.
3. Smoking can also contribute to joint pain due to peripheral vascular injury.

D. Review of systems.

1. Specific symptoms to ask patients with joint pain.
   a. Fever.
   b. Weight loss.
   c. Night sweats.
   d. Rash.
   e. Nodules.
   f. Neuropathy.
   g. Joint swelling.
   h. Joint erythema.
   i. Tenderness.
   j. Warmth around the joint.
   k. Inability to use the joint.
   l. Eye pain.
   m. Eye dryness.
   n. Recent infection.
   o. Recent tick bite.
   p. Recent exposure to sexually transmitted infection (STI).
   q. Recent joint injection or surgery.
   r. History of immunosuppression.

E. Joint pain may represent a vast number of problems. The following questions can help direct clinical decision-making and narrow down the differential diagnosis:

1. Localize the complaint anatomically (articular vs. nonarticular).
2. Determine the extent of the involvement (monoarticular, polyarticular vs. widespread). Is one joint affected or many joints affected?

a. One joint: Monoarticular.
b. Two to four joints: Oligoarticular.
c. More than five joints: Polyarticular.
   i. If polyarticular, which joints are mostly involved? For example:
     1) OA: Distal interphalangeal (DIP), carpometacarpal (CMC), hip, or knee joints.
     2) RA: Symmetric involvement of proximal interphalangeal (PIP), metacarpophalangeal (MCP), or metatarsophalangeal (MTP) joints.

3. Determine the nature of the pathologic process (inflammatory vs. noninflammatory).

4. Determine chronology of symptoms (acute vs. chronic).

5. Are there systemic symptoms?

6. Formulate a differential diagnosis, with the most common disorders being considered first.

7. Attainable plan may include an accurate diagnosis, timely intervention or therapy, and avoidance of unnecessary diagnostic tests.

PHYSICAL EXAMINATION

A. Complete history and physical examination is appropriate for all patients presenting with joint pain since this symptom may be the initial manifestation of a systemic illness.

B. The following findings on physical examination could indicate a more serious pathogenesis of joint pain:

1. General survey: Level of patient's pain and ability to carry out activities of daily living (ADLs).

2. Vital signs: Fever.

3. Eye: Keratoconjunctivitis sicca, uveitis, conjunctivitis, and episcleritis.

4. Neck: Lymphadenopathy.

5. Mouth: Parotid enlargement and oral ulcerations.

6. Cardiovascular: Murmur, pericardial, or pleural friction rubs.

7. Lungs: Fine inspiratory rales (secondary to interstitial lung disease).

8. Skin: Skin lesions may suggest that the joint symptoms are due to PsA, SLE, viral infection, or Still disease.

9. Musculoskeletal: Swollen, erythematous, warm joints, joint deformities, and ROM of joints. Quantify the level of pain elicited by palpation or movement. Active and passive ROM should be assessed in all planes with contralateral comparison.

10. Neurovascular: Muscle tone, muscle strength, sensory perceptions, and gait.

DIAGNOSTIC TESTS

A. Arthrocentesis (aspiration) and examination of synovial fluid to include a cell count, Gram stain, crystal analysis, and culture.

1. Noninflammatory synovial fluid is usually clear and viscous, with white blood cell (WBC) count of less than 2,000/mcL and mostly mononuclear cells.

2. Inflammatory synovial fluid is usually turbid and yellow and WBC count is elevated between 2,000/mcL and 50,000/mcL and polymorphonuclear leukocytes (PMNs; >75%).

a. Gout: Monosodium urate crystals seen.
b. Pseudogout: Calcium pyrophosphate dihydrate crystals.

3. Septic synovial fluid is usually opaque and purulent and WBC count is elevated at greater than 50,000/mcL with predominance of PMNs (>75%).

B. Laboratory tests.

1. Complete blood count (CBC) with WBC count and differential.

2. Basic metabolic panel (BMP).

3. Liver function test (LFTs).

4. Erythrocyte sedimentation rate (ESR).

5. C-reactive protein (CRP).

6. Serum uric acid.

7. Antinuclear antibody (ANA).

8. RF.

9. Cyclic citrullinated peptide (CCP) antibodies.

10. Lyme.

C. Radiologic imaging of affected joint(s).

1. Plain radiographs (x-rays) helps aid in the diagnosis and staging of articular disorders.

2. Ultrasonography is useful in the detection of soft tissue abnormalities, for example, tenosynovitis.

3. CT scan provides detailed visualization of the axial skeleton and may help with the diagnosis of low back pain (LBP) syndromes.

4. MRI provides advanced assistance when evaluating complex musculoskeletal disorders. MRI generates multiplanar images with great anatomic detail. It is more sensitive than arthrography or CT especially with soft tissue injuries.

D. Tissue biopsy.

DIFFERENTIAL DIAGNOSIS

A. Adult Still disease.

B. Ankylosing spondylitis (AS).

C. Avascular necrosis.

D. Bone cancer.

E. Certain types of arthritis.

1. OA.

2. Juvenile RA.

3. PsA.

4. ReA.

5. RA.

6. Septic arthritis.

F. Fractured bone.

G. Bursitis.

H. Complex regional pain syndrome.

I. Dislocation.

J. Gonococcal arthritis.

K. Gout.

L. Hypothyroidism.

M. Leukemia.

N. Lupus.

O. Lyme disease.
P. Osteomyelitis.
Q. Paget bone disease.
R. Polymyalgia rheumatica.
S. Pseudogout.
T. Rickets.
U. Sarcoidosis.
V. Sprains and strains.
W. Tendinitis.

EVALUATION AND MANAGEMENT PLAN

A. General plan.
 1. Alleviate pain to the affected joint and minimize loss of physical function, which may include a multimodality approach including nonpharmacotherapy and pharmacologic elements.
  a. Avoid activities that precipitate pain.
  b. Use ice for 15 to 20 minutes of each hour.
  c. Redistribute load across the joint with a brace/compressive wrap and/or splint.
  d. Unload the joint during weight-bearing with crutches/cane or walker.
 2. Specific treatments targeted to each individual diagnosis may include but not limited to:
  a. Physical therapy.
  b. Pharmacologic intervention (see the following section).
  c. Surgical management.
B. Patient/family teaching points.
 1. Exercise and weight loss are highly effective in relieving joint pain.
 2. Start with low-impact exercises that do not irritate the joint, such as swimming or cycling.
 3. Short-term joint pain can be relieved with rest, ice, compressing with a wrap, and elevating the joint above the level of the heart.
C. Pharmacotherapy.
 1. Analgesic medications.
  a. Acetaminophen (Tylenol) or nonsteroidal anti-inflammatory drugs (NSAIDs) are first-line agents.
   i. Acetaminophen dosing is 1 g up to four times a day. Do not exceed 4 g daily due to liver toxicity.
   ii. Oral NSAID dosing varies, but must be taken with food due to high rates of gastrointestinal side effects. They are nephrotoxic and should not be used in patients with kidney disease. Overall, there is about a 30% improvement in pain with NSAIDs compared with high-dose acetaminophen.
  b. Cyclooxygenase 2 (COX-2) inhibitors.
   i. May increase cardiovascular (CV) events and are not appropriate long-term treatment choices especially for high-risk heart disease or stroke patients.
  c. Opiates.
   i. High side effect profile including dizziness, sedation, nausea/vomiting, constipation,

urinary retention, and pruritus. Use sparingly and with caution due to respiratory and central nervous system (CNS) depression.
 2. Oral corticosteroids.
 3. Intra-articular injections:
  a. Steroids or hyaluronans.
 4. Disease-modifying antirheumatic drugs (DMARDs).
D. Surgical interventions.
 1. Total hip arthroplasty (THA) and total knee arthroplasty (TKA) are highly effective elective procedures for patients who suffer from hip and knee pain which is mainly due to joint deterioration from OA.
  a. THA and TKA can relieve pain, restore function, and improve quality of life by replacing the diseased articular surfaces with synthetic material.
  b. Discharge criteria.
   i. Stable vital signs and afebrile for more than 24 hours postoperatively.
   ii. Wound incision clean, dry, and intact.
   iii. Hip and knee pain well-managed and controlled.
   iv. No signs and symptoms of infection, such as fever, hip erythema, and warmth.
   v. No signs and symptoms of blood clot, such as hip or leg swelling, and calf tenderness.
  c. Activity.
   i. Full weight-bearing status with physical therapy.
   ii. Walker and crutch training will be provided prior to hospital discharge.
   iii. Patient can resume most daily activities within a few weeks after surgery.
   iv. After a posterior THA, patients may need to adhere to hip precautions for 6 weeks.
    1) Avoid bending and flexing hips greater than 90 degrees.
    2) Avoid twisting the leg in or out (internal or external rotation).
    3) Avoid crossing the legs at the knee or ankle.
    4) Avoid allowing the legs to cross midline.
    5) Avoid raising the knee higher than the hip.
    6) Avoid allowing the toes to point inward (pigeon-toe) or to rotate outward (duck-walking).
    7) Always lie on the back while resting in bed, and place a pillow between the thighs if lying on one's side.
    8) Sit on chairs higher than knee height.
    9) Avoid low beds.
    10) Avoid pivoting on the operated leg and take small steps when turning.
    11) Before standing, scoot to the edges of beds and chairs.
   v. After a TKA, the following measures are needed to protect a new knee joint:

1) Place a pillow between the thighs if lying on one's side.
2) Avoid kneeling or squatting.
3) Avoid twisting the new knee.
d. Diet.
   i. Patients are not able to eat or drink until fully recovered from anesthesia.
   ii. To avoid nausea after surgery, start patients slowly on a clear liquid diet.
   iii. Once clear liquid diets are tolerated, patients may be offered solid foods.
   iv. Since narcotics should not be mixed with alcohol, limit alcohol consumption.
   v. Eat healthy foods and watch weight.
   vi. Obesity can add more stress to the new joint.
e. Medications.
   i. Used for postoperative pain management, the multimodal perioperative pain protocol (MP3) consists of high-dose Tylenol, short-acting opioids, oral nonsteroidal anti-inflammatory COX-2 inhibitor NSAIDs, intravenous (IV) NSAIDs, and neuropathologic agents.
   ii. Oxycodone 5 mg one to two tablets every 4 to 6 hours as needed.
   iii. Gabapentin 100 mg TID for 1 week.
   iv. Celebrex 200 mg BID for 4 weeks.
   v. Tylenol 1,000 mg Q8H for 4 weeks.
   vi. Toradol 7.5 mg IV Q6H as needed (do not exceed 5 days).
   vii. Hydromorphone 2 mg IV every 2 to 3 hours as needed for breakthrough pain only and should be stopped within 24 hours after surgery.
f. Wound care.
   i. Always keep the surgical wound clean and dry.
   ii. Unless instructed to do otherwise, do not apply any lotions, creams, oils, ointments, or powders to the surgical wound area.
   iii. Leave the dressing in place for 14 days postoperatively.
   iv. Dressing will be removed by a provider in the office or at rehab or can be removed by a home health nurse.
   v. Two weeks from the day of surgery, at the first orthopedic follow-up appointment, staples or sutures will be removed, along with a wound check.
   vi. Patient may shower but the incision must be well-covered. Do not scrub the incision.
g. Follow-up.
   i. Patients are instructed to follow up with the surgeon within 2 to 6 weeks postoperatively or immediately for any concerning signs or symptoms.
   ii. Discuss with patients concerning signs or symptoms to monitor for, including:

1) Difficulty breathing, shortness of breath, dyspnea, or pleuritic chest pain.
2) Persistent nausea or vomiting.
3) Persistent fever over 101°F/38.3°C, chills, and sweating.
4) Signs of a blood clot which include:
   a) Pain in the operative leg and calf tenderness.
   b) Tenderness and erythema of the operative leg.
   c) Unexplained swelling, which does not dissipate with elevation, of the operative limb.
5) Pain with rotation of the limb and worsening pain even after taking pain medicine.
6) Unexplained limb shortening or extreme rotation.
7) Wound drainage soaking through the bandage over the incision.
8) Intermittent claudication, which is walking-based thigh pain that clears quickly with sitting.
9) Signs of wound infection which include:
   a) Increased pain, swelling, warmth, or erythema around the incision.
   b) Pus fluid draining from the incision.
h. Intraoperative complications.
   i. Fracture.
   ii. Nerve injury.
   iii. Vascular injury.
i. Postoperative complications and readmission concerns.
   i. Deep vein thrombosis (DVT).
   ii. Pulmonary embolism (PE).
   iii. Septic arthropathy: Hip or knee.
   iv. Cellulitis.
   v. Hematoma.
   vi. Hip dislocation.
   vii. Periprosthetic fracture.
      1) Hip fractures.
         a) Femoral head fracture.
         b) Femoral neck fracture.
         c) Intertrochanteric fracture.
         d) Subtrochanteric fracture.
         e) Femoral shaft fracture.
         f) Distal femur fracture.
      2) Knee fractures and tendon ruptures.
         a) Patella fracture.
         b) Quadriceps tendon rupture.
         c) Patella tendon rupture.
         d) Tibial plateau fracture.
         e) Tibia and fibula shaft fracture.
   viii. Knee dislocation.
   ix. Aseptic loosening.
   x. Heterotrophic ossification.
   xi. Leg length discrepancy.
   xii. Foot drop due to peroneal nerve palsy.
   xiii. Quadriceps weakness due to femoral nerve palsy

FOLLOW-UP

A. Follow up with a provider when joint pain begins. Do not wait until the pain is intense and the joint becomes stiff.
B. Physical therapy can assist patients in relieving joint pain with exercises.

CONSULTATION/REFERRAL

A. Based on patient diagnosis, but may include:
  1. Primary care.
  2. Orthopedist.
  3. Rheumatologist.
  4. Infectious disease.

SPECIAL/GERIATRIC CONSIDERATIONS

A. Certain joint pain diagnoses are more frequent in adults older than 60 years.
  1. OA.
  2. Gout and pseudogout.
  3. Polymyalgia rheumatica.
  4. Osteoporotic fracture.
  5. Septic arthritis.

CASE SCENARIO: JOINT PAIN

A 62-year-old patient with a past medical history (PMHx) of type 2 diabetes, hypertension, hypersensitivity lung disease, and chronic kidney disease stage 3, as well as a smoking history and a family history of systemic lupus, presents with acute right hip pain that started about a week ago. He reports that his right hip feels extremely stiff and swollen. Prior to this episode, he could walk without any assistive devices but is now using a cane. He has taken acetaminophen with no relief. He denies any recent trauma. He denies fever or chills or recent weight loss. Vital signs are within normal range. His body mass index (BMI) is 32.1 and his hemoglobin A1C (HgA1C) is 5.7 on recent lab work. On exam, he walks with antalgic gait and has limited active and passive range of motion (ROM) of his right hip. A joint effusion is noticed with some warmth to palpation. No erythema or drainage is noted. Log roll test is negative, and there are good pulses distally, otherwise neurovascularly intact as well as the contralateral side.

1. Which diagnostic test would be best to use to evaluate his condition?
  A. Ultrasound-guided hip aspiration for synovial fluid analysis
  B. X-rays including anteroposterior pelvis and unilateral hip
  C. CT scan of the right lower extremity
  D. MRI of the right hip

2. Prior to this appointment, what would have been a good educational point for this patient and treatment suggestion for his joint pain?
  A. Patient should start nonsteroidal anti-inflammatory drug (NSAID) therapy.
  B. Patient should see an endocrinologist for diabetes management.
  C. Patient should try to lose weight as a way of relieving joint pain.
  D. Patient should engage in high-impact exercises.

3. A synovial fluid analysis was completed on this patient and showed a white blood cell count of 48,000/mcL and monosodium urate crystals, which confirm which diagnosis?
  A. Pseudogout
  B. Gout
  C. Psoriatic arthritis
  D. Septic arthritis due to bacteria

BIBLIOGRAPHY

Baer, A. N. (2016, December 26). *The approach to the painful joint*. In H. S. Diamond (Ed.), *Medscape*. https://emedicine.medscape.com/article/336054-overview

Cleveland Clinic. (2018, March 28). *Joint Pain: Symptoms, Causes, and Treatment*. Author. https://my.clevelandclinic.org/health/symptoms/17752-joint-pain

Joint Pain. (2016, February 26). *Mayo clinic*. http://www.mayoclinic.org/symptoms/joint-pain/basics/definition/sym-20050668

Longo, F. (2022). *Harrison's principles of internal medicine, Vol. 1 and 2; 18th Edition* (Revised ed ed., Vol. 2). McGraw Hill Education Books USA.

Papadakis, M. A., McPhee, S. J., & Rabow, M. W. (Eds.). (2016). *Current medical diagnosis & treatment 2016*. McGraw-Hill.

Plamer, T., & Toombs, J. D. (2004). Managing joint pain in primary care. *Journal of the American Board of Family Medicine, 17*(Suppl. 1), 32–42. https://doi.org/10.3122/jabfm.17.suppl_1.S32

Shmerling, R. H. (2019, March 7). *Evaluation of the adult with polyarticular pain*. In M. Ramirez Curtis (Ed.), *UpToDate*. https://www.uptodate.com/contents/evaluation-of-the-adult-with-polyarticular-pain

Villa-Forte, A. (2022, July 1). *Joint pain: Many joints*. Merck Manuals Consumer Version. https://www.merckmanuals.com/home/bone,-joint,-and-muscle-disorders/symptoms-of-musculoskeletal-disorders/joint-pain-many-joints

OSTEOARTHRITIS

Eric Jacala

DEFINITION

A. Osteoarthritis (OA) is defined as evident cartilage loss without inflammatory or crystal arthropathy, resulting in reactive changes in the bone and destruction of the associated joint (irrespective of whether the patient has symptoms).

INCIDENCE

A. OA is the most common type of joint disease, affecting more than 32 million individuals in the United States alone.
B. 90% of all people have radiographic evidence of OA in weight-bearing joints by age 40.

PATHOGENESIS

A. OA is characterized by degeneration of cartilage and by hypertrophy of the bone at the articular margins.
B. Cartilage, subchondral bone, and synovium have been found to all have key roles in disease pathogenesis.
C. OA can involve almost any joint but typically affects the hands, knees, hips, and feet.

PREDISPOSING FACTORS

A. Hereditary factors may be involved.

B. Obesity is a risk factor for OA as it increases the intra-articular load, subsequently causing wear and tear of weight-bearing articular cartilage.
C. Repetitive movements or overuse causes damage to joints, tendons, and ligaments, and may lead to progressive cartilage degeneration.
   1. Playing competitive contact sports increases the risk of developing OA.
   2. Jobs requiring frequent bending and carrying increase the risk of knee OA.
D. Previous injury in the form of fracture, ligament sprain, and/or instability of the surrounding ligaments increases the risk of OA.
E. Sex assigned at birth: Females have a higher incidence of OA.
F. Age: Symptomatic disease increases with age.

SUBJECTIVE DATA
A. Common complaints/symptoms.
   1. The onset is insidious.
   2. The disease process may start with articular stiffness or deep aching joint pain typically lasting less than 30 minutes; may be most prominent upon awakening.
B. Common/typical scenario.
   1. Reduced range of motion (ROM) and crepitus of the affected joint are frequently present.
   2. There are no systemic manifestations.
C. Review of systems.
   1. Elicit the onset, frequency, duration, and location of symptoms.
   2. Inquire if pain is worse during activity or at rest.
   3. Inquire about exacerbating factors.
   4. Inquire about presence and duration of morning stiffness.
   5. Determine if there are any systemic signs such as fever or associated rash/discolorations.

PHYSICAL EXAMINATION
A. Comprehensive musculoskeletal examination may reveal:
   1. Flexion contracture or varus deformity of the knee.
   2. Palpable osteophytes of the distal interphalangeal (DIP; Heberden nodes) and proximal interphalangeal (PIP; Bouchard nodes).
   3. Limited ROM of the affected joint or joints.
   4. Crepitus felt over the knee joint.
   5. Joint effusion and other articular signs of inflammation.

DIAGNOSTIC TESTS
A. Laboratory test are nonspecific.
B. Joint aspiration: Synovial fluid tends to be noninflammatory (i.e., low white blood cell [WBC] and polymorphonuclear leukocytes [PMN] count).
C. Imaging.
   1. Plain film radiographs of the affected joint may reveal:

    a. Narrowing of the joint space.
    b. Osteophyte formation.
    c. Lipping of marginal bone.
    d. Thickened, dense subchondral bone.
    e. Bone cysts.

DIFFERENTIAL DIAGNOSIS
A. Gout.
B. Pseudogout.
C. Rheumatoid arthritis (RA).
D. Psoriatic arthritis (PsA).
E. Reactive arthritis (ReA).
F. Septic arthritis.
G. Fibromyalgia.
H. Tendonitis.
I. Avascular necrosis.
J. Charcot joint.
K. Lyme disease.
L. Patellofemoral syndrome.
M. Prepatellar bursitis.

EVALUATION AND MANAGEMENT PLAN
A. Treatment.
   1. Nonpharmacologic.
    a. Supportive care with bracing or splinting, especially during strenuous activity.
    b. Use of assistive devices (e.g., a cane on the contralateral side) to decrease load bearing can improve functional status.
    c. Weight loss.
    d. Yoga/tai chi.
   2. Pharmacotherapy.
    a. Acetaminophen is first-line analgesic therapy (2.64 g/d orally).
    b. Nonsteroidal anti-inflammatory drugs (NSAIDs) provide more pain relief but have greater side effects of toxicity (e.g., increased risk for gastric ulcers, bleeding, acute kidney injury).
    c. Chondroitin sulfate and glucosamine, alone or in combination, are no better than placebo in reducing pain in patients with knee or hip OA. However, studies do show they may help decrease stiffness.
    d. Duloxetine, a serotonin norepinephrine reuptake inhibitor, has been shown to provide greater pain relief than placebo but may be difficult to tolerate due to its side effects.
    e. Intra-articular injections.
     i. Triamcinolone (2,040 mg) in patients with OA of the knee or hip may reduce the need for oral analgesics and can be repeated up to four times a year. The American College of Rheumatology does not recommend corticosteroid injections for OA of the hand.
     ii. Sodium hyaluronate produces moderate reduction in symptoms in some patients with OA of the knee.
    f. Opioids should be reserved for short-term use or when all other options have been exhausted.

3. Surgical intervention.

a. Total hip and knee replacements provide excellent symptomatic and functional improvement when involvement of that joint severely restricts walking or causes pain at rest.

b. Arthroscopic surgery for knee OA is ineffective.

4. Patient/family teaching points.

a. General education of patients regarding benefits of exercise and weight loss.

b. Exercise can strengthen muscles and reduce pain and potentially help patients avoid surgery.

c. Weight loss will reduce pressure on joints and slow down destruction of cartilage.

d. Avoid repetitive movements of an affected joint.

e. Use protective gear, such as joint padding, when playing sports to avoid injury.

FOLLOW-UP

A. Follow up with the provider on a regular basis until pain and mobility level are optimized.

B. The patient should call once joint pain starts for better management.

C. Follow up at least once a year with the provider once symptoms are controlled.

CONSULTATION/REFERRAL

A. Refer to an orthopedic surgeon when pain, loss of function, or both warrant consideration of hip or knee joint replacement surgery.

SPECIAL/GERIATRIC CONSIDERATIONS

A. OA may account for up to 70% of the geriatric population's joint pain.

B. OA places geriatric patients at a higher risk for falls.

C. Nonsurgical candidates should be considered for physical reconditioning and pharmacologic pain control.

CASE SCENARIO: OSTEOARTHRITIS

A new patient, 52 years of age, wishes to establish care and would like advice regarding her ongoing left knee pain. The patient's chart shows a medical history of hypertension, hyperlipidemia, atrial fibrillation chronically on apixaban, and body mass index (BMI) of 35.7. The patient reports that she injured her left knee anterior cruciate ligament (ACL) and meniscus playing basketball in college, which required surgical repair, but she was able to return to play after completing physical therapy. She has had no other injury to her knee since then. She works as a custodian in a nursing home and is on her feet for the majority of the day. Over the past 3 months, the patient has noted pain in her right knee while carrying her new puppy up the stairs, and since then has noticed similar pain and associated weakness in the same knee at work. She has been taking over-the-counter naproxen 500 mg BID for the past month and is thinking of adding glucosamine.

1. Which of the following is a nonmodifiable risk factor for the patient to develop osteoarthritis (OA)?

A. Obesity
B. Hyperlipidemia
C. Previous injury
D. Occupation

2. What imaging should be obtained first to support a clinical diagnosis of osteoarthritis (OA)?

A. MRI of the right knee
B. CT scan of the right knee with and without contrast
C. X-ray of the right knee
D. Joint aspiration

3. What pharmacologic therapy should be recommended to the patient?

A. Acetaminophen
B. Glucosamine
C. Naproxen
D. Oxycodone

BIBLIOGRAPHY

Chen, L., & Yu, Y. (2020). Exercise and osteoarthritis. *Advances in Experimental Medicine and Biology, 1228,* 219–231. https://doi.org/10.1007/978-981-15-1792-1_15

Katz, J. N., Arant, K. R., & Loeser, R. F. (2021). Diagnosis and treatment of hip and knee osteoarthritis: A review. *JAMA, 325*(6), 568–578. https://doi.org/10.1001/jama.2020.22171

Lozada, C. J. (2016, November 30). Arthritis. *Medscape.* http://emedicine.medscape.com/article/330487

Mandl, L. A. (2019). Osteoarthritis year in review 2018: Clinical. *Osteoarthritis and Cartilage, 27*(3), 359–364. https://doi.org/10.1016/j.joca.2018.11.001

Thomas, A. C., Hubbard-Turner, T., Wikstrom, E. A., & Palmieri-Smith, R. M. (2017). Epidemiology of posttraumatic osteoarthritis. *Journal of Athletic Training, 52*(6), 491–496. https://doi.org/10.4085/1062-6050-51.5.08

Wang, L. J., Zeng, N., Yan, Z. P., Li, J. T., & Ni, G. X. (2020). Post-traumatic osteoarthritis following ACL injury. *Arthritis Research & Therapy, 22*(1), 57. https://doi.org/10.1186/s13075-020-02156-5

Zhu, X., Sang, L., Wu, D., Rong, J., & Jiang, L. (2018). Effectiveness and safety of glucosamine and chondroitin for the treatment of osteoarthritis: a meta-analysis of randomized controlled trials. *Journal of Orthopaedic Surgery and Research, 13*(1), 170. https://doi.org/10.1186/s13018-018-0871-5

RHEUMATOID ARTHRITIS

Eric Jacala

DEFINITION

A. Rheumatoid arthritis (RA) is a chronic, inflammatory, symmetric polyarthritis that can have systemic effects on multiple organ systems with no clear etiology.

INCIDENCE

A. Prevalence of 1%, with a female-to-male ratio of 3:1.
B. Peak onset in women is in the fourth to fifth decade.
C. Peak onset in men is in the sixth to eighth decade.
D. Annual incidence is 40 per 100,000.
E. Increased frequency of the disease in first-degree relatives and monozygotic twins.

PATHOGENESIS

A. No clear cause has been identified for RA; however, genetics and environment appear to contribute to the development of RA. The best characterized genetic risk factor is inheritance of the HLA-DRB1 alleles encoding a "shared epitope."

B. Chronic synovitis and joint destruction are characteristic of RA.

C. Pannus, hyperplastic synovial tissue, is a distinctive feature of RA and destroys adjacent cartilage, bone, ligaments, and tendons.

PREDISPOSING FACTORS

A. Sex-specific risk factors.

    1. Women: Nulliparity and postpartum state can increase acute flare.

    2. Men: Below-normal testosterone levels.

B. Genetic predisposition.

C. Cigarette smoking, heavy caffeine consumption, and obesity, particularly in patients carrying the shared epitope.

D. Infection (both bacterial and viral) has been hypothesized to trigger RA. No specific bacterial or viral pathogens have been identified; however, porphyromonas gingivalis, a gram-negative oral anaerobe that commonly causes periodontitis, can trigger autoimmune responses/RA.

E. Autoantibody carriers, specifically rheumatoid factor (RF) and anticitrullinated peptide/protein antibodies (ACPA), increase the risk of development of RA.

F. Occupational exposures, including dust and silica, and air pollution.

SUBJECTIVE DATA

A. Common complaints/symptoms.

    1. Insidious onset of polyarticular inflammation and complaints of joint pain and stiffness are the most common presentation, but some patients may present with acute symptoms.

    2. Joint stiffness will last more than 30 minutes and is prominent in the morning, after periods of inactivity, and after strenuous activity.

    3. Systemic manifestations can also be present.

    4. Symptoms tend to be reported in the small joints of the hands, wrist, and forefoot. All joints of the extremities can be affected. Typically, the axial skeleton, except for the cervical spine, will not be involved.

B. Common/typical scenario.

    1. Systemic symptoms may include dryness of the eyes and mucous membranes, presence of rheumatoid nodules, pulmonary symptoms including cough and dyspnea, weight loss, fatigue, neuropathies, and depression.

    2. Felty syndrome is seen in advanced RA disease and is characterized by splenomegaly and neutropenia, and is often accompanied by thrombocytopenia and anemia.

C. Family and social history.

    1. Family history of RA.

    2. Social history.

        a. Smoking.

        b. Caffeine intake.

        c. Occupational exposures.

D. Review of systems.

    1. Joint pain and stiffness.

    2. Swelling.

    3. Presence of skin nodules.

    4. Changes in skin color.

    5. Dryness of mucous membranes.

    6. Cough.

    7. Dyspnea.

PHYSICAL EXAMINATION

A. Symmetrical, polyarticular swelling with pain and tenderness is characteristic.

B. "Boggy" feeling over the affected joints due to synovial thickening or effusion.

C. Palmar erythema may be present in acute flares.

D. Deformities are common in late disease and may be asymmetrical.

E. Decreased grip strength is noted in disease affecting the hands and can be an early indicator of disease.

F. Ulnar deviation, swan neck deformities (flexion of the distal interphalangeal [DIP] joint with extension of the proximal interphalangeal [PIP] joint), and Boutonniere deformities (hyperextension of the DIP joint with flexion of the PIP joint) of the fingers are common in chronic RA.

G. Tendon ruptures can occur.

H. Rheumatoid nodules are subcutaneous nodules found over bony prominences (most commonly), bursae, and tendon sheaths, and are found in 20% of patients.

I. Ocular findings include scleritis and episcleritis.

DIAGNOSTIC TESTS

A. Radiographs (most specific testing): Early images may be normal or show evidence of soft tissue swelling and juxta-articular demineralization. Later images will reveal joint space narrowing and erosions.

B. Elevated erythrocyte sedimentation rate (ESR) and C-reactive protein (CRP) levels: Elevated in acute phases.

C. Anticyclic citrullinated peptide (anti-CCP) antibodies and RF: Present in about three-fourths of patients with RA.

    1. RF specificity for RA is 60% to 85%, while the specificity of ACPA for RA is 85% to 99%.

    2. RF can be falsely elevated in patients with other autoimmune disease and also among older adults.

D. Synovial fluid analysis: Inflammatory effusion often performed to rule out septic arthritis.

DIFFERENTIAL DIAGNOSIS

A. Fibromyalgia.

B. Lyme disease.

C. Myelodysplastic syndrome.

D. Osteoarthritis (OA).

E. Sarcoidosis.

F. Systemic lupus erythematosus (SLE).

EVALUATION AND MANAGEMENT PLAN

A. General plan.
  1. Goals.
      a. Reduce pain and inflammation.
      b. Preserve function.
      c. Prevent deformity.
  2. Nonpharmacologic.
      a. Physical and occupational therapy.
      b. Diet and exercise.
      c. Smoking cessation.
      d. Osteoporosis screening and treatment.
      e. Immunizations to reduce risk of immunosuppressive therapies.

B. Patient/family teaching points.
  1. Similar to nonpharmacologic management.
  2. Diet.
  3. Exercise.
  4. Smoking cessation.
  5. Physical and occupational therapy.
  6. Routine screening and immunizations.

C. Pharmacotherapy.
  1. Nonsteroidal anti-inflammatory drugs (NSAIDs): For symptomatic relief, but not to be used as monotherapy.
  2. Corticosteroids.
      a. Used to bridge until disease-modifying antirheumatic drugs (DMARDs) are effective or during active disease.
      b. Will decrease inflammation and slow articular erosion.
      c. Recommended dose is prednisone 5 to 10 mg PO daily.
          i. Higher doses may be needed to treat extra-articular manifestations and should be tapered when discontinuing.
      d. Intra-articular corticosteroids may be helpful to treat one to two symptomatic joints but may not be administered more than four times per year.
      e. Recommended dose is triamcinolone 10 to 40 mg based on the size of the joint being treated.
  3. DMARDs.
      a. Begin as soon as RA is confirmed.
      b. More efficacious when used in combination than as a monotherapy.
      c. Most commonly used combination is methotrexate with a tumor necrosis factor (TNF) inhibitor.
          i. Methotrexate: Initial synthetic DMARD of choice (7.5 mg PO weekly); can see improvement in 2 to 6 weeks.
          ii. TNF inhibitors: Added when patients do not respond to methotrexate.
      d. Biomarkers are often used to monitor a patient's actual response to treatment.
      e. Before starting DMARDs, it is recommended to screen for latent tuberculosis, hepatitis B virus, and hepatitis C virus infections as the immunosuppression that occurs with DMARDs may reactivate infections.

D. Reconstructive surgery for severe cases.

FOLLOW-UP

A. Patients should follow up after starting or changes are made to medications.

CONSULTATION/REFERRAL

A. Rheumatology as early as possible to confirm diagnosis and manage disease.

SPECIAL/GERIATRIC CONSIDERATIONS

A. RA can be a debilitating disease that makes activities of daily living (ADLs) very difficult.

B. Geriatric patients may have increased risk associated with RA, such as:
  1. Cognitive impairment.
  2. Depression.
  3. Falls.
  4. Urinary incontinence.
  5. Malnutrition.

CASE SCENARIO: RHEUMATOID ARTHRITIS

A 56-year-old patient presents to the clinic for ongoing progressive left wrist, right index finger, and right ankle pain for the last 6 months. She denies any rash or weight loss but vaguely remembers roughly 4 days of fever and fatigue 2 months prior to when symptoms started. She states that she has been taking naproxen for her symptoms, which helps; however, she is concerned because she feels as if her symptoms keep returning and she is finding it increasingly difficult to get ready in the morning. Her medical history consists of celiac disease controlled with dietary modification and frequent gingival disease; otherwise, she does not take medications for any comorbidities. She admits to daily alcohol consumption with dinner, with occasional binge drinking on weekends when she and her friends visit wineries. She also admits to a 20 pack-year history of tobacco use.

1. Which lab finding would most support a diagnosis of rheumatoid arthritis (RA)?
   A. Positive rheumatoid factor (RF)
   B. Leukocytosis
   C. Elevated erythrocyte sedimentation rate (ESR) and C-reactive protein (CRP)
   D. Elevated anticitrullinated protein/peptide antibody (ACPA)

2. Why would a positive RF be less specific for this patient?
   A. RF can be falsely negative because she had a fever within the past year.
   B. RF can be falsely positive in those with other autoimmune disease (e.g., celiac disease).
   C. RF is not accurate in a patient who is postmenopausal.
   D. RF will be accurate only if a rash is present.

3. Methotrexate is the recommended first line of treatment for RA. However, what pertinent aspect of the patient's history would most defer starting methotrexate?

   A. Current tobacco use

   B. Age

   C. Heavy alcohol use

   D. Celiac disease

4. When discussing further treatment options, what education should be provided to the patient about treatment with nonsteroidal anti-inflammatory drugs (NSAIDs) versus disease-modifying antirheumatic drugs (DMARDs) for RA?

   A. NSAIDs, unlike DMARDs, do not inhibit progression of structural joint damage of those suffering from RA.

   B. NSAIDs have no benefit in relieving symptoms of RA compared with placebo.

   C. NSAIDs, although infrequently, can worsen RA as they can inadvertently increase inflammatory markers.

   D. DMARDs have no benefit in relieving symptoms of RA compared with placebo.

BIBLIOGRAPHY

Atzeni, F., Talotta, R., Masala, I. F., Bongiovanni, S., Boccassini, L., & Sarzi-Puttini, P. (2017). Biomarkers in rheumatoid arthritis. *The Israel Medical Association Journal: IMAJ, 19*(8), 512–516.

Giannini, D., Antonucci, M., Petrelli, F., Bilia, S., Alunno, A., & Puxeddu, I. (2020). One year in review 2020: Pathogenesis of rheumatoid arthritis. *Clinical and Experimental Rheumatology, 38*(3), 387–397.

Lin, Y. J., Anzaghe, M., & Schülke, S. (2020). Update on the pathomechanism, diagnosis, and treatment options for rheumatoid arthritis. *Cells, 9*(4), 880. https://doi.org/10.3390/cells9040880

Moreland, L. W., & Cannella, A. (2018, May 31). *General principles of management of rheumatoid arthritis in adults.* In P. L. Romain (Ed.), *UpToDate.* https://www.uptodate.com/contents/general-principles-of-management-of-rheumatoid-arthritis-in-adults?source=search_result&search=treatment%20rheumatoid%20arthritis&selectedTitle=1

Scherer, H. U., Häupl, T., & Burmester, G. R. (2020). The etiology of rheumatoid arthritis. *Journal of Autoimmunity, 110*, 102400. https://doi.org/10.1016/j.jaut.2019.10240

Venables, P. J. W. (2017, October 12). *Clinical manifestations of rheumatoid arthritis.* In P. L. Romain (Ed.), *UpToDate.* https://www.uptodate.com/contents/clinical-manifestations-of-rheumatoid-arthritis?source=search_result&search=rheumatoid%20arthritis&selectedTitle=2

Wasserman, A. (2018). Rheumatoid arthritis: Common questions about diagnosis and management. *American Family Physician, 97*(7), 455–462.

SPONDYLOARTHROPATHIES

Dolores Diana Zollo

DEFINITION

A. Spondyloarthropathies are a group of overlapping disorders that share certain genetic predisposing factors and clinical features.

B. Clinical characterizations of spondyloarthropathies include inflammatory back pain, dactylitis (inflammation of the entire digit), enthesitis (inflammation at sites where tendons, ligaments, or joint capsules attach to the bone), and extra-articular manifestations such as uveitis and dermatologic changes.

   1. Inflammatory back pain is their most characteristic feature.

C. Disorders included are ankylosing spondylitis (AS), psoriatic arthritis (PsA), reactive arthritis (ReA), undifferentiated spondylitis, and inflammatory bowel disease (IBD)-associated spondyloarthropathy.

D. Also known as seronegative spondyloarthropathies. Seronegative spondyloarthropathies share similarities in clinical manifestations and have a genetic makeup that suggests they share pathogenic mechanisms.

INCIDENCE

A. Males are more often affected than females.

   1. Ratio of about 2:1 or 3:1.

B. Onset is typically before age 40.

C. AS is common to manifest in late teens and early 20s.

PATHOGENESIS

A. The cause of spondyloarthropathies is not well-understood.

B. It appears to have a genetic relationship with HLA-B27.

   1. B27 composes more than half of the genetic component.

C. Some theories exist that attribute microbial exposure as a possible cause, for example, chlamydia-induced arthritis, PsA, and the development of arthritis in patients with IBD such as Crohn's disease and ulcerative colitis.

   1. Manifestations can be triggered by gastrointestinal bacterial species such as *Shigella, Salmonella, Yersinia*, and *Campylobacter*, as well as genital species including *Chlamydia trachomatis*.

PREDISPOSING FACTORS

A. Male sex assigned at birth.

B. Genetic predisposition.

C. Bacterial infections.

SUBJECTIVE DATA

A. Common complaints/symptoms.

   1. The initial symptom is dull back pain with insidious onset, felt deep in the lower lumbar or gluteal region, with duration of greater than 3 months.

     a. Back pain and physical findings mirror the "inflammatory pattern," often before 40 years of age. It improves with exercise but returns with rest. Nocturnal pain forces the patient to get out of bed and move.

     b. Specific findings include loss of spinal mobility, especially lumbar extension or anterior lateral flexion and chest expansion.

     c. Another characteristic can be relief of pain within 24 to 48 hours of taking nonsteroidal anti-inflammatory drugs (NSAIDs). Indomethacin is the treatment of choice.

   2. Peripheral arthritis will affect the knees and ankles predominantly and will often be asymmetrical, affecting one to three joints.

   3. Ocular complaints include redness, pain, and photophobia. These may be the first presenting symptoms of spondyloarthropathy.

B. Common/typical scenario.

1. AS will progress in cephalad or axial direction, with limited chest expansion.

2. Cardiac disease characterized by aortic and mitral root dilation, as well as conduction defects and regurgitation, will manifest in severe disease.

3. Constitutional symptoms are typically absent.

4. PsA may present with symmetric polyarthritis similar to rheumatoid arthritis (RA) due to being immune-mediated. Patients usually have psoriasis. Pitting of the nails and onycholysis are also common.

5. ReA (formerly Reiter syndrome) will present with oligoarthritis, conjunctivitis, urethritis, and often mouth lesions. Patients will often report a history of enteric or sexually transmitted infections (STIs).

  a. Systemic symptoms such as fever, malaise, and weight loss are more common.

  b. Extra-articular involvement is key, including the eyes, skin, nails, genitalia, and mucous membranes.

C. Family/social history.

1. Family history.

  a. Spondyloarthropathies.

  b. IBD.

2. Social history.

  a. Sexual activity.

  b. Exercise.

D. Review of systems.

1. Back pain.

2. Joint pain.

3. Swelling.

4. Eye pain.

5. Eye redness.

6. Mucosal ulcers.

7. Rashes.

8. Changes in nails.

9. Vomiting.

10. Bowel changes.

11. Diarrhea.

12. Dysuria.

13. Genital discharge.

14. Fever.

15. Weight loss.

PHYSICAL EXAMINATION

A. Musculoskeletal findings include the following:

1. Decreased range of motion (ROM) in the back over time.

2. Edema in peripheral arthritis.

3. Enthesitis or bony tenderness most commonly occurs in the heel or Achilles tendon, but can be seen in the following:

  a. Iliac crests.

  b. Greater trochanters.

  c. Epicondyles and tibial plateaus.

  d. Costochondral junctions of the sternum.

  e. Humeral tuberosities and manubrial-sternal joints.

  f. Occiput.

  g. Spinous processes.

4. Dactylitis is a characteristic feature of spondyloarthropathies, especially PsA and less frequently ReA. The physical finding is also known as "sausage toe or sausage finger" and is characterized by swelling of the entire digit without pain or tenderness.

5. Ocular findings include nonpurulent conjunctivitis and anterior uveitis.

6. Dermatologic findings include psoriasis and pitting nails, particularly in patients with peripheral joint manifestations.

DIAGNOSTIC TESTS

A. No laboratory tests are specific for spondyloarthropathies.

B. HLA-B27: 90% of patients with AS and 50% to 70% of patients with other types of spondyloarthropathies will be positive.

C. Negative test for rheumatoid factor (RF) or antinuclear antibodies. Anticyclic citrullinated peptide (anti-CCP) antibodies may be present in about 10% of cases.

D. Elevated erythrocyte sedimentation rate (ESR) and C-reactive protein (CRP) are elevated in about 50% of patients. They are also used to assess radiographic progression and response to therapy.

E. Uric acid levels may be high with PsA.

F. Synovial fluid cultures in ReA are negative.

G. Axial signs on radiographs: Findings of bilateral symmetric sacroiliitis, as well as erosions, ankylosis, changes in joint width, or sclerosis, of the spine are specific for spondyloarthropathies; however, it takes several years to be visible on radiograph. Syndesmophytes can develop on the spine, which are ossifications that can bridge the intervertebral space resulting in the "bamboo spine" pattern.

H. MRI can be useful in patients with nonradiographic evidence of spondyloarthropathies.

1. MRI is much more sensitive in detecting early intra-articular inflammation, changes in cartilage, and bone marrow edema in sacroiliitis than radiography.

I. Ultrasound has been used to confirm enthesitis and tendon sheath effusions.

DIFFERENTIAL DIAGNOSIS

A. Degenerative disc disease.

B. Kyphosis.

C. Spine fractures, dislocations, or history of trauma.

D. Osteoarthritis (OA).

E. Spinal stenosis.

EVALUATION AND MANAGEMENT PLAN

A. General plan.

1. Reduce swelling and pain by addressing the inflammatory reaction.

2. Treat infectious processes and skin disorders.

B. Patient/family teaching points.

1. Encourage home exercise program including spinal extension exercises.

2. Patient education, outpatient physical therapy, home exercise, and proper posturing can be helpful nonpharmacologic interventions.

C. Pharmacotherapy.

1. NSAID therapy is the first-line agent (use with caution in patients with IBD and patients with kidney disease).

2. Tumor necrosis factor (TNF) inhibitors have been used for NSAID-refractory cases of AS and methotrexate-refractory cases of PsA. Both may also be used in ReA.

3. Methotrexate is used in PsA to treat both cutaneous and prominent peripheral arthritic manifestations.

4. Monoclonal antibody therapy has been used in PsA patients who do not respond to TNF inhibitors.

5. Sulfasalazine is a second-line agent used when patients do not respond to NSAIDs or cannot tolerate them. It can be used for a short-term treatment in AS and is more effective with peripheral arthritis than axial involvement.

6. Psoralen and ultraviolet A (PUVA) therapy for psoriasis skin lesions.

7. Antibiotics may be needed to treat gastrointestinal (GI) or genitourinary infections in patients with ReA.

FOLLOW-UP

A. Interval follow-up is necessary to monitor medication safety and patient's response to therapy.

CONSULTATION/REFERRAL

A. Physical therapy for exercise regimens.
B. Dermatology for skin manifestations.
C. Gastroenterology for GI manifestations.
D. Ophthalmology for ocular manifestations.
E. Infectious disease for STIs or other infectious diseases.

SPECIAL/GERIATRIC CONSIDERATIONS

A. Markers of disease progression and treatment do not appear to be age-related.
B. Standard precautions in older adult patients related to pharmacokinetics still apply.

CASE SCENARIO: SPONDYLOARTHROPATHIES

A 25-year-old patient presents to the clinic with no significant medical history or surgical history but reports a distant family history of autoimmune diseases. He presents with a dull low back pain (LBP) that radiates into his gluteal regions bilaterally, which has been occurring for a couple of months. He reports that he feels extremely stiff in the morning but that the pain improves throughout the day when he moves around. He also reports that the pain wakes him up at night and that he took acetaminophen with no relief. He denies any recent trauma, fever or chills, or weight loss. Vitals are within normal range. On exam, he has limited extension and flexion of his spine. There is a soft diastolic murmur on auscultation and decreased chest expansion with inhalation. The lungs are clear. There is point tenderness on palpation of both sacroiliac (SI) joints and pain with range of motion (ROM) of both hips. He denies leg weakness or paresthesias.

1. Which diagnostic test should be ordered to better evaluate his condition?
A. Ultrasound-guided hip aspirations
B. X-rays, including anteroposterior (AP), of the pelvis and lumbar spine
C. Routine bloodwork, including C-reactive protein (CRP) and erythrocyte sedimentation rate (ESR)
D. Urinalysis and urine culture

2. What would be the first-line agent for treatment?
A. Steroid taper
B. Anti-tumor necrosis factor (TNF) therapy
C. Outpatient physical therapy
D. Nonsteroidal anti-inflammatory drugs (NSAID) therapy

3. What genetic component or laboratory study may help in the diagnosis of this patient's condition?
A. Human leukocyte antigen (HLA)-B27
B. Rheumatoid factor
C. Anticyclic citrullinated peptide (anti-CCP) antibodies
D. Serum uric acid

BIBLIOGRAPHY

Hannon, R. A., & Porth, C. M. (2017). *Porth pathophysiology: Concepts of altered health states* (2nd ed.). Wolters Kluwer.

Kataria, R. K., & Brent, L. H. (2004, June 15). *Spondyloarthropathies. American Academy of Family Physicians.* https://www.aafp.org/afp/2004/0615/afp20040615p2853.pdf

Longo, F. (2022). *Harrison's principles of internal medicine, Vol. 1 and 2; 18th Edition* (Revised ed ed., Vol. 2). McGraw Hill Education Books USA

Papadakis, M. A., McPhee, S. J., & Rabow, M. W. (2016). *Current medical diagnosis & treatment 2016.* McGraw Hill Education.

Yu, D. T., & van Tubergen, A. (2018, September 7). *Overview of the clinical manifestations and classification of spondyloarthritis.* In P. L. Romain (Ed.), *UpToDate.* https://www.uptodate.com /contents/overview-of-the-clinical-manifestations-and-classification-of-spondyloarthritis?source=search_result&search=spondyloarthropathy &selectedTitle=1

Yu, D. T., & van Tubergen, A. (2019, January 1). *Pathogenesis of spondyloarthritis.* In P. L. Romain (Ed.), *UpToDate.* https://www.uptodate.com /contents/pathogenesis-of-spondyloarthritis?source=search_result&

SYSTEMIC LUPUS ERYTHEMATOSUS

Monica Richey

DEFINITION

A. Systemic lupus erythematosus (SLE) is a chronic inflammatory disorder characterized by:
1. Multisystem involvement.
2. Presence of antinuclear antibodies.
B. It has a chronic relapsing nature.
C. The course of the disease is variable, alternating between periods of stable disease (remission) and/or flares with high disease activity.

INCIDENCE/EPIDEMIOLOGY

A. The incidence of SLE in the United States ranges from 2.0 to 7.6 cases per 100,000 persons per year.
B. Prevalence ranges from 14.6 to 68 cases per 100,000 persons.

C. Affects more females than males with a ratio of 9:1, with a higher incidence among women of childbearing age.

D. Disproportionately affects more Black women, with a three to four times higher prevalence than Whites.

E. There is a higher incidence of SLE among the Afro-Caribbean, Asian, American Indian, and Hispanic descent populations as compared with the White population.

F. Black, Asian, and Hispanic individuals with SLE tend to develop more severe disease, exhibit a greater number of manifestations, and rapidly accumulate damage from lupus. Even after considering socioeconomic factors, race/ethnicity remains a key determinant of poor outcomes.

G. Male patients tend to have severe manifestations at the time of diagnosis.

PATHOGENESIS

A. SLE can be set off by a combination of predisposing genetic traits, hormonal and environmental factors, or infectious agents.

B. These result in an abnormal immune response with dysregulation of B- and T-cells, resulting in the following:

1. Production and formation of autoantibodies.
2. Complement fixing.
3. Immune complexes that promote inflammation and tissue damage.

SUBJECTIVE DATA

A. Common complaints/symptoms.

1. Cutaneous manifestations: Petechiae, vasculitis, malar rash, Raynaud, and livedo reticularis.
2. Joint pain.
3. Fatigue.
4. Fever.
5. Chest pain and shortness of breath.
6. Leg swelling.
7. Lymphadenopathy.
8. Alopecia.
9. Memory loss.

B. Common/typical scenario.

1. Typically presents with fever, joint pain, and rash in women of childbearing age.

C. Family and social history.

1. More than 126 genes are involved in the development of lupus.
2. There are currently no screening or genetic tests available.
3. Children whose mothers have SLE have a 20% risk of developing lupus if they are female and 5% if they are male.

D. Review of systems.

1. Common questions.
   a. Onset of symptoms.
   b. Length of symptoms.
   c. New onset or previously experienced.
   d. Any triggers.
   e. Recent infections.
2. Constitutional.
   a. Fevers.
   b. Chills.
   c. Malaise.
   d. Weight loss.
3. Skin.
   a. Rashes.
   b. Photosensitivity.
4. Head, ear, eyes, nose, and throat (HEENT).
   a. Lymphadenopathy.
   b. Dry mouth/eye.
5. Cardiovascular.
   a. Chest pain.
   b. Palpitations.
6. Pulmonary.
   a. Shortness of breath.
   b. Pleuritic chest pain.
7. Peripheral vascular.
   a. Edema.
   b. Raynaud.
   c. Wounds.
8. Musculoskeletal.
   a. Joint pain or swelling.
   b. Muscle weakness.
   c. Joint deformities.
9. Gastrointestinal.
   a. Nausea.
   b. Vomiting.
   c. Changes in stools.
   d. Abdominal pain.

PHYSICAL EXAMINATION

A. Physical examination for SLE requires a full head-to-toe examination.

B. Cutaneous manifestations.

1. Cutaneous vasculitis: Palpable petechiae in dependent areas, cutaneous necrosis, ulceration, and gangrene.
2. Raynaud phenomenon: Red, white, and blue, independent of disease activity, ulceration, atrophy, and gangrene.
3. Livedo reticularis: Antiphospholipid syndrome (APS), blanchable red-purple ring, and lace-like.
4. Photosensitivity: Rashes, fever, malaise, adenopathy, and arthritis.
5. Malar rash: Erythematous, edematous, and spares the nasolabial folds.
6. Mucocutaneous lesions: Upper palate, may be painless, and sharply marginated.
7. Alopecia: Diffuse or patchy, reversible, or permanent.

C. Musculoskeletal manifestations.

1. Arthralgias.
2. Arthritis.
3. Myalgia and myositis.

D. Pulmonary manifestations.

1. Pleurisy.
2. Acute lupus pneumonitis: 80% mortality rate.
3. Interstitial lung disease ground glass or honeycomb.

4. Pulmonary embolus.

5. Pulmonary hemorrhage.

6. Pulmonary hypertension.

7. Shrinking lung syndrome.

E. Cardiac/peripheral vascular manifestations: Add imaging as needed.

　　1. Pericarditis (echo).

　　2. Myocarditis and myocardial dysfunction.

　　3. Myocardial infarction (MI).

　　4. Deep vein thrombosis (DVT).

　　5. Edema.

F. Central nervous system (CNS) manifestations (19 different manifestations).

　　1. Central.

　　　　a. Aseptic meningitis.

　　　　b. Cardiovascular (CV) disease.

　　　　c. Demyelinating syndrome.

　　　　d. Headache.

　　　　e. Movement disorder.

　　　　f. Myelopathy.

　　　　g. Seizure disorder.

　　　　h. Acute confusional state.

　　　　i. Anxiety disorder.

　　　　j. Cognitive dysfunction.

　　　　k. Mood disorder.

　　　　l. Psychosis.

　　　　m. CNS vasculitis: Fevers, seizures, meningismus, and altered behavior patterns.

　　2. Peripheral.

　　　　a. Guillain–Barré syndrome and autonomic neuropathy.

　　　　b. Mononeuropathy.

　　　　c. Myasthenia gravis.

　　　　d. Cranial neuropathy.

　　　　e. Plexopathy.

　　　　f. Polyneuropathy.

　　3. Hematologic manifestations.

　　　　a. Anemia.

　　　　b. Thrombocytopenia.

　　　　c. Leukopenia.

　　　　d. Pancytopenia.

　　4. Renal manifestations.

　　　　a. Proteinuria.

　　　　b. Elevated serum creatinine.

DIAGNOSTIC TESTS

A. The diagnosis of lupus is based on clinical presentation and laboratory analysis.

B. The clinician should suspect lupus if 2+ organ systems are involved.

　　1. Positive laboratory workup only with no symptoms does not give the diagnosis and does not require treatment.

C. Drug-induced SLE should be ruled out if there is presence of the following medications:

　　1. Anti-tumor necrosis factor (TNF).

　　2. Hydralazine.

　　3. Anticonvulsants.

　　4. Isoniazid.

　　5. Thorazine.

　　6. Procainamide.

　　7. Penicillamine.

　　8. Minocycline.

D. Laboratory workup for diagnosis.

　　1. Complete blood count (CBC)/comprehensive metabolic panel (CMP)/elevated erythrocyte sedimentation rate (ESR)/C-reactive protein (CRP)/antinuclear antibody (ANA).

　　2. Antihistone (if applicable).

　　3. ANA: Never to be ordered without full serologies.

　　4. Anti-double-stranded DNA (DsDNA).

　　5. C3.

　　6. C4.

　　7. Anti-Smith antibody.

　　8. Ribonucleoprotein (RNP).

　　9. Anti-Ro (SSa).

　　10. Anti-La (SSb).

　　11. Urine with microscopy.

E. Laboratory workup for flares.

　　1. CBC/CMP/ESR/CRP.

　　2. C3.

　　3. C4.

　　4. DsDNA.

　　5. Urine with microscopy.

F. Diagnostic criteria.

　　1. The 1997 update of the 1982 American College of Rheumatology revised the criteria for classification of SLE (Table 14.1).

　　2. 2019 European League Against Rheumatism/American College of Rheumatology classification criteria for SLE (Figure 14.2).

　　3. 2012 SLICC/ACR Damage Index for SLE (Table 14.2)

　　4. These criteria are used mostly in clinical trials and population studies rather than for diagnostic purposes.

DIFFERENTIAL DIAGNOSIS

A. Malignancies.

B. Infectious processes (cytomegalovirus [CMV], Epstein–Barr virus [EBV], HIV, and hepatitis).

C. Rheumatoid arthritis (RA).

D. Scleroderma.

E. Fibromyalgia.

F. Thrombotic thrombocytopenia purpura (TTP).

G. Multiple sclerosis.

H. Myositis/dermatomyositis.

EVALUATION AND MANAGEMENT PLAN

A. In 2019 the European Alliance of Associations for rheumatology released a new series of recommendation for the management of SLE.

　　1. Treatment in SLE should aim at remission or low disease activity and prevention of flares in all organs, maintained with the lowest possible dose of glucocorticoids (GCs).

　　2. Flares of SLE can be treated according to the severity of organ(s) involvement by adjusting ▶

TABLE 14.1 1997 UPDATE OF THE 1982 AMERICAN COLLEGE OF RHEUMATOLOGY REVISED CRITERIA FOR CLASSIFICATION OF SYSTEMIC LUPUS ERYTHEMATOSUS

Criterion	Definition
1. Malar rash	Fixed erythema, flat and raised, over the malar eminences, tending to spare the nasolabial folds
2. Discoid rash	Erythematous raised patches with adherent keratotic scaling and follicular plugging; atrophic scarring may occur in older lesions
3. Photosensitivity	Skin rash as a result of unusual reaction to sunlight, by patient history or physician observation
4. Oral ulcers	Oral or nasopharyngeal ulceration, usually painless, observed by physician
5. Nonerosive arthritis	Involving two or more peripheral joints, characterized by swelling, tenderness, or effusion
6. Pleuritis or pericarditis	Pleuritis: Convincing history of pleuritic pain or rubbing heard by a physician or evidence of pleural effusion OR Pericarditis: Documented by EKG, or rub or evidence of pericardial effusion
7. Renal disorder	Persistent proteinuria >0.5 g/d or >3+ if quantitation not performed OR Cellular casts: May be red cell, hemoglobin, granular, tubular, or mixed
8. Neurologic disorder	Seizures: In the absence of offending drugs or known metabolic derangements (e.g., uremia, ketoacidosis, electrolyte imbalance) OR Psychosis: In the absence of offending drugs or known metabolic derangements (e.g., uremia, ketoacidosis, electrolyte imbalance)
9. Hematologic disorder	Hemolytic anemia: With reticulocytosis OR Leukopenia: <4,000/mm³ on ≥2 occasions OR Lymphopenia: <1,500/mm³ on ≥2 occasions OR Thrombocytopenia: <100,000/mm³ in the absence of offending drugs
10. Immunologic disorder	Anti-DNA: Antibody to native DNA in abnormal titer OR Anti-Sm: Presence of antibody to Sm nuclear antigen OR Positive finding of antiphospholipid antibodies on: ■ An abnormal serum level of IgG of IgM anticardiolipin antibodies ■ A positive test result for lupus anticoagulant using a standard method, or ■ A false-positive test result for at least 6 months confirmed by *Treponema pallidum* immobilization or fluorescent treponemal antibody absorption test
11. Positive antinuclear antibody	An abnormal titer of antinuclear antibody by immunofluorescence or an equivalent assay at any time and in the absence of drugs

IgG, immunoglobulin M; IgM, immunoglobulin M.

ongoing therapies (GCs, immunomodulating agents) to higher doses, switching, or adding new therapies.

3. Treatment of SLE.

a. Hydroxychloroquine (HCQ) is recommended for all patients with SLE unless contraindicated, at a dose not exceeding 5 mg/kg.

b. In the absence of risk factors for retinal toxicity, ophthalmologic screening (by visual fields examination and/or spectral domain-optical coherence tomography) should be performed at baseline, after 5 years, and yearly thereafter.

c. GC can be used at doses and route of administration that depend on the type and severity of organ involvement.

d. Pulses of intravenous (IV) methylprednisolone (usually 250–1,000 mg/d, for 1–3 days) provide immediate therapeutic effect and enable the use of lower starting dose of oral GC.

Entry criterion
Antinuclear antibodies (ANA) at a titer or ≥1:80 on HEp-2 cells or an equivalent positive test (ever)

↓

If absent, do not classify as SLE
If present, apply additive criteria

↓

Additive criteria
Do not count a criterion if there is a more likely explanation than SLE.
Occurrence of a criterion on at least one occasion is sufficient.
SLE classification requires at least one clinical criterion and ≥10 points.
Criteria need not occur simultaneously.
Within each domain, only the highest weighted criterion is counted toward the total score§.

Clinical domains and criteria	Weight	Immunology domains and criteria	Weight
Constitutional		**Antiphospholipid antibodies**	
Fever	2	Anti-cardiolipin antibodies OR	
Hematologic		Anti-β2GP1 antibodies OR	
Leukopenia	3	Lupus anticoagulant	2
Thrombocytopenia	4	**Complement proteins**	
Autoimmune hemolysis	4	Low C3 OR low C4	3
Neuropsychiatric		Low C3 AND low C4	4
Delirium	2	**SLE-specific antibodies**	
Psychosis	3	Anti-dsDNA antibody OR	
Seizure	5	Anti-Smith antibody	6
Mucocutaneous			
Non-scarring alopecia	2		
Oral ulcers	2		
Subacute cutaneous OR discoid lupus	4		
Acute cutaneous lupus	6		
Serosal			
Pleural or pericardial effusion	5		
Acute pericarditis	6		
Musculoskeletal			
Joint involvement	6		
Renal			
Proteinuria >0.5g/24h	4		
Renal biopsy Class II or V lupus nephritis	8		
Renal biopsy Class III or IV lupus nephritis	10		

Total score:

↓

Classify as Systemic Lupus Erythematosus with a score of 10 or more if entry criterion fulfilled.

FIGURE 14.2 2019 European League Against Rheumatism/America College of Rheumatology classification criteria for systemic lupus erythematosus.

DsDNA, double-stranded DNA; SLE, systemic lupus erythematosus.

e. For chronic maintenance treatment, GC should be minimized to less than 7.5 mg/d (prednisone equivalent) and, when possible, withdrawn.

f. Prompt initiation of immunomodulatory agents can expedite the tapering/discontinuation of GC.

g. Immunosuppressive therapies.

i. In patients not responding to HCQ (alone or in combination with GC) or patients unable to reduce GC below doses acceptable for chronic use, addition of immunomodulating/immunosuppressive agents such as methotrexate, azathioprine, or mycophenolate should be considered.

ii. Immunomodulating/immunosuppressive agents can be included in the initial therapy in cases of organ-threatening disease.

TABLE 14.2   2012 SLICC/ACR DAMAGE[a] INDEX FOR SYSTEMIC LUPUS ERYTHEMATOSUS

Item	Score
Ocular (either eye, by clinical assessment) • Any cataract ever • Retinal change OR optic atrophy	1 1
Neuropsychiatric • Cognitive impairment (e.g., memory deficit, difficulty with calculation, poor concentration, difficulty in spoken or written language, impaired performance level) OR major psychosis • Seizures requiring therapy for 6 months • Cerebrovascular accident ever (score 2 of >1) • Cranial or peripheral neuropathy (excluding optic) • Transverse myelitis	1 1 1 (2) 1 1
Renal • Estimated or measured glomerular filtration rate <50% • Proteinuria ≥3.5 g/24 hr OR • End-stage renal disease (regardless of dialysis or transplantation)	1 1 3
Pulmonary • Pulmonary hypertension (right ventricular prominence, or loud P2) • Pulmonary fibrosis (physical and radiograph) • Shrinking lung (radiograph) • Pleural fibrosis (radiograph) • Pulmonary infarction (radiograph)	1 1 1 1 1
Cardiovascular • Angina OR coronary artery bypass • Myocardial infarction ever (score 2 if >1) • Cardiomyopathy (ventricular dysfunction) • Valvular disease (diastolic, murmur, or systolic murmur >3/6) • Pericarditis for 6 months OR pericardiectomy	1 1 (2) 1 1 1
Peripheral vascular • Claudication for 6 months • Minor tissue loss (pulp space) • Significant tissue loss ever (e.g., loss of digit or limb; score 2 if >1 site) • Venous thrombosis with swelling, ulceration, OR venous stasis	1 1 1 (2) 1
Gastrointestinal • Infarction or resection of bowel below the duodenum, spleen, liver, or gallbladder ever, for any cause (score 2 if >1 site) • Mesenteric insufficiency • Chronic peritonitis • Stricture OR upper gastrointestinal tract surgery ever	1 (2) 1 1 1
Musculoskeletal • Muscle atrophy or weakness • Deforming or erosive arthritis (including reducible deformities, excluding avascular necrosis) • Osteoporosis with fracture or vertebral collapse (excluding avascular necrosis) • Avascular necrosis (score 2 if >1) • Osteomyelitis	1 1 1 1 (2) 1
Skin • Scarring chronic alopecia • Extensive scarring or panniculus other than scalp and pulp space • Skin ulceration (excluding thrombosis) for >6 months	1 1 1
Premature gonadal failure	1
Diabetes (regardless of treatment)	1
Malignancy (exclude dysplasia; score 2 if >1 site)	1 (2)

[a]Damage (nonreversible change, not related to active inflammation) occurring since onset of lupus, ascertained by clinical assessment and present for at least 6 months unless otherwise stated. Repeat episodes must occur at least 6 months apart to score 2. The same lesion cannot be scored twice.

iii. Cyclophosphamide can be used for severe organ-threatening or life-threatening SLE as well as "rescue" therapy in patients not responding to other immunosuppressive agents.

h. Biologics.

i. In patients with inadequate response to standard of care (combinations of HCQ and GC with or without immunosuppressive agents), defined as residual disease activity not allowing tapering of GC and/or frequent relapses, add-on treatment with belimumab should be considered.

ii. In organ-threatening disease refractory or with intolerance/contraindications to standard immunosuppressive agents, rituximab can be considered.

i. Specific manifestations.

i. Skin disease.

1) First-line treatment of skin disease in SLE includes topical agents (GC, calcineurin inhibitors antimalarials [HCQ, quinacrine]) and/or systemic GC.

2) In nonresponsive cases or cases requiring high-dose GC, methotrexate, retinoids, dapsone, or mycophenolate can be added.

ii. Neuropsychiatric disease.

1) Attribution to SLE—as opposed to non-SLE-related neuropsychiatric manifestationsis essential and can be facilitated by neuroimaging, investigation of cerebrospinal fluid (CSF), consideration of risk factors (type and timing of the manifestation in relation to the onset of lupus, patient age, nonneurologic lupus activity, presence of antiphospholipid antibodies [aPL]), and exclusion of confounding factors.

2) Treatment of SLE-related neuropsychiatric disease includes GCs/immunosuppressive agents for manifestations considered to reflect an inflammatory process and antiplatelet/anticoagulants for atherothrombotic/aPL-related manifestations.

iii. Hematologic disease.

1) Acute treatment of lupus thrombocytopenia includes high-dose GC (including pulses of IV methylprednisolone) and/or intravenous immunoglobulin G (IVIG).

2) For maintenance of response, immunosuppressive/GC-sparing agents such as mycophenolate, azathioprine, or cyclosporine can be used.

3) Refractory cases can be treated with rituximab or cyclophosphamide.

iv. Renal disease.

1) Early recognition of signs of renal involvement and when present performance of a diagnostic renal biopsy is essential to ensure optimal outcomes.

2) Mycophenolate and low-dose IV cyclophosphamide are recommended as initial (induction) treatment as they have the best efficacy to toxicity ratio. In patients at high risk for renal failure (reduced glomerular filtration rate, histologic presence of fibrous crescents or fibrinoid necrosis, or tubular atrophy/interstitial fibrosis), similar regimens may be considered, but high-dose IV cyclophosphamide can also be used.

a) For maintenance therapy, mycophenolate or azathioprine should be used.

b) In cases with stable/improved renal function but incomplete renal response (persistent proteinuria >0.8–1 g/24 hours after at least 1 year of immunosuppressive treatment), repeat biopsy can distinguish chronic from active kidney lesions. Mycophenolate may be combined with a low dose of a calcineurin inhibitor in severe nephrotic syndrome or incomplete renal response in the absence of uncontrolled hypertension, high chronicity index on kidney biopsy, and/or reduced glomerular filtration rate (GFR).

v. Comorbidities.

1) APS.

a) All patients with SLE should be screened at diagnosis for aPL.

b) Patients with SLE with high-risk aPL profile (persistently positive medium/high titers or multiple positivity) may receive primary prophylaxis with antiplatelet agents, especially if other atherosclerotic/thrombophilic factors are present, after balancing the bleeding hazard.

c) For secondary prevention (thrombosis, pregnancy complication/loss), the therapeutic approach should be the same as for primary APS.

vi. Infectious diseases.

1) Patients with SLE should be assessed for general and disease-related risk factors for infections, such as advanced age/frailty, diabetes mellitus, renal involvement, immunosuppressive/biological therapy, and use of GC.

2) General preventive measures (including immunizations) and early recognition and treatment of infection/sepsis are recommended.

vii. CV disease.

1) Patients with SLE should undergo regular assessment for traditional and disease-related risk factors for CV disease, including persistently active disease, increased disease duration, medium/high titers of aPL, renal involvement (1b/B; especially persistent proteinuria and/or GFR).

viii. Management of lupus flares.

TABLE 14.3 PHARMACOTHERAPY FOR SLE

Medications	Uses	Side Effects
Topical steroids: For example, hydrocortisone, triamcinolone, fluocinolone	Can be used to treat lupus rashes and skin lesions—short-term use	
NSAIDs	Can be used to help treat arthralgias, polyarthritis, and myalgias Must add PPI Clinician should watch blood count and creatinine To be avoided if kidney involvement is present Never for long-term use	
Antimalarial drugs: The mainstay of SLE treatment and the most prescribed medication is HCQ at a dose 6.5 mg/kg up to a maximum of 400 mg daily; has less ocular and GI reactions than chloroquine	Modulate the immune system, reducing flares by as much as 50% May prevent activation of plasmacytoid dendritic cells Many benefits to the use of hydroxychloroquine, including maintaining remission and protecting against vascular and thrombotic events Is safe to use during pregnancy and while breastfeeding Protects against UV light and may improve skin lesions Can improve muscle and joint pain, pericarditis, pleuritis, fatigue, and fever	Prevalence of retinal toxicity was <2% during the first 10 years of use, but increased to ~20% after 20 years of routine HCQ use Patients to get an eye exam by an ophthalmologist prior to initiation and annually after 5 years of regular HCQ use Nausea and diarrhea: Most common side effects Skin rashes; bluish like color Cardiomyopathy (rare)
GC oral, IV, and topical forms Acthar Gel: Repository corticotropin injection; activates the adrenal gland to produce GCs; has the same effect and side effects as GCs.	Dose dependent on severity and complication Should be avoided as long-term treatment High-dose therapy to be reserved for organ-threatening presentation such as LN, hemolytic anemia, etc.	Decreased bone density, infections, sodium retention, edema, hypertension, glucose intolerance, hypokalemia, insomnia, euphoria, depression, and mania Osteonecrosis, moon face and buffalo hump, glaucoma, and cataracts
Methotrexate	Antimetabolite and cytotoxic agent, reduces antigen-dependent T-cell proliferation, and suppresses inflammation Dose varies in SLE patients from 10 to 25 mg weekly with folic acid or folinic acid supplementation Mostly used to treat joint pain, can be used or treat some skin manifestations of SLE	Anemia and neutropenia Stomatitis and oral ulcers (can be prevented or alleviated by folate) Nodulosis, hepatic fibrosis, pulmonary fibrosis, lethargy, fatigue, and renal insufficiency Hair loss Contraindicated in pregnancy, considered a teratogenic agent Should be given under cover of two forms of contraception
Mycophenolate mofetil	Inhibits B- and T-cell proliferation Used for organ-threatening disease such as LN Patients typically started at 500 mg/d, with maintenance target of 2–3 g/d No consistent data on the tapering schedule during maintenance phase	Serious infections and GI manifestations Contraindicated in pregnancy due to increased risk of birth defects and miscarriage Should be given under cover of two forms of contraception Stop at least 12 weeks before planned pregnancy

(continued)

TABLE 14.3   PHARMACOTHERAPY FOR SLE (*CONTINUED*)

Medications	Uses	Side Effects
Azathioprine (off-label use)	A prodrug that is converted to 6-mercaptopurine, its active metabolite Blocks T-lymphocytes Prior to initiation of treatment, patients to be screened for TPMT (enzyme) Takes 3 to 4 months for complete effectiveness Blood counts and liver function to be monitored every 1–3 months Dose varies from 50 to 150 mg daily (weight-based)	GI tract toxicity, oral ulcers, nausea, vomiting, diarrhea, and epigastric pain, dose-related toxicity to the bone marrow can lead to leukopenia, thrombocytopenia, and anemia Increased risk of lymphoma after 3 years of therapy Safe for use during pregnancy
Cyclophosphamide	Potent immunosuppressive and alkylating agent that depletes B- + T-cells Used to treat severe manifestations of autoimmune/inflammatory diseases Has a well-established efficacy in LN and is given in lower doses than typically prescribed for cancer chemotherapy Due to a high rate of clinical relapse, sometimes requires a repeated course of treatment Established efficacy in patients with LN	Nausea, vomiting, and hair loss (reversible) Increased risk of common and opportunistic infections Teratogenicity, sterility, and secondary hematologic malignancy Toxicity to the urinary bladder, including hemorrhagic cystitis and bladder cancer
Belimumab	Blocks the activity of B-cell lymphocytes Available in both subcutaneous and IV formulations Currently approved to be used in treatment of LN in addition to standard treatment Moderate efficacy in serologically active patients with skin and joint involvement	Infections, headaches, and depression
Rituximab (off-label use)	A chimeric anti-CD20 mAb that blocks B lymphocytes that are CD20 receptor-positive Used in refractory disease	Opportunistic infections and leukopenia, in rare cases Progressive multifocal leukoencephalopathy
Voclosporin	A next-generation calcineurin inhibitor approved in 2019 to be used in combination therapy for treatment of LN Is structurally like CsA but has increased potency and faster elimination Does not require drug levels to be checked	Opportunistic infections, GI disorders, kidney dysfunction, hyperkalemia, diabetes, and increase in blood pressure
Anifrolumab	Interferon type 1 blocker	Upper respiratory infections, urinary infection, bronchitis, herpes zoster, and opportunistic infections

CsA, cyclosporine A; GC, glucocorticoid; GI, gastrointestinal; HCQ, hydroxychloroquine; IV, intravenous; LN, lupus nephritis; mAb, monoclonal antibody; NSAIDs, nonsteroidal anti-inflammatory drugs; PPI, proton pump inhibitor; SLE, systemic lupus erythematosus; TPMT, thiopurine S-methyltransferase.

1) GC: Patients with organ disease require high doses of prednisone (1 mg/kg; up to 60 mg daily) or equivalent for 4 to 6 weeks, followed by taper of 10% per week.

2) Flares presenting with synovitis, fevers, rashes, or serositis are managed with lower doses (10–20 mg daily) with quick taper.

3) Long-term therapy with corticosteroids can lead to myopathy, osteoporosis, hypertension, diabetes, cataracts, atherosclerotic vascular disease, avascular necrosis of the bone, and infections.

B. Patient/family teaching points.

1. Exercise and healthy lifestyle may be important factors in mitigating symptoms.

2. The disease is lifelong, and the goal of care is to reduce flare-ups and attain low disease activity.

3. Medication compliance and discussion of possible side effects should be discussed with the patient and family.

C. Pharmacotherapy (Table 14.3).

FOLLOW-UP

A. Patient should always be referred to a rheumatologist as soon as possible for follow-up and further treatment decisions.

CONSULTATION/REFERRAL

A. Rheumatologist.

B. Other specialties as needed, including dermatology, nephrology, and cardiology.

C. Social work.

D. Physical/occupational therapy.

SPECIAL/GERIATRIC CONSIDERATIONS

A. Infections.

1. Patients with SLE/lupus nephritis (LN) are at increased risk of infections.

2. They should be encouraged to receive all inactivated vaccines, following the Centers for Disease Control and Prevention (CDC) recommendations for patients who are immunosuppressed.

B. Heart disease.

1. SLE patients have a 7.5-fold increase in coronary artery disease (CAD).

2. Routine care for patients with SLE should include:

a. Screening for CV risk factor.

b. Counseling for lifestyle modification, such as smoking cessation, encouraging physical activity, and weight loss.

c. Screening for symptoms suggestive of heart disease.

C. Contraception.

1. Contraceptive options and education should be offered to all women with SLE.

2. Intrauterine devices containing levonorgestrel are among the safest and most effective options.

3. Progesterone-only pills are also effective in long-term contraception.

4. Intense screening of risk factors for thrombotic events in women with SLE is important when prescribing contraceptives.

D. Osteoporosis.

1. Recommendations for patients taking GC for more than 3 months include smoking cessation, regular exercise, and the administration of calcium (1,200–1,500 mg) and vitamin D (800–1,000 international units).

2. All patients starting on chronic treatment with GC for more than 5 mg/d should be started on a bisphosphonate if there are no contraindications.

E. Pregnancy concerns.

1. SLE patients have worse outcomes with increased rates of the following:

a. Preeclampsia.

b. Fetal loss.

c. Preterm delivery (higher rates of delivery <34 weeks).

d. Fetal growth retardation (FGR).

e. Infants small for gestational age.

2. Blood pressure control is of utmost importance in managing SLE/LN patients during pregnancy.

3. Angiotensin-converting enzyme (ACE) inhibitors and angiotensin receptor blockers (ARBs) are contraindicated during all three trimesters of pregnancy.

a. Switch patients to other agents safer to use (if the potential benefits justify the potential risk to the fetus), such as methyldopa, labetalol, or nifedipine.

4. Due to immunosuppressants' fetal toxicity, only GCs, azathioprine, and HCQ can be used safely during pregnancy.

5. They should be managed by a high-risk obstetrician in a tertiary center with a multidisciplinary team approach.

CASE SCENARIO: SYSTEMIC LUPUS ERYTHEMATOSUS

A 25-year-old patient presents with 3 months of fever, weight loss of more than 20 lb, skin rashes, joint pain, and swelling. She reports fever of up to 102°F/38.8°C to 103°F/39.4°C that can last all day, with temporary relief from Tylenol. The patient takes Advil for joint pain and swelling, with minimal response, and reports being unable to care for her children due to loss of function of multiple joints, including the hands and shoulders. Facial rash is mildly pruritic and tender and is worse when exposed to sunlight. Symptoms started after the birth of the patient's second child. The patient reports a family history of rheumatoid arthritis (RA) in her mother and one cousin with systemic lupus erythematosus (SLE). Social history reveals no smoking, no alcohol, or substance use. Her blood pressure is 90/60, temperature 102.5°F/39.2°C, pulse 100 beats per minute, and weight 130 lb. Labs done at the urgent care center reveal the following: White blood cell count (WBC) 2.0, hemoglobin (HgB) 9, hematocrit (Hct) 26, and platelet (Ptl) 70; comprehensive metabolic panel (CMP): normal; erythrocyte sedimentation rate (ESR) 80, normal (0–20); C-reactive protein (CRP) 10, normal (0–4); and 2022 antinuclear antibody (ANA) 1:2560, homogeneous. She is referred to rheumatology and rheumatology labs show the following: C3 30; C4 10; double-stranded (DsDNA): negative; Smith: positive; ribonucleoprotein (RNP): negative; SSA: positive; SSB: negative. The diagnosis is SLE as per American College of Rheumatology, Systemic Lupus International Collaborating Clinics, and European League Against Rheumatism criteria. The patient is started on prednisone 40 mg daily, and hydroxychloroquine started at 200 mg daily as per her current weight. Follow-up with labs at 1 month shows the following: WBC 4.5, HgB 10.5, Plt 150, ESR 30, and CRP 4. Prednisone is tapered by 10 mg every 3 weeks; slow taper of prednisone is necessary as hydroxychloroquine can take up to 2 months to achieve therapeutic effect. At follow-up after 2 months, the patient is still on hydroxychloroquine 200 mg and prednisone 10 mg, and complete blood count (CBC)/CMP and ESR/CRP are normalized. Her DsDNA is 300, C3 40, and C4 12. It is normal to see variations in the levels of DsDNA, C3, and C4. DsDNA will always be positive despite disease activity, but in cases of severe variations can predict flares or worsening disease and organ-threatening disease. After 3 months, the patient has regained 20 lb. Hydroxychloroquine dose is increased to 400 mg daily. Prednisone is tapered to 5 mg daily, joint pain is persistent, and methotrexate 10 mg weekly with folic acid daily is started in addition to hydroxychloroquine (Plaquenil). Pregnancy planning and birth control in the setting of methotrexate is discussed with the patient. After 1 month, the patient reports minimal joint pain but no swelling. Her malar rash has resolved and she has no fevers. Treatment of SLE requires high doses of prednisone depending on disease activity and is tapered slowly. Monitoring of complications such as hypertension, diabetes, and weight gain is necessary. Patients usually require more than one medication to control SLE, usually hydroxychloroquine in combination with either disease-modifying antirheumatic drugs (DMARDs) or immunosuppressives and biologics.

1. What clinical labs should be ordered when systemic lupus erythematosus (SLE) is suspected?

A. Antinuclear antibody (ANA), complete blood count (CBC), comprehensive metabolic panel (CMP)

B. Erythrocyte sedimentation rate (ESR), C-reactive protein (CRP) urine

C. ANA, double-stranded DNA (DsDNA), ESR, CRP

D. ANA, DsDNA, Smith, ribonucleoprotein (RNP), SSA/SSBA, and complements, alongside CBC and CMP

2. How much prednisone should patients be prescribed?
A. 10 mg
B. 60 mg
C. 100 mg
D. 20 to 60 mg

3. What is the role of the primary care provider in the care of SLE?

A. None; the rheumatologist provides care

B. Works with the rheumatologist to treat complications of treatment and uses preventive care

C. Prescribes antimalarial drugs

D. Calls the rheumatologist periodically to check on the patient

BIBLIOGRAPHY

American College of Rheumatology Ad Hoc Committee on Systemic Lupus Erythematosus Guidelines. (1999). Guidelines for referral and management of systemic lupus erythematosus in adults. *Arthritis and Rheumatology, 42*(9), 1785–1796.

Aringer, M., Costenbader, K., Daikh, D., Brinks, R., Mosca, M., Ramsey-Goldman, R., Smolen, J. S., Wofsy, D., Boumpas, D. T., Kamen, D. L., Jayne, D., Cervera, R., Costedoat-Chalumeau, N., Diamond, B., Gladman, D. D., Hahn, B., Hiepe, F., Jacobsen, S., Khanna, D. ... Johnson, S. R. (2019). 2019 European league against rheumatism/American College of rheumatology classification criteria for systemic lupus erythematosus. *Arthritis & Rheumatology, 71*(9), 1400–1412.

Bailey, T., Rowley, K., & Bernknopf, A. (2011). A review of systemic lupus erythematosus and current treatment options. *Formulary, 46*, 178–194.

Bramham, K., Hunt, B. J., Bewley, S., Germain, S., Calatayud, I., Khamashta, M. A., & Nelson-Piercy, C. (2011). Pregnancy outcomes in systemic lupus erythematosus with and without previous nephritis. *The Journal of Rheumatology, 38*(9), 1906–1913.

Buckley, L., Guyatt, G., Fink, H. A., Cannon, M., Grossman, J., Hansen, K. E., Humphrey, M. B., Lane, N. E., Magrey, M., Miller, M., Morrison, L., Rao, M., Robinson, A. B., Saha, S., Wolver, S., Bannuru, R. R., Vaysbrot, E., Osani, M., Turgunbaev, M. ... McAlindon, T. (2017). 2017 American College of rheumatology guideline for the prevention and treatment of glucocorticoid-Induced osteoporosis. *Arthritis & Rheumatology, 69*(8), 1521–1537.

Chakravarty, E. F. (2008). What we talk about when we talk about contraception. *Arthritis & Rheumatology, 59*(6), 760–761.

Fanouriakis, A., & Bertsias, G. (2019). Changing paradigms in the treatment of systemic lupus erythematosus. *Lupus Science & Medicine, 6*(1), e000310.

Fanouriakis, A., Kostopoulou, M., Alunno, A., Aringer, M., Bajema, I., Boletis, J. N., Cervera, R., Doria, A., Gordon, C., Govoni, M., Houssiau, F., Jayne, D., Kouloumas, M., Kuhn, A., Larsen, J. L., Lerstrøm, K., Moroni, G., Mosca, M., Schneider, M. ... Boumpas, D. T. (2019). 2019 update of the EULAR recommendations for the management of systemic lupus erythematosus. *Annals of the Rheumatic Diseases, 78*(6), 736–745.

Faurschou, M., Mellemkjaer, L., Starklint, H., Kamper, A. L., Tarp, U., Voss, A., & Jacobsen, S. (2011). High risk of ischemic heart disease in patients with lupus nephritis. *The Journal of Rheumatology, 38*(11), 2400–2405.

Fava, A., & Petri, M. (2019). Systemic lupus erythematosus: Diagnosis and clinical management. *Journal of Autoimmunity, 96*, 1–13.

Gladman, D., Ginzler, E., Goldsmith, C., Fortin, P., Liang, M., Urowitz, M., Bacon, P., Bombardieri, S., Hanly, J., Hay, E., Isenberg, D., Jones, J., Kalunian, K., Maddison, P., Nived, O., Petri, M., Richter, M., Sanchez-Guerrero, J., Snaith, M. ... Zoma, A. (1996). The development and initial validation of the systemic lupus international collaborating clinics/American College of Rheumatology damage index for systemic lupus erythematosus. *Arthritis & Rheumatism: Official Journal of the American College of Rheumatology, 39*(3), 363–369.

Grossman, J. M., Gordon, R., Ranganath, V. K., Deal, C., Caplan, L., & Chen, W. (2010). American College of Rheumatology 2010 recommendations for the prevention and treatment of glucocorticoid-induced osteoporosis. *Arthritis Care & Research (Hoboken), 62*(11), 1515–1526.

Hahn, B. H., McMahon, M. A., Wilkinson, A., Wallace, W. D., Daikh, D. I., & Fitzgerald, J. D. (2012). American College of rheumatology guidelines for screening, treatment, and management of lupus nephritis. *Arthritis Care & Research (Hoboken), 64*(6), 797–808.

Hahn, B. H., & Wallace, D. J. (Eds.). (2013). B. H. Hahn& D. J. Wallace (Eds.), *Dubois' lupus erythematosus and related syndromes*, Elsevier/Saunders.

Hochberg, M. C. (1997). Updating the American College of rheumatology revised criteria for the classification of systemic lupus erythematosus. *Arthritis and Rheumatism, 40*(9), 1725. https://doi.org/10.1002/art.1780400928

Märker-Hermann, E., & Fischer-Betz, R. (2010). Rheumatic diseases and pregnancy. *Current Opinion in Obstetrics & Gynecology, 22*(6), 458–465. https://doi.org/10.1097/GCO.0b013e3283404d67

Markowitz, G. S., & D'agati, V. D. (2007). The ISN/RPS 2003 classification of lupus nephritis: an assessment at 3 years. *Kidney International, 71*(6), 491–495.

Michalski, J. P., & Kodner, C. (2010). Systemic lupus erythematosus: Safe and effective management in primary care. *Primary Care, 37*(4), 767–778. https://doi.org/10.1016/j.pop.2010.07.006

Morand, E. F., Furie, R., Tanaka, Y., Bruce, I. N., Askanase, A. D., Richez, C., Bae, S.-C., Brohawn, P. Z., Pineda, L., Berglind, A., Tummala, R., & for the TULIP-2 Trial Investigators. (2020). Trial of anifrolumab in active systemic lupus erythematosus. *New England Journal of Medicine, 382*(3), 211–221.

Mosca, M., Tani, C., Aringer, M., Bombardieri, S., Boumpas, D., & Brey, R. (2010). European League against rheumatism recommendations for monitoring patients with systemic lupus erythematosus in clinical practice and in observational studies. *Annals of the Rheumatic Diseases, 69*(7), 1269–1274. https://doi.org/10.1136/ard.2009.117200

TABLE 14.4   CLASSIFICATION OF VASCULITIS

Variable Vessel	Large Vessel	Medium Vessel	Small Vessel
Behçet disease Essential cryoglobulinemia	Takayasu arteritis Giant cell/temporal arteritis	Polyarteritis nodosa Kawasaki disease Buerger disease Primary angiitis of the central nervous system	Henoch–Schönlein purpura (IgA vasculitis) ANCA-associated disorders • Granulomatosis with polyangiitis • Microscopic polyangiitis • Eosinophilic granulomatosis with polyangiitis

ANCA, antineutrophil cytoplasmic antibodies; IgA, immunoglobulin A.

Podymow, T., August, P., & Akbari, A. (2010). Management of renal disease in pregnancy. *Obstetrics and Gynecology Clinics of North America*, 37(2), 195–210. https://doi.org/10.1016/j.ogc.2010.02.012

Rahman, A., & Isenberg, D. A. (2008). Systemic lupus erythematosus. *The New England Journal of Medicine*, 358(9), 929–939. https://doi.org/10.1056/NEJMra071297

Rovin, B. H., Teng, Y. O., Ginzler, E. M., Arriens, C., Caster, D. J., Romero-Diaz, J., Gibson, K., Kaplan, J., Lisk, L., Navarra, S., Parikh, S. V., Randhawa, S., Solomons, N., & Huizinga, R. B. (2021). Efficacy and safety of voclosporin versus placebo for lupus nephritis (AURORA 1): A double-blind, randomised, multicentre, placebo-controlled, phase 3 trial. *The Lancet*, 397(10289), 2070–2080.

Stojan, G., & Petri, M. (2018). Epidemiology of systemic lupus erythematosus: An update. *Current Opinion in Rheumatology*, 30(2), 144.

Tan, E. M., Cohen, A. S., Fries, J. F., Masi, A. T., McShane, D. J., & Rothfield, N. F. (1982). The 1982 revised criteria for the classification of systemic lupus erythematosus. *Arthritis and Rheumatism*, 25(11), 1271–1277. https://doi.org/10.1002/art.1780251101

Tunnicliffe, D. J., Singh-Grewal, D., Kim, S., Craig, J. C., & Tong, A. (2015). Diagnosis, monitoring, and treatment of systemic lupus erythematosus: A systematic review of clinical practice guidelines. *Arthritis Care & Research*, 67(10), 1440–1452. https://doi.org/10.1002/acr.22591

Turano, L. (2013). Premature atherosclerotic cardiovascular disease in systemic lupus erythematosus: Understanding management strategies. *Journal of Cardiovascular Nursing*, 28(1), 48–53. https://doi.org/10.1097/JCN.0b013e3182363e3b

Wallace, D. J. (2008). *Lupus: The essential clinician's guide* (1st ed., pp. 78–80). Oxford University Press.

VASCULITIS: VARIABLE VESSEL

Paul Kashmanian

DEFINITION

A. Part of a group of disorders that result from inflammatory changes to the walls of veins and arteries, causing damage to the mural structures, which ultimately may cause tissue ischemia and necrosis.

B. Nomenclature is changing for the specific forms of vasculitis based on the 2012 Revised Chapel Hill Consensus Conference (CHCC).

C. Two main types:

1. Behçet disease.
2. Essential cryoglobulinemia.

INCIDENCE

A. More common in patients of Asian, Turkish, and Middle Eastern descent.

B. Prevalence similar in men and women.

C. Commonly afflicts patients 20 to 40 years of age.

D. Disease is more severe in young male patients from Middle East or Far Eastern Asia.

PATHOGENESIS

A. Vasculitis can be a primary pathology or can be secondary to another underlying disease process (Table 14.4).

B. Direct injury to the vessel, infectious agents, or immune processes are known to cause vasculitis.

C. Secondary vascular injury may occur from physical agents such as cold and irradiation, mechanical injuries, and toxins.

1. Behçet disease.
   a. Affects both arteries and veins of all sizes.
2. Essential cryoglobulinemia.
   a. Cold-precipitated,immune-complex-mediated.
   b. Occurs in chronic underlying infection (hepatitis C most commonly), connective tissue disease, and lymphoproliferative disorders.

PREDISPOSING FACTORS

A. First-degree relative with Behçet disease increases risk of the disease.

B. Essential cryoglobulinemia is associated with chronic hepatitis C infection.

SUBJECTIVE DATA

A. Common complaints/symptoms.

1. Constitutional symptoms are common with all-size vessel vasculitis and include fever, weight loss, malaise, and arthralgias/arthritis.
2. Behçet disease.
   a. Aphthous lesions of mouth and genitals.
   b. Tender, erythematous popular lesions which ulcerate.
   c. Knee and ankle arthritis.
   d. Posterior uveitis and hypopyon.
   e. Neurologic conditions including sterile meningitis, cranial nerve palsies, seizures, encephalitis, mental status changes, and spinal cord lesions.
   f. Hypercoagulable states.
3. Essential cryoglobulinemia.
   a. Palpable purpura.
   b. Peripheral neuropathy.
   c. Abdominal pain.
   d. Digital gangrene.

e. Pulmonary disease.

f. Glomerulonephritis.

B. Common/typical scenario.

  1. Essential cryoglobulinemia.

    a. Purpura.

    b. Weakness.

    c. Arthralgia.

  2. Behçet disease.

    a. Recurrent, painful ulcers of mouth and genitals.

    b. Follicular rash.

    c. Uveitis.

    d. Sterile pustules at needlestick sites.

    e. Arthritis.

C. Family and social history.

  1. Essential cryoglobulinemia.

    a. Sexual history.

    b. Intravenous (IV) drug use.

    c. Family history of Behçet disease.

D. Review of systems.

  1. Essential cryoglobulinemia.

    a. Abdominal pain.

    b. Sensitivity to cold.

    c. Skin changes.

    d. Paresthesias.

    e. Weakness.

  2. Behçet disease.

    a. Mucosal ulcers.

    b. Skin nodules.

    c. Skin rashes.

    d. Joint pain.

    e. Eye pain.

    f. Photophobia.

    g. Eye redness.

    h. Visual changes.

    i. Headache.

    j. Weakness.

    k. Mental status changes.

    l. Chest pain.

    m. Dyspnea.

PHYSICAL EXAMINATION

A. Behçet disease.

  1. Aphthous ulcers of mouth and genitals.

  2. Follicular rash.

  3. Erythema nodosum-like lesions.

  4. Hypopyon.

B. Essential cryoglobulinemia.

  1. Palpable purpura.

  2. Peripheral sensorimotor deficits.

  3. Raynaud phenomenon.

DIAGNOSTIC TESTS

A. Behçet disease.

  1. Elevated erythrocyte sedimentation rate (ESR) and C-reactive protein (CRP).

  2. No definitive tests.

  3. Positive pathergy test: At least a 2-mm papule will develop 24 to 48 hours after needle insertion to the skin.

B. Essential cryoglobulinemia.

  1. Elevated liver enzymes.

  2. Positive cryoglobulins.

  3. Low C4 level.

DIFFERENTIAL DIAGNOSIS

A. Hepatitis B.

B. Hepatitis C.

C. HIV.

D. Connective tissue disease.

E. Lymphoproliferative disorders.

F. Other types of vasculitis.

EVALUATION AND MANAGEMENT PLAN

A. General plan.

  1. Based on cause and severity of the vasculitis.

  2. Alleviation of symptoms.

B. Patient/family teaching points.

  1. Regular follow-up is necessary to monitor condition.

  2. Patients should also be educated on side effects of medications used for treatment.

C. Pharmacotherapy.

  1. Behçet disease.

    a. Colchicine 0.6 mg one to three times per day and thalidomide 100 mg daily.

    b. Apremilast for oral ulcers.

    c. Corticosteroids or azathioprine for severe disease.

    d. Infliximab, cyclosporine, or cyclophosphamide for ocular and neurologic disease.

  2. Essential cryoglobulinemia.

    a. Corticosteroids and rituximab or cyclophosphamide for 2 to 4 months.

    b. Hepatitis C treatment.

FOLLOW-UP

A. Regular follow-up determined based on severity and cause of vasculitis.

CONSULTATION/REFERRAL

A. Based on cause and course of disease.

B. Consider:

  1. Ophthalmology.

  2. Dermatology.

  3. Infectious disease.

SPECIAL/GERIATRIC CONSIDERATIONS

A. Progression of these diseases is unpredictable and can affect basically all body systems.

B. Treatment is symptomatic alleviation.

BIBLIOGRAPHY

Hannon, R. A., & Porth, C. M. (2017). *Porth pathophysiology: Concepts of altered health states* (2nd ed.). Wolters Kluwer.

Merkel, P. A. (2019, March 1). *Overview of and approach to the vasculitides in adults*. In M. Ramirez Curtis (Ed.), *UpToDate*. https://www.uptodate.com/contents/overview-of-and-approach-to-the-vasculitides-in-adults/print

Papadakis, M. A., McPhee, S. J., & Rabow, M. W. (2016). *Current medical diagnosis & treatment 2016*. McGraw Hill Education.

Smith, E. L., & Yazici, Y. (2018, November 13). *Clinical manifestations and diagnosis of Behçet syndrome*. In M. Ramirez Curtis (Ed.), *UpToDate*. https://www.uptodate.com/contents/clinical-manifestations-and-diagnosis-of-behcets-syndrome

VASCULITIS: SMALL VESSEL

Paul Kashmanian

DEFINITION

A. Part of a group of disorders that result from inflammatory changes to the walls of veins and arteries, causing damage to the mural structures, which ultimately may cause tissue ischemia and necrosis.

B. Nomenclature is changing for the specific forms of vasculitis based on the 2012 Revised Chapel Hill Consensus Conference (CHCC).

C. There are several main types of small vessel vasculitis.

  1. Henoch–Schönlein purpura (immunoglobulin A [IgA] vasculitis).

  2. Antineutrophil cytoplasmic antibody (ANCA)-associated disorders.

    a. Granulomatosis with polyangiitis (formerly Wegener granulomatosis).

    b. Microscopic polyangiitis.

      i. Most common cause of pulmonary-renal syndromes.

      ii. Does not cause chronic upper respiratory tract disease.

      iii. Does not have granulomatous inflammation on biopsy.

    c. Eosinophilic granulomatosis with polyangiitis (formerly Churg–Strauss syndrome).

INCIDENCE

A. Henoch–Schönlein purpura (IgA vasculitis).

  1. 90% of cases occur in pediatric population.

  2. Most common systemic vasculitis of childhood.

B. ANCA-associated disorders.

  1. Granulomatosis with polyangiitis (formerly Wegener granulomatosis).

    a. 12 cases in 1 million people annually.

    b. Not sex-specific.

    c. Age of onset commonly fourth to fifth decades.

  2. Microscopic polyangiitis.

    a. Most common cause of pulmonary-renal syndromes.

  3. Eosinophilic granulomatosis with polyangiitis (formerly Churg–Strauss syndrome).

    a. Mean age of onset is 40 years.

    b. No sex specificity.

    c. Possibility of genetic predisposition.

PATHOGENESIS

A. Vasculitis can be a primary pathology or can be secondary to another underlying disease process.

B. Direct injury to the vessel, infectious agents, or immune processes are known to cause vasculitis.

C. Secondary vascular injury may occur from physical agents such as cold and irradiation, mechanical injuries, and toxins.

D. Small vessel vasculitis may also be associated with ANCA.

  1. Henoch–Schönlein purpura (IgA vasculitis): Associated with IgA subclass 1 deposition in vessel walls.

  2. ANCA-associated disorders.

    a. Granulomatosis with polyangiitis (formerly Wegener granulomatosis).

      i. Characterized by upper and lower respiratory tract disease and glomerulonephritis.

      ii. Fatal if not treated.

    b. Microscopic polyangiitis: Caused by necrotizing vasculitis.

    c. Eosinophilic granulomatosis with polyangiitis (formerly Churg–Strauss syndrome): Idiopathic in patients with asthma.

PREDISPOSING FACTORS

A. Henoch–Schönlein purpura (IgA vasculitis): Recent upper respiratory tract infections such as group A streptococcus account for approximately 50% of cases.

B. ANCA-associated disorders: Systemic diseases such as systemic lupus erythematous, rheumatoid conditions, and polychondritis can predispose patients.

  1. Granulomatosis with polyangiitis (formerly Wegener granulomatosis).

  2. Microscopic polyangiitis.

  3. Eosinophilic granulomatosis with polyangiitis (formerly Churg–Strauss syndrome).

SUBJECTIVE DATA

A. Common complaints/symptoms.

  1. Small vessel vasculitis will often present with purpura, vesiculobullous lesions, urticaria, glomerulonephritis, alveolar hemorrhage, cutaneous extravascular necrotizing granulomas, splinter hemorrhages, uveitis, episcleritis, and scleritis.

    a. Henoch–Schönlein purpura (IgA vasculitis).

      i. Palpable purpura usually on lower extremities, arthralgias of knees and ankles, abdominal pain, and hematuria.

    b. ANCA-associated disorders.

      i. Granulomatosis with polyangiitis (formerly Wegener granulomatosis).

        1) Upper respiratory tract: Nasal congestion, crusting, ulceration, bleeding, septal perforation, "saddle nose," sinusitis, otitis media, mastoiditis, gingival edema, stridor, and subglottic stenosis.

        2) Lower respiratory tract: Cough, dyspnea, and hemoptysis.

        3) Renal system: Hematuria, often not evident until disease is advanced (urinary tract disease [UTD]).

        4) Other systems: Arthritis, ocular manifestations such as proptosis, scleritis, episcleritis, conjunctivitis, skin lesions, and neuropathy.

        5) Deep vein thrombosis (DVT) and pulmonary embolism (PE) are also common.

ii. Microscopic polyangiitis.
   1) Palpable purpura.
   2) Ulcers.
   3) Splinter hemorrhages.
   4) Vesicular bullous lesions.
   5) Interstitial lung fibrosis.
   6) Pulmonary-renal syndromes.
iii. Eosinophilic granulomatosis with polyangiitis (formerly Churg–Strauss syndrome).
   1) Allergic rhinitis.
   2) Asthma.

B. Review of systems.
   1. Fever.
   2. Fatigue.
   3. Weight loss.
   4. Arthralgias.
   5. Respiratory symptoms (rhinorrhea, cough).
   6. Skin changes.
   7. Eye pain.
   8. Eye redness.
   9. Hematuria.

PHYSICAL EXAMINATION

A. Henoch–Schönlein purpura (IgA vasculitis).
   1. Palpable purpura most commonly noted along lower extremities and buttock.
B. ANCA-associated disorders.
   1. Granulomatosis with polyangiitis (formerly Wegener granulomatosis).
      a. Nasal examination will reveal the following:
         i. Congestion.
         ii. Crusting.
         iii. Ulceration.
         iv. Bleeding.
         v. Septal perforation.
      b. "Saddle nose" deformity is a late finding.
      c. Otitis media.
      d. Proptosis.
      e. Conjunctivitis.
      f. Scleritis.
      g. Episcleritis.
      h. Signs of DVT.
         i. Calf swelling.
         ii. Erythema.
         iii. Tenderness.
   2. Microscopic polyangiitis.
      a. Palpable purpura.
      b. Ulcers.
      c. Splinter hemorrhages.
      d. Vesiculobullous lesions.
      e. Pneumonitis.
   3. Eosinophilic granulomatosis with polyangiitis (formerly Churg–Strauss syndrome).
      a. Skin and lung involvement.
         i. Wheezing.
         ii. Rhinitis.
         iii. Macular rash.
         iv. Urticaria.
         v. Palpable purpura.

DIAGNOSTIC TESTS

A. Henoch–Schönlein purpura (IgA vasculitis).
   1. Skin biopsy will reveal leukocytoclastic vasculitis with IgA deposition. Kidney biopsy reserved for cases with severe kidney involvement if otherwise unclear presentation.
B. ANCA-associated disorders.
   1. Granulomatosis with polyangiitis (formerly Wegener granulomatosis).
      a. Leukocytosis, thrombocytosis, normocytic, and normochromic anemia.
      b. Elevated creatinine.
      c. Elevated C-reactive protein (CRP) and elevated erythrocyte sedimentation rate (ESR).
      d. Positive ANCA.
      e. Red cell casts and proteinuria.
      f. Lung biopsy more likely to show granulomas.
      g. Chest CT.
   2. Microscopic polyangiitis.
      a. 75% will be positive.
      b. Microscopic hematuria, proteinuria, and red blood cell casts.
      c. Renal biopsy for necrotizing glomerulonephritis.
   3. Eosinophilic granulomatosis with polyangiitis (formerly Churg–Strauss syndrome).
      a. Eosinophilia in peripheral blood smear.
      b. Positive ANCA.

DIFFERENTIAL DIAGNOSIS

A. Other types of vasculitis.
B. Infection.
C. Malignancy.
D. Atherosclerosis.
E. Thromboembolic disease.
F. Congenital/hereditary disorders.
G. Hypercoagulable states.
H. Inflammatory disorders (may want to consider making this a general differential diagnosis for all forms of vasculitis).

EVALUATION AND MANAGEMENT PLAN

A. General plan.
   1. Henoch–Schönlein purpura (IgA vasculitis).
      a. Corticosteroids have been controversial and have not demonstrated reduction in long-term complications.
   2. ANCA-associated disorders.
      a. The disease process involves multiple systems. Treatment is symptomatic.
B. Patient/family teaching points.
   1. Requires regular examinations and tests to monitor for complications of the disease process.
   2. Take medications as indicated.
C. Pharmacotherapy.
   1. Henoch–Schönlein purpura (IgA vasculitis).
      a. Nonsteroidal anti-inflammatory drugs (NSAIDs) and Tylenol for treatment of pain; corticosteroids are reserved for refractory pain.

▶

2. ANCA-associated disorders.

a. Granulomatosis with polyangiitis (formerly Wegener granulomatosis).

   i. Induction of remission.

   1) Corticosteroids plus methotrexate preferred for initial nonsevere disease.

   2) Cyclophosphamide (2 mg/kg/d orally adjusted for renal disease and age >70) plus corticosteroids (1 mg/kg/d).

   3) Rituximab and corticosteroids.

   4) Bactrim for prophylaxis of opportunistic infections if using cyclophosphamide.

   ii. Maintenance of remission.

   1) Azathioprine (up to 2 mg/kg/d orally) if no evidence of thiopurine methyltransferase deficiency is confirmed.

   2) Methotrexate (20–25 mg/wk orally or intramuscularly [IM]) if no renal insufficiency.

   3) Rituximab (500 mg intravenously [IV]) at remission, repeat on day 14, and then three times every 6 months.

b. Microscopic polyangiitis (treatment is the same as granulomatosis with polyangiitis [formerly Wegener granulomatosis]).

c. Eosinophilic granulomatosis with polyangiitis (formerly Churg–Strauss syndrome).

   i. Mepolizumab plus corticosteroids preferred for nonsevere disease.

   ii. Prednisone 0.5 to 1.5 mg/kg/d.

   iii. Cyclophosphamide for severe disease.

FOLLOW-UP

A. Interval follow-up based on severity of disease.

CONSULTATION/REFERRAL

A. Refer to rheumatology.

B. Consider consultation based on course of illness.

1. Nephrology for renal disease.

2. Pulmonology for pulmonary disease.

SPECIAL/GERIATRIC CONSIDERATIONS

A. The presence of comorbid diseases as commonly found in the geriatric population can impact care or obscure diagnosis.

B. Infection is a prominent cause of morbidity and mortality in vasculitis patients and particularly with geriatric patients whose immune system may be compromised by other conditions and age.

C. Influenza can be potentially life-threatening and there is no evidence that immunization has a negative impact on vasculitis patients.

D. Recommend all geriatric vasculitis patients receive annual influenza vaccination.

E. Use of glucocorticoids as treatment for vasculitis can cause osteoporosis and may lead to increased risk of falls and fractures.

BIBLIOGRAPHY

Chung, S. A., Langford, C. A., Maz, M., Abril, A., Gorelik, M., Guyatt, G., Archer, A. M., Conn, D. L., Full, K. A., Grayson, P. C., Ibarra, M. F., Imundo, L. F., Kim, S., Merkel, P. A., Rhee, R. L., Seo, P., Stone, J. H., Sule, S., Sundel, R. P., . . . Mustafa, R. A.. (2021). 2021 American College of Rheumatology/Vasculitis Foundation guideline for the management of antineutrophil cytoplasmic antibody-associated vasculitis. *Arthritis & Rheumatology, 73*(8), 1366–1383. https://doi.org/10.1002/art.41773

Dedeoglu, F., & Kim, S. (2021, May 14). *IgA vasculitis (Henoch-Schönlein purpura): Management*. In E. TePas (Ed.), *UpToDate*. https://www.uptodate.com/contents/henoch-schonlein-purpura-immunoglobulin-a-vasculitis-management

Falk, R. J., Merkel, P. A., & King, T. E., Jr. (2019, January 23). *Granulomatosis with polyangiitis and microscopic polyangiitis: Clinical manifestations and diagnosis*. In A. Q. Lam & M. Ramirez Curtis (Eds.), *UpToDate*. https://www.uptodate.com/contents/clinical-manifestations-and-diagnosis-of-granulomatosis-with-polyangiitis-and-microscopic-polyangiitis

Hannon, R. A., & Porth, C. M. (2017). *Porth pathophysiology: Concepts of altered health states* (2nd ed.). Wolters Kluwer.

King, T. E., Jr. (2018, November 29). *Treatment and prognosis of eosinophilic granulomatosis with polyangiitis (Churg-Strauss)*. In H. Hollingsworth (Ed.), *UpToDate*. https://www.uptodate.com/contents/treatment-and-prognosis-of-eosinophilic-granulomatosis-with-polyangiitis-churg-strauss

Merkel, P. A. (2021, March 30). *Overview of and approach to the vasculitides in adults*. In M. Ramirez Curtis (Ed.), *UpToDate*. https://www.uptodate.com/contents/overview-of-and-approach-to-the-vasculitides-in-adults

Papadakis, M. A., McPhee, S. J., & Rabow, M. W. (2016). *Current medical diagnosis & treatment 2016*. McGraw Hill Education.

VASCULITIS: MEDIUM VESSEL

Paul Kashmanian

DEFINITION

A. Part of a group of disorders that result from inflammatory changes to the walls of veins and arteries, causing damage to the mural structures, which ultimately may cause tissue ischemia and necrosis.

B. Nomenclature is changing for the specific forms of vasculitis based on the 2012 Revised Chapel Hill Consensus Conference (CHCC).

C. Several different types.

1. Polyarteritis nodosa.

2. Kawasaki disease (more common in peds).

3. Buerger disease (thromboangiitis obliterans).

4. Primary angiitis of the central nervous system (CNS).

INCIDENCE

A. Polyarteritis nodosa.

1. Not common: 30 cases per 1 million people.

2. Males affected more than females; common age presentation is in sixth decade.

B. Buerger disease (thromboangiitis obliterans).

1. Typical patient is a young, male smoker using raw tobacco.

C. Primary angiitis of the CNS.

1. Rare disorder with male predominance.

2. Can occur at any age, with median age being 50 years.

PATHOGENESIS

A. Vasculitis can be a primary pathology or can be secondary to another underlying disease process.

B. Direct injury to the vessel, infectious agents, or immune processes are known to cause vasculitis.

C. Secondary vascular injury may occur from physical agents such as cold and irradiation, mechanical injuries, and toxins.

D. Polyarteritis nodosa.

    1. First form of vasculitis reported.

    2. Predilection for vessels of skin, peripheral nerves, mesenteric vessels, renal vessels, heart, and brain.

    3. 10% of cases caused by hepatitis B infection.

E. Buerger disease (thromboangiitis obliterans).

    1. Highly cellular and inflammatory occlusive thrombus affecting the extremities.

F. Primary angiitis of the CNS.

    1. Vasculitis affecting brain and spinal cord.

PREDISPOSING FACTORS

A. Male sex assigned at birth.

B. Use of raw tobacco for Buerger disease.

SUBJECTIVE DATA

A. Common complaints/symptoms.

    1. Polyarteritis nodosa.

        a. Arthralgia, myalgia, and neuropathy.

        b. Skin manifestations include lower extremity malleoli skin ulcerations (most common), digital gangrene, livedo reticularis, and subcutaneous nodules.

        c. Acute abdomen presentation when abdominal vessels are affected, including abdominal pain, nausea, and vomiting.

        d. Hypertension when renal vessels are affected.

    2. Buerger disease (thromboangiitis obliterans).

        a. Distal extremity ischemia, ischemic digit ulcers, digit gangrene, and migratory phlebitis.

    3. Primary angiitis of the CNS.

        a. Weeks to months of headaches, encephalopathy, and multifocal strokes.

B. Common/typical scenario.

    1. Patients will complain of various symptoms upon presentation that may be mistaken for other diseases.

    2. In polyarteritis nodosa, patients commonly present with acute abdominal pain.

    3. In Buerger disease, patients present with pain in their extremities; in primary angiitis, patients may present with strokes.

C. Family and social history.

    1. Buerger disease: Use of raw tobacco.

D. Review of systems.

    1. Arthralgias.

    2. Myalgias.

    3. Paresthesias.

    4. Skin changes.

    5. Abdominal pain.

    6. Nausea and vomiting.

    7. Headaches.

    8. Ataxia.

PHYSICAL EXAMINATION

A. Polyarteritis nodosa.

    1. Ulcerations on malleoli.

    2. Motor and sensory deficits.

    3. Digital gangrene.

B. Kawasaki disease (more common in peds).

    1. Bilateral conjunctivitis without exudate.

    2. Lip and oral erythema.

    3. Cervical lymphadenopathy.

    4. Rash.

    5. Edema of hands and feet.

C. Buerger disease (thromboangiitis obliterans).

    1. Superficial phlebitis.

    2. Digit ischemia.

D. Primary angiitis of the CNS.

    1. Motor and sensory deficits.

DIAGNOSTIC TESTS

A. Polyarteritis nodosa.

    1. Anemia and leukocytosis.

    2. Antineutrophil cytoplasmic antibody (ANCAs) negative.

    3. Elevated C-reactive protein (CRP) and elevated erythrocyte sedimentation rate (ESR).

    4. Hepatitis B screening.

    5. Skin biopsy and angiogram of vessels and organs.

B. Buerger disease (thromboangiitis obliterans).

    1. Normal CRP, ESR, immunologic panel, hypercoagulability screen, and toxicology screen.

    2. Positive anticardiolipin antibodies.

    3. Consider arteriogram of upper and lower extremities and aorta.

C. Primary angiitis of the CNS.

    1. Cerebrospinal fluid (CSF): Leukocytosis with increased protein.

    2. Angiograms: String of beads pattern.

    3. Positive brain biopsy.

    4. Clinical diagnosis made by ruling out infection, neoplasm, metabolic disorder, and cocaine use.

DIFFERENTIAL DIAGNOSIS

A. Other forms of vasculitis.

B. Thromboembolic events.

EVALUATION AND MANAGEMENT PLAN

A. General plan.

    1. Symptom management.

    2. Exercise and healthy lifestyle changes.

    3. Buerger disease (thromboangiitis obliterans).

        a. Smoking cessation is the cornerstone of treatment.

        b. Local wound care.

        c. Pneumatic compression and spinal cord stimulation for pain due to ischemia.

B. Patient/family teaching points.

    1. Treatment of vasculitis with corticosteroids or other immunocompromising medications causes an immunocompromised state.

2. Corticosteroids can lead to complications with diabetes, weight gain, or osteoporosis.

C. Pharmacotherapy.

1. Polyarteritis nodosa.

a. Methotrexate or azathioprine plus corticosteroids preferred for nonsevere disease.

b. Methylprednisolone 1,000 mg IV daily for 3 days for the critically ill and severe disease.

c. Immunosuppressive agents such as cyclophosphamide for moderate to severe disease.

2. Buerger disease (thromboangiitis obliterans).

a. Calcium channel blockers for vasospasm.

3. Primary angiitis of the CNS.

a. Corticosteroids and cyclophosphamide.

FOLLOW-UP

A. Interval follow-up based on severity of disease.

CONSULTATION/REFERRAL

A. Refer to rheumatology.

SPECIAL/GERIATRIC CONSIDERATIONS

A. There are no specific age-related considerations in vasculitis-medium vessel.

BIBLIOGRAPHY

Chung, S. A., Gorelik, M., Langford, C. A., Maz, M., Abril, A., Guyatt, G., Archer, A. M., Conn, D. L., Full, K. A., Grayson, P. C., Ibarra, M. F., Imundo, L. F., Kim, S., Merkel, P. A., Rhee, R. L., Seo, P., Stone, J. H., Sule, S., Sundel, R. P. ... Mustafa, R. A. (2021). 2021 American College of Rheumatology/Vasculitis Foundation guideline for the management of Polyarteritis Nodosa. *Arthritis & Rheumatology, 73*(8), 1384–1393. https://doi.org/10.1002/art.41776

Hajj-Ali, R. A., & Calabrese, L. H. (2017, July 3). *Primary angiitis of the central nervous system in adults.* In M. Ramirez Curtis (Ed.), *UpToDate.* https://www.uptodate.com/contents/primary-angiitis-of-the-central-nervous-system-in-adults

Hannon, R. A., & Porth, C. M. (2017). *Porth pathophysiology: Concepts of altered health states* (2nd ed.). Wolters Kluwer.

Merkel, P. A. (2019, March 1). *Overview of and approach to the vasculitides in adults.* In M. Ramirez (Ed.), *UpToDate.* https://www.uptodate.com/contents/overview-of-and-approach-to-the-vasculitides-in-adults

Olin, J. W. (2018, September 20). *Thromboangiitis obliterans (Buerger's disease).* In K. A. Collins (Ed.), *UpToDate.* https://www.uptodate.com/contents/thromboangiitis-obliterans-buergers-disease

Papadakis, M. A., McPhee, S. J., & Rabow, M. W. (2016). *Current medical diagnosis & treatment 2016.* McGraw Hill Education.

Sundel, R. (2018, November 13). *Kawasaki disease: Clinical features and diagnosis.* In E. TePas (Ed.), *UpToDate.* https://https://www.uptodate.com/contents/kawasaki-disease-clinical-features-and-diagnosis

VASCULITIS: LARGE VESSEL

Paul Kashmanian

DEFINITION

A. Part of a group of disorders that result from inflammatory changes to the walls of veins and arteries, causing damage to the mural structures, which ultimately may cause tissue ischemia and necrosis.

B. Nomenclature is changing for the specific forms of vasculitis based on the 2012 Revised Chapel Hill Consensus Conference (CHCC).

C. Two main types:

1. Takayasu arteritis.

2. Giant cell arteritis/temporal arteritis.

INCIDENCE

A. Takayasu arteritis.

1. Common in patients of Asian descent.

2. Women are typically more affected than men.

3. Age of onset tends to be early adulthood.

B. Giant cell arteritis/temporal arteritis.

1. Most common vasculitis (UTD).

2. Afflicts more females than males; age older than 50 years, with the most common presenting age between 70 and 79 years.

3. Common in Scandinavian descent.

PATHOGENESIS

A. Vasculitis can be a primary pathology or can be secondary to another underlying disease process.

B. Direct injury to the vessel, infectious agents, or immune processes are known to cause vasculitis.

C. Secondary vascular injury may occur from physical agents such as cold and irradiation, mechanical injuries, and toxins (P).

D. Takayasu arteritis.

E. Granulomatous vasculitis of aorta and its major branches (C).

F. Possible immunogenetic predisposition (U).

G. Giant cell arteritis/temporal arteritis.

1. Chronic inflammatory disease of cranial branches of carotid arteries.

PREDISPOSING FACTORS

A. Female sex assigned at birth and age typically older than 60 years.

B. Some familial pattern.

SUBJECTIVE DATA

A. Common complaints/symptoms.

1. Constitutional symptoms are common with all-size vessel vasculitis and include fever, weight loss, malaise, and arthralgias/arthritis.

2. Large vessel vasculitis will often present with limb claudication, asymmetric blood pressures, absence of pulses, bruits, and aortic dilatation.

3. Takayasu arteritis.

a. Decreased pulses.

b. Unequal upper extremity blood pressures.

c. Carotid and subclavian artery bruits.

d. Limb claudication and hypertension.

4. Giant cell arteritis/temporal arteritis.

a. Headache and scalp tenderness.

b. Visual changes, such as amaurosis fugax.

c. Jaw claudication.

d. Throat pain.

e. Temporal artery tenderness.

B. Common/typical scenario.

1. See previous sections for common/typical scenario.

C. Family and social history.

1. Inquire about family history of vasculitis.

D. Review of systems.
  1. See previous sections for review of systems.

PHYSICAL EXAMINATION

A. Cardiology.
  1. Decreased pulses.
  2. Unequal upper extremity blood pressures.
  3. Carotid and subclavian artery bruits.
B. Limb claudication and hypertension.
C. Headache and scalp tenderness.
D. Visual changes, such as amaurosis fugax.
E. Jaw claudication.
F. Throat pain.
G. Temporal artery tenderness.

DIAGNOSTIC TESTS

A. Takayasu arteritis.
  1. Elevated C-reactive protein (CRP) and elevated erythrocyte sedimentation rate (ESR).
  2. MRI or CT angiography (CTA) of affected vessels.
B. Giant cell arteritis/temporal arteritis.
  1. Normochromic anemia, normal leukocytes, decreased serum albumin, elevated liver enzymes, and elevated CRP and ESR.
  2. Best diagnostic test to confirm is temporal artery biopsy (UTD).
  3. In patients with normal temporal artery biopsy, consider magnetic resonance angiography (MRA) or CTA for confirmation.

DIFFERENTIAL DIAGNOSIS

A. Other forms of vasculitis.
B. Nonarteritic anterior ischemic optic neuropathy (NAAION).

EVALUATION AND MANAGEMENT PLAN

A. General plan.
  1. Giant cell arteritis: Early intervention is necessary to prevent blindness, which can become permanent.
B. Pharmacotherapy.
  1. Takayasu arteritis.
    a. Prednisone 1 mg/kg orally for 1 month, then tapered over several months to 10 mg orally daily.
    b. Methotrexate and mycophenolate mofetil may also be helpful.
  2. Giant cell arteritis/temporal arteritis.
    a. Glucocorticoids are the mainstay.
    b. Tocilizumab recently approved; can be monotherapy or in addition to steroids.
    c. Must be initiated quickly to avoid permanent blindness; therefore, if clinically suspected begin treatment.
    d. Visual loss present at time of diagnosis: Intravenous (IV) methylprednisolone 1,000 mg IV daily for 3 days followed by oral steroids (UTD).
    e. Prednisone 60 mg PO daily × 1 month, then taper dose.
    f. Low-dose aspirin, 81 mg PO daily.
C. Surgical management can be considered for progression of disease or failure of immunosuppressives.

FOLLOW-UP

A. Giant cell arteritis.
  1. Follow-up should be monthly for 6 months if possible and then spaced accordingly.
  2. Consider ophthalmology consult for visual symptoms.
B. Takayasu arteritis.
  1. Requires regular monitoring.

CONSULTATION/REFERRAL

A. Refer to rheumatology.
B. Refer to vascular surgery

SPECIAL/GERIATRIC CONSIDERATIONS

A. Chronic steroid use can cause osteoporosis so consideration should be made to treat osteoporosis.

CASE SCENARIO: VASCULITIS

A 6-year-old patient is brought to the pediatrician's office by his parents for a chief complaint of "spots of bruising" that the parents have noticed diffusely develop over the patient's lower extremities the past 2 days, along with knee and ankle pain. The parents have not witnessed any falls or noticeable trauma that may have preceded the "bruising." Of note, they were recently seen in the office and diagnosed with confirmed strep throat infection and have just completed a 10-day course of amoxicillin for treatment. The parents are unsure if this is a medication reaction because this is the first exposure the child has had to amoxicillin. Examination shows that the skin manifestations are along both the lower legs as well as the buttocks. The skin lesions are slightly raised and do not blanch when pressed. Further examination reveals fairly normal-appearing mucosa of the oropharynx, no murmurs, and lung sounds clear to auscultation. Review of systems does not display any coughing. Vital signs are as follows: Temperature (oral): 100.6°F/38.1°C; heart rate: 119 beats per minute; respiratory rate: 30 breaths per minute; oxygen saturation: 98%.

1. What is the most likely diagnosis based on the information presented?
  A. Eosinophilic granulomatosis with polyangiitis
  B. Henoch–Schönlein purpura (immunoglobulin A [IgA] vasculitis)
  C. Microscopic polyangiitis
  D. Kawasaki disease

2. What is the appropriate test for a definitive diagnosis of this condition?
  A. Urinalysis
  B. Ultrasound of lower extremities
  C. Complete blood count (CBC) with peripheral blood smear
  D. Biopsy

3. What is the appropriate initial treatment for the diagnosis?
  A. Colchicine
  B. Rituximab
  C. Nonsteroidal anti-inflammatory drugs (NSAIDs) and Tylenol
  D. Corticosteroids

4. What classification of vasculitis does this condition belong to?

A. Variable vessel

B. Small vessel

C. Medium vessel

D. Large vessel

BIBLIOGRAPHY

Docken, W. P. (2022, March 8). *Treatment of giant cell arteritis*. In M. Ramirez Curtis (Ed.), *UpToDate*. https://www.uptodate.com/contents/treatment-of-giant-cell-temporal-arteritis?source=see_link

Hannon, R. A., & Porth, C. M. (2017). *Porth pathophysiology: Concepts of altered health states* (2nd ed.). Wolters Kluwer.

Maz, M., Chung, S. A., Abril, A., Langford, C. A., Gorelik, M., Guyatt, G., Archer, A. M., Conn, D. L., Full, K. A., Grayson, P. C., Ibarra, M. F., Imundo, L. F., Kim, S., Merkel, P. A., Rhee, R. L., Seo, P., Stone, J. H., Sule, S., Sundel, R. P., & R. A, ... Mustafa. (2021). 2021 American College of Rheumatology/Vasculitis Foundation guideline for the management of giant cell arteritis and Takayasu arteritis. *Arthritis & Rheumatology, 73*(8), 1349–1365. https://doi.org/10.1002/art.41774

Merkel, P. A. (2021, March 30). *Overview of and approach to the vasculitides in adults*. In M. Ramirez Curtis (Ed.), *UpToDate*. https://www.uptodate.com/contents/overview-of-and-approach-to-the-vasculitides-in-adults

Papadakis, M. A., McPhee, S. J., & Rabow, M. W. (2016). *Current medical diagnosis & treatment 2016*. McGraw Hill Education.

Salvarani, C., & Muratore, F. (2021, December 22). *Diagnosis of giant cell arteritis*. In M. Ramirez Curtis (Ed.), *UpToDate*. https://www.uptodate.com/contents/diagnosis-of-giant-cell-arteritis?topicRef=8240&source=related_link#H18

Salvarani, C., Muratore, F., & Rosenbaum, J. T. (2021, June 30). *Clinical manifestations of giant cell arteritis*. In M. Ramirez Curtis (Ed.), *UpToDate*. https://www.uptodate.com/contents/clinical-manifestations-of-giant-cell-temporal-arteritis

KNOWLEDGE CHECK: CHAPTER 14

1. What are the patient's signs and symptoms when presenting with disc herniation pain?

   A. Pain is constant and dull, unrelieved by rest, and worse at night, often awakening the patient.

   B. Pain is relieved by rest and forward flexion and is worsened by activities such as walking, prolonged standing, and back extension.

   C. Pain is greater in intensity and radiates from the spine to the leg in a specific nerve root distribution.

   D. Pain is worsened by coughing, Valsalva maneuver, and sitting and is relieved by lying in the supine position.

2. What is the gold standard study for suspected spinal infection, neoplasm, and epidural compression syndromes?

   A. CT scan

   B. MRI scan

   C. Plain x-ray films

   D. Lumbar puncture or spinal tap

3. Which compartment is the most common location of acute coronary syndrome (ACS) during intracranial pressure (ICP) measurement of the lower leg?

   A. Anterior compartment

   B. Lateral compartment

   C. Superficial posterior compartment

   D. Deep posterior compartment

4. What is the indicated time for an absolute fasciotomy?

   A. Arterial ischemic time greater than 6 hours

   B. Arterial ischemic time greater than 4 hours

   C. Venous ischemic time greater than 8 hours

   D. Venous ischemic time greater than 10 hours

5. What condition would best describe a patient who presents with chronic joint pain with symmetrical polyarticular involvement, especially in the proximal interphalangeal (PIP), metacarpophalangeal (MCP), and metatarsophalangeal (MTP) joints?

   A. Osteoarthritis (OA)

   B. Rheumatoid arthritis (RA)

   C. Fibromyalgia

   D. Gout

6. After a posterior approach total hip arthroplasty (THA), what activities would increase the likelihood of dislocation in the first 6 weeks?

   A. Keeping the legs slightly abducted with a pillow between the legs while sleeping

   B. Bending the knee to the hip

   C. Hip flexion to 90 degrees

   D. Crossing the legs over midline

7. Which of the following is not an appropriate non-pharmacologic management for OA?

   A. Weight loss

   B. Physical therapy

   C. Inactivity of affected joint

   D. Tai chi practice

8. What is Felty syndrome?

   A. Scleritis and fever occasionally seen in advanced stages of RA

   B. "Boggy" feeling over affected joints due to synovial thickening or effusion in early stages of RA

   C. Triad of RA, splenomegaly, and neutropenia

   D. Urinary incontinence seen in older adult patients with RA

9. Why is it important to screen for hepatitis B and C infections before starting a patient on a disease-modifying antirheumatic drugs (DMARD)?

   A. DMARDs may cause tendon ruptures in patients with hepatitis B.

   B. DMARDs are immunosuppressants and may reactivate hepatitis B and/or C.

   C. DMARDs may cause QTc prolongation in patients with hepatitis C.

   D. It is not important to screen for hepatitis B or C before starting a patient on a DMARD.

10. What are the common symptoms and clinical findings associated with reactive arthritis (ReA)?

    A. Polyarthritis, Crohn's disease, and chronic uveitis

    B. Polyarthritis, nail pitting, and dactylitis

    C. Oligoarthritis, urethritis, and conjunctivitis

    D. Low back pain, aortic regurgitation, and acute uveitis

(See answers next page.)

1. **D) Pain is worsened by coughing, Valsalva maneuver, and sitting and is relieved by lying in the supine position.**

   Disc herniation is worsened by coughing, Valsalva maneuver, and sitting and is relieved by lying in the supine position. The spinal canal has limited space, which is inadequate for the spinal nerve and the displaced herniated disc fragment. Due to this displacement, the disc presses on the spinal nerves, often producing pain that may be severe.

2. **B) MRI scan**

   MRI scan is the gold standard study in cases of suspected spinal infection, neoplasm, and epidural compression syndromes. MRI is favored over CT due to the advantages of sagittal images and the clarity of the anatomic relationships between the discs and the nerve roots. MRI also excludes herniations at other sites or unsuspected tumors.

3. **A) Anterior compartment**

   The most common location of acute coronary syndrome (ACS) is the anterior compartment or anterior tibial compartment of the lower extremity.

4. **B) Arterial ischemic time greater than 4 hours**

   An absolute indication for fasciotomy is an arterial ischemic time greater than 4 hours. Neurologic injury is reversible if the fasciotomy is performed within 4 hours.

5. **B) Rheumatoid arthritis (RA)**

   RA is a chronic inflammatory disease that is polyarticular and involves the proximal interphalangeal (PIP), metacarpophalangeal (MCP), and metatarsophalangeal (MTP) joints. Osteoarthritis is usually a chronic noninflammatory arthritis that involves the distal interphalangeal (DIP), carpometacarpal (CMC), and hip/knee joints. Fibromyalgia is a nonarticular condition, and gout is an acute, not chronic, inflammatory condition.

6. **D) Crossing the legs over midline**

   After a total hip arthroplasty (THA), the patient should avoid allowing the legs to cross midline. Postoperative THA patients may need to adhere to hip precautions for 6 weeks to avoid hip dislocation. Patients should avoid bending and flexing the hips to greater than 90 degrees, avoid twisting the leg in or out (internal or external rotation), avoid crossing the legs at the knee or ankle, and avoid raising the knee higher than the hip.

7. **C) Inactivity of affected joint**

   Inactivity will lead to increased symptoms of osteoarthritis (OA). Weight loss, physical therapy, and practice of yoga or tai chi have well-documented benefits in persons with knee OA. Tai chi and yoga have been shown to be beneficial in managing OA.

8. **C) Triad of RA, splenomegaly, and neutropenia**

   Felty syndrome is the rare triad of RA, splenomegaly, and neutropenia seen in advanced stages of RA. Felty syndrome is often accompanied by anemia and thrombocytopenia.

9. **B) DMARDs are immunosuppressants and may reactivate hepatitis B and/or C.**

   Before starting disease-modifying antirheumatic drugs (DMARDs), it is recommended by the American College of Rheumatology to screen for latent tuberculosis, hepatitis B virus, and hepatitis C virus infections because the immunosuppression that occurs with DMARDs may reactivate infections. Additionally, a false-positive result on rheumatoid factor (RF) antibody testing may occur in the setting of chronic infections.

10. **C) Oligoarthritis, urethritis, and conjunctivitis**

    Reactive arthritis (ReA) clinical manifestations include oligoarthritis, urethritis, conjunctivitis, and mucosal lesions, which can be triggered by either gastrointestinal or genital infections. Polyarthritis, Crohn's disease, and chronic uveitis are associated with inflammatory bowel disease (IBD)-associated spondyloarthritides. Polyarthritis, nail pitting, and dactylitis are associated with psoriatic arthritis (PsA). Low back pain, aortic regurgitation, and acute uveitis are associated with aortic stenosis (AS).

11. Psoriatic arthritis (PsA) is treated with which medication to inhibit progression of joint disease?

- **A.** Tumor necrosis factor (TNF) inhibitors
- **B.** Methotrexate
- **C.** Nonsteroidal anti-inflammatory drugs (NSAIDs)
- **D.** Psoralen and ultraviolet A (PUVA)

12. What medication(s) is(are) used to treat lupus nephritis?

- **A.** Hydroxychloroquine
- **B.** Mycophenolate, cyclophosphamide, and glucocorticoids
- **C.** Anifrolumab and glucocorticoids
- **D.** Nonsteroidal anti-inflammatory drugs

13. What is the most common side effect of immunosuppressants?

- **A.** Constipation
- **B.** Opportunistic infection
- **C.** Diarrhea
- **D.** Headache

14. What is the mode of action of anifrolumab?

- **A.** Calcineurin inhibitor
- **B.** T-cell blocker
- **C.** Interferon type 1 blocker
- **D.** B-cell activation blocker

15. What would be found in the physical examination of a patient recently diagnosed with Behçet disease?

- **A.** Otitis media
- **B.** Painful aphthous ulcers of the mouth and genitals
- **C.** Palpable purpura on lower extremities
- **D.** Pallor and coolness of distal hand digits

16. What is the most appropriate initial treatment for Behçet disease in preventing painful recurrent oral and genital ulcers?

- **A.** Colchicine
- **B.** Apremilast
- **C.** Steroids
- **D.** Cyclophosphamide

17. All of the following are antineutrophil cytoplasmic antibody (ANCA)-associated disorders with the EXCEPTION of:

- **A.** Granulomatosis with polyangiitis
- **B.** Henoch–Schönlein purpura
- **C.** Microscopic polyangiitis
- **D.** Eosinophilic granulomatosis with polyangiitis

18. Which of the following is a known predisposing factor for Henoch–Schönlein purpura?

- **A.** Recent group A streptococcus infection
- **B.** Lupus
- **C.** Rheumatoid arthritis (RA)
- **D.** Polychondritis

19. Which class of antihypertensives is used for treatment of vasospasm in Buerger disease?

- **A.** Calcium channel blockers
- **B.** Loop diuretics
- **C.** Beta-blockers
- **D.** Alpha-1 blockers

20. What is the most common vasculitis among all types (mixed, small, medium, and large vessel)?

- **A.** Henoch–Schönlein purpura
- **B.** Giant cell arteritis/temporal arteritis
- **C.** Takayasu arteritis
- **D.** Kawasaki disease

(*See answers next page.*)

11. A) tumor necrosis factor (TNF) inhibitors

TNF inhibitors, such as etanercept, have been shown to control disease activity and inhibit progression of joint destruction. Methotrexate has efficacy in rheumatoid arthritis, but in psoriatic arthritis (PsA) has not shown effectiveness in halting erosive joint disease. Nonsteroidal anti-inflammatory drugs (NSAIDs) symptomatically treat swelling and pain in PsA but do not inhibit joint disease. Psoralen and ultraviolet A (PUVA) is used only to treat skin manifestations of PsA.

12. B) Mycophenolate, cyclophosphamide, and glucocorticoids

As per the American College of Rheumatology guidelines, immunosuppressants should be used for treatment of lupus nephritis, based on classification and severity of the disease.

13. B) Opportunistic infection

The most common side effects of immunosuppressants are opportunistic infections, upper respiratory infection (URI), and viral infections.

14. C) Interferon type 1 blocker

Anifrolumab was approved in 2020 and is a type 1 interferon blocker. Opportunistic infections are the most common side effect.

15. B) Painful aphthous ulcers of the mouth and genitals

A distinct hallmark of Behçet disease is painful ulcerations of the mouth and genital regions.

16. A) Colchicine

Colchicine is used to prevent ulcers of both oral and genital regions, whereas apremilast is used only for preventing oral ulcers, and steroids are used only for severe disease.

17. B) Henoch–Schönlein purpura

Henoch–Schönlein purpura is an immunoglobulin A (IgA) vasculitis and is not antineutrophil cytoplasmic antibody (ANCA)-associated.

18. A) Recent group A streptococcus infection

Group A streptococcus throat infections in pediatric populations are common predisposing factors in Henoch–Schönlein purpura, whereas lupus, rheumatoid arthritis (RA), and polychondritis are more common in antineutrophil cytoplasmic antibody (ANCA)-associated disorders.

19. A) Calcium channel blockers

Calcium channel blockers such as nifedipine and verapamil are the mainstay and the only antihypertensive class of medication used in the treatment of vasospasm.

20. B) Giant cell arteritis/temporal arteritis

Giant cell arteritis is the most common vasculitis. Henoch–Schönlein purpura is the most common vasculitis only in the pediatric population. Takayasu arteritis and Kawasaki disease are less common.

CHAPTER 15

DERMATOLOGY GUIDELINES

Kelley Scott

ATOPIC DERMATITIS

DEFINITION

A. Dermatitis refers to inflammation of the skin. A broad description, referring to an abnormal finding of the skin.
B. Causes of dermatitis may be mechanical, environmental, allergic, viral, bacterial, fungal, parasitic, inflammatory, autoimmune (drug, lupus, psoriasis), neoplastic, and occasionally a combination.
C. Treatment includes removing the offending agent and decreasing inflammation to allow the skin to recover.
D. Approach to diagnosis of skin eruptions begins with consideration of all-inclusive differentials narrowed by obtaining a thorough history, which includes key clinical features of the skin eruption. The acute care advanced practice provider (APP) must make the determination of whether a skin finding is acute, chronic, and/or emergent. This determination is largely dependent on the presenting characteristics of the eruption. An eruption may be painful, pruritic, draining, and/or have characteristic pattern and distribution features, or be associated with systemic symptoms. If the condition is determined to be emergent, for example, presenting with anaphylaxis (severe swelling), fever, or toxic appearance, a prompt consult for emergency care is warranted.
E. Atopic dermatitis (AD), also called eczema, is a chronic relapsing, pruritic, inflammatory skin disease. It is clinically diagnosed based on the pattern and distribution of the eruptions. It is common with immunoglobulin E (IgE)-associated disorders such as allergic rhinitis, rhinoconjunctivitis, asthma, and food allergies.

INCIDENCE

A. AD may occur at any age.
  1. Estimated one in five children will develop AD; the condition may continue throughout the life span.
  2. Approximately 10% of adults are affected by AD.
B. In developed countries, and in approximately 60% of cases, onset of disease occurs in the first year of life.
C. AD has a greater incidence at higher latitudes, which may be related to decreased sun exposure and lower humidity levels.
D. Peaks during cold dry weather.

PATHOGENESIS

A. A defective skin barrier susceptible to xerosis and environmental irritants and allergens leads to inflammation and pruritus.

B. Pruritus is a major cause of breakdown of the skin barrier. A complex, disordered, and overactive immune response involves the immunologic release of cytokines, activation of skin neuroinflammatory sensors, and associated histamine and serotonin release from mast cells resulting in intense histaminergic itch.

PREDISPOSING FACTORS

A. Family history of AD.
  1. Genetic variations are likely associated with the development of AD, although they are not yet definitively linked to the disorder. A suspected mutation of the gene responsible for the protein filaggrin. Filaggrin provides a healthy, protective barrier on the outer layer of the skin.
B. Breakdown of skin.
  1. Dry skin.
  2. Abrasion or injury.
  3. Contact dermatitis (allergies, irritants).
  4. Seasonal, environmental, or food allergies.
  5. Dry weather.
  6. Heat.
  7. Stress.

SUBJECTIVE DATA

A. Characteristic/distribution and onset of eruption.
  1. Intense pruritus, often interrupting sleep.
  2. Dry skin patches with distribution on the face, trunk, and flexural folds of the neck, arms, legs, wrists, and ankles.
B. Common/typical scenario.
  1. Chronic relapsing rash.
    a. Worse in cooler months; better in summer.
    b. Triggers with exposure to allergens or stress.
C. Family and social history.
  1. Family or personal history of AD or of the atopic triad.
    a. AD/eczema.
    b. Asthma.
    c. Allergies.
  2. Frequent hand washer or bather.
D. Review of systems.
  1. Condition often limited to skin.
  2. Seasonal allergic symptoms.
  3. Psychological complaints of anxiety and depression related to disordered sleep patterns and chronicity of skin condition.

PHYSICAL EXAMINATION

A. Dry pruritic, erythematous, and sometimes hyperpigmented patches.

B. Oozing and crusting of eruptions lead to thickening and hardening of the skin, which is referred to as lichenification.

C. Eruptions can occur with and without infection; lesions with infection are referred to as impetiginized.

D. Distribution tends to be on face and trunk, flexural folds of the neck, arms, legs (especially antecubital and popliteal fossae), wrists, and ankles (Figure 15.1A,B).

DIAGNOSTIC TESTS

A. Diagnostic biomarker is not available for AD.

B. Laboratory testing is not routinely necessary. If secondary bacterial infection is suspected, a culture for isolation of specific bacterial organism (e.g., *Staphylococcus or Streptococcus*) and for antibiotic sensitivity is indicated. A viral polymerase chain reaction (PCR) for superinfection with herpes simplex virus for diagnosis of eczema herpeticum may be necessary.

C. A complete blood count (CBC) with differential may support the diagnosis of infection if elevated white blood cell count or if differential has a left shift; if eosinophilia is present, indicate allergic component; if thrombocytopenia is present, it may indicate Wiskott–Aldrich syndrome, which can mimic presentation of AD.

D. Serum IgE testing for specific antigens.

E. Skin biopsy: New lesions are preferred over older lesions. Older skin lesions often have either been lichenified or "burnt out"; hyperpigmented macules and patches may represent postinflammatory hyperpigmentation and not active rash.

F. Potassium hydroxide (KOH) preparation should be negative to exclude tinea corporis.

DIFFERENTIAL DIAGNOSIS

A. Tinea (corporis, cruris, versicolor, manuum, pedis).

B. Seborrheic dermatitis.

C. Allergic contact dermatitis.

D. Stasis dermatitis.

E. Scabies.

F. Psoriasis.

G. Molluscum contagiosum.

H. Mycosis fungoides/cutaneous T-cell lymphoma.

EVALUATION AND MANAGEMENT PLAN

A. General plan.

  1. Avoid triggers.

  2. Avoid exacerbations (dry heat, hot showers, excessive washing/bathing, contact with irritants, or use of irritants).

  3. Maintain skin integrity through moisturization and decreasing inflammation.

B. Patient/family teaching points.

  1. Practice gentle skin care.

    a. Limit bathing to 5 minutes once daily at the most.

    b. Limit soap use.

    c. Use gentle nonsoap cleansers only.

    d. Do not use loofah or washcloth; use only hands to wash body.

    e. Wash only "dirty" areas: Face, axilla, genitalia, groin, hands, and feet.

    f. When drying after bathing pat skin, dry gently; do not rub.

    g. For flares, apply topical medications within 5 minutes of leaving shower/bath.

    h. For nonflared areas and daily maintenance, apply emollient/moisturizer within 5 minutes of leaving shower/bath.

    i. Avoid wool clothing.

    j. Use hypoallergenic laundry detergents, hand soaps, body soaps, facial cleansers, and moisturizers.

    k. Use a humidifier.

  2. Decrease stress.

  3. Avoid scratching.

  4. Treat early onset to limit the duration of steroid needed.

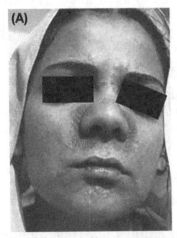

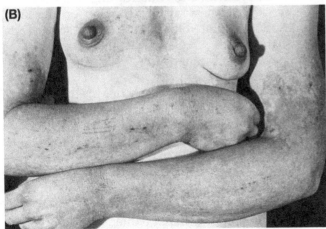

FIGURE 15.1   Examples of atopic dermatitis on the **(A)** face and **(B)** arms/trunk.

Sources: Image A from Zaidi, Z., Hussain, K., & Sudhakaran, S. (2018). Eczema. In: *Treatment of skin diseases* Springer, Cham.; image B courtesy of Centers for Disease Control and Prevention.

C. Pharmacotherapy.

  1. Topical emollients or moisturizers.

    a. Preparations.

      i. Lotions: Tend to not hold moisture in skin, despite containing more water than creams and ointments.

      ii. Creams: Effectively lock in moisture and are preferred over lotions. Examples include Aveeno cream, Cetaphil cream, CeraVe cream, Eucerin cream, Lubriderm cream, and Vanicream.

      iii. Barrier creams: Zinc oxide (may provide antiseptic protection).

      iv. Ointments: Help lock in moisture better than creams. Examples include Vaseline and petroleum jelly.

  2. Topical steroid reduces local skin inflammation. Suggested topically twice daily for 2 consecutive weeks. Topical corticosteroids are associated with cutaneous atrophy, telangiectasias, striae, and worsening of disease after discontinuation (rebound phenomenon).

    a. Low potency for face, neck, groin, inner thighs, and buttocks.

    b. Medium potency for other areas such as extremities and trunk.

    c. High potency for hands and feet.

  3. Topical calcineurin inhibitors (TCIs) are an alternative treatment for acute flares (tacrolimus [approved for moderate to severe disease] or pimecrolimus [approved for mild to moderate disease] applied two to three times weekly [daily if nonresponsive to topical corticosteroids or if unable to use topical corticosteroids]).

  4. Oral steroid: Prednisone, typically 20 to 30 mg daily. Treatment with oral corticosteroids is discouraged without specialty dermatology consultation due to potential for rebound flare with discontinuation of therapy and the associated side effects of the medication.

  5. Topical Phosphodiesterase-4 (PDE4) inhibitors: PDE4, mainly present in immune cells, epithelial cells, and brain cells, manifests as an intracellular nonreceptor enzyme that modulates inflammation and epithelial integrity. Eucrisa (crisaborole) is a topical PDE4 inhibitor nonsteroidal topical treatment 2% ointment applied twice daily to the affected area.

  6. Antihistamines.

    a. Low to medium strength.

      i. Nonsedating (Claritin, Zyrtec).

      ii. Sedating (Benadryl).

    b. Medium to high strength.

      i. Hydroxyzine.

  7. Phototherapy: Refer to specialty dermatology.

  8. Biologics: Refer to specialty dermatology. Multiple topical and oral biologic agents are available. Emerging biologic therapies are targeted to inhibit key inflammatory molecules that are involved in the pathogenesis of chronic inflammatory disorders as well as physiologic immune responses.

  9. Treat secondary infections with oral therapy (viral, bacterial). Treat bacterial infections with systemic antibiotics (e.g., cephalexin, or if resistant organism is suspected, sulfamethazole-trimethoprim). Carefully diluted bleach baths (up to daily) and nasal mupirocin (for nasal colonization) may also be necessary to clear frequent skin infections.

D. Discharge instructions.

  1. If systemic develop or signs of toxicity, prompt referral to ED.

FOLLOW-UP

A. Primary care provider (PCP) in 1 week.

B. Dermatology in 1 to 3 months, depending on severity.

CONSULTATION/REFERRAL

A. If condition persists or worsens despite treatment, consult or refer to dermatology.

B. If diffuse, always refer to dermatology to rule out cutaneous lymphoma or another erythroderma. Cutaneous T-cell lymphoma, also known as mycosis fungoides, is a malignancy of the T-helper (CD4+) cells. Diagnosis is difficult early in the course of this disease because it mimics other skin disorders, including AD.

SPECIAL/GERIATRIC CONSIDERATIONS

A. Controlling allergen exposure is essential.

B. Poor compliance and poor education will likely lead to longer duration of flares and increased intensity of flares; consistent early treatment is best.

C. Older adult patients all develop drier and thinner skin with age, making it harder to clear and prevent flares.

D. *Staphylococcus aureus* colonization seen in more than 90% of AD patients. *S. aureus* may contribute to the inflammation of AD lesions and lead to secondary infection and impetiginization.

E. Individuals with AD have an increased risk of developing other conditions.

  1. Inflammatory conditions such as inflammatory bowel disease, rheumatoid arthritis, and hair loss caused by a malfunctioning immune reaction, such as alopecia areata, and potentially an increased risk of malignancy.

  2. Behavioral/psychiatric disorders, such as attention deficit hyperactivity disorder (ADHD), depression, and suicidal ideation, have been reported.

BIBLIOGRAPHY

Albrecht, J. (2022, May 25). The power of topical steroids. *JAMA Dermatology.* https://doi.org/10.1001/jamadermatol.2022.0816

Bernd, W. M., Arents, E. J., van Zuuren, S., Vermeulen, J., Schoones, W., & Fedorowicz, Z. (2022). Global guidelines in dermatology mapping project (GUIDEMAP), a systematic review of atopic dermatitis clinical practice guidelines: Are they clear, unbiased, trustworthy and evidence based. *British Journal of Dermatology, 186*(5), 792–802. https://doi-org.ezproxy2.library.drexel.edu/10.1111/bjd.20972

Clinical overview, eczema and atopic dermatitis. (2022). *Elsevier Point of Care.* https://www-clinicalkey-com.ezproxy2.library.drexel.edu/#!/content/clinical_overview/67-s2.0-1d298cb2-646a-43ec-b159-3f390fd22162

Drucker, A. M., Eyerich, K., deBruin-Weller., S. M., Thyssen, J. P., Spuls, P. I., Irvine, A. D., Girolomoni, G., Dhar, S., Flohr, C., Murrell, D. F., Paller, A. S., & Guttman-Yassky, E. (2018). Use of systemic corticosteroids for atopic dermatitis: International Eczema Council consensus statement. *The British Journal of Dermatology, 178*(3), 768–775. https://doi.org/10.1111/bjd.15928

Girolomoni, G., & Busà, V. M. (2022). Flare management in atopic dermatitis: From definition to treatment. *Therapeutic Advances in Chronic Disease, 13*, 20406223211066728. https://doi.org/10.1177/20406223211066728

Hawerkamp, H. C., Fahy, C. M. R., Fallon, P. G., & Schwartz, C. (2022). Break on through: The role of innate immunity and barrier defense in atopic dermatitis and psoriasis. *Skin Health and Disease, 2*(2), e99–n/a. https://doi.org/10.1002/ski2.99

Li, H., Zuo, J., & Tang, W. (2018). Phosphodiesterase-4 inhibitors for the treatment of inflammatory diseases. *Frontiers in Pharmacology, 9*, 1048. https://doi.org/10.3389/fphar.2018.01048

Mendes, C. R., Dilarri, G., Forsan, C. F., Sapata, V. M. R., Lopes, P. R. M., de Moraes, P. B., Montagnolli, R. N., Ferreira, H., & Bidoia, E. D. (2022). Antibacterial action and target mechanisms of zinc oxide nanoparticles against bacterial pathogens. *Scientific Reports, 12*, 2658. https://doi.org/10.1038/s41598-022-06657-y

Mohney, L. A., Singh, R., & Feldman, S. R. (2022). Review of ruxolitinib in the treatment of atopic dermatitis. *Annals of Pharmacotherapy*, 1–10. https://doi-org.ezproxy2.library.drexel.edu/10.1177/10600280221103282

Roediger, B., & Schlapbach, C. (2022). T cells in the skin: Lymphoma and inflammatory skin disease. *Journal of Allergy and Clinical Immunology, 149*(4), 1172–1184. https://doi.org/10.1016/j.jaci.2022.02.015

Sahni, V. N., Balogh, E. A., Strowd, L. C., & Feldman, S. R. (2022). The evolving atopic dermatitis management landscape. *Expert Opinion on Pharmacotherapy, 23*(4), 517–526. https://doi.org/10.1080/14656566.2021.1999412

Zhu, Y., Wang, H., He, J., Yang, L., Zhou, X., Li, Z., Zhou, H., Zhao, H., & Li, Y. (2022). Atopic dermatitis and skin cancer risk: A systematic review. *Dermatologic Therapy (Heidelb), 12*, 1167–1179. https://doi.org/10.1007/s13555-022-00720-2

CELLULITIS

DEFINITION

A. Cellulitis is a bacterial infection of the deep dermis that often extends into the subcutaneous tissues.

B. Characteristic symptoms of cellulitis include tenderness, poorly demarcated erythematous margins, with warmth, and swelling.

C. Cellulitis can result from any condition or injury that disrupts the integrity of the normal flora of the skin barrier which provides protection from microbial pathogens.

D. Nonpurulent and purulent infections.

 1. Nonpurulent infection forms include cellulitis and erysipelas.

 2. Purulent infection forms include abscess.

E. Erysipelas, similar to cellulitis, is a tender, erythematous bacterial infection but with sharply demarcated borders. Erysipelas often lies within the upper dermis extending into the superficial cutaneous lymphatics, common to the face and lower.

INCIDENCE

A. 14 million cases occurring in the United States annually.

B. Occurs at any age; more common in middle age and in older males.

C. Typically in extremities, especially lower extremities.

D. Highly seasonal, more likely to occur during warmer summer months.

PATHOGENESIS

A. Bacterial invasion of the epidermis triggers a cascade of cytokine and neutrophil activity. The cytokine and neutrophil recruitment leads to an epidermal response. Antimicrobial peptides and keratinocyte proliferation produce the characteristic spreading erythema, warmth, edema, and tenderness which are commonly present. Cellulitis is typically polymicrobial.

B. Gram-positive bacteria (*S. aureus* and streptococci) such as group A *beta-hemolytic streptococcus* or methicillin-susceptible *Staphylococcus aureus* (MSSA), most commonly:

 1. Group A *beta-hemolytic streptococcus* is most common with erysipelas.

 2. *Streptococcus pyogenes* often presents with lymphangitis.

  a. Virulence factors such as pyrogenic exotoxins (A, B, C, and F) and streptococcal superantigen are suspected in more invasive disease.

 3. *Methicillin-resistant Staphylococcus aureus* (MRSA), often associated with the purulent form of cellulitis. May include pustular eruption or purulent collection.

 4. *Erysipelothrix rhusiopathiae* contact with raw meat (poultry, fish, other meat), typically seen in butchers or other handlers.

 5. Anaerobes such as Peptostreptococcus or Clostridium perfringens attributed to gas gangrene infections.

C. Gram-negative pathogens (*Proteus mirabilis, Escherichia coli, Klebsiella pneumoniae, Pseudomonas aeruginosa*).

 1. *P. aeruginosa* is commonly found in freshwater environment. Common infections include folliculitis, pneumonia, and otitis externa, and also with infected puncture wounds leading to osteomyelitis. Immunocompromised individuals are often affected. Increased antibiotic resistance patterns have been identified.

 2. Vibrio species from marine injuries, saltwater swimming, sea urchin impalement, or contact with raw seafood.

 3. *Aeromonas hydrophilia* from fresh water swimming.

 4. *Pasteurella multocida* from animal bite or injury.

PREDISPOSING FACTORS

A. Injury or disruption of integument (abrasion, laceration, surgical incision, intravenous [IV] drug abuse, insect/animal bites, and so forth).

B. History of cellulitis.

C. Decreased mobility or sedentary lifestyle.

D. Impairment of the vascular–lymphatic system.

 1. Venous insufficiency.

 2. Lymphedema due to impaired lymphatic drainage.

 3. Lymph node resection.

 4. Prior radiation treatments to the affected area.

E. Chronic comorbid conditions.

 1. Malnourishment, obesity, diabetes, chronic kidney disease, chronic liver disease, alcohol abuse.

2. Immunosuppression (HIV, cancer, taking immunosuppressive agents).

3. Tinea pedis, or any other dermatitis, such as intertrigo, or intertriginous dermatitis (a common inflammatory condition of the skin folds characterized by moist erythema, malodor, weeping, pruritus, and tenderness).

SUBJECTIVE DATA

A. Common complaints/symptoms.
   1. Elicit onset and duration of symptoms.
   2. Edema.
   3. Erythema, usually expanding or spreading.
   4. Tenderness or pain.
   5. With or without drainage or collection.
B. Common/typical scenario.
   1. Expanding, painful, erythematous, edematous area affecting the lower extremity for 1 to 2 days, possibly associated recent wound or injury.
C. Family and social history.
   1. Alcohol abuse.
   2. IV drug abuse.
   3. Any trauma to or near the affected area.
   4. Previous infection. Annual recurrence of cellulitis occurs in about 8% to 20% of patients, with overall reoccurrence rates projected to be as high as 49%.
D. Review of systems.
   1. May have malaise.
   2. Fever.
   3. Chills.
   4. Regional lymphadenopathy.
   5. Decreased mobility due to pain or swelling.

PHYSICAL EXAMINATION

A. Often one extremity (if bilateral less likely to be cellulitis. Stasis dermatitis is often bilateral and frequently misdiagnosed as cellulitis).
B. Poorly demarcated area of erythema (a sharply demarcated indurated border increases likelihood of erysipelas).
C. Painful.
D. Mild to moderate swelling.
E. Sometimes regional lymphadenitis (tender or enlarged lymph nodes) or lymphangitis (proximally streaking erythema).
F. Rarely blisters and/or necrosis.
G. Calf swelling, pain, warmth, and erythema; rule out deep vein thrombosis (DVT).
H. If exquisite tenderness and rapid progression occurs, rule out necrotizing fasciitis (emergent surgical evaluation).
I. Systemic signs of toxicity: Fever, hypotension, and tachycardia require a higher level of care.

DIAGNOSTIC TESTS

A. Imaging is not routinely recommended. The Infectious Diseases Society of America practice guidelines recommend imaging if febrile neutropenia is present.
B. Culture.

1. Culture of the affected site only when purulent discharge is present. Often cannot be cultured unless abscess is present for incision and drainage.
2. Blood cultures are recommended if exhibiting signs of systemic toxicity, persistent cellulitis despite adequate antibiotic treatment, if immunocompromised, or in the case of an immersion injury or animal bite.
C. Biopsy may lead to prolonged healing and offers low diagnostic yield.
D. Lab.
   1. Elevated sedimentation rate and/or C-reactive protein inflammatory markers.
   2. Complete blood count (CBC) with differential for leukocytosis, left shift.
   3. Procalcitonin is an inflammatory response protein, which when elevated can be associated with bacterial infections.

DIFFERENTIAL DIAGNOSIS

A. Stasis dermatitis.
B. Lipodermatosclerosis.
C. DVT.
D. Folliculitis.
E. Insect bite reaction.
F. Contact dermatitis.
G. Erysipelas.
H. Necrotizing fasciitis.

EVALUATION AND MANAGEMENT PLAN

A. General plan.
   1. Antibiotics coverage for either gram-positive (most common), MRSA, or gram-negative.
   2. Keep affected extremity elevated to limit edema and inflammation.
   3. Treatment of underlying conditions (such as edema or underlying cutaneous disorders).
   4. Maintaining hydrated skin to avoid dryness and cracking without encouraging interdigital maceration.
   5. Mark borders to monitor improvement or worsening.
   6. Point-of-care ultrasound to differentiate abscess from cellulitis (which usually has cobblestone appearance).
   7. Patients with drainable abscess should undergo incision and drainage. In addition, antibiotic therapy may be warranted if clinical criteria are met, especially for those at high risk for poor outcomes related to infective endocarditis.
   8. If systemic symptoms are present, prompt evaluation for treatment with systemic IV antibiotics and blood cultures.
   9. Hospitalization for IV antibiotics.
      a. Systemic symptoms present.
      b. Failure of outpatient therapy with oral antibiotics.
      c. Immunocompromised.
      d. Rapid progression of erythema.
      e. Unable to tolerate oral antibiotics.
      f. Cellulitis over or near an indwelling medical device.

B. Patient/family teaching points.
1. Elevate affected extremity.
2. Keep area clean with gentle soap and water.
3. Do not squeeze or irritate area.
4. Worsening pain or erythema warrants immediate follow-up.

C. Pharmacotherapy.
1. Empiric antimicrobial therapy is modified as indicated based on:
   a. Local resistance patterns (refer to local antibiogram).
   b. Known pathogen.
   c. Underlying conditions (such as diabetes and/or immunocompromise).
   d. Special circumstances:
      i. Animal bites.
      ii. Immersion or water exposure.
      iii. Perioral/perirectal abscess.
      iv. Associated pressure ulcer, or skin necrosis.
2. Duration of antimicrobial therapy: The treatment duration of antimicrobial therapy should be considered on a case-by-case basis. Antibiotic therapy is routinely prescribed from 5 to 14 days. The consensus of evidence recommends empiric antibiotic therapy for 1 week. Duration of antibiotic treatment may vary depending on:
   a. Clinical presentation.
   b. Comorbidity.
   c. Causative factors.
   d. Progression of clinical response.
3. Antibiotic coverage: With all antibiotic treatments, consider the need for renal dosing and for the potential of associated gastrointestinal side effects, including the risk of *Clostridioides difficile* infection.
4. Coverage against beta-hemolytic streptococci and methicillin-sensitive *Staphylococcus aureus* (MSSA) for mild disease with no risk factors for MRSA: Oral amoxicillin–clavulanic acid or oral fluoroquinolone antibiotics, such as Cipro and Levaquin.
5. Moderate cellulitis without hypotension or rapid deterioration may require IV therapy with ceftriaxone or equivalent beta-lactam.
6. Antibiotics for MRSA coverage include trimethoprim–sulfamethoxazole (TMP/SMX) DS, clindamycin, doxycycline, and minocycline; alternative treatments include linezolid, tedizolid, delafloxacin, or omadacycline.
7. Parenteral MRSA coverage options include linezolid, tedizolid, daptomycin, ceftaroline, or ceftobiprole. Dalbavancin is indicated for mild-moderate suspected MRSA cellulitis. Dalbavancin has low drug–drug interactions and a long half-life (up to 14days). Dalbavancin can be administered in a single shot of the total dose or in two administrations once weekly for 2 weeks.
8. Severe cellulitis is treated with broad-spectrum antibiotic coverage including linezolid or daptomycin with or without clindamycin with piperacillin–tazobactam or imipenem–cilastatin.
   a. In severe circumstance, a diagnostic workup including surgical evaluation to exclude necrotizing fasciitis.
9. History of episode of MRSA or known colonization, or lack of response to antibiotic regimen that does not cover for MRSA, consider empiric treatment with vancomycin or daptomycin.
10. Coverage for gram-positive and gram-negative bacteria and anaerobes requires vancomycin or daptomycin in combination with another antibiotic(s).
11. IV antibiotics should be initiated to cover against group A strep. If no risk factors for MRSA, treat with IV cefazolin, and when able de-escalate to cephalexin for a total of at least 5 days of treatment. If risk factors for MRSA are present, initiate therapy with vancomycin with subsequent antibiotic de-escalation to trimethoprim–sulfamethoxazole.
12. In immunocompromised patients requiring hospitalization for parenteral antibiotics, broad-spectrum antimicrobial coverage may be necessary with vancomycin plus piperacillin-tazobactam or a carbapenem.
   a. Indicated for systemic signs of toxicity (e.g., fever >100.5°F/38°C, hypotension, or sustained tachycardia).
   b. Rapid progression of erythema.
   c. Progression of clinical findings after 48 hours of oral antibiotic therapy.
   d. Inability to tolerate oral therapy.
   e. Proximity of the lesion to an indwelling medical device (e.g., prosthetic joint or vascular graft).
   f. Extensive skin involvement.
13. Oral corticosteroids. There is conflicting evidence with regard to the addition of an oral corticosteroid in the treatment of cellulitis. Corticosteroids may reduce inflammation for some individuals. Oral corticosteroids are not routinely recommended due to lack of scientific support and the potential for adverse outcomes especially for individuals with underlying conditions such as diabetes and those with invasive infection.

D. Discharge instructions.
1. Complete course of antibiotic.
2. Review common side effects of antibiotic treatment (nausea, diarrhea, rash, and *Candida* infections, including symptoms of *C. difficile* infection).
3. Keep affected extremity elevated.
4. Warm compress to the affected area.
5. Avoid Neosporin due to risk of allergic contact dermatitis.
6. If condition worsens, seek immediate evaluation.

FOLLOW-UP

A. Primary care provider (PCP) in 1 to 2 days.
B. Infectious disease or dermatologist within 3 days.
C. If worsening or signs of systemic toxicity develop, emergent treatment is suggested.

CONSULTATION/REFERRAL

A. Infectious disease or specialty dermatology consult.
  1. If periorbital or orbital cellulitis.
  2. If no improvement within 24 to 48 hours of starting antibiotic therapy.
  3. If recurrent infection, up to 49% of patients with cellulitis report at least one prior episode; recurrences occur in approximately 14% of cellulitis cases within 1 year and 45% of cases within 3 years, usually in the same location.

SPECIAL/GERIATRIC CONSIDERATIONS

A. Many patients with cellulitis have comorbidities.
B. Immunosuppressed individuals have higher risk for complications such as necrotizing fasciitis, lymphangitis, gangrene, and severe sepsis.
C. Use extra caution with patients who have prosthetic joints or who have had recent surgeries.
D. If patient has history of another known skin rash such as psoriasis and AD, may be best to consult specialty dermatology.

BIBLIOGRAPHY

Brown, B. D., & Hood Watson, K. L. (2021). Cellulitis. In *StatPearls [Internet]*. StatPearls Publishing. https://www.ncbi.nlm.nih.gov/books/NBK549770/

Dinulos, J. (2019). Bacterial infections. In J. Dinulos (Ed.), *Habif's Clinical Dermatology. A color guide to diagnosis and therapy* (9th ed., pp. 331–375.e1). Elsevier Inc.

Edwards, G., Freeman, K., Liewelyn, M. J., & Hayward, G. (2020). What diagnostic strategies can help differentiate cellulitis from other causes of red legs in primary care? *British Medical Journal, 368*, m54. https://doi.org/ 10.1136/bmj.m54

Emilio, B., & Almudena, B. (2022). Current international and national guidelines for managing skin and soft tissue infections. *Current Opinion in Infectious Diseases, 35*(2), 61–71. https://doi.org/ 10.1097/QCO.0000000000000814

Lida, B., Neslihan, O. S., Gizem, K. E., Zahide, M. Z., Nevin, H., Sami, H., Figen, B. P., Ulviye, Y., Mesut, D., & Ali, B. (2022). Preseptal and orbital cellulitis. *The Pediatric Infectious Disease Journal, 41*(2), 97–101. https://doi.org/10.1097/INF.0000000000003382

Russo, A., Vena, A, & Bassetti, M. (2022). Antibiotic treatment of acute bacterial skin and skin structure infections. *Current Opinion in Infectious Diseases, 35*(2), 120–127. https://doi.org/10.1097/QCO.0000000000000822

Shaukat, M. Y. (2021). Erysipelas. In *StatPearls [Internet]*. StatPearls. https://www.ncbi.nlm.nih.gov/books/NBK532247/

Sullivan, T., & de Barra, E. (2018). Diagnosis and management of cellulitis. *Clinical medicine, 18*(2), 160–163. https://doi.org/10.7861/clinmedicine.18-2-160

Tartaglia, K. (2022). Can't miss infections. *Medical Clinics of North America, 106*(3), 537–543.

NECROTIZING FASCIITIS

DEFINITION

A. Life-threatening infection.
B. Aggressive infection that spreads quickly along the fascial planes resulting in necrosis of the muscle fascia and subcutaneous tissues.
C. Deep fascial involvement in early stages initially spares overlying tissues, potentially delaying diagnosis until advanced stages.
D. Rapid progression may lead to septic shock.
E. Toxin-producing virulent bacteria are responsible for destruction of local tissue, causing "flesh-eating" effect.
F. May occur idiopathically.
G. 80% of cases are a result of bacterial infection from a breach in skin integrity.
H. Associated with high morbidity and the potential for long-lasting, significant functional deficits.
I. Mortality rate may be affected by patient age, patient comorbidity, type of organism, and the rapidity of diagnosis and treatment.

INCIDENCE

A. Estimated cases in the United States are 700 to 1,150 cases each year.
B. Male and female patients are equally affected.
C. All ages from 1 to 95 years.
D. Estimated to be misdiagnosed 15% to 34% of the time, leading to delay in care and an increase in the risk of mortality.
E. Increased incidence in alcoholism, hepatitis C infection, diabetes mellitus, cancer, chemotherapy, intravenous (IV) drug use, HIV infection, corticosteroid use, and with radiation therapy.

PATHOGENESIS

A. Often caused by gram-positive cocci, *Streptococcus pyogenes*, referred to as group A streptococcus (GAS). May be polymicrobial.
B. Four groups based on the microbiological spectrum:
  1. Type I (most common 80%–90% of cases) infection is polymicrobial with aerobic and anaerobic organisms and often affects immunocompromised individuals.
  2. Type II infections often involve group A beta-hemolytic streptococci and can be combined with staphylococcal bacteria, which typically has a rapid progression within hours.
  3. Type III necrotizing fasciitis is a monomicrobial gram-negative infection such as with *Vibrio vulnificus*, a species found in saltwater.
  4. Type IV infections are caused by fungal invasion primarily affecting immunocompromised or burn patients.
C. The pathogenic appearance of erythema, swelling, and edema and bullae formation commonly associated with gas gangrene are a result of toxic bacterial infiltration of the horizontal fascial planes. Platelet aggregation leads to the development of microthrombi, resulting in infarction of nutrient vessels, leading to necrosis.

PREDISPOSING FACTORS

A. Risk factors include trauma, recent surgery, or any process that compromises skin integrity.
  1. Increased risk in diabetic patients managing their diabetes with sodium-glucose cotransporter-2 (SGLT2) inhibitors, a class of diabetes medication that excretes glucose through the urine. These infections often occur in the perineum.
B. Poor prognosis with:
  1. Resistant organism.
  2. Advanced age.

3. Malignancy.
4. Uncontrolled diabetes.
5. Immunosuppression (increased mortality from disseminated infection).
6. Delayed diagnosis/intervention.
7. Altered level of consciousness.
8. Respiratory distress such as acute respiratory distress syndrome.
9. Renal impairment.

SUBJECTIVE DATA
A. History of breach of skin integrity.
B. Presenting with progressive intense pain, fever, body aches, malaise, and gastroenteritis.
C. Report painful cutaneous erythema.
D. Pain, disproportionate in relation to clinical finding.

PHYSICAL EXAMINATION
A. Rapid progression of infection (over hours to days). Erythema, swelling, and tissue necrosis and pain.
B. Systemic findings of fever, tachycardia and hemodynamic instability, subcutaneous hemorrhage, hemorrhagic bullae, necrosis, and purpura.

DIAGNOSTIC TESTS
A. Surgical consultation and intervention should not be delayed awaiting for laboratory and/or diagnostic studies.
B. Diagnosis established via surgical exploration of the soft tissue, subcutaneous tissue, fascial planes, and muscle.
C. Serum complete blood count (CBC).
D. Serum C-reactive protein and/or erythrocyte sedimentation rate (ESR).
E. Serum chemistries, including renal function.
F. Serum glucose.
G. Blood cultures (two sets).
H. Liver function.
I. Serum coagulation studies.
J. Serum creatinine kinase (CK).
K. Serum lactic acid.
L. Serum procalcitonin.
M. CT has a negative predictive value of 100%.
N. Point-of-care ultrasound (POCUS) of the affected area.

DIFFERENTIAL DIAGNOSIS
A. Cellulitis.
B. Deep vein thrombosis (DVT).
C. Abscess.
D. Pyomyositis.
E. Pyoderma gangrenosum.
F. Gas gangrene.

EVALUATION AND MANAGEMENT PLAN
A. A high index of suspicion should prompt immediate surgical consultation in patients with erythema, disproportionate pain, and hemodynamic instability.

B. Positive outcomes have been associated with early surgical intervention with prompt debridement of devitalized tissue, hydration, and broad-spectrum antibiotics.
C. Treatment.
1. Pain control (subjective).
2. Prompt surgical exploration and debridement.
3. Prompt initiation of IV antibiotics.
4. Aggressive fluid resuscitation with isotonic fluids.
5. Inotropic support for hypotension.
6. Postoperative nutritional support to support negative protein balance that occurs as a result of catabolism.
D. Patient/family teaching points.
1. Provide patient and family support with regard to progression of infection and consequences of antibiotic use.
2. Provide support with regard to adjustment of daily activities and roles associated with potential functional limitations.
3. Anticipate need for emotional support.
E. Pharmacotherapy.
1. Prompt administration of IV antibiotics.
2. Antibiotic coverage, including coverage for both gram-positive, gram-negative, and anaerobic bacteria, with a broad-spectrum beta-lactam such as piperacillin–tazobactam.
3. Additional considerations should include (case by case):
  a. Local susceptibility patterns.
  b. Individual comorbid factors.
  c. Progression of infectious process.
4. Aminoglycosides should be reserved for broadening spectrum in case of septic shock.
5. Clindamycin combination in suspected GAS infection.
  a. Limb infection.
  b. Streptococcal toxic shock.
  c. Absence of comorbidities.
  d. Blunt trauma.
  e. Absence of chronic skin lesions.
  f. Homelessness.
  g. Injectable drug use.
  h. Nonsteroidal anti-inflammatory drug use.
6. No clear guidelines exist regarding treatment duration. IV antibiotic therapy is recommended at least 48 to 72 hours after surgical intervention if there is clinical improvement. The total duration of antibiotic therapy is generally recommended from 7 to 15 days.
F. Discharge instructions.
1. Rehab support for functional deficits.
2. Case management for home care.
3. Family support.

CONSULTATION/REFERRAL
A. Early surgical consult for intervention/debridement and for soft tissue reconstruction as needed.
B. Specialty wound care services.
C. Infectious disease consult.
D. Physical therapy consult.
E. Nutrition consult.
F. Case management consult.

SPECIAL/GERIATRIC CONSIDERATIONS

A. Management of comorbid conditions to optimize organ function.

B. Continued interdisciplinary collaboration at discharge with surgery, physical therapy nursing, infectious disease, and dietary and case management.

C. The geriatric population has been associated with both increased risk and the potential for poor outcomes. Early identification and intervention is essential in this population.

BIBLIOGRAPHY

Diab, J., Bannan, A., & Pollitt, T. (2020). Necrotizing fasciitis. *British Medical Journal (Online), 369*, m1428. https://doi.org/https://doi.org/10.1136/bmj.m1428

Fay, K., Onukwube, J., Chochua, S., Schaffner, W., Cieslak, P., Lynfield, R., Muse, A., Smelser, C., Harrison, L. H., Farley, M., Petit, S., Alden, N., Apostal, M., Snippes Vagnone, P., Nanduri, S., Beall, B., & Van Beneden, C. A. (2021). Patterns of antibiotic nonsusceptibility among invasive group A *Streptococcus* infections—United States, 2006–2017. *Clinical Infectious Diseases, 73*(11), 1957–1964. https://doi-org.ezproxy2.library.drexel.edu/10.1093/cid/ciab575

Fujinaga, J., Kuriyama, A., Ilegami, T., & Onodera, M. (2021). Laboratory risk indicator for necrotizing fasciitis score and patient outcomes. *Journal of Emergencies, Trauma and Shock, 14*(1), 38–41.

Group A streptococcal (GAS) disease. (2022). *Centers for disease control and prevention.* U.S. Department of health & Human Services. https://www.cdc.gov/groupastrep/diseases-public/necrotizing-fasciitis.html#:~:text=CDC%20tracks%20necrotizing%20fasciitis%20caused%20by%20group%20A%20strep%20with,year%20in%20the%20United%20States

Hamada, S., Nakajima, M., Kaszynski, R. H., Otaka, S., Goto, H., Matsui, H., Fushimi, K., Yamaguchi, Y., & Yasunaga, H. (2022). Association between adjunct clindamycin and in-hospital mortality in patients with necrotizing soft tissue infection due to group A *Streptococcus*: A nationwide cohort study. *European Journal of Clinical Microbiology & Infectious Disease, 41*, 263–270. https://doi-org.ezproxy2.library.drexel.edu/10.1007/s10096-021-04376-2

Kang-Auger, G., Chasse, M., Quach, C., Ayoub, A., & Auger, N. (2021). Focus: Rare disease, necrotizing fasciitis: Association with pregnancy-related risk factors early in life. *Yale Journal of Biology and Medicine, 94*(4), 573–584.

Kjaldgaard, L., Cristall, N., Gawaziuk, J. P., Kohja, Z., & Logsetty, S. (2021). Predictors of mortality in patients with necrotizing Fasciitis: A literature review and multivariate analysis. *Plastic Surgery*, 1–8. https://doi-org.ezproxy2.library.drexel.edu/10.1177/22925503211034830

Lahham, S., Shniter, I., Desai, M., Andary, R., Saadat, S., Fox, J.C.., & Pierce, S. (2022). Point of care ultrasound in the diagnosis of necrotizing fasciitis. *The American Journal of Emergency Medicine, 51*, 397–400. https://doi.org/10.1016/j.ajem.2021.10.033

McGee, S. A., Barnum, M., & Nesbit, R. D. (2022). The Epidemiology of necrotizing fasciitis at a rural level 1 trauma center during the COVID-19 pandemic. *The American Surgeon*, 31348221074251. https://doi.org/10.1177/00031348221074251

Ravins, M., Ambalavanan, P., Biswas, D., Tan, R. Y. M., Lim, K. X. Z., Kaufman, Y., Anand, A., Sharma, A., & Hanski, E. (2022). Murine soft tissue infection model to study group A Streptococcus (GAS) pathogenesis in necrotizing fasciitis. In O. Gal-Mor (Ed.), *Bacterial virulence. Methods in molecular biology* (p. 2427). Humana. https://doi.org/10.1007/978-1-0716-1971-1_16

Tartaglia, K. (2022). Can't miss infections. *Medical Clinics of North America, 106*(3), 537–543.

Urbina, T., Razazi, K., Ourghanlian, C., Woerther, P. L., Chosidow, O., Lepeule, R., & de Prost, N. (2021). Antibiotics in necrotizing soft tissue infections. *Antibiotics, 10*, 1104. https://doi.org/10.3390/antibiotics10091104

Wallace, H. A., & Perera, T. B. (2021). Necrotizing fasciitis. In *StatPearls [Internet]*. StatPearls Publishing. https://www.ncbi.nlm.nih.gov/books/NBK430756/

Wladis, E. J. (2022). Periorbital necrotizing fasciitis. *Survey of Ophthalmology, 67*(5), 1547–1552. https://doi.org/ 10.1016/j.survophthal.2022.02.006

Xu, L. Q., Zhao, X. X., Wang, P. X., Yang, J., & Yang, Y. M. (2019). Multidisciplinary treatment of a patient with necrotizing fasciitis caused by *Staphylococcus aureus*: A case report. *World Journal Clinical Cases, 7*(21), 3595–3602. https://doi.org/10.12998/wjcc.v7.i21.3595 PMID: 31750343; PMCID: PMC6854421

SEBORRHEIC DERMATITIS

DEFINITION

A. Chronic and relapsing inflammatory skin condition.

B. Sebaceous rich areas of the scalp, face (Figure 15.2), and skin folds of the body.

INCIDENCE

A. Approximately 5% of the general population.

B. All ethnic groups and all regions globally.

C. Peak incidences among infants in the first 3 months of life, adolescents at puberty, and adults aged 30–50 years.

D. 35% of HIV and 85% of AIDS population.

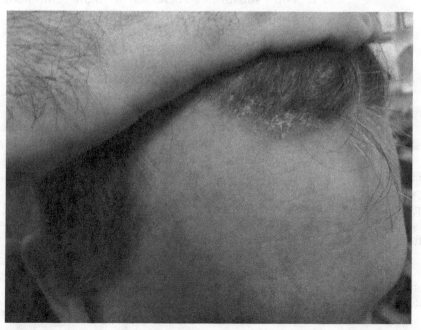

FIGURE 15.2 Seborrheic dermatitis.

Source: From Lyons, F., & Ousley, L. (2015). *Dermatology for the advanced practice nurse.* Springer Publishing Company.

PATHOGENESIS

A. Disruption of the skin's microbiota.
B. *Malassezia* yeasts trigger inflammatory and hyperproliferative epidermal responses compromising the stratum corneum.
C. Disruption of cutaneous neurotransmitters.
D. Abnormal shedding of keratinocytes.

PREDISPOSING FACTORS

A. Age.
B. Male sex.
C. Stress.
D. Increased sebaceous gland activity.
E. Diabetes.
F. Polycystic ovarian syndrome.
G. Immunocompromise: Lymphoma, transplant, and HIV-AIDS.
H. Neuropsychiatric disorders: Parkinson, Alzheimer dementia, major depression, autonomic dysfunction, and cerebrovascular accident.
I. Drug therapy: Immunosuppressants, dopamine antagonists, and lithium.
J. Low humidity, low temperature environments.

SUBJECTIVE DATA

A. Common complaints/symptoms.
  1. Pruritus.
  2. Scaling and flaking skin.
  3. Oily hair.
B. Common/typical scenario.
  1. Erythematous, greasy, pruritic, burning, with dryness in a symmetric distribution pattern affecting the scalp and the face (particularly the nasolabial folds, eyebrows, and ears).
  2. Improves with more frequent hair washing.
  3. Worse in the summer months.
  4. Sudden severe onset should be a red flag for the presence of HIV-AIDS.
C. Family and social history.
  1. May be familial.
D. Review of systems.
  1. Typically limited to skin complaints.

PHYSICAL EXAMINATION

A. Folliculocentric salmon-colored papules and plaques with a fine white scale.
B. A yellowish crust often described as a greasy scale crust may be present.
C. Less scaling on flexural surfaces with lesions with poorly defined margins.
D. Mostly found on the scalp (see Figure 15.2), brows, nasolabial folds, nasal alae, conchal bowls, and postauricular, and sometimes on the neck, chest, axillae, or groin folds.
E. Darker skin presentations may be persistent dyschromia with variable hyper/hypopigmentation.

DIAGNOSTIC TESTS

A. Diagnostic evaluation is not routinely recommended and may be indicated to confirm or evaluate another process.

B. If sudden, severe onset, HIV serology should be expedited.
C. Syphilis testing (venereal disease research laboratory [VDRL]).
D. Serum zinc level.
E. Antinuclear antibodies (ANA); if positive, obtain extractable nuclear antigen antibodies (ENA).
F. ESR.
G. Potassium hydroxide (KOH) skin scraping preparation will demonstrate hyphae.
H. Fungal culture, if suspicion for tinea is in differential diagnosis.
I. Skin biopsy, helpful in overlapping presentations with other dermatoses.

DIFFERENTIAL DIAGNOSIS

A. Tinea (capitis, corporis, cruris, versicolor).
B. Pityriasis rosacea.
C. Psoriasis.
D. Contact dermatitis.
E. Drug eruption.
F. Lupus erythematous.
G. In children, consider acrodermatitis enteropathica or transient neonatal zinc deficiency.

EVALUATION AND MANAGEMENT PLAN

A. General plan.
  1. Decrease oil on scalp and affected areas.
  2. Decrease scale and itch.
  3. Management variables.
    a. Age.
    b. Distribution of dermatitis.
    c. Severity.
  4. Clinical features of Parkinson's disease require evaluation in older adult patients.
  5. Review of current daily medications.
B. Patient/family teaching points.
  1. Wash scalp frequently, focus on scalp more than hair.
  2. Soap substitute such as a light emollient moisturizer.
C. Pharmacotherapy.
  1. Seborrheic dermatitis responds to a variety of immunosuppressive and antifungal therapies, but there is no cure. Combination treatment rotation may be more effective and associated with fewer adverse reactions as compared with monotherapy.
  2. Topical antifungal and anti-inflammatory agents are mainstay treatments. New novel approaches such as with topical calcineurin inhibitors (TCIs) with immunomodulator properties have been promising. Examples include tacrolimus and pimecrolimus.
  3. Topical creams, ointments, and lotions (face and body).
    a. 2% salicylic acid + 2% sulfur in sorbolene cream or emulsifying ointment.
    b. 2% ketoconazole cream.
    c. 1% clotrimazole + 1% hydrocortisone cream.
    d. 10% sulfacetamide + 5% sulfur lotion.

e. Betamethasone dipropionate 0.05% lotion.
f. 0.03% and 0.1% tacrolimus ointment.
4. Shampoos (scalp).
   a. 1% zinc pyrithione.
   b. 1% to 0.5% selenium sulfide.
   c. 2% ketoconazole.
   d. 1% ciclopirox.
   e. 5% coal tar + 2% salicylic acid.
   f. 0.1% and 0.03% tacrolimus.
5. Oral medications.
   a. Itraconazole.
   b. Fluconazole.
   c. Terbinafine.
      i. Oral treatment for generalized or refractory disease, but may have systemic consequences. Itraconazole can worsen heart failure. Fluconazole should be adjusted for renal impairment. Itraconazole has the greatest anti-inflammatory effect, while oral terbinafine may be more effective than oral fluconazole.
D. Discharge instructions.
1. Discuss risks of prolonged topical steroid use: Atrophy of skin, hypopigmentation of skin, risk of glaucoma if use is near the eyes or hands are not washed after use.
2. May take a few weeks to improve.

FOLLOW-UP
A. Dermatology in the next 1 to 3 months.

CONSULTATION/REFERRAL
A. If persists or worsens, consult/refer to dermatology.

SPECIAL/GERIATRIC CONSIDERATIONS
A. Nursing home patients may have difficulty adhering to washing regimen.
B. Eyelids are prone to secondary bacterial infections, especially during acute flares.
C. The diaper region is particularly prone to overgrowth with *Candida*.
D. New evidence suggests high fruit intake diet may be associated with a 25% lower risk of seborrheic dermatitis.

BIBLIOGRAPHY
Azizzadehm, M., Pahlevan, D., & Bagheri, B. (2021). The efficacy and safety of pimecrolimus 1% cream vs. sertaconazole 2% cream in the treatment of patients with facial seborrhoeic dermatitis: A randomized blinded trial. *Clinical and Experimental Dermatology*, 47(5), 926–931. https://doi-org.ezproxy2.library.drexel.edu/10.1111/ced.15067
Dhawan, G. K., & Coulson, I. H. (2022). Seborrheic eczema. In M. G. Lebwohl, W. R. Heymann, I. H. Coulson, De. F. Murrell (Eds.), *Treatment of skin disease* (pp. 792–795). Elsevier Ltd.
Heath, C. R., & Usatine, R. P. (2021). Seborrheic dermatitis. *Journal Family Practice*, 70(9), E3–E4. https://doi.org/10.12788/jfp.0315 PMID: 34818158
Seborrhoeic Dermatitis Market Size, Epidemiology, Treatment, Therapies and Companies by DelveInsight. (2022). *M2 Presswire, gale general one-file*. link.gale.com/apps/doc/A707360458/ITOF?u=drexel_main&sid=bookmark-ITOF&xid=5ada43f9
Tao, R., Wang, R., Wan, Z., Song, Y., Wu, S., & Li, R. (2022). Ketoconazole 2% cream alters the skin fungal microbiome in seborrhoeic dermatitis: A cohort study. *Clinical and Experimental Dermatology*, 47(6), 1088–1096. https://doi-org.ezproxy2.library.drexel.edu/10.1111/ced.15115
Tucker, D., & Masood, S. (2022). Seborrheic dermatitis. In *StatPearls [Internet]*. StatPearls Publishing. https://www.ncbi.nlm.nih.gov/books/NBK551707/

STASIS DERMATITIS

DEFINITION
A. Also known as stasis eczema; dermatitis primarily of the lower extremities due to chronic venous insufficiency.
B. Eczema-like inflammation of the lower extremities is associated with impairment of the vascular–lymphatic system.
C. According to the Clinical, Etiologic, Anatomic, Pathophysiologic (CEAP) classification of venous disorders, venous stasis is classified as the following:
   1. C4: Changes in the skin and subcutaneous tissue secondary to venous disease.
      a. C4a: Pigmentation or eczema.
      b. C4b: Lipodermatosclerosis or atrophie blanche, which accompanies stasis dermatitis.

INCIDENCE
A. 6.2% among individuals older than 65 years.
B. Up to 20% of women.
C. Up to 17% of men.

PATHOGENESIS
A. Venous hypertension and chronic inflammatory changes are attributed to the development of stasis dermatitis.
B. Dysfunctional venous valves lead to hypertension as a result of:
   1. Obstruction of venous flow. *AND/OR*
   2. Incompetent valves, leading to valvular reflux.
C. Leucocytes accumulate in the areas of high venous pressure, migrate to the surrounding tissues releasing damaging proteolytic enzymes, resulting in inflammatory cutaneous changes.
D. Cellular accumulation of inflammatory T cells and macrophages combined with extravasation of red blood cells (RBCs) in the affected skin occurs as a result of venous hypertension.
E. Extravasation of the RBCs leads to the breakdown of hemoglobin, causing excessive iron to accumulate in the tissue.
F. Iron is stored as hemosiderin in the tissue.
G. Classic clinical exam findings are attributed to epidermal spongiotic changes, papillary structure alternation, and capillary proliferation.
H. Lesions vary in relation to valvular dysfunction and often extend proximally with progression.

PREDISPOSING FACTORS
A. Advanced age, female sex.
B. Malnourishment, obesity, sedentary lifestyle, prolonged standing occupation.
C. Elevated estrogen levels, pregnancy.
D. Trauma: History of bone fracture, history of deep vein thrombosis (DVT).

E. Impairment of the vascular–lymphatic system.
  1. Venous insufficiency.
  2. Lymphedema due to impaired lymphatic drainage.
  3. Lymph node resection.
  4. Prior radiation treatments to the affected area.
F. Chronic comorbidity conditions.
  1. Diabetes, congestive heart failure, hypertension, chronic kidney disease, chronic liver disease, alcohol abuse.
  2. Immunosuppression: HIV, cancer, taking immunosuppressive agents.
  3. Tinea pedis or other dermatitis affecting skin integrity.

SUBJECTIVE DATA

A. Common complaints/symptoms.
  1. Symptoms related to chronic venous insufficiency.
    a. Pruritus.
    b. Poorly demarcated erythematous plaques.
    c. Hyperpigmented patches.
    d. Scaly.
    e. Atrophic skin.
    f. Ulceration.
    g. Edema or swelling.
    h. Often bilateral lower extremities, especially medial malleolus.
B. Common/typical scenario.
  1. Erythematous scaly eruption on one lower leg at the ankle (medial malleolus) spreading proximally and bilaterally.
  2. Pruritus.
  3. Evolving over several weeks to months.
  4. Pain or symptoms of discomfort, described as a fullness or heaviness, dragging or aching, or frank pain that is exacerbated by standing, increases throughout the day, and is relieved by rest when the limb is elevated.

C. Family and social history.
  1. Smoking.
  2. Family history of vascular disorder.
D. Review of systems.
  1. Limited to the skin.

PHYSICAL EXAMINATION

A. Hyperpigmented and/or erythematous dry patches of the skin with or without scale.
B. Unilateral or bilateral extremities, worse on the ankles (Figure 15.3).
C. Mild to moderate swelling.
D. Rarely blisters, necrosis.
E. If palpate warmth, need to rule out DVT.
F. If exquisite tenderness and rapid progression occurs, rule out necrotizing fasciitis.
G. Chronic stasis dermatitis characterized by hyperpigmented and lichenified plaques.

DIAGNOSTIC TESTS

A. Culture: Usually negative, but may present with secondary infection especially if purulent discharge is present. Cannot be cultured unless drainage is present.
B. Biopsy: Not usually indicated due to poor healing and low diagnostic yield.
C. Doppler ultrasound (if DVT is suspected).
D. Serology may be indicated if another process such as an infection is suspected.

DIFFERENTIAL DIAGNOSIS

A. Cellulitis.
B. Contact dermatitis.
C. Purpuric dermatoses.
D. Lipodermatosclerosis.
E. DVT.
F. Venous ulcer.
G. Insect bite reaction.
H. Skin cancer (squamous cell carcinoma).

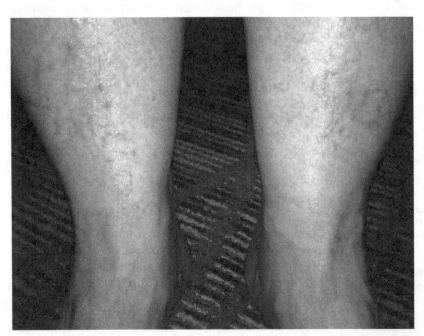

FIGURE 15.3 Example of stasis dermatitis.

Source: From Lyons, F., & Ousley, L. (2015). *Dermatology for the advanced practice nurse.* Springer Publishing Company.

I. Erysipelas.
J. Necrotizing fasciitis.

EVALUATION AND MANAGEMENT PLAN
A. General plan.
 1. Maintain skin integrity.
 2. Increase venous return.
B. Patient/family teaching points.
 1. Stress the importance of management of underlying comorbid conditions.
 2. Elevate legs daily for 30 minutes four to five times daily, especially at night.
 3. Compression stockings during daytime activities.
 4. Participate in regular exercise, especially walking.
 5. Avoid skin irritants.
 6. Use a fragrance-free emulsion to keep dry skin moist.
 7. Avoid harsh soaps.
 8. Maintain a healthy weight.
 9. Stay well-hydrated.
 10. Limit dietary salt intake.
C. Pharmacotherapy.
 1. Topical steroids are indicated for erythema, pruritus, vesiculation, and oozing. Petroleum-based topical corticosteroids such as triamcinolone ointment or fluocinolone ointment without additives are best to minimize the risk of sensitization.
 a. High- to mid-potency corticosteroids in an ointment formulation applied to the affected skin area once or twice daily for 1 to 2 weeks.
 b. Prolonged use of high-potency corticosteroids should be avoided as they may induce skin atrophy, increasing the risk of breakdown and atrophy.
 2. Corticosteroids: If topical steroids are ineffective or if worsening inflammatory symptoms, consider the possibility of secondary allergic contact dermatitis or the possibility of autosensitization. In these patients, they may benefit from a short course of corticosteroids, such as prednisone 20 to 30 mg once daily for 5 to 7 days or a single dose or triamcinolone 40 mg intramuscularly.
 3. Antibiotic therapy.
 a. Topical antibiotic may be indicated if secondary bacterial impetiginized lesions present. Topical mupirocin is indicated if *Staphylococcus* or *Streptococcus* is suspected. If drainage is present, consider culture of lesion.
 b. Oral antibiotics are not recommended unless secondary bacterial infection is present. Cellulitis misdiagnosis has been associated with the unnecessary use of oral antibiotics which have been attributed to unnecessary hospitalization, increased healthcare costs, and potential for patient harm.
D. Discharge instructions (if standard accepted guidelines exist, please use discharge template).

FOLLOW-UP
A. Dermatology.
B. Follow up in 1 to 3 months.

CONSULTATION/REFERRAL
A. If persists or worsens, consult/refer to dermatology.

SPECIAL/GERIATRIC CONSIDERATIONS
A. Older adult populations with comorbid conditions are at higher risk of venous insufficiency. Key strategies include:
 1. Management of comorbid diseases.
 2. Encouraging an active lifestyle for venous return.
 3. Management of an acute flare.
 4. Educating the patient on when to seek immediate care.

CASE SCENARIO: DERMATOLOGY

A 66-year-old patient presents with left lower extremity erythema accompanied by mild swelling and pruritus. He first noticed symptoms approximately 2 months ago and reports the symptoms are now worse. He notes the eruption has gradually worsened and is now spreading up the anterior aspect of his lower extremity. He denies fever or dyspnea. He denies new product or drug exposure or injury. His medical history is significant for hypertension, for which he reports is stable on losartan 100 mg daily. On examination, an area of poorly demarcated erythema appearing mildly edematous with scaling and mild serous oozing is observed on the mid-distal anterior and medial aspect of the left lower extremity. No other abnormal findings were noted on physical exam. He reports he applied Vaseline to the area with mild improvement of symptoms "a few weeks ago." He is afebrile. Temperature is 98.2°F/36.7°C, blood pressure is 150/98, and heart rate is 76.

1. Which of the following is the *least likely* of the differentials?
 A. Drug reaction dermatitis
 B. Contact dermatitis
 C. Deep vein thrombosis (DVT)
 D. Chronic stasis dermatitis

2. What is this patient's condition most often misdiagnosed as?
 A. DVT
 B. Cellulitis
 C. Poison ivy dermatitis
 D. Contact dermatitis

3. Which of the following medications would be the best treatment?
 A. Hydrocortisone 1% cream topically
 B. Triamcinolone 0.1% ointment
 C. Benadryl 50 mg PO QID
 D. Zyrtec 10 mg PO daily.

BIBLIOGRAPHY
Agnihothri, R., & Shinkai, K. (2021). Stasis dermatitis. *JAMA Dermatology, 157*(12), 1524. https://doi.org/10.1001/jamadermatol.2021.3475
Fransway, A., Fowler, J., & Corona, R. (2022). *Stasis dermatitis*. UptoDate. https://www.uptodate.com/contents/stasis-dermatitis
Hashimoto, T., Kursewicz, C. D., Fayne, R. A., Nandam, S., Shah, S. M., Nattkemper, L., Yokozeki, H., & Yosipovitch, G. (2019). Mechanisms of itch in stasis dermatitis: Significant role of IL-31 from macrophages. *Journal of Investigative Dermatology, 140*(4), 850–859.e3. https://doi.org/10.1016/j.jid.2019.09.012
Kilinc, F., Akbas, A., Sener, S., & Hayran, Y. (2021). Cutaneous findings in patients with chronic venous insufficiency. *Journal of Cosmetic Dermatology, 21*(5), 2106–2112.
Piyush, K., Khan, A. K., Das, A., & Shah, H. (2022). Chronic venous disease. Part 1: Pathophysiology and clinical features. *Clinical and experimental dermatology, 47*(7), 2106–2112. https://doi-org.ezproxy2.library.drexel.edu/10.1111/ced.15143
Zegarra, T. I., & Tadi, P. (2022). CEAP classification of venous disorders. In *StatPearls [Internet]*. StatPearls Publishing. https://www.ncbi.nlm.nih.gov/books/NBK557410/

KNOWLEDGE CHECK: CHAPTER 15

1. An adult patient with a history of asthma reports chronic eruption, greater in the flexor folds of the extremities, neck, and "sometimes" the periorbital region. The patient shows a solid understanding of the preferred skin care regimen when stating:

   A. "I take three to four bleach baths per day."
   B. "I limit daily bathing to only essential 'dirty' areas."
   C. "I avoid moisturizers without scents."
   D. "I use baby powder daily."

2. A patient notes that an eruption in the left elbow is erythematous and tender. The patient reports that the area is now draining a "cloudy yellow fluid." A secondary bacterial infection is suspected. What findings would be expected in the complete blood count?

   A. Elevated eosinophil count
   B. Elevated white blood cell count
   C. Elevated platelet count
   D. Low white blood cell count

3. If a secondary bacterial infection is suspected, what is the best treatment option?

   A. Treatment with an oral antibiotic
   B. Topical emulsion to affected areas
   C. Medium-potency topical steroids to affected areas
   D. The finding is chronic; no treatment necessary at this time

4. An older adult with type 2 diabetes controls their blood sugar with empagliflozin (Jardiance). The patient presents to the clinic with a tender erythematous eruption in the genital region. They report feeling fatigued and "chilled" and note persistent symptoms for 2 days. The patient has not noticed any drainage from the site. Necrotizing fasciitis of the perineum, also known as Fournier gangrene, is suspected. Priority treatment for this patient should include:

   A. Prompt referral to diabetic educator to review diabetic diet
   B. Treatment with oral antibiotics and return to the clinic in 1 week for reevaluation
   C. Referral to inpatient care because this infection can be life-threatening
   D. High-potency topical steroids to control inflammation

5. A 40-year-old patient with no medical conditions presents with a tender erythematous eruption of their left leg. The patient reports that 1 week ago they were injured at work when a piece of sheet metal punctured the skin of their left lower leg. The patient notes that the area was healing "fine" but now has become painful and erythematous. The patient has no fever and offers no complaints of other systemic symptoms. The patient has no history of skin infection. On exam, a scabbed area is noted on the left lower leg that has poorly demarcated erythematous margins. The area is mildly tender, feels hot to touch, and is mildly swollen. No drainage or collection has been identified. What condition may be suspected?

   A. Contact dermatitis from metal puncture
   B. Cellulitis
   C. Necrotizing fasciitis
   D. Stasis dermatitis

6. What is the best treatment option for a patient with cellulitis?

   A. Oral amoxicillin-clavulanic acid
   B. Oral amoxicillin
   C. Oral azithromycin
   D. Oral nitrofurantoin

7. A patient reports erythematous, greasy, pruritic, dry skin in a symmetric distribution pattern affecting the scalp and the face (particularly the nasolabial folds, eyebrows, and ears). They report that the condition has been ongoing and "sometimes gets really bad." What condition is suspected?

   A. Cellulitis
   B. Contact dermatitis
   C. Seborrheic dermatitis
   D. Atopic dermatitis

8. The best treatment option for seborrheic dermatitis is:

   A. Topical 1% clotrimazole + 1% hydrocortisone cream
   B. Topical mupirocin
   C. Oral clindamycin
   D. Oral amoxicillin-clavulanic acid

(See answers next page.)

1. B) "I limit daily bathing to only essential 'dirty' areas."

It is suggested that bathing is kept to a minimum, focusing on daily essential areas.

2. B) Elevated white blood cell count

A complete blood count with differential may support the diagnosis of an infection if there is an elevated white blood cell count or if the differential has a left shift. Eosinophilia would indicate an allergic component; if thrombocytopenia is present, it may indicate Wiskott–Aldrich syndrome, which can mimic presentation of atopic dermatitis.

3. A) Treatment with an oral antibiotic

Secondary infections should be treated with oral therapy. Systemic antibiotics may be necessary in combination with carefully diluted bleach baths (up to daily) and nasal mupirocin (for nasal colonization) to clear frequent skin infections.

4. C) Referral to inpatient care because this infection can be life-threatening

Patients with suspected necrotizing fasciitis of the perineum should be treated promptly and aggressively. Symptoms include tenderness, redness, often swelling of the genitals or the area from the genitals back to the rectum, and a fever above 100.4°F/38°C, or a general feeling of being unwell. These symptoms can worsen quickly and can be aggressive and life-threatening.

5. B) Cellulitis

Cellulitis is a bacterial infection of the deep dermis that often extends into the subcutaneous tissues, often caused by a break in skin integrity. Characteristic symptoms of cellulitis include tenderness, poorly demarcated erythematous margins, with warmth, and swelling.

6. A) Oral amoxicillin–clavulanic acid

Coverage against beta-hemolytic streptococci and methicillin-sensitive *Staphylococcus aureus* for mild disease with no risk factors for methicillin-resistant *Staphylococcus aureus* (MRSA) would include oral amoxicillin–clavulanic acid or oral fluoroquinolone antibiotics.

7. C) Seborrheic dermatitis

Seborrheic dermatitis is erythematous, greasy, pruritic, burning skin with dryness in a symmetric distribution pattern. It affects the scalp and the face (particularly the nasolabial folds, eyebrows, and ears). It is a chronic and relapsing inflammatory skin condition.

8. A) Topical 1% clotrimazole + 1% hydrocortisone cream

Topical antifungal and anti-inflammatory agents are the mainstay of treatment. Seborrheic dermatitis responds to a variety of immunosuppressive and antifungal therapies, but there is no cure. Combination treatment rotation may be more effective and associated with fewer adverse reactions as compared with monotherapy.

CHAPTER 16

GERIATRIC GUIDELINES

DELIRIUM

Abimbola Farinde

DEFINITION

A. Delirium includes five key characteristics as described in the *Diagnostic and Statistical Manual of Mental Disorders* (Fifth Edition; *DSM-5*; American Psychiatric Publishing; needed for diagnosis).

  1. A disturbance of attention and awareness.

  2. Developed over hours to a few days, with a change in baseline functioning. May fluctuate in severity with time of day.

  3. Additional changes in cognition.

  4. Not influenced by an existing neurocognitive disorder or state of arousal (e.g., coma).

  5. Reasonable suspicion the change is caused by a medical condition, substance addiction or withdrawal, medication side effect, or due to multiple etiologies.

B. Additional features.

  1. Hyperactivity, hypoactivity, or mixed level of activity with alterations in sleep.

  2. Emotional disturbance and possible illusions or hallucinations.

  3. Extremes of mood, including agitation.

  4. Disorganized thinking, rambling, irrelevant, or incoherent speech.

  5. Psychomotor disturbances, including restlessness and lethargy.

C. The terms *acute confusional state* or *delirium* are often used interchangeably.

INCIDENCE

A. Age: More common in the aged, but can occur with any illness.

B. Incidence:

  1. Up to 50% of older surgical patients can experience delirium.

  2. Highest rates found among ICU patients (45%–87%), followed by ED and hospice.

  3. The prevalence of delirium tends to be highest among hospitalized older individuals.

C. Frequency: While once considered only a temporary condition common in ill patients, delirium is now associated with increased length of stay, rate of complications, and cost of hospitalization, and more importantly in hospital mortality rates. There can be variability of presentation based on a person's characteristics, type of health setting, and sensitivity to the detection method.

PATHOGENESIS

A. Multifactorial.

  1. Difficult to study in already ill patients.

  2. Affects arousal and attention.

    a. Arousal and attention are affected by the reticular activation system (RAS).

    b. The nondominant parietal and frontal lobes govern attention.

    c. Cortical functions are needed for insight and judgment.

  3. May be related to drug toxicity, inflammation from trauma, sepsis, surgery, neuronal injury, and environmental factors.

PREDISPOSING FACTORS

A. Increase baseline vulnerability.

  1. Underlying brain disease.

  2. Advanced age.

  3. Sensory impairment.

  4. Use of restraints.

  5. Urinary retention.

  6. Constipation.

  7. Anticholinergic medications.

  8. Pain.

B. Precipitate the disturbance.

  1. Polypharmacy.

  2. Infection.

  3. Dehydration.

  4. Immobility.

  5. Malnutrition.

  6. Bladder catheters.

  7. Hypo- and hyperglycemia.

  8. Electrolyte imbalances.

SUBJECTIVE DATA

A. Common complaints/symptoms.

  1. Feeling confused.

  2. Hallucinations.

3. Difficulty maintaining attention and focus.
B. Common/typical scenario.
  1. Patient with delirium is not able to give information or accurate details.
  2. Family or caregivers will often seek medical attention for the patient, or the patient is brought in through emergency services.
C. Family and social history.
  1. Inquire if the patient uses drugs or drinks alcohol, particularly how often and how much.
  2. Inquire about medications and recent travel.
D. Review of systems.
  1. Inquire about disturbances of consciousness.
    a. Change in level of awareness.
    b. Inability to focus.
    c. Loss of mental clarity.
    d. Family member may report "not acting like herself" or "not acting right."
    e. Distractible, usually noted in conversation.
    f. May have decreased level of consciousness (typical) or be hypervigilant (some situations like withdrawal).
    g. Day/night reversal.
  2. Inquire about altered cognition.
    a. Memory loss.
    b. Disorientation.
    c. Difficulty with language and speech.
    d. Perceptual disturbances.
      i. Delusions.
      ii. Hallucinations: Visual, auditory, or somatosensory.
      iii. Lack of insight.
  3. Medications.
    a. Changes in medication regimen, particularly initiation of new medications, dose changes, brand changes, or medication additions.
  4. Changes in health status.
  5. Note time of acute onset, fluctuation of symptoms, changes in consciousness, and decline.
  6. Identify modifiable risk factors.
    a. Sensory impairment.
    b. Immobilization.
    c. Concurrent disease or illness.
    d. Metabolic derangements.
    e. Environment.
    f. Pain.
    g. Sleep deprivation.
  7. Identify nonmodifiable risk factors.
    a. Dementia.
    b. Age older than 65 years.
    c. Multiple comorbidities.
    d. Renal or hepatic disease.

PHYSICAL EXAMINATION
A. Sometimes difficult with the delusional patient.
B. Be alert for signs that may point to a cause of the delirium.
  1. Diaphoresis may be postfebrile, indicating possible infection.

2. Jaundice, indicating hepatic failure or pancreatitis.
3. Stigmata of drug use.
4. Smell of alcohol.
5. Indication of postictal state.
6. Indication of sepsis.
7. Signs of fatigue, tiredness, difficulty concentrating, or other indicators of kidney impairment.
C. Neurologic examination is typically very difficult and can sometimes be misleading. Should assess:
  1. Attention.
  2. Arousal.
  3. Motor function.
  4. Senses.
  5. Deep tendon reflexes.
  6. Higher cognitive functioning.
  7. Thought cohesiveness.

DIAGNOSTIC TESTS
A. Confusion Assessment Method (CAM; see Exhibit 16.1).
  1. Standard screen for delirium.
  2. Takes 5 minutes.
  3. Has a method especially for ICU patients, including vented patients, called the CAM-ICU.
B. Intensive care delirium screening checklist (ICDSC) is also used in the ICU setting (see Exhibit 16.2).
C. Mini-Mental State Examination is not useful for this population.
D. Use history and physical examination to guide additional diagnostic testing.
  1. Labs for fluid/electrolyte disturbances, infections, toxicities, metabolic disorders, shock states, and postoperative status.
  2. Arterial blood gas (ABG).
  3. Liver function test (LFT), thyroid, and B_{12} as with dementia.
  4. EKG.
E. Medication review is very important as toxicities are culprits in 30% of all cases of delirium.
F. If no cause is found, further diagnostics are necessary.
  1. CT/MRI head.
  2. EEG.
  3. Lumbar puncture as indicated.

DIFFERENTIAL DIAGNOSIS
A. Medical issues; determine if patient has a masked baseline dementia.
B. Treat sundowning as delirium until all medical issues are ruled out.
C. Wernicke aphasia, bitemporal dysfunction, Anton syndrome, tumors, or trauma in the frontal region.
D. Subacute brain lesions, stroke, or inflammation; head injuries.
E. Nonconvulsive status epilepticus.
F. Dementia or primary psychiatric illness.

EVALUATION AND MANAGEMENT PLAN
A. General plan.
  1. Treat the underlying cause.
  2. Supportive care.

EXHIBIT 16.1   Confusion Assessment Method

Confusion Assessment Method for the ICU (CAM-ICU)
Worksheet
Instructions: To evaluate for the presence of delirium in your patient, complete this clinical assessment <u>every</u> shift (8–12 hours).
CAM-ICU is a valid and reliable delirium assessment tool recommended by the Society of Critical Care Medicine (SCCM) in its 2013 Pain, Agitation, and Delirium (PAD) guidelines.

CAM-ICU	Criteria	✓ Present
FEATURE 1: Alteration/Fluctuation in Mental Status		
▪ Is the patient's mental status different than his/her baseline? **OR** ▪ Has the patient had any fluctuation in mental status in the past 24 hours as evidenced by fluctuation on a sedation scale (e.g., RASS, GCS), or previous delirium assessment?	If Yes for either question ▶	☐
FEATURE 2: Inattention 1: Alteration/Fluctuation in Mental Status		
Letters Attention Test:		
Tell the patient *"I am going to read to you a series of 10 letters. Whenever you hear the letter 'A,' squeeze my hand."*	If number of errors >2 ▶	☐
SAVEAHAART		
Count errors (each time patient fails to squeeze on the letter "A" and squeezes on a letter other than "A").		
FEATURE 3: Altered LOC		
▪ Present if the RASS score is anything <u>other than</u> Alert and Calm (zero) OR ▪ If SAS is anything <u>other than</u> Calm (4).	If RASS ≠ 0 **OR** SAS ≠ 4 ▶	☐
FEATURE 4: Disorganized Thinking		
Yes/No Questions: Ask the patient to respond: 1. Will a stone float on water? 2. Are there fish in the sea? 3. Does 1 pound weigh more than 2 pounds? 4. Can you use a hammer to pound a nail? Count errors (each time patient answers incorrectly). **Commands:** Ask the patient to follow your instructions: a. *"Hold up this many fingers."* (Hold two fingers up in front of the patient.) b. *"Now do the same thing with the other hand."* (Do **not** demonstrate the number of fingers this time.) ▪ If unable to move both arms, for part "b" of command ask patient to "Hold up one more finger." **Count errors if patient is unable to complete the entire command.**	If combined number of errors >1 ▶	☐
If Features 1 <u>and</u> 2 are both present and either Features 3 <u>or</u> 4 are present:	**Delirium present**	☐
CAM-ICU is positive, delirium is present.	**Delirium absent**	☐

Copyright 2002, E. Wesley Ely, MD, MPH, and Vanderbilt University, all rights reserved. Adapted with permission.
CAM-ICU, confusion assessment method for the ICU; GCS; Glasgow Coma Scale; LOC, level of consciousness.

B. Patient/family teaching points.
   1. Treat pain issues.
   2. Encourage movement.
   3. Avoid overstimulation.
   4. Manage behaviors.
   5. Family might need a sitter to assist with care.
C. Pharmacotherapy.
   1. Pharmacologic treatment of delirium depends on cause.
      a. Removing medications may be the treatment.
      b. All medications should be evaluated for polypharmacy interactions.
   2. Use the Beers criteria for prescribing medications for older adults.
      a. Behavioral control.
         i. Haloperidol.
         ii. Risperidone.
         iii. Quetiapine.
      b. Agitation.
         i. Haloperidol (first line).

EXHIBIT 16.2 Intensive Care Delirium Checklist for Screening

Intensive Care Delirium Screening Checklist (ICDSC)
Worksheet

- Score your patient over the entire shift. Components don't all need to be present at the same time.
- Components #1 through #4 require a focused bedside patient assessment. This cannot be completed when the patient is deeply sedated or comatose (i.e., SAS = 1 or 2; RASS = –4 or –5).
- Components #5 through #8 are based on observations throughout the entire shift. Information from the prior 24 hr (i.e., from prior 1–2 nursing shifts) should be obtained for components #7 and #8.

			NO	0	1	Yes
1.	**Altered Level of Consciousness**					
	Deep sedation/coma over entire shift [SAS= 1, 2; RASS = –4, –5]	= Not assessable				
	Agitation [SAS = 5, 6, or 7; RASS= 1–4] at any point	= 1 point				
	Normal wakefulness [SAS = 4; RASS = 0] over the entire shift	= 0 points				
	Light sedation [SAS = 3; RASS = –1, –2, –3]	= 1 point (if no recent sedatives)				
		= 0 points (if recent sedatives)				
2.	**Inattention**		NO	0	1	Yes
	Difficulty following instructions or conversation; patient easily distracted by external stimuli. Will not reliably squeeze hands to spoken letter A: **SAVEAHAART**					
3.	**Disorientation**		NO	0	1	Yes
	In addition to name, place, and date, does the patient recognize ICU caregivers? Does patient know what kind of place he or she is in (list examples: Dentist's office, home, work, hospital)?					
4.	**Hallucination, delusion, or psychosis**		NO	0	1	Yes
	Ask the patient if he or she is having hallucinations or delusions (e.g., trying to catch an object that isn't there). Is the patient afraid of the people or things around him or her?					
5.	**Psychomotor agitation or retardation**		NO	0	1	Yes
	Either: (a) Hyperactivity requiring the use of sedative drugs or restraints in order to control potentially dangerous behavior (e.g., pulling IV lines out or hitting staff) OR (b) Hypoactive or clinically noticeable psychomotor slowing or retardation					
6.	**Inappropriate speech or mood**		NO	0	1	Yes
	Patient displays: Inappropriate emotion; disorganized or incoherent speech; sexual or inappropriate interactions; is either apathetic or overly demanding					
7.	**Sleep-wake cycle disturbance**		NO	0	1	Yes
	Either: Frequent awakening/< 4 hr sleep at night OR sleeping during much of the day					
8.	**Symptom fluctuation**		NO	0	1	Yes
	Fluctuation of any of the previous symptoms over a 24 hr period.					
	TOTAL SHIFT SCORE:		(0–8)			

	Score	Classification
	0	Normal
	1–3	Subsyndromal delirium
	4–8	Delirium

Source: Adapted from Bergeron, N., Dubois, M. J., Dumont, M., Dial, S., & Skrobik, Y. (2001). Intensive care delirium screening checklist: Evaluation of a new screening tool. *Intensive Care Medicine, 27,* 859–864; Ouimet, S., Riker, R., Bergeron, N., Cossette, M., Kavanagh, B., & Skrobik, Y. (2007). doi.org/10.1007/s001340100909
Subsyndromal delirium in the ICU: Evidence for a disease spectrum. *Intensive Care Medicine, 33,* 1007–1013. doi.org/10.1007/s00134-007-0618-y

ii. Olanzapine (oral only).
iii. Risperidone.
c. Anxiolytics-benzodiazepine, such as lorazepam.
d. Cholinesterase inhibitor, such as donepezil.
D. Discharge instructions.
  1. Behavioral management.
    a. Reorient patient frequently.
    b. Use large, visible clocks.
    c. An outside-facing window is preferable.
    d. Keep nighttime noise to a minimum.
    e. Try to provide uninterrupted sleep overnight.
    f. Limit napping during the day.
    g. Try to make the hospital room more like home.
    h. Allow family visits and support.
  2. Safety.
    a. Consider a sitter to stay with the patient during the course of the delirium.

FOLLOW-UP

A. Delirium usually subsides as the acute illness resolves.
B. If delirium persists, additional diagnostics should be considered.

CONSULTATION/REFERRAL

A. Geriatric psychiatry may be consulted if the patient has behavioral issues or is unusually aggressive.
B. Consult case management if placement outside the home will be required.
C. Consult social work if there is any concern for drugs or alcohol or evidence of abuse or neglect.

SPECIAL/GERIATRIC CONSIDERATIONS

A. It may take geriatric patients 6 to 8 weeks to fully recover from a delirious event and they are at high risk of persistent delirium even if the cause has been eliminated or treated.

CASE SCENARIO: DELIRIUM

A 79-year-old man is transported to the ED by his daughter due to reports of being confused, agitated, and lacking awareness of surroundings. While in the ED, the man's status becomes much worse. It is first observed that he is hyperactive and restless, and then he becomes even more confused and agitated. The man does not listen to the instructions that are being given by his assigned nurse and proceeds to wander all over the ED. It is important for the provider to evaluate for any potential source of infection in this patient or any evidence of any recent trauma. The practice expectation is that there can be use of medicine and nonmedicine interventions in order to help address delirium and ensure patient safety.

1. Which of the following is the most appropriate initial intervention for a patient with delirium?
  A. Environmental intervention
  B. Somatic intervention
  C. Psychiatric intervention
  D. Medical intervention

BIBLIOGRAPHY

Adamis, D., Macdonald, A., McCarthy, G., Morandi, A., Bellelli, G., & Meagher, D. (2022). Towards understanding the nature and need of delirium guidelines across nations and cultures. *Aging Clinical and Experimental Research*, *34*(3), 633–642. https://doi.org/10.1007/s40520-021-01978-w

Ali, M. A., Hashmi, M., Ahmed, W., Raza, S. A., Khan, M. F., & Salim, B. (2021). Incidence and risk factors of delirium in surgical intensive care unit. *Trauma Surgery & Acute Care Open*, *3*(6), e000564. https://doi.org/10.1136/tsaco-2020-000564, PMID: 33748426; PMCID: PMC7931752

American Psychiatric Association. (2013). *Diagnostic and statistical manual of mental disorders* (5th ed.). Author.

Burton, J. K., Craig, L. E., Yong, S. Q., Siddiqi, N., Teale, E. A., Woodhouse, R., Barugh, A. J., Shepherd, A. M., Brunton, A., Freeman, S. C., Sutton, A. J., & Quinn, T. J. (2021). Non-pharmacological interventions for preventing delirium in hospitalised non-ICU patients. *The Cochrane Database of Systematic Reviews*, *7*(7), CD013307. https://doi.org/10.1002/14651858.CD013307.pub2

Egbert, A., Alan, H., Zierre, G., & Mattace-Raso, F. (2021). Antipsychotics and lorazepam during delirium: Are we harming older patients? A real life data study. *Drugs Aging*, *38*(1), 53–62.

Guthrie, P. F., Rayborn, S., & Butcher, H. K. (2018). Evidence-based practice guideline: Delirium. *Journal of Gerontological Nursing*, *44*(2), 14–24. https://doi.org/10.3928/00989134-20180110-04

Jung, P., Puts, M., Frankel, N., Syed, A. T., Alam, Z., Yeung, L., Malik, U., Rosario, C., Ayala, A. P., Hudson, J., & Alibhai, S. (2021). Delirium incidence, risk factors, and treatments in older adults receiving chemotherapy: A systematic review and meta-analysis. *Journal of Geriatric Oncology*, *12*(3), 352–360. https://doi.org/10.1016/j.jgo.2020.08.011

Oh, E. S., Fong, T. G., Hshieh, T. T., & Inouye, S. K. (2017). Delirium in older persons: Advances in diagnosis and treatment. *JAMA*, *318*(12), 1161–1174. https://doi.org/10.1001/jama.2017.12067

DEMENTIA

Abimbola Farinde

DEFINITION

A. Major neurocognitive disorder in which the patient exhibits a significant cognitive decline in one or more of the areas described in the *Diagnostic and Statistical Manual of Mental Disorders* (Fifth Edition; *DSM-5*).
  1. Complex attention.
  2. Executive function.
  3. Language.
  4. Learning and memory.
  5. Perceptual-motor function.
  6. Social cognition.
B. The *DSM-5* also states the impairment should be acquired and a decline from the patient's normal functioning, inhibits independence and activities of daily living (ADLs), and not be occurring during bouts of delirium or as a function of another mental condition (e.g., depression or schizophrenia).
C. Alzheimer disease (AD) accounts for most cases of dementia, with an estimated 6.2 million Americans aged 65 and older living with Alzheimer dementia. While the term is often used interchangeably with dementia, AD only represents a single subtype of neurodegenerative dementia. Neurodegenerative dementias are progressive and exhibit an insidious onset.

INCIDENCE

A. Age: Typically over the age of 65; however, early-onset dementia accounts for 40 to 100 cases per 100,000 people in the developed world.

B. Incidence: Alzheimer dementia affects more than five million individuals over the age of 65, accounting for 80% of dementia cases, with vascular dementia second.

PATHOGENESIS

A. Dementia can be influenced by multiple pathologies and is disease-specific.

B. Types of dementia and selected pathophysiology:

1. Neurodegenerative (Alzheimer, dementia with Lewy bodies, and Parkinson disease).

2. Vascular diseases (vascular, cerebral amyloid angiopathy, and angiitis).

3. Infectious diseases (prion disease such as Creutzfeldt–Jakob disease [CJD; mad cow], herpes encephalitis, and neurosyphilis).

4. Inflammatory and autoimmune (multiple sclerosis, para- and nonparaneoplastic, autoimmune diseases).

5. Neurometabolic disorders.

6. Other (traumatic encephalopathy, alcohol abuse, and Wilson and Huntington diseases).

a. Genetic.

b. Malnutrition.

PREDISPOSING FACTORS

A. Age (frequency increases with age).

B. Positive family history.

C. Female sex assigned at birth (could be related to life span).

D. History of head trauma or cerebrovascular accident (CVA).

E. Low education level.

F. Environmental factors: Aluminum, mercury, and viruses.

G. Physical condition and other medical factors (e.g., diabetes, hypertension, and hypercholesterolemia).

SUBJECTIVE DATA

A. Common complaints/symptoms.

1. While memory is a problem, it is usually not mentioned by the patient, but by the significant other or family.

2. Frequently cannot pinpoint the condition's onset; years may have passed with problems, but until a major change happens, such as needing to stop driving or a hospital admission, the patient may be mostly functional in their familiar environment.

3. Signs and symptoms.

a. Difficulty maintaining new information or task.

b. Inability to manage complex task, such as balancing a checkbook.

c. Lapses in reasoning.

d. Becoming lost in familiar places.

e. Word finding issues.

f. Changes in behavior over time.

B. Common/typical scenario.

1. Patients typically present with subtle short-term memory changes, frequent forgetfulness, difficulty finding the right words, or difficulty completing tasks.

2. The patient may progress over months and years before coming to a provider.

C. Family and social history.

1. Family history and first-degree relatives may be important in AD.

2. Obesity and chronic sedentary lifestyle may increase risk.

3. Smoking, alcohol, and drug abuse increase risk of dementia.

D. Review of systems.

1. Neurologic: Ask about memory and any confusion or deficits in calculation and abstraction.

2. Psychological: Ask about depressed mood, hopelessness, or suicide tendencies or changes in personality.

3. Inquire about rate of onset of changes.

4. History from a reliable source, including medications.

PHYSICAL EXAMINATION

A. Assessment and physical examination change with the type of dementia that is presented. Motor, somatosensory, and visual functions may remain intact until later in the disease process.

1. Disorder of motion.

2. Eye movement.

3. Primary memory.

4. Performance on cognitive assessments.

DIAGNOSTIC TESTS

A. Cognitive function evaluation.

1. Mini-Mental State Examination (maximum score 30; <24 indicates possible dementia).

a. Concentration.

b. Language.

c. Orientation.

d. Memory.

e. Attention.

2. Montreal Cognitive Assessment (maximum score 30; <25 indicates possible dementia).

3. Clinical Dementia Rating (includes a caregiver).

4. Mini-Cog (clock draw and recall test).

5. Informant interview to ask caregivers about the patient's functioning.

a. Issues with judgment.

b. Lack of interest in usual activities.

c. Repetition of questions, statements, and stories.

d. Difficulty learning new tools or household appliances.

e. Inability to remember the month or year.

f. Loss of ability to manage finances.

g. Missing appointments.

h. Persistent issues with thinking or memory.

B. Physical examination.

1. Full and comprehensive neurologic examination. ▶

2. General physical examination to identify any medical illness that could account for deficits.

3. Motor examination to identify prior stroke or evidence of Parkinson disease or autoimmune issues.

4. Evaluation of sleeping habits.

C. Lab studies (*as recommended by the American Academy of Neurology).

1. Screen for B$_{12}$ deficiency*.

2. Hypothyroidism*.

3. Rapid plasma reagin (RPR) screening*.

4. Complete blood count (CBC).

5. Comprehensive metabolic panel (CMP).

6. Liver function test (LFT).

7. Immune/autoimmune workup.

8. Cerebrospinal fluid (CSF) analysis if infective cause is suspected.

D. Imaging: Neuroimaging (as recommended by the American Academy of Neurology), including CT or MRI and possibly electrophysiologic testing.

E. Brain biopsy not recommended unless in vasculitis, cancers, or infection.

F. Genetic testing is not recommended except for specific diseases in family history (e.g., Huntington disease).

DIFFERENTIAL DIAGNOSIS

A. Treatable: Thyroid, vitamin deficiencies, tumor, drug and medication intoxication, chronic infection, and severe depression. Once these are ruled out, the differential is among the types of dementia.

B. Structural: Cortical and hippocampus atrophy leads to AD.

C. Psychiatric history with pharmacologic treatment may be drug-related.

D. Associated: Gait disturbances could be vascular or Lewy body, including Parkinson, which may be based on time of onset.

E. Rapid onset could be CJD or frontotemporal dementia.

F. For early onset (under the age of 65), there is a much broader list of differentials and requires more extensive testing.

EVALUATION AND MANAGEMENT PLAN

A. General plan.

1. Includes finding and correcting any reversible causes.

  a. Vitamin or thyroid replacements.

  b. Discontinuing contributing medications or starting medications for contributing conditions such as depression.

  c. Treating any structural dysfunction, such as neoplasms or increased intracranial pressure.

  d. Treating any infections contributing to mental status.

2. When no correctable cause is found, supportive care for the patient and the caregiver is warranted.

3. Diet.

  a. Patients with dementia often have decreased appetite for a variety of reasons.

  b. When possible, provide food to support adequate nutrition.

  c. Supplement any deficiencies.

  d. Adequate overall intake may be preferred over following a strict low cholesterol/glucose/fat/sodium diet.

4. Other therapies/considerations.

  a. Provide utmost safety for the patient and the caregiver while maintaining some form of independence for the patient.

  b. Modify environment.

  c. Maintain a routine.

  d. Treat occult conditions that could contribute to behavioral problems (like toothache or constipation).

  e. Provide simple physical activities.

  f. Provide caregiver respite as needed.

B. Patient/family teaching points.

1. Patient teaching is more geared toward the caregiver.

2. Many changes must be made in the patient's life, including relinquishing some independence for the sake of safety.

3. When considering activities such as driving, safety for both the patient and the public should be considered.

C. Pharmacotherapy.

1. U.S. Food and Drug Administration (FDA)-approved for AD: Cholinesterase inhibitors, which are available in different formulations.

  a. Donepezil.

  b. Rivastigmine.

  c. Galantamine.

2. FDA-approved for AD: N-methyl-D-aspartate (NMDA) receptor antagonist.

  a. Memantine.

3. Pharmaceutical therapy for symptom control.

  a. Phenothiazine.

  b. Benzodiazepines.

  c. Second-generation antipsychotics: Risperidone, quetiapine, and olanzapine.

  d. Anticholinergics or sedatives.

  e. Antidepressants, especially selective serotonin reuptake inhibitors (SSRIs).

FOLLOW-UP

A. Patient should be seen at regularly scheduled appointments dependent on several factors.

1. Physical needs of the patient.

2. Mental status and rate of decline.

3. Emotional status.

4. Ability of caregiver to maintain the safety, welfare, and health of the patient.

B. Follow-up assessments include efficacy of medication, with changes, additions, and discontinuance as needed.

C. Monitor for correctable physical factors that may contribute to behavioral issues, both becoming withdrawn and outburst.

D. Assess for additional resources needed by the patient and the caregiver, including ability of the patient to function with safety as the determining factor when discussing activity limitations.

CONSULTATION/REFERRAL

A. Neuropsychologist.

B. Social workers/case managers.

C. Cognitive rehab can help maintain memory and cognitive functioning while also providing some respite to the caregiver.

D. Exercise programs.

E. Occupational therapy.

SPECIAL/GERIATRIC CONSIDERATIONS

A. Comorbid conditions.

B. Family support.

C. Daily care.

D. End-of-life plans.

CASE SCENARIO: DEMENTIA

An 85-year-old woman is referred to the memory clinic by her primary care physician for an assessment of memory impairment. She presents to the clinic with her daughter. Based on the administration of the Mini-Mental State Examination, her score is 12, which is indicative of moderate dementia. Her daughter reports that she has experienced significant deterioration in aspects of her cognition over the last 10 months. The patient also indicates that she has experienced memory issues in the past and believes that her short memory may be an issue for her.

1. Which of the following combination of medications can be initiated in this patient?

    A. Donepezil and rivastigmine

    B. Galantamine and donepezil

    C. Rivastigmine and donepezil

    D. Donepezil and memantine

BIBLIOGRAPHY

Alzheimer's Association. (n.d.). Know what to expect. https://www.alz.org/help-support/i-have-alz/know-what-to-expect

American Psychiatric Association. (2013). *Diagnostic and statistical manual of mental disorders (DSM-5)* (5th ed.). Author.

Arvanitakis, Z., Shah, R. C., & Bennett, D. A. (2019). Diagnosis and management of dementia: Review. *JAMA, 322*(16), 1589–1599. https://doi.org/10.1001/jama.2019.4782

Brosch, J. R., & Farlow, M. R. (2018, June 8). *Early-onset dementia in adults.* In J. L. Wilterdink (Ed.), UpToDate. https://www.uptodate.com/contents/early-onset-dementia-in-adults

Cunningham, E. L., McGuinness, B., Herron, B., & Passmore, A. P. (2015). Dementia. *The Ulster Medical Journal, 84*(2), 79–87.

Duong, S., Patel, T., & Chang, F. (2017). Dementia: What pharmacists need to know. *Canadian Pharmacists Journal: CPJ = Revue des Pharmaciens du Canada: RPC, 150*(2), 118–129. https://doi.org/10.1177/1715163517690745

Fiest, K. M., Jetté, N., Roberts, J. I., Maxwell, C. J., Smith, E. E., Black, S. E., Blaikie, L., Cohen, A., Day, L., Holroyd-Leduc, J., Kirk, A., Pearson, D., Pringsheim, T., Venegas-Torres, A., & Hogan, D. B. (2016). The prevalence and incidence of dementia: A systematic review and meta-analysis. *The Canadian Journal of Neurological Sciences. Le journal Canadien des Sciences Neurologiques, 43*(Suppl 1), S3–S50. https://doi.org/10.1017/cjn.2016.18

Hui, E. K., Tischler, V., Wong, G., Lau, W., & Spector, A. (2021). Systematic review of the current psychosocial interventions for people with moderate to severe dementia. *International Journal of Geriatric Psychiatry, 36*(9), 1313–1329. https://doi.org/10.1002/gps.5554

Shaji, K. S., Sivakumar, P. T., Rao, G. P., & Paul, N. (2018). Clinical practice guidelines for management of dementia. *Indian Journal of Psychiatry, 60*(Suppl 3), S312–S328. https://doi.org/10.4103/0019-5545.224472

FALLS

Megan Hebdon

DEFINITION

A. The Agency for Healthcare Research and Quality (AHRQ) defines falls as an unplanned descent to the ground that may or may not result in injury to the patient. Consequences of falls may include lacerations, contusions, fractures, or internal bleeding, and contribute to increased healthcare utilization. About one-third of falls can be prevented, and falls with injury are reportable to The Joint Commission and are considered a "never event" by the Centers for Medicare and Medicaid Services. Up to 50% of older adults may not report history of falls to anyone for fear of being removed from the home.

B. Categories and classification of major fall injuries:

    1. Categories: Falls may be accidental (extrinsic, environmental factors), anticipated physiologic (confusion related to dementia), or unanticipated physiologic (acute stroke).

    2. Classification of major fall injuries: Major A (temporary functional impairment, major facial injury without internal injury, or disruption of a surgical wound), major B (cause long-term functional impairment and may increase mortality), and major C (well-established risk of mortality).

INCIDENCE

A. Inpatient falls.

    1. In the United States, 700,000 to 1,000,000 patients fall yearly. Approximately half of nursing home residents in the United States fall each year, with 10% of adverse events in skilled nursing facilities being falls with significant injuries.

    2. More than one-third of hospital falls result in injury, and length of stay may increase to as many as 6.7 additional inpatient hospital days.

    3. In the United States, the cost of nonfatal falls is about $50 billion annually, with $754 million for fatal falls.

B. Morbidity.

    1. Women are more likely to fall and sustain nonlife-threatening injuries than men, while men are more likely to die due to a fall.

    2. Falls are a contributing factor to admissions to rehabilitation centers, skilled nursing facilities, and ultimately nursing homes.

C. Mortality.
   1. Falls are the number one cause of death from unintentional injuries for adults 65 years or older in the United States.
   2. Falls can also be associated with an indirect cause of death.

PATHOGENESIS
A. Intrinsic factors.
   1. Decline in strength and mobility.
   2. Chronic health conditions.
   3. Medications.
   4. Low vitamin D.
B. Challenges to postural control.
   1. Environment.
   2. Changing positions.
   3. Normal activity.
C. Mediating factors.
   1. Risk-taking behaviors.
   2. Physical environmental hazards.

PREDISPOSING FACTORS
A. Medications.
   1. Anticholinergics.
   2. Antiarrhythmics.
   3. Antihypertensive medications.
   4. Narcotics.
   5. Muscle relaxants.
   6. Alcohol.
B. Incontinence: Urinary and fecal incontinence.
C. Health conditions.
   1. Alzheimer disease (AD): Patients have two times the probability of falling than those of the same age without the disease.
   2. Parkinson disease: 38% to 68% of patients with Parkinson disease fall due to gait disturbances.
   3. Diabetes: Women with diabetes are 1.6 times more likely to fall and two times more likely to suffer fall-related injuries than women without diabetes.
   4. Depression: There is a 2.2-fold increase in the risk of falls in this population of older adult patients.
D. Mobility impairments.
E. Medical history.
   1. Previous falls.
   2. Diabetes.
   3. Chronic obstructive pulmonary disease (COPD).
   4. Coronary artery disease (CAD).
   5. Arrhythmias.
   6. Dementia-related diseases, AD, vascular dementia (includes cerebrovascular accident [CVA]), Parkinson dementia, and so forth.
   7. Osteoarthritis.
   8. Joint replacements (knee surgeries especially susceptible).
   9. Chronic pain.
   10. Blindness.
   11. Macular degeneration.
   12. Glaucoma.
   13. Chronic kidney disease.
   14. Vestibular disease.

SUBJECTIVE DATA
A. Common complaints/symptoms.
   1. Dizziness when bending over or changing position.
   2. Unsteady gait/balance.
   3. Poor vision.
   4. Fatigue, weakness.
   5. Other signs and symptoms.
     a. Use of assistive equipment to ambulate.
     b. Use of walls or furniture to maintain balance.
     c. Use of assistive devices or medications for visual or hearing impairments related to aging.
B. Family and social history.
   1. Family history noncontributory in most cases.
   2. Social history: Important to note the presence of family caregivers to provide assistance with mobility.
C. Review of systems.
   1. Review all medications.
   2. Use risk assessment tools (Morse Fall Scale, STRATIFY Risk Assessment Tool).
     a. History of falls.
     b. Mental status.
     c. Vision.
     d. Toileting.
     e. Transfer and mobility.
     f. Head, ear, eyes, nose, and throat (HEENT).
       i. Dizziness.
       ii. Poor vision.
       iii. Loss of peripheral vision.
       iv. Depth perception.
     g. Musculoskeletal.
       i. Unsteady gait.
       ii. Uses walls to maintain balance.
     h. Neurologic.
       i. Neuropathy.
       i. General.
       i. Overall hazards in the home (rugs).

PHYSICAL EXAMINATION
A. Perform a head-to-toe physical examination.
   1. Neurologic examination.
     a. Glasgow Coma Scale.
     b. National Institutes of Health (NIH) Stroke Scale.
     c. Detailed neurologic examination if indicated, cranial nerves, gait, and balance testing.
   2. Mentation status.
     a. Mini-Mental State Examination.
     b. Confusion Assessment Method (CAM) or other delirium screening tool.
     c. Thorough review of medications for offending medications.
   3. Cardiovascular examination.
     a. Murmurs/arrhythmias.
     b. Carotid bruits.
     c. Pulses weak/thready.
     d. Evaluate for edema.
     e. Orthostasis.
   4. Pulmonary examination.
     a. Oxygen saturation (SpO$_2$)

b. Breath sounds.

c. Accessory muscle use.

5. Integumentary.

a. Bruising, scrapes, and lacerations over the knees, shoulders, forearms, shins, ankles, and toes. This indicates the patient is bumping into furniture or walls, which may indicate unaddressed balance issues or are defensive in nature.

b. Excoriation in perianal area: This may indicate urinary or fecal incontinence related to diet, medications, or infection.

6. Gastrointestinal.

a. Abdominal bruits.

b. Pain.

c. Nodules or skin changes.

d. Look for ecchymosis and signs of bleeding.

7. Genitourinary.

a. Incontinence, urgency, frequency, and dysuria (less common in older adults, new-onset delirium can be a sign of a urinary tract infection [UTI]).

DIAGNOSTIC TESTS

A. Depends upon the etiology of the fall, health history, current medications, and physical examination findings.

B. CT of the head to rule out bleeding, due to stroke or as a result of the fall. Some cranial bleeds that are not related to a CVA can be spontaneous if a patient is on anticoagulation therapy. CT angiography (CTA) or MRI/magnetic resonance angiography (MRA) may be indicated.

C. X-rays to rule out fractures in suspicious areas where there is evidence of impact from the fall.

D. Other diagnostics as indicated by patient history of present illness, health history, and physical examination.

1. Metabolic panel.

2. Carotid Doppler study.

3. Complete blood count (CBC) with differential.

4. EKG.

5. Echocardiogram (heart murmurs).

6. Evaluate for vitamin deficiencies, serum 25-hydroxyvitamin D level, B12, thiamine.

7. Guaiac stools if indicated.

8. MRA (suspect thrombus, hemorrhage).

9. MRI (gait disturbances, neurologic deficits).

10. Tilt table test.

11. Urinalysis to rule out infection.

12. Dix–Hallpike test (if physically feasible for suspected benign paroxysmal positional vertigo).

E. Review diagnostic test results.

1. Laboratory findings.

2. Radiologic examinations.

DIFFERENTIAL DIAGNOSIS

A. Anemia.
B. Arrhythmia.
C. Arthritis.
D. Carotid stenosis.
E. Dehydration.
F. AD or other dementias.
G. Depression.

H. Electrolyte deficiencies (severe hyponatremia) and vitamin deficiencies.
I. Frailty.
J. Hypoglycemia/hyperglycemia.
K. Infection/sepsis.
L. Labyrinthitis or benign paroxysmal positional vertigo.
M. Malnutrition.
N. Orthostatic/postural hypotension.
O. Peripheral neuropathy.
P. Peripheral vascular disease.
Q. Neurologic disorders, such as stroke, seizure, or Parkinson disease.
R. Uncorrected farsightedness/nearsightedness or poor vision from macular degeneration, glaucoma, underlying infection, or diabetic retinopathy.
S. Medications that contribute to delirium.

1. Alcohol.
2. Antiarrhythmics.
3. Antidepressants.
4. Antihypertensives.
5. Antipsychotics.
6. Diuretics.
7. Hypnotics.
8. Neuroleptics.
9. Sedatives.

EVALUATION AND MANAGEMENT PLAN

A. General plan.

1. Best to start with prevention activities to reduce fall risk and fall sequelae.

2. Perform a full medication review and use the Beers and screening tool of older persons' prescriptions (STOPP)/screening tool to alert to right treatment (START) criteria to determine medications that are contraindicated in older adults.

3. Perform multidisciplinary rounds in patients at moderate and higher fall risk, all patients over 75 years of age, and those who are frail.

4. Evaluate nutritional status, and order nutritional consult if indicated.

5. Evaluate for safe discharge on admission utilizing case management and a social worker to collaborate with family and caregivers. Include nurses, advanced practice nurses (APNs), physical therapists (PT), occupational therapists (OT), dietitian and nutritional support staff, pharmacists, and physicians.

6. Request fall risk alerts for patient safety to include an order for bed and chair alarms.

7. Correct underlying medical etiology or physical deficit if possible, which may include medication revisions, correction of vision/hearing with assistive devices, and use of ambulatory devices to aid with balance.

8. Place on telemetry, especially if there is evidence or history of cardiac disease.

B. Patient/family teaching points.

1. Discuss with patient/caregiver.

a. Signs and symptoms to monitor.

b. Common occurrences.

c. Readmission concerns.

C. Discharge instructions.

1. Evaluate for safe transfer of care from initiated unit: ICU to floor, floor to home, or other institution.

2. Accurate discharge summary of events including chief complaint and events leading up to admission and during hospitalization.

3. Copy of discharge summary to the family or caregivers, primary care provider, and specialists to ensure communication and history of recent events are transferred to community providers. Inpatient providers should state the patient's condition upon discharge and the patient's ability to transfer to the next level of care.

4. Thorough medication evaluation and reconciliation, including the Beers and STOPP/START criteria; ensure obsolete medications are removed from medication list and the patient has prescriptions and access to any medication initiated during hospitalization.

5. Separate education for medication reconciliation regarding discontinued medications, new medications, and administration.

6. Education for signs and symptoms of worsening condition, what is expected to happen, and readmission concerns.

7. Discharge education regarding follow-up appointments; medications and instructions on medications; any medical treatments that require an explanation, including physical therapy or wound care therapy; and breathing treatment or injections, to name but a few.

8. Use of any new assistive devices, walkers, canes, or braces.

9. Education on making the patient's environment safe from falls, such as removing rugs, having a clear walkway between rooms, keeping lights on, using nonskid shoes, and use of durable medical equipment such as grab bars, shower chairs, and raised toilet seats.

FOLLOW-UP

A. Follow-up depends on the cause of the fall and the sequelae of the fall.

B. For falls caused by cardiac disease, the patient should follow up with cardiology.

C. If a patient has an injury due to the fall, the patient should follow up with the appropriate services, such as orthopedics or neurosurgery.

CONSULTATION/REFERRAL

A. Case management and social workers ensure safe discharge to appropriate level of care.

B. Arrange for delivery of any durable medical equipment to the patient's assisted living, adult living, group home, or home.

C. Considerations of insurance coverage and deductible amounts are important for elders on fixed budgets.

D. Financial resources and availability of social support through appropriate government resources are important for safe transition, especially to independent living and home.

1. Medications: Ensure insurance is available for medications and durable medical equipment necessary for safe patient discharge.

2. If possible, arrange for first follow-up medical appointments with appropriate physicians and/or specialists.

3. If home therapy is utilized for wound or physical/occupational therapy, ensure setup and appointments for home visits are arranged.

4. If indicated, a home health visit can be set up to provide support and help arrange first appointments.

CASE SCENARIO: FALLS

Juno is a 72-year-old patient admitted to the hospital following a fall at home. The patient sustained a right wrist fracture and head injury and was admitted to the ICU for observation due to new-onset syncope and loss of consciousness following the fall. Telemetry shows a normal sinus rhythm, and CT scan in the ED shows no intracranial bleeding. Lab work is evaluated for infection, dehydration, and nutritional status. Juno's albumin is low and social evaluation notes that Juno is food-insecure. Following transfer to the medical–surgical floor, the patient is assessed by a multidisciplinary team.

1. Which of the following would be important for the management of Juno's health and prevention of future falls?

A. Medication reconciliation by pharmacist

B. Evaluation by physical therapy and occupational therapy

C. Nutritional evaluation by a dietitian

D. Resource support by social work

E. All of the above

BIBLIOGRAPHY

The 2019 American Geriatrics Society (AGS) Beers Criteria® Update Expert Panel. (2019). American geriatrics society 2019 updated AGS Beers Criteria® for potentially inappropriate medication use in older adults. *Journal of the American Geriatrics Society, 00*(00), 1–21. https://doi.org/10.1111/jgs.15767

Agency for Healthcare Research and Quality. (2013). Preventing falls in hospitals. https://www.ahrq.gov/patient-safety/settings/hospital/fall-prevention/toolkit/overview.html

Agency for Healthcare Research and Quality. (2021). Tool 3H: Morse fall scale for identifying fall risk factors. Content last reviewed March 2021 https://www.ahrq.gov/patient-safety/settings/hospital/fall-prevention/toolkit/morse-fall-scale.html

Burns, Z., Khasnabish, S., Hurley, A. C., Lindros, M. E., Carroll, D. L., Kurian, S., Alfieri, L., Ryan, V., Adelman, J., Bogaisky, M., Adkison, L., Yu, S. P., Scanlan, M., Herlihy, L., Jackson, E., Lipsitz, S. R., Christiansen, T., Bates, D. W., & Dykes, P. C. (2020). Classification of injurious fall severity in hospitalized adults. *Journals of Gerontology— Series A Biological Sciences and Medical Sciences, 75*(10), e138–e144. https://doi.org/10.1093/gerona/glaa004

Centers for Disease Control and Prevention. (2016). Falls are leading cause of injury and death in older Americans. https://www.cdc.gov/media/releases/2016/p0922-older-adult-falls.htm

Centers for Disease Control and Prevention. (2020). Cost of older adult falls. https://www.cdc.gov/falls/data/fall-cost.html

Currie, L. (2008, April). Fall and injury prevention. Patient safety and quality: An evidence-based handbook for nurses. In R. G. Hughes (Ed.), *Agency for healthcare research and quality (US). Chapter 10.* https://www.ncbi.nlm.nih.gov/books/NBK2653/

Morris, R., & O'Riordan, S. (2017). Prevention of falls in hospital. *Clinical Medicine Journal*, 17(4), 360–362. https://doi.org/10.7861/clinmedicine.17-4-360

O'Mahony, D., O'Sullivan, D., Byrne, S., O'Connor, M. N., Ryan, C., & Gallagher, P. (2015, March). STOPP/START criteria for potentially inappropriate prescribing in older people: version 2. *Age and Ageing*, 44(2), 213–218. https://doi.org/10.1093/ageing/afu145

Patient Safety Network. (2019). *Falls.* https://psnet.ahrq.gov/primer/falls

Rubenstein, L. Z. (2021). Falls in older people. *Merck Manual.* https://www.merckmanuals.com/professional/geriatrics/falls-in-older-people/falls-in-older-people

URINARY INCONTINENCE

Megan Hebdon

DEFINITION

A. Urinary incontinence in men and women is defined as an involuntary leakage of urine. Incontinence is further broken down into types of urinary leakage as follows:

1. Urge incontinence is loss of urine associated with a sense of an urgency to void. This may present suddenly. This is the most common type of urinary incontinence in older adults and may be exacerbated by use of diuretics or atrophic vaginitis in women.

2. Stress incontinence occurs when there is an abrupt change in intra-abdominal pressure, such as exertion, sneezing, or coughing.

3. Mixed incontinence is the most common type of urinary incontinence for women. It includes features of both urgency and stress incontinence.

4. Functional incontinence is related to personal and environmental factors that prevent an individual from reaching the bathroom in time to void.

5. Postvoid incontinence is associated with postvoid residual (PVR) urine in the urethra which leaks out after voiding.

6. Incomplete urinary emptying (overflow) incontinence relates to incomplete emptying of the bladder due to an impaired detrusor contractility or a bladder outlet obstruction.

7. Reflex incontinence etiology is related to neurologic dysfunction of the central nervous system (CNS).

8. Transient incontinence is often self-limited and causes can be identified with the pneumonic **DIAPPERS** (**D**elirium, **I**nfection, **A**trophic urethritis and vaginitis, **P**harmaceuticals, **P**sychiatric disorders, **E**xcess urine output, **R**estricted mobility, and **S**tool impaction).

9. Overactive bladder is associated with frequency, urgency, and nocturia. This may or may not have incontinence associated with it.

INCIDENCE AND PREVALENCE

A. Urinary incontinence affects about 15% of older men and 30% of older women. About 70% of long-term care residents experience urinary incontinence.

B. Prevalence in men:

1. Increases with age, but men are half as likely as women to seek care.

C. Prevalence in women:

1. Approximately 10% of adult women experience urinary incontinence.

2. This increases to 40% in women 70 years and older.

3. Of the types of incontinence, stress is most commonly seen in women who are younger than 65 years old. However, urge incontinence and mixed are more common among women older than 65 years. Stress incontinence affects both young and older women at a rate of 15% to 60%, respectively.

PATHOGENESIS

A. Urge incontinence can be related to an uninhibited detrusor activity.

B. Stress incontinence is generally due to an increase in intra-abdominal pressure, which exerts pressure on the bladder. This can happen with coughing, sneezing, laughing, heavy lifting, jumping, or vigorous exercise.

1. Radical prostatectomy surgery is the most common cause in men due to damage to the prostatic apex. Transurethral resection of the bladder has less incidence of damage to the external sphincter.

2. In women, stress incontinence is due to weakening of the pelvic floor muscles.

C. Overflow incontinence is the least common cause of incontinence due to impaired detrusor contractility and/or a bladder outlet obstruction. Impaired detrusor contractility is usually related to neurogenic etiologies. These include neuropathies such as mitral stenosis (MS), diabetes mellitus, meningomyelocele, lumbosacral nerve disease from tumors, prolapsed intravertebral discs, and higher spinal cord injuries.

D. Mixed incontinence is a combination incontinence of stress and urge; this is most common in women. The bladder outlet is weak and the detrusor is overactive. This may also include urethral hypermobility coupled with detrusor instability.

E. Transient incontinence refers to a temporary loss of urine due to causes that could be reversible, such as delirium, infection, atrophic vaginitis or urethritis, pharmaceuticals, or a psychological etiology related to excess fluid intake. Impaired mobility, endocrine disorders, medications, fecal impaction, atrophic urethritis or vaginitis, infections, and delirium are also included in the etiologies of transient incontinence.

F. Reflex incontinence for specific neurologic disease processes include, but are not limited to, MS and demyelinating plaques of the frontal lobe or lateral columns. Cerebrovascular accident (CVA) or vascular compromise of particular areas of the brain may result in lower urinary tract dysfunction.

PREDISPOSING FACTORS

A. Older age and comorbid health conditions.

B. Aging process.
  1. Atrophic vaginitis or urethritis.
  2. Prostate enlargement.
C. Gastrointestinal system dysfunction.
  1. Constipation.
  2. Fecal impaction.
D. Cancer.
  1. Pelvic organs.
  2. Pelvic radiation within 6 months.
  3. Prostate cancer (tumor status; urge/stress).
  4. Prostate surgery or radiation.
E. CNS or spinal cord disorders.
  1. Delirium or dementia.
  2. Normal pressure hydrocephalus.
  3. Neuropathies.
F. Connective tissue disorders.
G. Medications: Oral estrogens, alpha-blockers, sedative-hypnotics, antidepressants, antipsychotics, angiotensin-converting enzyme (ACE) inhibitors, loop diuretics, nonsteroidal anti-inflammatory drugs, and calcium channel blockers.
H. Obesity.
I. Pelvic organ prolapse (uterus/bladder).
J. Chronic obstructive pulmonary disease (COPD).
K. Impaired mobility.
L. Sleep apnea.
M. Urinary stones or urinary tract infection (UTI), more than two episodes a year.

SUBJECTIVE DATA

A. Common complaints/symptoms.
  1. Sudden onset of the need to urinate.
  2. Urine leakage after emptying bladder.
  3. Unable to make it to the bathroom with the urge to urinate.
  4. Feeling of incomplete emptying of the bladder with urination.
  5. Burning with urination.
  6. Flu-like symptoms.
  7. Other health issues related to incontinence.
    a. Cellulitis.
    b. Skin irritation and sores.
    c. Falls and subsequent fractures.
    d. Perineal candida infections.
    e. Pressure injuries.
    f. Sleep deprivation.
  8. Psychosocial morbidity related to incontinence.
    a. Depression and anxiety.
    b. Poor self-esteem.
    c. Sexual dysfunction.
    d. Social isolation.
    e. Work impairment.
    f. Reduced quality of life.
    g. Increased caregiver burden.
  9. Urine leakage.
  10. Hygiene issues.
  11. Need for assistance with activities of daily living (ADLs).
B. Common/typical scenario.
  1. Patients may have difficulty discussing incontinence, but will report varying degrees of urine urgency, frequency, or pain when urinating which may be minor, situational, or even debilitating.
C. Family and social history.
  1. Family history is noncontributory.
  2. Social history: Determine if there is a family caregiver or multiple family caregivers involved in patient care.
D. Review of systems.
  1. Dermatologic: Ask about skin infections, itchiness, redness, and pressure sores.
  2. Psychological: Ask about social involvement, sexual functioning, mood, and sleep habits.
  3. Genitourinary: Ask about moisture felt in the underwear, leakage issues, itching, burning during urination, frequency, urinating at night, and perineal irritation.
  4. Gastrointestinal: What is the typical bowel pattern? Are there complaints of constipation or impaction?

PHYSICAL EXAMINATION

A. General.
  1. Appearance.
  2. Signs of depression, distress, or anxiety.
B. Gastrointestinal.
  1. Abdominal distention.
C. Musculoskeletal.
  1. Joint stiffness.
  2. Mobility.
  3. Range of motion (ROM).
  4. Use of assistive devices.
D. Neurologic.
  1. With emphasis on cognition, functional status, and pyramidal and extrapyramidal symptoms.
  2. Integrity of sacral roots S2, S3, and S4; anal tone; and anal wink reflex.
  3. Evaluate for peripheral neuropathy.
E. Male.
  1. Visual examination of the penis, enlarged prostate, and scrotum.
  2. Review medical history for prostate issues.
F. Female.
  1. Visual examination for prolapse of pelvic organs and perineal irritation.
G. Transgender.
  1. Thorough history to understand sex at birth, gender, hormonal use, and surgical history. Physical exam of the perineal area appropriate to the patient's history.

DIAGNOSTIC TESTS

A. Laboratory.
  1. Metabolic panel and complete blood count (CBC).
  2. Prostate-specific antigen (PSA) level.
  3. Urinalysis with cytology and microscopy.
B. Radiology.
  1. PVR bladder scan.

▶

2. Renal ultrasound (US) if indicated by abnormal renal laboratory studies.

3. Additional imaging as indicated by history and physical exam.

DIFFERENTIAL DIAGNOSIS

A. CNS or spinal cord disorders.
B. Connective tissue disorders.
C. Constipation or fecal impaction.
D. Medication-induced.
E. Normal pressure hydrocephalus.
F. Neuropathy, diabetic neuropathy.
G. Obesity.
H. Pelvic organ prolapse (uterus/bladder).
I. Sleep apnea.
J. Urinary tract stones.
K. UTI.

EVALUATION AND MANAGEMENT PLAN

A. General plan.
  1. Perform a full medication review using the Beers and STOPP/START criteria and reconciliation.
  2. Perform multidisciplinary rounds in geriatric patients and include continence strategies for those who are incontinent, all patients over 75 years of age, and those who are frail. Include pharmacist, dietitian, radiation therapy (RT), physical therapist (PT), occupational therapist (OT), dietitian and nutritional support staff, pharmacists, and physicians.
  3. Evaluate nutritional status; order nutritional consult if indicated.
  4. Patient safety.
    a. Modify inpatient environment; include toileting into hourly rounds, place call light within reach, use lights at night, and clear the walkway to bathroom/bedside commode.
    b. Patient/family caregiver education on use of the call light for assistance.
    c. Evaluate for safe discharge on admission utilizing case management and social worker to collaborate with family and caregivers. Include nurses, advanced practice nurses (APNs), PT/OT, dietitian, pharmacist, and physicians.
    d. Request toileting rounds for patient safety to include an order for bed and chair alarms for those older adult patients with urgency and frequency.
    e. Urinals at bedside for male patients and bedpans for those unable to ambulate or get up to use a commode.
  5. Correct underlying medical etiology or physical deficit if possible, which may include medication revisions, treatment of infection, correction of vision/hearing with assistive devices, and use of ambulatory devices.
B. Patient/family teaching points.
  1. Pelvic floor exercises.
  2. How to use absorbent products.
  3. Toileting schedules and removal of environmental barriers.
  4. Modifications to diet and lifestyle may help patient control incontinence.
C. Pharmacotherapy.
  1. Medications depend upon the type of urinary incontinence being treated.
  2. Medications may not be effective in stress incontinence.
  3. Anticholinergics (antimuscarinics) block cholinergic receptors of the bladder and decrease contractility.
    a. All antimuscarinics are contraindicated in narrow angle glaucoma, gastric retention, and if PVR is greater than 150 L. Educate for side effects. Costs vary.
    b. Consider the Beers criteria and assess patient fall risk with anticholinergic medications.
  4. Benign prostatic hypertrophy (BPH)-related incontinence: Alpha-blockers have extensive precautions for administration. Orthostatic hypotension, hypotension, bradycardia, vertigo, priapism, cautious administration, and lab surveillance in patients with hepatic impairment should be considered.
  5. UTI: Antibiotic-focused therapy, either oral or intravenous (IV), depending upon the severity and hemodynamic status of the patient.
  6. Other treatments.
    a. Barrier creams.
    b. Oral multivitamins with zinc.
    c. Absorbent undergarments.
    d. Pelvic floor exercises.
    e. Bladder retraining.
    f. Biofeedback.
    g. Transient incontinence; treat the underlying cause: Infection, obstruction, environmental barriers, mobility issues, and so forth.
    h. Surgical interventions as indicated.
D. Discharge instructions.
  1. Evaluate for safe transfer of care from initiated unit: ICU to floor, floor to home, or other institution.
  2. Provider to provider report.
  3. Accurate discharge summary of events including chief complaint and events leading up to admission and medical nursing care during hospitalization.
  4. Copy of discharge summary to the family or caregivers, primary care provider, and specialists to ensure communication and history of recent events are transferred to community providers. Inpatient providers should state the patient's condition upon discharge and the patient's ability to transfer to the next level of care.
  5. Thorough medication reconciliation, including attention to the Beers and STOPP/START criteria; ensure obsolete medications are removed from medication administration record (MAR) and home medication list. Ensure the patient has prescriptions and access to any medication initiated during hospitalization.

6. Separate education for medication reconciliation regarding discontinued medications, new medications, and administration.

7. Education for signs and symptoms of worsening condition, what is expected to happen, and readmission concerns.

8. Discharge education regarding physician follow-up; medications and instructions on medications; and any medical treatments that require an explanation, including physical or occupational therapy, wound care therapy, or medication application.

9. Use of any new assistive devices, walkers, canes, braces, or hearing devices.

10. Education on making the incontinent patient's home safe from falls *AND* removing environmental barriers for toileting. Clear lighting, removing area rugs, clearing the walkway, and use of durable medical equipment for sitting, standing, and transfers.

FOLLOW-UP

A. Patient should follow up with the provider in 2 weeks to assess progress in treatment plan.

CONSULTATION/REFERRAL

A. Urology or gynecology.
B. Primary care provider/gerontologist.
C. Wound care, if indicated.
D. Physiotherapist: Pelvic floor exercises, bladder training, and strategies to maintain continence.

SPECIAL/GERIATRIC CONSIDERATIONS

A. Case management and social worker are used to ensure safe discharge to appropriate level of care.
B. Arrange for delivery of any durable medical equipment to the patient's assisted living, adult living, group home, or home. Considerations of insurance coverage and deductible amounts are important for older adults on fixed budgets. Financial resources and availability of social support through appropriate government resources are important for safe transition, especially to independent living and home.

1. Medications: Ensure insurance is available for medications and durable medical equipment necessary for safe patient discharge, such as bedside commode and so forth.

2. If possible, arrange first follow-up medical appointments with appropriate physicians and/or specialists.

3. If home therapy is needed for wound therapy or medication management, ensure appointments for home visits are set up.

C. If indicated, set up home health visit to provide appropriate support in arranging first appointments.

D. Discuss with patient, caregiver, and/or family.
1. Signs and symptoms to monitor.
2. Common occurrences.
3. Readmission concerns.

CASE SCENARIO: URINARY INCONTINENCE

Diane is a 73-year-old patient admitted to the hospital for a total right hip arthroplasty. She has done well with recovery following the surgery but is having difficulty maintaining urinary continence. She is starting to develop skin irritation in her perineal area. She reports having difficulty in the past with getting to the toilet in time and leaking urine when she coughs or sneezes.

1. Which steps can the multidisciplinary team take to support Diane and her urinary incontinence while she is in the hospital?

A. Make frequent rounds and offer to assist the patient to the toilet.

B. Provide mobility aids and transfer assistance for toileting.

C. Provide barrier cream to help the patient with skin breakdown.

D. All of the above.

BIBLIOGRAPHY

The 2019 American Geriatrics Society (AGS) Beers Criteria® Update Expert Panel. (2019). American Geriatrics Society 2019 updated AGS Beers Criteria® for potentially inappropriate medication use in older adults. *Journal of the American Geriatrics Society*, 00(00), 1–21. https://doi.org/10.1111/jgs.15767

Clemens, J. Q. (2022). Urinary incontinence in men. https://www.uptodate.com/contents/urinary-incontinence-in-men.

Davis, N. J., Wyman, J. F., Gubitosa, S., & Pretty, L. (2020, January). CMSRN Urinary incontinence in older adults. *American Journal of Nursing*, 120(1), 57–62. https://doi.org/10.1097/01.NAJ.0000652124.58511.24

Lukacz, E. S. (2022). Female urinary incontinence: Evaluation https://www.uptodate.com/contents/female-urinary-incontinence-evaluation

Milsom, I., & Gyhagen, M. (2018). The prevalence of urinary incontinence. *Climacteric*, 22(3), 217–222. https://doi.org/10.1080/13697137.2018.1543263

O'Mahony, D., O'Sullivan, D., Byrne, S., O'Connor, M. N., Ryan, C., & Gallagher, P. (2015, March). STOPP/START criteria for potentially inappropriate prescribing in older people: Version 2. *Age and Ageing*, 44(2), 213–218. https://doi.org/10.1093/ageing/afu145

Panesar, K. (2014). Drug-induced urinary incontinence. *US Pharm*, 39(8), 24–29.

Shenot, P. J. (2021). Urinary incontinence in adults. *Merck Manual*. https://www.merckmanuals.com/professional/genitourinary-disorders/voiding-disorders/urinary-incontinence-in-adults

Vassavada, S. P. (2021). *What is the pathophysiology of reflex urinary incontinence?* In E. D. Kim (Ed.), *Medscape*. https://www.medscape.com/answers/452289-172381/what-is-the-pathophysiology-of-reflex-urinary-incontinence

KNOWLEDGE CHECK: CHAPTER 16

1. Which of the following statements are TRUE when it comes to symptom presentation of delirium?

   A. The disturbance can occur over months to years.
   B. The disturbance develops over hours to a few days.
   C. The essential feature of delirium is disturbance of mental health or awareness.
   D. The presence of mood alterations is not a component of the condition.

2. Which of the following factors can increase the risk of developing delirium?

   A. Infections
   B. History of falls
   C. Use of multiple medications, especially those with psychoactive properties
   D. All of the above

3. Delirium can be associated with increased risk of decline, hospitalization, and possible mortality. Which of the following is NOT considered a modifiable risk factor for delirium?

   A. Use of drugs with psychoactive properties
   B. Environment
   C. Fall status
   D. Kidney impairment

4. The Beers criteria are designed to help prevent inappropriate prescribing of certain medications in the older population and can serve as a major guide when it comes to prescribing of medications in this age group. When would it be deemed appropriate to use a benzodiazepine, lorazepam, in an older adult with delirium?

   A. When the patient has failed all other therapies
   B. When the patient is in a confusional state
   C. When the patient is not also taking antipsychotics
   D. All of the above

5. Based on the types of dementia, which of the following can be associated with both motor movement issues and visual hallucinations?

   A. Vascular dementia
   B. Alzheimer dementia
   C. Frontotemporal dementia
   D. Lewy body dementia

6. The Mini-Mental State Examination (MMSE) and the Montreal Cognitive Assessment are tools that are commonly used to identify dementia symptoms. Which of the following elements of diagnosis are important to recognize when it comes to dementia?

   A. Frequency of activity
   B. Level of alertness
   C. Increased forgetfulness
   D. Visual impairment

7. The development of dementia can present with cognitive decline, and with the progression of the disease the goal is to slow the occurrence. Which of the following medications can be used in conjunction with cholinesterase inhibitors as the disease progresses?

   A. Anticholinergics
   B. Benzodiazepines
   C. N-methyl-D-aspartate (NMDA) receptor antagonist
   D. Antidepressants

8. Which of the following is TRUE about falls in older adults?

   A. They are costly.
   B. They can be directly or indirectly associated with death.
   C. Women are more likely to have nonlife-threatening injuries from falls than men.
   D. All of the above.

9. Which of the following would increase a 75-year-old male patient's risk of falls?

   A. Age
   B. Having diabetes
   C. Being physically active
   D. None of the above

10. An 83-year-old female patient takes the following medications: Furosemide, gabapentin, metoprolol, and vitamin D. Which of these does not increase her fall risk?

   A. Vitamin D
   B. Furosemide
   C. Metoprolol
   D. Gabapentin

(See answers next page.)

1. **B) The disturbance develops over hours to a few days.**
The development of delirium can arise over hours to a few days, with a reflection of a change from a person's baseline of attention and awareness and with fluctuations being observed during the course.

2. **D) All of the above**
There is an increased risk of development of delirium in the presence of functional impairments as well as in the context of infections, history of falls, and multiple drugs, particularly those with psychoactive properties that can have an impact.

3. **D) Kidney impairment**
When it comes to the modifiable risk factors for delirium, there are elements that can be changed, such as an individual's environment, the potential for falls by implementing preventive measures, and decreasing the use of medications of psychoactive medications when not necessary. However, once organ decline or impairment occurs in an individual, this can prove to be more difficult to reverse.

4. **C) When the patient is not also taking antipsychotics**
The use of antipsychotics in conjunction with lorazepam has been shown to increase the risk of poor outcomes so it is important for clinicians to be careful when prescribing these medications to older patients with delirium. Additional investigation is needed to further clarify this association.

5. **D) Lewy body dementia**
Lewy body dementia can present with the classic symptoms of memory loss, but individuals may also present with movement or balance issues, along with visual hallucinations, which tend to occur early on in the disease.

6. **B) Level of alertness**
Dementia can be associated with gradual memory loss that leads to individuals forgetting to complete daily activities of living. The tendency to forget can start to lead to significant impairment over time.

7. **C) N-methyl-D-aspartate (NMDA) receptor antagonist**
As Alzheimer disease (AD) progresses from mild to moderate and then to severe, adjunctive medications can be included in the regimen. Memantine is an NMDA receptor antagonist that can be used in conjunction with cholinesterase inhibitors for moderate to severe AD.

8. **D) All of the above**
Falls are frequent and costly in older adults. They can increase risk of mortality both directly and indirectly. Women are more likely to sustain nonlife-threatening injuries from falls than men, although men may be more likely to die from a fall than women.

9. **B) Having diabetes**
Having diabetes increases fall risk due to the potential for neuropathy and hypoglycemia. Aging is not a direct risk factor, but a decline in strength and mobility that may occur with age can increase someone's fall risk. Being physically active may be protective by promoting conditioning and muscle strength.

10. **A) Vitamin D**
Diuretics, antihypertensives, and neuroleptics all increase fall risk. Vitamin D may be used as treatment in individuals who have low vitamin D levels.

11. Causes of transient incontinence can be remembered by which mnemonic?

   A. DIAPPERS
   B. KEEP DRY
   C. STOPP
   D. BEERS

12. An 85-year-old female patient is hospitalized for a kidney infection. Her presenting symptom is confusion. On day 2 of hospitalization, she tells her nurse about the difficulty she has at home of getting to the restroom in time to urinate. She uses a walker for ambulation, lives alone, and reports having a house "full of stuff." Which of the following health issues should be assessed for that are often associated with urinary incontinence?

   A. Sleep deprivation
   B. Perineal *Candida* infections
   C. Pressure injuries
   D. All of the above

13. Before discussing a prescription for an anticholinergic with an older adult patient, the multidisciplinary team recognizes the need to assess the patient for:

   A. Medication allergies
   B. Blood pressure
   C. Fall risk
   D. None of the above

(See answers next page.)

11. A) DIAPPERS

DIAPPERS can be used to remember the following causes of transient incontinence: **D**elirium, **i**Infection, **A**trophic urethritis and vaginitis, **P**harmaceuticals, **P**sychiatric disorders, **E**xcess urine output, **R**estricted mobility, and **S**tool impaction.

12. D) All of the above

Other health conditions associated with urinary incontinence include cellulitis, skin irritation and sores, falls and subsequent fractures, perineal *Candida* infections, pressure injuries, and sleep deprivation.

13. C) Fall risk

Fall risk is an important factor to consider in older adults before prescribing anticholinergic medications. Talking through the risks and benefits of the medication with patients and their caregivers will help with shared decision-making.

CHAPTER 17

TRAUMA GUIDELINES

CHEST TRAUMA

Susan F. Galiczynski

DEFINITION

A. Any mechanism that causes injury to the bony or soft tissue in the thorax.

B. In a very short period of time, any of these injuries alone or in combination can be devastating and life-threatening to the patient.

INCIDENCE

A. Accounts for up to 25% of all trauma-related deaths.

B. Approximately 70% of all cases of chest trauma will be related to blunt trauma.

C. Approximately 80% to 85% of patients with chest trauma will experience at least one rib fracture.

D. Fractures of scapula, first/second rib, or sternum: Mortality can be as high as 35%.

E. Gunshot wounds (GSWs) to the chest tend to be more fatal.

F. Approximately 5% to 10% of chest trauma will involve sternal fractures.

G. Death rates among falls in the older adults are up by 3%. Chest injuries can account for up to 23%.

PATHOGENESIS

A. Related to mechanism of injury.

B. Common mechanisms for blunt chest trauma include (a) direct blunt trauma to the chest, (b) acceleration–deceleration/shearing forces, (c) compressive forces, and (d) blast injury.

PREDISPOSING FACTORS

A. Higher incidence in younger males who may engage in high-risk behaviors.

B. Falls in the geriatric population.

C. Osteopenia is common in older adults. Presence of rib fractures may increase the incidence of pneumonia and mortality.

SUBJECTIVE DATA

A. Common complaints/symptoms.

   1. Chest wall and back pain, worse with movement, coughing, and breathing.

   2. Radiating shoulder pain is common in the presence of rib fracture.

   3. Shortness of breath.

   4. Increased pain with palpation.

B. Common/typical scenario.

   1. Other signs and symptoms.

     a. Crepitus in the presence of fractures.

     b. Splinting or shallow breathing.

     c. Decreased breath sounds on the affected side (pneumothorax).

     d. Beck triad: Muffled, distant heart sounds (cardiac tamponade), jugular venous distention, and narrowed pulse pressures.

     e. Cyanosis to the lips and fingers.

     f. Dyspnea/tachypnea.

     g. Tachycardia.

     h. Tracheal deviation (late sign).

     i. Diaphoresis.

     j. Signs of respiratory distress.

     k. Signs of shock (hypoperfusion).

C. Review of systems.

   1. Ask the patient about the events surrounding the injury. With falls, ask if the patient tripped or passed out. Evaluate for need for syncopal workup.

   2. If motor vehicle collisions (MVCs) occur, ask the patient about seat belt use. Was there a steering wheel deformity? Were the airbags deployed?

   3. Ask about prior chest trauma and cardiac history. (Chest trauma can lead to arrhythmias.)

   4. Assess for chest pain. Location? Characteristics? Reproducible?

PHYSICAL EXAMINATION

A. Aimed at identifying the most life-threatening injury first.

B. Advanced trauma life support (ATLS) guidelines provide a quick but thorough approach to patient assessment.

C. If there is concern for pneumothorax, a tube thoracostomy must be considered.

DIAGNOSTIC TESTS

A. FAST (focused assessment with sonography for trauma) examination may show cardiac tamponade and can be used to determine the presence of a pneumothorax without the use of chest x-ray (CXR).

B. Plain radiograph of the chest to identify fractures, atelectasis, pneumothorax, or widened mediastinum (possible aortic injury).

C. CT and CT angiogram help to identify specific bony, organ, and vascular injuries.

D. EKG and centralized telemetry to monitor for arrhythmias.

E. Arterial blood gas (ABG) may show respiratory acidosis related to hypoventilation as a result of pain and splinting.

F. Cardiac enzymes.

DIFFERENTIAL DIAGNOSIS

A. Common traumatic chest injuries.

1. Bony injuries.
   a. Rib fractures.
      i. Definition: Fractures of one or more ribs. Can be located bilaterally or may be displaced, and can stand alone or result in injury to underlying structures, such as the lungs, subclavian vessels, or organs such as the spleen and liver.
         1) Flail chest: Occurs when at least two adjacent ribs are broken in multiple places, creating a free-moving segment, allowing that segment of the chest wall to move independently. If fractures are near the sternum, there can be a free-floating segment of the sternum, as well as rib. This can be a life-threatening condition.
   b. Sternal fractures.
      i. Definition: Fractures of the manubrium or sternal body. Persons older than 65 years will have increased risk of death (10%–12%) with one rib fracture. The rate increases by 5% with each additional rib fracture. Other bony injuries may include posterior scapula and thoracic spine fractures.
      ii. Management.
         1) Rule out underlying injury to other tissues or organs.
         2) Cardiac echo will determine if there is a cardiac contusion or other heart-related injury.
         3) Pain management.
         4) Aggressive pulmonary hygiene. Encourage incentive spirometer.
         5) Supplemental oxygen.
         6) Displaced rib fractures or flail segments may require operative intervention for stabilization.

2. Lung injuries.
   a. Pulmonary contusion.
      i. Definition.
         1) Bruising to the lung parenchyma.
         2) Clinical course: Tend to worsen in the first 24 to 48 hours. Can lead to atelectasis, infiltrate, effusions, or empyema.
         3) Frequently associated with rib fractures.
      ii. Management.
         1) Supplemental oxygen.
         2) May require intubation and supported ventilation.
         3) Analgesia.
         4) Chest physiotherapy.
   b. Pneumothorax.
      i. Definition.
         1) Accumulation of air in the pleural space, resulting in partial or complete collapse of the lung.
         2) Tension pneumothorax: Life-threatening condition. As air accumulates in the pleural space, it exerts an increased pressure on the heart; mediastinal shift to the unaffected side can lead to circulatory collapse.
   c. Hemothorax.
      i. Definition.
         1) Blood accumulates in the pleural space.
         2) Considered "massive hemothorax" when drainage exceeds 1.5 L in less than 2 hours after injury, necessitating emergent thoracotomy.
      ii. Physical examination findings of pneumothorax or hemothorax.
         1) Decreased breath sounds on the affected side.
         2) Deviated trachea is a late sign.
         3) Respiratory distress, hypoxia, tachycardia, or hypotension may be present.
      iii. Other physical findings.
         1) Cyanosis.
         2) Diaphoresis.
         3) Chest pain.
         4) Altered mental status.
         5) Subcutaneous emphysema.
         6) Signs of shock and hypovolemia.
      iv. Management.
         1) Small pneumothorax or hemothorax can be managed conservatively by observation and repeat CXR.
         2) Tension pneumothorax is a clinical diagnosis based on hemodynamics and respiratory distress. Chest needle decompression may be required as an emergent intervention until a chest tube is placed.
         3) Pneumothorax greater than 20% requires thoracostomy tube (chest tube) insertion.
         4) Massive hemothorax with drainage of more than 1.5 L in 2 hours may require thoracotomy and repair of lung injury.
         5) Retained hemothorax (RH) is a complication of traumatic chest injury where residual blood clots in the pleural space cannot be drained by a traditional chest tube and is diagnosed using chest CT. This condition can lead to empyema (infection) and pneumonia. Treatment options include video-assisted thoracoscopic surgery (VATS) and use of fibrinolytic agents, instilled into the pleural space, to help dissolved retained clot.
   d. Cardiac tamponade.
      i. Definition.
         1) Accumulation of blood or fluid in the pericardial sac, causing a compression of the heart muscles. This leads to decreased cardiac output, which is life-threatening.
      ii. Physical examination findings.

1) Beck triad: A constellation of findings suggestive of tamponade.
  a) Jugular vein distention.
  b) Hypotension with narrowing pulse pressures.
  c) Distant or muffled heart sounds.
iii. Other physical findings.
  1) Tachycardia.
  2) Pulsus paradoxus.
  3) Altered mentation.
  4) Oliguria.
  5) Signs of impending shock.
iv. Management.
  1) Pericardiocentesis.
  2) Management of shock.
e. Great vessel injuries.
  i. Definition.
    1) Interruption of the wall of any of the great vessels is a life-threatening event. Injuries to the aorta, internal vena cava, or subclavian vessels can be the result of laceration from bony segments or shearing or compressive forces. These require operative intervention. These may require operative intervention.
  ii. Physical findings.
    1) Chest or back pain, shortness of breath, weakness.
    2) Hypotension.
    3) Variations in blood pressure (BP) in both upper extremities.
    4) Shock.
  iii. Management.
    1) Thoracotomy with repair to affected vessels; may require cardiopulmonary bypass.
    2) Mechanical ventilation.
    3) Replacement of blood volume with transfusion; may require massive transfusion protocols.
    4) May require hemodynamic support with vasopressors and volume resuscitation.
    5) Other chest injuries to be suspicious for may include traumatic diaphragmatic tears/lacerations and tracheobronchial injuries, which may require prompt surgical intervention.

EVALUATION AND MANAGEMENT PLAN
A. General plan.
  1. Identify specific injuries and treat accordingly.
  2. Primary goals of therapy.
    a. Pain management.
    b. Prevention of atelectasis and pneumonia.
    c. Weaning of supplemental oxygen.
    d. Consulting appropriate services based on injuries.
  3. Explain expectant course with patient and family.
  4. Consider adding cardiac enzymes to workup to rule out underlying stress to the heart.

5. May require multiple radiographs to evaluate the course of healing.
6. For patients with chest tubes, document the output and consistency of drainage and whether an air leak is present. Daily CXRs for evaluation of the presence of pneumothorax.
B. Patient/family teaching points.
  1. Cough and deep breathing exercises.
  2. Incentive spirometry or other airway clearance devices.
  3. Incisional wound care.
  4. Early ambulation.
C. Pharmacotherapy.
  1. When indicated, vasopressors to support hemodynamics.
  2. Multimodal pain management using opioids only when indicated.
    a. Nonsteroidal anti-inflammatory drugs (NSAIDs) and Tylenol for mild pain.
    b. Lidocaine patch for localized pain.
    c. Intravenous (IV) Toradol and Tylenol with supplemental opioid for moderate pain.
    d. Muscle relaxers for spasms.
    e. For severe pain, consider:
      i. Epidural pain medication.
      ii. Intercostal nerve block.
      iii. Patient-controlled analgesia (PCA) pain management.
      iv. Oral opioids.
  3. Bronchodilator treatments when indicated.
  4. If evidence of infection is noted, use appropriate antibiotic therapies.

FOLLOW-UP
A. Follow-up should be dictated by the level of injury and hospital course.
B. For minor injuries, patients may follow up with the primary care provider in 1 to 2 weeks.
C. Postsurgical follow-up may be indicated in a 7- to 14-day period for wound checks, repeat imaging, or suture/staple removal.

CONSULTATION/REFERRAL
A. Patients with severe injury should always be referred to a designated trauma center if the institution does not have the resources to treat the patient.
B. Refer any additional injuries requiring specialist consultation.

SPECIAL/GERIATRIC CONSIDERATIONS
A. Morbidity associated with rib fractures increases with age and is the highest in older adult patients.

CASE SCENARIO: CHEST TRAUMA
A 68-year-old restrained driver presents following a motor vehicle collision (MVC) involving crashing into a tree. The patient presents with ecchymosis and pain on the right side of the chest and reports a steering wheel deformity. Physical exam findings include shortness of breath, decreased breath sounds on the right chest, and tachycardia.

Pulse oximetry is 86% on 2-L nasal cannula. Injuries include right posterior rib fractures 5 to 9, with moderate pneumothorax and bilateral pulmonary contusions. The patient also has a right clavicle fracture and multiple thoracic spine fractures.

1. The acute care nurse practitioner (NP) should prepare for which of the following actions?

   A. Video-assisted thoracoscopic surgery (VATS) procedure
   B. Follow-up chest x-ray (CXR) in 6 hours
   C. Placement of thoracostomy tube (chest tube)
   D. Syncope workup

2. Fracture of one or more adjacent ribs, broken in multiple places, is known as:

   A. Beck triad
   B. Flail chest
   C. Sternal fracture
   D. Crepitus

3. Accumulation of blood or fluid in the pericardial sac is known as:

   A. Pneumothorax
   B. Hemothorax
   C. Pleural effusion
   D. Cardiac tamponade

4. Which life-threatening condition occurs with a rapidly expanding or untreated pneumothorax leading to deviated trachea, decreased venous return, and compromise of the opposite lung?

   A. Rib fractures
   B. Pulmonary contusion
   C. Tension pneumothorax
   D. Sternal fracture

BIBLIOGRAPHY

Alisha, C., Gajanan, G., & Jyothi, H. (2015). Risk factors affecting the prognosis in patients with pulmonary contusion following chest trauma. *Journal of Clinical Diagnostic Research, 9*(8), OC17–OC19. https://doi.org/10.7860/JCDR/2015/13285.6375

Alwatari, Y., Simmonds, A., Ayalew, D., Khoraki, J., Wolfe, L., Leichtle, S. W., Aboutanos, M. B., & Rodas, E. B. (2022, January 27). Early video-assisted thoracoscopic surgery (VATS) for non-emergent thoracic trauma remains underutilized in trauma accredited centers despite evidence of improved patient outcomes. *European Journal of Trauma and Emergency Surgery, 48*(4), 3211–3219. https://doi.org/10.1007/s00068-01881-7

American College of Surgeons. Committee on Trauma. (2018). *Advanced trauma life support: Student course manual* (10th ed.). American College of Surgeons.

Bozzay, J. D., & Bradley, M. J. (2019). Management of post-traumatic retained hemothorax. *Trauma, 21*(1), 14–20. https://doi.org/10.1177/1460408617752985

Bulger, E. M., Arneson, M. A., Mock, C. N., & Jurkovich, G. J. (2000). Rib fractures in the elderly. *Journal of Trauma and Acute Care Surgery, 48*(6), 1040–1047.

Chan, K. K., Joo, D. A., McRae, A. D., Takwoingi, Y., Prenji, Z. A., Lang, E., & Wakai, A. (2020, July). Chest ultrasonography v. supine chest radiography for diagnosis of pneumothorax in trauma patient in the emergency department. *The Cochrane Database System Review, 7*(7), CD013031. https://doi.org/10.1002/14651858.CDO13031.pub2

Chou, Y. P., Lin, H. L., & Wu, T. C. (2015). Video-assisted thoracoscopic surgery for retained hemothorax in blunt chest trauma. *Current Opinion in Pulmonary Medicine, 21*(4), 393–398. https://doi.org/10.1067/MCP.0000000000000173

Dennis, B. M., Belliser, S. A., & Guillamondegui, O. D. (2017, October). Thoracic trauma. *Surgical Clinics of North America, 97*(5), 1047–1064. https://doi.org/10.1016/j.scc2017.06.009

Dogrul, B. N., Kiliccalan, I., Asci, E. S., & Peker, S. C. (2020, June). Blunt trauma related chest wall and pulmonary injuries: An overview. *Chinese Journal of Traumatology, 23*(3), 125–138. https://doi.org/10.1016/j.cjtee.2020.04.003. Epub 2020, April 20; PMID: 32417043; PMCID: MD7296362.

DuBose, J., Inaba, K., Demetriades, D., Scalea, T. M., O'Connor, J., Menaker, J., Morales, C., Konstantinidis, A., Shiflet, A., & Copwood, B. (2012, January). Management of post-traumatic retained hemothorax: A prospective, observational, multicenter AAST study. *Journal of Trauma and Acute Care Surgery, 72*(1), 11–22. https://doi.org/10.1097/TA.0b013e318242e368

Marro, A., Chan, V., Haas, B., & Ditkofsky, N. (2019, October). Blunt chest trauma: Classification and management. *Emergency Radiology, 26*(5), 557–566. https://doi.org/10.1007/s10140-019-01705-z. Epub 2019, July 6; PMID: 31280427.

Martin, C. S., Lu, N., Inouye, D. S., Nakagawa, K., Ng, K. Yu, M, & Hayashi, M. S. (2021, September 27). Delayed respiratory failure after blunt chest trauma. *American Surgery, 87*(9), 1468–1473. https://doi.org/10.1177/00031348096627. Epub 2020, December 27; PMID: 33356435.

Sawa, J., Green, R., Thoma, B., Erdogan, M., & Davis, P. (2017, August 11). Risk factors for adverse outcomes in older adults with blunt chest trauma: A systematic review. *Canadian Journal of Emergency Medicine, 20*(4), 1–9. https://doi.org/10.1017/cem.2017.377

Senn-Reeves, J. N., & Stafileno, B. A. (2013). Long term outcomes after blunt injury to the boney thorax. *Journal of Trauma Nursing, 20*(1), 56–64. https://doi.org/10.1097/JTN.0b013e318286629b

Stewart, D. J. (2014). Blunt chest trauma. *Journal of Trauma Nursing, 21*(6), 282–286. https://doi.org/10.1097/JTN.0000000000000079

PENETRATING CHEST INJURIES

Susan F. Galiczynski

DEFINITION

A. A penetrating chest injury is one in which the projectile enters the thorax in any area below the level of the clavicle to the diaphragm.

B. Structures at risk for injury include the chest wall, ribs, lungs and pleura, esophagus, trachea, diaphragm, thoracic blood vessels, thoracic spine, heart, and mediastinal structures.

C. Penetrating trauma occurs less often than blunt trauma but carries higher mortality.

INCIDENCE

A. Thoracic injuries account for approximately 20% to 25% of all traumatic deaths.

B. Approximately 16,000 deaths annually in the United States can be attributed to thoracic injury.

C. Increase in number with the increase in the number of violent crimes.

D. Much of the research in thoracic trauma comes from military experiences.

E. Firearm injuries are a leading cause of traumatic deaths in the United States and have increased by approximately 20% since 2014.

F. Penetrating/firearm trauma is a public health crisis in the United States.

PATHOGENESIS

A. A bullet or projectile object can enter the body at any location, but if it travels into the thoracic cavity any of the structures there are at risk for injury.

PREDISPOSING FACTORS

A. Males are more at risk than females.
B. Males older than 65 years.
C. Single people are more at risk than married people.
D. City resident.
E. Lower income individuals.
F. Drug and alcohol use.
G. History of depression.
H. History of suicide attempts.
I. History of gunshot wounds (GSWs).

SUBJECTIVE DATA

A. Common complaints/symptoms.
　1. Most patients with penetrating chest wounds will be brought to the ED via emergency medical services.
　2. These patients complain of chest pain and shortness of breath. If the patient is in a state of shock, they may be minimally responsive to answering questions.
B. Common/typical scenario.
　1. Penetrating injuries are often described in terms of kinetic energy/velocity. High-velocity injuries are most often associated with riffles/long barrel guns. Hand guns are often considered medium-energy/velocity injuries.
　2. Low-velocity injuries are seen with stab wounds and impalements.
　3. Penetrating injuries, both individual and mass casualty incidents, are increasing in numbers and need to be viewed as a public health crisis.
C. Family and social history.
　1. Unlike chronic diseases, family history is noncontributory to the patient presentation.
　2. Penetrating chest injuries occur more frequently in violent areas, large metropolitan areas, and areas of conflict.
D. Review of systems.
　1. Neurologic: Ask about dizziness, lightheadedness, and loss of consciousness (LOC).
　2. Cardiac: Heart racing, palpitations, and chest pain.
　3. Respiratory: Shortness of breath, breathing difficulties, and airway obstructions.
　4. Integumentary: Areas of bleeding or bruising.
　5. If known, ask patient the caliber of weapon, distance from weapon to the site of injury, and the number of shots fired.

PHYSICAL EXAMINATION

A. Assess chest, back, and abdomen for additional wounds.
B. Integumentary: The physical examination requires a thorough investigation of the skin for breaks, redness, or discoloration, with particular attention to the chest, back, abdomen, axillae, and buttocks.
C. Neurologic: Assess cognition and responsiveness (Glasgow Coma Scale [GCS]).
D. Cardiac: Monitor blood pressure BP and heart rate (HR).

E. Respiratory: Assess quality of breath sounds and respiratory rate, as well as equal rise and fall of the chest. Look for tracheal deviation.
F. Assess pain: Location, severity, characteristics, and responses to medications.
G. Preserve evidence. Paper bags may be applied to cover hands. Do not cut through any holes in patient clothing when removing it. Do not dispose of any bullet fragments found on or removed from the patient.
H. Follow strict chain of custody protocols when handing off evidence.

DIAGNOSTIC TESTS

A. CT.
B. Supine chest radiograph can help to identify foreign bodies, such as bullets.
C. Ultrasound FAST exam.
D. Appropriate labs.

DIFFERENTIAL DIAGNOSIS

A. Location of injury, trajectory of penetrating object, size of object and velocity of entry, and patient report may help focus assessment for identifying potential injuries.
B. Lung lacerations, pneumothorax, and hemothorax.
C. Cardiac injuries.
D. Great vessel injuries.
E. Thoracic spine injuries.
F. Combine thoracoabdominal injuries.

EVALUATION AND MANAGEMENT PLAN

A. General plan.
　1. The primary approach to penetrating trauma to the thorax is to answer the question of whether the patient needs lifesaving operative intervention.
　2. Goals of treatment are aimed at controlling hemorrhage, maintaining adequate perfusion, promptly addressing airway compromise, and maintaining adequate oxygenation.
　3. Criteria for operative intervention and resuscitative thoracotomy:
　　a. Hemodynamic instability: BP less than 90 or HR greater than 120.
　　b. Hypotension despite fluid resuscitation.
　　c. Altered mental status without obvious head injury.
　　d. Metabolic acidosis, in combination with other altered vital signs (VS) or pulmonary embolism (PE) findings.
　　e. Significant findings on diagnostic studies.
　　f. Severe shock or cardiac arrest.
　4. For the patient presenting in extremis, an ED thoracotomy, performed by a trained provider, may be necessary as an immediate lifesaving effort.
　5. Recommendations for chest tube placement:
　　a. **Small-bore** (18–24 F)/pigtail catheters can be used for simple pneumothorax and pleural effusions.

b. **Large-bore** (28–3 6F) tubes may be used for hemothorax to avoid retained hemothorax (RH) and subsequent empyema.

6. The need for subsequent video-assisted thoracoscopy or intrapleural fibrinolytic therapy may be necessary to evacuate RH.

B. Patient/family teaching points.

1. Patient and family education should be geared toward anticipated patient needs as discharge nears.

2. Some examples include wound care, tracheotomy care, physical medicine, and rehab goals.

C. Pharmacotherapy.

1. In the acute phase of care, interventions may include:

a. Hemodynamic support: Blood transfusions and vasopressors may be necessary to reduce risks of hypotension related to hypovolemia and shock states.

b. Use of tranexamic acid (TXA) is indicated in hemorrhagic shock to decrease bleeding and need for transfusion. TXA reduces blood loss by inhibiting the enzymatic breakdown of fibrin.

c. Sedation and pain management with continuous infusions to keep the patient comfortable may be indicated.

d. Prophylactic antibiotic treatment for penetrating thoracic trauma has been shown to demonstrate reduced risk of infection with tube thoracostomy and postoperative prophylaxis.

e. Patients with suspected or documented infection should have antibiotic therapy narrowed to specific organisms, once identified.

FOLLOW-UP

A. Many of these patients have a long critical care and hospital course and will become deconditioned. Preparing the patient and family for potential rehabilitation needs is key.

B. If the patient has multiple injuries not related to just one organ system, education about follow-up with those injury-specific specialty groups is recommended.

C. Physical medicine and rehab may have a very active role in postdischarge care.

CONSULTATION/REFERRAL

A. Trauma.

B. Cardiothoracic surgery.

C. Other necessary consultants, based on injury.

D. Physical medicine and rehab services.

E. Psychiatry for self-inflicted wounds/suicide attempts.

F. Trauma counselors for posttraumatic stress disorder (PTSD).

SPECIAL/GERIATRIC CONSIDERATIONS

A. Indicators of poor outcomes/higher mortality include:

1. Lower GCS on arrival.

2. Increased age.

3. Suicide attempt (self-inflicted).

4. Coagulopathy.

5. Multiple comorbidities.

CASE SCENARIO: INTRACRANIAL PENETRATING TRAUMA

An 18-year-old male with no medical history presents to the trauma center with a single gunshot wound (GSW) to the lower chest, just left of midline. On presentation, the patient was lethargic, pale, and had weak peripheral pulses. Vital signs revealed heart rate (HR) of 130, blood pressure (BP) of 80/40, and respiratory rate (RR) of 10. During the initial survey, a bedside FAST exam demonstrated a left-sided hemothorax. A 32-F chest tube was placed. Chest radiography showed hemothorax with chest tube in good position and displaced rib fractures 8 to 10. Massive transfusion protocol was initiated, and the patient was transfused with 2 units of packed red blood cells (RBCs) as he was prepared for transport to the operating room. In the operating room, a lung laceration was repaired and the shattered spleen was removed. In total, the patient received one dose of intravenous (IV) tranexamic acid (TXA) of 1 g, followed by a continuous infusion of 1 g over the next 8 hours. In addition, 6 units of packed RBCs, two packs of fresh frozen plasma, and two platelets were given. The patient remained intubated postoperatively and was admitted to the shock trauma ICU on fentanyl and propofol infusions for sedation.

1. Retained hemothorax (RH) is:

A. Blood that has drained from the pneumothorax.

B. Instrument used in thoracotomy.

C. Blood that has not been drained using traditional tube thoracostomy.

D. Not seen with trauma thoracic injuries.

2. Indications for emergent surgical intervention in trauma chest injuries include:

A. Glasgow Coma Scale (GCS) score of 15 with normal vital signs (VS).

B. Immediate chest tube output less than 500 mL.

C. Negative diagnostic studies with complaints of pain at injury site.

D. Hemodynamic instability with blood pressure (BP) less than 90 and heart rate (HR) greater than 120.

3. Groups at higher risk for penetrating thoracic injury include:

A. Farmers and country dwellers.

B. Urban dwelling, young males.

C. Infants under age 1.

D. Females over 65 years of age.

4. Firearm injuries are considered:

A. Rare occurrences, limited to military events.

B. High-energy injuries.

C. Low-energy mechanisms.

D. Equal to blunt trauma in both incidence and injury patterns.

BIBLIOGRAPHY

American College of Surgeons. Committee on Trauma. (2018). *Advanced trauma life support: Student course manual* (10th ed.). American College of Surgeons.

Bauchner, H., Rivara, F. P., Bonow, R. O., Bressler, N. M., Disis, M. L., Heckers, S., Josephson, S. A., Kibbe, M. R., Piccirillo, J. F., Redberg, R. F., Rhee, J. S., & Robinson, J. K. (2017). Death by gun violence—A public health crisis. *JAMA*, *318*, 1763–1764. https://doi.org/10.1001/jama.2017.16446

Berg, R. J., Karamanos, E., Inaba, K., Okoye, O., Teixeira, P. G., & Demetriades, D. (2014, February). The persistent diagnostic challenge of thoracoabdominal stab wounds. *Journal of Trauma and Acute Care Surgery, 76*(2), 418–423. https://doi.org/10.1097/TA.0000000000000120

Bouzat, P., Raux, M., David, J. S., Tazarourte, K., Galinski, M., Desmettre, T., Garrigue, D., Ducros, L., Michelet, P., Expert's, group., Freysz, M., Savary, D., Rayeh-Pelardy, F., Laplace, C., Duponq, R., Monnin Bares, V., D'Journo, X. B., Boddaert, G., Boutonnet, M., & Vardon, F. (2017, April). Chest trauma: First 48 hours management. *Anaesthesia Critical Care Pain Medicine, 36*(2), 135–145. https://doi.org/10.1016/j.accpm.2017.01.003 Epub 2017 January 16. PMID: 28096063

Chan, K. K., Joo, D. A., McRae, A. D., Takwoingi, Y., Prenaji, Z. A., Lang, E., & Wakai, A. (2020, July). Chest ultrasonography versus supine chest radiography for diagnosis of pneumothorax in trauma patients in the emergency department. *The Cochrane Database of Systematic Reviews, 7*(7), CD013031. https://doi.org/10.1002/14651858.CD013031.pub2

Davis, J. S., Satahoo, S. S., Butler, F. K., Dermer, H., Naranjo, D., Julien, K., Van Haren, R. M., Namias, N., Blackbourne, L. H., & Schulman, C. I. (2014, August). An analysis of prehospital deaths: Who can we save? *Journal of Trauma and Acute Care Surgery, 77*(2), 213–218. https://doi.org/10.1097/TA.0000000000000292

Dennis, B. M., Bellister, S. A., & Guillamondegui, O. D. (2017, October). Thoracic trauma. *Surgical Clinics of North America, 97*(5), 1047–1064. https://doi.org/10.1016/j.suc.2017.06.009

Grinshteyn, E., & Hemenway, D. (2019, June). Violent death rates in the US compared to those of other high-income countries, 2015. *Preventative Medicine, 123*, 20–26. https://doi.org/10.1016/j.ypmed.2019.02.026

Hicks, J. L., Nelson, J., Fidles, J., Kuhls, D., Eastman, A., & Dries, D. (2020, February). Triage, trauma and today's mass violent events. *Journal of the American College of Surgeons, 230*(2), 251–256. https://doi.org/10.1016/j.jamcollsurg.2019.10.011

Kamarova, M., & Kendall, R. (2017, December). 13 Prophylactic antibiotics for penetrating injury: A review of practice at a major trauma centre, literature review and recommendations. *Emergency Medicine Journal, 34*(12), A869. https://doi.org/10.1136/emermed-2017-207308.13

Klein, J., Prabhakaran, K., Latifi, R., & Rhee, P. (2022). Firearms: The leading cause of years of potential life lost. *Trauma Surgery and Acute Care Open, 7*(1), e000766. https://doi.org/10.1136/tsaco-2021-000766

Krestan, C., & Greitbauer, M. (2020, July). Trauma an Brustwirbelsäule und knöchernem Thorax [Trauma to the thoracic spine and chest]. *Radiologe, 60*(7), 610–623. https://doi.org/10.1007/s00117-020-00712-3. German PMID: 32601929.

Madden, B. P. (2017, January). Evolutional trends in the management of tracheal and bronchial injuries. *Journal of Thoracic Disease, 9*(1), E67–E70. https://doi.org/10.21037/jtd.2017.01.43

Mollberg, N. M., Tabachnik, D., Farjah, F., Lin, F. J., Vafa, A., Abdelhady, K., Merlotti, G. J., Wood, D. E., & Massad, M. G. (2013, August). Utilization of cardiothoracic surgeons for operative penetrating thoracic trauma and its impact on clinical outcomes. *Annals of Thoracic Surgery, 96*(2), 445–450. https://doi.org/10.1016/j.athoracsur.2013.04.033

Moore, H. B., Moore, E. E., Burlew, C. C., Biffl, W. L., Pieracci, F. M., Barnett, C. C., Bensard, D., Jurkovich, G. J., & Fox, C. J. (2016, July). Establishing benchmarks for resuscitation of traumatic circulatory arrest: Success-to-rescue and survival among 1,708 patients. *Journal of the American College of Surgeons, 223*(1), 42–50. https://doi.org/10.1016/j.jamcollsurg.2016.04.013

O'Connor, J. V., Muran, B., Galvagno, S. M. Jr., Deane, M., Feliciano, D. V., & Scalea, T. M. (2020, April). Admission physiology vs blood pressure: Predicting he need for operating room thoracotomy after penetrating thoracic trauma. *Journal of the American College of Surgeons, 230*(4), 494–500. https://doi.org/10.1016/j.jamcollsurg.2019.12.019

Ranney, M. L. (2021, March 30). We must treat gun violence as a public health crisis. These 4 steps will help to reduce deaths. *Time.*

Schwab-Reese, L. M., & Peek-Asa, C. (2019). Factors contributing to homicide-suicide: Differences between firearm and non-firearm deaths. *Journal of Behavioral Medicine, 42*, 681–690. https://doi.org/10.1007/s10865-019-00066-9

Seamon, M. J., Haut, E. R., VanArendonk, K., Barbosa, R. R., Chiu, W. C., Dente, C. J., Fox, N., Jawa, R. S., Khwaja, K., Lee, J. K., Magnotti, L. J., Mayglothling, J. A., McDonald, A. A., Rowell, S., To, K. B., Falck-Ytte, Y., & Rhee, P. (2015, July). An evidence-based approach to patient selection for emergency department thoracotomy: A practice management guideline from the Eastern Association for the Surgery of Trauma. *Journal of Trauma and Acute Care Surgery, 79*(1), 159–173. https://doi.org/10.1097/TA.0000000000000648

PENETRATING INTRACRANIAL INJURIES

Susan F. Galiczynski

DEFINITION

A. A penetrating intracranial injury is one in which the projectile enters the cranium.
B. Penetrating trauma to the head is less common than blunt injury but carries a worse prognosis.
C. Gunshot wounds (GSWs) are high-energy, high-velocity injuries that can cause extensive damage as the object enters the body.
D. GSWs carry a higher mortality than other penetrating wounds. They are almost always fatal if the bullet crosses the midline, crosses both hemispheres, or lodges in the brain.
E. The blast energy of a bullet can be as high as 30 to 40 times the diameter of the bullet and can cause increased tissue damage as the bullet travels and displaces surrounding tissue.
F. Stab wounds and impalements are considered low impact and the focus is more on the immediate tissue injury and area of impact.

INCIDENCE

A. Head injuries are the leading cause of trauma-related deaths in the United States.
B. Affects almost two million people annually.

PATHOGENESIS

A. A bullet or projectile object crosses the skull barrier and enters the brain parenchyma.
B. Degree of injury is related to (a) location of injury, (b) energy and speed of projectile, and (c) size and type of object.

PREDISPOSING FACTORS

A. Males greater than females.
B. Males older than 65 years of age.
C. Single people are at higher risk than married people.
D. City resident.
E. Lower income individuals.
F. Drug and alcohol use.
G. History of depression.
H. History of suicide attempts.
I. History of GSW.

SUBJECTIVE DATA

A. Common complaints/symptoms.
  1. Patients will typically come in via emergency services, but will occasionally walk in or be driven by friends or family with a foreign object that has penetrated the skull.

B. Family and social history (pertinent findings—positive/negative).

    1. Family history is noncontributory. Penetrating head injuries occur more frequently in violent areas, large metropolitan areas, and areas of conflict.

C. Review of systems (pertinent findings—positive/negative).

    1. Neurologic: Ask about headaches, dizziness, vertigo, and decreased sensation.

    2. Head, ear, eyes, nose, and throat (HEENT): Blurry vision, double vision, loss of vision, changes in smell, and bleeding from anywhere on the head. Ask patient if they have a salty taste in their mouth as this can be indicative of a cerebrospinal fluid (CSF) leak.

    3. Musculoskeletal: Any weakness in the arms or legs or numbness/tingling.

PHYSICAL EXAMINATION

A. Perform a Glasgow Coma Scale (GCS) score (see Table 17.1). The score ranges from 3 to 15. If the patient is intubated, that is notated by the use of the letter "T" after the number, such as 8T, to indicate GCS score of 8 in an intubated patient.

B. Patient requires detailed cranial nerve (CN) assessment including CN I, olfactory nerve.

C. Assess for signs of other injuries by completely undressing the patient. Axillae, groin, and buttocks are areas that require inspection, as stab wounds and GSWs are often found in these locations.

D. Assess ears and nose for any evidence of blood or CSF. If blood is present, perform halo test.

E. Assess the head, scalp, and face for contusions, lacerations, or hematoma.

TABLE 17.1   GLASGOW COMA SCALE
Eye Opening (E)   Spontaneous 4   To voice 3   To pain 2   No response 1
Verbal Response (V)   Oriented conversation 5   Confused/disoriented 4   Incomprehensible words 3   Incomprehensible sounds 2   No response 1
Motor Response (M)   Moves all extremities 6   Localizes to pain 5   Withdraws to pain 4   Decorticate posture 3   Decerebrate posture 2   No response 1
Total GCS = E + V + M

GCS, Glasgow Coma Scale score.

F. A detailed neuro examination is performed when possible to determine baseline neurologic function. This should include full motor exam to look for deficits.

DIAGNOSTIC TESTS

A. CT: Noncontrast of head and cervical spine as indicated.

B. Flat plate of skull can be done to identify foreign bodies (e.g., bullets).

C. CT angiogram of head and neck to look for vascular infarcts.

DIFFERENTIAL DIAGNOSIS

A. Subarachnoid hemorrhage.

B. Subdural hemorrhage.

C. Epidural hemorrhage.

D. Intracranial hemorrhage.

E. Open skull/facial bone fractures.

F. Epidural hematoma.

G. Cervical spine injury.

EVALUATION AND MANAGEMENT PLAN

A. General plan.

    1. These patients are often critically ill and have a higher mortality.

    2. Goals of treatment are geared toward preventing secondary brain injury by maintaining adequate perfusion and oxygenation to the brain.

    3. Intracranial pressure (ICP) monitoring, including bolt placement and/or ventriculostomy.

    4. Objects that penetrate the intracranial compartments and remain partially visible (as in cases of stab wound or impalement) must be left in place until vascular and neurosurgical consultation and plan has been completed.

    5. If ophthalmology is consulted, clear with neurosurgery prior to dilated fundoscopic exam.

    6. Surgical craniotomy or craniectomy (bone flap removal) may be necessary.

    7. Brain death exam.

    8. Discussions around organ donation.

B. Patient/family teaching points.

    1. Patient and family education should be geared toward anticipated patient needs as discharge nears.

    2. Some examples include wound care, tracheotomy care, physical medicine, and rehab goals.

    3. Speech therapy for communication and cognitive evaluations.

    4. Discussion with family to emphasize functional outcomes can vary.

C. Pharmacotherapy.

    1. In the acute phase of care, interventions may include:

        a. Hemodynamic support: Blood transfusions and vasopressors may be necessary to reduce risks of hypotension related to hypovolemia and shock states.

b. Seizure prophylaxis is indicated for severe brain injury and may include Keppra, Dilantin, or fosphenytoin.

c. Sedation and pain management with continuous infusions are used to keep the patient comfortable and avoid elevations in increased ICP.

d. Antibiotic treatments that cross the blood–brain barrier, such as ceftriaxone, are warranted for open fractures and for any ICU-related infections.

e. Osmotic diuretics, such as mannitol and hypertonic saline, help to reduce ICP.

FOLLOW-UP

A. If the patient survives, follow up with neurosurgeon in 10 to 14 days post discharge is recommended.

B. If the patient had any additional injuries (multiple GSWs often do), follow-up with injury-specific specialty groups is recommended.

C. Physical medicine and rehab may have a very active role in postdischarge care. Most head traumas will require rehabilitative care and potentially neurologic cognitive testing, evaluation, and management.

CONSULTATION/REFERRAL

A. Trauma is consulted on all trauma cases.

B. Neurosurgery will be consulted on penetrating injuries to the brain.

C. Other necessary consultants are selected based on the type and extent of injury.

D. Physical medicine and rehab services are needed for discharge assessment and planning.

E. Refer to psychiatry for self-inflicted wounds/suicide attempts.

SPECIAL/GERIATRIC CONSIDERATIONS

A. Indicators of poor outcomes/higher mortality include:

1. Lower GCS score on arrival.
2. Increased age.
3. Suicide attempt (self-inflicted).
4. Transcranial injury.
5. Perforated brain injury (entrance and exit wounds).
6. Coagulopathy.
7. Any episode of hypoxia prehospital or during hospitalization.
8. Multiple comorbidities.

B. Neurologic pulmonary edema.

1. Neurologic pulmonary edema is a rare clinical syndrome that can occur with any neurologic insult to the brain. It is characterized by acute onset of pulmonary edema and evidence of stunning of the heart, without history of cardiac or respiratory disease. Although the exact etiology is unknown, it is thought to be caused by an intense trigger of the sympathetic nervous system, leading to a surge of catecholamines, resulting in cardiopulmonary dysfunction. Onset of this syndrome can begin within minutes of injury up to the first 24 hours postinjury. Morality may be as high as 50%.

CASE SCENARIO: PENETRATING INTRACRANIAL INJURIES

A 22-year-old male presented to the trauma center with a single gunshot wound (GSW) to the left occiput. On arrival, he had a Glasgow Coma Scale (GCS) score of 6, with eyes open but no verbal or motor noted. Pupils were 2 mm and sluggish. On arrival, vital signs included temperature of 96.8°F/36°C, blood pressure (BP) of 80/30, and heart rate (HR) of 56. Agonal respirations were noted. Pulse oximetry was 88%. The patient initially had no extremity movement. The patient was immediately intubated, but during intubation the patient vomited. FAST exam demonstrated a stunned left ventricle with minimal movement. There were no signs of tamponade or effusion. The patient remained hypotensive and massive transfusion protocol was initiated. CT demonstrated GSW to the left posterior parietal area terminating in the anterior frontal lobe.

1. The Glasgow Coma Scale (GCS) is:

A. Meaningful only in awake and alert patients.

B. A quick, simple, and objective assessment of neurologic exam.

C. A diagnostic tool to measure degree of hemorrhage in trauma patients.

D. An assessment tool used to distinguish types of traumatic brain injury (TBI).

2. Using the Glasgow Coma Scale (GCS) score, coma is defined as:

A. 13 to 15.

B. 0.

C. 9 to 12.

D. Less than 8.

3. Cerebral perfusion pressure (CPP) is defined as:

A. Mean arterial pressure (MAP)–CPP.

B. MAP–intracranial pressure (ICP).

C. Blood pressure (BP)–heart rate (HR).

D. Systolic BP–diastolic BP.

4. Gunshot wounds (GSWs) to the head are considered:

A. Low-energy, low-impact injuries.

B. Lower mortality than blunt trauma.

C. High-energy, high-velocity injuries.

D. Low risk for seizure activity.

BIBLIOGRAPHY

Aarabi, B., Tofighi, B., Kufera, J. A., Hadley, J., Ahn, E. S., Cooper, C., Malik, J. M., Naff, N. J., Chang, L., Radley, M., Kheder, A., & Uscinski, R. H. (2014, May). Predictors of outcome in civilian gunshot wounds to the head. *Journal of Neurosurgery*, 120(5), 1138–1146. https://doi.org/10.3171/2014.1.JNS131869

American College of Surgeons. Committee on Trauma. (2018). *Advanced trauma life support: Student course manual* (10th ed.). American College of Surgeons.

Burgess, P., Sullivent, E., Sasser, S., Wald, M., Ossmann, E., & Kapil, V. (2010). Managing traumatic brain injury secondary to explosions. *Journal of Emergencies, Trauma and Shock*, 3(2), 164–172. https://doi.org/10.4103/0974-2700.62120

Carney, N., Totten, A. M., O'Reilly, C., Ullman, J. S., Hawryluk, G. W., Bell, M. J., Bratton, S. L., Chestnut, R., Harris, O. A., Kissoon, N., Rubiano, A. M., Shutter, L., Tasker, R. C., Vavilala, M. S., Wilberger, J., Wrigth, D. W., & Ghajar, J. (2017, January 1). Guidelines for the management of severe traumatic brain injury, fourth edition. *Neurosurgery*, 80(1), 6–15. https://doi.org/10.1227/NEU.0000000000001432

Davidson, D. L., Terek, M., & Chawla, L. S. (2012). Neurogenic pulmonary Edema. *Critical Care*, 16(2), 212. https://doi.org/10.1186/cc11226

Folio, L., Solomon, J., Biassou, N., Fischer, T., Dworzak, J., Raymont, V., Sinaii, N., Wassermann, E. M., & Grafman, J. (2013, March). Semi-automated trajectory analysis of deep ballistic penetrating brain injury. *Military Medicine*, 178(3), 338–345. https://doi.org/10.7205/MILMED-D-12-00353

Mac Donald, C. L., Johnson, A. M., Cooper, D., Nelson, E. C., Werner, N. J., Shimony, J. S., Snyder, A. Z., Raichle, M. E., Witherow, J. R., Fang, R., Flaherty, S. F., & Brody, D. L. (2011, June 2). Detection of blast-related traumatic brain injury in U.S. military personnel. *The New England Journal of Medicine*, 364(22), 2091–2100. https://doi.org/10.1056/NEJMoa1008069

Paiva, W. S., de Andrade, A. F., Amorim, R. L., Figueiredo, E. G., & Teixeira, M. J. (2012, October). Brainstem injury by penetrating head trauma with a knife. *British Journal of Neurosurgery*, 26(5), 779–781. https://doi.org/10.3109/02688697.2012.655809

Rajagopal, R., Ganesh, S., & Vetrivel, M. (2017, May). Neurogenic pulmonary Edema in traumatic brain injury. *Indian Journal of Critical Care Medicine*, 21(5), 329–331. https://doi.org/10.4103/ijccm.IJCCM_431_16

Saito, N., Hito, R., Burke, P. A., & Sakai, O. (2014). Imaging of penetrating injuries of the head and neck: Current practice at a level I trauma center in the United States. *The Keio Journal of Medicine*, 63(2), 23–33. https://doi.org/10.2302/kjm.2013-0009-RE

SHOCK

Rose Milano

DEFINITION

A. Shock is a life-threatening condition resulting from acute peripheral circulatory failure.

B. Acute peripheral circulatory failure results in impaired cellular and tissue oxygenation leading ultimately to systemic hypoxemia.

C. If not managed in its early stages, systemic hypoxemia results not only in cellular and tissue damage, but potentially systemic multiorgan dysfunction and death.

D. Types of shock (Table 17.2):

1. Hypovolemic: Inadequate circulating volume that leads to decreased cardiac preload and decreased cardiac output, resulting in decreased perfusion of vital organs.

2. Cardiogenic: Severe impairment of cardiac function, leading to decreased cardiac output, end-organ hypoperfusion, and hypoxia.

3. Distributive: Loss of peripheral vascular tone causing decreased blood flow and damage to vital organs.

In addition, the capillary wall becomes permeable, allowing fluids to leak out into the surrounding tissues.

4. Obstructive: An impedance of adequate cardiac filling, either by preventing blood from entering the right heart during diastole (e.g., tension pneumothorax or pericardial tamponade) or preventing the heart from ejecting blood during systole (e.g., pulmonary embolism or left ventricular outflow obstruction).

INCIDENCE

A. 15.7% of shock states are hypovolemic.

B. 16.7% of shock states are cardiogenic.

C. 62% of shock states are distributive in nature and due to sepsis, and 4% are distributive in nature from causes other than sepsis.

D. 2% of shock states are obstructive.

PATHOGENESIS (CELLULAR)

A. Inadequate oxygen delivery changes cell metabolism from aerobic to anaerobic.

B. Anaerobic metabolism leads to lactic acid production, causing the cell to cease function and swell.

C. Once the cell swells, the membrane becomes permeable, allowing electrolytes and fluids to seep in, causing the sodium and potassium pumps to fail.

D. This pump failure leads to inadequate energy production and metabolic failure.

E. This inadequate energy production and metabolic failure lead to mitochondrial damage and cell death.

PREDISPOSING FACTORS

A. Hypovolemic.
1. Hemorrhage.
2. Vomiting.
3. Diarrhea.
4. Poor oral intake.
5. Burns.
6. Diabetic insipidus.
7. Ascites.
8. Diuresis.

B. Cardiogenic.
1. Myopathic: Myocardial ischemia.
2. Valvular/mechanical failure.
3. Prolonged cardiopulmonary bypass.

TABLE 17.2 HEMODYNAMIC PROFILE OF SHOCK

Types of Shock	HR	CO	Ventricular Filling Pressure	SVR	Pulse Pressure	SVO$_2$
Cardiogenic	↑	↓	↑	↑	↓	↓
Hypovolemic	↑	↓	↓	↑	↓	↓
Distributive	↑	↑ or ↓	↓	↓	↑	↑
Obstructive	↑	↓	↑ or normal	↑	↓	↓

CO, cardiac output; HR, heart rate; SVO$_2$, mixed venous oxygen saturation; SVR, systemic vascular resistance.
Source: Data from Bergeron, N., Dubois, M.J., Dumont, M., Dial, S., & Skrobik, Y. (2001). Intensive care delirium screening checklist: Evaluation of a new screening tool. *Intensive Care Medicine*, 27, 859–864. https://doi.org/10.1007/s001340100909.

4. Preexisting myocardial damage.
5. Cardiac arrhythmias.
6. Drug overdose/poisoning.
7. Heart failure.
C. Distributive.
  1. Sepsis.
  2. Anaphylaxis.
  3. Adrenal insufficiency.
  4. Neurogenic.
  5. Liver failure.
  6. Fat embolism.
D. Obstructive.
  1. Cardiac tamponade.
  2. Pulmonary embolism (PE).
  3. Tension pneumothorax.
  4. Constrictive pericarditis.
  5. Traumatic diaphragmatic injury.

SUBJECTIVE AND OBJECTIVE DATA

A. Common complaints/symptoms.
  1. Vital sign changes.
    a. Hypotension.
      i. Systolic blood pressure (SBP) less than 90 mmHg.
      ii. Mean arterial pressure (MAP) less than 60 mmHg.
      iii. Change is SBP greater than 40 mmHg.
      iv. Widening pulse pressure.
    b. Tachycardia.
    c. Bradycardia in neurodistributive shock.
    d. Tachypnea.
  2. Neurologic changes.
    a. Obtunded.
    b. Altered mental status.
  3. Genitourinary changes.
    a. Oliguria.
    b. Anuria.
  4. Integumentary changes.
    a. Cold, clammy extremities.
    b. Mottled skin.
    c. Poor capillary refill.
  5. Lactic acidosis (anion gap acidosis).
B. Additional specific shock state complaints/symptoms.
  1. Hypovolemic shock.
    a. Hypotension/tachycardia.
    b. Pallor.
    c. Flattened jugular veins (patient at 45-degree angle).
  2. Cardiogenic shock.
    a. Chest pain.
    b. Narrow pulse pressure.
    c. Distended jugular veins (patient at 45-degree angle).
    d. Fluid in the lungs (crackles).
    e. Significant arrhythmias.
  3. Distributive shock.
    a. Sepsis: Symptoms associated with infectious cause.
    b. Anaphylaxis: Hypotension, flushing, hives, wheeze, and stridor.

    c. Adrenal crisis: Hypotension, tachycardia, hypoglycemia, mental status changes, and seizures.
    d. Neurogenic: Hypotension, bradycardia, warm/flushed skin, and low central venous pressure (CVP).
  4. Obstructive shock.
    a. Cardiac tamponade: Chest pain, distant heart sounds, distended neck veins (patient at 45-degree angle), decreased pulse pressure, and dyspnea.
    b. PE: Chest pain, tachycardia, hypotension, cough, sudden onset dyspnea, and hemoptysis.
    c. Tension pneumothorax: Tachypnea, distended jugular veins (patient at 45-degree angle), decreased/absent breath sounds on the side of the tension pneumothorax, and tracheal deviation away from the side of the tension pneumothorax.
    d. Constrictive pericarditis: Distended jugular veins (patient at 45-degree angle), pulsus paradoxus, Kussmaul respirations, peripheral edema, ascites, cachexia, and pulsatile hepatomegaly.
C. Family/social history.
  1. Further history needs to be obtained, as well as a more thorough assessment.
  2. Does the patient have a history that is significant for cardiac problems?
  3. Does the patient have a history that is significant for exposure to infectious sources?
  4. Does the patient have a significant history of allergies?
  5. Does the patient have a history of a recent traumatic event?
  6. Does the patient have a history of substance abuse?
  7. Does the patient have a history of diabetes?

PHYSICAL EXAMINATION

A. Does the patient's skin feel cool and clammy, warm, or normal?
B. If the patient has cool and clammy skin, significant cardiac history, or new chest pain, avoid fluids and start workup by obtaining a stat echo.
C. Is skin warm or normal to touch? 62% of patients in shock will be distributive/septic in nature. Start treatment for presumed sepsis until otherwise noted.
  1. Fluid bolus of 30 mL/kg of isotonic fluids within the first 3 hours.

DIAGNOSTIC TESTS

A. For all forms of shock, obtain lab work and additional data points as quickly as possible.
  1. Complete blood count (CBC).
  2. Arterial blood gas (ABG).
  3. Lactate.
  4. Comprehensive metabolic panel (CMP).
  5. Blood cultures.
  6. Urine culture.
  7. Sputum culture.

8. Wound culture (if appropriate).
9. Coagulation panel.
10. Chest x-ray (CXR).
B. EKG/echocardiogram
C. Helical CT scan.
D. Central venous oxygen saturation (ScVO$_2$; if central access is in place).
E. CVP can be monitored with minimally invasive monitoring through the arterial line.
F. Obtaining additional parameters such as passive leg raise, fluid challenges against stroke volume measurements, or variations in systolic pressures, pulse pressure, or stroke volume changes while on mechanical ventilation should be considered when applicable.
G. For all forms of shock, start vasopressors if patient is unresponsive to fluid.
    1. If patient is unresponsive to vasopressor support and history is suggestive, consider obstructive shock and implement treatment quickly. This is often referred to as pressor refractory shock.
H. Once data points are back, identify correct diagnosis and treat appropriately (see Table 17.2).

DIFFERENTIAL DIAGNOSIS
A. Myocardial infarction.
B. Thyroid storm.
C. Acute pancreatitis.
D. PE.
E. Sepsis.
F. Toxic/metabolic syndrome.
G. Coagulopathy.
H. Poisoning.

EVALUATION AND MANAGEMENT PLAN
A. General plan.
    1. Correct underlying process.
    2. Fluids.
      a. Bolus.
        i. 10 to 30 mL/kg depending on the type of shock encountered.
        ii. The Surviving Sepsis Campaign recommends 30 mL/kg intravenous (IV) fluids within the first 3 hours of diagnosis of septic shock.
      b. Types of fluids.
        i. Isotonic fluids.
          1) Lactated Ringer's.
          2) Normal saline.
          3) Plasma-Lyte A.
        ii. Blood products: Replacement of blood products should be based on the individual patient's laboratory values. Advanced trauma life support (ATLS) guidelines recommend massive transfusion protocol with universal red blood cells (RBCs) and plasma platelet pool for each 6 units of RBCs. Some trauma centers use a 1:1:1 ratio of packed RBCs, plasma, and platelets as a resuscitation mixture.
    3. Vasopressor support.
      a. Terminology.
        i. Chronotropic: To change heart rate (HR).
        ii. Inotropic: To change the force of the heart contraction. Positive inotropes increase the force of the contraction and negative inotropes weaken the force of contraction, otherwise known as squeeze.
      b. Norepinephrine.
        i. Endogenous catecholamine.
        ii. Acts as an excitatory neurotransmitter.
        iii. Alpha receptor-mediated peripheral vasoconstriction.
        iv. Weak beta-1 receptor agonist.
        v. Dose: 0.01 to 1 mcg/kg/min and titrate to effect.
        vi. Side effects: Local tissue necrosis.
        vii. First-line pressor for septic shock.
      c. Epinephrine.
        i. Endogenous catecholamine.
        ii. Most potent beta-1 agonist.
        iii. Both alpha and beta properties.
        iv. Potent inotropic and chronotropic.
        v. Dose: 0.01 to 1 mcg/kg/min.
        vi. Second pressor choice in septic shock.
      d. Phenylephrine.
        i. Pure alpha receptor agonist.
        ii. Produces widespread vasoconstriction.
        iii. Dose: 0.1 to 5 mcg/kg/min.
        iv. Side effects.
          1) Bradycardia.
          2) Low cardiac output.
          3) Hypoperfusion to kidneys and bowel.
        v. Not recommended in septic shock.
      e. Vasopressin.
        i. Antidiuretic hormone (ADH)/osmoregulatory hormone.
        ii. Acts through V1 receptors to produce vasoconstriction.
        iii. Dose: 0.03 units/min.
        iv. Typically not titratable.
        v. Not recommended as single agent.
        vi. Use with norepinephrine to decrease dose or to improve perfusion by increasing MAP.
B. Treatment of specific shock states.
    1. Hypovolemic.
      a. Fluids.
      b. Vasopressor support.
      c. Control cause of fluid loss.
        i. Stop ongoing bleeding.
        ii. Stop ongoing emesis or diarrhea.
    2. Cardiogenic.
      a. Improve myocardial function—percutaneous coronary intervention (PCI).
      b. Treat arrhythmias.
      c. Vasopressors plus inotropes.
    3. Obstructive.
      a. Relief of obstruction.
    4. Distributive.
      a. Fluids.
      b. Vasopressors.

c. Treatment of cause.
  i. Early cultures prior to antibiotic administration.
  ii. Antibiotics initiated within the first hour.
  iii. Removal of source of infection (source control).

FOLLOW-UP

A. Resolution of hypotension, tachycardia, and tachypnea.
B. Resolution of oliguria/anuria.
C. Lactic acid: Trend until the level falls below 2.
D. Resolution of cause of shock.

CONSULTATION/REFERRAL

A. Consult critical care team for management of shock.
B. Consult appropriate service for type of shock.
  1. Consider cardiac surgery consult for cardiogenic shock or interventional radiology for obstructive shock (PE, pericardial tamponade, and tension pneumothorax).
  2. Consider infectious disease consult for distributive (infectious disease) source of shock.
  3. Consider general surgery consult for distributive (burn or abdominal infection) and hypovolemic (traumatic hemorrhage) source of sepsis.
  4. Consider neurology consult for distributive (neurogenic) source of sepsis.
  5. Consider internal medicine consult for distributive (diabetes, adrenal crisis, substance overdose, anaphylaxis) and hypovolemic (excessive diuresis, nausea, vomiting, diarrhea, poor oral intake) source of sepsis.

SPECIAL/GERIATRIC CONSIDERATIONS

A. Consider age-related changes in geriatric patients.
B. Response to treatment may occur much more slowly than in younger patients.
C. Signs of shock may go unrecognized early on in geriatric patients due to loss of compensatory mechanisms that are common with aging.
D. Also, medications such as beta-blockers may diminish the body's ability to compensate.

CASE SCENARIO: A 32-YEAR-OLD IN A MOTOR VEHICLE CRASH

A 32-year-old male is transported to a level 1 trauma center after being involved in a motor vehicle crash. He complains of pain to his chest, abdomen, and left hip, and shortness of breath. He presents with the following vital signs: blood pressure (BP) of 86/42, heart rate (HR) of 118, respiratory rate (RR) of 28, temperature of 98.8°F/37.1°C, and oxygen saturation of 88% on 2-L nasal cannula. Primary survey findings demonstrate that the airway is intact, breathing is symmetric, circulation is intact in all four extremities, and his Glasgow Coma Score Scale (GCS) score is 13 on presentation, E3V4M6. Significant physical exam findings include skin that is pale, cool, and clammy, left clavicular/chest wall tenderness, flat jugular veins, left upper/lower quadrant abdominal tenderness, and left hip/pelvis tenderness. The patient is diagnosed with the following injuries: (a) grade III splenic laceration, (b) chest contusion with small left pneumothorax, and (c) shattered left kidney. Initial management of this patient includes 2 L of lactated saline and 2 units of packed red blood cells (RBCs) to stabilize his vital signs. He is then taken to the interventional radiology department for coiling and embolization of his left main renal arteries. He has a repeat angiogram prior to discharge which demonstrates no further extravasation after the embolization. All of his other injuries are nonoperative. The patient recovers and is discharged home in 6 days with his family.

1. Upon presentation to the trauma center, which classification of shock does this patient fall under?
  A. Hypovolemic
  B. Cardiogenic
  C. Distributive
  D. Obstructive

BIBLIOGRAPHY

Angus, D., & van der Poll, T. (2013). Severe sepsis and septic shock. *The New England Journal of Medicine, 369*, 840–851. https://doi.org/10.1056/NEJMra1208623

Beck, V., Chateau, D., & Bryson, G. L. (2014). Timing of vasopressor initiation and mortality in septic shock: A cohort study. *Critical Care, 18*(3), R97. https://doi.org/10.1186/cc13868

Bisschop, M., & Bellou, A. (2012). Anaphylaxis. *Current Opinion in Critical Care, 18*, 308–317. https://doi.org/10.1097/MCC.0b013e3283557a63

The Committee on Trauma. (2018). *Advanced trauma life support* (10th ed.). American College of Surgeons.

Dalton, T., Rushing, M., Escott, M., & Monroe, B. (2015, November 2). Complexities of geriatric trauma patients. *Journal of Emergency Medical Services, 40*. http://www.jems.com/articles/print/volume-40/issue-11/features/complexities-of-geriatric-trauma-patients.html?c=1

DeBacker, D., Biston, P., Devriendt, J., Madl, C., Chochrad, D., Aldecoa, C., Brasseur, A., Defrance, P., Gottignies, P., & Vincent, J. L. (2010). Comparison of dopamine and norepinephrine in the treatment of shock. *The New England Journal of Medicine, 362*(9), 779–789. https://doi.org/10.10.1056/NEJMoa0907118

Dellinger, R., Levy, M., Rhodes, A., Annane, D., Gerlach, H., Opal, S. M., Sevransky, J. E., Sprung, C. L., Douglas, I. S., Jaeschke, R., Osborn, T. M., Nunnally, M. E., Townsend, S. R., Reinhart, K., Kleinpell, R. M., Angus, D. C., Deutschman, C. S., Machado, F. R., Rubenfeld, G. D. . . . Moreno, R. (2013). Surviving sepsis campaign: International guidelines for management of severe sepsis and septic shock: 2012. *Critical Care Medicine, 41*(2), 580–637. https://doi.org/10.1097/CCM.0b013e31827e83af

Gutierrez, G., Reines, H., & Wulf-Gutierrez, M. (2004). Clinical review: Hemorrhagic stroke. *Critical Care, 8*, 373–381. https://doi.org/10.1186/cc2851

Haseer Koya, H., & Paul, M. (2022, January). Shock. In *StatPearls* [Internet]. StatPearls Publishing. https://www.ncbi.nlm.nih.gov/books/NBK531492

Imazio, M., & DeFerrari, G. M. (2021). Cardiac tamponade: An educational review. *European Heart Journal: Acute Cardiovascular Care, 10*, 102–109. https://doi.org/10.1177/2048872620939341

Kadri, S., Rhee, C., Strich, J., Morales, M., Hohmann, S., Menchaca, J., Suffredini, A. F., Danner, R. L., & Klompas, M. (2017). Estimating ten year trends in septic shock incidence and mortality in United States Academic Medical Centers using clinical data. *Chest, 151*(2), 278–285. https://doi.org/10.1016/j.chest.2016.07.010

Klein, T., & Ramani, G. (2012). Assessment and management of cardiogenic shock in the emergency department. *Cardiology Clinics, 30*, 651–664. https://doi.org/10.1016/j.ccl.2012.07.004

Kumar, A., Tremblay, V., Vasquez-Grande, G., & Parillo, J. E. (2019). Shock: Classification, pathophysiology and approach to management. In R. P. Dellinger & J. E. Parillo (Eds.), *Critical care medicine: Principles of diagnosis and management in the adult* (pp. 288–310). Elsevier.

Maier, R. V. (2001). Approach to the patient with shock. In J. Jameson, A. S. Fauci, D. L. Kasper, S. L. Hauser, D. L. Longo, & J. Loscalzo (Eds.), *Harrison's principles of internal medicine* (20th ed.). McGraw-Hill.

Moore, A. J., Wachsmann, J., Chamarthy, M. R., Panjikaran, L., Tanabe, Y., & Rajiah, P. (2018). Imaging of acute pulmonary emboli: An update. *Cardiovascular Diagnostics and Therapy, 8*(3), 225–243. https://doi.org/10.21037/cdt.2017.12.01

Moranville, M., Mieure, K., & Santayana, E. (2011). Evaluation and management of shock states: Hypovolemic, distributive and cardiogenic. *Journal of Pharmacy Practice, 24*(1), 44–60. https://doi.org/10.1177/0897190010388150

Pandit, V., Rhee, P., Hashmi, A., Kulvatunyou, N., Tang, A., Khalil, M., O'Keeffe, T., Green, D., Friese, R. S., & Joseph, B. (2014). Shock index predicts mortality in geriatric trauma patients: An analysis of the National Trauma Data Bank. *Journal of Trauma and Acute Care Surgery, 76*(4), 1111–1115. https://doi.org/10.1097/TA.0000000000000160

Pauler, P., Newell, M., Hildebrandt, D., & Kirkland, L. (2017). Incidence, etiology and implications of shock in therapeutic hypothermia. *Journal of the Minneapolis Heart Institute Foundation, 1*, 19–23. https://doi.org/10.21925/2475-0204-1.1.19

Reynolds, H., & Hochman, J. (2008). Cardiogenic shock: Current concepts and improving outcomes. *Circulation, 117*, 686–697. https://doi.org/10.1161/CIRCULATIONAHA.106.613596

Rhee, C., Murphy, M. V., & Li, L. (2015). Lactate testing in suspected sepsis: Trends and predictors of failure to measure levels. *Critical Care Medicine, 43*(8), 1669–1676. https://doi.org/10.1097/CCM.0000000000001087

Richards, J., & Wilcox, S. (2014). Diagnosis and management of shock in the emergency department. *Emergency Medicine Practice, 16*(3), 1–22.

Silva, J., Concalves, L., & Sousa, P. (2018). Fluid therapy and shock: An integrative review. *British Journal of Nursing, 27*(8), 449–454. https://doi.org/10.12968/bjon.2018.27.8

Sobol, J., & Louro, J. (2017). Advanced perioperative crisis management: Obstructive shock. In M. McEvoy & C. M. Furse (Eds.), *Oxford Medicine Online*. https://doi.org/10.1093/med/9780190226459.001.0001

Taghavi, S., & Askari, R. (2021). Hypovolemic shock. In *StatPearls* [Internet]. StatPearls Publishing.

Vahdatpout, C., Collins, D., & Goldberg, S. (2019). Cardiogenic shock. *Journal of the American Heart Association, 8*(8), 1–12. https://doi.org/10.1161/JAHA.119.01.011991

Welch, T. D. (2018). Constrictive pericarditis: Diagnosis, management and clinical outcomes. *Heart, 104*(9), 725–732. https://doi.org/10.1136/heartjnl-2017-31683

Weyker, P. D., Webb, C. A.-J., & Brentjens, T. E. (2017). Advanced perioperative crisis management: Hypovolemic shock. In M. McEvoy & C. M. Furse (Eds.), *Oxford Medicine Online*. https://doi.org/10.1093/med/9780190226459.001.0001

SPINAL CORD INJURIES

Susan F. Galiczynski

DEFINITION

A. Spinal cord injury (SCI) is any damage to the spinal cord that causes temporary or permanent changes disrupting normal function. This includes changes to motor, sensory, or autonomic function in the body below the level of the SCI.

B. Complete SCI results in total loss of all motor and sensory functions below the level of injury and is most often bilateral. Up to 50% of SCIs are complete.

C. Incomplete SCI will retain some function below the primary level of the injury and may affect one side more than the other.

D. The American Spinal Injury Association (ASIA) uses the following letter grading scale to describe the severity of the injury. The more severe the injury, the less likely a recovery will occur.

1. ASIA A: Injury is complete SCI with no sensory or motor function preserved.

2. ASIA B: A sensory incomplete injury with complete motor function loss.

3. ASIA C: A motor incomplete injury, where there is some movement, but less than half the muscle groups are antigravity (can lift against the force of gravity with a full range of motion).

4. ASIA D: A motor incomplete injury with more than half of the muscle groups are antigravity.

5. ASIA E: Normal.

INCIDENCE

A. Can affect up to 750 people per million annually.

B. In the United States, there are approximately 10,000 to 12,000 new traumatic SCIs per year.

C. Approximately 280,000 people are presently living with SCI in North America.

D. Up to 60% of injuries include the cervical spine.

E. For the geriatric population, majority of injuries are incomplete.

F. For the geriatric patient, mortality and morbidity are significantly higher.

G. Higher incidence of central cord injuries occurs in the geriatric population.

H. It is estimated up to 25% of patients with spinal injury have at least a mild brain injury.

I. Up to 10% of patients with a cervical spine fracture have a second, noncontiguous vertebral column fracture.

PATHOGENESIS

A. SCIs are considered high-impact injuries, often resulting from high-speed motor vehicle crashes or falls from significant heights.

B. Other mechanisms may include:

1. Hyperextension injury with or without longitudinal ligament tear.

2. Vertical column loading (axial load) compression.

3. Distraction injuries (seen with hangings).

4. Penetrating injuries.

5. Pathologic fractures (seen more commonly in older adults).

PREDISPOSING FACTORS

A. Male.

B. Persons between 15 and 24 years of age.

C. Increasing occurrence in persons over the age of 65.

SUBJECTIVE DATA

A. Common complaints/symptoms.

1. Neck or back pain.

2. Numbness.

3. Loss of limb function.

4. Paresthesia.

B. Common/typical scenario.

1. Other signs and symptoms.

a. Bowel and bladder dysfunction.

b. Priapism.

c. Hyperesthesia/pain.

C. Family and social history.

1. Emergency medical support (EMS) report may give significant information regarding the scene and how the patient was found.

2. If possible, ask the patient about the history of events: Mechanism? Motor vehicle collision (MVC)? Location in car? Restrained? Ejected? Mechanical fall or syncope? Fall from height? How far?

3. Blunt versus penetrating.

4. Distraction injury to spine? Hyperextension, hyperflexion, hyperrotation?

5. Ask the patient about pain, sensation, and ability to move extremities after injury (Figure 17.1).

6. Assess for drug or alcohol use as this may impact examination.

PHYSICAL EXAMINATION

A. Primary survey (advanced trauma life support [ATLS]) to assess for life-threatening injuries.

B. Pay particular attention to respiratory status as level of injury can impact spontaneous breathing.

1. Injuries above C3 result in respiratory arrest.

2. Injuries at C5 to C6 spare the diaphragm, and diaphragm breathing is seen.

3. Injuries below T1 to the level of L2 can affect the intercostals.

C. Motor and sensory assessment to assess level of injury.

1. Turn off or pause sedation and opioid gastric transit times for accurate neuro assessment.

D. Cardiovascular changes seen with SCI: SCI can impact the sympathetic pathways leading to alterations in blood pressure (BP), heart rate (HR), and temperature regulation.

E. Gastrointestinal (GI) changes associated with SCI may include loss of bowel function, development of an ileus, or obstruction.

F. Genitourinary: Urinary incontinence and retention.

G. Always have a heightened suspicion for other injuries.

DIAGNOSTIC TESTS

A. CT.

B. MRI.

C. Plain films (x-rays) can help identify fractures.

DIFFERENTIAL DIAGNOSIS

A. Central cord syndrome.

B. Anterior cord syndrome.

C. Posterior cord syndrome.

D. Brown-Sequard syndrome (often seen with penetrating trauma).

E. Cord contusion.

F. Cord concussion.

EVALUATION AND MANAGEMENT PLAN

A. General plan.

1. Interventions in SCI are aimed at preventing secondary injury.

2. Earlier surgical intervention, when indicated, has been shown to improve neurologic recovery.

3. Maintain adequate airway and respirations.

4. Cervical spine immobilization.

5. Thoracic and lumbar bracing if necessary.

6. Maintain adequate circulation.

7. Ongoing neurologic assessment.

8. Assess for signs of neurogenic shock and support hemodynamics.

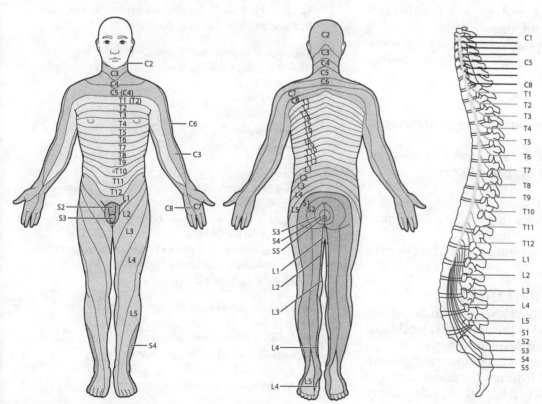

FIGURE 17.1 Dermatome map.

9. Aggressive bowel regimen to prevent constipation.

10. Monitor urine with either a Foley catheter or self-catheterization as needed.

11. Evaluate for blunt carotid vascular injury (BCVI).

B. Patient/family teaching points.

1. Patients need to be taught how to monitor and assess their skin for any breakdown.

2. Depending on the level of the SCI, patients may have bowel, bladder, and sexual dysfunction.

3. Teach patients and caregivers to recognize a life-threatening condition called autonomic dysreflexia, which can be caused by bladder spasms, urinary tract infections, or even external factors, such as too tight clothing, belts, or shoes.

4. Physical and occupational therapy will be necessary for reducing muscle contractures and atrophy.

C. Pharmacotherapy.

1. Use of glucocorticoids, specifically methylprednisolone, after acute traumatic SCI has been a controversial concept. The recommendations were to use methylprednisolone for either 24 or 48 hours, depending on whether it was started 3 or 8 hours after injury, respectively.

  a. Many studies are showing early surgical intervention with decompression is preferable to steroid use.

2. Other pharmacologic agents used in human clinical trials include tirilazad, naloxone, GM ganglioside, and riluzole. Recent neuroprotection agents involved in clinical trial include BA-120 (Cethrin) and minocycline.

3. Antibiotics for penetrating injuries.

4. GI prophylaxis and aggressive bowel regimen.

5. Early assessment and med administration for neuropathic pain.

6. Stabilization of BP secondary to SCI with vasopressor agents and/or midodrine.

7. Correction of bradycardia secondary to autonomic dysreflexia with the use of atropine, aminophylline, and/or beta-blockers.

FOLLOW-UP

A. SCI patients have a long course of physical medicine and rehabilitation.

B. Neurosurgery, orthopedics, and any other specialty groups may be involved in the patient's care.

CONSULTATION/REFERRAL

A. Neurosurgery/orthopedics (bony injuries) for management and possible fixation/fusion.

B. Prompt transfer to a level I trauma center needs to be prioritized.

SPECIAL/GERIATRIC CONSIDERATIONS

A. SCI is an ever-increasing challenge with an annual incidence of 750 per million in the developed world and even higher incidence in the developing world.

B. Pathophysiology of SCI involves primary and secondary injury mechanisms with future treatment strategies and emphasis on preventing or reversing secondary injury.

C. Medical management of SCI patients is in accordance with the ATLS guidelines. Surgery for acute SCI within 24 hours of injury as a treatment option is not associated with any increased risk of complications and may provide a neurologic benefit.

D. Patients with an unstable spinal column with incomplete SCI should be considered for acute stabilization as soon as possible after obtaining necessary imaging studies.

E. Spinal cord injury without radiographic abnormality (SCIWORA) refers to objective clinical signs of traumatic SCI without evidence of fracture or subluxation on radiographs or CT of the spine. More often seen in pediatric population.

F. Neurogenic shock: Loss of vasomotor tone and sympathetic innervation to the heart. Usually occurs with SCI of cervical spine and upper thoracic spine (above the level of T6).

G. Spinal shock refers to the loss of muscle tone (flaccidity) and reflexes that occur immediately postinjury.

CASE SCENARIO: SPINAL CORD INJURIES

A 20-year-old male with no medical history presented to the trauma center with a single gunshot wound (GSW) to the back at the midthoracic level. On presentation, he was not moving his lower extremities. Injuries included ballistic T8 spinous process fracture, ballistic T8 lamina propria and vertebral body fracture—ballistic vertebral body fracture and ballistic right eighth rib fracture. He also had a right hemopneumothorax and a left pneumothorax (from needle decompressed in the field).

1. Which grading system is used to describe severity of spinal cord injury?

  A. Glasgow Coma Scale (GCS)

  B. American Spinal Injury Association (ASIA)

  C. Clinical Institute Withdrawal Assessment (CIWA)

  D. Neuromuscular Recovery Scale (NRS)

2. In addition to spine immobilization, focused assessment of which of the following is important during the initial assessment?

  A. Urinary retention

  B. Constipation

  C. Skin integrity

  D. Respiratory effort

3. Spinal shock is:

  A. Loss of vasomotor tone and sympathetic innervation to the heart.

  B. Injury to the motor and sensory pathways in the anterior part of the spinal cord.

  C. Flaccidity (loss of muscle tone) and loss of reflexes that occur immediately after spinal cord injury.

  D. Found in L1 burst fracture.

4. Spinal cord injury without radiographic abnormality (SCIWORA) is:

  A. Rehab admission criteria.

  B. Classification of spinal cord injury (SCI).

  C. ICU sedation algorithm.

  D. Medication for spasmatic movements.

BIBLIOGRAPHY

American College of Surgeons. (2018). *Advanced trauma life support: Student course manual.* (10th ed.). Author.

Bracken, M. B., Shepard, M. J., Collins, W. F., Jr, Holford, T. R., Baskin, D. S., Eisenberg, H. M., Flamm, E., Leo-Summers, L., Maroon, J. C., & Marshall, L. F. (1992). Methylprednisolone or naloxone treatment after acute spinal cord injury: 1-Year follow-up data. Results of the second national acute spinal cord injury study. *Journal of Neurosurgery, 76*(1), 23–31. https://doi.org/10.3171/jns.1992.76.1.0023

Bracken, M. B., Shepard, M. J., Collins, W. F., Jr, Holford, T. R., Young, W., Baskin, D. S., Eisenberg, H. M., Flamm, E., Leo-Summers, L., & Maroon, J. (1990). A randomized, controlled trial of methylprednisolone or naloxone in the treatment of acute spinal-cord injury. Results of the second national acute spinal cord injury Study. *The New England Journal of Medicine, 322*(20), 1405–1411. https://doi.org/10.1056/NEJM199005173222001

Bracken, M. B., Shepard, M. J., Holford, T. R., Leo-Summers, L., Aldrich, E. F., Fazl, M., & Young, W. (1997). Administration of methylprednisolone for 24 or 48 hours or tirilazad mesylate for 48 hours in the treatment of acute spinal cord injury: Results of the third national acute spinal cord injury randomized controlled trial. *Journal of the American Medical Association, 277*(20), 1597–1604. https://doi.org/10.1001/jama.1997.03540440031029

Cengiz, S. L., Kalkan, E., Bayir, A., Ilik, K., & Basefer, A. (2008). Timing of thoracolumbar spine stabilization in trauma patients; impact on neurological outcome and clinical course. A real prospective (RCT) randomized controlled study. *Archives of Orthopaedic and Trauma Surgery, 128*(9), 959–966. https://doi.org/10.1007/s00402-007-0518-1

Cheung, V., Hoshide, R., Bansal, V., Kasper, E., & Chen, C. (2015). Methylprednisolone in the management of spinal cord injuries: Lessons from randomized, controlled trials. *Surgical Neurology International, 6*, 142. https://doi.org/10.4103/2152-7806.163452

Conrad, B. P., Horodyski, M., Wright, J., Ruetz, P., & Rechtine, 2nd, R. (2007). Log-rolling technique producing unacceptable motion during body position changes in patients with traumatic spinal cord injury. *Journal of Neurosurgery Spine, 6*(6), 540–543. https://doi.org/10.3171/spi.2007.6.6.4

DeVivo, M. J. (1997). Causes and costs of spinal cord injury in the United States. *Spinal Cord, 35*(12), 809–813. https://doi.org/10.1038/sj.sc.3100501

Fassett, D. R., Harrop, J. S., Maltenfort, M., Jeyamohan, S. B., Ratliff, J. D. Anderson., G, D., Hilibrand, A. S., Albert, T. J., Vaccaro, A. R., & Sharan, A. D. (2007). Mortality rates in geriatric patients with spinal cord injuries. *Journal of Neurosurgery Spine, 7*(3), 277–281. https://doi.org/10.3171/SPI-07/09/277

Fehlings, M. G., & Perrin, R. G. (2006). The timing of surgical intervention in the treatment of spinal cord injury: A systematic review of recent clinical evidence. *Spine (Phila Pa 1976), 31*(Suppl. 11), S28–S35. https://doi.org/10.1371/journal.pone.0032037

Fehlings, M. G., & Sekhon, L. (2000). Cellular, ionic, and biomolecular mechanisms of the injury process. In C. H. Tator & E. Benzel (Eds.), *Contemporary management of spinal cord injury: From impact to rehabilitation* (pp. 33–50). American Association of Neurological Surgeons. https://doi.org/10.1097/01.brs.0000217973.11402.7f

Fehlings, M. G., Vaccaro, A., Wilson, J. R., Singh, A., Cadotte, W. D., Harrop, J. S., Aarabi, B., Shaffrey, C., Dvorak, M., Fisher, C., Arnold, P., Massicotte, E. M., Lewis, S., & Rampersaud, R. (2012). Early versus delayed decompression for traumatic cervical spinal cord injury: Results of the surgical timing in acute spinal cord injury study (STASCIS). *PLOS ONE, 7*(2), e32037. https://doi.org/10.1371/journal.pone.0032037

Hadley, M. N., Walters, B. C., Grabb, P. A., Oyesiku, N. M., Przybylski, G. J., Resnick, D. K., & Ryken, T. C. (2002a). Blood pressure management after acute spinal cord injury. *Neurosurgery, 50*(Suppl. 3), S58–S62. https://doi.org/10.1097/00006123-200203001-00012

Hadley, M. N., Walters, B. C., Grabb, P. A., Oyesiku, N. M., Przybylski, G. J., Resnick, D. K., & Ryken, T. C. (2002b). Treatment of subaxial cervical spinal injuries. *Neurosurgery, 50*(Suppl. 3), S156–S165. https://doi.org/10.1097/00006123-200203001-00024

Hagen, S. (1999). *CBO memorandum: Projections of expenditures for long-term care services for the elderly.* Congressional Budget Office.

Hamamoto, Y., Ogata, T., Morino, T., Hino, M., & Yamamoto, H. (2007). Real-time direct measurement of spinal cord blood flow at the site of compression: Relationship between blood flow recovery and motor deficiency in spinal cord injury. *Spine, 32*(18), 1955–1962. https://doi.org/10.1097/BRS.0b013e3181316310

Katoh, S., el Masry, W. S., Jaffray, D., McCall, I. W., Eisenstein, S. M., Pringle, R. G., & Ikata, T. (1996). Neurologic outcome in conservatively treated patients with incomplete closed traumatic cervical spinal cord injuries. *Spine, 21*(20), 2345–2351. https://doi.org/10.1097/00007632-199610150-00008

La Rosa, G., Conti, A., Cardali, S., Cacciola, F., & Tomasello, F. (2004). Does early decompression improve neurological outcome of spinal cord injured patients? Appraisal of the literature using a meta-analytical approach. *Spinal Cord, 42*(9), 503–512. https://doi.org/10.1038/sj.sc.3101627

Levi, L., Wolf, A., & Belzberg, H. (1993). Hemodynamic parameters in patients with acute cervical cord trauma: Description, intervention, and prediction of outcome. *Neurosurgery, 33*(6), 1007–1016. https://doi.org/10.1227/00006123-199312000-00008

Liverman, T. C., Altevogt, B. M., Joy, E. J., & Johnson, T. R. (Eds.). (2005). *Spinal cord injury: Progress, promise, and priorities.* National Academy of Sciences.

McKinley, W., Meade, M. A., Kirshblum, S., & Barnard, B. (2004). Outcomes of early surgical management versus late or no surgical intervention after acute spinal cord injury. *Archives of Physical Medicine and Rehabilitation, 85*(11), 1818–1825. https://doi.org/10.1016/j.apmr.2004.04.032

Oyinbo, C. A. (2011). Secondary injury mechanisms in traumatic spinal cord injury: A nugget of this multiply cascade. *Acta Neurobiologiae Experimentalis, 71*(2), 281–299.

Pointillart, V., Petitjean, M. E., Wiart, L., Vital, J. M., Lassié, P., Thicoipé, M., & Dabadie, P. (2000). Pharmacological therapy of spinal cord injury during the acute phase. *Spinal Cord, 38*(2), 71–76. https://doi.org/10.1038/sj.sc.3100962

Pollard, M. E., & Apple, D. F. (2003). Factors associated with improved neurologic outcomes in patients with incomplete tetraplegia. *Spine, 28*(1), 33–39. https://doi.org/10.1097/00007632-200301010-00009

Rahimi-Movaghar, V. (2005). Efficacy of surgical decompression in the setting of complete thoracic spinal cord injury. *Journal of Spinal Cord Medicine, 28*(5), 415–420. https://doi.org/10.1080/10790268.2005.11753841

Rowland, J. W., Hawryluk, G. W., Kwon, B., & Fehlings, M. G. (2008). Current status of acute spinal cord injury pathophysiology and emerging therapies: Promise on the horizon. *Neurosurgical Focus, 25*(5), E2. https://doi.org/10.3171/FOC.2008.25.11.E2

Sapkas, G. S., & Papadakis, S. A. (2007). Neurological outcome following early versus delayed lower cervical spine surgery. *Journal of Orthopaedic Surgery, 15*(2), 183–186. https://doi.org/10.1177/230949900701500212

Sekhon, L. H., & Fehlings, M. G. (2001). Epidemiology, demographics, and pathophysiology of acute spinal cord injury. *Spine, 26*(Suppl. 24), S2–S12. https://doi.org/10.1097/00007632-200112151-00002

Tanhoffer, R. A., Yamazaki, R. K., Nunes, E. A., Pchevozniki, A. I., Pchevozniki, A. M., Nogata, C., Aikawa, J., Bonatto, S. J., Brito, G., Lissa, M. D., & Fernandes, L. C. (2007). Glutamine concentration and immune response of spinal cord-injured rats. *Journal of Spinal Cord Medicine, 30*(2), 140–146. https://doi.org/10.1080/10790268.2007.11753925

Tator, C. H., Duncan, E. G., Edmonds, V. E., Lapczak, L. I., & Andrews, D. F. (1987). Comparison of surgical and conservative management in 208 patients with acute spinal cord injury. *The Canadian Journal of Neurological Sciences, 14*(1), 60–69. https://doi.org/10.1017/S0317167100026858

Velmahos, G. C., Toutouzas, K., Chan, L., Tillou, A., Rhee, P., Murray, J., & Demetriades, D. (2003). Intubation after cervical spinal cord injury: To be done selectively or routinely? *The American Surgeon, 69*(10), 891–894.

Waters, R. L., Meyer, P. R., Jr., Adkins, R. H., & Felton, D. (1999). Emergency, acute, and surgical management of spine trauma. *Archives of Physical Medicine and Rehabilitation, 80*(11), 1383–1390. https://doi.org/10.1016/S0003-9993(99)90248-4

Wyndaele, M., & Wyndaele, J. J. (2006). Incidence, prevalence and epidemiology of spinal cord injury: What learns a worldwide literature survey? *Spinal Cord, 44*(9), 523–529. https://doi.org/10.1038/sj.sc.3101893

Xu, K., Chen, Q.-X., Li, F.-C., Chen, W.-S., Lin, M., & Wu, Q. (2009). Spinal cord decompression reduces rat neural cell apoptosis secondary to spinal cord injury. *Journal of Zhejiang University Science B, 10*(3), 180–187. https://doi.org/10.1631/jzus.B0820161

TRAUMATIC BRAIN INJURY

Susan F. Galiczynski

DEFINITION

A. Traumatic brain injury (TBI) is an insult to the brain caused by direct physical force that may produce a diminished or altered state of consciousness, which may result in an impairment of cognitive abilities or physical functioning.
B. These impairments may be temporary or permanent, depending on the degree of injury.

INCIDENCE

A. Leading cause of trauma-related death in persons under age 45.
B. Often occurs during the most productive years.
C. Represents approximately 200 cases per 100,000 injuries annually in the United States.
D. Responsible for approximately 12% to 30% of all traumatic deaths.
E. Motor vehicle collisions (MVCs) are the leading cause of TBI.

PATHOGENESIS

A. Although there are many mechanisms that can result in traumatic injury, brain injuries are often classified as blunt or penetrating trauma. Blunt injuries result from a blunt or concussive forces and are usually localized to the area of impact. Although these may result in lacerations at the area of impact, there is not an associated penetrating injury. Examples of blunt injury are motor vehicle accidents, assaults, falls, and sports-related injuries.
B. Two main forces are associated with TBI.
  1. Impact loading is the direct force against the skull, causing disruption of brain tissue, vascular, and nerve structures.
  2. Impulsive loading is sudden movement without direct impact as seen with acceleration–deceleration injury.
C. In patients with TBIs, 75% are mild injuries, 15% moderate, and 10% severe.
  1. Mild Glasgow Coma Scale (GCS) score 13 to 15.
  2. Moderate GCS score 9 to 12.
  3. Severe GCS score less than 8.

PREDISPOSING FACTORS

A. Infants/children, newborns to age 4.
B. Young adults ages 15 to 25.
C. Adults over age 65.
D. Males, in any age group.
E. Drug and alcohol use.
F. Athletic participants.
G. Military and industrial workers.
H. City residents.
I. Lower income individuals.
J. Drug and alcohol use.
K. History of previous TBIs.

SUBJECTIVE DATA

A. Common complaints/symptoms.
  1. ±Loss of consciousness (LOC).
  2. Nausea and/or vomiting.
  3. Headache and/or dizziness.
  4. Amnesia to events surrounding trauma.
  5. Visual disturbances/changes.
B. Common/typical scenario.
  1. Other signs and symptoms.
    a. Altered mentation.
    b. Increased lethargy.
    c. Slurred speech.
    d. Combative behavior.
    e. History of seizures.
    f. Compromised airway.
C. Family and social history.
  1. Ask patient to describe events leading up to trauma. What is the last thing the patient remembers? What symptoms are they experiencing? Nausea? Vomiting? Headache? Dizziness? Photophobia? Does the patient have pain? Location? Characteristics?
  2. Ask the patient about recent drug and alcohol use.
  3. Ask the patient about medical history. Seizures? Concussions?
  4. Determine if the patient is on any anticoagulants or antiplatelet medications.

PHYSICAL EXAMINATION

A. The American College of Surgeons has developed the advanced trauma life support (ATLS) guidelines to provide a quick but systematic approach to assessment to help identify those injuries that can be life-threatening as soon as possible. Using the mnemonic **ABCDE** (**A**irway, **B**reathing, **C**irculation, **D**isability, and **E**xposure), the primary survey must be completed before the secondary survey can be started and a plan of care established (Table 17.3).
B. If any potentially life-threatening issue is identified during the primary survey, it needs to be addressed before moving onto the next assessment. For example, if the patient has decreased breath sounds (B) on the right side and has sustained chest trauma, a pneumothorax should be suspected. A chest tube should be placed before moving on with assessment to circulation (C). The secondary survey is a complete head-to-toe evaluation of the patient, looking for other potential injuries, once it is determined that the patient is stable at the end of the primary survey.
C. Perform a GCS (see Table 17.1).
D. Assess for signs of other injuries by completely undressing the patient.
E. Assess head, scalp, and face for contusions, lacerations, or hematoma.

DIAGNOSTIC TESTS

A. For trauma to the head, the standard diagnostic tool is the noncontrast CT scan. If other injuries are suspected, additional studies, such as the cervical spine, chest/abdomen, and pelvis, can be imaged as well. CT chest, abdomen, and pelvis are with contrast.

TABLE 17.3 PRIMARY SURVEY

System	Assessment Points
A: Airway	Is it patent? Is the patient talking? Normal voice? Hoarse? Is airway occluded by debris? Blood? Vomit? Teeth? Could there be an airway injury given the mechanism? Is the cervical spine immobilized?
B: Breathing	Is the patient breathing? Are there breath sounds bilaterally? Are the lungs clear?
C: Circulation	Does the patient have pulses? Is there active hemorrhage?
D: Disability	What is the GCS score? Is the patient awake and following commands? Is the patient confused? Is the patient conscious?
E: Exposure	Undress the patient completely. Look for any holes, lacerations, unusual bruising, or marks.

GCS, Glasgow Coma Scale.

B. CT angiography (CTA) to rule out blunt carotid vascular injury (BCVI).
C. Labs including blood glucose.

DIFFERENTIAL DIAGNOSIS

A. Concussion: Transient, nonfocal neurologic disturbance that often includes LOC. The patient may experience amnesia to events, headache, dizziness, photophobia, nausea, and vomiting. It is usually self-limiting.
B. Cerebral contusion: Fairly common and can be found with other brain injuries. Most are found in the frontal and temporal areas. These can worsen before they get better and can result in hemorrhage, requiring surgical intervention.
C. Coup-contrecoup injuries: Usually refers to two separate injuries in the brain. The coup injury is under the point of impact. The contrecoup injury occurs on the opposite side of impact.
D. Epidural hematoma: Relatively uncommon. Often located in the temporal area and are usually arterial in origin. These have a biconvex or lenticular shape as they push the dura away from the skull. Classic presentation involves a lucid period, followed by neurologic deterioration.
E. Subdural hematoma: More common than epidural hematomas. Related to shearing of small surface blood vessels or bridging veins in the cerebral cortex. These have a flatter appearance as they conform to the contours of the brain.
F. Subarachnoid hematoma (SAH) is bleeding into the subarachnoid space, the area between the arachnoid membrane and the pia mater surrounding the brain. Symptoms may include a rapidly developing severe headache, change in mental status, vomiting, and neck pain.
G. Mass lesions (may have prompted fall): These can be brain abscesses or tumors.
H. Diffuse axonal injury: Scattered areas of microtears in the white and gray matter. This can be a cause of prolonged coma and can result in residual injury and neurologic impairment.
I. Significant scalp laceration, with or without underlying skull fractures.

EVALUATION AND MANAGEMENT PLAN

A. General plan.
　1. The primary goal of treatment of TBI is to prevent secondary injury by maintaining adequate perfusion (blood pressure) and oxygenation of the brain tissue.
　　NOTE: The mortality for TBI patients who present with hypotension is more than double the patients who do not have hypotension. Hypoxia with hypotension will increase the risk of death for TBI patients.
　2. For the severely injured patient, you must:
　　a. Complete a thorough exam; identify other potential injuries.
　　b. Ensure adequate airway with intubation and support breathing.
　　c. Avoid hypotension and hypoxia. Treat shock aggressively with isotonic solutions without dextrose (can increase cerebral edema).
　　d. In severe brain injury, be suspicious for other injuries. Do a thorough exam.
　　e. When moderate to severe injuries are identified, call for emergent neurosurgical consult.
　　f. Determine need to transfer to high-level facility.
　3. For less life-threatening concussion, treatment is symptom-based.
　4. Scalp lacerations can result in significant blood loss. Monitor complete blood count (CBC) for acute blood loss anemia. Transfusion may be necessary.
　5. Assess for drug and alcohol use, which may place the patient at risk for withdrawal.
　6. Capnography.
B. Patient/family teaching points.
　1. Monitoring for postconcussive syndrome is important.
　2. Follow-up with concussion clinic may be advised based on the degree of concussion and residual symptoms.
　3. Neuropsychology depending on severity of symptoms.
C. Pharmacotherapy.
　1. Try to avoid opioids.
　2. For more severe head injury, seizure prophylaxis may be indicated for up to 10 days. Length depends ▶

on whether the patient presents with a seizure or has any seizure activity during hospitalization.

3. For severe head injury, osmotic diuretics and/or hypertonic saline may be used to reduce edema.

4. Patients may need to be kept sedated in the initial period after injury to allow for brain rest.

5. Bromocriptine may be considered in patient with TBI-induced hyperthermia.

6. Propranolol should be considered in TBI-induced tachycardia.

FOLLOW-UP

A. No contact sports for minimum of 6 weeks.

B. Physical therapy (PT)/occupational therapy (OT) and speech consults for cognition evaluation.

C. Neurosurgical evaluation 10 to 14 days postdischarge. May need repeat CT head at that time.

CONSULTATION/REFERRAL

A. Inpatient referrals: Trauma and neurosurgery.

B. May need rehab referral.

C. Outpatient concussion follow-up for postconcussive syndrome.

SPECIAL/GERIATRIC CONSIDERATIONS

A. For persons with repeated concussion, a discussion regarding cessation of sports is imperative. Repeated concussions have been shown to have a residual effect.

B. For patients on anticoagulation or antiplatelet therapy, risk of injury and complications needs to be discussed. Will need discussion surrounding resumption of antiplatelet/anticoagulant medications prior to discharge (risk vs. benefit discussion).

C. If the Glasgow Coma Scale (GCS) score is less than 8, intubation should be considered as the patient may not be awake enough to maintain a patent airway.

CASE SCENARIO: TRAUMATIC BRAIN INJURY

A 17-year-old female, with no known medical history, presents as an unrestrained rear-seat passenger who was found partially ejected from the front windshield. There was prolonged extrication. On scene, the Glasgow Coma Scale (GCS) score was 3 and the patient was unresponsive. Paramedics intubated the patient before transporting to the trauma center. On arrival, the patient remained unresponsive. CT of the head reveals multiple areas of subarachnoid hemorrhage and subdural hemorrhage. CT of the cervical spine demonstrates atlanto-occipital dislocation with ligamentous disruption of C1 to C2. In addition, the patient was found to have multiple facial fractures, bilateral rib fractures, and a right-sided internal carotid artery (ICA) dissection. The patient was admitted to the trauma ICU. Subsequent MRI of the brain to evaluate prolonged unresponsive state (coma) revealed diffuse axonal injury and bilateral middle cerebral artery (MCA) infarcts.

1. This patient arrives at the ED, intubated and unconscious. One of the first actions should be to:

A. Notify family of patient arrival.

B. Insert Foley for adequate intake and output (I&O).

C. Ensure correct placement of endotracheal tube.

D. Obtain urinalysis for pregnancy test.

2. The primary goal in treatment of traumatic brain injury (TBI) is to:

A. Prevent secondary injury.

B. Start planning for TBI rehab.

C. Start tube feeding in the first 24 hours as nutrition helps healing.

D. Do nothing. The brain will heal on its own.

3. As part of the treatment plan in moderate to severe TBI, it is recommended to:

A. Start antibiotic therapy immediately.

B. Order a 7- to 10-day course of antiseizure medication.

C. Infuse dextrose 5% in water (D5W) for maintenance fluid while patient is NPO.

D. Order chest radiography every 4 hours to monitor oxygenation.

4. Which of these is a symptom of concussion?

A. Timing and location of injury

B. Neck and back pain

C. Nausea, vomiting, and headache

D. Ambulation with steady gait

BIBLIOGRAPHY

American College of Surgeons. (2018). *Advanced trauma life support: Student course manual* (10th ed.). Author.

Carney, N., Totten, A., O'Reilly, C., Ullman, J., Hawryluk, G., Bell, M., & Ghajar, J. (2016). Guidelines for the management of severe traumatic brain injury, fourth edition. *Neurosurgery, 80*, 1–10. https://doi.org/10.1227/NEU.0000000000001432

Esterov, D., & Greenwald, B. D. (2017, August 11). Autonomic dysfunction after mild traumatic brain injury. *Brain Sciences, 7*(8), e100. https://doi.org/10.3390/brainsci7080100

Haring, R. S., Narang, K., Canner, J. K., Asemota, A. O., George, B. P., Selvarajah, S., & Schneider, E. B. (2015, January 15). Traumatic brain injury in the elderly: Morbidity and mortality trends and risk factors. *The Journal of Surgical Research, 195*, 1–9. https://doi.org/10.1016/j.jss.2015.01.017

Steyerberg, E. W., Mushkudiani, N., Perel, P., Butcher, I., Lu, J., McHugh, G. S., & Maas, A. I. (2008, August 5). Predicting outcome after traumatic brain injury: Development and international validation of prognostic scores based on admission characteristics. *PLOS Medicine, 5*(8), e165. https://doi.org/10.1371/journal.pmed.0050165

Teasdale, G., & Jennett, B. (1974). Assessment of coma and impaired consciousness. *Lancet, 2*, 81–84. https://doi.org/10.1016/S0140-6736(74)91639-0

Teasdale, G., & Jennett, B. (1976). Assessment and prognosis of coma after head injury. *Acta Neurochirurgica, 34*, 45–55. https://doi.org/10.1007/BF01405862

Thompson, D. O., Hurtado, T. R., Liao, M. M., Byyny, R. L., Gravitz, C., & Haukoos, J. S. (2011, November). Validation of the simplified motor score in the out-of-hospital setting for the prediction of outcomes after traumatic brain injury. *Annals of Emergency Medicine, 58*(5), 417–425. https://doi.org/10.1016/j.annemergmed.2011.05.033

Tian, H. L., Geng, Z., Cui, Y. H., Hu, J., Xu, T., Cao, H. L., & Chen, H. (2008, August 14). Risk factors for posttraumatic cerebral infarction in patients with moderate or severe head trauma. *Neurosurgical Review, 31*, 431–436. https://doi.org/10.1007/s10143-008-0153-5

SECTION II

PERIOPERATIVE CONSIDERATIONS

CHAPTER 18

PREOPERATIVE EVALUATION AND MANAGEMENT

William A. Edwards, Jr.

SCOPE OF CHAPTER

The advanced practice provider (APP) frequently evaluates patients prior to surgery. The APP must be aware of acute and chronic patient history, medications, surgical and anesthesia history, and any surgical and anesthetic complications, along with being aware of any pre-, intra-, and postsurgical risk factors, appropriate testing needed to be completed, evaluation of these test results, and the correlating American Society of Anesthesiologists (ASA) classification, in order to make an informed decision of a patient's readiness for surgery. This chapter explores what the APP needs to know to make these decisions.

CONSIDERATIONS

RISK FACTORS

A. Age: There is an increased surgical risk with age as a result of increased incidence of varied comorbidities, changes in end-organ reserves, increased incidence of cognition impairments, decreased functional capacities, increased incidence of hemodynamic instability, and increased incidence of pathologic processes.
B. Exercise capacity.
　1. Ability to perform four or more metabolic equivalents (METs) reduces the risk of cardiovascular complications associated with surgery. Examples include:
　　a. Walking up a flight of stairs.
　　b. Mowing the lawn.
　　c. Walking at ground level at 4 mi/hr.
　　d. Performing heavy work around the house.
　2. Inability to perform four or more METs is associated with increased length of stay and perioperative complications.
　　a. Preoperative evaluation by physical therapy for rehabilitation and cardiology for cardiac testing can be beneficial in higher surgical/procedural risk patients.
C. Nutritional.
　1. *Nutrition* can be defined as a state between patient intake and regulatory/metabolic needs of the said patient to facilitate proper hormone, protein, cell, and energy synthesis to promote and maintain homeostasis. If out of balance, a patient can be considered malnourished,

leading to metabolic derangements, impaired physiologic functions, and weight changes, either lost or gained.
　2. Malnutrition can be assessed and evaluated with standardized tools and correlated with a patient's clinical picture, including physical assessment and lab values (e.g., albumin, prealbumin, etc.). Such tools that have been considered the gold standard for sensitivity and specificity in malnutrition are the Nutritional Risk Screening (NRS)-2002, Malnutrition Universal Screening Tool (MUST), Short Nutritional Assessment Questionnaire (SNAQ), and Malnutrition Screening Tool (MST). The NRS-2002 and SNAQ) tools have been considered superior, yet either tool can be used alone or in conjunction with each other.
　3. Malnutrition prior to surgery is associated with:
　　a. Increased infection risk.
　　b. Poor wound healing.
　　c. Intestinal bacterial overgrowth.
　　d. Increased hospital length of stay: Increases postoperative complications; for example, hypoxia from apnea and decreased respiratory function, changes in drug pharmacokinetics and dynamics, and anastomotic leak from enterocutaneous fistula formation, to name a few.
　4. Obesity is one of the most prominent causes of morbidity and mortality in the postoperative period. Obesity is a risk factor for cardiopulmonary complications, poor airway patency, periods of apnea, and pulmonary thromboembolism, as well as an increased incidence of wound infections, pneumonia, and other clinical derangements.
D. Pulmonary.
　1. Obstructive sleep apnea: Increases risk of postoperative hypoxemia, intubation/reintubation, and ICU admission.
　2. Smoking: Increases risk of wound complications, infections, pulmonary complications, and ICU admissions.
E. Alcohol: Screen for the possibility of malnutrition, as well as developing withdrawal and/or delirium tremens, in the postoperative period. May impact dosing of medications pre-, intra-, and postoperatively, as well as hemodynamics intraoperatively and postoperatively.

F. Illicit drug use and prescription drug abuse: Screen for opioid narcotics, benzodiazepines, marijuana, and amphetamine use, as perioperative and postoperative pain control may prove to be difficult. Withdrawal may also occur and would need to be assessed. There may also be a needed adjustment in medication doses and incorporation of pain management protocols and/or consults.

G. Endocrine disorders: Diabetes increases risk of surgical site infection, hemodynamic instability, as well as perioperative cardiac events. Patient history of hypothyroidism may need to be considered with presentation of increased sedation and decreased airway patency postprocedure. Adrenal suppression may need to be considered with use of etomidate during the intraoperative period and/or if the patient is on chronic steroid therapy. The latter two can be risk factors for intractable hypotension and/or other cardiopulmonary derangements.

H. Medication use.

1. A full medication reconciliation should be obtained before surgery, including the use of over-the-counter medications, such as aspirin, ibuprofen, and other non-steroidal anti-inflammatory drugs (NSAIDs), which are associated with an increased risk of perioperative bleeding.

2. Alternative, herbal, and natural supplement use should also be assessed and documented due to drug interactions, possible complications, and risk of bleeding.

3. Anticoagulants should be evaluated and stopped per prescriber recommendations and/or surgical consultations.

I. Personal/family history of anesthetic complications, such as malignant hyperthermia (MH), should be evaluated, along with personal history of difficult airway management and postoperative nausea and vomiting (PONV).

CALCULATING RISK OF PERIOPERATIVE COMPLICATIONS

A. American College of Surgeons Surgical Risk Calculator: riskcalculator.facs.org/RiskCalculator.

1. Factors that can affect surgical risk.

a. Age.

b. Sex assigned at birth.

c. Functional status.

d. ASA classification.

e. Diabetes, hypertension (HTN), and/or congestive heart failure (CHF).

f. Smoking and/or history of chronic obstructive pulmonary disease (COPD).

g. Renal disease and/or on dialysis.

h. Steroid use for chronic conditions.

i. Hepatic disease and/or presence of ascites.

j. Disseminated cancer.

k. Emergency surgery.

BIBLIOGRAPHY

Assadi, F. (2010, July). Hypophosphatemia: An evidence-based problem-solving approach to clinical cases. *Iranian Journal of Kidney Diseases, 4,* 195–201. https://pubmed.ncbi.nlm.nih.gov/20622306/

Cohen, M. E., Liu, Y., Ko, C. Y., & Hall, B. L. (2017). An examination of American College of Surgeons NSQIP surgical risk calculator accuracy. *Journal of the American College of Surgeons, 224*(5), 787–795. https://doi.org/10.1016/j.jamcollsurg.2016.12.057

Dindo, D., Muller, M. K., Weber, M., & Clavien, P. A. (2003). Obesity in general elective surgery. *Lancet, 361*(9374), 2032–2035. https://doi.org/10.1016/S0140-6736(03)13640-9

Fan, Y., Yao, Q., Liu, Y., Jia, T., Zhang, J., & Jiang, E. (2022). Underlying causes and co-existence of malnutrition and infections: An exceedingly common death risk in cancer. *Frontiers in Nutrition, 9,* 814095. https://doi.org/10.3389/fnut.2022.814095

Fiaccadori, E., Coffrini, E., Fracchia, C., Rampulla, C., Montagna, T., & Borghetti, A. (1994). Hypophosphatemia and phosphorus depletion in respiratory and peripheral muscles of patients with respiratory failure due to COPD. *Chest, 105*(5), 1392–1398. https://doi.org/10.1378/chest.105.5.1392

Fleisher, L. A., Fleischmann, K. E., & Auerbach, A. D. (2014). ACC/AHA guideline on perioperative cardiovascular evaluation and management of patients undergoing noncardiac surgery: A report of the American College of Cardiology/American heart association task force on practice guidelines. *Journal of the American College of Cardiology, 64*(22), e77–e137. https://doi.org/10.1016/j.jacc.2014.07.945

Grønkjr, M., Eliasen, M., & Skov-Ettrup, L. S. (2014). Preoperative smoking status and postoperative complications: A systematic review and meta-analysis. *Annals of Surgery, 259*(1), 52–71. https://doi.org/10.1097/SLA.0b013e3182911913

Gropper, M. A., & Miller, R. D. (2020). *Miller's anesthesia* (9th ed.). Elsevier.

Hines, R. L., & Marschall, K. E. (2018). *Stoelting's anesthesia and co-existing disease* (7th ed.). Elsevier.

Juby, A. G., & Mager, D. R. (2019). A review of nutrition screening tools used to assess the malnutrition-sarcopenia syndrome (MSS) in the older adult. *Clinical Nutrition ESPEN, 32,* 8–15. https://doi.org/10.1016/j.clnesp.2019.04.003

Kaw, R., Pasupuleti, V., Walker, E., Ramaswamy, A., & Foldvary-Schafer, N. (2012). Postoperative complications in patients with obstructive sleep apnea. *Chest, 141*(2), 436–441. https://doi.org/10.1378/chest.11-0283

Kleinwächter, R., Kork, F., & Weiss-Gerlach, E. (2010). Improving the detection of illicit substance use in preoperative anesthesiological assessment. *Minerva Anestesiologica, 76*(1), 29–37.

Nagelhout, J., & Elisha, S. (2018). *Nurse anesthesia* (6th ed.). Elsevier.

Oresanya, L. B., Lyons, W. L., & Finlayson, E. (2014). Preoperative assessment of the older patient: A narrative review. *Journal of the American Medical Association, 311*(20), 2110–2120. https://doi.org/10.1001/jama.2014.4573

Palace, M. R. (2017). Perioperative management of thyroid dysfunction. *Health Services Insights, 10,* 117863291668967. https://doi.org/10.1177/1178632916689677

Sidney, M. J. K., & Blumchen, G. (1990). Metabolic equivalents (METs) in exercise testing, exercise prescription, and evaluation of functional capacity. *Clinical Cardiology, 13,* 555–565. https://doi.org/10.1002/clc.4960130809

Tønnesen, H., Nielsen, P. R., Lauritzen, J. B., & Møller, A. M. (2009). Smoking and alcohol intervention before surgery: Evidence for best practice. *British Journal of Anaesthesia, 102*(3), 297–306. https://doi.org/10.1093/bja/aen401

Türkoğlu, I., Ilgaz, F., Aksan, A., Çerçi, A., Yalçın, T., Yürük, A. A., Gökmen-Özel, H., Akal-Yıldız, E., & Samur, G. (2015). Mon-PP155: Comparison of four nutritional screening tools to assess malnutrition risk in hospitalized adult patients. *Clinical Nutrition, 34.* https://doi.org/10.1016/s0261-5614(15)30587-2

CARE PRINCIPLES

TESTING IN THE PERIOPERATIVE SETTING

A. The ASA recommends against routine preoperative laboratory testing in the absence of clinical indications.

1. Testing should occur depending on the patient's age, facility policy and procedures, medical history, underlying disease(s), increased perioperative risk, and/or high-risk surgery. Common testing includes:

a. Complete blood count (CBC).

   i. Hemoglobin/hematocrit.

      1) Both cardiac and noncardiac surgical patients should have a hemoglobin greater than 7 g/dL to reduce cardiovascular complications as a result of surgery. Patients may require packed red blood cell (PRBC) transfusion(s) for hemoglobin value of 7 or less.

      2) Patients with anemia or thrombocytopenia prior to major surgery may need to be seen and cleared by hematology.

   ii. Platelet count.

      1) Greater than 50,000 per microliter for most major surgeries.

      2) Greater than 100,000 per microliter for neurosurgery/ocular surgery.

      3) Greater than 80,000 per microliter for epidural and/or spinal anesthesia.

      4) Greater than 20,000 to 50,000 per microliter for endoscopy.

b. Coagulation studies.

   i. Only obtain if clinically indicated by physical examination and/or patient history of coagulopathies and/or liver impairment. Tests to obtain may include the following:

      1) Prothrombin time (PT) and partial thromboplastin time (PTT).

      2) International ratio (INR) may be variable. If less than 2.0, there is minimal indication that the patient will have more than normal tissue oozing.

        a) If a patient is taking warfarin, the medication should be stopped and the level should predictably drop to less than 1.5 within 4 to 5 days.

        b) In older adult patients, the reversal of warfarin may be longer and presents with increased risk of a thromboembolic event. In these cases, patients may need to be covered with therapeutic low molecular weight heparin or unfractionated heparin.

      3) Thromboelastography (TEG) may be useful (if available) to identify any hemostasis dysfunction(s) in the perioperative period to reduce thrombotic complications and reduce unnecessary blood product transfusion.

c. Basic metabolic profile (BMP).

   i. It is recommended to obtain routine BMP results.

   ii. Patients with type 2 diabetes mellitus (DM) taking oral antihypoglycemic agents should be converted to sliding scale insulin until oral medications can be resumed postoperatively. Monitor for hypoglycemia and lactic acidosis if metformin is still taken by patients preoperatively despite preoperative instructions not to do so.

   iii. Patients with a history of type 1 DM should have a perioperative insulin plan depending on the type of insulin they are using and the type of surgical procedure they are undergoing.

   iv. Due to the risk of diabetic ketoacidosis, patients with type 1 DM must have basal insulin supplied at all times.

   v. Renal function: Obtain serum creatinine in patients over the age of 50 if undergoing intermediate- or high-risk surgery.

d. Urine pregnancy test for all women of childbearing years.

e. EKG.

   i. Routine screening in asymptomatic patients undergoing low-risk surgery is not recommended.

   ii. In intermediate- or high-risk surgeries, patients with known coronary disease, peripheral vascular disease, cerebrovascular disease, dysrhythmias, and/or other structural heart disease should have at least a preoperative 12-lead EKG performed per facility guidelines prior to procedure, for example, 30 to 90 days preoperatively. Consultation with anesthesiology and/or cardiology for further testing recommendations (such as cardiac stress testing or echocardiogram) may be needed depending on the underlying cardiac conditions and the type of procedure the patient is undergoing.

f. Chest radiography.

   i. Unless the type of procedure, patient condition, and/or history warrant preoperative radiograph, routine screening is not indicated.

g. Pulmonary function testing.

   i. May be required for lung surgery, if patient has underlying history of COPD or if surgery is dependent on lung volume measurements.

   ii. Not indicated for routine screening.

AMERICAN SOCIETY OF ANESTHESIOLOGISTS CLASSIFICATIONS

A. Physical status classification system.

  1. Simple classification system to predict perioperative risk of increased morbidity and mortality associated with anesthesia and surgery.

  2. Six-tiered system.

   a. ASA 1: Healthy patient: No acute or chronic diseases and normal body mass index (BMI) percentile per age.

   b. ASA 2: Mild systemic disease: Asymptomatic cardiovascular disease, asthma without exacerbation, well-controlled DM, abnormal BMI per age $(30 < BMI < 40)$, current smoker, social alcohol drinker, and pregnancy.

   c. ASA 3: Severe systemic disease: Uncorrected stable cardiovascular disease, morbid obesity, malnutrition, poorly controlled DM, renal failure, asthma with exacerbation, difficult airway, and history of myocardial infarction (MI), cerebrovascular accident (CVA), transient ischemic attack (TIA), and coronary artery disease (CAD), with or without stents.

   d. ASA 4: Severe systemic disease that is a constant threat to life: Recent MI, CVA, and CAD with or without stents within 3 months of surgery, ▶

severe cardiac valve dysfunction, sepsis, and disseminated intravascular coagulation (DIC).

e. ASA 5: Moribund patient who is not expected to survive without the procedure: Ruptured abdominal/thoracic aneurysm, massive trauma, intracranial bleed with mass effect, and multiple organ/system failure.

f. ASA 6: Declared brain-dead patient who is undergoing organ procurement.

B. Mallampati classification.

1. Used to predict ease of intubation.

2. May help predict obstructive sleep apnea.

3. Simple test done during physical examination.

a. Patient should sit upright with head in neutral position.

b. Ask patient to open their mouth and extend their tongue *without* speaking or making noise.

4. Scoring.

a. Class 1: Complete visualization of the soft palate.

b. Class 2: Complete visualization of the uvula (Figure 18.1).

c. Class 3: Visualization of the base of the uvula.

d. Class 4: Soft palate not visible at all.

NUTRITION AND FLUIDS

A. Preoperative nutritional considerations.

1. Preoperative nutritional assessment.

a. NRS (2002) tool.

i. This score is calculated from two variables.

1) Impaired nutritional status: Recent weight loss, decreased food intake, and BMI ≤ 18.5 kg/mg^2.

2) Severity of illness.

ii. A score 3 or more would indicate need for nutritional supplementation/support prior to surgery.

b. Protein status.

i. Serum albumin, transferrin, and prealbumin have all been studied, but there are conflicting data on utility, although serum albumin could be evaluated/considered for drug dosing and bioavailability purposes.

ii. Only a serum albumin less than 2.2 g/dL has shown to be the most predictive of poorer patient outcomes with regard to nutrition status.

c. Patients with severe preoperative malnutrition may benefit from nutritional support prior to surgery.

i. Options include oral supplementation with high-protein shakes, tube feedings with indwelling feeding tube, total parenteral nutrition (TPN), and/or albumin infusion(s) for drug bioavailability and fluid status purposes if clinically warranted.

d. ASA fasting guidelines for lowest risk of aspiration perioperatively.

i. Clear liquids up to 2 hours before surgery.

ii. Nonclear fluids and breast milk (pediatrics) up to 4 hours before surgery.

iii. A light meal (toast and clear liquids), non-human milk, and infant formula up to 6 hours before surgery.

iv. A regular meal (fried food, high-fat foods, and meat) up to 8 hours before surgery.

B. Fluid considerations.

1. Patients may be nil per os (NPO) for up to 12 hours before surgery whether inpatient or outpatient.

a. Inpatient.

i. Dextrose-containing fluids should be started when NPO to prevent lean muscle catabolism if indicated by care team, patient history, and type of procedure (e.g., may be contraindicated in intracranial surgery).

b. Outpatient.

i. Fluid status should be assessed and intravenous (IV) fluid(s) administered accordingly.

BIBLIOGRAPHY

American Society of Anesthesiologists. (2014). ASA Physical status classification system. https://www.asahq.org/resources/clinical-information/asa-physical-status-classification-system

American Society of Anesthesiologists Committee. (2011). Practice guidelines for preoperative fasting and the use of pharmacologic agents to reduce the risk of pulmonary aspiration: Application to healthy patients undergoing elective procedures: An updated report by the American Society of Anesthesiologists Committee on Standards and Practice Parameters. *Anesthesiology, 114*(3), 495–511. https://doi.org/10.1097/ALN.0b013e3181fcbfd9

Anesthesiology. (2017). Practice guidelines for preoperative fasting and the use of pharmacologic agents to reduce the risk of pulmonary aspiration: Application to healthy patients undergoing elective procedures. *Anesthesiology, 126*(3), 376–393. https://doi.org/10.1097/aln.0000000000001452

Apfelbaum, J. L., & Connis, R. T. (2012). Practice advisory for preanesthesia evaluation: An updated report by the American Society of Anesthesiologists Task Force on Preanesthesia Evaluation. *Anesthesiology, 116*(3), 522–538. https://doi.org/10.1097/ALN.0b013e31823c1067

Chee, Y. L., Crawford, J. C., Watson, H. G., & Greaves, M. (2008). Guidelines on the assessment of bleeding risk prior to surgery or invasive procedures. British Committee for Standards in Haematology. *British Journal of Haematology, 140*(5), 496–504. https://doi.org/10.1111/j.1365-2141.2007.06968.x

Committee on Economics. (2020, December 13). *ASA Physical Status Classification System/American Guidelines, Statements, Clinical Resources.* https://www.asahq.org/standards-and-guidelines/asa-physical-status-classification-system

Fleisher, L. A., Fleischmann, K. E., & Auerbach, A. D. (2014). 2014 ACC/AHA guideline on perioperative cardiovascular evaluation and management of patients undergoing noncardiac surgery: A report of the American College of Cardiology/American Heart Association Task Force on Practice Guidelines. *Journal of the American College of Cardiology, 64*(22), e77–e137. https://doi.org/10.1016/j.jacc.2014.07.945

García-Miguel, F. J., Serrano-Aguilar, P. G., & López-Bastida, J. (2003). Preoperative assessment. *Lancet, 362*(9397), 1749–1757. https://doi.org/10.1016/S0140-6736(03)14857-X

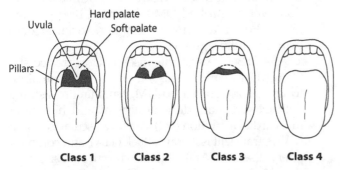

FIGURE 18.1 Mallampati classification. Visualization used to predict ease of intubation.

Kaplan, E. B., Sheiner, L. B., & Boeckmann, A. J. (1985). The usefulness of preoperative laboratory screening. *Journal of the American Medical Association, 253*(24), 3576–3581. https://doi.org/10.1001/jama.1985.03350480084025

Kondrup, J., Rasmussen, H. H., Hamberg, O., & Stanga, Z. (2003). Nutritional risk screening (NRS 2002): A new method based on an analysis of controlled clinical trials. *Clinical Nutrition, 22*(3), 321–336. https://doi.org/10.1016/S0261-5614(02)00214-5

Kumar, A., Mhaskar, R., & Grossman, B. J. (2015). Platelet transfusion: A systematic review of the clinical evidence. *Transfusion, 55*(5), 1116–1127. https://doi.org/10.1111/trf.12943

Lawrence, V. A., Dhanda, R., Hilsenbeck, S. G., & Page, C. P. (1111). Risk of pulmonary complications after elective abdominal surgery. *Chest, 110*(3), 744–750. https://doi.org/10.1378/chest.110.3.744

Macpherson, D. S. (1993). Preoperative laboratory testing: Should any tests be "routine" before surgery? *The Medical Clinics of North America, 77*(2), 289–308. https://doi.org/10.1016/S0025-7125(16)30252-8

Mallampait, S. R. (1985). A clinical sign to predict difficult tracheal intubation: A prospective study. *Canadian Anaesthetists' Society Journal, 32*(4), 429–434. https://doi.org/10.1007/BF03011357

McClave, S. A., Kozar, R., Martindale, R. G., Heyland, D. K., Braga, M., Carli, F., Drover, J. W., Flum, D., Gramlich, L., Herndon, D. N., Ko, C., Kudsk, K. A., Lawson, C. M., Miller, K. R., Taylor, B., & Wischmeyer, P. E. (2013). Summary points and consensus recommendations from the North American Surgical Nutrition Summit. *Journal of Parenteral and Enteral Nutrition, 37*(5 Suppl. 1), 99S–105S. https://doi.org/10.1177/0148607113495892

Nagelhout, J., & Elisha, S. (2018). *Nurse anesthesia* (6th ed.). Elsevier.

O'Neill, F., Carter, E., Pink, N., & Smith, I. (2016). Routine preoperative tests for elective surgery: Summary of updated NICE guidance. *British Medical Journal, 354*, i3292. https://doi.org/10.1136/bmj.i3292

van Stijn, M. F., Korkic-Halilovic, I., Bakker, M. S., van der Ploeg, T., van Leeuwen, P. A., & Houdijk, A. P. (2013). Preoperative nutrition status and postoperative outcome in elderly general surgery patients: A systematic review. *Journal of Parenteral and Enteral Nutrition, 37*(1), 37–43. https://doi.org/10.1177/0148607112445900

MEDICATION MANAGEMENT

PREOPERATIVE MEDICATION MANAGEMENT

A. Anticoagulation.

1. Risk of bleeding versus risk of thromboembolism must be assessed and reasonably estimated when deciding to stop anticoagulation due to the following conditions:

a. A thromboembolic event.

  i. Atrial fibrillation poses an estimated 0.2% to 1.2% risk based on three major studies.

   1) RE-LY.

   2) Rocket AF.

   3) ARISTOTLE.

  ii. Prosthetic heart valves increase the risk of a thromboembolic event of anticoagulation by 3.7-fold.

  iii. Recent thromboembolic event (venous or arterial) within the last 3 months.

   1) Elective surgery should be delayed if possible.

   2) Venous thromboembolism risk of anticoagulation.

    a) Within the first month of occurrence, risk is 50%.

    b) Between the first and third month of occurrence, risk decreases to 8% to 10%.

    c) After 3 months, risk decreases to 4% to 5%.

   3) Arterial embolism risk of anticoagulation.

    a) 0.5% per day within the first month after occurrence.

    b) Estimate risk of bleeding with continuation versus cessation of anticoagulation agent based on complexity of surgery, patient condition/history, and recommendations per anesthesiology, prescriber of anticoagulation, and surgical team.

  iv. High bleeding risk 2% to 4%.

   1) Coronary bypass surgery.

   2) Procedures greater than 45 minutes.

   3) Procedures in compartments that can increase the severity of bleeding complications, such as intracranial, pericardial, and intraocular compartments.

  v. Low bleeding risk 0% to 2%.

   1) Procedures less than 45 minutes.

   2) Carpal tunnel surgery.

   3) Hysterectomy.

2. Determine timing of anticoagulation holding/cessation.

a. Low bleeding risk surgeries may not require anticoagulation cessation.

  i. Cutaneous procedures such as skin biopsy.

  ii. Cardiac implantable device.

  iii. Endovascular procedures.

  iv. Certain dental procedures.

b. For surgeries with a moderate to high risk of bleeding, consider the following:

  i. Warfarin.

   1) Stop 5 days prior to surgery.

   2) Check the INR the day before.

    a) If greater than 1.5, administer 1 to 2 mg oral vitamin K.

    b) OK for surgery if 1.4 or less.

   3) Resume 12 to 24 hours after surgery due to prolonged action of onset. Full therapeutic effect may take up to 5 days. Should also consider bridging with heparin infusion or low molecular weight heparin (LMWH) subcutaneous injection therapy due to hospital policy/protocol/individualized patient clinical picture.

  ii. Direct thrombin inhibitor: Dabigatran.

   1) Stop 2 to 3 days prior to surgery.

   2) May need to stop longer if:

    a) Patient has renal insufficiency.

    b) Surgery has high risk for bleeding.

   3) Rapid onset of action.

    a) Delay restarting for 1 day after surgery with procedures that are low risk for bleeding.

b) Delay restarting for 2 to 3 days after surgery with procedures that are high risk for bleeding.

iii. Direct factor Xa inhibitors: Rivaroxaban, apixaban, and edoxaban.

1) Stop 2 to 3 days prior to surgery.
2) May need to stop longer if:
   a) Patient has renal insufficiency.
   b) Surgery has high risk for bleeding.
3) Rapid onset of action.
   a) Delay restarting for 1 day after surgery with procedures that are low risk for bleeding.
   b) Delay restarting for 2 to 3 days after surgery with procedures that are high risk for bleeding.

3. Determine if anticoagulation agent bridge is needed.
   a. Used mainly in patients with a high risk of thromboembolic event due to atrial fibrillation, mechanical heart valve, and/or personal history of a thromboembolic event.
   b. When to consider bridging (Table 18.1).
   c. Bridging preoperatively versus postoperatively, or both.
      i. Use the Thrombosis Canada Tool to determine if bridging is required preoperatively,

postoperatively, or both: https://thrombosiscanada.ca/tools/?calc=perioperativeAnticoagulantAlgorithm.
   d. Inferior vena cava (IVC) filter.
      i. Consider temporary IVC filter if patient is unable to restart anticoagulation for 3 to 4 weeks after surgery.

4. Case example: A 74-year-old patient with nonvalvular atrial fibrillation and ischemic stroke on warfarin who needs a total knee replacement.
   a. Stop warfarin 5 days before surgery.
   b. Preoperative bridging with LMWH starting 3 days before surgery and stopped the day of surgery.
   c. Resume warfarin within 24 hours of surgery.
   d. Resume LMWH within 24 hours of surgery and continue until INR is therapeutic.

B. Antiplatelet medications.
   1. Common examples include:
      a. Aspirin: Can be continued through *most* surgeries. However, patient clinical picture, individual risk of bleeding versus a thromboembolic event, and institutional policies/protocols may also impact aspirin continuation.
      b. Clopidogrel and ticagrelor: Should be discontinued at least 5 days before surgery.
      c. Prasugrel: Should be discontinued at least 7 days before surgery.

TABLE 18.1   PERIOPERATIVE BRIDGING: WHEN IT IS APPROPRIATE TO BRIDGE IN THE PERIOPERATIVE PERIOD

High Risk (Consider Bridging)	Moderate Risk (Case by Case)
Atrial Fibrillation	**Atrial Fibrillation**
Recent (<3 months) stroke/TIA CHADS$_2$ 5–6 Rheumatic heart	CHADS$_2$ = 3–4 mechanical heart valves Bileaflet aortic valve + risk factor
Mechanical Heart Valve	**VTE**
Ball or tilting disc valve Mitral valve Recent (<3 months) stroke/TIA	VTE 3–12 months prior cancer
VTE	**Low Risk (Consider NOT Bridging)**
Recent (<3 months) VTE Severe thrombophilia	**Atrial Fibrillation**
	CHADS$_2$ 0–2 mechanical heart valves Bileaflet aortic valve + risk factor
	VTE
	VTE >12 months ago

CHADS, congestive heart failure/hypertension/age/diabetes/prior stroke; TIA, transient ischemic attack; VTE, venous thromboembolism.
Source: Data from Douketis, J. D., Spyropoulos, A. C., Spencer, F. A., Mayr, M., Jaffer, A. K., Eckman, M. H., & Kunz, R. (2012). Perioperative management of antithrombotic therapy: Antithrombotic therapy and prevention of thrombosis, 9th ed. American College of Chest Physicians evidence-based clinical practice guidelines. *Chest, 141*, e326. https://doi.org/10.1378/chest.11-2298.

d. Ticlopidine: Should be discontinued at least 10 days before surgery.

e. Cilostazol: Discontinued 3 to 5 days before surgery.

2. Nonsteroidal anti-inflammatory drugs (NSAIDs) can cause decreased platelet function and should be discontinued for a minimum of 3 days before surgery.

C. Diabetic medications.

1. DM type 1.

a. Patients with type 1 DM are prone to ketosis, acidosis, and extremes of blood glucose during surgery.

b. Take extreme caution in regulating fluid and electrolyte balance as well as blood sugar levels.

c. Goal blood sugar is between 110 and 180 mg/dL.

d. Start dextrose-containing solution during procedure at 75 to 125 mL/hr if clinically indicated.

e. Check blood sugar every hour.

f. Short procedures less than 2 hours.

   i. Discontinue/hold short- or rapid-acting insulin on the morning of surgery.

   ii. If a patient takes two types of insulin only in the morning, give one-half to two-thirds of intermediate- or long-acting insulin on the day of surgery to prevent complications with ketosis.

   iii. If a patient takes insulin multiple times per day, give one-third to one-half total morning dose of intermediate- or long-acting insulin.

   iv. May allow patient's indwelling insulin pump to remain infusing if present and clinically warranted.

   v. Endocrine and/or insulin prescriber should be consulted for complex patients and those sensitive to small adjustments to insulin regimen, also known as "brittle diabetics."

g. Long procedures.

   i. Start IV insulin infusion if clinically indicated and indwelling insulin pump not present.

2. DM type 2.

a. In patients who manage their diabetes with diet alone, no additional therapy is required.

b. Oral hypoglycemics and noninsulin injectables.

   i. Should be held the morning of surgery.

   ii. Sliding scale insulin regimen can be used to manage excessive preoperative and elevated postoperative hyperglycemia if needed.

c. Insulin: Should give one-third to one-half the regular morning dose on the day of surgery if clinically warranted. Recommendations are to keep the same dose the night before.

d. If patient inadvertently took oral antihyperglycemic agent and/or full dose of insulin, assess for signs and symptoms of hypoglycemia and/or lactic acidosis as clinically indicated.

D. Glucocorticoids.

1. No need for perioperative stress dose corticosteroids if:

a. Any dosing less than 3 weeks.

b. Less than 5 mg/d, or less than 10 mg every other day.

2. Stress dose corticosteroids indicated if:

a. Greater than 20 mg/d for more than 3 weeks.

b. Cushingoid appearance.

c. Use of etomidate intraoperatively/on intubation, and/or intractable hypotension with prior use of steroid therapy.

d. Stress dose glucocorticoid therapy is typically hydrocortisone 100 mg IV Q8H.

e. Adrenocorticotropic hormone (ACTH) stimulation testing should be performed for any patient with a question of hypothalamic–pituitary–adrenal (HPA) axis suppression.

E. Cardiovascular medications.

1. Most commonly prescribed medications should be continued perioperatively and include:

a. Beta-blockers.

b. Angiotensin-converting enzyme (ACE) inhibitors and angiotensin receptor blockers (ARBs), although data and literature conflict regarding this. Advise patients to communicate these medications to anesthesia and surgical teams to be aware of possible vasoplegia syndrome and corresponding intractable hypotension intraoperatively.

c. Calcium channel blockers.

d. Statins: Exceedingly imperative to maintain therapy to decrease patient morbidity and mortality during the perioperative period.

F. Preoperative checklist for APP provision: See Table 18.2.

TABLE 18.2 PREOPERATIVE CHECKLIST

Risk factors	1. 2. 3.
American College of Surgeons risk score	(score)
Preoperative testing	Test—Result Test—Result
ASA classification	(class)
Nutritional considerations	(NRS-2002 score), nutritional support type
Medications	Drug—why on—when to stop—plan Drug—why on—when to stop—plan

ASA, American Society of Anesthesiologists; NRS-2002, Nutritional Risk Screening 2002.

Source: Data from DeLamar, L. M. (2005). Preparing your patient for surgery. *Topics in Advanced Practice Nursing eJournal,* 5(1). https://www.medscape.com/viewarticle/500887_2.

BIBLIOGRAPHY

Caldeira, D., Canastro, M., Barra, M., Ferreira, A., Costa, J., Pinto, F. J., & Ferreira, J. J. (2015). Risk of substantial intraocular bleeding with novel oral anticoagulants. *JAMA Ophthalmology, 133*(7), 834. https://doi.org/10.1001/jamaophthalmol.2015.0985

DeLamar, L. M. (2005). Preparing your patient for surgery. *Topics in Advanced Practice Nursing eJournal, 5*(1). https://www.medscape.com/viewarticle/500887_2

Douketis, J. D., Spyropoulos, A. C., Spencer, F. A., Mayr, M., Jaffer, A. K., Eckman, M. H., & Kunz, R. (2012). Perioperative management of antithrombotic therapy: Antithrombotic therapy and prevention of thrombosis, 9th ed American College of Chest Physicians evidence-based clinical practice guidelines. *Chest, 141*, e326. https://doi.org/10.1378/chest.11-2298

Douketis, J. D., Woods, K., Foster, G. A., & Crowther, M. A. (2005). Bridging anticoagulation with low-molecular-weight heparin after interruption of warfarin therapy is associated with a residual anticoagulant effect prior to surgery. *Thrombosis and Haemostasis, 94*, 528. https://doi.org/10.1160/TH05-01-0064

Dunn, A. S., Spyropoulos, A. C., & Turpie, A. G. (2007). Bridging therapy in patients on long-term oral anticoagulants who require surgery: The Prospective Peri-operative Enoxaparin Cohort Trial (PROSPECT). *Journal of Thrombosis and Haemostasis, 5*(11), 2211–2218. https://doi.org/10.1111/j.1538-7836.2007.02729.x

Fleisher, L. A., Fleischmann, K. E., Auerbach, A. D., Barnason, S. A., Beckman, J. A., & Bozkurt, B. (2014). 2014 ACC/AHA guideline on perioperative cardiovascular evaluation and management of patients undergoing noncardiac surgery: A report of the American College of Cardiology/American Heart Association Task Force on Practice Guidelines. *Circulation, 130*, e278. https://doi.org/10.1161/CIR.0000000000000105

Garcia, D., Alexander, J. H., Wallentin, L., Wojdyla, D. M., Thomas, L., Hanna, M., & Lopes, R. D. (2014). Management and clinical outcomes in patients treated with apixaban vs warfarin undergoing procedures. *Blood, 124*(25), 3692–3698. https://doi.org/10.1182/blood-2014-08-595496

Gropper, M. A., & Miller, R. D. (2020). *Miller's anesthesia* (9th ed.). Elsevier.

Hines, R. L., & Marschall, K. E. (2018). *Stoelting's anesthesia and co-existing disease* (7th ed.). Elsevier.

Healey, J. S., Eikelboom, J., Douketis, J., Wallentin, L., Oldgren, J., Yang, S., Themeles, E., Heidbuchel, H., Avezum, A., Reilly, P., Connolly, S. J., Yusuf, S., & Ezekowitz, M. (2012). Periprocedural bleeding and thromboembolic events with dabigatran compared with warfarin: Results from the randomized evaluation of long-term anticoagulation therapy (RE-LY) randomized trial. *Circulation, 126*(3), 343. https://doi.org/10.1161/CIRCULATIONAHA.111.090464

Liu, H., Yu, L., Yang, L., & Green, M. S. (2017). Vasoplegic syndrome: An update on perioperative considerations. *Journal of Clinical Anesthesia, 40*, 63–71. https://doi.org/10.1016/j.jclinane.2017.04.017

Marik, P. E., & Varon, J. (2008). Requirement of perioperative stress doses of corticosteroids: A systematic review of the literature. *Archives of Surgery, 143*(12), 1222–1226.

Nagelhout, J., & Elisha, S. (2018). *Nurse anesthesia* (6th ed.). Elsevier.

Nouthe, B., Ngongang Ouankou, C., Spaziano, M., & Sia, Y. T. (2020). Ace-inhibitors and Vasoplegia in the post CABG population/valvular surgery population: An updated systematic review and meta-analysis. *Circulation, 142*(Suppl. 3), https://doi.org/10.1161/circ.142.suppl_3.16264

Rotruck, S., Suzan, L., Vigersky, R., Rotruck, J., Brown, C., Capacchione, J., & Todd, L. A. (2018, June). Should continuous subcutaneous insulin infusion (CSII) pumps be used during the perioperative period? Development of a Clinical Decision Algorithm. *AANA Journal, 86*, 194–200. https://www.aana.com/docs/default-source/aana-journal-web-documents-1/should-continuous-subcutaneous-insulin-infusion-pumps-be-used-during-the-perioperative-period-development-of-a-clinical-decision-algorithm-june-2018.pdf?sfvrsn=a5cb58b1_8

Sherwood, M. W., Douketis, J. D., Patel, M. R., Piccini, J. P., Hellkamp, A. S., Lokhnygina, Y., Spyropoulos, A. C., Hankey, G. J., Singer, D. E., Nessel, C. C., Mahaffey, K. W., Fox, K. A. A., Califf, R. M., Becker, R. C., & ROCKET AF Investigators. (2014). Outcomes of temporary interruption of rivaroxaban compared with warfarin in patients with nonvalvular atrial fibrillation: Results from the rivaroxaban once daily, oral, direct Factor Xa inhibition compared with vitamin K antagonism for prevention of stroke and embolism trial in atrial fibrillation. *Circulation, 129*(18), 1850–1859. https://doi.org/10.1161/CIRCULATIONAHA.113.005754

Thompson Bastin, M. L., Baker, S. N., & Weant, K. A. (2014). Effects of etomidate on adrenal suppression: A review of intubated septic patients. *Hospital Pharmacy, 49*(2), 177–183. https://doi.org/10.1310/hpj4902-177

Thrombosis Canada. (n.d.). Anticoagulant dosing in atrial fibrulation. http://thrombosiscanada.ca/tools/?calc=perioperativeAnticoagulantAlgorithm

Umpierrez, G. E., Smiley, D., Jacobs, S., Peng, L., Temponi, A., Mulligan, P., & Rizzo, M. (2011). Randomized study of basal-bolus insulin therapy in the inpatient management of patients with type 2 diabetes undergoing general surgery (RABBIT 2 surgery). *Diabetes Care, 34*, 256. https://doi.org/10.2337/dc10-1407

Van den Berghe, G., Wilmer, A., Hermans, G., Meersseman, W., Wouters, P. J., Milants, I., Van Wijngaerden, E., Bobbaers, H., & Bouillon, R. (2006). Intensive insulin therapy in the medical ICU. *The New England Journal of Medicine, 354*, 449–461. https://doi.org/10.1056/NEJMoa052521

Van den Berghe, G., Wouters, P., Weekers, F., Verwaest, C., Bruyninckx, F., Schetz, M., & Bouillon, R. (2001). Intensive insulin therapy in critically ill patients. *The New England Journal of Medicine, 345*, 1359–1367. https://doi.org/10.1056/NEJMoa011300

CHAPTER 19

PERIOPERATIVE AND INTRAOPERATIVE MANAGEMENT

William A. Edwards, Jr.

SCOPE OF CHAPTER

This chapter is not meant to be exhaustive in teaching the advanced practice provider (APP) how to function in the intraoperative setting. Rather, this chapter is included to provide an overview of the process that occurs while patients are in surgery, as well as to help the APP in the postoperative period understand why certain complications occur. For instance, patient positioning may impact postoperative atelectasis, or a difficult airway may delay extubation. By understanding the general concepts of anesthesia care and delivery, the APP will be knowledgeable in how to optimize physiologic parameters and combat physiologic derangements.

CONSIDERATIONS

DELIVERY OF ANESTHESIA

A. Primary goal.
  1. Maintain homeostasis and optimize physiologic response to surgical insult.
B. Secondary goal.
  1. Provide patient amnesia, anxiolysis, sedation, and anesthesia.
    a. Minimizing the memory of the operative and perioperative experience.
    b. Commonly used medications include:
      i. Benzodiazepines.
      ii. Propofol.
      iii. Ketamine.
      iv. Volatile (inhalational) anesthetics.
  2. Provide patient analgesia.
    a. Multimodal approach should be used to limit the adverse effects of opioids and includes:
      i. Opioid/narcotic medications.
      ii. Nonsteroidal anti-inflammatory drugs (e.g., ketorolac).
      iii. Local/regional anesthetics (inclusive to epidural and spinal anesthesia; extremity or abdominal nerve blockade).
  3. Monitored anesthesia care (MAC).
    a. Site-specific local anesthesia with combined sedation and analgesia.

      i. Patient-controlled analgesia may be used postoperatively.
      ii. Continuous intravenous (IV) infusion or boluses of sedation agent (e.g., midazolam, propofol, ketamine, dexmedetomidine).
    b. Deemed first choice of anesthesia delivery in many types of procedures.
      i. Colonoscopy.
      ii. Bronchoscopy.
      iii. Minor procedures and surgeries less than 2 hours.
      iv. Extremity procedures with concurrent regional anesthesia (e.g., arthroplasties).
      v. Many, if not most, outpatient procedures.
    c. Used in patients who can protect their airways without the assistance of a supraglottic airway or endotracheal tube.
      i. Bispectral index (BIS) monitor can be used to assess a patient's level of consciousness and confirm level of sedation.
    d. Goal of MAC.
      i. Safe sedation.
      ii. Control of patient anxiety.
      iii. Decrease awareness of procedure.
      iv. Minimize pain during and after procedure.
    e. Medications.
      i. Midazolam: Short-acting benzodiazepine without analgesic effect. Can cause respiratory depression especially in conjunction with other sedatives and/or opioids.
      ii. Propofol: Rapidly acting sedative with antiemetic effects, without analgesic effects, and can be used to transition to general anesthesia with dose increases if needed.
      iii. Opioids.
        1) Fentanyl: Short-acting opioid.
        2) Remifentanil: Ultrashort-acting opioid typically given as an infusion.
      iv. Dexmedetomidine: Bolus and/or infusion agent with sedative, anxiolytic, antishivering, and analgesic effects. Does not cause respiratory depression.
      v. Ketamine: Significant analgesic and sedative agent with minimal respiratory depression. Can reduce the need for opioids.

▶

4. Neuromuscular blockade (NMB).
   a. Used for optimal intubation conditions and optimal operative conditions to keep patients still during surgery.
   b. Common medications include:
      i. Depolarizing agents.
         1) Succinylcholine.
            a) Faster onset, shorter acting.
            b) Side effects include bradycardia, hyperkalemia, fasciculations, rhabdomyolysis, and malignant hyperthermia (MH) for those with a genetic disposition to it.
            c) Primarily used for rapid sequence intubation and only a few other indications.
      ii. Nondepolarizing agents.
         1) Longer acting, can use as a bolus or infusion.
         2) Provide sustained blockade as opposed to succinylcholine.
         3) Typical neuromuscular blocking (NMB) agents used.
         4) Examples:
            a) Rocuronium.
            b) Vecuronium.
            c) Cisatracurium.
            d) Mivacurium.
         5) Side effects include increased histamine release (mivacurium), rash, bronchospasm, anaphylactic/anaphylactoid reactions, respiratory depression/apnea, critical illness myopathy, peripheral vascular resistance, tachycardia, and hypotension.
5. Maintenance of hemostasis and hemodynamic stability.
   a. Fluids: Goals of fluid therapy during surgery are normovolemia and normotension; avoid liberal or constricted volume approaches to fluid replacement.
      i. Crystalloids (e.g., Ringer's lactate, PlasmaLyte) used instead of 0.9% and 0.45% normal saline to avoid hypernatremia and metabolic acidosis. The goal is to maintain intravascular fluid volume with balanced electrolytes.
         1) Most commonly used therapy to maintain normotension in perioperative period.
         2) Avoid large volumes of fluid to prevent poor patient outcomes from overload.
         3) Use of goal-directed fluid therapy (GDFT) modalities by anesthesiology and critical care helps limit fluid overload with concurrent vasopressor agents.
      ii. Colloids (e.g., human albumin) known to expand vascular fluid volume. Can be used with concurrent IV fluid therapy and can be considered to minimize infusing large volumes of fluid.
      iii. Blood products: Replace intraoperative blood loss, may positively impact fluid status (all products), and promote tissue oxygenation (packed red blood cells [PRBCs]). May help with intraoperative and postoperative bleeding (fresh frozen plasma, cryoprecipitate, and platelets).
      iv. Hemodynamic parameters, patient response to fluids versus vasopressors, and anticipated blood loss will guide fluid replacement quantities and type (especially with GDFT utilization).
   b. Vasopressors.
      i. Phenylephrine: Usually given in bolus doses and can be used as an infusion.
      ii. Norepinephrine: May be used as an infusion if infusing prior to procedure or as a later option (noncardiac procedures). Often given in cardiothoracic surgeries.
      iii. Epinephrine: May be used in the event of anaphylaxis, profound bradycardia, or bronchospasm in bolus doses. May be used as an infusion if currently infusing or as a later option (noncardiac procedures). Often used in cardiothoracic procedures (e.g., coronary artery bypass grafting [CABG], valve repair).
      iv. Ephedrine: Usually given in bolus doses. Increases heart rate and has a tachyphylaxis effect.
      v. Dobutamine: May be used in cardiac surgery as an infusion, although milrinone is typically the medication of choice over dobutamine in cardiac surgery. May be used as a vasopressor in sepsis management, but may not be a first-line agent due to side effects.
   c. Transfusions.
      i. PRBCs: Transfusion should be considered at hemoglobin concentrations of 7 g/dL or less and/or with excessive intraoperative blood loss.
      ii. Fresh frozen/thawed plasma: Given to correct coagulopathy, reverse the effects of warfarin, decrease a high international normalized ratio (INR) result, and/or combat known coagulation factor deficiencies.
      iii. Platelets: May be given in suspected platelet dysfunction, proper thromboelastography (TEG) interpretation with indication, and presence of antiplatelet agents and bleeding. Indicated if serum platelet count falls below 50,000 per microliter in the presence of excessive bleeding.
      iv. Cryoprecipitate: Administered when serum fibrinogen is less than 80 to 100 mg/dL in the presence of excessive bleeding and fibrinolysis. Also used in von Willebrand disease with or without DDAVP.
      v. Indications for autotransfusion: Same as PRBC indications. Patients are transfused their own blood lost during the procedure or if the blood was previously provided weekly up to 5 days prior to surgery. Most hospitals ▶

hold donor and autologous blood for a limited period of time, usually 35 to 40 days due to its shelf-life sustainability and cell life span.

    vi. Pharmacologic treatments.

        1) DDAVP (desmopressin): Facilitates platelet adhesion and aggregation; especially indicated in von Willebrand disease.

        2) Tranexamic acid (TXA): Typically administered for prophylaxis of excessive bleeding before and/or during a procedure and postoperatively in cardiothoracic surgery.

        3) Coagulation factor concentrates: Can be beneficial in varied surgeries for emergency reversal of novel oral anticoagulants (NOAC) therapy and warfarin (e.g., prothrombin complex concentrate). Off-label use for microvascular bleeding has also been performed due to coagulation factor deficiencies. These agents can increase risk of thromboembolic events.

        4) Thrombin gel: Used for hemostasis intraoperatively.

6. Postoperative nausea and vomiting (PONV) prevention.

    a. Highest risk within the first 24 hours after surgery, with an incidence of 30% to 40% of patients.

    b. Risks of PONV include history of PONV and/or motion sickness, longer duration of surgery, use of volatile anesthetics, laparotomies and laparoscopic procedures, gynecologic procedures, ear/nose/throat procedures, and breast and plastic surgeries.

    c. Prevention.

      i. Scopolamine patch at least 2 hours prior to anesthesia induction to start taking effect.

      ii. Dexamethasone 4 to 8 mg IV after anesthesia induction.

      iii. Ondansetron 4 mg IV at the conclusion of surgery.

      iv. Propofol bolus of 15 to 20 mg IV at the end of surgery or as a low-dose infusion of 10 to 20 mcg/kg/min during surgery.

      v. Avoid the use of volatile anesthetics.

    d. Other alternative treatments.

      i. Promethazine 6.25 to 12.5 mg IV at anesthesia induction.

      ii. Prochlorperazine 5 to 10 mg IV at the conclusion of surgery.

7. Reversal of neuromuscular blockade.

    a. Used to restore patient functions of breathing, movement, and reflexes at the end of a surgery during a process called *emergence*. IV and volatile anesthetics are turned off prior to this and do not need to be reversed. Neuromuscular blockade during the procedure needs to be reversed at this time.

    b. Neuromuscular reversal agents.

      i. Neostigmine: Used in conjunction with glycopyrrolate to indirectly reverse paralysis at the neuromuscular junction.

      ii. Sugammadex: Works directly on nondepolarizing neuromuscular blocking agents (e.g., rocuronium and vecuronium) to bind to the medication and block its effect at the neuromuscular junction. This is more effective than several agents above. Of note, patients taking birth control should be counseled, educated, and encouraged to consume alternative agents due to sugammadex impacting the efficacy of birth control agents.

ANESTHETIC CONSIDERATIONS

A. Local infiltration anesthesia, also known as local anesthesia.

    1. Indications: Provides anesthesia and analgesia to a specified location that will be focused on during the surgery or procedure (e.g., extremity procedure, skin procedure). Often given by a surgeon.

    2. Duration of action can be increased when mixed with epinephrine. Of note, be cautious of tissue necrosis if epinephrine is used in a local anesthetic infiltration technique.

    3. Most common medications used are as follows:

      a. Lidocaine (0.5%, 1%, and 2%).

        i. Onset: 2 to 5 minutes, typically seen faster anecdotally.

        ii. Duration: 30 to 120 minutes (180 minutes when mixed with epinephrine).

        iii. Maximum doses.

          1) With epinephrine: 7 mg/kg (no more than 350 mg to be administered).

          2) Without epinephrine: 4 mg/kg (no more than 350 mg to be administered).

      b. Bupivacaine (0.125%, 0.25%).

        i. Onset: 5 to 20 minutes.

        ii. Duration: Up to 6 to 8 hours.

        iii. Maximum doses.

          1) With epinephrine: 3 mg/kg (no more than 175 mg to be administered).

          2) Without epinephrine: 2 mg/kg (no more than 175 mg to be administered).

      c. Liposomal bupivacaine (also known as Exparel).

        i. Onset: 5 to 20 minutes.

        ii. Duration: Up to 8 to 18 hours.

        iii. Maximum dose 3.8 mg/kg, or no more than 266 mg to be administered.

        iv. Not mixed with epinephrine.

    4. Complications of local anesthetic administration.

      a. Toxicity.

        i. Cardiovascular system.

          1) Lidocaine is a class I antiarrhythmic medication and can cause cardiac disturbances, such as:

            a) Bradycardia.

            b) Decreased inotropy.

            c) Atrioventricular block. ▶

d) Vasodilation.
e) Dysrhythmias.
f) Cardiac arrest.
ii. Central nervous system.
1) Seizures.
2) Paresthesias.
3) Tinnitus.
4) Decreased level of consciousness.
B. Regional anesthesia: Peripheral nerve blocks.
  1. Locations.
    a. Upper extremity nerve blocks.
      i. Interscalene block: Indicated for shoulder and upper arm surgery. Pneumothorax can occur during procedure and this block misses ulnar nerve distribution (the lateral forearm and fifth digit will feel pain), which is the most significant concern for this block. Watch for signs and symptoms, as well as for Horner syndrome.
      ii. Supraclavicular block: Indicated for all types of upper extremity surgeries except for shoulder surgery. Pneumothorax can occur with this procedure. Phrenic nerve block and Horner syndrome may also occur during this procedure. Watch for signs and symptoms.
      iii. Infraclavicular block: Indicated for elbow, forearm, wrist, and hand surgeries. Risk of pneumothorax is low with this procedure; however, be mindful of signs and symptoms of it.
      iv. Axillary nerve block: Indicated for procedures below the elbow. A complication may be arterial puncture. This block misses the musculocutaneous nerve and this may need to be blocked for lateral forearm desensitization/anesthetization.
    b. Lower extremity blocks.
      i. Sciatic block: Indicated for multiple lower extremity procedures and commonly combined with other blocks below. Approach is not performed often and requires a needle length of 150 mm.
      ii. Femoral block: Indicated for anterior thigh procedures. Was very common in the previous years for total knee arthroplasty for postoperative analgesia. Patient loses motor function with this block and most providers perform adductor canal block instead to avoid this.
      iii. Adductor canal block: A purely sensory nerve block indicated for knee procedures and arthroplasties. Blocks obturator and saphenous nerve and allows motor function for quicker mobility and better outcomes.
      iv. Fascia iliaca nerve block: Indicated for hip and thigh surgeries, often performed for hip fractures. It is another alternative of the femoral nerve block and impacts femoral and lateral femoral nerves.
      v. Lumbar plexus nerve block: Achieves blockade of the entire lumbar plexus inclusive to femoral, obturator, and lateral femoral cutaneous nerves.
      vi. Popliteal block: Indicated for surgeries distal to the knee (calf, ankle, and foot). Often combined with adductor canal block for knee or foot surgery.
      vii. Ankle block: Indicated for foot surgery. Four out of five nerves are blocked, excluding the saphenous nerve (blocked with adductor canal block).
  2. Contraindications to peripheral regional anesthesia.
    a. Body habitus may make regional blockade difficult due to equipment limitations and patient positioning.
    b. Active infection at the site of injection.
    c. Coagulopathy and noncompressive site of injection.
    d. Preexisting neural and/or motor deficits in the dermatomal distribution of the block.
    e. Hemidiaphragm paralysis.
    f. Laryngeal nerve paralysis.
    g. Patient refusal.
  3. Complications of regional anesthesia.
    a. Prolonged paresthesias/paralysis.
    b. Pneumothorax.
    c. Vascular puncture.
    d. Phrenic nerve injury.
    e. Local anesthetic systemic toxicity (LAST): Rare but often fatal occurrence. This complication of local anesthesia is due to the sodium channels of cardiac muscle binding to the local anesthetic; in essence, heart blockade occurs, and the heart is refractory to normal function and normal interventions of CPR. Seizure activity is also noted with local anesthetic toxicity and has deleterious effects as well. Treatment is with intralipid therapy and should follow the LAST intralipid protocol as follows:
      i. Initially administer intralipid 20% at a dose of 1.5 mL/kg over 1 minute.
      ii. Follow immediately with an infusion at a rate of 0.25 mL/kg/min.
      iii. Continue chest compressions (lipid must circulate to be effective).
      iv. Repeat bolus every 3 to 5 minutes up to 3 mL/kg total dosage until circulation is restored.
      v. Continue infusion until hemodynamic stability is restored.
      vi. Increase the rate to 0.5 mL/kg/min if blood pressure declines.
      vii. A maximum total dose of 12 mL/kg is recommended. Provide life-sustaining measures during this process as well.

C. Regional anesthesia: Spinals.
  1. Indications.
    a. Lower extremity procedures (e.g., total hip/knee arthroplasties, knee arthroscopy).
    b. A 2-hour or less anticipated surgery duration for surgeries/procedures below the umbilicus (e.g., Cesarean sections, cystoscopy with/without stenting).
    c. Patients with a high risk for general anesthesia complications needing surgeries distal to the umbilicus.
    d. Patients with spinal cord injuries, where autonomic dysreflexia could occur during surgery/procedure.
    e. Those who may have genetic dispositions to MH.
    f. Often combined with sedation for procedure toleration.
D. Regional anesthesia: Epidurals.
  1. Indications.
    a. Longer surgical procedures.
    b. Unknown duration of surgery.
    c. Help with intraoperative and postoperative pain management.
    d. Thoracic, abdominal, and extremity surgeries for patients at increased risk of complications for general anesthesia.
    e. Patients with spinal cord injuries, where autonomic dysreflexia could occur during surgery/procedure.
    f. Those who may have genetic dispositions to MH.
    g. Parturients for labor and delivery.
    h. Often combined with sedation for procedure toleration.
  2. Contraindications to epidural/spinal anesthesia.
    a. Hypovolemia: May cause spinal shock from sympathectomy and vascular dilation to further cause intractable hypotension if performed.
    b. Coagulopathy: May cause epidural hematoma and/or cauda equina syndrome.
    c. Increased intracranial pressure: Risk of herniation.
    d. Abscess: Nullifies the effect of local anesthetic. Can cause further infection and/or sepsis if performed.
  3. Complications of epidural/spinal anesthesia.
    a. Hypotension: Causes sympathectomy from the level of anesthesia placement down, dilates corresponding vessels, and decreases blood return.
    b. High or "total" spinal: Life-threatening event of anesthetic traveling cephalad that is associated with cardiovascular and respiratory compromise, loss of consciousness, and/or cardiopulmonary arrest.
E. The three phases of general anesthesia provision.
  1. Induction of anesthesia.
    a. Often achieved with a combination of IV and inhaled anesthetics, but may be done with either agent alone.

    b. Rapid administration (<2 minutes) of agents to prepare patient for procedure/surgery, with or without intubation.
    c. IV medications.
      i. Propofol.
      ii. Etomidate.
      iii. Ketamine.
      iv. Midazolam.
      v. Opioid narcotics, for example, fentanyl or remifentanil.
      vi. Neuromuscular blocking agent(s).
    d. Inhalational anesthetics.
      i. Adult patients.
        1) Commonly used for quicker induction.
        2) May have an unpleasant smell.
        3) May have increased risk of PONV.
        4) May be considered over IV induction in higher risk patients who have a low cardiac ejection fraction.
      ii. Pediatric and/or intellectually/cognitively impaired patients.
        1) May be preferred over IV induction due to fear and/or patient compliance with induction process and following directions.
  2. Maintenance of general anesthesia.
    a. Considered the phase where patient is maintained during surgery/procedure after anesthesia induction, for example, vitals, sedation level, adequate analgesia, adequate patient paralysis, and adequate hemodynamic status within specified parameters per patient norms and per procedure requirements.
    b. Inhalational agents.
      i. Sevoflurane: Agent that facilitates a moderate to quick induction and emergence during general anesthesia provision. Is used for those spontaneously breathing during the procedure with a supraglottic airway device and is also used to prevent bronchospasm during maintenance and emergence of general anesthesia.
      ii. Desflurane: Agent that facilitates quick induction and emergence during general anesthesia. May cause bronchoconstriction/bronchospasm as well as tachycardia.
      iii. Nitrous oxide: Agent that facilitates the quickest induction and emergence of general anesthesia. Increases risk of PONV and is contraindicated in many bowel, intraocular, and intracranial procedures. Can facilitate hypoxemia and diffusion hypoxia.
    c. IV agents.
      i. Propofol.
      ii. Neuromuscular blocking agents.
      iii. Opioids.
        1) Fentanyl.
        2) Sufentanil.
        3) Remifentanil.
  3. Emergence of general anesthesia.
    a. A restoration of patient breathing, movement, and reflexes at the end of a ▶

surgery/procedure with a subsequent increased level of consciousness.

b. Many variables determine timing of emergence and level of arousal; depends on IV and/or inhaled anesthetics, specified type(s) of agents used, duration of procedure, patient's medical history, and patient's physiology.

c. Timing is critical during emergence and can occur in a stepwise approach.

    i. Discontinue anesthetic agents.

    ii. Administer antiemetic(s).

    iii. Administer reversal of neuromuscular blocking agent(s).

    iv. Assess adequacy of analgesia: For example, indicators involving blood pressure, heart rate, and respiratory rate parameters and regularity.

    v. Assess adequacy of tidal volume and minute ventilation of spontaneous respiration by observing values on the anesthesia machine.

    vi. Assess level of anesthesia and return of reflexes.

       1) Some providers emerge patients to a point of being fully awake and following commands, while others maintain a level of sedation, and patients maintain their respiratory status and intermittently follow commands.

       2) Either technique can be performed and is deemed safe.

       3) Extubation or removal of supraglottic airway is performed when patient is deemed able to maintain their airways without assistance, all reflexes are present, and tidal volumes are adequate per individual patient norms.

F. Complications of general anesthesia.

  1. MH.

    a. Potentially fatal occurrence due to a genetic predisposition. Occurs with patient exposure of any inhalational anesthetic agent and/or succinylcholine. Hallmark signs are masseter muscle tension, biting on the endotracheal tube, entire body musculature rigidity, sharp and immediate increase in end-tidal carbon dioxide, and sharp increase of body temperature up to 104°F/40°C. Treatment is to call the MH hotline IMMEDIATELY and to quickly administer dantrolene or Ryanodex per MH protocol. May occur up to 12 hours postsurgery so it should be considered in a differential diagnosis.

  2. Laryngospasm and bronchospasm.

    a. Occurs with an increased level of anesthesia and occurs with either closing of the vocal cords (laryngospasm) or constriction of the bronchus (bronchospasm).

    b. Hallmark signs for both are impaired respirations, impaired ventilation, possible oxygen desaturation, and ineffective or absent tidal volumes.

    c. Laryngospasm typically presents with an inspiratory stridor, while bronchospasm presents with

difficulty or inability to assist patient with respirations due to bronchial constriction. Both can be life-threatening or can increase morbidity if not reversed.

  3. Nausea and/or vomiting.

  4. Agitation and/or delirium: Often in the pediatric, posttraumatic stress disorder (PTSD), and older adult populations. Can be avoided with midazolam or dexmedetomidine administration prior to emergence, or midazolam during presentation.

  5. Urinary retention.

  6. Hypotension.

BIBLIOGRAPHY

Berde, C. B. (1993). Toxicity of local anesthetics in infants and children. *The Journal of Pediatrics, 122*(5 Pt. 2), S14–S20. https://doi.org/10.1016/S0022-3476(11)80004-1

Borgeat, A., Ekatodramis, G., Kalberer, F., & Benz, C. (2001). Acute and nonacute complications associated with interscalene block and shoulder surgery: A prospective study. *Anesthesiology, 95*(4), 875–880. https://doi.org/10.1097/00000542-200110000-00015

Caironi, P., Tognoni, G., Masson, S., Fumagalli, R., Pesenti, A., Romero, M., Fanizza, C., Caspani, L., Faenza, S., Grasselli, G., Iapichino, G., Antonelli, M., Parrini, V., Fiore, G., Latini, R., & Gattinoni, L. (2014). Albumin replacement in patients with severe sepsis or septic shock. *New England Journal of Medicine, 370*(15), 1412–1421. https://doi.org/10.1056/nejmoa1305727

Cascella, M., Bimonte, S., & Muzio, M. R. (2018). Towards a better understanding of anesthesia emergence mechanisms: Research and clinical implications. *World Journal of Methodology, 8*(2), 9–16. https://doi.org/10.5662/wjm.v8.i2.9

Dubin, A., Lattanzio, B., & Gatti, L. (2017). The spectrum of cardiovascular effects of dobutamine—From healthy subjects to septic shock patients. *Revista Brasileira De Terapia Intensiva, 29*(4), 490–498. https://doi.org/10.5935/0103-507x.20170068

El-Boghdadly, K., Pawa, A., & Chin, K. J. (2018). Local anesthetic systemic toxicity: Current perspectives. *Local and Regional Anesthesia, 11*, 35–44. https://doi.org/10.2147/lra.s154512

Gropper, M. A., & Miller, R. D. (2020). *Miller's anesthesia* (9th ed.). Elsevier.

Liu, H., Kendrick, J. B., Kaye, A. D., Tong, Y., Belani, K., Urman, R. D., & Hoffman, C. (2019). Goal-directed fluid therapy in the perioperative setting. *Journal of Anaesthesiology Clinical Pharmacology, 35*(5), 29. https://doi.org/10.4103/joacp.joacp_26_18

Masuda, Y. (2019). Total spinal block (TSB). In K. Ohseto, H. Uchino, & H. Iida (Eds.), *Nerve blockade and interventional therapy* (pp. 285–287). Springer. https://doi.org/10.1007/978-4-431-54660-3_72

Nagelhout, J., & Elisha, S. (2018). *Nurse anesthesia* (6th ed.). Elsevier.

New York School of Regional Anesthesia. (n.d). *Spinal anesthesia*. http://www.nysora.com/techniques/neuraxial-and-perineuraxial-techniques/landmark-based/3423-spinal-anesthesia

NYSORA. (2022, February 1). Local anesthetic systemic toxicity. https://www.nysora.com/topics/complications/local-anesthetic-systemic-toxicity/

Pollard, R. J., Coyle, J. P., Gilbert, R. L., & Beck, J. E. (2007). Intraoperative awareness in a regional medical system: A review of 3 years' data. *Anesthesiology, 106*(2), 269–274. https://doi.org/10.1097/00000542-200702000-00014

Thwaites, A., Edmends, S., & Smith, I. (1997). Inhalation induction with sevoflurane: A double-blind comparison with propofol. *British Journal of Anaesthesia, 78*(4), 356–361. https://doi.org/10.1093/bja/78.4.356

Urman, R. D., & Ehrenfeld, J. M. (2021). *Pocket anesthesia* (4th ed.). Wolters Kluwer.

Weinberg, G., Rupnik, B., Aggarwal, N., Fettiplace, M., & Gitman, M. (2020). Local anesthetic systemic toxicity (LAST) revisited: A paradigm in evolution. *APSF Newsletter, 35*(10). https://doi.org/https://www.apsf.org/article/local-anesthetic-systemic-toxicity-last-revisited-a-paradigm-in-evolution/

White, P. F., Kehlet, H., & Neal, J. M. (2007). The role of the anesthesiologist in fast-track surgery: From multimodal analgesia to perioperative medical care. *Anesthesia and Analgesia, 104*(6), 1380–1396. https://doi.org/10.1213/01.ane.0000263034.96885.e1

CARE PRINCIPLES

POSITIONING

A. Goals of proper patient positioning.
   1. Maintain airway.
   2. Provide adequate surgical exposure.
   3. Allow for proper patient monitoring.
   4. Prevent vascular compression and ischemia.
   5. Prevent nerve injuries.
   6. Maintain skin integrity.
   7. Keep patient comfortable and keep as many body parts as possible in a neutral position.

B. Each surgical procedure has specific anesthetic and positioning considerations.

C. Typical positioning in the operating room.
   1. Supine: This position causes minimal effects on circulation and perfusion of the lungs. Hips and knees can be slightly flexed to increase venous return. May need to assess sacral skin integrity for prolonged procedures and observe for s/s of brachial plexus injury if arms are abducted greater than 90 degrees (Figure 19.1).
   2. Prone: This position places pressure on the ventral aspect of the head and body. Corneal abrasions, postoperative vision loss, as well as hypotension intraoperatively due to increased intrathoracic and intra-abdominal pressure from position can occur if not addressed preemptively. Temporary facial swelling may be present postprocedure due to patient being in a face-down position with fluid pooling to dependent facial structures (Figure 19.2).
   3. Lateral: This position leads to possible complications of ventilation-perfusion (V/Q) mismatch with unequal lung perfusion, corneal abrasions, and/or brachial plexus injuries. Even with adequate support, venous hypertension in the dependent arm is almost inevitable due to outflow obstruction. Padding and pillows should be placed between the legs to prevent damage to both the common peroneal and saphenous nerves (Figure 19.3).

   4. Lithotomy: This position may impair pulmonary function as it may impair respiratory mechanics. Common peroneal nerve injury and palsy is possible if pressure on the nerve over the fibula is not protected by adequate padding and/or positioning. Hyperflexion of the hip joint can cause femoral and lateral femoral cutaneous nerve injury and palsy. Obturator and saphenous nerve injuries are also complications of lithotomy position (Figure 19.4).
   5. Trendelenburg: This position provides better surgical exposure to lower intra-abdominal organs for specified procedures. Arms should be padded and tucked at sides or well-secured if they are to remain out and untucked per surgeon request. While supine and before converting to Trendelenburg position, padded shoulder blocks are placed superior to the acromioclavicular (AC) joints and fit snug on the operating room table. Brachial plexus, ulnar nerve, and common peroneal nerve injuries may occur in this position. Facial swelling may occur especially in a steep-angle Trendelenburg position and prolonged surgery in this position. This position can also cause decreased perfusion of the lower extremities, increased mean arterial pressure (MAP) of the vessels supplying the head, decreased cardiac output, decreased lung compliance, decreased vital capacity, decreased functional residual volume, increased V/Q mismatch subcutaneous emphysema, and possible pulmonary congestion and/or edema. Airway edema is also a concern and should be evaluated to prevent subsequent reintubation (Figure 19.5).
   6. Reverse Trendelenburg: This position is the complete opposite position of the Trendelenburg position, with the head of the OR table angled upward. This position provides better surgical exposure to upper intra-abdominal organs for specified procedures. Arms should be padded and tucked at sides ▶

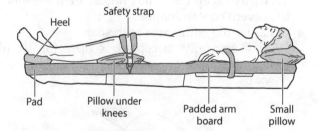

FIGURE 19.1 Supine position.

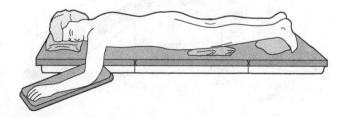

FIGURE 19.2 Prone position.

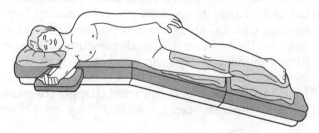

FIGURE 19.3 Lateral position.

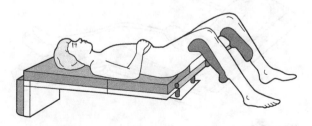

FIGURE 19.4 Lithotomy position.

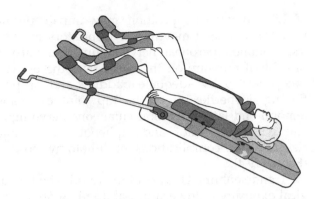

FIGURE 19.5 Trendelenburg position.

or well-secured if they are to remain out per surgeon request. While supine and before converting to revere Trendelenburg position, the patient's feet must be firmly and securely resting on the padded footboard to prevent the patient from sliding down or off the table. Brachial plexus, ulnar nerve, and common peroneal nerve injuries may occur in this position. Remarkable hypotension may occur in this position due to venous pooling and decreased venous return, especially when in a steep-angle reverse Trendelenburg position.

7. Sitting position/beach chair position: This position is primarily used for shoulder surgeries and intracranial procedures. Complications in this position may include hypotension and hemodynamic instability due to decreased venous return, risk of venous air embolism, quadriplegia in rare cases resulting from cervical spine ischemia with neck and head hyperflexion, sciatic nerve injury from extreme flexion of the hip, as well as tongue and facial swelling from extreme neck flexion (Figure 19.6).

8. Jackknife position: This position is typically used for anorectal procedures and places pressure on the ventral aspect of the head and body, similar to the prone position. Additionally, this position causes decreased venous return due to blood pooling cephalad and distally to the feet, possibly causing hypotension. Corneal abrasions and postoperative vision loss can occur due to facial pressure. Decreased lung volume and expansion may also occur due to increased intrathoracic and intra-abdominal pressure from this position and restricted diaphragm movement. Temporary facial swelling may be present

postprocedure due to patient being in a face-down position with fluid pooling to dependent facial structures (Figure 19.7).

D. Complications of patient positioning.

1. Compression nerve injuries: Specific nerve compression is dependent on the position used and the adequacy of optimal positioning and the optimal and accurate use of padding.

2. Pressure injuries: May start to occur in as little as 60 minutes if patient is not positioned and/or padded adequately and correctly.

3. Cerebral perfusion: Head malpositioning may cause decreased cerebral perfusion and can result in anoxic brain injuries if not properly prevented and/or addressed.

4. Upper airway edema: Particularly occurs when patient is in a steep Trendelenburg position due to fluid dependence and blood pooling cephalad. May necessitate reintubation if severe and clinically indicated.

5. Atelectasis and decreased lung expansion: May occur from most positions apart from the supine position (although it can rarely occur in this position as well). Oxygen desaturation may indicate this. Positive end-expiratory pressure (PEEP) and/or recruitment breaths could be provided prior to extubation to avoid this, and incentive spirometry, coughing, and deep breathing are performed postoperatively.

PRINCIPLES OF ASEPTIC TECHNIQUE

A. Surgical scrub of the surgical team prior to surgery.

  1. Length.

    a. 3 to 5 minutes.

    b. Stroke count method.

  2. Area.

    a. 5 cm above the elbow to the fingertips.

  3. Procedure.

    a. Remove all jewelry from the hands.

    b. Use nail file to clean under the nails.

    c. Always keep the hands higher than the elbow to prevent contamination.

    d. Lather the entire area with soap.

      i. Commonly accepted soaps for scrub: Chlorhexidine or povidone-iodine-containing soaps.

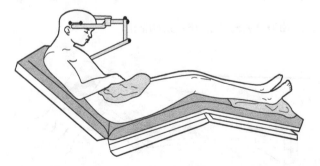

FIGURE 19.6 Sitting/beach chair position.

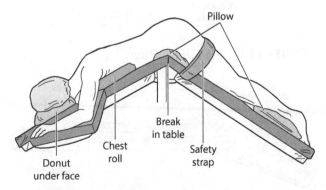

Pillow

Break in table

Chest roll

Safety strap

Donut under face

FIGURE 19.7 Jackknife position.

e. Use warm water. Hot water can destroy a healthy layer of protective skin.

f. Start the scrub from the fingertips and work to the elbows.

i. Rinse from the fingers to the elbow in one direction only.

ii. Scrub each side of the finger and back/front of the hand for 2 minutes (total time).

iii. Scrub from the wrist to the elbow on each arm for 1 minute.

iv. Repeat the process on the other hand and arm.

v. Rinse the hands and arms by passing them through the water in one direction only.

g. Proceed to the operating room with hands up and above the elbows.

h. Once in the operating room, the hands and arms should be dried with a sterile towel and aseptic technique prior to placing on the gown and gloves.

B. Personal sterile field area designation in the operating room.

1. From nipple line to waist: Above or below this area is considered "nonsterile."

2. Only in the front of a person: Anything behind a person is considered "nonsterile."

3. Neck can be contaminated by mask and is not considered a sterile part of the field.

C. Prepping the surgical patient.

1. Skin antisepsis.

a. Decreases the burden of skin flora and reduce the incidence of surgical site infections.

b. Common agents used for antisepsis preparation:

i. Chlorhexidine: The preferred scrub prep for surgeons and assistants.

ii. Povidone-iodine: Must be used when prepping an open wound or mucous membrane, for example, the vagina or rectum.

iii. Iodine and isopropyl alcohol.

iv. Iodine-impregnated adhesive covering (usually applied after another surgical prep agent is applied to the area).

2. Draping.

a. Sterile draping of the surgical field is performed by the surgeon and the surgical assistants/physician assistant/registered nurse first assist in order to:

i. Provide a sterile field.

ii. Provide adequate surgical area exposure.

iii. Cover all nonsterile areas to maintain sterility of the operative field.

WOUND CLASSIFICATIONS

A. Clean: Uninfected wounds without inflammation. This wound is classified clean by not having any breaks in sterility during wound insult, as well as wound not entering and/or progressing into any underlying organs.

B. Clean-contaminated: Controlled entering of the viscus during the sterile procedure with minimal to no contact with pathogens. These wounds have entered an organ(s) with minimal to no spillage of the said organ's contents.

C. Contaminated: Nonsterile wounds that likely have come in contact with pathogens that can cause infection. Examples include:

1. Acute, open wounds from trauma.

2. Major breaks in sterile techniques and/or surgical field.

3. Gross spillage of viscous contents.

D. Dirty: Old, traumatic wounds that often have retained devitalized tissue, pathogen exposure with possible replication, retained foreign objects, or fecal contamination.

WOUND HEALING

A. Primary intention.

1. Used for clean incisions that are not wide in diameter.

2. These wounds are elective and not a result of a traumatic injury.

3. Suturing is performed early, usually within 4 to 8 hours of wound insult.

4. Tissue granulation is promoted due to tension closure of the wound.

5. Minor cosmetic scar will be present postwound closure.

6. These wounds are classified as either clean or clean-contaminated wounds as described above.

B. Secondary intention.

1. Used for wider wounds as well as wounds that will remain fully or partially open without approximation from a provider.

2. Allows granulation tissue to fill the base of the wound with or without later suturing.

a. The key to healing is through granulation of the tissue as opposed to full immediate wound approximation.

3. Larger cosmetic scar present postwound closure.

4. These wounds are a concern for postinsult infections.

5. These wounds are often classified as either contaminated or dirty wounds as described above.

C. Tertiary intention.

1. Used for irregular wounds and can be considered a delayed primary intention.

2. Allows granulation tissue to fill the base of the wound as superficial layers are left open to allow edema and/or infection to run its course and resolve before closure.

3. Used intently to prevent subsequent evisceration and dehiscence if closed before edema and/or infection is still fulminant.

4. Usually larger cosmetic scar(s) will be present postwound closure.

ROLE OF THE FIRST ASSISTANT

A. The main role of a surgical first assistant is to provide support to the primary surgeon(s) during a surgical procedure.

B. The first assistant's scope of practice will vary from state to state and by surgical facility. These roles can be dictated by the surgeon and/or the institution and can include any or all of the following:

1. Providing exposure.
2. Hemostasis.
3. Surgical tying and suturing.
4. Suctioning.

C. First assistants are generally positioned opposite of the surgeon's preferred side or based on the side of the procedure being performed.

DOCUMENTATION REQUIREMENTS

A. What to include in brief operative notes:

1. Procedure: State the actual procedure that was done in completion (can include multiple and/or unintended aspects).
2. Complications: State any and all complications that occurred during the procedure.
3. Intake and output: Document the total fluid administered and the totaled urinary output postprocedure.
4. Estimated blood loss (EBL): Document the communicated EBL that was totaled by the surgeon/proceduralist at the end of the procedure. The EBL can often be a subjective estimation due to totaling lap pads and sponges with blood as well as blood that is mixed with irrigation that is suctioned. Consider underestimation in a hypotensive patient.
5. Postoperative vital signs: Document vital signs at the end of the procedure. Document any interventions that were performed if vitals were not within typical parameters for the patient, case, and level of consciousness.
6. Postoperative checks: Document any specific physical examinations that were completed, that is, assess and document sensation and motor function postspinal procedure.

BIBLIOGRAPHY

Anderson, K., & Hamm, R. (2012). Factors that impair wound healing. *Journal of the American College of Clinical Wound Specialists*, 4(4), 84–91. https://doi.org/10.1016/j.jccw.2014.03.001

Berríos-Torres, S. I., Umscheid, C. A., Bratzler, D. W., Leas, B., Stone, E. C., Kelz, R. R., Reinke, C. E., Morgan, S., Solomkin, J. S., Mazuski, J. E., Dellinger, E. P., Itani, K. M. F., Berbari, E. F., Segreti, J., Parvizi, J., Blanchard, J., Allen, G., Kluytmans, J. A. J. W., Donlan, R., . . . For the Healthcare Infection Control Practices Advisory Committee. (2017). Centers for disease control and prevention guideline for the prevention of surgical site infection. *JAMA Surgery*, 152(8), 784–791. https://doi.org/10.1001/jamasurg.2017.0904

Gardner, D., & Anderson-Manz, E. (2001). How to perform surgical hand scrub. *Infection Control Today*. http://www.infectioncontroltoday.com/articles/2001/05/how-to-perform-surgical-hand-scrubs.aspx

Goodman, T., & Spry, C. (2017). *Essentials of perioperative nursing* (6th ed.). Jones & Bartlett.

Gropper, M. A., & Miller, R. D. (2020). *Miller's anesthesia* (9th ed.). Elsevier.

Jaffe, R. A., Schmiesing, C. A., & Golianu, B. (2020). *Anesthesiologist's manual of surgical procedures*. Wolters Kluwer.

Leaper, D. J. (2006). Traumatic and surgical wounds. *British Medical Journal*, 332(7540), 532–535. https://doi.org/10.1136/bmj.332.7540.532

Nagelhout, J., & Elisha, S. (2018). *Nurse anesthesia* (6th ed.). Elsevier.

Salcido, R. (2017). Healing by intention. *Advances in Skin & Wound Care*, 30(6), 246–247. https://doi.org/10.1097/01.asw.0000516787.46060.b2

Urman, R. D., & Ehrenfeld, J. M. (2021). *Pocket anesthesia* (4th ed.). Wolters Kluwer.

MEDICATION MANAGEMENT

PREOPERATIVE ANTIBIOTICS

A. Antimicrobial prophylaxis to prevent surgical site infections depends on several factors.

1. Type of surgical specialty and/or specific procedure.
2. Safety.
3. Pharmacokinetic and pharmacodynamic profiles.
4. Bactericidal activity.
5. Cost.

B. Given within 60 to 90 minutes of surgical incision to have optimal tissue concentration depending on the antibiotic used, per national standards.

C. Common examples.

1. First-generation cephalosporin: Cefazolin (most widely used antibiotic for surgeries).
2. Second-generation cephalosporin (broader gram-negative coverage): Cefuroxime, cefoxitin, and cefotetan.
3. Penicillin-allergy alternatives: Vancomycin and clindamycin.
4. Metronidazole is often added in bowel cases.

BIBLIOGRAPHY

Anderson, D. J., Podgorny, K., Berríos-Torres, S. I., Bratzler, D. W., Dellinger, E. P., Greene, L., Nyquist, A.-C., Saiman, L., Yokoe, D. S., Maragakis, L. L., & Kaye, K. S. (2014). Strategies to prevent surgical site infections in acute care hospitals: 2014 update. *Infection Control & Hospital Epidemiology*, 35(6), 605–627. https://doi.org/10.1086/676022

Berríos-Torres, S. I., Umscheid, C. A., Bratzler, D. W., Leas, B., Stone, E. C., Kelz, R. R., Reinke, C. E., Morgan, S., Solomkin, J. S., Mazuski, J. E., Dellinger, E. P., Itani, K. M. F., Berbari, E. F., Segreti, J., Parvizi, J., Blanchard, J., Allen, G., Kluytmans, J. A. J. W., Donlan, R., & For the Healthcare Infection Control Practices Advisory Committee. (2017). Centers for disease control and prevention guideline for the prevention of surgical site infection, 2017. *JAMA Surgery*, 152(8), 784–791. https://doi.org/10.1001/jamasurg.2017.0904

Bratzler, D. W., Dellinger, E. P., Olsen, K. M., Perl, T. M., Auwaerter, P. G., Bolon, M. K., Fish, D. N., Napolitano, L. M., Sawyer, R. G., Slain, D., Steinberg, J. P., & Weinstein, R. A. (2013). & American Society of Health-System Pharmacists; Infectious Disease Society of America; Surgical Infection Society. Clinical practice guidelines for antimicrobial prophylaxis in surgery. *Surgical Infections*, 14(1), 73–156. https://doi.org/10.1089/sur.2013.9999

Heuer, A., Kossick, M. A., Riley, J., & Hewer, I. (2017, August). *Update on guidelines for perioperative antibiotic selection and administration from the Surgical Care Improvement Project (SCIP) and American Society of health-system pharmacists*. AANA Journal, 85(4), 293–299. https://pubmed.ncbi.nlm.nih.gov/31566549/

Spruce, L., & Van Wicklin, S. (2014). Back to basics: Positioning the patient. *AORN Journal*, 100, 299–303. https://doi.org/10.1016/j.aorn.2014.06.004

CHAPTER 20

POSTOPERATIVE EVALUATION AND MANAGEMENT

William A. Edwards, Jr.

SCOPE OF CHAPTER

The postoperative period is a vulnerable time for the patient. The advanced practice provider (APP) must perform a timely physical assessment, anticipate postoperative complications, manage surgical wounds, and treat pain. This section provides an overview on managing patients during this time frame.

OUTCOMES

A. Patient assessment.
B. Postoperative complications.
C. Wound healing.
D. Pain management.

PATIENT ASSESSMENT

A. Patient assessment.
  1. Physical examination.
  2. Vital signs.
  3. Skin integrity.
  4. Pain management.
B. Two phases of the recovery process and the postanesthesia care unit (PACU).
  1. Phase I: Patient assessment ensuring that a patient recovers fully from anesthetic agents, has an appropriate level of arousal, maintains reflexes, and has return of normal vital signs; includes pain management and monitoring for postoperative complications.
  2. Phase II: Focuses on wound assessment, patient comfort, review of medications, maintaining normal and appropriate functioning and reflexes, urine output, control of bleeding, and discharge home if an outpatient procedure was performed or hand-off to the nurse from an inpatient unit.
C. Hand-off communication.
  1. Communication between the operating room (OR) and PACU is critical and should contain the following elements at minimum:
    a. Type of anesthesia used during the procedure.
    b. Type of procedure performed and duration.
    c. Medications given in the OR.
    d. Positioning of patient.

e. Intake and output, including the amount of estimated blood loss and the desired urinary status.
    f. Complications or unusual events during the procedure.
    g. Wound closure status, type, and/or device used for closure.
    h. Types of dressings, lines, and monitoring devices.
    i. Clinical presentation, care directives, and orders listed immediately below.
D. Postoperative orders for inpatient stays.
  1. Admit to team, physician, and type of unit.
  2. Diagnosis and procedure performed.
  3. Postoperative condition.
  4. Allergies.
  5. Vital signs and frequency.
  6. Activity.
  7. Any specific nursing procedures, such as wound care, when to notify house officer and/or surgeon, and incentive spirometry.
  8. Deep vein thrombosis (DVT) prophylaxis.
  9. Intake and output, intravenous (IV) fluids, and drains with maintenance care, for example, chest tubes.
  10. Medications.
  11. Any special laboratory tests and when they should be drawn.
  12. Radiology per surgeon and/or team for postoperative evaluations of procedure.
  13. Pain management types(s) frequency and/or consult.
  14. Enhanced recovery after surgery (ERAS) guidelines.
    a. Diet: Patients should be advanced to oral nutrition within the first 24 hours of uncomplicated surgery. Consider oral supplements with meals if unable to tolerate food.
    b. Early intake of oral fluids: Offer day of surgery.
    c. Early removal of urinary catheters and discontinuing IV fluids.
    d. Early ambulation: Ambulate patient day of surgery as tolerated.
    e. Multimodal approach to pain management: Provide opioid-sparing pain control and mitigate nausea and vomiting; use additional classes of medications and other pain management modalities (e.g., blocks, positioning).
    f. Early discharge when possible.

▶

15. Oxygen requirements and type of delivery.
16. Consults such as physical therapy, social work, and dietitian.

COMMON POSTOPERATIVE COMPLICATIONS
A. Pulmonary.
  1. Tachypnea (respiratory rate >30 breaths per minute).
    a. Inadequate pain control.
      i. Supplemental analgesia if inadequate pain control.
    b. Laryngospasm.
      i. Jaw thrust/chin lift and sustained positive pressure ventilation to promote airflow. Notify anesthesia and/or respiratory for additional assistance.
    c. Airway edema.
      i. May need to be intubated/reintubated for airway protection.
    d. Negative pressure pulmonary edema.
      i. Provide positive pressure ventilation and possibly furosemide 20 to 40 mg IV.
    e. Pulmonary embolism.
      i. Management depends on cardiopulmonary compromise and anticoagulation status.
    f. Fever.
      i. Add fluids and antipyretics as needed. Assess for signs and symptoms (s/s) of infection if clinically indicated.
  2. Bradypnea (respiratory rate <8 breaths per minute).
    a. Oversedated from anesthesia, benzodiazepine, or opioid use; typically seen in PACU setting.
      i. Consider adding opioid and/or benzodiazepine reversal agents if oversedated (naloxone and/or Romazicon, respectively).
B. Cardiovascular.
  1. Hypotension (systolic blood pressure <90 mmHg, mean arterial pressure [MAP] <65 mmHg).
    a. Most often due to volume depletion, anesthetic medications (opioids, benzodiazepines, propofol), regional anesthesia techniques, and drug reactions to antibiotics.
    b. Management: Give crystalloid bolus, may start with 250 mL to 500 mL, and reassess blood pressure. Repeat as needed to maintain adequate blood pressure and urine output. May need to add vasopressors if nonresponsive to fluids. Review anesthesia record for accurate reflection of intake and output, current medications the patient is on (especially angiotensin-converting enzyme [ACE] inhibitors, angiotensin receptor blockers [ARB] inhibitors, and steroids), as well as baselines in blood pressure and the use of vasopressors intraoperatively.
  2. Hypertension.
    a. Most commonly due to inadequate pain control and agitation emerging from anesthesia.
    b. Management: Provide analgesia to maintain blood pressure within defined parameters and possibly provide an agent for agitation, such as midazolam or dexmedetomidine.
    c. Review current and home medications, including antihypertensives. Evaluate the efficacy and accuracy of medication therapies to determine if this may contribute to postoperative hypertension.
  3. Dysrhythmias.
    a. Tachycardia (heart rate >100 beats per minute).
      i. Typically due to pain, hypovolemia, fever, or anemia from blood loss.
    b. Bradycardia (heart rate <40 beats per minute).
      i. Usually due to reversal agent for neuromuscular blockade, such as neostigmine, dexmedetomidine, or regional anesthesia techniques.
      ii. Hypoxemia and myocardial infarction can also cause bradycardia. Assess for s/s.
    c. Atrial fibrillation, atrial flutter, and ventricular tachycardia should be managed by advanced cardiac life support (ACLS) algorithms and/or cardiology consult, especially if new onset. For more information, refer to Chapter 3.
C. Gastrointestinal.
  1. Nausea/vomiting.
    a. Most common postoperative complication.
    b. Often rated worse than pain by patients.
  2. Management with head of bed elevation, fluids, and antiemetic agents.
  3. Antiemetic medication options.
    a. Serotonin receptor agonists: Ondansetron 4 mg IV.
    b. Glucocorticoids: Dexamethasone 4 to 8 mg IV.
    c. Anticholinergics: Scopolamine patch, ideally at least 2 hours prior to surgery.
    d. Phenothiazines: Promethazine 6.25 to 12.5 mg IV.
    e. Butyrophenones: Droperidol 0.625 mg IV or Haldol 1 to 2 mg IV.
D. Genitourinary.
  1. Acute renal failure.
    a. Persistent oliguria and elevated creatinine.
    b. Management.
      i. May need diuretics if fluid overloaded.
      ii. Need to balance effective circulating volume with output.
      iii. Avoid nephrotoxic agents.
      iv. Avoid contrast agents.
      v. Consider hemodialysis or continuous renal replacement therapy (CRRT) if clinically indicated to prevent further renal injury, remove fluid from overload, manage electrolytes, and prevent further patient compromise.
  2. Urinary infection.
    a. Management.
      i. Early removal of urinary catheter.
      ii. Maintain adequate hydration.
      iii. Early ambulation.

iv. Antibiotic coverage per organism sensitivity and/or infectious disease consult.

3. Postoperative urinary retention (POUR).
   a. Risk greater in patients who:
      i. Have neuropathy or neurologic damage.
      ii. Have chronic constipation.
      iii. Take anticholinergic medications.
      iv. Had bladder or anorectal procedures.
      v. Had long duration of anesthesia.
      vi. Use of opioid medications.
      vii. Male sex assigned at birth.
   b. Strategies to reduce risk:
      i. Adequate hydration perioperatively.
      ii. Early mobilization.
      iii. Use of commode.
      iv. Consider cessation of offending agent if applicable.
      v. May consider use of alpha-1 antagonist (e.g., tamsulosin).

4. Metabolic derangements.
   a. Monitor and replace electrolytes to maintain normal values.
      i. Potassium.
      ii. Magnesium.
      iii. Phosphorous.
   b. Maintain acid base balance.
   c. Observe IV fluid type and quantity administered.
   d. Observe serum lactate level.

E. Postoperative pain control.
   1. Early intervention, multimodal management, and optimal pain management provisions are essential.
   2. Untreated surgical pain can limit cough and deep breathing, which contribute to a decrease in alveolar ventilation and increase in atelectasis.
   3. Inadequate relief may result in psychological derangements such as:
      a. Minor to severe depression.
      b. Pain-related catastrophizing.
      c. Chronic postsurgical pain syndromes.

F. Neuropsychiatric.
   1. Transient ischemic attack or stroke.
      a. Avoid ischemia: DVT prophylaxis and anticoagulation as indicated.
      b. Avoid hypotension or hypertension: Address pain and hemodynamic status.
   2. Delirium during emergence is highest during the first hour postanesthesia.
      a. Management.
         i. Reassurance with familiar family/friends at the bedside.
         ii. Assess for signs of uncontrolled pain and treat.
         iii. Consider low-dose benzodiazepine for anxiolysis and/or disorientation.
   3. Discharge from PACU.
      a. Postanesthetic Discharge Scoring System (PADSS): Score of 9 or greater can be safely discharged to the accepting unit (Box 20.1).

G. Fever.
   1. Fever is a common complication after surgery that can be attributed to many different causes. Always consider the following with associated "Ws":
      a. Fever immediately after surgery.
         i. Atelectasis ("Wind").
         ii. Medication reactions ("Wonder drugs").
         iii. Endocrine emergencies ("Wonky glands").
      b. Fever 48 to 72 hours after surgery.
         i. Urinary tract infection ("Water").
         ii. Wound infection ("Wound").
         iii. DVT ("Walking").
         iv. Alcohol or drug reactions ("Withdrawal").

H. DVT.
   1. Patients should be encouraged to ambulate as early and as often as safely possible.
      a. Improves mobility and pulmonary function, prevents atelectasis, and prevents DVT.

BOX 20.1 POSTANESTHETIC DISCHARGE SCORING SYSTEM

Vital Signs

0 = Blood pressure and pulse ≥40% preoperative baseline
1 = Blood pressure and pulse 20%–40% preoperative baseline
2 = Blood pressure and pulse <20% preoperative baseline

Activity

0 = Unable to ambulate

1 = Requires assistance

2 = Ambulates without assistance, no dizziness

Nausea and Vomiting

0 = Severe/continuous despite treatment

1 = Moderate/treated with parenteral medications

2 = Minimal/treated with oral medications

Pain Controlled With Oral Analgesics and Acceptable by Patient

1 = No

2 = Yes

Surgical Bleeding

0 = Severe, or ≥3 dressing changes

1 = Moderate, or up to 2 dressing changes

2 = Minimal, or no dressing changes

Source: Reproduced with permission from Chung, F., Ghan, V. W. S., & Ong, D. (1995). A post-anesthetic discharge scoring system for home readiness after ambulatory surgery. *Journal of Clinical Anesthesia, 7*, 500–506. https://doi.org/10.1016/0952-8180(95)00130-A.

2. Optimal timing for pharmacologic thromboprophylaxis in nonorthopedic patients is unknown and should be individualized.

3. If risk of bleeding is low, pharmacologic agents can begin 2 to 12 hours preoperatively.

4. Initiate pharmacologic treatment for DVT prevention in patients not considered suitable for preoperative pharmacologic thromboprophylaxis or who have a high risk of bleeding 2 to 72 hours postoperatively.

    a. Low-dose unfractionated heparin.

    b. Low molecular weight heparin.

    c. Factor Xa inhibitors and direct thrombin inhibitors are used less commonly for DVT prophylaxis and more frequently in patients with allergy to heparin or in some vascular patients for full treatment.

5. Sequential compression devices (SCDs) or compression stockings can/should be used per individualized clinical presentation and/or hospital policy/protocol.

6. The Modified Caprini Risk Assessment Score provides an individualized risk assessment for DVT prevention (Table 20.1).

BIBLIOGRAPHY

Aarts, M. A., Okrainec, A., Glicksman, A., Pearsall, E., Victor, J. C., & McLeod, R. S. (2012). Adoption of enhanced recovery after surgery (ERAS) strategies for colorectal surgery at academic teaching hospitals and impact on total length of hospital stay. *Surgical Endoscopy, 26*(2), 442–450. https://doi.org/10.1007/s00464-011-1897-5

Apfel, C. C., Korttila, K., & Abdalla, M. (2004). A factorial trial of six interventions for the prevention of postoperative nausea and vomiting. *The New England Journal of Medicine, 350*(24), 2441–2451. https://doi.org/10.1056/NEJMoa032196

TABLE 20.1   MODIFIED CAPRINI RISK ASSESSMENT SCORE

1 Point	2 Points	3 Points	4 Points
Age 41–60 years	Age 61–74 years	Age ≥75 years	Stroke within 1 month
Minor surgery	Arthroscopic surgery	History of VTE	Elective arthroplasty
BMI ≥25	Major open surgery	Family history of VTE	Pelvis, hip, or leg fracture
Swollen legs	Laparoscopic surgery	Genetic clotting disorder	Acute spinal cord injury
Varicose veins	Malignancy		
Pregnancy/postpartum	Confined to bed >72 hours		
History of spontaneous abortion	Lower extremity immobilization		
Oral hormone medication	Central venous access		
History of sepsis <1 month			
Underlying lung disease			
Abnormal pulmonary function			
History of AMI			
CHF			
History of IBD			

Score	Surgical Risk	Intervention for DVT Prevention
0	Very low	Early mobilization
1–2	Low	Early mobilization + mechanical compression devices
3–4	Moderate	Pharmacologic prophylaxis
≥5	High	

AMI, acute myocardial infarction; BMI, body mass index; CHF, congestive heart failure; DVT, deep vein thrombosis; IBD, inflammatory bowel disease; VTE, venous thromboembolism.
Sources: Data from Caprini, J. A. (2005). Thrombosis risk assessment as a guide to quality patient care. *Disease-a-Month, 51,* 70–78. https://doi.org/10.1016/j.disamonth.2005.02.003; Kearon, C., Akl, E., Ornelas, J., Blaivas, A., Jimenez, D., Bounameaux, H., Huisman, M., King, C. S., Morris, T. A., Sood, N., Stevens, S. M., Vintch, J. R. E., Wells, P., Woller, S. C., & Moores, L. (2016). Antithrombotic therapy for VTE disease. CHEST Guideline and expert panel report. *Chest, 149,* 315–352. https://doi.org/10.1016/j.chest.2015.11.026.

Apfelbaum, J. L., Silverstein, J. H., & Chung, F. F. (2013). Practice guidelines for postanesthetic care: An updated report by the American Society of Anesthesiologists task force on postanesthetic care. *Anesthesiology, 118*(2), 291–307. https://doi.org/10.1097/ALN.0b013e31827773e9

Caprini, J. A. (2005). Thrombosis risk assessment as a guide to quality patient care. *Disease-a-Month, 51*, 70–78. https://doi.org/10.1016/j.disamonth.2005.02.003

Caprini, J. A. (2010). Risk assessment as a guide for the prevention of the many faces of venous thromboembolism. *American Journal of Surgery, 199*(Suppl. 1), S3–S10. https://doi.org/10.1016/j.amjsurg.2009.10.006

Chung, F., Ghan, V. W. S., & Ong, D. (1995). A post-anesthetic discharge scoring system for home readiness after ambulatory surgery. *Journal of Clinical Anesthesia, 7*, 500–506. https://doi.org/10.1016/0952-8180(95)00130-A

Gan, T., Tramer, M., Watcha, M., Krenke, P., Kovac, A., Habib, A., & Diemunsch, P. (2014). Consensus guidelines for the management of postoperative nausea and vomiting. *Anesthesia & Analgesia, 118*(3), 689. https://doi.org/10.1213/ane.0000000000000140

Gould, M. K., Garcia, D. A., Wren, S. M., Karanicolas, P. J., Arcelus, J. I., Heit, J. A., & Samama, C. M. (2012). Prevention of VTE in non-orthopedic surgical patients antithrombotic therapy and prevention of thrombosis, 9th ed: American College of Chest Physicians evidence-based clinical practice guidelines. *Chest, 141*(2), e227S–e277S. https://doi.org/10.1378/chest.11-2297

Heuer, A., Kossick, M. A., Riley, J., & Hewer, I. (2017, August). *Update on guidelines for perioperative antibiotic selection and administration from the Surgical Care Improvement Project (SCIP) and American Society of health-system pharmacists. AANA Journal.* https://pubmed.ncbi.nlm.nih.gov/31566549/

Kearon, C., Akl, E., Ornelas, J., Blaivas, A., Jimenez, D., Bounameaux, H., Huisman, M., King, C. S., Morris, T. A., Sood, N., Stevens, S. M., Vintch, J. R. E., Wells, P., Woller, S. C., & Moores, L. (2016). Antithrombotic therapy for VTE disease. CHEST Guideline and expert panel report. *Chest, 149*, 315–352. https://doi.org/10.1016/j.chest.2015.11.026

Macario, A., Weinger, M., Carney, S., & Kim, A. (1999). Which clinical anesthesia outcomes are important to avoid? The perspective of patients. *Anesthesia and Analgesia, 89*(3), 652–658.

Maday, K. R., Hurt, J. B., Harrelson, P., & Porterfield, J. (2016). Evaluating postoperative fever. *Journal of the American Academy of PAs, 29*(10), 23–28. https://doi.org/10.1097/01.JAA.0000496951.72463.de

Nagelhout, J., & Elisha, S. (2018). *Nurse anesthesia* (6th ed.). Elsevier.

Whitlock, E. L., Vannucci, A., & Avidan, M. S. (2011). Postoperative delirium. *Minerva Anesiologica, 7*(4), 448–456.

WOUND MANAGEMENT

INFECTION PREVENTION

A. Surgical site infections (SSI).

  1. Can be superficial (skin/subcutaneous tissue), deep (muscle/fascia), or organ- and surrounding space-specific.

  2. Occurs within 30 days of surgery.

  3. Majority of cases of SSI superficial infections (83%), deep infections (7%), and the rest are organ-specific infections.

  4. Factors associated with SSI:

    a. Previous surgery.

    b. Prolonged surgery time.

    c. Hypoalbuminemia.

    d. History of chronic obstructive pulmonary disease (COPD).

    e. Obesity.

    f. Diabetes.

    g. American Society of Anesthesiologists (ASA) score.

    h. Wounds classified as "dirty."

    i. Type of surgical procedure, such as bowel surgery, may increase risk of infection.

  5. Organisms associated with SSI:

    a. Staphylococci.

    b. Streptococci.

    c. Enteric bacilli, enterococci.

    d. *Pseudomonas*.

    e. Clostridia.

    f. *Mycobacterium tuberculosis*.

    g. Multidrug-resistant organisms.

  6. Prevention strategies:

    a. Standard precautions.

    b. Perioperative antibiotics.

      i. Administer within 60 to 90 minutes of skin incision dependent on type of antibiotic.

      ii. Discontinue within 24 hours, as clinically indicated.

    c. Clip operative site and avoid shaving.

    d. Control of perioperative glucose values greater than 180 mg/dL.

    e. Aseptic technique.

B. Classification of surgical wounds.

  1. Class I: Clean—uninfected operative wound.

  2. Class II: Clean-contaminated—operative wound in which respiratory, alimentary, genital, or urinary tracts are entered under controlled conditions.

  3. Class III: Contaminated—open, fresh, accidental wounds; major breaks in sterile technique; gross spillage from gastrointestinal tract; incisions in acute nonpurulent inflammation is encountered.

  4. Class IV: Dirty/infected—old traumatic wounds with retained devitalized tissue and those that involve existing clinical infection or perforated viscera; organisms present before procedure.

C. Wound healing.

  1. Classified by etiology.

    a. Surgical.

    b. Traumatic.

  2. Classified by initial presentation.

    a. Closed wound (preferred).

    b. Open wound (based on amount of tissue lost).

  3. Types of wound healing.

    a. Primary intention: Wound is clean; little loss of tissue.

      i. Preferred technique.

      ii. Heals quickly with minimal scarring.

    b. Secondary intention: Occurs in open wounds due to difficulty of reapproximating edges secondary to the amount of tissue loss.

      i. Granulation tissue fills the defect.

      ii. Healing takes longer.

      iii. Results in more scarring.

        1) May inhibit normal physiologic function in that area.

c. Tertiary intention.
    i. Delayed primary closure.
    ii. Cannot close wound due to concern for infection and/or edema.
    iii. Wound remains open until resolution of infection and/or edema.
    iv. Increased granulation and inflammatory reaction compared with primary intention.

4. Factors that delay wound healing.
  a. Age.
  b. Immunosuppressed states.
    i. HIV/AIDS.
    ii. Diabetes.
    iii. Cancer.
  c. Autoimmune disorders.
  d. Altered nutritional status.
  e. Smoking.
  f. Anemia.
  g. Inadequate oxygenation (e.g., COPD).
  h. Vascular disease.

5. Medications that impair wound healing.
  a. Anticoagulants.
  b. Anti-inflammatory agents (aspirin, nonsteroidal anti-inflammatory drugs [NSAIDs]).
  c. Steroids.
  d. Colchicine.

6. Herbal medicines that may impair wound healing.
  a. Ephedra: Increases heart rate and blood pressure.
  b. Feverfew: Inhibits platelet activity.
  c. Garlic: Inhibits platelet aggregation.
  d. Gingko: Inhibits platelet activation.
  e. Nicotine: Impairs oxygen delivery.

D. Wound assessment.
  1. Dressings.
    a. Applied under sterile conditions in the operating room (OR).
    b. Prevent contamination of wound.
    c. Protect wound from further trauma.
    d. Absorb exudate.
    e. Provide physical support.
    f. Assist in wound closure (e.g., wound vacuum-assisted closure [VAC]).
  2. High-risk patients may require wound care consult.
  3. Compressive wraps must not impair blood flow.
    a. Assess for:
      i. Pulses.
      ii. Cyanosis.
      iii. Capillary refill.
      iv. Temperature of body around dressing.
  4. Types of dressings.
    a. Primary intention closure.
      i. Transparent polyurethane dressings.
        1) Protect wound.
        2) Check incision site without disturbing the dressing.
        3) Can be left in place for 3 to 5 days.

      ii. Semipermeable films.
        1) Provides a barrier against bacteria.
      iii. Surgical glue.
    b. Secondary intention closure.
      i. Alginates.
        1) Maintain moist wound surface.
        2) Removal of cellular debris.
      ii. Polyurethane foams.
        1) Absorbent.
        2) Maintain optimum healing environment.
        3) Reduce trauma during dressing changes.
      iii. Hydrocolloids.
        1) Absorbent.
        2) Maintain moist wound surface.
      iv. Hydrogels.
        1) Rehydration of tissues.
        2) Some absorbency.
      v. Low-adherent wound contact layers.
        1) Minimize risk of trauma on wound surface.
        2) Decrease pain during dressing change.
      vi. Antimicrobial carrying dressings.
        1) Stimulate the immune system for wound healing.

BIBLIOGRAPHY

Anderson, K., & Hamm, R. (2012). Factors that impair wound healing. *Journal of the American College of Clinical Wound Specialists, 4*(4), 84–91. https://doi.org/10.1016/j.jccw.2014.03.001

Berríos-Torres, S. I., Umscheid, C. A., Bratzler, D. W., Leas, B., Stone, E. C., Kelz, R. R., Reinke, C. E., Morgan, S., Solomkin, J. S., Mazuski, J. E., Dellinger, E. P., Itani, K. M. F., Berbari, E. F., Segreti, J., Parvizi, J., Blanchard, J., Allen, G., Kluytmans, J. A. J. W., Donlan, R., . . . for the Healthcare Infection Control Practices Advisory Committee. (2017). Centers for disease control and prevention guideline for the prevention of surgical site infection. *JAMA Surgery, 152*(8), 784–791. https://doi.org/10.1001/jamasurg.2017.0904

Dumville, J., Gray, T., Walter, C., Sharp, C., Page, T., Macefield, R., Blencowe, N., Milne, T. K., Reeves, B. C., & Blazeby, J. (2016). Dressings for the prevention of surgical site infection. *Cochrane Database of Systematic Reviews, 2016*(12). https://doi.org/10.1002/14651858.CD003091.pub4

Heuer, A., Kossick, M. A., Riley, J., & Hewer, I. (2017, August). *Update on guidelines for perioperative antibiotic selection and administration from the Surgical Care Improvement Project (SCIP) and American Society of health-system pharmacists. AANA Journal.* https://pubmed.ncbi.nlm.nih.gov/31566549/

Maver, T., Maver, U., Kleinschek, S., Smrke, D., & Kreft, S. (2015). A review of herbal medicines in wound healing. *International Journal of Dermatology, 54*(7), 740–751. https://doi.org/10.1111/ijd.12766

Mu, Y., Edwards, J. R., Horan, T. C., Berrios-Torres, S. I., & Fridkin, S. K. (2011). Improving risk-adjusted measures of surgical site infection for the National Healthcare Safety Network. *Infection Control & Hospital Epidemiology, 32*(10), 970–986. https://doi.org/10.1086/662016

National Collaborating Centre for Women's and Children's Health (UK). (2008). *Surgical site infection: Prevention and treatment of surgical site infection.* RCOG Press.

National Healthcare Safety Network, Centers for Disease Control and Prevention. (2019, January). *Surgical site infection (SSI) event.* http://www.cdc.gov/nhsn/pdfs/pscmanual/9pscssicurrent.pdf

Salcido, R. (2017). Healing by intention. *Advances in Skin & Wound Care, 30*(6), 246–247. https://doi.org/10.1097/01.asw.0000516787.46060.b2

MEDICATION MANAGEMENT

PAIN MANAGEMENT

A. Should be a multimodal approach.

B. Types of pain.

  1. Nociceptive pain.

    a. Somatic pain: Associated mostly with surgery; results from damage to connective tissue, muscle, bone, and skin.

    b. Visceral pain: Associated with pain in internal organs.

  2. Can be described as aching, pressure, or sharp.

  3. Associated with periosteum, joints, muscle injury, colic, and muscle spasm.

  4. Can have effects on various systems such as:

    a. Cardiovascular: Increased heart rate and blood pressure.

    b. Pulmonary: Decreased deep breathing, increased atelectasis, and increased oxygen demand.

    c. Endocrine: Decreased insulin production and fluid retention.

    d. Metabolic: Increased blood sugar.

    e. Gastrointestinal: Delayed gastric emptying, nausea, decreased motility, and potential for ileus.

  5. Neuropathic pain: May result from injury to the nerves during surgery.

  6. Psychogenic pain: May be due to psychological factors that exaggerate pain response.

C. Assessment of pain.

  1. Wong–Baker Visual Analog Scale: Uses pictures to help patients express how much pain they are in.

  2. Numerical Rating Scale: Rating scale that rates pain from 0 to 10, with 0 being no pain and 10 being the worst pain imaginable.

  3. Verbal Rating Scale: Patient reports pain on four possible points: No pain, mild pain, moderate pain, and severe pain.

  4. Elements of pain assessment:

    a. Onset and pattern of pain.

    b. Location.

    c. Quality of pain.

    d. Intensity of pain.

    e. Aggravating or relieving factors.

    f. Previous treatment.

    g. Effect on physical function and emotional distress.

    h. Consider barriers that might affect reliability of pain assessment.

D. Nonpharmacologic management of pain.

  1. Relaxation therapy.

  2. Hypnosis.

  3. Cold or heat.

  4. Splinting of wounds.

  5. Compression binders.

  6. Teach patient about benefits of transcutaneous electrical nerve stimulation (TENS unit) and acupuncture in the outpatient setting.

E. Pharmacologic management of pain.

  1. World Health Organization (WHO) analgesic ladder.

    a. Mild pain: Nonopioids.

    b. Moderate pain: Use weak opioids with or without nonopioids.

    c. Severe pain: Use strong opioids with or without nonopioids.

  2. Pain medication options.

    a. Nonopioids.

      i. NSAIDs: Use cautiously due to their antiplatelet effect, concern for delayed bone healing, and an occurrence of acute renal failure. Caution in older adults; may need to adjust doses.

      ii. NSAIDs such as ketorolac are commonly used after major orthopedic surgery and spine surgery. They are highly effective but carry the perceived risk of increased bleeding. To date there are NO human studies that exist to support this belief, only animal studies. NSAID use remains controversial after surgery.

        1) Ketorolac: 15 to 30 mg every 6 × 48 hours.

        2) Ibuprofen: 800 mg Q8H.

        3) Diclofenac: 50 mg Q8H.

      iii. Acetaminophen: 1,000 mg Q6H; maximum dosage per day is 4 g in a patient without liver dysfunction.

      iv. Adjuvant medications.

        1) Steroids such as dexamethasone.

        2) Antidepressants such as nortriptyline, desipramine, and amitriptyline.

        3) Anticonvulsants: Gabapentin, pregabalin, and carbamazepine.

        4) N-methyl-D-aspartate (NMDA) receptor antagonists for neuropathic pain: Ketamine boluses and/or infusion.

        5) Cannabinoids.

        6) Lidocaine patch.

        7) Lidocaine infusion.

        8) Magnesium bolus infusions.

    b. Opioids: Weak.

      i. Codeine oral 30 mg every 4 to 6 hours.

      ii. Tramadol oral 50 to 100 mg every 4 to 6 hours.

      iii. Propoxyphene oral 100 mg Q4H.

      iv. Oxycodone low-dose oral 5 mg every 4 to 6 hours.

      v. Hydrocodone oral 5 to 10 mg every 4 to 6 hours.

        1) Contains acetaminophen and needs to be calculated in 4 g/d limit.

    c. Opioids: Strong.

      i. Morphine IV 2 to 10 mg Q3H.

      ii. Fentanyl IV 25 mg per hour for breakthrough pain.

iii. Hydromorphone IV 1 to 2 mg Q3H.
  1) In opioid-naïve and older patients, consider starting with 0.25 to 0.5 mg.
iv. Oxycodone high-dose oral: 10 to 15 mg Q4H.
d. Special considerations of opioid use in older adults.
  i. Start with low doses.
  ii. Consider longer dosing intervals.
  iii. Slow titration to find optimal dose.
e. Interventional therapy.
  i. Nerve blocks.
  ii. Epidural analgesia with or without opioids.
  iii. Spinal analgesia (intrathecal opioid).

F. Delivery of pain medications.
  1. Oral is the preferred route of delivery for patients who can take oral medications.
    a. Scheduled.
    b. As needed (PRN).
  2. Subcutaneous.
    a. Good absorption.
    b. Onset more rapid.
    c. Can have longer duration of action.
    d. Be aware that absorption may be unpredictable, especially if the peripheries are poorly perfused.
  3. Intravenous (IV) push.
    a. Scheduled.
    b. PRN.
  4. Patient-controlled analgesia (PCA) pumps.
    a. Used when parenteral route is needed for systemic analgesia for more than a few hours.
    b. Avoid basal rate in opioid-naïve adults.

c. Dosed until pain is relieved or patient becomes symptomatic: Increased somnolence, apnea, hypoxemia, and/or hypotension.

BIBLIOGRAPHY

American Society of Anesthesiologists Task Force on Acute Pain Management. (2012). Practice guidelines for acute pain management in the perioperative setting: An updated report by the American society of anesthesiologists task force on acute pain management anesthesiology. *Anesthesiology*, 116(2), 248–273. https://doi.org/10.1097/ALN.0b013e31823c1030

Buvanedran, A., & Kroin, J. S. (2009). Multimodal analgesia for controlling acute postoperative pain. *Current Opinion Anesthesiology*, 22(5), 588–593. https://doi.org/10.1097/ACO.0b013e328330373a

Dahl, J. B., Nielsen, R. V., Wetterslev, J., Nikolajsen, L., Hamunen, K., Kontinen, V. K., Hansen, M. S., Kjer, J. J., & Mathiesen, O. (2014). & Scandinavian Postoperative Pain Alliance (ScaPAlli). Postoperative analgesic effects of paracetamol, NSAID's, glucocorticoids, gabapentinoids and their combination: A topical review. *Acta Anaesthesiologica Scandinavica*, 58(10), 1165–1181. https://doi.org/10.1111/aas.12382

DeCosmo, G. (2015). The use of NSAIDs in the postoperative period: Advantages and disadvantages. *Journal of Anesthesia & Critical Care*, 3(4), 00107. https://doi.org/10.15406/jaccoa.2015.03.00107

Do, S.-H. (2013). Magnesium: A versatile drug for anesthesiologists. *Korean Journal of Anesthesiology*, 65(1), 4. https://doi.org/10.4097/kjae.2013.65.1.4

Garimella, V., & Cellini, C. (2013). Postoperative pain control. *Clinics Colon Rectal Surgery*, 26(3), 191–196. https://doi.org/10.1055/s-0033-1351138

Nagelhout, J., & Elisha, S. (2018). *Nurse anesthesia* (6th ed.). Elsevier.

Roden, A., & Sturman, E. (2009). Assessment & management of patients with wound-related pain. *Nursing Standard*, 23(45), 53–62. https://doi.org/10.7748/ns.23.45.53.s52

Shin, H.-J., Na, H.-S., & Do, S.-H. (2020). Magnesium and pain. *Nutrients*, 12(8), 2184. https://doi.org/10.3390/nu12082184

World Health Organization. (2009). *WHO's pain relief ladder*. http://www.who.int/cancer/palliative/painladder/en

World Union of Wound Healing Societies. (2007). *Principles of best practice: Minimizing pain at wound dressing-related procedures. A consensus document*. WoundPedia.

SECTION III

PROCEDURES

- Ankle Brachial Index Measurement
- Arterial Lines
- Bone Marrow Aspiration and Biopsy
- Bronchoscopy
- Central Venous Access
- Chest Tube Insertion
- Chest Tube Removal
- Digital Nerve Blocks
- Extracorporeal Membrane Oxygenation
- Endotracheal Intubation
- Endotracheal Extubation
- External Ventricular Drain
- Intraosseous Vascular Access
- Long Leg Casting
- Lumbar Puncture
- Peripherally Inserted Central Catheter Placement
- Reduction of the Ankles
- Reduction of the Fingers
- Reduction of the Hips
- Reduction of the Patella
- Reduction of the Shoulder
- Splinting
- Synovial Fluid Aspiration
- Thoracentesis
- Transpyloric Feeding Tube Placement

ANKLE BRACHIAL INDEX MEASUREMENT

Cara Staley

DESCRIPTION
A. A tool used to objectively detect the presence of lower extremity peripheral arterial disease (PAD).
B. Compares the blood pressure measured in the ankles with that of the arms.

INDICATIONS
A. Primary care setting.
  1. Used in a symptomatic patient to diagnose PAD.
  2. Used in an asymptomatic patient to assess the vascular risk for PAD.
B. Emergency or trauma setting.
  1. Useful to evaluate patients at risk of lower extremity arterial injury, as follows:
    a. An ankle brachial index (ABI) less than 0.90 suggests a need for further vascular imaging: Angiography in a stable patient and operative exploration in an unstable patient.
    b. An ABI greater than 0.90 decreases the likelihood of an arterial injury; thus, the patient may be observed with serial ABI assessments or may undergo a vascular study on a delayed basis.

PRECAUTIONS
A. ABI measurement is contraindicated in the following patients:
  1. Patients with deep vein thrombosis. Obtaining an ABI measurement could lead to a thrombus dislodgement.
  2. Patients with excruciating pain in their legs.

EQUIPMENT REQUIRED
A. Blood pressure cuff: Appropriate size for upper and lower extremities.
B. Sphygmomanometer.
C. Doppler device.
D. Ultrasound transmission gel.
E. Examination table.

PROCEDURE
A. Place the patient in the supine position with the arms and legs at the same level as the heart, for a minimum of 10 minutes before measurement.
B. Obtain brachial systolic pressures of both arms using the Doppler device.
C. Choose the higher of the two values as the "brachial systolic pressure."
D. Obtain the posterior tibial and dorsalis pedis systolic pressures of the extremity in question and choose the higher of the two values as the "ankle pressure measurement" (Figure III.1).
E. Divide the ankle pressure by the brachial artery pressure; the result is the ABI.

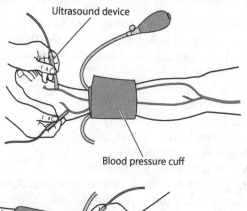
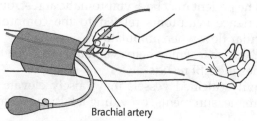

FIGURE III.1 Ankle brachial index test.

EVALUATION AND RESULTS
A. Values obtained for the ABI are interpreted in Table III.1.

CLINICAL PEARLS
A. Patients who are unable to remain supine for the duration of the examination are not candidates for an adequate ABI.

TABLE III.1 INTERPRETATION OF VALUES OBTAINED FOR ABI

ABI Reading	Interpretation of ABI for PAD
1.00–1.29	Normal
0.91–0.99	Borderline
0.41–0.90	Mild to moderate disease: Sufficient to cause claudication
≤0.40	Severe disease: Sufficient to cause resting pain or gangrene
≥1.30	Noncompressible disease: Severely calcified vessel

ABI, ankle brachial index; PAD, peripheral arterial disease.
Source: Data from Rooke, T. W., Hirsch, A. T., Misra, S., Sidawy, A. N., Beckman, J. A., Findeiss, L. K., Golzarian, J., Gornik, H. L., Halperin, J. L., Jaff, M. R., Moneta, G. L., Olin, J. W., Stanley, J. C., White, C. J., White, J. V., & Zierler, R. E. (2011, November 1). 2011 ACCF/AHA focused update of the guideline for the management of patients with peripheral artery disease (updating the 2005 guideline): A report of the American College of Cardiology Foundation/American Heart Association Task Force on Practice Guidelines. *Journal of the American College of Cardiology,* *58*(19), 2020–2045. https://doi.org/10.1016/j.jacc.2011.08.023.

B. Any form of sedative or anesthetic may affect the accuracy of the examination due to its effect on blood pressure.

C. Patients with an ABI less than 0.90 have a higher risk of coronary artery disease, stroke, and death and therefore should be referred to a credentialed vascular laboratory for further testing.

D. Claudication is a specific, but not a sensitive, finding in patients with PAD.

    1. One study reports that up to 90% of patients with a documented ABI of less than 0.90 did not report claudication as a symptom.

E. An ABI of 0.91 to 0.99 is borderline.

    1. The patient may be asymptomatic at rest, but may experience symptoms related to the compromised vascular flow when ambulating.

    2. Exercise test may help evaluate a patient who has borderline ABI results.

F. Heavily calcified vessels may falsely elevate ankle pressure measurements, providing a false positive.

BIBLIOGRAPHY

Bailey, M. A., Griffin, K. J., & Scott, D. J. (2014, December). Clinical assessment of patients with peripheral arterial disease. *Seminars in Interventional Radiology, 31*(4), 292–299. https://doi.org/10.1055/s-0034-1393964

Davies, J. H., Kenkre, J., & Williams, E. M. (2014, April 17). Current utility of the ankle-brachial index (ABI) in general practice: Implications for its use in cardiovascular disease screening. *BMC Family Practice, 15*, 69. https://doi.org/10.1186/1471-2296-15-69

Ferket, B. S., Spronk, S., Colkesen, E. B., & Hunink, M. G. (2012). Systematic review of guidelines on peripheral artery disease screening. *The American Journal of Medicine, 125*(2), 198. https://doi.org/10.1016/j.amjmed.2011.06.027

Rooke, T. W., Hirsch, A. T., Misra, S., Sidawy, A. N., Beckman, J. A., Findeiss, L. K., Golzarian, J., Gornik, H. L., Halperin, J. L., Jaff, M. R., Moneta, G. L., Olin, J. W., Stanley, J. C., White, C. J., White, J. V., Zierler, R. E., & Society for Cardiovascular Angiography and Interventions; Society of Interventional Radiology; Society for Vascular Medicine; Society for Vascular Surgery. (2011, November 1). 2011 ACCF/AHA focused update of the guideline for the management of patients with peripheral artery disease (updating the 2005 guideline): A report of the American College of Cardiology Foundation/American Heart association task force on practice guidelines. *Journal of the American College of Cardiology, 58*(19), 2020–2045. https://doi.org/10.1016/j.jacc.2011.08.023

ARTERIAL LINES

Dominick Osipowicz

DESCRIPTION
A. Insertion of arterial catheter.
  1. Radial.
  2. Brachial.
  3. Femoral.
  4. Dorsalis pedis.
  5. Axillary.
B. Techniques.
  1. Inserted using physical landmarks and palpation of pulse.
  2. Inserted using direct visualization of artery with ultrasound.

INDICATIONS
A. Frequent arterial blood gas sampling: Useful in patients with respiratory distress or metabolic derangements.
B. Frequent sampling of blood for diagnostic labs when no other intravenous access is readily available.
C. Continuous blood pressure monitoring.
  1. Shock.
  2. Patients on vasopressors or antihypertensive medication infusions.
D. Continuous monitoring of cardiac output and stroke volume.

PRECAUTIONS
A. Pain at the insertion site may cause the patient to pull away or move the arm, placing them at increased risk of complications.
B. Bleeding can occur with arterial punctures and multiple attempts, especially if the patient is on anticoagulants or antiplatelet medications; holding pressure with the arm elevated is often required to achieve hemostasis.
C. Any puncture through the skin can increase the risk for potential infection.

D. Hematomas can occur at the insertion site.
  1. Greater likelihood of occurrence with multiple attempts; avoid more than three attempts at a single site.
E. Approach:
  1. If using landmarks to insert the catheter, palpate the pulse while advancing the needle.
  2. If using ultrasound guidance to insert the catheter, visualize the artery the entire time while advancing the needle.
F. Be cautious of nerves that run lateral to the artery (Figures III.2 and III.3).

EQUIPMENT REQUIRED
A. Sterile gloves.
B. Sterile gauze/towels.
C. Sterile drape.
D. Sterile transparent occlusive adhesive dressing.
E. Chlorhexidine/Betadine for skin preparation.
F. Appropriate catheter size for cannulation of the artery. The most commonly used catheter is 20 G.
G. Sutures.
H. Adhesive tape.
I. Arm board.
J. Pressure tubing.
K. 500 to 1,000 mL 0.9% normal saline solution (NSS) bag.
L. Pressure bag for 0.9% NSS bag.
M. 1% lidocaine 5-mL vial with 25-G, ¾-in. needle and 5-mL syringe.
N. Pressure tubing.
O. Transducer.

PROCEDURE
A. Arterial line placement is typically done at the bedside while the patient is in a supine position.
B. Prior to any arterial line placement, collateral blood flow to the limb should be checked; for example, perform ▶

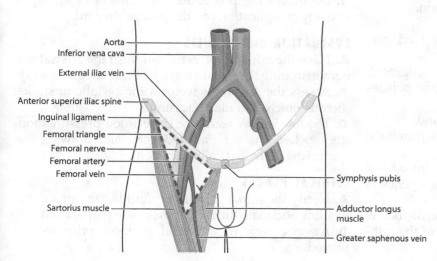

FIGURE III.2 Femoral anatomy.

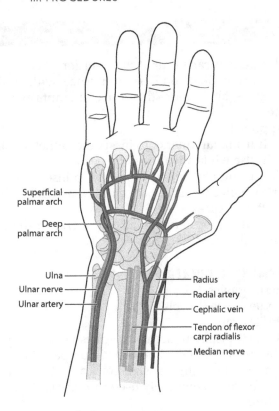

FIGURE III.3   Radial anatomy.

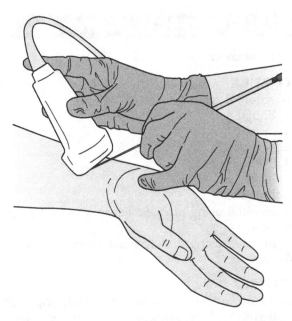

FIGURE III.4   Ultrasound-guided insertion of a radial arterial catheter.

the Allen test to ensure adequate ulnar artery perfusion prior to radial artery cannulation.

C. Explain the procedure to the patient and/or family.

D. Obtain informed consent unless the procedure is performed on an urgent/emergent need.

E. Perform hand hygiene.

F. Perform a universal protocol with the nursing staff.

G. Ensure extremity is supinated.

H. Position patient arm with tape and arm board if required for the approach.

I. Sterilize the area with chlorhexidine/Betadine as per protocol.

J. Open all equipment needed for cannulation.

K. Place sterile drape over the extremity.

L. Have a pressure bag/saline/transducer cord prepared by the RN for monitoring.

M. Don sterile gloves, personal protective equipment, and goggles/face shield as per facility-specific policies and procedures.

N. Palpate pulse and visualize with ultrasound.

O. Inject around the site with 1% lidocaine to numb the area.

P. Using the appropriate catheter with an introducer needle, hold the dominant hand as if holding a pencil at a less than 35-degree angle to the extremity.

Q. If using landmark approach, insert the needle below the area of palpation and view the window of the catheter for a flash of blood.

R. If using ultrasound guidance, insert the needle below the ultrasound probe and visualize needle advancement into the vessel lumen (Figure III.4).

S. After obtaining a flash of blood, using the nondominant hand, advance the wire to secure the position of the catheter (the wire should advance smoothly).

T. Slowly advance the catheter over the wire/needle into the vessel.

U. Remove the wire/needle; place thumb over the catheter opening to avoid excess bleeding.

V. Attach pressure tubing and evaluate the monitor for an appropriate waveform.

W. Once confirmed, suture the catheter in place and cover the insertion site with sterile transparent adhesive dressing.

X. Remove the sterile drape and dispose of all sharps in a sharps container.

Y. Document the procedure, the number of attempts, and any complications on the patient's record.

EVALUATION AND RESULTS

A. Have the nurse level, zero, and flush the arterial line demonstrating the square wave test and adequate whip.

B. Assess the arterial waveform for systolic upstroke, dicrotic notch, and diastolic runoff.

C. The line is now ready for close blood pressure monitoring, trending arterial blood gas, and drawing frequent labs in the critically ill patient.

CLINICAL PEARLS

A. Notify the nurse prior to performing the procedure to allow adequate time for appropriate preparation.

B. Always perform universal protocol prior to any procedure.

C. Have all of the equipment needed for the procedure set up and opened before donning sterile gloves.
D. Hold firm pressure or cover the catheter opening with thumb, preventing pulsatile blood from coming out of the catheter before attaching pressure tubing.
E. If hematoma occurs, hold firm pressure and apply pressure dressings and continue to monitor for bleeding.
F. Always start at the most distal place on the extremity if possible.

BIBLIOGRAPHY

Koyfman, A., Radwine, Z., & Sawyer, J. L. (2018, March 16). *Arterial line placement*. In V. Lopez Rowe (Ed.), *Medscape*. https://emedicine.medscape.com/article/1999586-overview

Tegtmeyer, K., Brady, G., Lai, S., Hodo, R., & Braner, D. (2006). Placement of an arterial line. *The New England Journal of Medicine, 354*, e13. https://doi.org/10.1056/NEJMvcm044149

Theodore, A. C., Gilles, C., & Dalton, A. (2022). *Intra-arterial catheterization for invasive monitoring: Indications, insertion techniques, and interpretation*. UpToDate. https://www.uptodate.com/contents/intra-arterial-catheterization-for-invasive-monitoring-indications-insertion-techniques-and-interpretation

BONE MARROW ASPIRATION AND BIOPSY

Pamela B. Dudkiewicz

DESCRIPTION

A. Bone marrow.

   1. A spongy or viscous tissue that is found inside the bones. Primary location of hematopoiesis consisting of hematopoietic stem cells, which produce red blood cells, white blood cells, and platelets.

   2. Found in the axial bones, including the sternum, ribs, vertebrae, clavicles, scapulae, skull, and pelvis, as well as the proximal ends of the femur and humerus.

B. Used for the diagnosis, staging, and treatment of various hematologic disorders and malignancies, such as aplastic anemia, multiple myeloma, leukemias, and lymphomas.

C. Bone marrow examination includes the assessment of bone marrow cellularity (age-dependent), cellular morphology, and maturation.

D. Ancillary tests are often performed on a bone marrow specimen.

   1. Cytogenetics.

   2. Fluorescent in situ hybridization (FISH).

   3. Molecular testing.

   4. Flow cytometry.

INDICATIONS

A. Diagnostic purposes: Cytopenia, aplastic anemia, lymphoma, leukemia, multiple myeloma, fever of unknown origin, or any suspected hematologic disease.

B. Treatment follow-up: Treatment response, treatment of isolated cytopenia, and marrow injury (e.g., radiation therapy, medication).

C. Tumor staging: Lymphoproliferative disorder and nonhematologic malignancies (neuroblastoma).

PRECAUTIONS

A. Primary risks of the procedure are bleeding and infections.

B. Absolute contraindications include uncorrected coagulopathies.

   1. Disseminated intravascular coagulopathy.

   2. Severe hemophilia.

C. Thrombocytopenia is not a contraindication regardless of severity; however, platelet transfusions can be given prior to the procedure if clinically warranted.

D. The only relative contraindication is anticoagulation.

   1. Withholding anticoagulation is not routinely recommended; however, it should be considered on a case-by-case basis (if clinically appropriate) prior to procedure.

   2. Bone marrow biopsy and aspiration are considered low-risk procedures; therefore, the risks of withholding may outweigh the benefits.

   3. Several guidelines for management of periprocedural anticoagulation are listed in Table III.2.

E. Patients with suspected multiple myeloma should *never* undergo sternal aspiration due to bone fragility and risk of sternal perforation.

F. Assess for allergies to anesthetics (e.g., lidocaine).

EQUIPMENT REQUIRED

A. Bone marrow aspiration/biopsy kits should contain most if not all required materials, as noted in the following:

   1. Equipment required for the procedure.

      a. Sterile gloves.

      b. Drape for sterile field.

      c. Iodine or chlorhexidine solution.

      d. 1% or 2% buffered or plain lidocaine with or without epinephrine.

      e. Scalpel blade #11.

      f. Luer lock syringes.

         i. 5-mL syringe for local anesthesia.

         ii. 10- or 20-mL syringe for aspiration.

      g. Needles for local anesthesia.

         i. 25-G × ⅝-in. needle for subcutaneous administration.

         ii. 20-G × 1-½-in. needle for deep administration.

      h. Sterile gauze and bandages.

      i. Bone marrow needle with stylet.

      j. Trephine biopsy needle.

         i. Jamshidi biopsy needle (traditional method; Figure III.5).

         ii. Combined aspiration/biopsy needle (powered driver method; Figure III.6).

   2. Equipment required to obtain specimens.

      a. All tubes and slides should be labeled with patient information.

      b. Labeled collection tubes.

      c. Labeled glass slides and coverslips.

      d. Formalin or other fixative container for biopsy and clot specimen.

PROCEDURE

A. Can be performed on the posterior superior iliac crest (most common), anterior iliac crest, sternum, or tibia (rarely). As bone marrow aspiration and biopsy on sites other than the posterior iliac crest are not commonly performed, the focus of the procedure will be on the preferred site of the posterior iliac crest.

   1. Posterior superior iliac crest: Most common location. Provides adequate marrow away from anatomic structures which are subject to injury. Used for both aspiration and core biopsy.

   2. Anterior iliac crest: Same advantages as the posterior iliac crest, but the cortical bone is thicker.

TABLE III.2   GUIDELINES FOR HOLDING ANTICOAGULATION PRIOR TO BONE MARROW PROCEDURE

Guideline	Bleeding Risk Category	Recommendations
Thrombosis Canada: NOACs/DOACs Preoperative Management	Moderate	Stop NOAC/DOAC 1 day prior to the procedure.
Thrombosis Canada: Warfarin Perioperative Management	Low/moderate	Selected procedures with large-bore needles (e.g., bone marrow biopsy) may need warfarin interruption. Stop warfarin 5 days before the procedure and consider bridging for high-risk groups.
MD Anderson Periprocedure Management of Anticoagulants	Low	Do not interrupt anticoagulation.
2016 Focused Update of the Canadian Cardiovascular Society Guidelines for the Management of Atrial Fibrillation	Low	Low-risk procedures are generally safe to perform without interrupting antithrombotic therapy, provided the INR is not supratherapeutic in the case of warfarin.
Society of Interventional Radiology Consensus Guidelines for the Periprocedural Management of Thrombotic and Bleeding Risk in Patients Undergoing Percutaneous Image-Guided Interventions—Part II: Recommendations	Low	Do not withhold anticoagulation. Target INR ≤3.0. Consider bridging for high thrombosis risk cases. Exception: Withhold glycoprotein IIb/IIIa inhibitors 4–8 hours before the procedure.
Manuals from the Canterbury District Health Board—Protocol for Bone Marrow Aspirate and Trephine Biopsy	Not specified	Warfarin interruption is not required.
Bleeding Risk Assessment for Bedside and Interventional Radiology Guided Procedures: Consensus Guidelines and Beyond	BM aspiration without biopsy: Low risk BM biopsy: Moderate to high risk	Stop DOAC 1–2 days prior to the procedure. Target INR <1.8 for high-risk procedures.

BM, bone marrow; DOACs, direct oral anticoagulants; INR, international normalized ratio; NOACs, novel oral anticoagulants.

3. Sternum: Provides ample material for aspiration but is only 1-cm thick. Core biopsies are contraindicated. Increased risk of damaging the heart or great vessels. Not to be performed with powered driver.
B. Some facilities use ultrasound- or CT-guided aspirations/biopsies; however, the procedure is commonly done with palpation alone.
C. The procedure:
  1. Explain the procedure to the patient and family and obtain informed consent.
  2. Wash hands/perform hand hygiene.
  3. Perform a proper time-out. All present in the room must identify the patient and agree on the correct procedure and the correct site of the procedure.
  4. Position the patient in prone (recommended) or lateral decubitus (Figure III.7) position.
  5. Palpate for posterior iliac crest.
  6. Select and mark the site.
    a. Approximately three finger widths from the midline and two finger widths (Figure III.8) inferior to the posterior iliac crest.

    b. Avoid areas concerning for skin or soft tissue infection (e.g., erythema or induration).
7. Using sterile technique, open the bone marrow tray and inspect all components.
8. Cleanse the marked area with povidone-iodine solution or chlorhexidine and drape the sterile field.
9. Anesthetize the skin and subcutaneous tissue of the marked site with 1% or 2% lidocaine solution using a 25-G needle.
10. Perform aspiration.
  a. Place the middle finger and index finger on either side of the marked site.
  b. Insert a 20-G needle into the marked site between the fingers and advance to the periosteum at a perpendicular angle.
  c. Anesthetize the periosteum by continually injecting small amounts of lidocaine on the bone surface (approximately a quarter-sized area).
  d. Make note of the angle of the needle and the landscape of the bone (particularly flat areas).

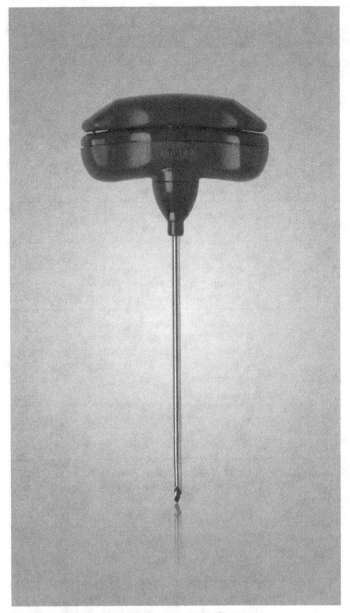

FIGURE III.5   Jamshidi biopsy needle.

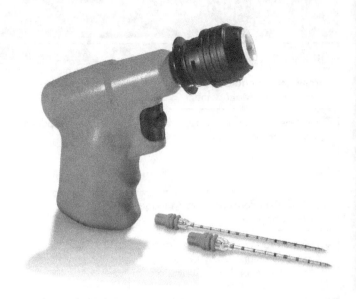

FIGURE III.6   Combined aspiration/biopsy needle (powered driver method).

i. Once the needle enters the marrow space, a "give" is felt, and the patient may note discomfort.

j. Ensure the needle is anchored in the bone and detach the driver from the needle if used and remove the stylet.

k. Attach a 10- or 20-mL syringe to the aspiration needle.

l. Aspirate 1 to 2 mL of marrow initially for smears and the clot section.

m. Additional aspirates will be required for ancillary testing (e.g., flow cytometry, cytogenetics, molecular testing). An assistant should handle the smears while the proceduralist continues to aspirate.

n. In general, it is not recommended to aspirate greater than 5 mL at a time as the contents may clot.

11. Perform biopsy (if required).

a. Using the same site, advance a Jamshidi needle into the cortical bone with a steady twisting motion until the needle is firmly lodged (see Figure III.7).

b. Remove the stylet.

c. Advise the patient that they should anticipate a dull, aching pressure.

d. Advance the needle 1 to 2 cm with a rotating motion applying pressure.

e. Once an adequate core biopsy depth is attained, rotate the needle 360 degrees in both directions

e. Allow 2 to 3 minutes for local anesthesia to take effect. In the meantime, prepare the bone marrow tray.

f. Insert the bone marrow needle with stylet in place perpendicular to the marked site (see Figure III.8) with the same approach and angle as the anesthetic needle.

g. Gently approach the periosteum and ensure that the area is anesthetized (patient should only experience dull sensations).

h. Steadily rotate the needle back and forth in a twisting motion to advance through the bone cortex. If using a powered driver, slowly press the driver through the bone cortex.

(A)

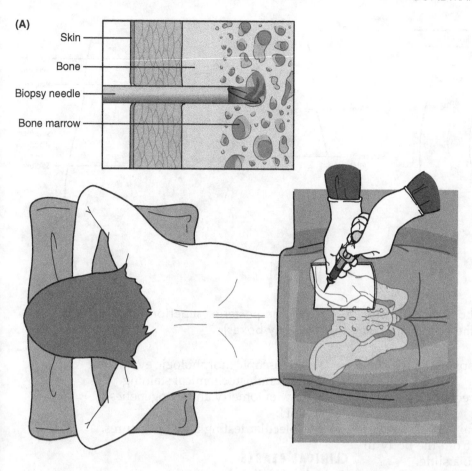

Skin

Bone

Biopsy needle

Bone marrow

(B)

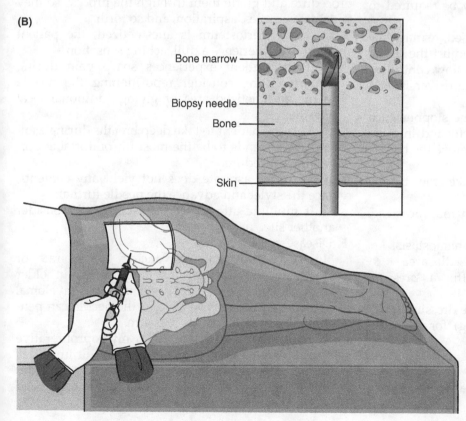

Bone marrow

Biopsy needle

Bone

Skin

FIGURE III.7 Position of the patient for bone marrow aspiration and biopsy. (**A**) prone position and (**B**) lateral decubitus position.

Source: From Healthwise, Incorporated.

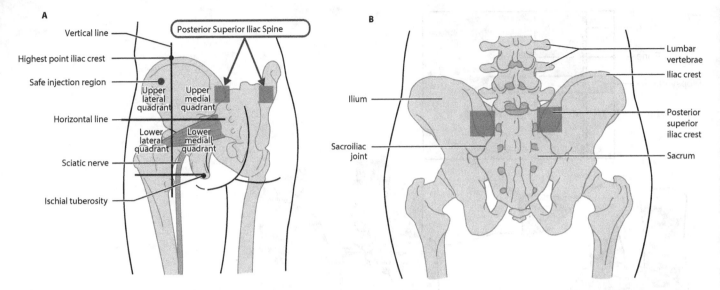

FIGURE III.8 **(A)** Pelvic anatomy for bone marrow procedures. **(B)** The posterior superior iliac crest is a bony prominence located superolateral to the coccyx (indicated by the gray boxes).

several times to separate the biopsy from the surrounding tissue.

f. Slowly remove the biopsy specimen by gently pulling and rotating the needle.

g. Insert the stylet into the distal end of the needle after it has been removed from the body to expel the biopsy specimen onto a slide.

h. Inspect the biopsy specimen for adequate size (1–2 cm). A second attempt may be required to obtain a complete specimen.

i. If a powered driver is being used, reattach the driver (stylet remains out) and adjust the depth gauge to a desired depth, and in a slow, controlled and continuous motion push the driver in and out.

j. Insert the tip of needle into the stopper, turn upside down, and insert the ejector rod into the opposite end of the stopper to remove the biopsy core.

k. The assistant will then make the biopsy imprints and place in fixative.

l. Send all specimens to pathology for processing.

12. Apply dressing.

a. Hold pressure over the site for hemostasis.

b. Use alcohol prep pads to cleanse the area.

c. Apply sterile gauze and affix a pressure bandage.

d. Advise the patient to leave the dressing intact and dry (no bathing/swimming) for 24 or 48 hours (if biopsy is performed).

EVALUATION AND RESULTS

A. Evaluation of the bone marrow aspiration and biopsy includes the following:

1. Microscopic morphologic evaluation.
2. Immunohistochemical staining.
3. Flow cytometry and cytogenetics.
4. FISH.
5. Molecular testing and/or cultures.

CLINICAL PEARLS

A. Maintain dialog with the patient throughout the procedure and guide them through the process so they anticipate needles, aspiration, and so forth.

B. Once the periosteum is anesthetized, the patient should only experience a dull, aching sensation.

1. If the patient experiences sharp pain during the procedure, consider repositioning the needle to the anesthetized area or giving additional local anesthetic.

C. Instruct the patient to take deep breaths during aspiration, as this tends to be the most uncomfortable portion of the procedure.

D. If the initial aspirate does not yield any contents, replace the stylet and advance the needle further.

1. If multiple attempts are unsuccessful, consider another site.

E. Disease-specific issues.

1. Use caution when advancing the aspirate or biopsy needle through the bony cortex in older adult patients or patients with multiple myeloma. Osteoporotic bone is weak, and the needle can penetrate the bone with little pressure.

2. Aspiration for patients with myeloproliferative disorders (e.g., myelofibrosis) may result in a "dry tap" due to increased marrow fibrosis. Consider repositioning the needle to another anesthetized site.

BIBLIOGRAPHY

Bain, B. J. (2001, September). Bone marrow aspiration. *Journal Clinical Pathology, 54*(9), 657–663.

Moore, C., & Kotchetkov, R. (2021). Anticoagulation and bone marrow biopsy: Is it safe to proceed? *Hematology, 26*(1), 206–209. https://doi.org/10.1080/16078454.2021.1880762

Patel, I. J., Davidson, J. C., Nikolic, B., Salazar, G. M., Schwartzberg, M. S., Walker, T. G., Saad, W. A., & Standards of Practice Committee, with Cardiovascular and Interventional Radiological Society of Europe (CIRSE). (2012). Consensus guidelines for periprocedural management of coagulation status and hemostasis risk in percutaneous image-guided interventions. *Endorsement, 23*(6), 727–736. https://doi.org/10.1016/j.jvir.2012.02.012

Pudusseri, A., & Spyropoulos, A. C. (2014). Management of anticoagulants in the periprocedural period for patients with cancer. *Journal of the National Comprehensive Cancer Network, 12*(12), 1713–1720. https://doi.org/https://doi.org/10.6004/jnccn.2014.0173

Radhakrishnan, N. (2017). *Bone marrow aspiration and biopsy*. In E. C. Besa (Ed.), *Medscape.* https://emedicine.medscape.com/article/207575-overview

Rindy, L. J., & Chambers, A. R. (2022, January). *Bone marrow aspiration and biopsy*. NCBI Bookshelf. A service of the National Library of Medicine, National Institutes of Health. https://www.ncbi.nlm.nih.gov/books/NBK559232/

Spyropoulos, A. C., & Douketis, J. D. (2012). How I treat anticoagulated patients undergoing an elective procedure or surgery. *Blood, 120*(15), 2954–2962. https://doi.org/10.1182/blood-2012-06-415943

Tomasian, A., & Jennings, J. W. (2022). Bone marrow aspiration and biopsy: Techniques and practice implications. *Skeletal Radiology, 51*, 81–88.

BRONCHOSCOPY

E. Moneé Carter-Griffin

DESCRIPTION

A. Direct visualization of the lower airways (e.g., trachea, bronchi, and bronchioles) with a scope containing a camera.

B. Most institutions have a bronchoscopy cart with all the required equipment, including a video screen to allow for visualization.

C. Typically, a respiratory therapist and/or a nurse will assist with the procedure.

INDICATIONS

A. Identifying the cause of hemoptysis or other symptoms that indicate endobronchial disease.

  1. Literature indicates bronchoscopy is not an optimal tool for diagnostic evaluation of hemoptysis.

B. Obtaining samples for pathology of abnormal spots or lesions noted on imaging.

C. Diagnosis and staging of lung carcinomas.

D. Removal of excessive secretions, mucus plugs, and so forth.

E. Removal of foreign objects.

F. Assistance with difficult intubations and to verify endotracheal tube placement.

G. Use during and post procedure (e.g., dilation and stent placement in tracheal stenosis).

H. Postoperative assessment of lung transplants.

PRECAUTIONS

A. Patients with coagulopathies or severe bleeding disorders: Aggressive suctioning or endobronchial interventions can cause bleeding.

B. Avoid in patients with severe hypoxemia and/or those requiring increased ventilatory support (e.g., acute respiratory distress syndrome [ARDS]), if possible.

C. Can cause irritation to the vocal cords and airways, leading to laryngospasm and bronchospasm, respectively.

EQUIPMENT REQUIRED

A. Bronchoscopy cart, if available.

B. Bronchoscope with light source and image processor to display any images onto a screen.

C. Bite block (only placed in intubated patients prior to bronchoscope insertion).

D. Swivel adapter for the bronchoscope.

E. Water-soluble lubricant.

F. Gauze (used to wipe secretions from the bronchoscope).

G. Suction tubing and suction device (e.g., wall suction unit or device on bronchoscopy cart).

H. Sterile bowl.

I. 10- to 20-mL syringes (2–3).

J. Saline (nonbacteriostatic).

K. Sputum trap if collecting a specimen.

L. Gloves, mask, and eye protection.

M. Moderate sedation medications.

N. Additional equipment may be required, such as biopsy forceps, bronchial brush, and so forth, if obtaining tissue samples.

PROCEDURE

A. Explain the procedure to the patient and family.

B. Always identify the patient and obtain informed consent.

C. Ensure the patient has intravenous (IV) access and hemodynamic monitoring (e.g., blood pressure, oxygen saturations) throughout the entirety of the procedure.

D. Assemble all equipment prior to the procedure.

E. Ensure the light source is working on the bronchoscope.

F. Connect suction tubing to the bronchoscope and a suction device.

G. Add saline to the sterile bowl.

H. Fill the syringes with saline prior to starting the procedure. The saline can be used to help with secretion clearance and for collection of a bronchoalveolar lavage (BAL).

I. Determine the entry route for the bronchoscope.

  1. Nonintubated patient: The nose is the preferred entry site.

  2. Intubated patient: The bronchoscope will enter through the existing endotracheal tube.

J. If the patient has a preexisting endotracheal tube, adjust the ventilator setting by increasing the fraction of inspired oxygen to 100% and placing the patient on assist control. Connect the swivel adapter to the endotracheal tube.

K. If the patient is not receiving mechanical ventilation, then an oxygen source is typically applied (e.g., nasal cannula).

L. Prior to procedure initiation, don a gown, gloves, mask, and eye protection.

M. Instruct the assistant to administer moderate sedation to assist with comfort and tolerance of the procedure.

N. Apply the water-soluble lubricant to the bronchoscope.

O. In a nonintubated patient, insert the bronchoscope through the nose. In an intubated patient, insert the bronchoscope through the swivel adapter connected to the endotracheal tube (Figure III.9).

P. Advance the bronchoscope through the trachea and into the lungs.

  1. Assessment of the vocal cords, trachea, and entire airway should be performed throughout the procedure.

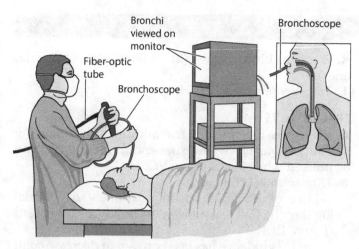

Bronchi viewed on monitor.
Fiber-optic tube
Bronchoscope
Bronchoscope

FIGURE III.9   The bronchoscopy procedure.

2. The indications for performing bronchoscopy will determine what interventions are completed (e.g., aspiration of secretions, biopsy of a lesion, and removal of foreign objects).

3. Prior to removing the bronchoscope, inspect the lungs for hemostasis or evidence of possible complications from the procedure.

Q. Once the procedure is complete, remove the bronchoscope.

R. Send a specimen collected in sputum trap to pathology and/or microbiology.

S. Obtain a chest x-ray post procedure to assess the lungs.

T. Document the procedure, indication, diagnostics sent, any complications, and the patient's tolerance of the procedure.

EVALUATION AND RESULTS

A. Results will vary on the rationale for performing the procedure.

B. Results could include clearance of secretions and mucus plugs, resulting in better oxygenation, identification of lesions for appropriate treatment, and so forth.

CLINICAL PEARLS

A. If using a traditional bronchoscope, the intubated patient will need at least a 7.5-mm endotracheal tube to pass the bronchoscope into the lungs.

B. The use of saline can help remove thick secretions from the airway.

BIBLIOGRAPHY

Du Rand, I. A., Blaikley, J., Booton, R., Chaudhuri, N., Gupta, V., Khalid, S., Mandal, S., Martin, J., Mills, J., Navani, N., Rahman, N. M., Wrightson, J. M., Munavvar, M., &British Thoracic Society Bronchoscopy Guideline Group. (2013, August). British Thoracic Society guideline for diagnostic flexible bronchoscopy in adults: Accredited by NICE. *Thorax, 68*(Suppl. 1), i1–i44. https://doi.org/10.1136/thoraxjnl-2013-203618

Mahmoud, N., Vashisht, R., Sanghavi, D., & Kalanjeri, S. (2022). *Bronchoscopy*. StatPearls Publishing. https://www.ncbi.nlm.nih.gov/books/NBK448152/#_NBK448152_pubdet_

Paradis, T. J., Dixon, J., & Tieu, B. H. (2016). The role of bronchoscopy in the diagnosis of airway disease. *Journal of Thoracic Disease, 8,* 3826–3837. https://doi.org/10.21037/jtd.2016.12.68

CENTRAL VENOUS ACCESS

Dominick Osipowicz

DESCRIPTION

A. A central venous catheter (CVC), also called a central line, is a thin, flexible catheter which is percutaneously placed terminating in central circulation (Figure III.10).
B. The ideal location for the tip of the catheter is the superior vena cava (SVC) at the cavoatrial junction.

INDICATIONS

A. Rapid administration of intravenous (IV) fluids (in the setting of sepsis, trauma, shock, burns) or blood products.
B. Inadequate peripheral access.
C. Emergent venous access.
D. Administration of medications with potential to cause vascular damage when administered peripherally, including:
    1. Vasopressors.
    2. Inotropes.
    3. Chemotherapy.
    4. Total parenteral nutrition.
    5. Hypertonic saline solutions such as 3%, 7.5%, and 23.4% saline.
E. Administration of incompatible drugs.
F. Access for placement of pulmonary artery catheters (PACs), hemodialysis catheters, and plasmapheresis catheters.
G. Hemodynamic monitoring, including central venous pressure (CVP) measurement.
H. Measurement of central venous oxygen saturation (SVO$_2$).
I. Cardiac pressures via PAC including CVP, pulmonary artery systolic and diastolic pressures, and pulmonary artery wedge pressure.
J. Measurement of mixed SVO$_2$ from a PAC.

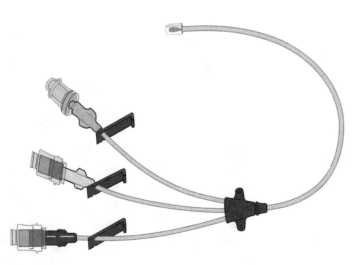

FIGURE III.10 A central venous catheter.

K. Frequent blood draws (in patients without arterial lines).
L. Transvenous cardiac pacing.

PRECAUTIONS

A. In order to help prevent complications, the following precautions, taken by an experienced provider, should be utilized when inserting a CVC.
B. Ultrasound (US) guidance.
    1. Use of US guidance for placement of internal jugular (IJ) CVCs is now considered gold standard (Figure III.11).
        a. US guidance has been proven to decrease complications, especially arterial cannulation.
        b. US guidance for insertion of central venous access in subclavian and femoral veins has less evidence and requires further research.
C. Manometry is a method of measuring pressure during CVC insertion in order to ensure venous rather than arterial puncture is obtained.
    1. Once the provider has inserted the needle into a vessel and has blood return, a sterile tube is connected to the hub of the needle or catheter.
    2. Tubing should then be filled with blood. This is done by lowering the sterile tubing below the level of the vein.
    3. The tubing is then held vertically over the patient. This allows for the blood level to equilibrate with venous pressure.
        a. If the needle is in an artery, the blood will continue to rise up the tube.
        b. If the needle is in the vein, the blood will begin to travel back down the column.
D. Providers should choose US guidance and pressure manometry (Figure III.12) as techniques to reduce complications. While dynamic US guidance helps reduce the risk of arterial sticks, pressure manometry reduces the risk of arterial cannulation.
E. Additional precautions.
    1. The nurse must be present during all portions of the procedure.
    2. The provider must confirm correct catheter tip location via chest x-ray prior to use.
    3. Antibiotic impregnated CVCs are sometimes used when available; the provider should check institutional policies.
    4. Prior to donning sterile gloves, the practitioner should use an antimicrobial soap or alcohol sanitizer.
    5. Antimicrobial site preparation.
        a. Prior to draping a patient, a sterile solution of chlorhexidine or betadine should be applied to the site by scrubbing for 30 seconds.
        b. The site should then be allowed to air-dry for at least 2 minutes.

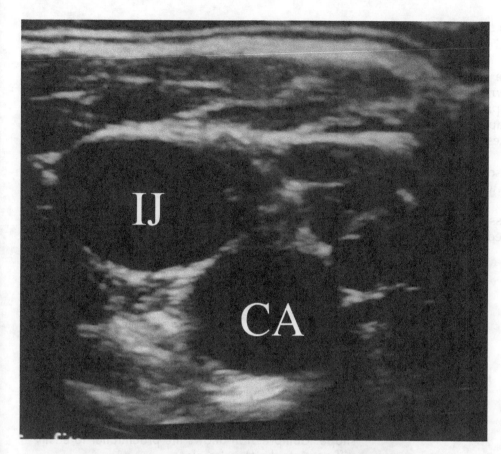

FIGURE III.11 Ultrasound showing internal jugular (IJ) and carotid artery (CA).

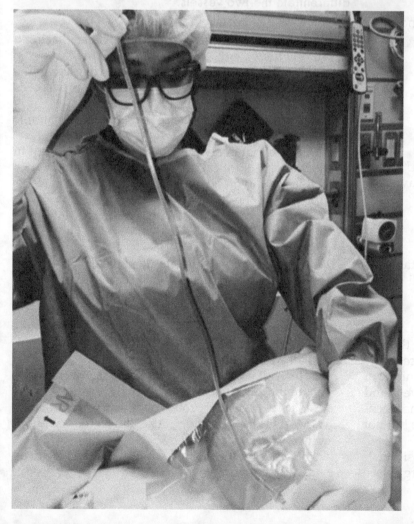

FIGURE III.12 An advanced practice provider demonstrating pressure manometry on a manikin.

6. Maximal barrier precautions.
   a. A full body drape should be placed over the patient.
   b. All those performing the procedures should wear a mask, cap, sterile gown, and sterile gloves.
   c. Any additional persons present in the room should wear a mask and a cap.
7. Timely removal of CVC is desired when deemed no longer necessary.
8. Femoral vein insertion is associated with greater risk of infection as compared with the subclavian vein or jugular vein.
F. Multiple complications are associated with CVC placement, including but not limited to:
   1. Catheter-related infection.
   2. Catheter-related thrombosis.
   3. Arterial puncture.
   4. Arterial cannulation.
   5. Vascular injury.
   6. Arrhythmia.
   7. Bleeding.
   8. Venous air embolism.
   9. Pneumothorax.
   10. Hemothorax.
   11. Infection.

EQUIPMENT REQUIRED

A. CVC kit.
B. Caps and mask for everyone present in the room.
C. Sterile gown for all providers.
D. Extra pair of sterile gloves.
E. Sterile full body drape.
F. Sterile US probe cover.
G. Chlorhexidine.
H. Sterile saline.
I. Pressure tubing for manometry.
J. Central line dressing.
K. If the provider does not have access to an US, consider alternate sites for insertion, such as subclavian or femoral.

PROCEDURE

A. Placement of IJ CVC.
   1. Explain the procedure to the patient and family.
   2. Obtain consent for CVC placement based on the institution's policy.
   3. Perform hand hygiene.
   4. Perform universal protocol. All present in the room must identify the patient and agree on the correct procedure and the correct site of the procedure.
   5. US patient anatomy prior to positioning of patient. Using US guidance identify the IJ vein and the carotid artery. The IJ is compressible when gentle pressure is applied. The artery is pulsatile but not compressible (Figure III.13).
   6. Place the patient in the Trendelenburg position. If the patient cannot tolerate the Trendelenburg, place

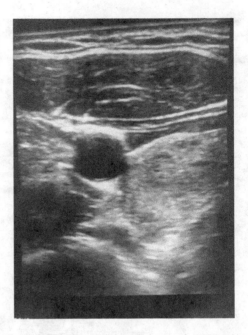

FIGURE III.13 The internal jugular is being compressed with gentle pressure as evidenced by the oblong shape that is formed from the previous circular shape in Figure III.11. The muscles around the carotid artery make it much more difficult to compress the carotid artery; therefore, it maintains its shape. Compression allows the practitioner to easily differentiate the two vessels.

the patient as flat as possible or consider placing a femoral line.
   7. Have the patient turn their head 45 degrees in the opposite direction of the side where the provider is placing the catheter (Figure III.14).
   8. If not using an US, please see section on anatomic landmarks below.
   9. Ensure that everyone who will remain present in the room has surgical cap and mask on.
10. Place a cap on the patient.
11. Open up the CVC tray.
12. Prepare the skin with chlorhexidine, per Centers for Disease Control and Prevention (CDC) guidelines.
13. Don sterile gown and sterile gloves.
14. Remove the sterile full body drape from the central line kit and drape it over the patient. There will be a hole, which should be placed over the site previously identified.
15. Set up a sterile kit in an orderly fashion. Ensure that all equipment is within arm's reach.
16. Flush all ports of the catheter with sterile saline to ensure they are functioning properly.
17. Place a sterile US probe cover on the US probe.
18. Most kits provide 1% lidocaine without epinephrine.
   a. Draw up the desired amount of lidocaine in an available syringe.

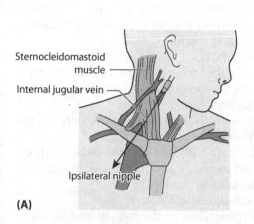
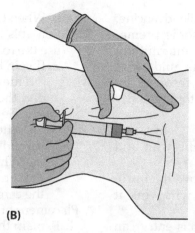

Sternocleidomastoid muscle

Internal jugular vein

Ipsilateral nipple

(A)　　　　　(B)

FIGURE III.14 Landmarks for accessing the internal jugular vein. **(A)** Aim the needle toward the ipsilateral nipple. **(B)** Insert the needle at the apex of the sternocleidomastoid muscle.

b. Replace the needle used to draw up lidocaine with a subcutaneous needle.
c. Using the US, identify the IJ vein and center it in the middle of the screen.
d. While watching the US screen to identify the needle, make an initial stick with the needle.
e. Prior to injecting lidocaine, draw back to ensure you do not have blood return.
f. Inject lidocaine into the subcutaneous tissue.
19. Maintain visualization of the IJ in the center of the US field.
20. Continue to hold the US probe in the nondominant hand while picking up the introducer needle with the dominant hand.
21. With the bevel up, insert the needle at a 30- to 40-degree angle to the patient directed at the ipsilateral nipple (Figure III.15). *Aspirate* the syringe the entire time the needle is being advanced.
22. Maintain visualization of the carotid artery and IJ vein on the US screen.

23. If one does not immediately aspirate venous blood:
a. Slightly withdraw the needle, without withdrawing the needle from the skin, and attempt to angle more laterally.
b. If this position also does not result in blood return, withdraw the needle again and attempt to angle more medially.
24. Once venous blood is aspirated, disconnect the syringe while securely holding the needle. Place a finger over the needle hub in order to reduce the risk of air embolism.
25. Attach tubing for pressure measurement as discussed earlier.
26. If the carotid artery is accessed, remove the needle and hold pressure for 10 to 15 minutes.
27. After venous entry is confirmed, remove the pressure tubing and insert the guide wire through the needle.
a. It should advance with minimal resistance.
b. While advancing the guide wire, watch the telemetry monitor for signs of ectopy.

a
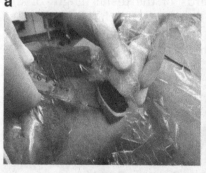
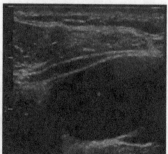

b
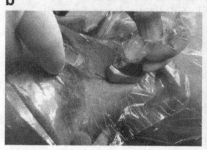
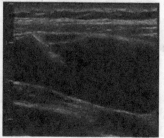

FIGURE III.15 Accessing the internal jugular with ultrasound. **(A)** Direct the needle toward the center of the ultrasound probe. **(B)** Advance the needle forward and look for penetration of the needle into the vessel.

Source: Reproduced with permission from Saugel, B., Scheeren, T. W. L., & Teboul, J.-L. (2017). Ultrasound-guided central venous catheter placement: A structured review and recommendations for clinical practice. *Critical Care, 21,* 225. https://doi.org/10.1186/s13054-017-1814-y.

c. Pay attention to telemetry alarms while advancing.

d. Patients may often experience some premature ventricular contractions or intermittent runs of ventricular tachycardia if the guide wire is advanced too far. This can be resolved by retracting the guide wire until all ectopic activity ceases.

E. If the patient develops ventricular tachycardia without resolution, completely remove the wire and reassess.

28. While holding the guide wire, remove the introducer needle. Never let go of the guide wire while it is in the patient.

29. An additional confirmation of venous entry can be performed by obtaining a transverse view via US of the IJ vein and following the guide wire down to the vein.

30. Once the introducer needle has been removed, make a small nick in the skin at the site of entry while continuing to hold the guide wire. The nick should be made with the scalpel facing away from the provider and should be a small inout stabbing motion.

31. Now, pass the dilator over the guide wire while continuing to hold the guide wire.

32. Dilate and retract the dilator while continuing to hold the guide wire.

33. Make sure the distal port of the CVC does not have a cap on it so the guide wire can pass through.

34. Pass the catheter over the guide wire. The guide wire will come out the distal port.

35. Continue advancing the catheter while holding the guide wire.

a. Once the guide wire can be seen coming out of the distal port of the catheter, grasp the guide wire.

B. Finish advancing the catheter until the appropriate depth is reached.

36. While holding the catheter in place, pull out the guide wire. It should be removed without any resistance. Place the thumb over the open port to avoid risk of air embolism.

37. Aspirate and flush each port to confirm blood return.

38. Suture the central line into place at the insertion site.

39. Apply Biopatch over the insertion site.

40. Place a sterile dressing over the insertion site.

41. Obtain a chest x-ray for radiograph placement and to rule out a pneumothorax.

42. Proper placement on chest x-ray will demonstrate the tip of the catheter in the SVC at the cavoatrial junction.

43. Document the procedure appropriately on the patient's record.

44. Anatomic landmarks for CVC placement without US guidance.

a. US guidance for placement of IJ CVCs is considered the gold standard. However, not all facilities have access to bedside US.

b. When US is not readily available for CVC insertion, it is important that an experienced provider use the following anatomic markings:

c. IJ vein landmarks.

i. Identify the triangle formed by the sternum and the two heads of the sternocleidomastoid muscle (SCM).

ii. After identifying this triangle, palpate the carotid pulse.

iii. While palpating the carotid pulse, pull on the carotid medially and insert needle lateral to the carotid. Refer to step 23.

B. Placement of subclavian CVC.

1. Explain the procedure to the patient and family.

2. Obtain consent for CVC placement based on the institution's policy.

3. Perform hand hygiene.

4. Perform universal protocol. All present in the room must identify the patient and agree on the correct procedure and the correct site of the procedure.

5. US guidance is rarely used in subclavian catheter placement due to the obstruction of the view of the vein by the clavicle.

6. Place the patient in the Trendelenburg position. If the patient cannot tolerate the Trendelenburg, place the patient as flat as possible or consider placing a femoral line.

7. Have the patient turn their head 45 degrees in the opposite direction of the side where the provider is placing the catheter.

8. Prior to beginning the procedure, identify the landmarks (Figure III.16).

a. Subclavian vein landmarks:

i. Identify the sternal notch.

ii. Find the curve of the clavicle, which is generally two-thirds of the distal length of the clavicle from the sternal notch (Figure III.17).

iii. Palpation of the subclavian artery is not possible due to obstruction by the clavicle.

iv. Visualization with US is not possible due to the clavicle obstructing the view.

9. Ensure that everyone who will remain present in the room has surgical cap and mask on.

10. Place a cap on the patient.

11. Open up the CVC tray.

12. Prepare the skin with chlorhexidine.

13. Don sterile gown and sterile gloves.

14. Remove the sterile full body drape from the central line kit and drape it over the patient. There will be a hole, which should be placed over the site previously identified.

15. Set up a sterile kit in an orderly fashion. Ensure that all equipment is within arm's reach.

16. Flush all ports of the catheter with sterile saline to ensure they are functioning properly.

17. Most kits provide 1% lidocaine without epinephrine.

(A)   (B)

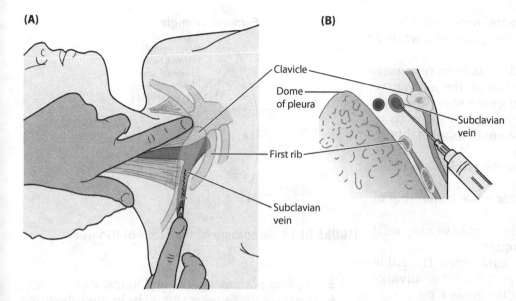

FIGURE III.16   (A) Advancing the needle in subclavian access. **(B)** Direct the tip of the needle toward the sternal notch.

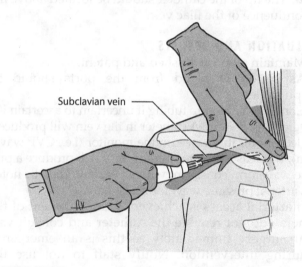

FIGURE III.17   Accessing the subclavian vein.

a. Draw up the desired amount of lidocaine in an available syringe.

b. Replace the needle used to draw up lidocaine with a subcutaneous needle.

c. Advance the subcutaneous needle into the subcutaneous tissue at the clavicular angle.

d. Prior to injecting lidocaine, draw back to ensure you do not have blood return.

e. Inject with lidocaine.

18. To access the subclavian vein, pick up the introducer needle with the dominant hand.

19. While maintaining the above described landmarks with the nondominant hand, use the dominant hand to insert the introducer needle at a shallow 10- to 20-degree angle to the curve of the clavicle directed at the sternal notch. Once the needle hits the clavicle, use the thumb of the nondominant hand to gently drive the needle tip underneath the clavicle. Avoid raising the angle of approach while under the clavicle, as this increases the likelihood of causing a

pneumothorax. Aspirate the syringe the entire time the needle is being advanced.

20. If one does not immediately aspirate venous blood:

a. Slightly withdraw the needle, without withdrawing the needle from the skin, and attempt to angle more cephalad.

b. If this position also does not result in blood return, withdraw the needle again and attempt to angle more caudal.

21. Once venous blood is aspirated, carefully disconnect the syringe from the needle, while securely holding the needle. Place a finger over the needle hub in order to reduce the risk of air embolism.

22. Attach tubing for pressure measurement as discussed earlier.

23. If the subclavian artery is accidentally accessed, remove the needle and hold pressure for 10 to 15 minutes. The clavicle makes it difficult or impossible to hold direct pressure over the subclavian artery. Call a stat vascular consult if bleeding cannot be controlled or the patient develops signs of hemodynamic instability.

24. After venous entry is confirmed, remove the pressure tubing and insert the guide wire through the needle.

a. It should advance with minimal resistance.

b. While advancing the guide wire, check the telemetry monitor for signs of ectopy.

c. Pay attention to telemetry alarms while advancing.

d. Patients may often experience some premature ventricular contractions or intermittent runs of ventricular tachycardia if the guide wire is advanced too far. This can be resolved by retracting the guide wire until all ectopic activity ceases.

e. If the patient develops ventricular tachycardia without resolution, completely remove the wire and reassess.

25. While holding the guide wire, remove the introducer needle. Never let go of the guide wire while it is in the patient.

26. Once the introducer needle has been removed, make a small nick in the skin at the site entry while continuing to hold the guide wire. The nick should be made with the scalpel facing away from the provider and should be a small inout stabbing motion.

27. Now, pass the dilator over the guide wire while continuing to hold the guide wire.

28. Dilate and retract the dilator while continuing to hold the guide wire.

29. Make sure the distal port does not have a cap on it so the guide wire can pass through.

30. Pass the catheter over the guide wire. The guide wire will come out the distal port. Continue advancing the catheter while holding the guide wire.

  a. Once the guide wire can be seen coming out of the distal port of the catheter, grasp the guide wire.
  b. Finish advancing the catheter until the appropriate depth is reached.

31. While holding the catheter in place, pull out the guide wire. It should be removed without any resistance. Place the thumb over the open port to avoid risk of air embolism.

32. Connect saline flush with cap to open port, aspirate and flush to confirm blood return.

33. Aspirate and flush each remaining port to confirm blood return.

34. Suture the central line into place at the insertion site.

35. Apply Biopatch over the insertion site.

36. Place a sterile dressing over the insertion site.

37. Obtain a chest x-ray for radiographic confirmation of placement and to evaluate for complications such as a pneumothorax.

38. Proper placement on a chest x-ray will demonstrate the tip of the catheter in the SVC at the cavoatrial junction.

39. Document the procedure appropriately on the patient's record.

C. Placement of femoral vein CVC.

  1. Identify the femoral triangle created by the inguinal ligament, sartorius muscle, and adductor longus muscle in the inguinal femoral area (see Figure III.18). Whenever possible, use US to access the vein using these landmarks.

  2. Palpate the femoral artery.

  3. The femoral vein will be medial to the femoral artery, and the bladder is in the pelvis medial to the vein. Use the femoral artery as a guide to avoid being too medial and inserting the needle into the bladder.

  4. Insert the needle with a 20- to 30-degree angle with the skin toward the umbilicus.

Femoral Triangle

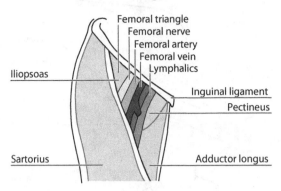

FIGURE III.18 Anatomy of the femoral triangle.

  5. Confirm placement with abdominal x-ray.
  6. The tip of the catheter should be located above the confluence of the iliac vein.

EVALUATION AND RESULTS
A. Maintain all ports flushed and patent.
B. Aspiration of blood from the ports should be nonpulsatile.
C. Connect to pressure tubing if uncertain to ascertain if a waveform is present. A catheter in the vein will produce a single nonpulsatile wave on the monitor (i.e., CVP waveform), whereas a catheter in the artery will produce a pulsatile waveform consistent with a peak and dicrotic notch (i.e., arterial pressure waveform).
D. If arterial access is achieved with placement of the catheter, do not remove the catheter and consult vascular surgery immediately as this is an emergency requiring intervention. Notify staff to not use the catheter.

CLINICAL PEARLS
A. Always maintain sterile technique; the presence of a nurse will help ensure sterility is maintained.
B. Always use US guidance if available.
C. Choose a method of pressure measurement and use it along with US guidance.
D. Always confirm line placement with a chest x-ray for IJ and subclavian lines, and abdominal x-ray for femoral lines.
E. Never hesitate to ask for help or supervision when first learning to perform central lines.

BIBLIOGRAPHY
American Society of Anesthesiologists Task Force on Central Venous Access., Rupp, S. M., Apfelbaum., J. L., Blitt, C., Caplan, R. A., Connis, R. T., Domino, K. B., Fleisher, L. A., Grant, S., Mark, J. B., Morray, J. P., Nickinovich, D. G., & Tung, A. (2012). Practice guidelines for central venous access: A report by the American Society of anesthesiologists task force on central venous access. *Anesthesiology, 116*(3), 539–573. https://doi.org/10.1097/ALN.0b013e31823c9569

CENTRAL VENOUS ACCESS **563**

CAE Healthcare. (n.d.). *Gen I central venous access ultrasound training model tissue insert*. http://www.bluephantom.com/product/Gen-I-Central-Venous-Access-Ultrasound-Training-Model-Tissue-Insert.aspx?cid=562

Institute of Healthcare Improvement. (n.d.). *Central line insertion team checklist*. http://www.ihi.org/resources/Pages/Tools/CentralLineInsertionCareTeamChecklist.aspx

Marino, P. L., & Sutin, K. M. (2006). *The ICU book* (3rd ed., pp. 107–128). Lippincott Williams & Wilkins.

Reichman, E. F. (Ed.). (2013). *Emergency medicine procedures* (2nd ed.). McGraw-Hill/Medical. https://accessemergencymedicine.mhmedical.com/content.aspx?bookid=683&sectionid=45343634

Saugel, B., Scheeren, T. W. L., & Teboul, J. L. (2017). Ultrasound-guided central venous catheter placement: A structured review and recommendations for clinical practice. *Critical Care, 21*, 225. https://doi.org/10.1186/s13054-017-1814-y

CHEST TUBE INSERTION

E. Moneé Carter-Griffin

DESCRIPTION

A. The insertion of a chest tube into the pleural space to drain collected fluid or air.

B. Chest tube insertion is also known as thoracostomy.

INDICATIONS

A. Any fluid collection in the pleural space.
1. Pleural effusion.
2. Hemothorax (blood collection).
3. Empyema (pus collection).
4. Hydrothorax (serous fluid collection).
5. Chylothorax (lymphatic fluid collection).

B. Pneumothorax (air collection).

C. Postoperative drainage of the thoracic cavity.

PRECAUTIONS

A. Assess coagulation profile. A patient with a coagulopathy may have excessive bleeding during and post insertion.

B. Avoid areas with adhesions or lung adherence to the pleura.

C. Careful consideration should be given to differentiate between pulmonary bullae and a pneumothorax.

EQUIPMENT REQUIRED

A. Personal protective equipment.
1. Sterile gloves, gown, and drape.
2. Cap, mask, and protective eyewear.

B. Chest tube drainage system with a water seal.

C. Suction tubing and connector.

D. Various thoracostomy tube sizes: Size used depends on the collection being drained.
1. Usually smaller bore chest tubes <24 Fr are used for a pneumothorax and may also be appropriate for certain fluid collections within the pleural space.
2. Larger bore chest tubes >24 Fr may be more appropriate for more viscous fluid collections, such as blood.
3. There is an ongoing debate about the appropriate size of a chest tube based on the indication for chest tube placement.

E. Antiseptic solution with chlorhexidine or povidone-iodine.

F. Lidocaine 1% with or without epinephrine for local anesthesia.

G. A 5- and 10-mL syringe.

H. 25-G, ⅝- to 1-in. needle.

I. 20- to 23-G, 1½-in. needle.

J. Chest tube insertion tray.
1. 4 × 4 sterile gauze.
2. Hemostats (2).
3. Kelly clamps (2—large and medium).

4. #10 scalpel.
5. Suture scissors.
6. Needle driver.
7. Nylon or silk suture.

K. Occlusive dressing: Vaseline gauze, 4 × 4s, and tape.

L. Surgical marker: Not required but helpful in identifying the point of entry.

PROCEDURE

A. Explain the procedure to the patient and family.

B. Always identify the patient and obtain informed consent.

C. Ensure the patient has intravenous (IV) access and hemodynamic monitoring (e.g., blood pressure, oxygen saturations).

D. Choose a chest tube size. A smaller chest tube, <24 Fr, can typically be used for pneumothoraces, and a larger chest tube, >24 Fr, is indicated for fluid collections.

E. Wash hands/perform hand hygiene.

F. Place the patient in the supine position with the ipsilateral arm raised above the head (Figure III.19).

G. Verify the location for chest tube placement.
1. Use a marker to identify the location/point of entry.
2. Locate the fourth to fifth intercostal space and midaxillary line.
3. The incision is typically made in between the anterior and midaxillary lines.

H. Don sterile attire and prepare sterile field prior to initiating the procedure: Can also be completed with the help of an assistant after the provider has donned sterile attire.
1. Ensure all equipment is available in the chest tube insertion tray.
2. The chest tube may be added during setup or the assistant can add it to the sterile field.

I. Administer moderate sedation.

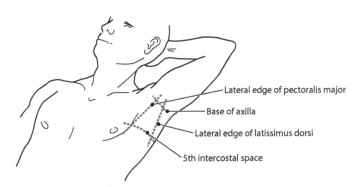

FIGURE III.19 Patient positioning for chest tube insertion.

J. Cleanse the area with chlorhexidine or a povidone-iodine solution. Allow to passively dry.

K. Use the larger Kelly clamp to grasp the proximal end of the chest tube and place it to the side within the sterile field.

L. Perform a time-out.

M. Cleanse the area again with chlorhexidine or a povidone-iodine solution.

N. Drape the identified area with the sterile drape.

O. Use the 25-G, ⅝-in. needle and the 5-mL syringe to inject a small wheal of lidocaine.

P. Use the 20-G, 1½-in. needle and the 10-mL syringe to infiltrate lidocaine into a wide area of subcutaneous tissue, periosteum, and pleura.

Q. Make an incision with a #10 scalpel in the same direction as the rib and below the desired entry level. The incision should be slightly larger than the chest tube size.

R. Insert the medium Kelly clamp downward through the incision, creating a tunnel by opening and closing the clamp (blunt tissue dissection). Create the tunnel tack over the fifth rib. Aim toward the superior aspect until the pleura of the fourth intercostal space is reached.

S. Once the pleura is reached, close the clamp, advance through the parietal pleura into the pleural space, then open/close the clamp to widen the hole.

T. Insert a finger into the tract to widen the tract and to ensure it ends at the upper border of the rib above the incision (Figure III.20).

   1. Remove the medium Kelly clamp but a finger should remain in place to avoid losing the tract.

U. Grasp the other Kelly clamp with the chest tube connected.

1. Advance the proximal end into the pleural space toward the apex of the lung, remove the Kelly clamp, and guide the tube further into the pleural space.

   2. Air and/or fluid may be in the space.

V. Connect the chest tube to the drainage system and have the assistant connect to suction. Typical suction setting is −20 cm H_2O, but the provider will indicate the desired amount of suction.

W. Suture chest tube in place to the chest wall using a purse string technique and wrap additional suture around the chest tube.

X. Place petroleum gauze around the test tube, add 4 × 4, and secure with tape.

Y. Dispose of all equipment.

Z. Obtain a chest x-ray immediately following placement.

AA. Document the procedure, indication, complications, and postprocedure imaging.

EVALUATION AND RESULTS

A. Depending on indication for placement, expect air or fluid removal.

B. Reexpansion of the lung tissue should occur.

CLINICAL PEARLS

A. In order for thoracostomy tubes to function properly, all of the fenestrations in the tube must be within the thoracic cavity. The last side-hole in a thoracostomy tube is indicated by a gap in the radiopaque line; if it is not within the thoracic cavity or there is evidence of subcutaneous air, the tube may not have been completely inserted.

B. Ultrasound guidance is beneficial for identification of fluid accumulation and may reduce risk of complications; however, it requires a competent operator.

C. Continuous bubbles indicate there is a leak within the patient or the chest tube system. Small fluctuations during inspiration and expiration are normal and expected.

BIBLIOGRAPHY

Dezube, R. (2019). *How to do a surgical tube thoracostomy.* Merck Manual Professional Version. https://www.merckmanuals.com/professional/pulmonary-disorders/how-to-do-pulmonary-procedures/how-to-do-surgical-tube-thoracostomy

Kwaitt, M., Tarbox, A., Seamon, M. J., Swaroop, M., Cipolla, J., Allen, C., Hallenbeck, S., Davido, H. T., Lindsey, D. E., Doraiswamy, V. A., Galwankar, S., Tulman, D., Latchana, N., Papadimos, T. J., Cook, C. H., & Stawicki, S. P. (2014). Thoracostomy tubes: A comprehensive review of complications and related topics. *International Journal of Critical Illness and Injury Science, 4,* 143–155. https://doi.org/10.4103/2229-5151.134182

Ravi, C., & McKnight, C. L. (2021). *Chest tube.* StatPearls Publishing. https://www.ncbi.nlm.nih.gov/books/NBK459199/

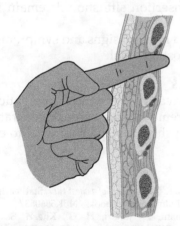

FIGURE III.20 Illustration demonstrating the index finger inserted into the tract.

CHEST TUBE REMOVAL

E. Moneé Carter-Griffin

DESCRIPTION

A. Removal of a chest tube from the pleural space when it is no longer needed for drainage of air or fluids.

INDICATIONS

A. Reexpansion of the lung tissue.

B. Resolution of air leaks (continuous bubbling) for at least 24 hours.

C. Pleural effusions: Tubes should have output less than 200 mL for greater than 24 hours prior to removal.

D. Cardiac surgery: Tubes can be removed once the fluid has changed from sanguineous to serosanguineous, no air leak is present, and less than 100 mL of fluid observed in the preceding 8 hours.

PRECAUTIONS

A. Avoid the introduction of air or contaminants during the removal to minimize further complications.

EQUIPMENT REQUIRED

A. Gloves, gown, mask, and eye protection.

B. Waterproof pad(s) to place under the removal site/area.

C. Suture removal kit.

D. Chlorhexidine or povidone-iodine antiseptic swabs/solution.

E. Kelly clamps (2).

F. Petrolatum gauze.

G. 4 × 4 gauzes.

H. Steri-Strips or some other form of elastic closure device.

I. Tape.

PROCEDURE

A. Prior to removal, verify there is no air leak and/or chest tube output.

B. Review imaging and assess respiratory status.

C. Explain the procedure to the patient and family.

D. Always identify the patient and obtain informed consent.

E. Ensure the patient has intravenous (IV) access and hemodynamic monitoring (e.g., blood pressure, oxygen saturations).

F. Wash hands/perform hand hygiene.

G. Don clean gloves.

H. Place the patient in a semi-Fowler position with waterproof pads directly under the patient and the chest tube site.

I. Gather all supplies. Open the suture removal kit, petrolatum gauze, and 4 × 4 gauzes.

J. Remove the suction from the drainage system. Assess for an air leak.

    1. Often, providers will remove suction hours prior to removal of the chest tube, especially in those with a chest tube due to a pneumothorax.

K. Remove dressing/tape and cleanse the area with chlorhexidine.

L. Clip and remove the sutures. Ensure the chest tube is free from sutures.

M. Pleural chest tubes: Cover the insertion site with the petrolatum gauze and the mediastinal chest tube site with 4 × 4 gauzes.

N. Clamp chest tube with Kelly clamps.

O. Instruct the patient to take a deep breath and to hold it for removal of each chest tube.

    1. Historically, providers remove the chest tube during expiration. Literature is mixed on the findings as to whether there is a difference between removal during inspiration and expiration.

P. Remove the chest tube quickly and smoothly in one rapid motion. Immediately apply pressure once the tube is removed.

Q. Secure the dressing in place.

R. Assess the patient's respiratory and hemodynamic status immediately following procedure.

S. Dispose of all equipment.

T. Obtain a chest x-ray 1 to 2 hours following removal.

U. Document the procedure, indications, complications, and patient tolerance.

EVALUATION AND RESULTS

A. Lung tissue should remain expanded post tube removal.

B. Chest tube insertion site should remain infection-free.

C. Patient should have no signs and symptoms of respiratory distress post removal.

CLINICAL PEARLS

A. Patients on invasive mechanical ventilation should have chest tube removed during peak inspiration.

B. Examine each chest tube post removal to ensure the tube is intact.

BIBLIOGRAPHY

Merkle, A., & Cindass, R. (2021). *Care of a chest tube*. StatPearls Publishing. https://www.ncbi.nlm.nih.gov/books/NBK556088/

Paydar, S., Ghahramani, Z., Johari, H. G., Khezri, S., Ziaeian, B., Ghayyoumi, M. A., Fallahi, M. J., Niakan, M. H., Sabetian, G., Abbasi, H. R., & Bolandparvaz, S. (2015). Tube thoracostomy (chest tube) removal in traumatic patients: What do we know? What can we do? *Bulletin of Emergency and Trauma, 3*, 37–40. https://www.ncbi.nlm.nih.gov/pmc/articles/PMC4771264/#__ffn_sectitle

Ravi, C., & McKnight, C. L. (2021). *Chest tube*. StatPearls Publishing. https://www.ncbi.nlm.nih.gov/books/NBK459199/

DIGITAL NERVE BLOCKS

Dominick Osipowicz

DESCRIPTION

A. A method of anesthetizing a finger or toe (digit) providing a large area of regional anesthesia.
B. Performed by injecting a prescribed amount of anesthetic into the subcutaneous space, forming a ring around the proximal portion of the affected digit.
C. Anesthetic can be:
   1. A short-acting medication, such as lidocaine 2%.
   2. A long-acting medication, such as bupivacaine 0.5%.
   3. A 50:50 mixture of both medications to provide both short and longer action.
D. Nerve block is not the same as local anesthesia of a wound; it eliminates the distortion effect on a laceration site encountered with the infiltration of a large amount of liquid.

INDICATIONS

A. The need for local anesthesia to the distal portion of a digit in order to perform a short, painful procedure, for example suturing a laceration.

PRECAUTIONS

A. Avoid injecting more than 4 mL total into any digit as it will increase the risk of compartment syndrome.
B. As with any blind injections, aspirate syringe prior to installation of medication in an effort to avoid injecting anesthetic into a blood vessel.

EQUIPMENT REQUIRED

A. Povidone-iodine or chlorhexidine preparation for cleansing the injection site.
B. 22- to 30-G needle for injection.
C. Separate 18- to 20-G blunt needle for drawing up anesthetic medication.
D. 2- to 3-mL syringes.
E. Vial of selected anesthetic (e.g., lidocaine, bupivacaine).
F. Sterile or clean gloves.

PROCEDURE

A. The purpose of injection is to surround the nerves in a bath of anesthetic (not reach nerves directly).
B. Perform hand hygiene.
C. Don clean gloves.
D. Prepare the skin with an antimicrobial solution.
E. Using a blunt or 18- to 22-G needle and syringe, draw up the desired amount of anesthetic.
F. Change needle to a smaller gauge for injection of anesthetic into the affected digits.
G. Make one to three punctures on the palmar surface (bottom) of the base of the digit (Figure III.21).
   1. Fan punctures out in a circumferential manner.

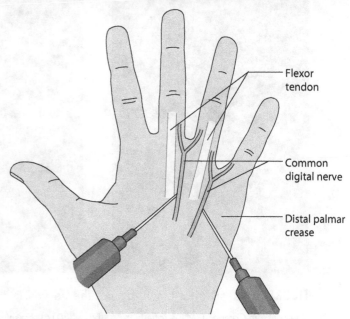

FIGURE III.21   The digital nerve block.

   2. Instill a maximum of 4 mL into the space around the proximal phalange.
H. Make two punctures on the dorsal surface (top) of the base of the digit (Figure III.22).
   1. One into the web spacing on each side of the phalange/phalanx.

EVALUATION AND RESULTS

A. Test areas of effectiveness prior to beginning the intended painful procedure.
B. If required, administer additional anesthetic (maximum 4 mL total per digit).

CLINICAL PEARLS

A. If attempting a single puncture, withdraw the needle to the base of the skin before redirecting toward the other side of the bone to get the maximum distribution of anesthetic from one puncture.
B. If using multiple puncture sites, instill anesthetic to the opposite surface, attempting to numb the intended site of the second puncture to minimize pain associated with the second puncture.
C. If the intended procedure will be performed immediately (e.g., suturing), then lidocaine alone may prove sufficient.
D. If the patient will be anesthetized and then sent for radiologic imaging for an extended period of time, then a 50:50 mixture of lidocaine and bupivacaine is preferred due to the extended duration of anesthesia.

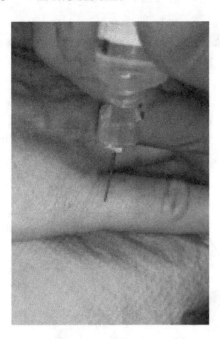 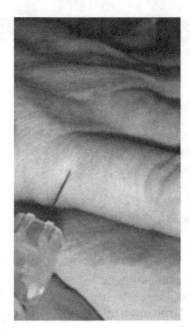 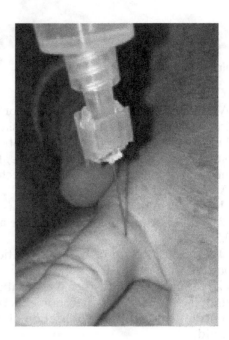

FIGURE III.22   Digital block around the nerves.

Source: From Campo, T. M., & Lafferty, K. A. (Eds.). (2016). *Essential procedures for emergency, urgent, and primary care settings* (2nd ed.). Springer Publishing Company.

BIBLIOGRAPHY

Baldor, R., & Mathes, B. (2020). Digital nerve block. *UpToDate.* https://www.uptodate.com/contents/digital-nerve-block

Okur, O. M., Şener, A., Kavakli, H. Ş., Çelik, G. K., Doğan, N. Ö., Içme, F., & Günaydin, G. P. (2017). Two injection digital block versus single subcutaneous palmar injection block for finger lacerations. *European Journal Trauma and Emergency Surgery, 43,* 863. https://doi.org/10.1007/s00068-016-0727-9

EXTRACORPOREAL MEMBRANE OXYGENATION

Nicole Cavaliere

DESCRIPTION

A. Extracorporeal membrane oxygenation (ECMO) is the use of a mechanical device that evolved from a cardiopulmonary bypass circuit for specialized life support.

B. The most common configurations of ECMO is veno-venous (VV) ECMO and veno-arterial (VA) ECMO.

  1. VV ECMO is used for oxygenation in patients with acute respiratory failure, such as severe acute respiratory distress syndrome (ARDS), and does not provide hemodynamic support.

  2. VA ECMO supports cardiac output in addition to providing oxygenation.

C. Although this procedure is outside the scope of practice for an advanced practice provider (APP), the APP may assist with the procedure and manages the system after cannulation.

INDICATIONS

A. Hypoxemic respiratory failure.
B. Pneumonia.
C. ARDS.
D. Pulmonary contusions.
E. Smoke inhalation.
F. Status asthmaticus.
G. Aspiration.
H. Bridge to lung transplant.
I. Refractory cardiogenic shock attributed to:
  1. Myocarditis.
  2. Acute myocardial infarction (MI).
  3. Acute cor pulmonale from massive pulmonary embolism.
  4. Intractable arrhythmias.
  5. Acute exacerbation of chronic heart failure.
J. Bridge to left ventricular assist device (LVAD).
K. Bridge to heart transplant.

PRECAUTIONS

A. Many ECMO centers adhere to strict criteria for patient selection for ECMO therapy due to limited resources and predictors of mortality.

B. ECMO cannulation is considered a surgical procedure and is to be performed only by a cardiovascular or thoracic surgeon with the assistance of an experienced surgical team. The presence of an ECMO-trained surgical team and a multidisciplinary team trained in management of ECMO following cannulation reduces the risks of complications. The surgical team includes:

  1. Cardiovascular or thoracic surgeon or interventional cardiologist trained for cannulation.

  2. ECMO-trained physician.

  3. Cardiac anesthesiologist.
  4. Respiratory therapist to manage ventilator settings.
  5. ECMO-trained critical care nurse.
  6. Cardiovascular perfusionist.
  7. Surgical scrub tech/nurse.
  8. Circulating nurse.
  9. ECMO-trained acute care nurse practitioner or physician assistant may or may not be present during cannulation. However, APPs play a vital role in the management of the critically ill ECMO patient after cannulation.

C. After a proper time-out has been completed, the patient should be sedated and paralyzed prior to placement of the venous cannula.

D. Patient should be typed and crossmatched for blood products.

  1. Whether cannulation is taking place at bedside or in the operating room, vital signs, telemetry, and pulse oximetry must be continuously monitored.

  2. Equipment and medications are needed for treatment of arrhythmias and bradycardia.

  3. Aortic dissection (during VA ECMO) or vessel rupture will result in the need for emergent sternotomy. Proper equipment and personnel should be available.

E. Complications of ECMO.
  1. Aortic dissection due to arterial cannulation.
  2. Venous rupture.
  3. Acute anemia due to blood loss.
  4. Venous spasm: Prevented by avoiding excessive manipulation.
  5. Arrhythmias.
  6. Bradycardia 2/2 to stimulation of vagus nerve.
  7. Distal extremity thrombosis and ischemia.

EQUIPMENT REQUIRED

A. Sterile gowns and gloves.
B. Sterile saline.
C. Syringes and needles.
D. Povidone-iodine solution.
E. Povidone-iodine ointment.
F. Semipermeable transparent membrane-type dressing.
G. Absorbable gelatin sponge.
H. Surgical lubricant.
I. Blood.
  1. Emergency situation: Uncrossmatched blood should be available.
  2. Difficult cannulation: 10 to 20 mL/kg of blood is often required for appropriate resuscitation.
J. Surgical caps and masks.
K. Electrocautery.

L. Wall suction.
M. Tubing clamps.
N. Pump (roller or centrifugal).
O. Membrane oxygenator.
P. ECMO cannulas.
 1. Patient's oxygenation is directly related to blood flow.
 2. To allow for maximal blood flow, the largest possible internal diameter should be utilized.

PROCEDURE

A. Discuss the procedure with the patient and/or family and obtain consent.
B. Select the cannula (decided by the primary operator: cardiovascular or thoracic surgeon); cannula size and selection directly affect the support patient is receiving from ECMO circuit.
C. Perform a time-out.
D. Sedate the patient; may also be paralyzed depending on surgeon preference.
E. Prime ECMO circuit with albumin (12.5 g) and CaCl (1 g).
F. Venous access obtained with introducer/sheath. In emergency cannulation situations, the APP may be the first provider on scene and can initiate this step.
G. Two main percutaneous techniques performed for VV ECMO by a trained cardiovascular or cardiothoracic surgeon:
 1. Placement of two cannulae: Internal jugular and femoral vein, or bilateral femoral veins (Figure III.23).
  a. Cannula (23–29 Fr) placed for drainage of blood from the inferior vena cava (IVC) via the femoral vein.
  b. Cannula (21–23 Fr) placed for reinfusion of blood through the jugular vein.
 2. Double-lumen cannula is used to allow blood to drain from both the IVC and the superior vena cava (SVC). The cannula's internal membrane directs blood across the tricuspid valve to minimize recirculation, avoiding femoral vein cannulation, and allowing patients to be more mobile while on ECMO.
H. Femoral peripheral cannulation is the most common approach for VA ECMO.
 1. Venous cannula (20–24 Fr) placed for drainage of blood with the tip aiming to be in the mid-right atrium (SVC-right atrial [RA] junction is ideal).
 2. Arterial cannula (16–20 Fr) placed for reinfusion of blood and lies in the iliac artery.
 3. Distal perfusion catheter (6–8 Fr) is placed in the superficial femoral artery and spliced into the arterial cannula to ensure adequate perfusion of the limb distal to the flow of the arterial cannula.
I. Following cannulation, management of the patient on VV ECMO includes managing flow and ventilator settings, sedation, gas exchange, and anticoagulation, as well as oxygen saturation (SaO_2) and venous oxygen saturation (SvO_2) monitoring.

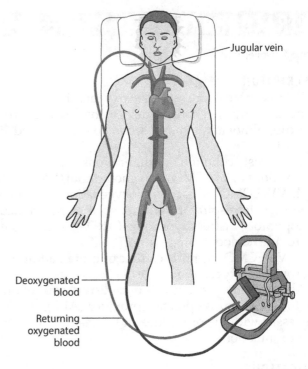

FIGURE III.23 Veno-venous extracorporeal membrane oxygenation internal jugular cannulation and circuit.

EVALUATION AND RESULTS

A. ECMO circuit.
 1. The primary purpose is exchange of both carbon dioxide (CO_2) and oxygen and mechanical circulatory support if cannulated with VA configuration (Figure III.24).
 2. Oxygenator is responsible for oxygenation and CO_2 elimination; has semipermeable membrane to allow diffusion by blood and gas flow in countercurrent directions.
 3. Determine if rate of diffusion occurs by adjusting gas sweep rate and blood flow rate.
  a. Gas sweep is the primary factor in CO_2 clearance.
   i. Other factors affecting CO_2 removal: Blood flow and total body surface area.
   ii. Sweep gas flow rate is measured in liters per minute.
   iii. Initial cannulation: Set at 2 to 4 L/min.
   iv. As rate of gas sweep increases, so does the rate of decarboxylation.
  b. Blood flow rate is the rate at which blood flows through ECMO circuit's oxygenator, one of the primary determinants of oxygenation.
   i. Other factors influencing oxygenation include fraction of inspired oxygen (FiO_2) and hemoglobin.
   ii. Measured in liters per minute and it is recommended that the blood flow rate be 3 mL/kg/min.

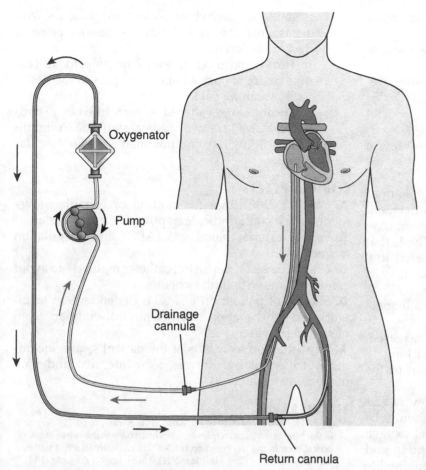

FIGURE III.24   Veno-arterial extracorporeal membrane oxygenation bifemoral peripheral cannulation.

B. Ventilator management for patients on ECMO.

   1. Varies from institution. Many centers practice ultra-protective ventilation for patients on ECMO to allow for lung rest; targets low tidal volumes, often 3 to 4 mL/kg/ideal body weight, and positive end-expiratory pressure (PEEP) of 10 to 15 cm H_2O while maintaining peak pressure less than 20 to 25 cm H_2O.

   2. Respiratory rates often set anywhere from 4 to 10 breaths per minute. Patients on ECMO are able to tolerate such low respiratory rates due to the high rate of CO_2 clearance provided by the ECMO circuit. As the ECMO circuit is responsible for fully oxygenated blood, FiO_2 settings on the ventilator can be minimal, often set to less than 30%.

C. Continuous management and monitoring.

   1. Required monitoring.

   a. Daily chest x-ray (CXR).

   b. Daily labs including:

   i. Complete blood count (CBC).

   ii. Lactate dehydrogenase (LDH).

   iii. D-dimer.

   iv. Comprehensive metabolic panel (CMP).

   v. Erythrocyte sedimentation rate (ESR).

   vi. Prothrombin time/international normalized ratio (PT/INR).

   vii. Fibrinogen level.

   c. Plasma free hemoglobin when there is concern for hemolysis.

d. Heparin is the gold standard anticoagulant to use while a patient is on ECMO. Based on institution, monitoring of heparin may vary and include activated partial thromboplastin time (APTT), activated clotting time (ACT), or heparin assays. These labs should be checked every 6 hours. Bivalirudin may be used as an alternative if a patient develops heparin-induced thrombocytopenia (HIT).

e. Blood cultures as indicated.

f. Electrolyte monitoring and repletion.

g. Thorough inspection of the entire circuit every shift.

h. Frequent pulse checks. Use of cerebral and lower extremity oximetry.

i. Monitoring of hematuria.

j. Maintain minimal ventilator settings.

   2. Suggested monitoring and management.

   a. Avoiding percutaneous procedures due to bleeding concerns.

   b. Avoiding subcutaneous injections due to bleeding concerns.

   c. Limiting invasive procedures to those that can be performed with a Bovie.

   d. Removing any excessive lines, which may lead to bleeding.

   e. Gentle suctioning and gentle placement of nasogastric (NG) and orogastric (OG) tubes.

f. Passive range of motion exercises to avoid contractures.

g. Providing full nutritional support as soon as possible.

h. Minimizing sedation while maintaining adequate pain control.

i. Safely obtaining neurologic exams on a daily basis.

j. Daily SvO_2 or central venous oxygen saturation ($ScvO_2$) monitoring.

3. Weaning ECMO.

a. Weaning trial should be performed often once there has been significant clinical improvement while on ECMO, as evidenced by sufficient oxygenation with gas flow rate of 0 L/min. Note that the ECMO blood flow cannot be decreased to 0 due to risk of thrombosis; only the gas flow is decreased to 0 L/min.

b. Increase ventilator settings to ensure adequate CO_2 removal during trial.

c. Once ventilator settings have been increased, slowly decrease gas flow rate until reaching 0 L/min; decrease rate is at the discretion of the attending physician.

d. For VV ECMO wean, while gas flow rate is maintained at 0 L/min, blood gas should be drawn and evaluated for a goal arterial oxygen pressure (PaO_2) of greater than 60 mmHg and a goal partial pressure of arterial carbon dioxide ($PaCO_2$) of 30 to 45 mmHg.

e. For VA ECMO wean, transesophageal echocardiogram (TEE) or transthoracic echocardiogram (TTE) can be utilized to assess for left ventricle (LV)/right ventricle (RV) function, while flow rate is decreased at intervals. Fluid challenge with a 250- to 500-mL bolus and/or inotropic glucose tolerance test (GTT) support may also be used during VA ECMO wean trial.

f. Each institution has varying requirements for weaning trials. Ensuring a patient is stable for anywhere from 4 to 24 hours with a gas flow rate of 0 L/min is desired prior to decannulation.

g. Turn heparin off at least 2 hours prior to cannula removal once a patient has passed the designated weaning trial.

h. Decannulation should be performed by experienced ECMO-trained medical staff due to significant bleeding risk and potential need for vascular repair.

CLINICAL PEARLS

A. Watch ECMO lines for clotting or cannula movement, which could indicate hypovolemia or anemia.

B. Follow arterial blood gas (ABG) and coagulation frequently.

C. Check the distal perfusion catheter regularly to avoid complications with limb ischemia.

D. Success of patient on ECMO is dependent on teamwork and collaboration among a multidisciplinary team of skilled providers.

E. Pay attention to details of the patient's care, including nutrition, daily diuresis, skin integrity, and pain management/sedation.

BIBLIOGRAPHY

Allen, S., Holena, D., McCunn, M., Kohl, B., & Sarani, B. (2011). A review of the fundamental principles and evidence base in the use of extracorporeal membrane oxygenation (ECMO) in critically ill adult patients. *Journal of Intensive Care Medicine, 26*(1), 13–26. https://doi.org/10.1177/0885066610384061

Brogran, T. V., Lequier, L., Lorusso, R., MacLaren, G., & Peek, G. (2017). *Extracorporeal life support: The ELSO red book* (5th ed.). Extracorporeal Life Support Organization.

Marasco, S. F., Lukas, G., McDonald, M., McMillan, J., & Ihle, B. (2008). Review of ECMO (extra corporeal membrane oxygenation) support in critically ill adult patients. *Heart, Lung and Circulation, 17*(Suppl. 4), S41–S47. https://doi.org/10.1016/j.hlc.2008.08.009

Sangalli, F., Patroniti, N., & Pesenti, A. (2014). *ECMO—Extracorporeal life support in adults.* Springer Publishing.

Short, B. L., Williams, L., (Eds.). (2010). *ECMO specialist training manual* (3rd ed.). Extracorporeal Life Support Organization.

ENDOTRACHEAL INTUBATION

E. Moneé Carter-Griffin

DESCRIPTION

A. Insertion of an endotracheal tube (ETT) into the airway to maintain patency, protection, delivery of oxygen, and/or ventilate a patient.

INDICATIONS

A. Inability to protect the airway (e.g., altered level or loss of consciousness).

B. Inadequate ventilation (e.g., hypercapnic respiratory failure).

C. Inadequate oxygenation (e.g., acute respiratory distress syndrome [ARDS], pneumonia).

D. Anticipated clinical decline/impending respiratory failure (e.g., septic shock).

E. Airway obstruction (e.g., facial trauma, burns, angioedema).

F. Ineffective ability or inability to clear secretions with high risk for aspiration.

G. Cardiac/respiratory arrest.

PRECAUTIONS

A. Surgical intervention is warranted in patients with total airway obstruction or loss of oropharyngeal landmarks.

EQUIPMENT REQUIRED

A. Ambu bag, mask, and oxygen source.

B. Sedatives and paralytics.

C. Laryngoscope handle and blade.

  1. Ensure light source works prior to intubation.

  2. Have more than one blade available.

  3. Standard blade sizes for adults are a 3 and 4.

  4. Know the differences between blades.

   a. A Macintosh is a curved blade.

   b. A Miller is a straight blade.

D. Use videolaryngoscope as alternative to allow for direct visualization of the oropharynx via camera (Figure III.25).

E. ETT.

  1. Varies in size: The size refers to the internal diameter of the tube.

  2. Size 7 to 7.5 mm for an average-sized female; size 8 mm is usually adequate for an average-sized male.

F. Stylet.

  1. Know the differences between the stylet used for traditional laryngoscopy and for videolaryngoscopy.

   a. Traditional laryngoscope uses a more flexible stylet.

   b. Videolaryngoscopy utilizes a stiffer stylet.

G. 10-mL syringe.

H. Water-soluble lubricant.

I. Suction catheter and source.

J. Oral airways.

K. End-tidal carbon dioxide (CO_2) detector and/or capnography.

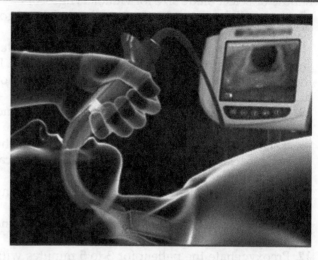

FIGURE III.25 GlideScope video-assisted laryngoscopy.

Source: From Campo, T. M., & Lafferty, K. (Eds.). (2016). *Essential procedures for emergency, urgent, and primary care settings: A clinical companion* (2nd ed.). Springer Publishing Company.

L. Bougie may be needed for difficult airways; keep at bedside.

M. ETT securing device/holder or tape postintubation.

N. Mask, eye protection, gloves, and gown.

PROCEDURE

A. Preparation.

  1. Explain the procedure to the patient and family.

  2. Obtain informed consent from the patient if possible or family if more appropriate.

  3. Inquire if the patient has a history of a difficult airway or prior upper airway or neck injuries, disorders, or surgeries that may make intubation difficult.

  4. Wash hands/perform hand hygiene.

  5. Don clean gloves.

  6. Assess oral cavity for oropharyngeal landmarks, dentures, missing teeth, or other potential obstructions.

  7. Ensure the patient has a functional intravenous (IV) line.

  8. The patient should have telemetry, blood pressure, respiratory, and oxygen saturation monitoring.

  9. Vital signs should be visible and checked frequently.

  10. Ensure all equipment is available.

B. Procedure.

  1. Choose appropriate-sized ETT.

  2. Check ETT cuff by attaching 10-mL syringe and inflating the cuff.

  3. Ensure there are no leaks and the cuff is inflating appropriately.

  4. Remove air from the cuff until it is completely deflated.

  5. Insert stylet into ETT ensuring it does not pass beyond the tip of the ETT. Lubricate deflated balloon with water-soluble lubricant.

▶

6. Choose blade size and attach it to laryngoscope handle or select blade size for videolaryngoscope.

7. Ensure light is working on traditional laryngoscope and camera on videolaryngoscope.

8. Prior to performing the procedure, the provider should obtain gloves, a mask, and eye protection. If there is concern for vomiting, copious secretions, or bleeding, then the provider may need a gown.

9. Position the patient with the head extended and the neck flexing forward ("sniffing position").

   a. The sniffing position may not be feasible if the patient has an underlying etiology (e.g., cervical trauma) preventing neck flexion.

10. Assess the patient's mouth and remove any dentures.

11. Suction mouth as needed for a clear view of the oropharynx.

12. Preoxygenate the patient for 3 to 5 minutes with 100% oxygen.

   a. If breathing, passive oxygenation with a mask is sufficient.

   b. If inadequate respirations or apnea, bagging is needed.

13. Administer ordered sedative first.

14. Administer ordered paralytic second.

   a. Administration of paralytic can be optional.

15. Use scissor-like motion to open mouth with the right hand.

16. Using the left hand, insert the laryngoscope at the right side of the mouth, moving midline while pushing the tongue to the left. This technique is usually not required for those using videolaryngoscopy.

17. Advance blade into the oropharynx past the base of the tongue toward the epiglottis using a "lift up and away" movement of the left hand until the vocal cords are visible (Figure III.26). Pending the type of blade, Macintosh versus Miller, will dictate the strategy for exposing the epiglottis.

   a. A Macintosh blade requires the provider to position the blade into the vallecula to expose the epiglottis.

   b. A Miller blade requires the provider to identify the epiglottis and lift up and away.

18. Use the right side of the mouth; under direct visualization, advance ETT into the oropharynx until the cuff passes through the cords. Advance an additional 1 to 2 cm.

19. Remove stylet and inflate cuff on ETT.

20. If the patient is observed to have a difficult airway, the provider may insert a bougie into the right side of the mouth and advance it through the cords. The ETT will be inserted over the bougie until it passes through the vocal cords. Once the ETT is through the vocal cords, the bougie is removed and the cuff inflated. The provider will continue the process with steps 21 to 23.

21. Attach CO_2 detector or capnography and observe for color change (gold indicates correct placement) or end-tidal CO_2 reading (a plateaued waveform, as shown in Figure III.27, with a value of at least 35 mmHg). Auscultate breath sounds over the stomach and over the lungs bilaterally.

22. Hold ETT carefully in place until securement device or tape has been applied.

23. Attach the patient to ventilator and immediately obtain chest x-ray to confirm placement.

EVALUATION AND RESULTS

A. Correct and secure placement of the ETT.

B. Adequate ventilation and oxygenation.

C. Secretion clearance.

CLINICAL PEARLS

A. If unable to get an adequate "sniffing position," place a roll under the patient's shoulders.

B. Ensure a patent airway prior to administering any paralytic.

C. Laryngoscope handle should always lift up and away from the provider doing the procedure.

D. Never lever the laryngoscope back in the oropharynx because it can cause trauma/damage to the teeth.

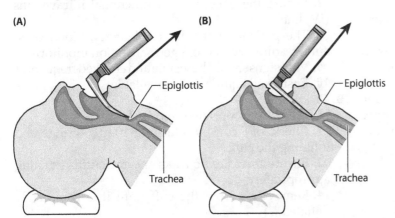

(A)   (B)

Epiglottis

Epiglottis

Trachea

Trachea

FIGURE III.26 The use of laryngoscope. **(A)** Macintosh blade. **(B)** Miller blade.

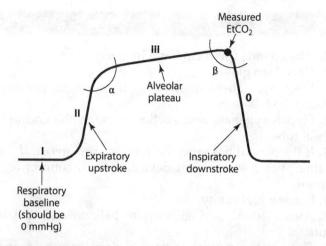

FIGURE III.27 The point of measured end-tidal carbon dioxide (EtCO₂).

BIBLIOGRAPHY

Al-Shaikh, B., & Stacey, S. (2013). *Essentials of anaesthetic equipment* (4th ed.). Churchill Livingstone/Elsevier.

Alvarado, A. C., & Panakos, P. (2021). *Endotracheal tube intubation techniques*. StatPearls Publishing. https://www.ncbi.nlm.nih.gov/books/NBK560730/

Bennett, L., & Cohen, F. M. (2017). Endotracheal intubation. In N. Multak (Ed.), *Clinical procedures for health professionals* (pp. 169–172). Jones & Bartlett.

Campo, T. M., & Lafferty, K (Eds.). (2016). *Essential procedures for emergency, urgent, and primary care settings: A clinical companion* (2nd ed.). Springer Publishing Company.

O'Connor, M. F., & Glick, D. B. (2015). Airway management. In J. B. Hall, G. A. Schmidt, & J. P. Kress (Eds.), *Principles of critical care* (4th ed., pp. 384–395). McGraw-Hill.

Salhi, B. A., Taylor, T. A., & Ander, D. S. (2017). Intubation and airway support. In S. C. McKean, J. J. Ross, D. D. Dressler, & D. B. Scheurer (Eds.), *Principles and practice of hospital medicine* (2nd ed., pp. 895–899). McGraw-Hill.

ENDOTRACHEAL EXTUBATION

E. Moneé Carter-Griffin

DESCRIPTION

A. Removal of an endotracheal tube, allowing the patient to breathe using their own upper airway.

INDICATIONS

A. Initial condition that led to the need for invasive mechanical ventilation has improved or resolved.
B. Hemodynamic stability has been obtained.
C. The patient can adequately protect their airway, clear secretions, and/or maintain minimal risk for aspiration.

PRECAUTIONS

A. Ensure the patient has met the parameters usually outlined in a protocol or by the provider prior to extubation to avoid need for reintubation.

EQUIPMENT REQUIRED

A. Gloves, eye protection, and mask.
B. Oxygen delivery device (e.g., nasal cannula, face mask) and source.
C. Suction catheter and source.
D. 10-mL syringe.
E. Scissors for patients with an endotracheal tube secured with tape.
F. Ambu bag and mask connected to oxygen source.
G. Supplies for endotracheal intubation in case emergent reintubation is required.

PROCEDURE

A. Explain the procedure to the patient and/or family and obtain informed consent.
B. Assess the patient's readiness for extubation, hemodynamic status, and ability to cough.
C. Ensure the patient has a functional intravenous (IV) line.
D. The patient should have telemetry, blood pressure, respiratory, and oxygen saturation monitoring.
E. Wash hands/perform hand hygiene.
F. Don clean gloves.
G. Place the patient in semi- or high-Fowler position prior to extubation.
H. Hyperoxygenate and suction through the endotracheal tube.
I. If the patient has tape, then use scissors to cut. If the patient has a securement device, then disconnect and remove.
J. Suction oral cavity.
K. Attach 10-mL syringe to pilot balloon and deflate cuff.
L. Instruct the patient to take a deep breath in and remove the endotracheal tube.
M. Once the tube has been removed, instruct the patient to take a deep breath and cough.
N. Suction mouth and apply supplemental oxygen.
O. Discard used supplies and equipment.
P. Document the procedure, indication, postextubation physical assessment, complications, and patient tolerance.

EVALUATION AND RESULTS

A. Stable respiratory status and oxygenation.
B. Atraumatic extubation.

CLINICAL PEARLS

A. Assessment of an air leak may be indicated in patients suspected of having ongoing upper airway edema.
B. A decreased air leak does not always suggest the patient will fail postextubation.

BIBLIOGRAPHY

Hyzy, R. (2019, February 6). *Extubation management in the adult intensive care unit*. In G. Finlay (Ed.), *UpToDate*. https://www.uptodate.com/contents/extubation-management
Saeed, F., & Lasrado, S. (2021). *Extubation*. StatPearls Publishing. https://www.ncbi.nlm.nih.gov/books/NBK539804/

EXTERNAL VENTRICULAR DRAIN

Catherine Harris

DESCRIPTION

A. External ventricular drains are tubes that are used to drain and monitor cerebrospinal fluid in the brain.

INDICATIONS

A. Reduce intracranial pressure by allowing cerebrospinal fluid to be removed from the lateral ventricles.

B. Monitor and measure cerebrospinal fluid chemistry and cytology.

C. Monitor intracranial pressure in the perioperative setting.

PRECAUTIONS

A. Any opening created in the skull increases chances of infection; strict sterile technique is mandatory.

B. Aggressive drilling can cause intracranial bleeding at the site; exercise caution past the second layer of compact bone.

EQUIPMENT REQUIRED

A. Ventriculostomy kit.

B. Cranial access kit: Drill, drill bit, scalp retractor, needles/syringes, forceps, and trochar.

C. Sterile gown, gloves, drapes, mask, and hat.

D. Betadine.

E. Hair clippers.

F. Lidocaine with epinephrine.

G. External ventricular setup.

PROCEDURE

A. Explain the procedure to the patient and/or family and obtain informed consent.

B. Wash hands/perform hand hygiene.

C. Place the patient supine with their head elevated 30 degrees.

D. Perform a proper time-out. All present in the room must identify the patient and agree on the correct procedure and the correct site of the procedure.

E. Clip hair around the site of drain insertion.

F. Pre-prep site with Betadine.

G. Mark superficial landmarks for the planned incision. Kocher's point: Found 10 to 11 cm back from nasion, as shown in Figure III.28A and B, and 2.5 to 3 cm lateral to the middle (midpupillary point).

H. Set up sterile field: Prep and drape site.

I. Infiltrate marked skin incision with 1% lidocaine with epinephrine.

J. Make a straight sagittal 1-in. incision with a #11 blade down to the bone.

K. Use self-retaining clamps to hold the skin back.

L. Use a handheld twist drill with a quarter-inch bit to create a burr hole down to the dura.

M. Once the dura has been exposed, puncture with a sharp spinal needle.

N. Advance the ventricular catheter about 5 cm into the lateral ventricle.

O. After catheter placement, remove the stylet and assess for cerebrospinal fluid.

   1. If present, record opening pressure.

   2. If not present, remove the catheter, then reintroduce the stylet and attempt a second pass.

P. Attach a trochar to the distal end of the catheter and tunnel it under the scalp about 3 cm away from the burr hole. *Do not move the intracranial catheter.*

Q. Once in place, confirm catheter position with flow of cerebrospinal fluid.

R. Attach plastic connector from the external drain system and secure with 3-0 silk tie.

S. Anchor the catheter to the scalp with 3-0 nylon to prevent dislodgment.

T. Confirm the catheter still drips cerebrospinal fluid.

U. Return to the initial incision, irrigate with saline, and achieve hemostasis.

V. Close the scalp wound with running 3-0 Monocryl suture. *Do not puncture the underlying catheter.*

W. Follow the institution's policy for dressing the drain site.

EVALUATION AND RESULTS

A. Confirmation of proper placement evidenced by return of cerebrospinal fluid.

CLINICAL PEARLS

A. If there is a lot of blood in the ventricle, clots may get into the holes of the catheter and impede spontaneous ▶

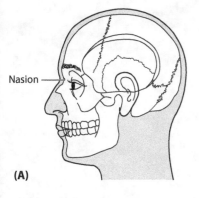

(A)

Nasion

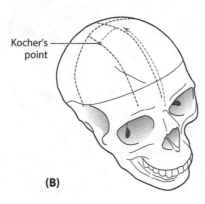

Kocher's point

(B)

FIGURE III.28   **(A)** Location of the nasion and **(B)** Kocher's point.

flow; the catheter may need to be repositioned, or another catheter may need to be placed.

B. Positioning the catheter toward landmarks is critical, but watch the trajectory of placement. If the ventricle is not entered after a couple of passes, seek expert guidance.

C. Do not go further than 7 cm deep. Critical brain structures may be damaged.

BIBLIOGRAPHY

Muirhead, W. R., & Basu, S. (2012). Trajectories for frontal external ventricular drain placement: Virtual cannulation of adults with acute hydrocephalus. *British Journal of Neurosurgery, 26,* 710–716. https://doi.org/10.3109/02688697.2012.671973

Toma, A. K., Camp, S., Watkins, L. D., Grieve, J., & Kitchen, N. D. (2009). External ventricular drain insertion accuracy: Is there a need for change in practice? *Neurosurgery, 65,* 1197–1200. https://doi.org/10.1227/01.NEU.0000356973.39913.0B

INTRAOSSEOUS VASCULAR ACCESS

Dominick Osipowicz

DESCRIPTION

A. Method for using noncollapsible venous plexuses through the bone marrow cavity to rapidly enter systemic circulation for fluid and medication administration.

B. Intraosseous (IO) access and infusion is possible due to the presence of veins that drain the medullary sinuses in the bone marrow of the long bones.

C. Any intravenous (IV) drug or routine resuscitation fluid can be administered safely by the IO route.

INDICATIONS

A. Acute, life-threatening emergency or medical necessity when standard venous access cannot be easily obtained.

B. During CPR, IO access can be considered as the first attempt in select patients.

PRECAUTIONS

A. Proximal ipsilateral fracture.

B. Ipsilateral vascular injury.

C. Severe osteoporosis.

D. Osteogenesis imperfecta.

EQUIPMENT REQUIRED

A. Commercially available and approved rapid IO drill device.

B. Standard bone aspiration needle or specialized IO infusion needle.

C. Standard precautions and safety equipment.

PROCEDURE

A. Explain the procedure to the patient and/or family and obtain informed consent if able; this can be performed as emergent if the patient and/or family is unavailable.

B. Perform hand hygiene.

C. Select site.

   1. The primary site in all age groups should be the proximal tibia, unless otherwise contraindicated.

   2. Landmark for proximal tibia.

   a. Aim insertion two finger breadths below the patella and 1 to 2 cm medial to the tibial tuberosity in adults.

   3. Other sites indicated with landmarks.

   a. Distal femur (under 12 months of age).

      i. Aim for the anterolateral surface, 3 cm above the lateral condyle.

   b. Distal tibia or fibula (over 12 months of age).

      i. Aim for 3 cm proximal to the most prominent aspect of the medial malleolus.

   c. Proximal humerus (over 18 years of age).

      i. Aim for approximately 1 cm above the surgical neck on the anterior shaft of the humerus, which is the greater tubercle.

   d. Manubrium (over 12 years of age).

      i. Superior one-third of the sternum may be accessed.

      ii. Requires a specialized device and training for insertion.

D. Place the patient in a comfortable position.

E. Don sterile gloves depending on hospital policy.

F. Ensure sterile preparation of the site using chlorhexidine solution or povidone-iodine.

G. Infiltrate the insertion site with 1% to 2% lidocaine if the patient is conscious; include the skin and the periosteum.

H. Stabilize extremity with nondominant hand.

I. Hold the IO needle in the dominant hand (Figure III.29).

J. Direct the needle perpendicular to the bone and away from joint spaces.

K. Twist if using manual IO needle or firmly press if using drill and apply constant pressure until sudden loss of resistance.

L. Remove the stylet.

M. Confirm placement by aspiration or infusion (IO access does not always provide blood return).

N. Secure placement with dressing.

EVALUATION AND RESULTS

A. Confirm placement and rule out procedure-induced fracture with x-ray.

B. Complications: Cellulitis, osteomyelitis, iatrogenic fracture, physeal plate injury, and fat embolism.

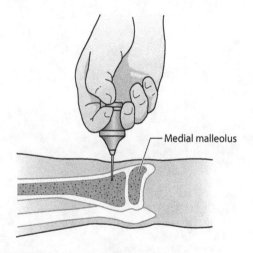

FIGURE III.29   Intraosseous needle insertion.

CLINICAL PEARLS

A. The 2005 American Heart Association (AHA) Guidelines for CPR and Emergency Cardiovascular Care recommend for the first time IO access over endotracheal drug administration during resuscitation.

BIBLIOGRAPHY

ECC Committee, Subcommittees and Task Forces of the American Heart Association. (2005). 2005 American Heart Association guidelines for cardiopulmonary resuscitation and emergency cardiovascular care. *Circulation*, *112*(24 Suppl), IV-1–IV-203.

Ngo, A., Oh, J., Chen, Y., Yong, D., & Ong, M. (2009). Intraosseous vascular access in adults using the EZ-IO in an emergency department. *International Journal of Emergency Medicine*, *2*(3), 155. https://doi.org/10.1007/s12245-009-0116-9

Perron, C. E. (2021). Intraosseous infusion. *UpToDate*. https://www.uptodate.com/contents/intraosseous_infusion

LONG LEG CASTING

Joanne Elaine Pechar

DESCRIPTION
A. Long leg cast is an immobilization device that covers and encases the entire circumference of the leg and foot.
B. Long leg cast is used to stabilize and hold anatomic structures in place until healing is achieved.

INDICATIONS
A. Immobilize and treat acute nondisplaced fractures, dislocations, and injured ligaments.
B. Allow earlier ambulation by stabilizing fractures of the lower extremity.
C. Improve function by stabilizing or positioning a joint.
D. Correct and treat congenital deformities, such as clubfoot and joint contractures.
E. Manage chronic foot and ankle ulcers.

PRECAUTIONS
A. Ensure sufficient gauze or other dressing material is applied to absorb blood if the cast is applied over a wound.
B. Before starting, ensure that adequate analgesia has been achieved.

EQUIPMENT REQUIRED
A. Stockinette.
　1. Stretchable, sock-like material in varying widths.
　2. Acts as a barrier between the skin and the cast padding.
　3. Pulled over rough edges of the cast to provide comfortable padded cast borders.
B. Fiberglass casting material.
　1. Comes in rolls of varying widths. 4- or 6-in. fiberglass is the preferred width.
　2. Commonly used (as opposed to plaster) due to its strength, durability, light weight, and ease of application.
　3. Begins to harden in 3 to 4 minutes. Fully hardens in 1 to 2 hours. Must be kept in its airtight foil package before application.
　4. Due to its sticky resin content, gloves should be worn when handling fiberglass.
C. Webril (cotton) or synthetic undercast padding.
　1. Available in 2-, 3-, 4-, 5-, and 6-in. widths, packaged in individual rolls.
　2. 3- or 4-in. padding is used on lower leg; 5- or 6-in. padding is used on upper leg.
D. Basin full of cool or room temperature water.
　1. Avoid lukewarm water: Can increase probability of exothermic reaction of cast materials, which can increase risk of thermal injury to the skin.
E. Bandage scissors.
F. Cast cutter and spreader.
G. Gloves and gown.

PROCEDURE
A. Position the patient.
　1. Supine, with the ankle over the edge of the table.
　2. Knee flexed to approximately 20 to 35 degrees to relax the gastrocnemius muscle and reduce possible hyperextension.
B. Apply stockinette.
　1. Support the leg (an assistant should support the leg to be casted).
　2. Measure the length of the stockinette (Figure III.30). Cut the stockinette to appropriate length with an extra 4 in. of stockinette on each end of the cast.
　3. Apply the stockinette, which is placed beyond the anticipated cast border.
　4. The proximal edge of the cast should lie below the greater trochanter on the lateral side and just below the groin on the medial side. The distal edge of the cast will be located at the level of the metatarsal heads, while the toes should remain free.
　5. Important positioning of foot: Plantigrade with toes pointing up (Figure III.31).
C. Apply Webril or synthetic undercast padding.
　1. Select appropriate cast padding size. Starting at distal border, gently roll and wind the padding, ▸

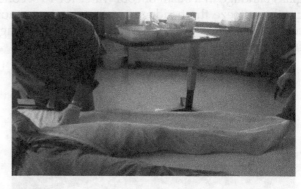

FIGURE III.30 An advanced practice provider measuring the length of the stockinette.

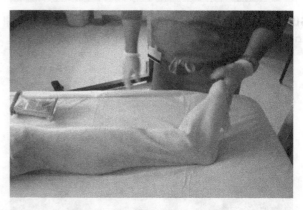

FIGURE III.31 Foot should be plantigrade, with the toes pointing up.

smoothly overlapping each time about 50% around the foot. Two to three padding layers are usually sufficient (Figure III.32).

2. To protect pressure points against pressure ulcers, apply additional Webril padding over the patella, malleoli, and heel.

3. When rolling padding, keep the roll in continuous contact with the extremity to avoid undesirable wrinkles that occur when the roll is lifted during application.

4. Wind cast padding toward the knee with an overlap of 50%, creating a double layer of padding.

5. Cast padding should extend slightly beyond the planned length of the cast, so that when the end of the stockinette is folded over the end of the cast will be well-padded.

6. Extend padding about 2 in. beyond the intended proximal and distal cast borders and add an additional two layers of padding at the proximal and distal borders of the cast (Figure III.33).

D. Apply fiberglass bandage.

1. Use 3- to 6-in. bandage rolls to provide sufficient time for molding.

2. Two or three layers of fiberglass are usually adequate, and construct a cast with uniform thickness.

3. Completely soak and immerse the roll of fiberglass bandage in a basin of cool water for 10 seconds, gently squeeze the bandage to remove excess moisture and water, and remove the fiberglass bandages from the water as soon as bubbling stops.

4. Starting with the bottom of the foot, roll the fiberglass bandage on smoothly around the ankle, overlapping each time by 50%.

5. In the same manner as Webril padding, pass the fiberglass bandage over the heel and then toward the knee with 50% overlap.

6. Where the first bandage ends, apply a second fiberglass bandage, continuing proximally toward the planned upper edge of the cast and then returning toward the foot.

7. As additional fiberglass bandages are required, they should begin at the end of the previous bandage to ensure even thickness of the cast.

8. Avoid wrinkling by folding or tucking fiberglass roll.

E. Form the proximal end of the cast.

1. Fold the loose end of the stockinette over the proximal edge of the cast.

2. Starting below the proximal edge, add another fiberglass bandage to secure the loose end of the stockinette and fiberglass (Figure III.34).

F. Form the distal end of the cast.

1. To create a padded and rolled edge border, pull the stockinette and cast padding over the distal end of the cast edge prior to rolling and securing the final layer of the fiberglass bandage.

G. Final molding.

1. While the fiberglass is still soft, mold the cast to the contour of the extremity by gently, but firmly, rubbing the cast between the palm of gloved hands.

2. To ensure the foot is plantigrade, apply gentle pressure to the sole of the forefoot.

3. Apply liquid soap for the fiberglass to harden.

4. Application of gentle pressure should be continued until the fiberglass hardens.

H. Completed cast.

1. Application of the long leg circular cast is now complete (Figure III.35).

2. Place a small pillow under the ankle until the cast is fully hard and dry.   ▶

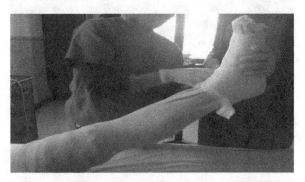

FIGURE III.32 Provide 3 to 4 layers of cotton webril padding before applying the cast material.

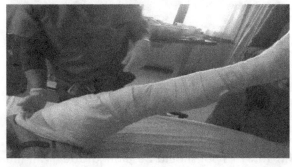

FIGURE III.33 Padding extends beyond the cast.

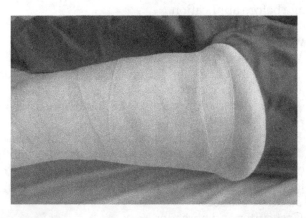

FIGURE III.34 Secure the loose ends of the stockinette and fiberglass.

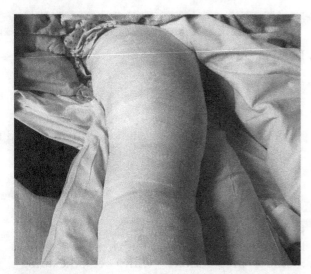

FIGURE III.35   Long leg cast completed.

3. Weight-bearing is restricted for 1 to 2 hours until the cast has fully hardened to avoid denting and cracking.

4. If the cast is to be used for walking, apply extra layers of padding and fiberglass bandage to the sole and heel areas. Finally, place a cast shoe for ambulation and that is typically full weight-bearing.

EVALUATION AND RESULTS

A. Ask the patient if the cast feels loose or tight to ensure comfortable fit.

B. Check if the cast extends to proper boundaries while not interfering with range of motion.

C. Check for any cast indentations or sharp edges. Trim sharp edges using a cast saw or bandage scissors.

D. Instruct the patient regarding:

1. Signs and symptoms of compression, such as swelling within the cast.

2. Required elevation of the injured extremity for 2 to 3 days.

3. Timing for being able to walk on the cast.

4. Weight-bearing and ambulation, which includes crutch or walker training.

5. Avoidance of insertion of any objects under the cast in an attempt to relieve itching.

6. Return to office for a cast check in 5 to 7 days.

7. Prompt notification for any tingling, numbness, weakness, skin ulcerations or discoloration, pallor, paresthesias, paralysis, or worsening pain in the casted extremity.

E. The following are common symptoms of a cast that is too tight:

1. Extremity numbness, tingling, or increased pain.

2. The toes turn to a different color (pale or bluish) than the color of the fingers or toes of the noninjured leg.

3. The toes become swollen.

SPECIAL CONSIDERATIONS IN PATIENTS WITH SPASTICITY

A. Serial casting involves the sequential application of casting material, either plaster or fiberglass, in a circumferential manner around the spastic joint.

B. Serial casting is discontinued when no incremental increase in range of motion is seen on two sequential castings. Patients are then transitioned to a bivalved cast as a long-term maintenance strategy.

C. The mechanism of spasticity reduction for this intervention is that casts minimize changes in muscle length and tension.

D. Potential complications of serial casting include skin breakdown, venous thrombosis, compartment syndrome, and decrease in bone mineral density.

CLINICAL PEARLS

A. In order to sufficiently protect the injured limb, the ideal cast must be thick and rigid.

B. During the setting process, do not place the patient at risk for thermal injury.

C. When supporting the extremity, be careful not to indent the cast with fingertips.

D. "Bivalve" (split) the cast immediately if unexpected swelling occurs in a long leg cast to avoid risk of acute compartment syndrome.

BIBLIOGRAPHY

Gravlee, J. R., & Van Durme, D. J. (2007, February 1). Braces and splints for musculoskeletal conditions. *American Family Physician, 75*(3), 342–348. https://www.aafp.org/afp/2007/0201/p342.html

Halanski, M., & Noonan, K. J. (2008, January). Cast and splint immobilization: Complications. *Journal of the American Academy of Orthopaedic Surgeons, 16*(1), 30–40. https://doi.org/10.5435/00124635-200801000-00005

Saulino, M., & Goldman, L. (2014). Spasticity. In I. B. Maitin & E. Cruz (Eds.), *CURRENT diagnosis & treatment: Physical medicine & rehabilitation*. McGraw Hill. https://accessmedicine.mhmedical.com/content.aspx?bookid=1180&sectionid=70376430

LUMBAR PUNCTURE

Dominick Osipowicz

DESCRIPTION

A. Commonly referred to as a spinal tap.
B. Performed in the lower lumbar spine to remove a sample of cerebrospinal fluid (CSF).

INDICATIONS

A. To obtain analysis of CSF for diagnostic purposes.
  1. Meningitis/encephalitis.
  2. Subarachnoid hemorrhage.
  3. Demyelinating diseases.
  4. Carcinomatous diseases.
B. To evaluate and treat various neurologic conditions.
  1. Guillain–Barré syndrome.
  2. Normal-pressure hydrocephalus.
  3. Pseudotumor cerebri.
C. To instill substances into the subarachnoid space.
  1. Chemotherapy.
  2. Contrast media.

PRECAUTIONS

A. Attempt to stay between L3 and L5 to avoid puncturing the spinal cord (ends around L1/L2). Identify the highest point of the iliac crest bilaterally with palpation to the site of L4 (Figure III.36).
B. Maintain sterility to prevent infection.
C. Be cautious with draining excessive CSF in an effort to avoid risk of cerebral herniation (20–40 mL of CSF can be safely removed).
D. Bleeding at the level of lumbar puncture could cause nerve irritation and damage to surrounding structures.

EQUIPMENT REQUIRED

A. Sterile gown, hat, gloves, and mask.
B. Lumbar puncture needle, 18 or 20 G × 3½ in. in length.

C. Lumbar puncture kit.
  1. 3-mL Luer lock syringe.
  2. 25-G, ⅝-in. needle.
  3. 22-G 1½-in. needle.
  4. Lidocaine 1%.
  5. Four specimen tubes with caps; tubes should be numbered 1 through 4.
  6. Sponge applicators.
  7. Three gauze pads.
  8. Fenestrated drape.
  9. Band-Aid.
  10. One stopcock: Three-way.
  11. Two-piece manometer with extension tubing.
D. Sterile preparation with chlorhexidine or povidone-iodine solution.

PROCEDURE

A. Explain the procedure to the patient and/or family, including indication and risk of complications, and obtain informed consent.
B. Perform hand hygiene.
C. Position the patient in either the lateral decubitus position with knees flexed or seated with their head bent forward.
D. Perform preprocedural universal protocol. All present in the room must identify the patient and agree on the correct procedure and the correct site of the procedure.
E. Palpate the highest level of iliac crests bilaterally to assess level of L3 to L4 or L4 to L5 interspace. Palpate the midline, in space between spinous processes (Figure III.37).
F. Prepare the skin in the usual sterile fashion.
G. Open the lumbar puncture kit.
H. Don sterile hat, mask, gown and gloves. Prepare the kit, arranging the tubes in numerical order and ▶

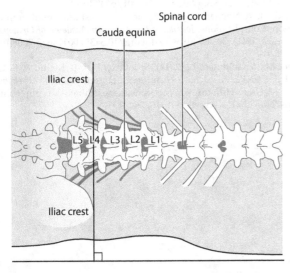

FIGURE III.36 Anatomic landmarks for lumbar puncture.

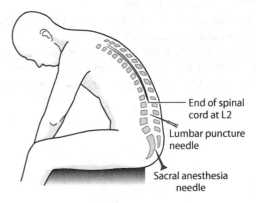

Lumbar puncture

FIGURE III.37 Placement of lumbar puncture needle.

Source: From Brown Emergency Medicine. *Lumbar puncture part 2: Pearls, pitfalls, and troubleshooting.* Brown University.

assembling the manometer including supplied extension tubing (optional). Apply sterile drape. Draw up lidocaine solution using supplied 3-mL syringe and supplied needle (filter or blunt needle).

I. The skin and fascia should be infiltrated with 1% lidocaine with a 25-G needle for superficial local anesthesia, then switch to 22-G needle for deeper local anesthesia.

J. Introduce spinal needle (including stylet) with the bevel *parallel to the spine* to separate the fibers longitudinally in an effort to avoid trauma to tissues.

K. Advance the needle parallel to the floor and perpendicular to the back of the patient, aiming toward the head with a 20- to 30-degree angle.

   1. Bone should be felt superiorly and the needle redirected in caudal direction.

   2. Slight resistance may be felt as the needle is advanced into the ligamentum flavum.

   3. Smooth pop may be felt as the needle penetrates the dural sac. (This may not be felt every time.)

   4. Advance the needle, periodically stop and remove the stylet to assess for drainage, replace the stylet, and advance further. Once CSF is obtained, stop advancing the needle.

L. Maintaining control of the spinal needle, remove the stylet, connect the manometer set up to measure the opening pressure, and record. Once complete, remove and place aside the manometer setup.

M. Use the collection tubes in the lumbar puncture kit to collect CSF. *Fill in numerical order.* The amount collected in each tube will vary depending on the patient and the purpose of the lumbar puncture. A minimum of 3 mL per vial should be obtained.

N. After CSF collection is completed, reinsert the stylet and remove the needle.

O. Hold pressure at the site and then place a Band-Aid or clear occlusive dressing with gauze over the puncture site.

P. Recommend the patient lie flat for 1 to 2 hours after the procedure in an effort to minimize postprocedural headaches.

EVALUATION AND RESULTS

A. Observe color and consistency of CSF.

B. Apply the manometer promptly to the needle in order to obtain an accurate opening pressure.

C. Record the opening pressure.

D. Document the volume of CSF collected and sent to the laboratory.

CLINICAL PEARLS

A. Lumbar puncture is a blind stick.

   1. It is possible to hit one of the nerves of the cauda equina.

   2. If patient complains of pain radiating down the left leg, reposition the needle right to stay central, and vice versa.

B. Positioning is one of the most important aspects of a successful lumbar puncture.

   1. If the interspace of spinal processes is difficult to palpate, ask the patient to arch the head and shoulders forward, while pulling up both knees up toward the chest.

   2. The more the knees are pulled up, the more the spinous processes will open up, making them easier to palpate.

C. A traumatic tap will be evidenced by blood in the CSF that diminishes in quantity collected in the specimen tubes. In patients who have a subarachnoid hemorrhage, the amount of blood will not vary significantly.

D. As blood breaks down over time, it becomes xanthochromic, which is characterized by a straw-yellow color of the CSF. This is indicative of blood being present for several hours. It is very important to get the specimen tubes to the laboratory as quickly as possible to distinguish between a traumatic tap (which will have no evidence of xanthochromia) and bleeding in the subarachnoid space, which may be caused by rupture of a vessel, such as an aneurysm.

BIBLIOGRAPHY

Burke-Doe, A. (n.d.). Ventricles and covergs of the brain. https://accessphysiotherapy.mhmedical.com/data/Multimedia/ grandRounds/ventricles/media/ventricles_print.html

Doherty, C., & Forbes, R. (2014). Diagnostic lumbar puncture. *Ulster Medical Journal, 83*(2), 93–102. https://www.ums.ac.uk/umj083/083(2)093.pdf

Fastle, R., & Bothner, J. (2018). *Lumbar puncture: Indications, contraindications, technique and complications in children.* In J. F. Wiley & II (Eds.), *UpToDate.* https://www.uptodate.com/contents/lumbar-puncture-indications-contraindications-technique-and-complications-in-children

PERIPHERALLY INSERTED CENTRAL CATHETER PLACEMENT

Catherine Harris

DESCRIPTION
A. A 3- to 6-Fr catheter is inserted into the upper arm via the basilic or brachial vessel until the tip reaches the superior vena cava junction.

INDICATIONS
A. According to the Centers for Disease Control and Prevention (CDC), the peripherally inserted central catheter (PICC) line is the safest central vascular catheter (CVC) capable of remaining indwelling for over a year.
B. Long-term antibiotics, total parenteral nutrition (TPN), vasopressors, and multiple incompatible medications.

PRECAUTIONS
A. Chronic kidney disease/end-stage renal disease (CKD/ESRD).
  1. Extended PICC line dwell time in peripheral vasculature can lead to stenosis of the brachial or basilic vessel due to intima hypertrophy/scarring; can complicate future fistula formation or graft placement.
  2. If renal replacement therapy (RRT) is imminent, nephrology should be consulted to decide if PICC would be suitable for the patient.
  3. Patient should receive tunneled jugular line placed by intervention radiology (IR) instead.
B. Bacteremia.
  1. Can result in central line-associated bloodstream infection (CLABSI). If cultures are pending, 48 hours of negative cultures or infectious disease approval is needed for PICC placement.
C. Permanent pacemaker.
  1. PICC lines should never occupy the same vessel as the pacemaker wires as this could potentially lead to wire displacement.
D. Coagulopathy.
  1. Cutoff for platelets, international normalized ratio (INR), partial thromboplastin time (PTT), and so forth will differ based on facility.
  2. Determine if static parameters should delay an intervention (e.g., a patient with disseminated intravascular coagulopathy will not improve and this could prohibit placement of PICC).

EQUIPMENT REQUIRED
A. Ultrasound.
B. Insertion kit with PICC line.
  1. One bag, bedside white 6⅗″ × 3½″ × 11¾″.
  2. One bag, poly, 7″ × 10″ × 2 Mil.
  3. One band bag, 36″ × 28″ clear.
  4. One basin, emesis, 700 mL.
  5. Two cups, 2 oz each.
  6. One drape, 53″ × 77¾″.
  7. One dressing, 4¾″ × 4.
  8. One forceps.
  9. 10 gauze 4″ × 4″.
  10. One gown.
  11. One needle, 18 G × 1½″ length.
  12. One pouch, 17¼″ × 22¾″.
  13. One scalpel #11.
  14. One scissor.
  15. One skin marker.
  16. Two syringes, 10 mL.
  17. One table cover, 44″ × 76″ × 3 Mil.
  18. Seven towels.
C. Probe cover.
D. Chlorhexidine solution.
E. Lidocaine 2%.
F. Extra wire.

PROCEDURE
A. Explain the procedure to the patient and/or family and obtain informed consent.
B. Perform a proper time-out. All present in the room must identify the patient and agree on the correct procedure and the correct site of the procedure.
C. Abduct the patient's arm to 90 degrees and proceed to identify vessel.
D. Measure from the insertion site to the right supraclavicular notch, then add 6 cm to the measurement.
E. Wash hands and open insertion tray.
F. Apply tourniquet to the procedure arm.
G. Don sterile gown and gloves.
H. Drape the patient's body with whole body drape.
I. Drape the patient's arm with window dressing.
J. Prepare the site with chlorhexidine for 30 seconds and allow 1 minute for dry time.
K. Flush all lumens of the PICC line.
L. Apply probe cover to ultrasound probe.
M. Inject lidocaine to the desired insertion site and wait 60 seconds.
N. Use ultrasound to identify target vessel and access the vessel with needle or angiocatheter.
O. Upon seeing flashback, proceed to walk the needle into the vessel.
P. Slide the wire into the needle, then remove the needle or angiocatheter.
Q. Undo tourniquet.
R. Slide peel-away introducer onto the wire, then remove the wire. The peel-away introducer allows the introducer to be peeled away and removed, leaving the catheter in place.
S. Confirm the insertion site is the same as measured in step C, then cut the catheter to that length.
T. Remove the introducer from the sheath, then insert the PICC into the sheath.

U. Continue to advance the catheter until the PICC is at the hub of the sheath.

V. Proceed to peel away the sheath.

W. Confirm blood return and flush all ports.

X. Place the probe on the jugular of the procedure side and flush the catheter. Ensure no sparkles appear on screen to confirm PICC is not in jugular.

Y. Apply occlusive dressing and discard sharps in appropriate container.

Z. Return patient room to preprocedure state.

AA. Page for x-ray for radiographic confirmation.

AB. Document the procedure on the patient's record.

CLINICAL PEARLS

A. In a difficult catheter advancement, additional wire could increase stiffness and increase success.

B. A j-looped wire could potentiate success as this can maneuver around a difficult anatomy.

C. Larger French equates to higher risk of upper extremity deep vein thrombosis (DVT). Catheter-associated DVTs are more likely to originate from the fibrin sheath that forms from decreased blood flow around the catheter due to decreased lumen size.

D. Using an angiocatheter for initial pads allows for catheter threading and decreased risk for unintentional posterior wall puncture.

BIBLIOGRAPHY

Kelly, L. (2013). A practical guide to safe PICC placement. *British Journal of Nursing, 22*(Suppl. 5), S13–S19. https://doi.org/10.12968/bjon.2013.22.Sup5.S13

O'Grady, N. P., Alexander, M., Dellinger, E. P., Gerberding, J. L., Heard, S. O., Maki, D. G., & Weinstein, R. A. (2002). *Guidelines for the prevention of intravascular catheter-related infections. MMWR Recommendations and Reports, 51*(RR-10), 1–26. https://www.cdc.gov/mmwr/preview/mmwrhtml/rr5110a1.htm?vm = r

Sansivero, G. E. (2000). The microintroducer technique for peripherally inserted central catheter placement. *Journal of Intravenous Nursing, 23*, 345–351.

Wallace, B. A., & Taylor, T. (n.d). *Ultrasound-guided venous access.* https://saem.org/cdem/education/online-education/m3-curriculum/bedside-ultrasonography/venous-access

REDUCTION OF THE ANKLES

Kathleen L. Collins

DESCRIPTION
A. Ankle dislocations seen after a traumatic or rotational injury.
B. May be associated with fracture/ligamentous injury.
C. Suspected ankle injuries confirmed on radiographic imaging.

INDICATIONS
A. Prompt reduction of ankle fractures reduces tension on skin, lessens soft tissue swelling, and minimizes pressure on neurovascular structures.
B. Most ankle fractures that require reduction will also require surgical intervention.
C. The goal of reduction is restoration of the ankle mortise or the normal anatomic relationship of the structures that make up the ankle.

EQUIPMENT REQUIRED
A. 18-G needle.
B. 10-mL syringe.
C. 1% lidocaine.
D. Facility-approved conscious sedation protocol, if needed.
E. U-shaped splint with well-padded posterior component.
F. Assistive device as needed (e.g., crutches).

PROCEDURE
A. Perform an initial examination of the patient.
    1. Focus on the soft tissue to look for open wounds, skin tenting, or skin blistering.
    2. Perform a thorough neurovascular examination with comparison with the uninjured extremity *prior to reduction*.
B. Explain the procedure to the patient and/or family and obtain informed consent.
C. Position the patient in the supine position with the affected limb flexed at the knee or flexed over the end of the bed.
    1. May perform intra-articular joint block of the affected ankle for pain control.
    2. Conscious sedation may be necessary to perform adequate reduction.
D. Perform a proper time-out. All present in the room must identify the patient and agree on the correct procedure and the correct site of the procedure.
E. Reduction for a given injury depends on fracture or dislocation pattern.
    1. Common techniques include internal rotation with supination or pronation while giving limb distal traction until audible or palpable reduction is achieved (Figure III.38).

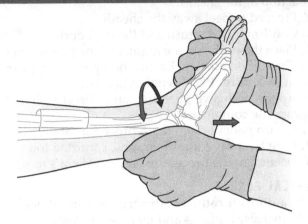

FIGURE III.38 Manual traction of the ankle.

F. Splint patient with lower extremity well-padded posterior and U-shaped splint with proper molding around the ankle joint for added stability.

EVALUATION AND RESULTS
A. Postreduction imaging to evaluate success of reduction and ensure no procedural injuries.
B. Perform postreduction neurovascular examination of bilateral lower extremities.
C. Provide patient with appropriate assistive device (crutches, cane, walker) and instruct no weight-bearing on the limb.
D. Follow up with orthopedics for surgical evaluation of fracture/dislocation.

CLINICAL PEARLS
A. Repeated forceful attempts at reduction can cause additional injury.
B. Failure of reduction after two to three attempts may warrant surgical intervention.
C. If a closed injury converts to an open injury, tetanus prophylaxis and antibiotic coverage should be administered. Open injuries warrant urgent orthopedic evaluation and intervention.

BIBLIOGRAPHY
Arnold, C., Fayos, Z., Bruner, D., & Arnold, D. (2017, December). Managing dislocations of the hip, knee, and ankle in the emergency department. *Emergency Medicine Practice, 19*(12), 1–28.
Court-Brown, C. M., Tornetta, P., McQueen, M. M., & Ricci, W. M, (Eds.). (2020). *Rockwood and green's fractures in adults.* Wolters Kluwer Health.
Egol, K. A., Koval, K. J., & Zuckerman, J. D. (2020). *Handbook of fractures.* Wolters Kluwer Health.
Melenevsky, Y., Mackey, R. A., Abrahams, R. B., Thomson, N. B., 3rd. (2015, May-June). Talar fractures and dislocations: A radiologist's guide to timely diagnosis and classification. *Radiographics, 35*(3), 765–779. https://doi.org/10.1148/rg.2015140156
Rammelt, S., & Goronzy, J. (2015, June). Subtalar dislocations. *Foot and Ankle Clinics, 20*(2), 253–264. https://doi.org/10.1016/j.fcl.2015.02.008
Wight, L., Owen, D., Goldbloom, D., & Knupp, M. (2017, October). Pure ankle dislocation: A systematic review of the literature and estimation of incidence. *Injury, 48*(10), 2027–2034. https://doi.org/10.1016/j.injury.2017.08.011

REDUCTION OF THE FINGERS

Kathleen L. Collins

DESCRIPTION

A. Loss of alignment of a digit joint: Distal interphalangeal (DIP), proximal interphalangeal (PIP), and metacarpophalangeal (MCP) joint.

INDICATIONS

A. Finger reduction is indicated when diagnosis of dislocation has been determined and fracture has been eliminated.

PRECAUTIONS

A. Prior to reduction, obtain imaging to rule out associated fracture.
B. Small wounds or scrapes can be concerning for open injuries connected to bone or joints.

EQUIPMENT REQUIRED

A. Lidocaine 1% or 2% without epinephrine for digital block (optional).
B. Finger splint.
C. Tape.

PROCEDURE

A. Explain the procedure to the patient and family and obtain informed consent.
B. Wash hands/perform hand hygiene.
C. Perform a proper time-out. All present in the room must identify the patient and agree on the correct procedure and the correct site of the procedure.
D. Administer digital block in the proximal aspect of the affected finger.
E. Reduction of dorsal dislocation.
　1. Apply axial traction with simultaneous flexion of the joint (Figure III.39).

2. If unsuccessful, try again but first hyperextend the distal portion to "unlock" the joint. Continue with axial traction and flexion.
3. DIP dorsal dislocation splint in full extension while allowing full range of motion of the PIP joint.
4. PIP dorsal dislocation splint with PIP in 20 degrees to 30 degrees of flexion.
F. Reduction of volar dislocation.
　1. Gently hyperflex while pushing the base of the dislocated phalanx into place (Figure III.40).
　2. Splint the PIP in 20 degrees to 30 degrees of flexion.
G. Reduction of lateral joint dislocation.
　1. Gently hyperextend the joint while correcting the ulnar or radial deformity (Figure III.41).
　2. DIP lateral dislocation splint in full extension.
　3. PIP lateral dislocation; apply dorsal splint with the PIP 20 degrees to 30 degrees of flexion.

EVALUATION AND RESULTS

A. Perform prereduction examination to evaluate capillary refill and rotational and angulatory deformity.
B. Perform postreduction imaging to evaluate the success of reduction and to ensure no procedural injuries.
C. Refer to orthopedic or hand surgeon if:
　1. Joint cannot be reduced (may require open reduction).
　2. Joint is unstable after reduction (may indicate soft tissue injury).
　3. Patient has fracture dislocation.
　4. Patient has open-fracture dislocation.

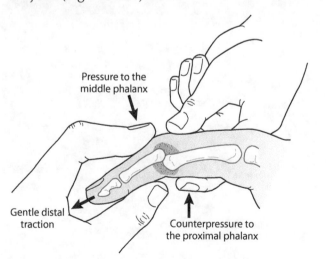

FIGURE III.39　Reduction technique of dorsal dislocation.

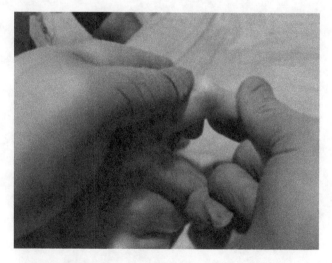

FIGURE III.40　Closed reduction of proximal interphalangeal joint dislocation.

Source: From Campo, T. M., & Lafferty, K. (Eds.). (2016). *Essential procedures for emergency, urgent, and primary care settings: A clinical companion* (2nd ed.). Springer Publishing Company.

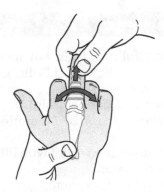

FIGURE III.41   Lateral joint dislocation.

CLINICAL PEARLS

A. An aggressive attempt at reducing fingers can cause a fracture of the joint being reduced or injury to the ligaments and soft tissue.

B. Infection is a concern if there is an open fracture.
C. Inadequate mobilization can lead to redislocation.
D. Nail plate alignment is inadequate to evaluate rotational deformity; rotation at one bone segment should be compared with the next distal segment.

BIBLIOGRAPHY

Campo, T. M., & Lafferty, K (Eds.). (2016). *Essential procedures for emergency, urgent, and primary care settings: A clinical companion* (2nd ed.). Springer Publishing Company.

Egol, K. A., Koval, K. J., & Zuckerman, J. D. (2020). *Handbook of fractures.* Wolters Kluwer Health.

Leggit, J. C., & Meko, C. J. (2006). Acute finger injuries: Part II. Fractures, dislocations, and thumb injuries. *American Family Physician, 73*, 827.

Muelleman, R. L., & Wadman, M. C. (2004). Injuries to the hand and digits. In J. E. Tintinalli, G. D. Kelen, & J. S. Stapczynski (Eds.), *Emergency medicine: A comprehensive study guide* (6th ed., pp. 1665–1673). McGraw-Hill.

REDUCTION OF THE HIPS

Kathleen L. Collins

DESCRIPTION

A. Displacement of the femoral head from the acetabulum.
B. Posterior dislocation more common than anterior dislocation.

INDICATIONS

A. All hip dislocations.
B. Less emergent in patients status post hip arthroplasty, as risk of osteonecrosis of femoral head is not present.

PRECAUTIONS

A. Contraindicated in patients with associated femoral neck fracture.
B. Native hip dislocations almost always result from high-energy trauma and 50% of patients sustain fractures elsewhere.
C. Prosthetic hip dislocations may warrant referral to orthopedics due to complexity of reduction and risk of periprosthetic fracture.

EQUIPMENT REQUIRED

A. Facility-approved conscious sedation protocol.
B. Second provider/assistant for traction.
C. Abduction pillow.

PROCEDURE

A. Explain the procedure to the patient and/or family and obtain informed consent.
B. Position the patient supine in bed.
C. Perform a proper time-out. All present in the room must identify the patient and agree on the correct procedure and the correct site of the procedure.
D. Place sheet around the proximal thigh of the affected limb.
E. Administer conscious sedation per facility protocol.
F. Stand on the patient's bed, straddling the lower extremities.
G. Use Allis method for posterior dislocations.
    1. Have a provider or assistant stabilize the pelvis by applying direct, downward (Figure III.42) pressure on the patient's bilateral anterior superior iliac spines (ASIS).
H. Apply traction in line with the femur.
I. While traction is maintained, slowly flex hip to 70 degrees (Figure III.43).
J. Combine traction with gentle rotation and slight adduction to help the femoral head clear the acetabular lip.
K. Continue traction and manipulation until palpable reduction is felt.
L. Place abduction pillow between the patient's legs to be worn in bed. Allow weight-bearing.

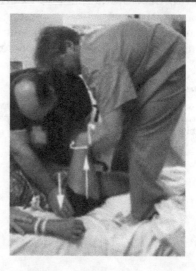

FIGURE III.42 Nurses performing the Allis technique on a patient.

Source: From Campo, T. M., & Lafferty, K. (Eds.). (2016). *Essential procedures for emergency, urgent, and primary care settings: A clinical companion* (2nd ed.). Springer Publishing Company.

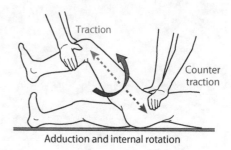

FIGURE III.43 Adduction and internal rotation of the hip.

EVALUATION AND RESULTS

A. Postreduction imaging to evaluate success of reduction and ensure no procedural injuries.
B. Postreduction CT scan of the hip recommended to verify concentric reduction as well as evaluate for intra-articular bony fragments.
C. Pre- and postreduction examinations with careful neurovascular examination are crucial.
D. Perform a full trauma survey evaluation on all patients with native hip dislocation due to the high-energy nature of these injuries.
E. Follow up with orthopedics for continued evaluation.

CLINICAL PEARLS

A. Another option for positioning the patient for a hip reduction is to place the patient on a backboard using a strap across the pelvis.
B. Make sure to use a steady sustained force during reduction.

C. If there is not any movement of the joint, try rocking back and forth with internal and external rotation at the hip.

D. Other common reduction methods include the Stimson gravity technique and the Bigelow and reverse Bigelow maneuvers.

BIBLIOGRAPHY

Campo, T. M., & Lafferty, K (Eds.). (2016). *Essential procedures for emergency, urgent, and primary care settings: A clinical companion* (2nd ed.). Springer Publishing Company.

Egol, K. A., Koval, K. J., & Zuckerman, J. D. (2020). *Handbook of fractures*. Wolters Kluwer Health.

Hendey, G. W., & Avila, A. (2011). The Captain Morgan technique for the reduction of the dislocated hip. *Annals of Emergency Medicine, 58,* 536–540. https://doi.org/10.1016/j.annemergmed.2011.07.010

Nordt, W. E., 3rd. (1999). Maneuvers for reducing dislocated hips: A new technique and literature review. *Clinical Orthopedic and Related Research, 360,* 260–264. https://doi.org/10.1097/00003086-199903000-00032

Waddell, B., Mohamed, S., Glomset, J., & Meyer, M. (2016). A detailed review of hip reduction maneuvers: A focus on physician safety and introduction of the Waddell technique. *Orthopedic Reviews, 8*(1), 6253. https://doi.org/10.4081/or.2016.6253

REDUCTION OF THE PATELLA

Kathleen L. Collins

DESCRIPTION
A. Loss of patellar alignment.
B. The most typical is lateral dislocation.

INDICATIONS
A. Lateral dislocations.
B. Unreduced dislocations need operative reduction.

PRECAUTIONS
A. Do not attempt closed reduction if there are associated injuries to dislocation.

EQUIPMENT REQUIRED
A. 18-G needle, optional.
B. 20-mL syringe, optional.
C. 5- to 10-mL lidocaine, optional.
D. Knee immobilizer brace.

PROCEDURE
A. Explain the procedure to the patient and/or family and obtain informed consent.
B. Traumatic hematoma present: Insert needle within the trochlear groove and aspirate to decompress hematoma and then exchange syringe to instill lidocaine.
C. Extend the affected knee (Figure III.44).
D. If extension alone does not relocate the patella, apply medially directed force to the laterally dislocated patella during extension.
E. Brace with knee immobilizer and allow weight-bearing.

EVALUATION AND RESULTS
A. Postreduction imaging to evaluate success of reduction and to ensure no procedural injuries.
B. Follow up with orthopedics and/or physical therapy.

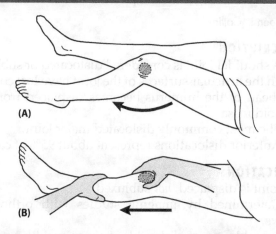

FIGURE III.44 Reduction of the patella. **(A)** Gently extend the lower leg to reduce the patella. **(B)** If needed, apply a medial force on the lateral patella while simultaneously extending the lower leg to relocate it into the trochlear groove.

CLINICAL PEARLS
A. Patellar dislocations are a common musculoskeletal injury.
B. Reductions of the patella typically do not require procedural sedation.
C. Recurrent dislocations warrant orthopedic referral for operative intervention.

BIBLIOGRAPHY
Davenport, M. (2017, April 13). *Reduction of patellar dislocation technique.* In E. Schraga (Ed.), *Medscape.* https://emedicine.medscape.com/article/109263-technique

Egol, K. A., Koval, K. J., & Zuckerman, J. D. (2020). *Handbook of fractures.* Wolters Kluwer Health.

Mehta, V. M., Inoue, M., Nomura, E., & Fithian, D. C. (2007, June). An algorithm guiding the evaluation and treatment of acute primary patellar dislocations. *Sports Medicine and Arthroscopy Review, 15*(2), 78–81. https://doi.org/10.1097/JSA.0b013e318042b695

Stefancin, J. J., & Parker, R. D. (2007, February). First-time traumatic patellar dislocation: A systematic review. *Clinical Orthopedics Related Research, 455,* 93–101. https://doi.org/10.1097/BLO.0b013e31802eb40a

REDUCTION OF THE SHOULDER

Kathleen L. Collins

DESCRIPTION

A. A shoulder joint is considered dislocated or subluxed when the articular surfaces of the joint have lost contact; the head of the humerus becomes displaced from the glenoid fossa.

B. The most commonly dislocated major joint.

C. Anterior dislocations represent about 95% of cases.

INDICATIONS

A. Joint is displaced, *not* subluxed.

B. Determined by imaging studies with orthogonal views.

C. Palpable or visual shoulder deformity with a mechanism of injury suggestive of dislocation; confirm with imaging to rule out fracture.

PRECAUTIONS

A. Obtain imaging of the shoulder prior to reduction to rule out evidence of fracture; require orthogonal views to adequately assess.

EQUIPMENT REQUIRED

A. Stretcher.

B. Weights (Stimson maneuver).

C. Analgesia (e.g., facility-approved conscious sedation protocol, or intra-articular block, if needed).

D. Shoulder immobilizer/sling.

PROCEDURE

A. Stimson technique (gravity-assisted reduction).

B. Explain the procedure to the patient and/or family and obtain informed consent.

C. Perform a proper time-out. All present in the room must identify the patient and agree on the correct procedure and the correct site of the procedure.

D. Administer analgesia, as indicated.

E. Perform neurologic examination of the bilateral upper extremities to include, but not limited to, function of axillary, musculocutaneous, median, radial, and ulnar nerves.

F. Place the patient prone on a stretcher with the dislocated extremity hanging off the side edge of the stretcher.

G. Have the assistant sit on the floor and apply gentle downward traction to the arm OR attach 5 to 15 lb of weight to the patient's arm (Stimson maneuver; Figure III.45).

H. While traction is performed, place the left thumb on the patient's acromion and left fingers on the front of the humeral head (Figure III.46).

I. Gently push the humeral head downward until it reduces into the glenoid fossa.

J. Brace the shoulder using immobilizer/sling.

EVALUATION AND RESULTS

A. Postreduction imaging to complete reduction with no procedural injuries.

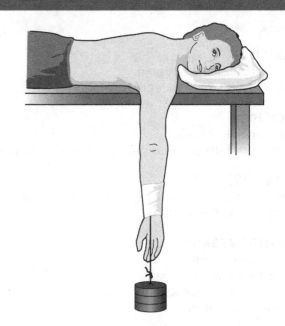

FIGURE III.45 The Stimson maneuver. The patient should lie prone on the table. A 5- to 15-lb weight should be attached to the affected arm, hanging off of the edge of the table as shown.

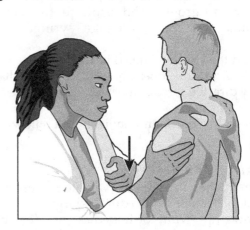

FIGURE III.46 The Cunningham technique. Face the patient diagonally and instruct them to relax and pull back their shoulders.

B. Perform postreduction bilateral upper extremity neurovascular examination and document findings.

C. Follow up with orthopedic surgeon for continued evaluation.

D. After appropriate immobilization period, refer for physical therapy/exercises for strength building and return of preinjury function.

CLINICAL PEARLS

A. Many shoulder dislocations can easily be reduced by medical professionals before muscles go into spasm.

B. Recurrent shoulder dislocations are common after the first injury.

C. Orthogonal radiographs include anteroposterior (AP), scapular Y, and axillary views; the Velpeau axillary view can replace standard axillary view if the patient does not tolerate the traditional imaging.

D. Other closed reduction techniques include Hippocratic, scapular manipulation, Milch, and Kocher.

BIBLIOGRAPHY

DeLee, J., Drez, D., & Miller, M. D (Eds.). (2003). *DeLee and Drez's orthopaedic sports medicine* (2nd ed., pp. 1038–1040). Elsevier Science.

Egol, K. A., Koval, K. J., & Zuckerman, J. D. (2020). *Handbook of fractures*. Wolters Kluwer Health.

Marinelli, M., & de Palma, L. (2009, March). The external rotation method for reduction of acute anterior shoulder dislocations. *Journal of Orthopedics and Traumatology, 10*(1), 17–20. https://doi.org/10.1007/s10195-008-0040-4

Westin, C. D., Gill, E. A., Noyes, M. E., & Hubbard, M. (1995, May-June). Anterior shoulder dislocation. A simple and rapid method for reduction. *American Journal of Sports Medicine, 23*(3), 369–371. https://doi.org/10.1177/036354659502300322

SPLINTING

Joanne Elaine Pechar

DESCRIPTION
A. Mechanism used to immobilize an injured extremity.
B. A splint is similar to a cast in that its function is to immobilize, but its main advantage is to allow for soft tissue swelling during the acute phase of an injury.
C. A splint is applied to suspected or confirmed fractures to avoid any further injury or damage to the surrounding muscles, skin, nerves, and vessels.

INDICATIONS
A. Immobilization of acute fractures.
B. Immobilization of dislocation after it has been reduced.
C. Treatment of soft tissue injuries not limited to sprains and strains.
D. Stabilize the joint above and below the suspected injury.

PRECAUTIONS
A. Do not place over broken, undressed skin/lacerations.
B. Ensure proper splint padding and placement to defer pressure sore.
C. Ensure the patient's proper position of function while splinted to avoid further injury.
D. The provider should reevaluate and document the limb's neurovascular status after any splinting procedure.
E. Soft tissue swelling can worsen after application, leading to potential significant neurovascular compromise if splint is tightly applied.

EQUIPMENT REQUIRED
A. Length- and width-appropriate prefabricated splint.
B. Additional padding.
C. Bucket of cool water.
D. Dry towel.
E. Elastic bandage wraps.

PROCEDURE
A. Short arm ulnar gutter (Figure II.47).
   1. To treat fractures of the fourth and fifth metacarpals and phalanges including the common "Boxer's fracture."
   2. Apply splint on the ulnar aspect of the upper extremity, from the tip of the little finger to just distal to the elbow, ending high on the forearm.
   3. The splint should be wide enough to encompass the fourth and fifth phalanges and metacarpals on the extensor and flexor aspects of the hands.
   4. Place wrist in 20-degree extension, the metacarpophalangeals (MCPs) flexed to 50 degrees, and the distal interphalangeal (DIP) and the proximal interphalangeal (PIP) joints in slight gentle flexion.
   5. Pad the upper extremity as indicated per patient presentation.
   6. Immerse the splint in a bucket of cool water.
   7. Remove excess water from the splint with towel.
   8. Apply the splint with the patient holding position of function, securing with All Cotton Elastic (ACE) bandages.
   9. Perform postsplint application neurovascular examination to bilateral upper extremities.
   10. Apply a sling for further immobilization.
B. Long arm posterior splint (Figure III.48).
   1. Used for acute immobilization of midforearm or proximal forearm fractures.
      a. It can also be used for fractures of the distal humerus.
   2. Place elbow in 90-degree flexion, with the forearm in neutral pronation or supination.
   3. Apply the splint to the ulnar aspect of the forearm, extending from the palmar crease to several inches above the elbow.
   4. Pad the upper extremity as indicated per patient presentation.
   5. Immerse the splint in a bucket of cool water.
   6. Remove excess water from the splint with a towel.
   7. Apply the splint with the patient holding the position of function, securing with ACE bandages.
   8. Perform a postsplint application neurovascular examination to the bilateral upper extremities.
C. Upper extremity sugar-tong splint (Figure III.49).
   1. Can be used for acute splinting of the wrist or distal forearm.

▶

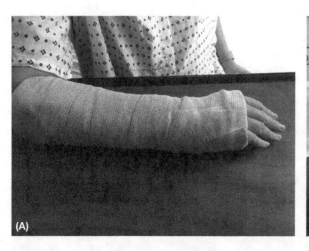

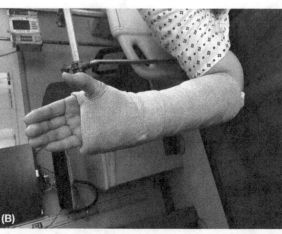

FIGURE III.47
Short arm ulnar gutter. **(A)** supine view and **(B)** prone view.

• Indications

- Distal humerus #

- Both-bone forearm #

- Unstable proximal radius or ulna # (sugar-tong better)

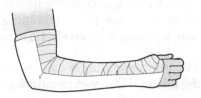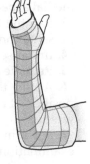

FIGURE III.48 Long arm posterior splint.

a. May provide more stability than a volar splint.
b. Prevents motion of wrist and elbow, including pronation–supination.

2. The splint begins at the palmar crease, moves along the volar forearm, moves around the elbow joint, and ends at the dorsal aspect of the MCP joints.

3. Pad the upper extremity as indicated per patient presentation.

4. Proper length of the sugar-tong dressing is important.

a. If too short, the splint will fail to immobilize the wrist.
b. If too long, it will impair motion of the MCP joints, leaving them stiff and making the fingers susceptible to swelling due to immobility.

5. Immerse the splint in a bucket of cool water.

6. Remove excess water from the splint with a towel.

7. Apply the splint with the patient holding the position of function, securing with ACE bandages.

8. Perform a postsplint application neurovascular examination to the bilateral upper extremities.

D. Volar wrist splint (Figure III.50).

1. Can be used for sprains of the wrist or for stable fractures of the distal radius and/or ulna.

2. The splint extends from the volar surface of the MCP joints to the proximal forearm.

3. Pad the upper extremity as indicated per patient presentation.

4. Immerse the splint in a bucket of cool water.

5. Remove excess water from the splint with a towel.

6. Apply the splint with the patient holding the position of function, securing with ACE bandages.

7. Perform a postsplint application neurovascular examination to the bilateral upper extremities.

E. Thumb spica splint (Figure III.51).

1. Used for sprains or fractures of the scaphoid, first metacarpal, or thumb proximal phalanx. The term *spica* applies to any dressing that encompasses the trunk in addition to one or more of its branches. In this case, the forearm plus the thumb.

2. The splint runs along the thumb from above the interphalangeal (IP) joint, along the radial aspect of the wrist to the forearm.

3. The wrist is splinted in the neutral position while the thumb is splinted slightly flexed: Have the patient oppose the thumb toward the index finger as if to make the "OK" sign. The goal is to preserve the thumb-to-index pinch function to minimize the patient's incapacitation. The neutral position of the wrist also avoids reproducing the position of injury in the case of scaphoid fracture, which is typically caused by forced dorsiflexion.

4. Pad the upper extremity as indicated per patient presentation.

5. Immerse the splint in a bucket of cool water.

6. Remove excess water from the splint with a towel.

7. Apply the splint with the patient holding the position of function, securing with ACE bandages.

8. Perform a postsplint application neurovascular examination to the bilateral upper extremities.

F. Short leg posterior splint (Figure III.52).

1. Used for acute immobilization of severe ankle sprains and fractures of the distal leg, ankle, and foot.

2. The splint is applied along the posterior aspect of the lower leg from 1 in. distal to the popliteal fossa to the distal ends of the toes.

3. Pad the lower extremity as indicated per patient presentation.

4. Immerse the splint in a bucket of cool water.

5. Remove excess water from the splint with a towel. ▶

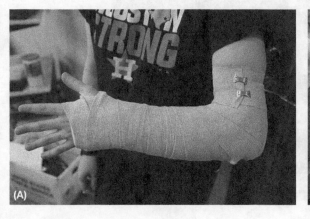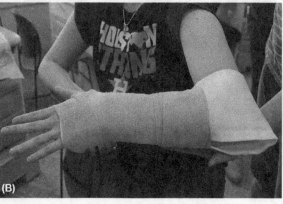

(A) (B)

FIGURE III.49 Upper extremity sugar-tong splint. **(A)** completed wrapping and **(B)** wrapped around the underlying pad.

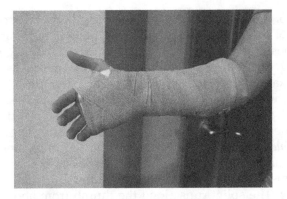

FIGURE III.50   Volar wrist splint.

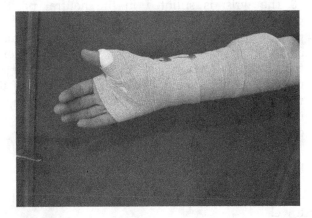

FIGURE III.51   Thumb spica splint.

6. Apply the splint with the patient holding the position of function, securing with ACE bandages.

7. Perform a postsplint application neurovascular examination to the bilateral lower extremities.

G. Lower leg sugar-tong splint.

  1. Can be used as an alternative to the short leg posterior splint when more stability is desired.

  2. It is a "U"-shaped splint starting at the lateral aspect of the knee, which goes under the proximal

foot and heel and moves upward, stopping at the medial aspect of the knee (Figure III.53).

  3. Pad the lower extremity as indicated per patient presentation.

  4. Immerse the splint in a bucket of cool water.

  5. Remove excess water from the splint with a towel.

  6. Apply the splint with the patient holding the position of function, securing with an elastic bandage wrap.

  7. Perform a postsplint application neurovascular examination to the bilateral lower extremities.

EVALUATION AND RESULTS

A. After splint placement, carefully assess to ensure the splint:

  1. Is in extension (not flexed).

  2. Does not interfere with range of motion of necessary joints.

  3. Does not have finger indentations or sharp edges puncturing the patient's skin.

B. The splint is never to be removed by the patient, only by a professional after follow-up with a specified specialist. ▶

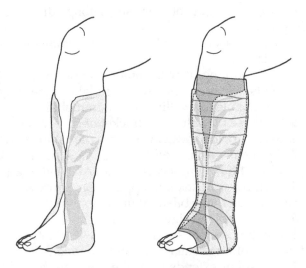

FIGURE III.53   Lower leg sugar-tong splint.

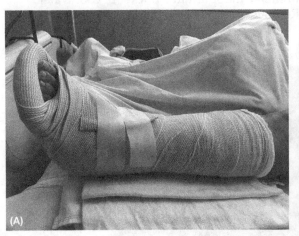

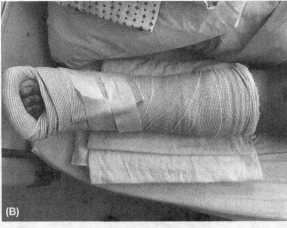

FIGURE III.52
Short leg posterior splint. **(A)** lateral view and **(B)** supine view.

C. If the splint is on the lower extremity, go over weight-bearing status with the patient and make sure they have sufficient and safe means of mobility (e.g., crutches, cane, walker).

D. The splint is to stay dry at all times. If the splint gets wet, a new splint needs to be placed.

E. Educate the patient that splints are usually temporary and they will most likely need to follow up with a specialist for continued care and treatment of the injury.

CLINICAL PEARLS

A. The extremities should be splinted in their correct anatomic position unless there is resistance or loss of circulation.

B. A poorly immobilized fracture can be more harmful than no splint at all.

C. When in doubt, splint an extremity even if it is not clear if there is a fracture.

BIBLIOGRAPHY

Do, T. (2017). Splinting. In E. D. Schraga (Ed.), *Medscape*. https://emedicine.medscape.com/article/1997864-overview

Egol, K. A., Koval, K. J., & Zuckerman, J. D. (2015). *Handbook of fractures* (5th ed., pp. 1–72). Wolters Kluwer.

Mayersak, R. J. (2020). Initial evaluation and management of orthopedic injuries. In J. E. Tintinalli, O. Ma, D. M. Yealy, G. D. Meckler, J. Stapczynski, D. M. Cline, & S. H. Thomas (Eds.), *Tintinalli's emergency medicine: A comprehensive study guide* (9th ed.). McGraw Hill. https://accessmedicine.mhmedical.com/content.aspx?bookid=2353&sectionid=222324221

Nackenson, J., Baez, A. A., & Meizoso, J. P. (2017). A descriptive analysis of traction splint utilization and IV analgesia by emergency medical services. *Prehospital and Disaster Medicine*, 32(6), 631–635. https://doi.org/10.1017/S1049023X17006859

SYNOVIAL FLUID ASPIRATION

Joanne Elaine Pechar

DESCRIPTION

A. Joint aspiration, also known as joint arthrocentesis, is a procedure to drain and remove fluid from the joint space using a needle and syringe.

B. Joint aspiration, commonly done under local anesthesia, offers both therapeutic and diagnostic benefits and is commonly done to relieve swelling or to obtain fluid for analysis.

INDICATIONS

A. Therapeutic.
　1. Hemarthrosis or bleeding into joint space.
　2. Symptomatic relief of joint effusion.
B. Diagnostic.
　1. Septic joint.
　2. Crystal-induced joint disease.
　3. Unexplained joint effusion.

PRECAUTIONS

A. Infection of overlying tissues is considered a relative contraindication.
　1. Skin overlying the affected joint should be free of cellulitis or impetigo to avoid contamination of the joint space during arthrocentesis.
B. In some cases, joint aspiration is still performed as it provides critical diagnostic information.
C. Anticoagulation should not be viewed as an absolute contraindication to arthrocentesis.
D. Arthrocentesis is typically a safe procedure in anticoagulated patients, including patients receiving direct oral anticoagulants.
E. For diagnostic workup and interpretation of results, orthopedics should be consulted before aspiration of the affected joint.

EQUIPMENT REQUIRED

A. Betadine swab.
B. Alcohol swab.
C. Ethyl chloride or cold anesthetic spray.
D. One pair of hemostats.
E. 16- or 18-G needle.
F. 10- to 60-mL syringe.
G. Gauze.
H. Tape.
I. Pen marker.
J. Three vacutainer lab tubes for joint fluid analysis (Gram stain, cell count, culture, and crystals).
K. Gloves.

PROCEDURE

A. Explain the procedure to the patient and/or family and obtain informed consent.
B. Use standard precautions to prep for the procedure.
C. Perform a proper time-out. All present in the room must identify the patient and agree on the correct procedure and the correct site of the procedure.

D. Assess for any evidence of infection or inflammation.
E. Place the patient supine and fully extend the knee. Make sure the quadriceps muscle is fully relaxed.
F. Identify the midpoint of the patella.
G. The knee joint can be entered either medial or lateral to the patella.
　1. Use medial approach when the effusion is small and lateral approach with larger effusions.
H. Identify bony landmarks, namely the superior pole and lateral edge of the patella and the soft spot approximately 1 to 2 cm below the lateral edge of the patella.
I. Mark entry site.
J. Prep site with Betadine and alcohol swab.
K. Ethyl chloride spray can be used to anesthetize the skin and soft tissues overlying the joint with a 25- to 30-G needle.
　1. Avoid intra-articular injection of anesthetic because it can inhibit bacterial growth and may result in a negative culture in early septic joint.
L. Lightly hold the patella between the thumb and the index finger.
M. Using an anteromedial or anterolateral approach, insert the needle into the joint space (Figure III.54). The insertion point of the needle is located approximately 1 cm inferior to the patella edge, either lateral or medial to the middle of the patella.
　1. In patients with large or obese knees, it may be necessary to use a needle larger than 1.5 in. to enter the joint space.
N. Once the needle enters the joint space, aspirate fluid. Advance the needle until synovial fluid is obtained (Figure III.55). ▶

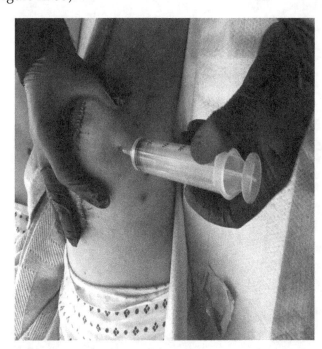

FIGURE III.54 Insertion of the needle into the joint space.

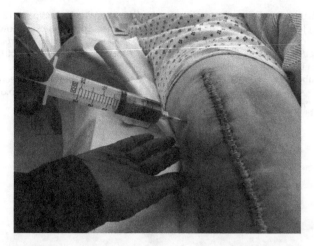

FIGURE III.55 Extraction of the synovial fluid.

O. Resistance to the flow of synovial fluid can be met at the joint capsule level.

P. Compression or milking applied to both sides (proximal and distal) of the joint space by an assistant to further facilitate aspiration of a small amount of synovial fluid.

Q. To maximize extraction of effusion or blood, directing the needle in multiple angles inside the joint space may be needed.

R. Remove as much synovial fluid as possible to obtain a good diagnostic sample and to relieve pain from joint capsule distention.

S. If the syringe becomes full of fluid, empty it by removing the syringe from the hub of the needle and replacing it with an empty syringe. Repeat aspiration until synovial fluid can no longer be aspirated or until knee effusion is no longer visible.

T. When the procedure is completed, hold direct pressure for at least 5 minutes.

U. Apply and cover with a 4 × 4 gauze dressing.

V. Promptly send aspirated fluid to the laboratory for culture, Gram stain, cell counts, and crystal analysis especially if infection or septic joint is suspected.

W. Instruct patients to avoid use of the joint for at least 1 day.

EVALUATION AND RESULTS

A. Review of the results of the synovial fluid (Table III.3).

B. Most purulent synovial fluid or effusions are due to septic arthritis.

C. Noninflammatory conditions include degenerative joint disease (DJD), osteochondritis dissecans, and neuropathic arthropathy.

D. Inflammatory conditions include rheumatoid arthritis (RA), gout, pseudogout, reactive arthritis, ankylosing spondylitis, and rheumatic fever.

E. Hemorrhagic conditions include hemarthrosis, hemophilia or other hemorrhagic diathesis, and trauma with or without fracture.

SPECIAL CONSIDERATIONS

A. Traumatic hemarthrosis.

   1. Associated with ligamentous injury or an intra-articular fracture.

   2. Effusion-caused trauma can range from small minor effusions to large painful fluid collection.

   3. Aspiration of very large traumatic effusions provides temporary relief and increases range of motion.

   4. Treatment includes immobilization, ice therapy, and elevation of the affected joint.

B. Spontaneous hemarthrosis.

   1. Indicates underlying systemic illness and should prompt consideration for primary or secondary coagulopathies.

   2. Hemophilias and von Willebrand disease should receive specific clotting factor replacement for hemarthrosis.

   3. Joint aspirations should only be performed after factor replacement.

CLINICAL PEARLS

A. If there is a suspicion of joint infection, cell count, culture, and Gram stain should be urgently sent for lab analysis.

B. Patients receiving anticoagulation at therapeutic levels can generally undergo arthrocentesis safely, but bleeding is to be expected.

TABLE III.3 SYNOVIAL FLUID FINDINGS

Findings	Normal Joint	Noninflammatory	Inflammatory	Septic	Hemorrhagic
Clarity	Transparent	Transparent	Translucent or cloudy	Opaque or turbid	Bloody
Color	Clear	Straw to yellow	Yellow	Yellow, green, purulent	Red
Fluid cell count: WBC	<200	<2,000	2,000–50,000	>50,000	200–2,000
Segmented neutrophils or PMNs	<25%	<25%	>70%	>90%	50%–75%
Fluid culture	Negative	Negative	Negative	Positive	Negative

PMN, polymorphonuclear leukocyte; WBC, white blood cell.

BIBLIOGRAPHY

Burton, J. H., & Fortuna, T. J. (2020). *Joints and bursae*. In J. E. Tintinalli, O. Ma, D. M. Yealy, G. D. Meckler, J. Stapczynski, D. M. Cline, & S. H. Thomas (Eds.), *Tintinalli's emergency medicine: A comprehensive study guide* (9th ed.). McGraw Hill. https://accessmedicine.mhmedical.com/content.aspx?bookid=2353&sectionid=222407706

Shlamovitz, G. (2019, February 28). *Knee arthrocentesis technique*. In E. D. Schraga (Ed.), *Medscape*. https://emedicine.medscape.com/article/79994-technique

Zhang, Q., Zhang, T., Lv, H., Xie, L., Wu, W., Wu, J., & Wu, X. (2012, July). Comparison of two positions of knee arthrocentesis: How to obtain complete drainage. *American Journal of Physical Medicine & Rehabilitation*, *91*(7), 611–615. https://doi.org/10.1097/PHM.0b013e31825a13f0

Zuber, T. J. (2002, October 15). Knee joint aspiration and injection. *American Family Physician*, *66*(8), 1497–1501. https://www.aafp.org/afp/2002/1015/p1497.html

THORACENTESIS

E. Moneé Carter-Griffin

DESCRIPTION
A. Needle insertion into the pleural space to remove excess fluid.

INDICATIONS
A. Therapeutic drainage of symptomatic pleural effusions.
B. Diagnostic evaluation of pleural fluid.

PRECAUTIONS
A. Patients with coagulopathies.
B. Avoid areas of skin infections on the chest wall.
C. Increased risk of pneumothorax in patients receiving positive pressure ventilation.
D. Patient's habitus or anatomy may hinder identifying landmarks.

EQUIPMENT REQUIRED
A. Sterile gloves, drape, and towels.
B. Antiseptic solution with chlorhexidine or povidone-iodine.
C. Lidocaine 1% with or without epinephrine for local anesthesia.
D. 25-G, ⅝- to 1-in. needle.
E. 20- to 22-G, 1½-in. needle.
F. 14- to 18-G needle.
G. 12- to 16-G catheter.
H. Pressure tubing.
I. Three-way stopcock.
J. Various syringe sizes, including 5-mL syringes up to 60-mL syringes.
　1. It is important to have at least a 10-, 20-, and 60-mL syringe.
K. Specimen vials and tubes, and aerobic/anaerobic media bottles.
L. Vacutainers, evacuated bottles, or drainage bag.
M. Pressure/connector tubing.
N. Sterile 4 × 4 gauze.
O. Adhesive dressing.

P. Keep a thoracostomy tray with supplies available in case of a pneumothorax.
　1. Chlorhexidine solution.
　2. Drapes.
　3. Gauze.
　4. Curved hemostat.
　5. Curved Kelly clamp.
　6. Scissors.
　7. Needle holder.
　8. Sterile thoracotomy tube.
　9. Scalpel.
　10. 4-0 silk suture on cutting needle.
　11. Petroleum-soaked gauze.
　12. Underwater sealed drainage system.

PROCEDURE
A. Explain the procedure to the patient and family and obtain informed consent.
B. Always identify the patient.
C. Wash hands/perform hand hygiene.
D. Ensure intravenous (IV) access and hemodynamic monitoring (e.g., blood pressure, oxygen saturations).
E. Position the patient (help of an assistant may be needed).
　1. Position the patient on the edge of the bed with feet on a solid surface (e.g., ground, stool).
　2. The assistant will stand in front of the patient or the patient will lean on a bedside table directly in front with the head on their arms.
F. Verify location for pleural drainage with ultrasound.
　1. If ultrasound is unavailable, utilize physical examination to locate area of effusion.
　2. The optimal site for needle insertion is posterolateral (midaxillary and midline) between the seventh and ninth intercostal space, 6 to 8 cm lateral to the spine (Figure III.56).
G. Don sterile attire.
H. Assemble all equipment and set up sterile field.

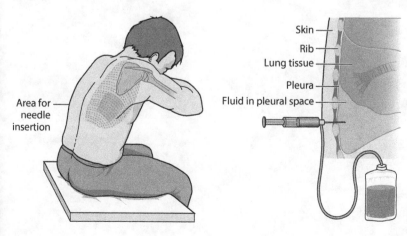

Area for needle insertion

Skin
Rib
Lung tissue
Pleura
Fluid in pleural space

FIGURE III.56 Insertion site.

I. Perform a proper time-out. All present in the room must identify the patient and agree on the correct procedure and the correct site of the procedure.

J. Cleanse the area again with chlorhexidine or a povidone-iodine solution.

K. Drape the identified area.

L. Use 25-G, ⅝-in. needle and 5-mL syringe to inject a small wheal of lidocaine.

M. Use 20-G, 1½-in. needle and 10-mL syringe to infiltrate lidocaine into a wide area of subcutaneous tissue, periosteum, and pleura.

N. For therapeutic thoracentesis, insert 14- or 18-G needle with a 20-mL syringe attached into anesthetized area until pleural fluid is obtained.

O. Remove the syringe and occlude the needle with a finger.

P. Insert 16- or 12-G catheter through gauged needle, positioned downward toward the diaphragm into the pleural space.

Q. Once the catheter is in place, remove the needle and attach the three-way stopcock and 60-mL syringe.

R. Fill 60-mL syringe with pleural fluid, turn the stopcock off to catheter, and remove the syringe. Fill each specimen vial with pleural fluid.

S. Attach pressure tubing to three-way stopcock and vacutainer.

T. Open stopcock to the vacutainer and allow pleural fluid to flow into the vacutainer. Limit drainage to 1 to 1.5 L to reduce risk of reexpansion pulmonary edema.

U. Remove the catheter and apply pressure to the puncture site.

V. Apply adhesive bandage and aid the patient back into bed.

W. Dispose of all equipment.

X. Obtain chest x-ray to evaluate for improvement in pleural effusion and to assess for complications (e.g., pneumothorax).

Y. Document the procedure, indication, amount of fluid removal, diagnostics sent, and the patient's tolerance of the procedure.

EVALUATION AND RESULTS

A. Resolution of pleural effusion and reexpansion of lung tissue.

B. Resolution of respiratory distress in patients with excess pleural fluid.

C. Etiology of pleural effusion determined based on pleural fluid analysis.

CLINICAL PEARLS

A. Ultrasound guidance to reduce complications and drainage location; however, this is dependent on the operator's competence with ultrasound.

B. Some institutions may have prepackaged thoracentesis kits.

C. If the patient is unable to sit up, have them lie in the lateral recumbent position on the unaffected side.

D. Coughing during and after a thoracentesis can be normal and does not necessarily imply the need to stop during the procedure.

E. Keep thoracostomy supplies available in case the patient develops a pneumothorax.

BIBLIOGRAPHY

Dimov, V., & Altaqi, B. (2005). *Thoracentesis: A step-by-step procedure guide with photos* [Blog post]. http://note3.blogspot.com/2004/02/thoracentesis-procedure-guide.html

Schildhouse, R., Lai, A., Barsuk, J. H., Mourad, M., & Chopra, V. (2017, April). Safe and effective bedside thoracentesis: A review of the evidence for practicing clinicians. *Journal of Hospital Medicine, 12*(4), 266–276. https://doi.org/10.12788/jhm.2716

Wiederhold, B. D., Amr, O., Modi, P., & O'Rourke, M. C. (2022). *Thoracentesis.* StatPearls Publishing. https://www.ncbi.nlm.nih.gov/books/NBK441866/

TRANSPYLORIC FEEDING TUBE PLACEMENT

Nicole Cavaliere

DESCRIPTION

A. Dobhoff tubes are flexible, nasogastric tubes used to administer nutrition and medications to patients unable to receive them by mouth.

B. The tube is inserted into the stomach via the nasal passages.

C. Dobhoff tubes are smaller in diameter than other nasogastric tubes, which allows for long-term use, more comfort for the patient, and postpyloric placement.

INDICATIONS

A. Sedated or mechanically ventilated patients who need to receive nutrition and/or medications.

B. Critical illness.

C. Severe malnutrition.

D. Prolonged anorexia.

E. Difficulty swallowing.

F. High risk of aspiration.

PRECAUTIONS

A. Improper setup and placement may result in placing tube in the lung, causing pneumothorax.

B. In patients with a basilar skull fracture, placement should be done with a clear visual pathway, typically performed with a scope by a member of the ear, nose, and throat (ENT) service. In very rare cases, a tube can circumnavigate to the brain without direct visualization.

C. Spinal cord fractures.

   1. Patient is typically encouraged to bend their neck forward for placement.

   2. Avoid this movement in patients with confirmed or suspected cervical spine fractures.

   3. Direct placement may be required.

D. Patients on a ventilator or who are sedated may have a decreased or absent cough reflex: Pay special attention to ANY changes in tidal volume, decrease in oxygen saturation, or persistent coughing.

E. Patients may be prone to naso-oropharyngeal bleeding if placement is traumatic and patient is anticoagulated.

EQUIPMENT REQUIRED

A. 10-Fr feeding tube with guide wire (Figure III.57).

B. Water-soluble lubricant.

C. 60-mL syringe.

D. Nasal strip tape to hold feeding tube in place.

E. Gloves.

PROCEDURE

A. Measure the tube from tip of the nose to the subxiphoid process (about 30 to 35 cm in most patients).

B. Have the patient sit upright and lean their head forward. If the patient is sedated, tilt the chin forward toward the chest.

C. Remove the feeding tube from the package and place some water-soluble lubricant on the tip to help facilitate passage of the tube through the nasal passages.

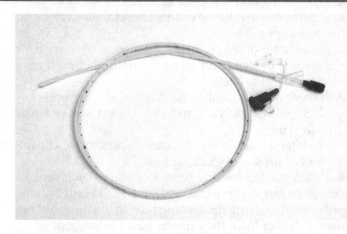

FIGURE III.57   10-Fr feeding tube with guide wire.

D. Place the tube through one naris and ask the patient to swallow as the tube passes down the oropharynx. The patient may gag but should not start coughing: Persistent coughing may be a warning sign that the tube is in the airway rather than the esophagus.

E. At 35 cm, STOP and confirm with chest x-ray that the tube is in the esophagus and not the mainstem bronchus.

   1. Confirmation is made if the feeding tube follows the path of the trachea straight below the carina.

   2. If placement is in the airway, the tube will curve into either the right or left mainstem bronchus; remove the feeding tube and start again.

F. Once x-ray confirms the feeding tube is in the esophagus, advance into the stomach.

G. Check placement by insufflating with air.

H. Advance the feeding tube to about 80 to 100 cm.

I. Leave the guide wire in place and obtain an abdominal x-ray (not chest).

J. If the tube is postpylorus, secure it and remove the wire; start feeds.

K. If the tube is not postpylorus, advance it further and obtain another abdominal x-ray.

L. Some institutions have adopted the use of a Cortrak device to assist with placement, which demonstrates real-time location of the Dobhoff tube (DHT), eliminating the two-step x-ray verification process (only x-ray for final placement confirmation at the end of the procedure).

EVALUATION AND RESULTS

A. Verify placement of the feeding tube with chest x-ray first to establish that the tube is below the carina and not in the right or left mainstem bronchus.

B. Verify placement of the feeding tube with abdominal x-ray once the tube is advanced and expected to be postpylorus.

C. Once visual placement is made, remove the wire and start tube feeds.

CLINICAL PEARLS
A. Positioning and setup are essential for success.
B. If patient is awake, have them bend their neck as far forward as possible.
C. Aim the tip of the feeding tube toward the very back of the nasal passage and allow the natural curvature of the tube to guide itself.
D. If there is significant resistance, try another naris.
  1. Strictures, polyps, and dried mucus may cause obstruction.
  2. After a couple of unsuccessful attempts, consult an ENT for direct visual approach.
E. When placing feeding tubes in patients on a ventilator, remember an endotracheal tube (ETT) cuff balloon will prevent placing the feeding tube in the lung, but not always. Never force the catheter past the balloon.
  1. Sometimes after hitting the ETT cuff balloon, the tube will curl back and come out of the patient's mouth.

2. After a couple of unsuccessful tries, consult an ENT for direct visual approach.
F. Do NOT rely on air insufflation to check correct position; always get an x-ray before beginning any tube feeds.
G. Postpyloric placement of a DHT reduces the risk of aspiration.

BIBLIOGRAPHY
Niv, E., Fireman, Z., & Vaisman, N. (2009). Post-pyloric feeding. *World Journal of Gastroenterology, 15*(11), 1281–1288. https://doi.org/10.3748/wjg.15.1281
Powers, J., Chance, R., Bortenschlager, L., Hottenstein, J., Bobel, K., Gervasio, J., & McNees, T. (2003). Bedside placement of small-bowel feeding tubes in the intensive care unit. *Critical Care Nurse, 23*(1), 16–24. http://ccn.aacnjournals.org/content/23/1/16.long
Simons, S. R., & Abdallah, L. M. (2012). Bedside assessment of enteral tube placement: Aligning practice with evidence. *The American Journal of Nursing, 112*(2), 40–46. https://doi.org/10.1097/01.NAJ.0000411178.07179.68

SECTION IV

SPECIAL TOPICS

- End-of-Life Considerations
- Palliative Care
- Health Prevention and Screening
- Hemodynamic Monitoring Devices
- Telemedicine in Acute Care
- Transitional Care
- Acute Care Billing

END-OF-LIFE CONSIDERATIONS

Jennifer Coates

INTRODUCTION

With life comes death. The dying process is not only an inevitable part of the life cycle, but it is also an important aspect of healthcare. Although discussions surrounding death and dying can be difficult for patients, caregivers, and even healthcare providers, these discussions are essential to ensure supportive and compassionate end-of-life care aligns with the patient's and the family's values and preferences.

Advances in healthcare treatment mean that people are living longer. Currently, life expectancy in the United States is 78.8 years. Annually, there are 823.7 deaths per 100,000 people. Increased life expectancy means that people are not only living longer in general but are also living longer with chronic diseases. Nearly 75% of all deaths in the United States are from the following 10 causes:

A. Heart disease.
B. Cancer.
C. Chronic lower respiratory diseases.
D. Unintentional injuries.
E. Stroke.
F. Alzheimer disease.
G. Diabetes.
H. Influenza and pneumonia.
I. Kidney disease.
J. Suicide.

Of these conditions, seven are chronic conditions. Of further note, two of these diseases (heart disease and cancer) together account for nearly 48% of all deaths. This information helps the advanced practice provider (APP) consider important aspects of discussing and providing end-of-life care, including the role of institutions and acute care during the death experience.

DISCUSSING THE DEATH EXPERIENCE

Discussing the death experience requires a shift in the healthcare provider's mind-set. Often, in tertiary care, the overall goal of care is to extend the patient's life in an attempt to delay death. However, the first step in planning and providing end-of-life care is an acceptance that death is the likely outcome. Specifically, the goal in acute care should be that the dying patient and their family are supported as the patient completes their life cycle.

Understanding the overall goal of end-of-life care prepares the APP to discuss the patient's and the family's preferences for end-of-life care and the dying experience. When entering into this discussion with a patient and their family, the APP should remember that *when* a patient will die is only one factor in the death experience. *Where* the patient will die and *how* they will die are also important aspects that need to be discussed. In general, where a patient dies has changed over time. In the early part of the 20th century, most people died at home;

however, today, most people will die in an institutional setting. The increased number of patients who experience cognitive impairment and dementia is one possible reason for this change. Some people have preferences about where they would like to die, so it is important to discuss this with the patient and their family.

DEFINING A "GOOD DEATH"

Another important factor to discuss is how the patient prefers to die. Every patient's experience with death is unique. To help the patient complete their life cycle in a way that is aligned with their preferences and beliefs, healthcare providers need to have a firm grasp on what a "good" death means for each patient. Defining a "good" death requires the APP to engage in an honest, open discussion that is focused on several important themes.

PREFERENCES FOR THE DYING PROCESS

Each patient has different preferences regarding where they prefer to die, the manner in which they will die, and who will be present when the patient completes their life cycle. In order to respect the patient's preferences, the APP should encourage the patient to express these preferences, both verbally in conversation and in written form, via an advance directive.

PAIN

Assessing and effectively managing pain are important in providing compassionate and comprehensive end-of-life care. Conversations about pain assessment and management will vary based on the patient's diagnosis. However, these discussions should center on how the patient's comfort level will be assessed and which interventions will be used to manage pain and side effects.

EMOTIONAL WELL-BEING AND SUPPORT SYSTEM

Another important part of completing one's life cycle is having the opportunity to discuss the meaning of death and to identify the role of a support system in death. The APP should be sure to allow the patient to discuss their personal wishes and ensure that an emotional support system is in place. People and organizations that are included in a patient's emotional support system vary, but may include the church, family, friends, a community, and/or beloved pets. In addition to identifying an emotional support system, the APP should also help the patient determine the role of their support system as the patient completes the life cycle. For example, how will the family and friends be involved in the process?

The APP plays an important role in emotionally supporting and preparing the patient's friends and family for the patient's death. The APP should help the patient's family and friends accept and prepare for the patient's death. This may include facilitating discussions, being available to answer questions, and providing resources as needed.

DIGNITY

Respecting all patients as individuals is central to providing end-of-life care. The APP can achieve this by empowering the patient to be independent and in control of their care. Dignity in death can take on many forms and is highly individualized. Asking the patient open-ended questions about what they feel is important will help the APP provide appropriate and respectful care during the patient's final months and days of life.

LIFE COMPLETION AND SPIRITUALITY

Saying goodbye and receiving religious/spiritual comfort are important aspects of life completion. When discussing this theme with the patient, the APP should be sure to inquire about the role of religion and spiritual comfort in the patient's life completion. During this discussion, the APP should also ask how they can help facilitate the opportunity for the patient to meet with clergy, if desired, and how they can help the patient see friends and family at life's completion. Chaplains are another important resource for the APP to consider in navigating spiritual needs.

TREATMENT PREFERENCES

As previously noted, the focus of treatments and interventions provided during end-of-life care shifts from life-prolonging to supporting the patient and the family as death approaches. During this time, the APP should take care to answer any questions the patient and their family may have. Often, the patient and their family want to know if all available treatments were offered and that they have control over treatment decisions.

QUALITY OF LIFE

The APP should be sure to discuss how they could help the patient maintain hope, pleasure, and gratitude as the patient completes their life cycle. Discussion should focus on how the disease is affecting the patient's physical mobility, emotional well-being, and social well-being. Conversation with the patient should center on strategies to help them feel that they have a life that is worth living.

RELATIONSHIP WITH TREATMENT TEAM

Building a strong relationship between the patient and the healthcare team is essential to providing supportive and comprehensive end-of-life care. The patient needs to trust as well as feel supported and comforted by the healthcare team. This relationship may be garnered in a variety of ways, but stems from the healthcare provider being comfortable with death and dying. Such a relationship will enable the patient to be at ease, which will in turn allow the patient to freely discuss their preferences, spiritual beliefs, and fears with the healthcare provider.

PORTABLE ORDERS FOR LIFE-SUSTAINING TREATMENT

As part of the ongoing discussion surrounding the type of death experience the patient desires, it is important that the APP also discusses the role of Portable Orders for Life-Sustaining Treatment (POLST) in ensuring the patient's desires are upheld. The title of this form varies between states. It is sometimes called Medical Orders for Life-Sustaining Treatment (MOLST) or Physician Orders for Life-Sustaining Treatment (POLST); this form provides standing medical orders that healthcare providers can act on immediately when the patient is in an acute situation. It outlines the type of care the patient wishes to receive or does not wish to receive during end of life. POLST topics include the patient's preferences concerning CPR, antibiotics, mechanical ventilation, and artificial nutrition. The POLST form is intended to help healthcare providers, including first responders, provide the type of treatment the patient wants if they are unable to communicate at the time care is provided. It has been shown to be more effective than traditional advance directives at limiting unwanted life-sustaining treatments.

The APP should initiate discussion about a POLST form with any patient with a serious or chronic illness who may not be expected to live past 1 year. Without a POLST form (Table IV.1), emergency responders will provide all appropriate medical interventions.

PAIN

Pain is the most common symptom a patient experiences at end of life. Effective pain control can be achieved by using a combination of several treatments. Nonpharmacologic treatments are those interventions that do not require the use of medications. This may include imagery, aromatherapy, relaxation, music therapy, massage, and distraction techniques. Pharmacologic treatments, or those that involve medications, may include the use of opioids and nonsteroidal anti-inflammatory agents, and acetaminophen. Ideal pain management at end of life can be achieved through a long-acting agent with the addition of an immediate-release agent for breakthrough pain.

DYSPNEA

Dyspnea is another common symptom during the end-of-life phase. The APP should aim to treat reversible causes, if possible. Nonpharmacologic interventions can also be especially helpful. These interventions can include providing reassurance, offering distraction techniques, and encouraging relaxation exercises.

ANXIETY

When a patient in an end-of-life situation experiences anxiety, it is important for the APP to first assess the cause of anxiety, identifying both physical and psychological contributors. Once the cause or causes have been identified, the APP should find ways to modify any anxiety contributors, if possible. Nonpharmacologic interventions include supportive counseling and reassurance. When considering pharmacologic interventions, the APP should use benzodiazepines cautiously as these may increase delirium in older adults.

TABLE IV.1 POLST

POLST	Medical Order
Who completes the POLST form?	Healthcare professionals such as MD, NP, or PA; who can sign the order varies by state
What does the form communicate?	Code status
Would the patient want CPR? (Check one.)	Attempt resuscitation/CPR Do not attempt resuscitation/DNR
What types of medical interventions are available? (Check one.)	Full treatment: No limitation in aggressive treatment options Limited treatment: Use medical treatment such as antibiotics, IV fluids, and cardiac monitor; no intubation, advanced airway interventions, or mechanical ventilation Comfort measures only: Comfort through symptom management
Artificially administered nutrition? (Check one.)	Long-term artificial nutrition by tube Defined period of artificial nutrition by tube No artificial nutrition by tube
Review	By healthcare professionals

DNR, do not resuscitate; IV, intravenous; NP, nurse practioner; PA, physician assistant; POLST, Portable Orders for Life-Sustaining Treatment.

FATIGUE

Fatigue may be caused by a number of medical problems. When considering the best intervention for fatigue, the APP should address any contributing medical problems. These may include anemia, electrolyte imbalances, infection, or hypoxemia. Depending on the cause of fatigue, nonpharmacologic and/or pharmacologic therapies may be indicated. Nonpharmacologic therapy may include energy conservation, frequent naps, occupational therapy, and physical therapy. Pharmacologic therapy may include considering corticosteroids and psychostimulants on a case-by-case basis.

DEPRESSION

Many patients will experience some degree of depression at the end of their life cycle. Some patients who experience depression at end of life may benefit from supportive psychotherapy. Pharmacologic therapy may be considered depending on the patient's life expectancy, since many antidepressants need several weeks to take effect.

CONSTIPATION

The APP should be sure to assess the end-of-life patient for constipation. Preventive treatment for constipation should be given to all patients taking opioid pain medicine. The patient may also benefit from increased consumption of prune juice as well as taking a pharmacologic stimulant or osmotic laxative.

DELIRIUM

The APP should identify underlying and reversible causes of delirium to determine the most appropriate interventions. Nonpharmacologic intervention primarily focuses on ensuring a calm environment with the family, friends, or caregivers at the bedside.

Pharmacologic interventions may be warranted if delirium is severe. Benzodiazepines should be avoided as these may worsen delirium.

HOSPICE CARE

Hospice care provides support and services to a patient with a terminal illness and focuses on providing comfort for the patient at the end of life, not curing the patient's illness. Hospice referral should occur when a prognosis of 6 months or less is suspected. In order to initiate hospice services, patients and their families elect to focus on the patient's comfort. In many cases, hospice occurs in the home, but may also occur in other settings, such as the hospital, a nursing home, or a residential living facility.

U.S. MEDICARE HOSPICE ELIGIBILITY

Hospice care is delivered by a multidisciplinary team and is covered under Medicare, Medicaid, and many private insurance plans. Those eligible for Medicare Part A include U.S. citizens or legal residents who are:
A. Eligible for Social Security or railroad retirement benefits and are over the age of 65.
B. Under the age of 65 and eligible for Medicare due to a long-term disability.

To be covered, a referral must be made to a hospice that is Medicare-certified by the Centers for Medicare and Medicaid Services. Certification from the healthcare provider should state that the patient has a terminal diagnosis and most likely has less than 6 months to live. If the patient outlives their estimated 6-month prognosis while on hospice, the benefit can be renewed indefinitely as long as there is clinical evidence of continued decline consistent with disease progression and limited life expectancy. Some examples of end-stage disease that would make patients candidates for hospice referral include cancer, dementia due to Alzheimer disease, heart disease, liver disease, pulmonary disease, renal disease, stroke, and amyotrophic lateral sclerosis.

DELIVERING BAD NEWS
When and How to Deliver Bad News
Caring for patients at the end of life may require the APP to communicate bad news to the patients and their families. *Bad news* is any information that has the potential to have a significant negative impact on an individual's view of the future. Sharing bad news is a complex communication task that requires more than just stating the words; it requires responding to a patient's emotions. The APP can achieve this by:
A. Identifying the important information.
B. Talking honestly and in a straightforward way.
C. Being willing to talk about death/dying.
D. Delivering bad news in an individualized way.
E. Listening.
F. Encouraging questions.
G. Being sensitive to patients when they want to talk about difficult issues.

SPIKES
SPIKES is a method for delivering bad news. It comprised six steps, which are outlined in the following:

Step 1: Setting Up the Interview
It is important to consider the setting where the news will be delivered as well as what will be said. Arrange for a place that will provide some privacy and involve significant others in the interview. It is also helpful to engage in a mental rehearsal of what will be said. During the interview, the APP should sit down with the patient, maintain eye contact, and effectively manage time constraints and interruptions.

Step 2: Assess the Patient's Perception
During the interview, use open-ended questions to ask the patient what they understand about the disease process. Listen to the patient's level of comprehension and be sure to correct any misinformation.

Step 3: Obtain the Patient's Invitation
It is important to assess how much or how little information the patient would like to have. Some people want to know detailed information, while other patients prefer not to know. Accept the patient's right not to know and offer to answer questions later, if needed.

Step 4: Giving Knowledge
When speaking to the patient, use vocabulary words and terminology that are aligned with the comprehension level of the patient. Giving information in small chunks and pausing in between each chunk can help increase the patient's understanding. It is also helpful to check in with the patient as you are giving information to ensure the patient understood what you said.

Step 5: Address the Patient's Emotions
When receiving difficult news, the patient may feel shock, isolation, and grief. It is important for the APP to acknowledge these feelings and to offer support. Give the patient time to express their feelings.

Step 6: Strategy and Summary
After speaking with the patient and answering any questions, it is important to close the meeting by discussing plans for the future or next steps.

FINAL DAYS AND HOURS OF LIFE
In the final days and hours of life, patients may experience several symptoms, including:
A. Loss of appetite.
B. Excessive fatigue and sleep.
C. Increased physical weakness.
D. Mental confusion or disorientation.
E. Labored breathing.
F. Social withdrawal.
G. Changes in urination (oliguria or anuria).
H. Swelling in the feet and ankles.
I. "Death rattle," which refers to a gurgling sound created by air moving through uncleared secretions in the trachea and vocal cords.

During this time, the APP should continue to provide compassionate care aligned with the patient's and the family's preferences. The patient and the family may ask questions about food and water intake, express fears of the unknown, and have concerns about symptom management. The APP should answer any questions the family and the patient have and provide continued support.

DEATH PRONOUNCEMENT
The following procedures should be followed during the clinical examination for pronouncing death:
A. Properly identify the patient using the identification (ID) bracelet.
B. Check the pupils for position and response to light.
C. Check response to tactile stimuli: Examine respectfully, refraining from sternal rubs or nipple pinches.
D. Check for spontaneous respiration for 1 minute.
E. Check for apical heart tones and pulses for 1 minute.
F. Record the time of death.
The following items should be included in the death note:
A. Date and time of death.
B. Name of provider pronouncing death.
C. Brief statement of the cause of death.
D. Documentation of the absence of a pulse, respiration, and pupil response.
E. Notation of family presence at the death and/or family notification of the death.
F. Document notification of attending physician, pastoral care staff, social work staff, or other staff as appropriate.
A death certificate needs to be filled out, with all marked sections completed using black ink. This is often the duty of the attending healthcare provider.

SUMMARY

It is important to remember that death is a natural part of life. When providing end-of-life care, the APP should remember that their primary role is to support the patient and the patient's family and to empower the patient to articulate the type of death they would like. This is achieved by facilitating open and honest communication, asking and answering questions, and eliciting information about the patient's specific priorities and goals.

CASE SCENARIO: END OF LIFE

A 63-year-old patient was diagnosed with nonsmall cell lung cancer last year. She has been receiving treatment as an outpatient. She also has type 2 diabetes, hypertension, and chronic obstructive pulmonary disease (COPD). She was admitted to the hospital yesterday with fatigue, confusion, and jaundice. Testing now shows that cancer has likely metastasized to both her brain and liver. The nurse practitioner is planning to discuss the results of the tests and provide treatment options. The patient has indicated that she would like her spouse to be present for this discussion.

1. Which of the following is considered NOT IMPORTANT when setting up a time and place to have this discussion with the patient?

A. Arrange a place that will provide privacy.

B. Sit down with the patient/family and maintain appropriate eye contact.

C. Effectively manage distractions, such as pagers/cell phones.

D. All of the above are important considerations.

2. Which question could be used to assess how much the patient knows about her current diagnosis/prognosis?

A. "Do you have a family history of breast cancer?"

B. "Were you ever a smoker? If so, how long ago did you quit?"

C. "What do you understand about what brought you into the hospital?"

D. "Are you planning on participating in pulmonary rehab after discharge?"

BIBLIOGRAPHY

Baile, W. F., Buckman, R., Lenzi, R., Glober, G., Beale, E. A., & Kudelka, A. P. (2000). SPIKES—A six-step protocol for delivering bad news: Application to the patient with cancer. *The Oncologist, 5*, 302–311. https://doi.org/10.1634/theoncologist.5-4-302

Bailey, F. A., & Williams, B. R. O. S. A. (2005). Preparation of residents for death pronouncement: A sensitive and supportive method. *Palliative & Supportive Care, 3*, 107–114. https://doi.org/10.1017/S1478951505050182

Bloomer, M. J., Moss, C., & Cross, W. M. (2011). End-of-life care in acute hospitals: An integrative literature review. *Journal of Nursing and Healthcare of Chronic Illness, 3*, 165–173. https://doi.org/10.1111/j.1752-9824.2011.01094.x

Buck, H. G., & Fahlberg, B. (2014). Using POLST to ensure patients' treatment preferences. *Nursing, 44*, 16–17. https://doi.org/10.1097/01.NURSE.0000443322.11726.91

Buckman, R. (1992). *How to break bad news: A guide for health care professionals* (p. 15). Johns Hopkins University Press.

Byock, I. (2004). *The four things that matter most: Essential wisdom for transforming your relationships and your life* (p. 240). Free Pr: S. & S.

Centers for Disease Control and Prevention. (n.d.). *Chronic disease overview*. https://www.cdc.gov/chronicdisease/pdf/nccdphp-overview-508.pd

Electronic Code of Federal Regulation. (2017, March 15). *U.S. government publishing office*. https://www.ecfr.gov/cgi-bin/ECFR?page=browse

Halter, J. B., Ouslander, J. G., Studenski, S., High, K. P., Asthana, S., Supaino, M. A., & Ritchie, C. S (Eds.). (2017). *Hazzard's geriatric medicine and gerontology* (7th ed.). McGraw-Hill.

Meier, E. A., Gallegos, J. V., Thomas, L. P. M., & Depp, C. A. (2016). Defining a good death (successful dying): Literature review and a call for research and public dialogue. *The American Journal of Geriatric Psychiatry, 24*, 261–271. https://doi.org/10.1016/j.jagp.2016.01.135

National Health Center for Statistics. (n. d). *Fact sheets*. https://www.cdc.gov/nchs/data/factsheets/nchs_overview.pdf

KNOWLEDGE CHECK

1. Which statement is TRUE about the Portable Order for Life-Sustaining Treatment (POLST)?

   A. It is used to ensure that the patient's end of life wishes are upheld.

   B. It is intended to be used by emergency responders, hospitals, and healthcare providers.

   C. It typically includes patients' preferences concerning CPR, antibiotics, mechanical ventilation, and artificial nutrition.

   D. All of the above are true.

2. Which of the following statements about hospice care is TRUE?

   A. Patients must have a terminal diagnosis.

   B. Hospice care is never covered by insurance.

   C. Hospice referral can be made when a patient is expected to live less than 12 months.

   D. Hospice care can only occur in the outpatient setting.

3. Which of the following should be included in the clinical exam to pronounce death?

   A. Properly identify the patient using the identification (ID) bracelet.

   B. Check pupils for position and response to light.

   C. Check for spontaneous respirations for 1 minute.

   D. All of the above.

(See answers next page.)

1. D) All of the above are true.

The Portable Orders for Life-Sustaining Treatment (POLST) is a form that provides standing medical orders that healthcare providers can act on immediately when the patient is in an acute situation. It outlines the type of care a patient wishes to receive or does not wish to receive during end of life. POLST topics include the patient's preferences concerning CPR, antibiotics, mechanical ventilation, and artificial nutrition. The POLST form is intended to help healthcare providers, including first responders, provide the type of treatment the patient wants.

2. A) Patients must have a terminal diagnosis.

Hospice referrals are made when the patient most likely has less than 6 months to live. This is typically covered by insurance and can occur in the inpatient or outpatient setting. Some examples of end-stage disease that would make patients candidates for hospice referral include cancer, dementia due to Alzheimer disease, heart disease, liver disease, pulmonary disease, renal disease, stroke, and amyotrophic lateral sclerosis.

3. D) All of the above

The following medical procedures should be followed during the clinical examination for pronouncing death: Properly identify the patient using the identification (ID) bracelet, check the pupils for position and response to light, check response to tactile stimuli (examine respectfully, refraining from sternal rubs), check for spontaneous respiration for 1 minute, check for apical heart tones and pulses for 1 minute, and record the time of death.

PALLIATIVE CARE

Caitlyn Moore

INTRODUCTION

Given the increasing prevalence and longevity of people living with chronic and life-limiting illnesses, the need for comprehensive, holistic palliative care (PC) has grown. PC is a nursing and medical specialty focused on improving the quality of life (QOL) of patients, families, and caregivers navigating serious illnesses (SIs). According to an international consensus definition authored by Radbruch et al. (2020, p. 754), "[p]alliative care is the active, holistic care of individuals across all ages with serious health-related suffering due to severe illness, especially those near the end of life. It aims to improve the QOL of patients, their families and their caregivers." It is commonly understood as an umbrella term with various functional and conceptual definitions. As of 2020, 83% of hospitals report having a PC team. PC clinicians often partner with primary and specialty teams to provide expert symptom management and assistance with complex medical decision-making. PC patients are not required to give up services or therapies to qualify. Notably, the appropriateness of PC referral for patients is not tied strictly to prognosis or age, as it is appropriate at any age or stage of an SI, from initial diagnosis up to end of life.

PC addresses the physical, emotional, spiritual, and psychosocial stress often associated with SI and is provided most effectively by an interdisciplinary team (IDT). It can be included along with curative or life-prolonging therapies. It provides an added layer of support for patients, their families, and caregivers. PC professionals are experts in symptom management and communication around complex medical decision-making. PC is a type of preventive care that prevents unnecessary suffering by matching treatments and plans of care to patient and family goals. PC can be provided across care settings, including home, outpatient, inpatient, and long-term care.

WHAT IS A SERIOUS ILLNESS?

SI has been defined by Kelley and Bollens-Lund (2018, p. S-7) as "a health condition that carries a high risk of mortality AND either negatively impacts a person's daily function or QOL, OR excessively strains their caregivers." SI is commonly associated with multiple chronic and life-limiting illnesses, including but not limited to, cancer, heart failure, chronic obstructive pulmonary disease, neurologic conditions such as stroke and dementia, kidney disease, and others. SI can have profound impacts on the QOL of individuals, families, and caregivers. Notably, SI is not distinctly defined by prognosis; instead, as the definition outlines, it is associated with function, QOL, and stress on caregivers. Understanding this definition allows the advanced practice provider (APP) to expand access to PC services by earlier recognition of patients who may benefit.

COMMON PALLIATIVE CARE CONSULT TRIGGERS

The APP may be uncertain regarding which patients may benefit from including specialist PC. There are specialty and population-specific trigger tools that can be implemented to aid in clinical decision-making. One nonspecific but sufficiently sensitive screening question is the "surprise question": "Would you be surprised if this patient died in the next year?" If the clinician would not be surprised that a patient could die within the next year, a PC consult should be strongly considered. If the APP would not be surprised that the patient could die within 6 months, hospice may be a more appropriate referral, although this will depend on patient and family goals of care (GOC). If those goals are unknown or not clear, then PC consult can help to clarify. Table IV.2 provides common PC specialist referral triggers the APP can consider.

PROGNOSTICATION

Prognosis is an important consideration for the APP that can guide clinical decision-making and discussions with patients and families regarding GOC and treatment options. PC teams are often consulted to assist patients with navigating prognostic information or determining hospice eligibility. Various tools exist that can aid the clinician in providing accurate information. A generalizable prognostic evaluation is the Palliative Performance Score (PPS), which evaluates a person's performance status, intake, and level of consciousness to provide a prognosis in the order of days, weeks, or months. Disease-specific prognostic tools include the Functional Assessment Staging Tool (FAST) for Alzheimer type dementia, the Model for End-Stage Liver Disease (MELD) score for liver disease, and the Acute Physiology and Chronic Health Evaluation (APACHE) for critically ill patients. A centralized repository of peer-reviewed prognostic information is available for open access online through ePrognosis (2022) from the University of California, San Francisco. Prognostic tools can be valuable decision aids but should always be considered in the context of the individual and included as part of larger, patient-centered GOC conversations.

Prognosis is not limited to measurements of time. Many individuals also desire prognostic information regarding potential cognitive or functional impairments, the ability to remain independent, the likelihood of recurrent hospitalizations, and so forth. Many treatment-related decisions may have long-term implications that can significantly impact the QOL of individuals. For example, treatments such as tracheostomy or feeding tube placement may require a skilled nursing facility or the use of restraints, which can impact decision-making. Both prognoses, in terms of time and trajectory, can have lasting impacts on decision-making and QOL. As with any prognosis discussion, it is critically important for the APP to ensure relevant stakeholders are present (the

TABLE IV.2 COMMON REFERRAL TRIGGERS FOR A SPECIALIST PALLIATIVE CARE CONSULTATION IN THE HOSPITAL SETTING

Recurrent or prolonged hospitalizations	Frequent hospital admissions or ED visits for the same condition within 3–6 months Long length of stay
Complex medical decision-making	Complex family dynamics OR challenging care decisions around life-sustaining therapies including tracheostomy or PEG tubes
Complex symptom management	Hospital admission for uncontrolled symptoms related to SI, such as cancer pain
Adult failure to thrive	A decline in functional status, weight, or ability to care for self
Family or caregiver distress	Family or caregiver stress, overwhelm, inability to meet the care needs of the patient Lack of caregiver support
Team or patient decisional conflict	Disagreement regarding the appropriateness of medical interventions between patients and families or with medical team members
Limited prognosis	The "surprise question" OR metastatic or locally advanced cancers, global cerebral ischemia after resuscitation, hip fracture with cognitive impairment, illness not responding to disease-directed therapies; see also "Prognostication."
Spiritual or psychosocial distress	Patients with limited psychosocial support, complex family dynamics, or spiritual/existential distress

PEG, percutaneous endoscopic gastrostomy; SI, serious illness.

Sources: Data from Dahlin, C., Coyne, P. J., & Ferrell, B. R. (2016). *Advanced practice palliative nursing.* Oxford University Press, Incorporated. http://ebookcentral.proquest.com/lib/philau/detail.action?docID=4413898; Swetz, K. M., & Kamal, A. H. (2018). Palliative care. *Annals of Internal Medicine, 168*(5), ITC33. https://doi.org/10.7326/AITC201803060; Wheeler, M. S. (2016). Primary palliative care for every nurse practitioner. *The Journal for Nurse Practitioners, 12*(10), 647–653. https://doi.org/10.1016/j.nurpra.2016.09.003.

patient and their chosen support people). It is recommended that the provider clarify what information the patient is willing or wants to know before disclosing it. Additionally, the APP should discuss prognostic information within the context of a GOC conversation (see also "Family Meeting and Determining Goals of Care").

INTERDISCIPLINARY TEAM

Having a working knowledge of the composition of PC teams allows the APP to recognize the breadth of services and benefits for patients. The PC team consists of interdisciplinary specialists working together to improve the QOL of patients with SI. The National Consensus Project for Quality Palliative Care identified eight domains of PC that incorporate the IDT at its core. Table IV.3 highlights these domains, as well as common role delineation and overlap of the PC IDT. Notably, the IDT works alongside the patient's primary medical and specialty teams to provide extensive support to patients and families. Each IDT member possesses a unique skill set that contributes to the optimal care of patients. Each PC team is composed of varying IDT members. Understanding the possible roles and potential impact of the IDT aids the APP in recognizing the totality of PC services.

LEVELS OF PALLIATIVE CARE

The growing need for PC continues to outpace the availability of providers. APPs comprise a significant portion

of the PC workforce, and there is much opportunity. The tenets and core principles of PC are integral to effective and holistic APP practice. The three main levels of PC are primary, secondary, and tertiary. Tertiary PC is commonly provided in academic medical centers, with an emphasis on research to advance the specialty. Secondary PC is provided by PC board-certified and specialist clinicians in consultation with complex cases. Primary PC is the incorporation of basic PC principles into the clinical practice of all providers outside the PC specialty. This includes an emphasis on the relief of suffering, engagement in GOC, and basic pain and symptom management. Despite the increasing availability of PC services, millions of Americans continue to face significant barriers to accessing PC, emphasizing the need for all APPs to possess primary PC competency. For example, many APPs are responsible for admitting patients into the hospital setting, and code status clarification is an essential component of this process. Additionally, basic pain and symptom management is the responsibility of the APP in various specialties. Primary PC skills are needed for APPs in any specialty.

PALLIATIVE CARE ACROSS SETTINGS

The provision of PC is not solely dependent on location and is available across settings in many regions. Access to PC remains a health disparity in various regions of the United States, particularly rural and underserved

TABLE IV.3   MEMBERS OF THE IDT AND THEIR ASSOCIATED SCOPE WITHIN PC

Consult Reason	Physician or APP	RN	Pharmacist	Social Worker	Chaplain	Therapy (PT/OT/SLT)
Complex symptom management	X	X	X			X
GOC	X	X		X	X	
Psychosocial distress	X	X		X	X	
Family or caregiver conflict	X	X		X	X	
Spiritual or existential distress	X	X			X	
Complex care coordination	X	X	X	X	X	X
End-of-life issues	X	X	X	X	X	X
Bereavement	X	X		X	X	

APP, advanced practice provider; GOC, goals of care; IDT, interdisciplinary team; OT, occupational therapist; PC, palliative care; PT, physical therapist; SLT, speech language therapist.

Source: Data from Tatum, P. E., & Mills, S. S. (2020). Hospice and palliative care: An overview. *The Medical Clinics of North America, 104*(3), 359–373. https://doi.org/10.1016/j.mcna.2020.01.001.

areas. As the availability of services continues to be considered and delivered more upstream within patient care, clinicians will encounter PC in various settings. PC services are available in acute, ambulatory, and community settings. Acute care settings include hospitals and long-term acute care (LTAC) facilities. Ambulatory practices include office-based and embedded specialty clinics (such as within oncology or heart failure practices). Community PC services can be provided in homes, nursing facilities, or assisted living facilities.

FAMILY MEETING AND DETERMINING GOALS OF CARE

Complex medical decision-making and recommendations for medical treatments should continually be assessed and discussed within GOC conversations. The APP will engage in family meetings across acute care settings. As with many medical procedures, following a structured approach to family meetings improves outcomes and allows for a patient- and family-centered approach. This process should prioritize the patient and include relevant support persons or surrogate decision-makers per the patient's request or if it is determined that the patient lacks the capacity for medical decision-making. One recommended framework for a family meeting can be reviewed in Table IV.4.

It is important to note that, especially for steps 4 and 5 in Table IV.4, the patient and the family should be doing most of the talking, and the role of the APP is to listen and understand. Common communication strategies for the APP to utilize during family meetings and potentially difficult conversations include "Ask-Tell-Ask" and using "I wish" and "I worry" statements. "Ask Tell Ask" allows the APP to assess the patient's or the surrogate's current knowledge, provide important clarifications or new prognostic and medical information, and then assess their understanding. Wish/worry statements allow clinicians to align with families while acknowledging the concerns of the clinical team. An example of a wish/worry statement is "I wish that your mother could come off the ventilator. I worry that it won't be possible without a tracheostomy and long-term weaning."

ADVANCE CARE PLANNING

Advance care planning (ACP) is a process that the APP should address across settings for all patients regardless of age or health status. For hospitalized patients, the APP should inquire about previous conversations with providers and surrogate decision-makers, in addition to the existence of previously created advance directive documents. It is a billable, iterative process that does not need to result in the completion of advance directives or medical orders (such as a Medical Orders for Life-Sustaining Treatment [MOLST] or Portable Orders for Life-Sustaining Treatment [POLST] form), although it certainly could. The APP should be familiar with state practice laws surrounding ACP and medical orders, particularly with vulnerable populations such as those with cognitive impairments, intellectual or developmental disabilities, or incarceration. If there is a concern regarding capacity, the APP should conduct a formal assessment and/or refer for indepth evaluation, such as psychiatry, as needed. ACP allows APPs to better understand their patient's goals and values while empowering them to advocate for goal-concordant care.

GENERAL SYMPTOM MANAGEMENT PRINCIPLES

Various symptom management considerations are provided throughout this textbook in relation to multiple disease processes. This section introduces symptom management principles and resources for patients

TABLE IV.4   STEPWISE FRAMEWORK FOR FAMILY MEETINGS

Step	Process
1. Preparation	Plan agenda, understand relevant clinical data, and determine meeting attendees and location.
2. Introductions and agenda setting	Introduce all present and their relationship to the patient and set agenda for meeting with input from patient/family.
3. Patient status and prognosis	Elicit views and perspectives of patient/family members, use "Ask-Tell-Ask" technique, validate emotions, and incorporate "I wish" and "I worry" statements.
4. Clarification of patient's GOC	Determine who the patient is as a person and what they determine to be QOL.
5. Discussion of treatment options and making recommendations	Summarize hopes and worries. Review options within outlined goals. Discuss reasonable treatments aligned with goals. Offer a recommendation.
6. Summary and next steps	Recap discussion. Review next steps. Clarify contact person or persons and discuss agenda for next meeting.
7. Debriefing	Review events with clinical team and discuss any changes to care plan. Discuss areas for improvement.

GOC, goals of care; QOL, quality of life.
Source: Adapted from Widera, E., Anderson, W. G., Santhosh, L., McKee, K. Y., Smith, A. K., & Frank, J. (2020). Family meetings on behalf of patients with serious illness. *New England Journal of Medicine, 383*(11), e71. https://doi.org/10.1056/NEJMvcm1913056.

with SI. Many conditions associated with SI have the potential to cause a variety of symptoms. All symptom presentations require a thorough history and physical examination. Additionally, a comprehensive review of medications is warranted. In many cases, further diagnostic workup may be required and will vary depending on the presenting symptom. In patients with SI presenting with new, uncontrolled, or worsening symptoms, the APP must always consider disease progression. Some of the most encountered symptoms in patients with an SI include pain, dyspnea, nausea, and constipation, among others.

There are many resources and clinical decision aids available to APPs to assist with symptom management. The Palliative Care Network of Wisconsin created "Palliative Care Fast Facts and Concepts" (2022) with web-based and mobile applications that serve as a quick reference guide to symptom management, GOC conversations, and much more. The Center to Advance Palliative Care (CAPC) offers online, self-paced symptom management courses for clinicians to learn the basic and essential elements. Many APPs also have access to institutional clinical decision aids and calculators to assist with pharmacologic considerations. Collaboration with the IDT, particularly pharmacists, can be of great benefit. Patients with uncontrolled or recurrent symptoms and SI should be considered for PC consultation to assist with complex symptom management. Complex pain may also require interventional or specialty pain management, depending on the situation and resources available. Uncontrolled or escalating symptom burden

often contributes to physical, emotional, spiritual, and psychosocial suffering, and vice versa. Addressing all aspects of suffering is crucial to improving patient outcomes.

HOLISTIC ASSESSMENT

The emphasis on holistic assessment within PC includes physical, emotional, spiritual, and social health. The psychological, emotional, spiritual, and financial impacts of multimorbidity and progressive SI are significant. The APP should assess all domains of health to inform patient care and incorporate the IDT appropriately. The assessment of emotional health and mental well-being should occur regularly as all patients with chronic illness are at risk of developing depression. The APP should consider both pharmacologic (e.g., selective serotonin reuptake inhibitors) and nonpharmacologic (e.g., counseling) interventions when managing emotional and mental health conditions associated with SI.

Many patients want their healthcare provider to engage with them regarding their spirituality. Not all patients identify as spiritual, but screening and assessment can facilitate holistic health. A validated, reliable, and widely implemented guide available to clinicians to assess spirituality in clinical practice is the Faith or Belief, Importance, Community, and Address in Care (FICA) Spiritual History Tool. The FICA tool (Table IV.5) offers clinicians a guide to gathering information regarding patients' spiritual care and preferences. While spirituality often informs decision-making and coping, it is critical that the APP recognize their own spiritual

PALLIATIVE CARE 621

TABLE IV.5 FICA SPIRITUAL HISTORY TOOL©

FICA[a]	Sample Questions
F: Faith, belief, meaning	"Do you consider yourself to be spiritual?" or "Is spirituality something important to you?" "Do you have spiritual beliefs, practices, or values that help you to cope with stress, difficult times, or what you are going through right now?" (contextualize to visit) "What gives your life meaning?"
I: Importance and influence	"What importance does spirituality have in your life?" "Has your spirituality influenced how you take care of yourself, particularly regarding your health?" "Does your spirituality affect your healthcare decision making?
C: Community	"Are you part of a spiritual community?" "Is your community of support to you and how?" For people who don't identify with a community consider asking "Is there a group of people you really love or who are important to you?" (*Communities such as churches, temples, mosques, family, groups of like-minded friends, or yoga or similar groups can serve as strong support systems for some patients.*)
A: Address/action in care	"How would you like me, as your healthcare provider, to address spiritual issues in your healthcare?" (*With newer models, including the diagnosis of spiritual distress, "A" also refers to the "Assessment and Plan" for patient spiritual distress, needs and or resources within a treatment or care plan.*)

[a]The acronym FICA can help to structure questions for healthcare professionals who are taking a spiritual history.
Source: From © Christina Puchalski, MD, and The George Washington University 1996 (updated 2022). All rights reserved. Adapted from: Puchalski, C., & Romer, A. L. (2000). Taking a spiritual history allows clinicians to understand patients more fully. *Journal of Palliative Medicine, 3*(1), 129–137.

beliefs, and neither impose them on patients nor assume people with similar beliefs will make the same medical decisions.

PALLIATIVE CARE AND HOSPICE

As previously discussed, PC is understood as an umbrella term. Included within this umbrella is hospice care. Hospice is a system of care delivery focused on providing comfort and dignity for patients at end of life (Table IV.6). There are key differences and commonalities that the APP must understand between PC and hospice. While there is an overlap in philosophy, there are key differences that can improve patient access and timely referral by the nurse practitioner (NP).

SUMMARY

PC is an interdisciplinary approach to patient care that focuses on improving QOL, relieving various types of suffering and stress associated with SI, and aligning the plan of care with patient and family goals and preferences. While an APP may choose to specialize in PC, all APPs play a vital role in the provision of PC at various levels. APPs are responsible for recognizing which patients are appropriate for PC consultation and the delivery of primary PC to all patients.

BIBLIOGRAPHY

Best, M., Butow, P., & Olver, I. (2015). Do patients want doctors to talk about spirituality? A systematic literature review. *Patient Education and Counseling, 98*(11), 1320–1328. https://doi.org/10.1016/j.pec.2015.04.017

Carroll, T., El-Sourady, M., Karlekar, M., & Richeson, A. (2019). Primary palliative care education programs: Review and characterization. *American Journal of Hospice and Palliative Medicine®, 36*(6), 546–549. https://doi.org/10.1177/1049909118809947
Center to Advance Palliative Care. (2022). *Reports and publications, center to advance palliative care.* https://www.capc.org/capc-reports-and-publications/
Center to Advance Palliative Care. (n.d.). *Symptom management courses.* https://www.capc.org/training/symptom-management/
Dahlin, C., Coyne, P. J., & Ferrell, B. R. (2016). *Advanced practice palliative nursing.* Oxford University Press, Incorporated. http://ebookcentral.proquest.com/lib/philau/detail.action?docID=4413898
DiBello, K. (2021). Underscoring the importance of advance care planning. *The Nurse Practitioner, 46*(9), 24–29. https://doi.org/10.1097/01.NPR.0000769740.05465.f1
Ferrell, B. R., Coyle, N., & Paice, J. (2015). *Oxford textbook of palliative nursing.* Oxford University Press, Incorporated. http://ebookcentral.proquest.com/lib/philau/detail.action?docID=1911601
Kamal, A. H., Wolf, S. P., Troy, J., Leff, V., Dahlin, C., Rotella, J. D., Handzo, G., Rodgers, P. E., & Myers, E. R. (2019). Policy changes key to promoting sustainability and growth of the specialty palliative care workforce. *Health Affairs, 38*(6), 910–918. https://doi.org/10.1377/hlthaff.2019.00018
Kelley, A. S., & Bollens-Lund, E. (2018). Identifying the population with serious illness: The "Denominator" challenge. *Journal of Palliative Medicine, 21*(Suppl 2), S-7–S-16. https://doi.org/10.1089/jpm.2017.0548
Palliative Care Network of Wisconsin. (2022). Fast facts and concepts. *Palliative Care Network of Wisconsin.* https://www.mypcnow.org/fast-facts/
Puchalski, C., & Romer, A. L. (2000). Taking a spiritual history allows clinicians to understand patients more fully. *Journal of Palliative Medicine, 3*(1), 129–137. https://doi.org/10.1089/jpm.2000.3.129
Quill, T. E., & Abernethy, A. P. (2013). Generalist plus specialist palliative care—Creating a more sustainable model. *New England Journal of Medicine, 368*(13), 1173–1175. https://doi.org/10.1056/NEJMp1215620
Radbruch, L., De Lima, L., Knaul, F., Wenk, R., Ali, Z., Bhatnaghar, S., Blanchard, C., Bruera, E., Buitrago, R., Burla, C., Callaway, M.,

TABLE IV.6   DIFFERENCES BETWEEN PALLIATIVE CARE AND HOSPICE CARE

	Palliative Care	Hospice Care
Patient population	Specialized care for patients with SI Holistic approach focused on comfort and enhanced QOL for patients and family	End-of-life care for people at end of life Holistic approach focused on comfort and enhanced QOL for patients and their family
Connection to prognosis	Provided at any age and at any stage of SI Not linked to prognosis	Provided to persons with a life expectancy measured in months rather than years Prognosis of <6 months if a disease were to continue its anticipated trajectory
Common criteria	Provided as an added layer of support alongside disease-directed therapies and specialists	Often requires patients to stop disease-directed or life-prolonging therapies (such as chemotherapies, radiation, surgery, and dialysis)[a]
Availability	Available across settings	Can occur in home or care facility, or a specialized inpatient hospice unit
Coverage	Covered by Medicare, Medicaid, and many private insurances; may have co-pays	Covered by Medicare, Medicaid, and most private insurances; often no co-pays

[a]There are exceptions, which may vary based on the disease process and ability of the hospice agency.
QOL, quality of life; SI, serious illness.
Source: Data from Tatum, P. E., & Mills, S. S. (2020). Hospice and palliative care: An overview. *The Medical Clinics of North America, 104*(3), 359–373. https://doi.org/10.1016/j.mcna.2020.01.001.

Munyoro, E. C., Centeno, C., Cleary, J., Connor, S., Davaasuren, O., Downing, J., Foley, K., Goh, C., … Pastrana, T. (2020). Redefining palliative care—A new consensus-based definition. *Journal of Pain and Symptom Management, 60*(4), 754–764. https://doi.org/10.1016/j.jpainsymman.2020.04.027

Swetz, K. M., & Kamal, A. H. (2018). Palliative care. *Annals of Internal Medicine, 168*(5), ITC33. https://doi.org/10.7326/AITC201803060

Tatum, P. E., & Mills, S. S. (2020). Hospice and palliative care: An overview. *The Medical Clinics of North America, 104*(3), 359–373. https://doi.org/10.1016/j.mcna.2020.01.001

Wheeler, M. S. (2016). Primary palliative care for every nurse practitioner. *The Journal for Nurse Practitioners, 12*(10), 647–653. https://doi.org/10.1016/j.nurpra.2016.09.003

Widera, E., Anderson, W. G., Santhosh, L., McKee, K. Y., Smith, A. K., & Frank, J. (2020). Family meetings on behalf of patients with serious illness. *New England Journal of Medicine, 383*(11).https://doi.org/10.1056/NEJMvcm1913056

HEALTH PREVENTION AND SCREENING

Michele DeCastro and Sara Van Craeynest

INTRODUCTION

Prevention and screening are important parts of providing comprehensive acute care. Appropriate prevention and screening can help keep diseases from occurring, detect diseases in their earliest stages, and improve healthcare outcomes. As such, it is of vital importance that the advanced practice provider (APP) in the acute care setting be familiar with the different levels of prevention and the different types of prevention. It is also important to understand common vaccinations and screening recommendations.

LEVELS OF PREVENTION

There are three main levels of prevention dispensed by the APP: Primary prevention, secondary prevention, and tertiary prevention. Primary prevention refers to interventions that focus on preventing disease from occurring. Examples of primary prevention include recommending smoking cessation to a patient to reduce their risk of lung cancer, administering influenza immunizations, and recommending a mastectomy for the breast cancer 1 (BRCA)-positive patient.

Secondary prevention focuses on interventions that detect disease early and prior to presentation of symptoms. Examples of secondary prevention include performing regular Pap smears on female patients to detect precancerous lesions and testing for HIV in at-risk populations even in the absence of symptoms. Tertiary prevention refers to anything that prevents diseases from becoming worse or decreases the complications from a particular disease process. Examples may include recommending that a patient use a beta-blocker after having a myocardial infarction (MI), or treating hypertension (HTN) and hyperlipidemia in diabetic patients. Ophthalmology examinations in patients with diabetes mellitus (DM) may also be considered a form of tertiary prevention.

TYPES OF PREVENTION

As mentioned previously, prevention can be provided in different ways. Common types of prevention include screening, immunization, and recommending lifestyle modifications to prevent disease.

For APPs in the acute care setting, understanding screening and immunizations is especially important, as many patients will present without access to these preventive measures. Knowing which high-risk conditions they are most at risk of developing can help with diagnosis, inpatient treatment, and posthospital care planning.

SCREENING

For APPs in the acute care setting, understanding screening guidelines is essential to practice. It is important to know which common conditions the patient should have been screened for based on their age and risk factors. Most screening recommendations used by healthcare providers in the United States are created by one of several expert groups. The U.S. Preventive Services Task Force (USPSTF) is the leading creator of screening recommendations. The USPSTF is an independent panel of nonfederal experts who specialize in prevention and evidence-based medicine and who come from a variety of fields. They complete thorough reviews of current research and make recommendations for primary care screening and prevention. In their review, the USPSTF assigns a letter grade to each of their recommendations based on the strength of evidence to support the recommendation and the balance of benefits against harms of the recommendation. The benefits of a recommendation must outweigh risks, and the USPSTF's focus is on overall health and quality of life of patients, not just on the identification of disease. Other expert bodies make prevention and screening recommendations on their clinical area of expertise. Some of these organizations include the American College of Cardiology (ACC), the American Heart Association (AHA), the American Cancer Society (ACS), and the American College of Physicians (ACP). Screening and prevention of the two leading causes of death in the United States, cardiovascular disease (CVD) and cancer, are discussed in further detail later in this section.

IMMUNIZATIONS

Another form of prevention is immunization. Immunizations may be indicated based on the patient's age, lifestyle, health factors, or risk factors. It is important for the APP to know immunization status and immunization needs in order to make an appropriate diagnostic assessment, create an inpatient plan, and coordinate and recommend any appropriate follow-up care. Age-appropriate immunization schedules are provided in Tables IV.7 and IV.8. The following sections outline other common immunizations that may be indicated for adult patients.

Haemophilus Influenzae Type B

Haemophilus influenzae type B (Hib) vaccine is administered to patients with anatomic or functional asplenia (including sickle cell disease). These patients, if immunized as children, are vaccinated by giving one dose of the immunization in adulthood. Patients undergoing hematopoietic stem cell transplant should also receive vaccination. Regardless of Hib vaccination history, the patient receives three doses (at least 4 weeks apart) beginning 6 to 12 months after transplant. Evidence of immunity occurs with documented vaccination.

Hepatitis A

Hepatitis A immunization is indicated for patients who use injection or noninjection illicit substances, men who ▶

have sex with men (MSM), persons who experience homelessness, persons who work in a laboratory with hepatitis A virus or in high-risk healthcare or institutional settings, patients who are pregnant and who are at risk of infection, and persons who work in or travel to areas of high endemic disease. For adults, two separate 1-mL vaccinations are done 6 to 12 months apart. Additionally, adults may receive a three-dose series of Hep A–Hep B immunization.

Hepatitis B

Immunization against hepatitis B may be indicated based on the patient's age or lifestyle. The following factors indicate immunization is recommended:
A. Persons age 60 years or older, also including those not at explicit risk for hepatitis B infection by identified risk factors below.
B. Patients with chronic liver disease.
C. Current or recent injection drug users.
D. Patients with HIV infection.
E. Healthcare personnel and public safety workers who are potentially exposed to blood or other infectious body fluids.
F. Household contacts and sex partners of hepatitis B surface antigen-positive persons.
G. Patients with end-stage renal disease on hemodialysis, peritoneal dialysis, and patients who are predialysis.
H. Incarcerated persons.
I. Persons working in institutional settings.
J. Patients with DM.
K. Persons traveling in countries with high or intermediate endemic hepatitis B.

Evidence of immunity occurs with documented administration of the vaccine for most patients.

Influenza

Although most adults in general good health will recover from influenza, certain populations, such as the very young, the very old, and those with immunocompromising conditions, may be especially susceptible to more severe infections with influenza. As such, the Centers for Disease Control and Prevention (CDC) recommend that all adults receive the influenza vaccination annually. Influenza vaccination is contraindicated in adults with a history of egg allergy more severe than hives, including difficulty breathing, respiratory distress, or angioedema. Patients who have only hives after exposure to egg should receive age-appropriate vaccine.

Measles, Mumps, and Rubella

Adult patients are immune to measles, mumps, and rubella (MMR) if:
A. They were born before 1957.
B. There is documentation of receipt of MMR.
C. There is laboratory evidence of immunity.

This immunization is contraindicated in patients who are pregnant, immunocompromised adults, or those having an anaphylactic reaction to neomycin.

The CDC recommends adult immunization to students in postsecondary education, those who work in healthcare, and patients who travel internationally. Patients should receive second immunizations, 28 days after the first.

Meningococcal Vaccines

There are two meningococcal vaccines that immunize against serogroups A, C, W, and Y meningococcal vaccine (Men-ACWY) and serogroup B meningococcal vaccine (MenB). MenACWY is given in either one or two doses and is indicated in patients who have:
A. Anatomic or functional asplenia (including sickle cell disease and other hemoglobinopathies).
B. HIV infection.
C. Persistent complement component deficiency.
D. Eculizumab use.
E. Travel to or live in countries where meningococcal disease is hyperendemic or epidemic.
F. At risk from a meningococcal disease outbreak attributed to serogroup A, C, W, or Y.
G. Microbiologists routinely exposed to *Neisseria meningitides*.
H. Military recruits.
I. First-year college students who live in residential housing.
J. MSM.

MenB can be given in a two- or three-dose series, depending on manufacturer, and is indicated in patients with the following characteristics:
A. Anatomic or functional asplenia (including sickle cell disease).
B. Persistent complement component deficiency.
C. Eculizumab use.
D. At risk from a meningococcal disease outbreak attributed to serogroup B.
E. Microbiologists routinely exposed to *N. meningitidis*.

Evidence of immunity occurs with documented administration of the vaccine for most patients.

Tetanus

The Td (tetanus and diphtheria toxoids)/Tdap (tetanus toxoid, reduced diphtheria toxoid, and acellular pertussis vaccine) vaccinations should be given once every 10 years to all patients 19 years and older. Tdap is generally recommended for all patients at approximately 11 years of age. If this was not completed, or status is unknown, all adults should receive Tdap once in adulthood, followed by Td immunization every 10 years. Adults with an unknown or incomplete history of a three-dose primary series with Td-containing vaccines should complete the primary series that includes one dose of Tdap. All pregnant women should receive one dose of Tdap regardless of previous immunization.

Pneumonia

There are two types of pneumococcal vaccines used to help prevent pneumonia. One is the pneumococcal ▶

TABLE IV.7 VACCINES FOR TEENAGERS 13 TO 18 YEARS

Age (Years)	Flu (Influenza)	Tdap	HPV	Meningococcal MenACWY	Meningococcal MenB	Pneumococcal	Hepatitis B	Hepatitis A	Polio	MMR	Chickenpox (Varicella)
11–12	Yearly	Vaccine recommended ×1	Vaccine recommended ×1	Vaccine recommended ×1	Vaccine for high risk recommended ×1	Vaccine for high risk recommended ×1	Catchup/ missed dose	Catchup/ missed dose	Catchup/ missed dose	Catchup/ missed dose	Catchup/ missed dose
13–15	Yearly	Catchup/missed dose	Catchup/missed dose	Catchup/missed dose	Vaccine for high risk recommended ×1	Vaccine for high risk recommended ×1	Catchup/ missed dose	Catchup/ missed dose	Catchup/ missed dose	Catchup/ missed dose	Catchup/ missed dose
16–18	Yearly	Catchup/missed dose	Catchup/missed dose	Booster at age 16	Optional vaccine	Vaccine for high risk recommended ×1	Catchup/ missed dose	Catchup/ missed dose	Catchup/ missed dose	Catchup/ missed dose	Catchup/ missed dose

Note: Yearly means that the vaccine is recommended every year. Catchup/missed dose indicates that the vaccine should be given if the patient is catching up on missed doses. Vaccine recommended for patients with certain health or lifestyle conditions that put them at risk of serious diseases. Optional vaccine is for patients who are not at increased risk but wish to be vaccinated after speaking with a healthcare provider.
HPV, human papillomavirus; MenACWY, serogroup A, C, W, and Y meningococcal vaccine; MenB, serogroup B meningococcal vaccine; MMR, measles, mumps, rubella; Tdap, tetanus, diphtheria, pertussis.

TABLE IV.8 VACCINES FOR ADULTS BY AGE: 19+ YEARS

Age (Years)	Flu (Influenza)	Td/Tdap	Shingles (Zoster)	Pneumococcal		Meningococcal	
				PCV13	PPSV23	MenACWY or MPSV4	MenB
19–21	Yearly	Recommended		May be recommended	May be recommended	May be recommended	May be recommended
22–26	Yearly	Recommended		May be recommended	May be recommended	May be recommended	May be recommended
27–59	Yearly	Recommended		May be recommended	May be recommended	May be recommended	May be recommended
60–64	Yearly	Recommended	Recommended	May be recommended	May be recommended	May be recommended	May be recommended
65+	Yearly	Recommended	Recommended	Recommended	Recommended	May be recommended	May be recommended
	Get flu vaccine every year.	Get Td booster every 10 years. You also need one dose of Tdap vaccine. Women should get Tdap vaccine during EVERY pregnancy.	You should get shingles vaccine if you are 60+ years even if you previously have had shingles.	You should get one dose of PCV13 and at least one dose of PPSV23 depending on your age and health condition.			

Vaccines for Adults by Health Condition

	Flu (Influenza)	Td/Tdap	Shingles (Zoster)	Pneumococcal		Meningococcal	
				PCV13	PPSV23	MenACWY or MPSV4	MenB
Pregnancy	Yearly	Recommended	DO NOT GET VACCINE		May be recommended	May be recommended	
Weakened immune system	Yearly	Recommended	DO NOT GET VACCINE	Recommended	Recommended	May be recommended	May be recommended
HIV: CD4 count less than 200	Yearly	Recommended	DO NOT GET VACCINE	Recommended	Recommended	Recommended	May be recommended

Condition	Flu (Influenza)	Td/Tdap	Shingles (Zoster)	Pneumococcal		Meningococcal	
				PCV13	PPSV23	MenACWY or MPSV4	MenB
HIV: CD4 count 200+	Yearly	Recommended	Recommended	Recommended	Recommended	Recommended	May be recommended
Kidney disease	Yearly	Recommended	Recommended	Recommended	Recommended	May be recommended	May be recommended
Asplenia	Yearly	Recommended	Recommended	Recommended	Recommended	Recommended	Recommended
Heart disease/ chronic lung disease/ alcoholism	Yearly	Recommended	Recommended	Recommended	Recommended	May be recommended	May be recommended
Diabetes (type 1 and 2)	Yearly	Recommended	Recommended	Recommended	Recommended	May be recommended	May be recommended
Chronic liver disease	Yearly	Recommended	Recommended	May be recommended	Recommended	May be recommended	May be recommended
	Get flu vaccine every year.	Get Td booster every 10 years. You also need one dose of Tdap vaccine. Women should get Tdap vaccine during EVERY pregnancy.	You should get shingles vaccine if you are 60+ years even if you previously have had shingles.	You should get one dose of PCV13 and at least one dose of PPSV23 depending on your age and health condition.			

	HPV						
	For Women	For Men	MMR	Chickenpox (Varicella)	Hepatitis A	Hepatitis B	Hib
	Recommended	Recommended	Recommended	Recommended	May be recommended	May be recommended	May be recommended
	Recommended	May be recommended	Recommended	Recommended	May be recommended	May be recommended	May be recommended

(continued)

TABLE IV.8 VACCINES FOR ADULTS BY AGE: 19+ YEARS (CONTINUED)

Flu (Influenza)	Td/Tdap	Shingles (Zoster)	Pneumococcal		Meningococcal	
			PCV13	PPSV23	MenACWY or MPSV4	MenB
Recommended			Recommended	May be recommended	May be recommended	May be recommended
			Recommended	May be recommended	May be recommended	May be recommended
			Recommended	May be recommended	May be recommended	May be recommended

MMR/HPV/Chickenpox/Hep A/Hep B: You should get this vaccine if you did not get it when you were a child. HPV: You should get HPV vaccine if you are a woman through the age of 26 or a man through the age of 21 and did not already complete the series.

HPV		MMR	Chickenpox (Varicella)	Hepatitis A	Hepatitis B	Hib
For Women	For Men					
Recommended		DO NOT GET VACCINE	DO NOT GET VACCINE	May be recommended	May be recommended	May be recommended
Recommended	Recommended	DO NOT GET VACCINE	DO NOT GET VACCINE	May be recommended	May be recommended	Recommended
Recommended	Recommended	DO NOT GET VACCINE	DO NOT GET VACCINE	May be recommended	Recommended	May be recommended
Recommended	Recommended	Recommended	Recommended	May be recommended	Recommended	May be recommended
Recommended	Recommended	Recommended	Recommended	May be recommended	May be recommended	May be recommended
Recommended	Recommended	Recommended	Recommended	May be recommended	May be recommended	
Recommended	Recommended	Recommended	Recommended	May be recommended	May be recommended	May be recommended

	Flu (Influenza)	Td/Tdap	Shingles (Zoster)	Pneumococcal		Meningococcal	
				PCV13	PPSV23	MenACWY or MPSV4	MenB
	Recommended	Recommended	Recommended	May be recommended	Recommended	May be recommended	
	Recommended	Recommended	Recommended	Recommended	Recommended	May be recommended	
	MMR/HPV/Chickenpox/Hep A/Hep B: You should get this vaccine if you did not get it when you were a child. HPV: You should get HPV vaccine if you are a woman through the age of 26 or a man through the age of 21 and did not already complete the series.				You should get Hib vaccine if you have sickle cell disease, had a bone marrow transplant, or you do not have a spleen.		

Hib, *Haemophilus influenzae* type B vaccine; HPV, human papillomavirus; MenACWY, serogroup A, C, W, and Y meningococcal vaccine; MenB, serogroup B meningococcal vaccine; MMR, measles, mumps, rubella; MPSV4, meningococcal polysaccharide vaccine; PCV13, pneumococcal conjugate vaccine; PPSV23, pneumococcal polysaccharide vaccine; Td, tetanus and diphtheria toxoids; Tdap, tetanus, diphtheria, pertussis.

polysaccharide vaccine (PPSV23) and the other is the pneumococcal conjugate vaccine (PCV20 and PCV15).

The APP should consider the patient's age, lifestyle, and any medical conditions the patient has to determine which vaccination to administer. Adults 65 and over should receive either one dose of PCV15 or one dose of PCV20. Adults who received PCV15 should receive one dose of PPSV23 at least 1 year after the initial PCV15 dose; PPSV23 is not recommended for people who have previously received a PCV20 vaccination. This same schedule applies for adults under 65 years with the following conditions or lifestyle factors:

A. Chronic heart or lung disease.
B. DM.
C. Alcoholism.
D. Chronic liver disease.
E. Adults who smoke cigarettes.
F. Diabetes.
G. Cerebrospinal fluid (CSF) leaks.
H. Cochlear implants.
I. Sickle cell disease or other hemoglobinopathies.
J. Congenital or acquired asplenia.
K. Congenital or acquired immunodeficiencies.
L. HIV infection.
M. Chronic renal failure.
N. Nephrotic syndrome.
O. Leukemia.
P. Lymphoma.
Q. Hodgkin disease.
R. Generalized malignancy.
S. Iatrogenic immunosuppression.
T. Solid organ transplant.
U. Multiple myeloma.

Only adults with an immunocompromised condition, cochlear implant, or CSF leak should decrease the wait time between PCV15 and PPSV23 to shorter than a year, and the wait time should be reduced to 8 weeks between doses.

PCV13 is no longer recommended for adults. Patients who previously received PCV13 vaccine should continue to previously recommended series of PCV13 followed by PPSV23; alternatively, if PPSV23 is not available, these adults should receive one dose of PCV20.

Varicella

All adults without evidence of immunity should receive two doses of the varicella vaccine, 4 weeks apart. Vaccination should be especially emphasized for those with high-risk contacts, such as healthcare workers, childcare workers, and workers in an institutional setting. This vaccination is contraindicated in pregnancy. Evidence of immunity includes the following:

A. Documentation of four doses at least 4 weeks apart.
B. United States-born before 1980, except healthcare workers and pregnant women.
C. History of herpes zoster.
D. Laboratory evidence of immunity.

Zoster

As of October 2017, recombinant zoster vaccine (RZV) is recommended for the prevention of herpes zoster and related complications for immunocompetent adults aged ≥50 years. RZV is a two-dose vaccine given 2 to 6 months apart. Prior to this variation of the vaccine, zoster vaccine live (ZVL) was the only vaccine available to prevent herpes zoster in adults over 50 years. It is recommended to administer two doses of RZV 2 to 6 months apart to adults who previously received ZVL at least 2 months after ZVL. CDC guidelines state that RZV is preferred over ZVL for prevention of herpes zoster and related complications. Both vaccines are contraindicated in patients who are pregnant or in patients with severe immunodeficiency, such as those with AIDS or who are undergoing cancer treatment. Evidence of immunity occurs with documented administration of the vaccine.

SCREENING AND PREVENTION FOR CARDIOVASCULAR DISEASE

The CDC reports that 659,000 deaths (1 in 4 deaths) annually are attributed to heart disease, making it the leading cause of death in the United States. There are many screening and prevention methods that the APP should consider when assessing and caring for patients who exhibit risk factors for CVD.

Use of Cardiovascular Risk Calculator

An appropriate initial step in screening patients for CVD is to use a cardiovascular (CV) risk calculator. The CV risk calculator that is based on the ACC/AHA 2013 Cholesterol Guidelines is the most commonly used and is available on the ACC's website. It is a form of pooled risk assessment that considers a patient's risk factors, including age, race, weight, cholesterol levels, and blood pressure. The calculator was based on multiple community-based population studies and considers risk of stroke and MI.

HYPERTENSION

There is clear evidence that controlling HTN will decrease one's risk of developing CVD. As such, it is vital to screen all adults who are 18 years and older for high blood pressure. The APP should recommend annual screening for those deemed at risk based on the results of the CVD risk calculator. Readings of blood pressure should be obtained outside of the clinic setting prior to definitive diagnosis. Please refer to Chapter 3 of this book for more information on the diagnosis and management of HTN.

CAROTID ARTERY STENOSIS

Approximately 15% of strokes are caused by large artery atherothrombotic disease, which includes carotid artery stenosis (CAS). The presence of asymptomatic CAS (>70% stenosis) in the population is estimated to be 1.7%. However, most ischemic strokes are not caused by CAS. Therefore, the burden of CAS causing stroke ▶

among the general population is low. The risks of intervention through performing a carotid endarterectomy (CEA) or carotid angioplasty and stenting (CAAS) are high, and include stroke, MI, pulmonary embolus, and death. Typically, screening for this occurs in patients by performing a carotid duplex ultrasonography. According to the USPSTF, the AHA, and the American Stroke Association, there is no clear benefit in screening via ultrasound or auscultation in asymptomatic patients. Patients who are at high risk for the disease include those with a carotid bruit heard on auscultation, those with confirmed atherosclerotic disease, and those age 65 years or older with a history of one or more of the following atherosclerotic risk factors: Coronary artery disease, smoking, or hypercholesterolemia. For these patients, it is a reasonable expectation to consider screening. However, for many of these patients, optimal medical therapy has already been initiated to treat their known atherosclerotic disease.

LIPIDS

Evidence has linked high cholesterol levels with increased risk of CVD. As such, the USPSTF recommends that adults 40 years and older be screened with a serum lipid profile. For patients with no history of CV events, there is no clear end date for when to END screening.

ELECTROCARDIOGRAM

There is no clear evidence that resting EKG is helpful for low- or high-risk patients in looking for coronary heart disease in asymptomatic patients. Therefore, the USPSTF does not recommend using an EKG as a method to screen for CVD in patients with no symptoms.

DIABETES

The APP should screen for diabetes as part of a CV risk assessment in all adults age 35 to 70 years who are overweight or obese. All patients with abnormal blood glucose results should be offered intensive behavioral counseling on diet and exercise and effective prevention interventions.

ABDOMINAL AORTIC ANEURYSM

It is recommended that men age 65 to 75 years who have ever smoked should undergo one-time screening for abdominal aortic aneurysm. Evidence seems to show a small benefit exists in screening men age 65 to 75 years who have never smoked; however, evidence is inconclusive regarding screening for women age 65 to 75 years who have ever smoked. It is not necessary to screen women age 65 to 75 years who have never smoked as there is a very low possibility of diagnosis.

TOBACCO USE

The U.S. Surgeon General reports that one-third of deaths from CVD are caused by smoking. It is important that the APP ask all adult patients about nicotine and tobacco use. All adult tobacco users and all pregnant women who use tobacco should be advised to stop. These patients should also be offered both pharmacologic and nonpharmacologic/behavioral interventions for tobacco cessation.

OBESITY

All adults should be screened for obesity. Clinicians should offer or refer patients with a body mass index (BMI) of 30 kg/m^2 or higher to intensive, multicomponent behavioral interventions. Weight loss can improve blood pressure, glycemic control, and decrease overall cardiovascular risk.

CANCER SCREENING AND PREVENTION

Cancer is attributed as the cause of 599,589 deaths annually, making it the second-leading cause of death in the United States. Cancers with the highest rates are cancer of the female breast, prostate cancer, lung and bronchus cancer, colon and rectal cancer, and corpus and uterine cancer. The greatest number of deaths from cancer is due to lung, colorectal, breast, and pancreatic cancers, respectively. Of these, pancreatic cancer has the highest mortality rate (6% survival rate in 5 years). The United States has not met the goals for screening for breast, cervical, prostate, and colorectal cancer as set by *Healthy People 2020*.

Cancer prevention includes measures such as tobacco cessation counseling for all patients due to its association with multiple cancers. The following sections outline the leading prevention and screening recommendations from the USPSTF, the ACS, and other expert recommendations for each type of the most common forms of cancer.

Breast

When considering which screening and prevention recommendation is appropriate, it is important for the clinician to determine the patient's risk of breast cancer. There are multiple models used to determine risk of developing breast cancer. One of the most commonly accepted and used tools for determining risk is the Breast Cancer Risk Assessment Tool as developed by the National Cancer Institute. Factors considered in this model include:

A. Family history.
B. Age.
C. Ethnicity.
D. History of abnormal breast biopsy.
E. Obstetric history.

Women with family or personal history of breast, ovarian, or peritoneal cancer, genetic predisposition, and women with a history of radiation to the chest are all considered higher risk.

U.S. Preventive Services Task Force Recommendation

The USPSTF recommends that in women 40 to 49 years the decision to screen should be an individual one. Screening should be considered in higher risk women. In women 50 to 74 years, screening reduces mortality and should be performed every 1 to 2 years. In women older than 75 years, evidence is insufficient to make a definitive screening recommendation.

American Cancer Society Recommendation

The ACS recommends that women age 40 to 44 years should have the opportunity to begin annual screening if they chose to and in discussion with a healthcare provider. Women with an average risk of breast cancer should undergo regular screening mammography starting at 45 years of age. Annual screening should continue in women until they are 54 years old. Women aged 55 years and older may transition to biennial screening or choose to continue screening annually. Women who have a life expectancy greater than 10 years and are in good health may continue screening with mammography. Women who are at high risk should undergo annual screening mammography and MRI starting at age 30 years. High-risk women are those with a known BRCA mutation; women who are untested, but have a first-degree relative with a BRCA mutation; or women with an approximately 20% to 25% or greater lifetime risk of breast cancer based on risk-estimation models.

Other Expert Recommendations

The ACP has the following age-specific recommendations for women of average risk:

A. 40 to 49 years: Discuss risks/benefits; biennial mammogram if informed woman requests.
B. 50 to 74 years: Biennial mammogram.
C. Younger than 40 years or older than 75 years OR life expectancy less than 10 years: No screening.

The American College of Obstetricians and Gynecologists (ACOG) recommends that women 40 years and older receive annual screening with mammogram.

Prevention

Mastectomy may be indicated as a preventive measure for very high-risk patients.

Cervical

U.S. Preventive Services Task Force Recommendation

The USPSTF recommends that women who are younger than 21 years do not need to be screened for cervical cancer. Women 21 to 29 years receive screening every 3 years with cytology (Pap alone). Women age 30 to 65 years should be screened every 5 years with cytology (Pap) in combination with human papillomavirus (HPV) testing. Women who are 65 years of age and have had adequate screening need no further testing. The APP should not screen women with hysterectomy who do not have a history of cervical cancer or high-grade precancerous lesion.

American Cancer Society Recommendation

The ACS does not recommend screening women who are 21 to 24 years. Women who are 30 to 65 years should have a Pap test with HPV every 5 years, or every 3 years with Pap alone. Women who are older than 65 years should no longer be screened for cervical cancer if they have had normal screening test results over a long period of time.

Other Expert Recommendations

The ACP does not recommend screening average-risk women younger than 21 years. Average-risk women should be screened for cervical cancer beginning at 21 years of age, and once every 3 years with cytology (Pap tests without HPV tests). Average-risk women should not be screened for cervical cancer with cytology more often than once every 3 years. Clinicians may choose to use a combination of Pap testing and HPV testing once every 5 years in average-risk women who are 30 years or older. However, clinicians should not perform HPV testing in average-risk women younger than 30 years.

The ACP recommendations are largely in line with the ACS recommendation. Women older than 65 years who have had three consecutive negative cytology results or two consecutive negative cytology plus HPV test results within 10 years, with the most recent test done within 5 years, should no longer be screened for cervical cancer. They do not recommend screening average-risk women of any age who have had a hysterectomy with removal of the cervix.

Prevention

The leading cause of cervical cancer is HPV. As such, preventing HPV infection is a primary form of prevention of cervical cancer. Interventions to prevent HPV infection may include:

A. Vaccinating against HPV (see Tables IV.7 and IV.8 for age-appropriate vaccination recommendations).
B. Encouraging the patient to use a barrier method during sexual intercourse.

Treatment and/or assessment of abnormal cells on cytology and treatment and/or assessment of HPV are also important preventive measures.

Colorectal

U.S. Preventive Services Task Force Recommendation

Patients age 50 to 75 years with an average risk should be screened for colorectal cancer. The test for screening chosen will determine the frequency of screening. Screening may begin earlier for patients with increased risk. Patients with a personal or family history of colon cancer are considered at increased risk. The APP should make an individualized decision on whether to screen patients older than 75 years. The overall health of the patient should be considered as well as the patient's ability to tolerate treatment, if diagnosed, and if previously screened. There is no superior test; however, if less invasive tests are positive, then direct visualization with colonoscopy is necessary.

Tests may also be indicated. Tests that detect cancer and colorectal polyps are as follows:

A. Colonoscopy: Perform every 10 years.
B. CT colonography: Perform every 5 years. If abnormal, proceed to colonoscopy.

▶

C. Flex sig: Perform every 5 years. If abnormal, proceed to colonoscopy.
D. Flex sig + fecal immunochemical test (FIT): Flex sig every 10 years plus FIT every year.

Tests that detect cancer are as follows:

A. Guaiac-based fecal occult testing: Perform annually. If abnormal, proceed to colonoscopy.
B. FIT: Perform annually. If abnormal, proceed to colonoscopy.
C. Stool DNA test: Perform every 1 to 3 years. If abnormal, proceed to colonoscopy.

American Cancer Society Recommendation
The ACS recommends that both men and women with average risk who are older than 45 years should start cancer screening. Refer to the USPSTF for type of testing recommendations.

Prevention
It is recommended that the APP perform early screening for abnormal tissue that could become cancer.

Lung
U.S. Preventive Services Task Force Recommendation
Current or former smokers age 50 to 80 years with a history of smoking 20 packs per year or quit within last 15 years should be screened annually for lung cancer. Screening includes a low-dose/helical CT (LDCT) scan of the lung. Informed and shared decision-making discussion should occur between the patient and the provider. Screening should stop once the patient has not smoked for 15 years or is no longer willing to undergo treatment with curative lung surgery.

American Cancer Society Recommendation
Current or former smokers age 50 to 74 years with a history of smoking 30 packs per year should be screened annually. Screening should include an LDCT scan of the lung. An informed and shared decision-making discussion should occur between the patient and the provider.

Other Expert Recommendations
The American Association for Thoracic Surgery recommends that patients who are 55 to 79 years old and who have a history of smoking 30 packs per year should be screened with LDCT annually. Lung cancer survivors should be screened with LDCT starting 5 years after treatment. Annual LDCT screening should be offered starting at 50 years of age and with a smoking history of 20 packs per year if they have an additional risk factor that produces a 5% risk of developing lung cancer over the next 5 years.

Prevention
Since cigarette smoking is the leading cause of lung cancer, smoking cessation is the primary form of prevention.

Prostate
U.S. Preventive Services Task Force Recommendation
The USPSTF recommends that for men age 55 to 69 the decision to screen for prostate cancer should be an individual one. The main modality for screening is a serum prostate-specific antigen (PSA) test. Before undergoing screening, men should have the chance to discuss the benefits of screening as well as weighing the risks of diagnosis and treatment. Complications of diagnosis and treatment include infection, erectile dysfunction, and incontinence. Prostate cancer is common. Many men have no symptoms of the disease and are only diagnosed through screening. Risk factors for the disease include men of older age, men who are African American, and men with a family history of prostate cancer. Only men who have been counseled on their own risk for the disease and on the risks and benefits of screening and treatment should be offered testing.

American Cancer Society Recommendation
Informed decision-making with a healthcare provider about whether to be screened for prostate cancer is indicated in patients considered to have average risk, are older than 50 years of age, and have at least a 10-year life expectancy. The APP should provide information to the patient about the potential benefits, risks, and uncertainties associated with prostate cancer screening. Screening should not happen in the absence of an informed decision-making process. Screening may be indicated in men who are 45 years and older who are at higher risk, including African American men and men with a first-degree family member (father or brother) who was diagnosed with prostate cancer before age 65 years.

Men who are 40 years and older should consider screening if they are at appreciably higher risk. These may include men who have had multiple family members diagnosed with prostate cancer before 65 years of age.

Other Expert Recommendations
The American Urological Association recommends against PSA screening in men younger than 40 years and also does not recommend screening in patients who are 40 to 54 years old who are at average risk.

They recommend that patients who are 55 to 69 years engage in the shared decision-making process (see also the Affordable Care Act [ACA] recommendation for this age range). For men who do elect screening after a shared decision-making process with their providers, screening should only occur at an interval of every 2 years or longer in between screenings. The American Urological Association does not recommend screening for patients who are older than 70 years or for any man with less than a 10- to 15-year life expectancy.

The ACP recommends that clinicians should have a one-time discussion (more if the patient requests them) with average-risk patients age 50 to 69 years who ▶

inquire about PSA-based prostate cancer screening. This discussion should inform the patient about the limited potential benefits and substantial harms of screening for prostate cancer using the PSA test. For men who have average risk and are 50 to 69 years of age who have not had an informed discussion and do not express a clear preference for screenings, no screening should be performed. Clinicians should not screen for prostate cancer using the PSA test in average-risk men younger than 50 years, those older than 69 years, or people whose life expectancy is less than 10 years.

SEXUALLY TRANSMITTED INFECTION SCREENING AND PREVENTION

The CDC and USPSTF have provided specific guidance on sexually transmitted infection (STI) screenings for adults based on risk and specific STIs. Understanding STI risk and prevention is especially important in caring for any patient who may present in the acute care setting with a new STI, be unaware of the source of infection, or have a complication from an STI. All STI prevention includes counseling patients on having protected intercourse with a condom and avoiding high-risk behaviors, such as sharing injection drug paraphernalia. The act of screening is also considered a prevention method as identifying asymptomatic patients and treating their infection will prevent the spread of disease to other persons.

Human Immunodeficiency Virus

Patients can present in the acute phase of HIV infection. However, they may also present with an opportunistic infection or complication of HIV, and HIV screening would be warranted. All adults between the ages of 13 and 65 should be screened for HIV at least once. Anyone who has unprotected intercourse and/or shares injection drug equipment should be screened for HIV annually. Sexually active gay and bisexual men should be screened for HIV more frequently (every 3–6 months).

All pregnant patients should also be screened for HIV. Also, sex partners of persons who are HIV-positive or are injection drug users should be screened.

Chlamydia and Gonorrhea

All sexually active women under the age of 25 should be screened for chlamydia and gonorrhea. Women 25 years and older who are at higher risk should also be routinely screened. At-risk women are those who have a new sex partner, more than one sex partner, a sex partner with concurrent partners, or a sex partner who has STI. Young men (younger than 25 years) who are presenting in a high-prevalence clinical setting should also be screened. MSM should be screened annually, or every 3 to 6 months for higher risk MSM if they or their partner(s) have multiple partners.

Hepatitis B

High-risk and women should be screened periodically. Those who are high risk include:

A. MSM.
B. Persons born in areas with high prevalence (≥2% population) of hepatitis B virus (HBV) infection.
C. Persons on immunosuppressant medications.
D. Patients on hemodialysis.
E. Patients who are HIV-positive.
F. Patients who are injection drug users.
G. Household contacts or sexual partners of persons with HBV infection.
H. Pregnant patients should also be screened at their first prenatal visit.

Hepatitis C

All men and women born between 1945 and 1965 should have a one-time screening for hepatitis C. Higher risk MSM should also be screened for hepatitis C. All patients with HIV should also be screened for hepatitis C annually. All pregnant patients should be screened during each pregnancy.

SUMMARY

The APP in acute care may not always be the clinician who is offering prevention and screening initiatives to their patients. However, many patients treated in the acute care setting will have limited access to healthcare and may not have been offered important screening and prevention measures. While the acute care environment is not the setting to offer many of these interventions, the clinicians working in these settings need to know which of these measures these patients have missed. This may help when both diagnosing current conditions and planning for any appropriate outpatient follow-up.

BIBLIOGRAPHY

American Cancer Society. (2021, April). *American Cancer Society recommendations for the early detection of cervical cancer.* https://www.cancer.org/cancer/cervical-cancer/detection-diagnosis-staging/cervical-cancer-screening-guidelines.html

American Cancer Society. (2021, August). *Can lung cancer be found early?* https://www.cancer.org/cancer/lung-cancer/detection-diagnosis-staging/detection.html#written_by

American Cancer Society. (2022, July). *American Cancer Society recommendations for the early detection of breast cancer.* https://www.cancer.org/cancer/breast-cancer/screening-tests-and-early-detection/american-cancer-society-recommendations-for-the-early-detection-of-breast-cancer.html

American College of Physicians. (2022, January). *Cervical cancer screening.* https://www.acponline.org/clinical-information/performance-measures/cervical-cancer-screening

American Diabetes Association. (2017). 3. Comprehensive medical evaluation and assessment of comorbidities. *Diabetes Care, 40*(Suppl. 1), S25–S32. https://doi.org/10.2337/dc17-S006

American Heart Association & American College of Cardiology. (n.d.). *2013 Prevention guidelines tools—CV risk calculator.* http://professional.heart.org/professional/GuidelinesStatements/PreventionGuidelines/UCM_457698_Prevention-Guidelines.jsp

Carter, H. B., Albertsen, P. C., Barry, M. J., Etzioni, R., Freedland, S., Greene, K., & Zietman, A. (2013). *Early detection of prostate cancer: AUA guideline.* https://www.auanet.org/education/guidelines/prostate-cancer-detection.cfm

Centers for Disease Control and Prevention. (2020, July). *Testing recommendations for hepatitis C virus infection.* https://www.cdc.gov/hepatitis/hcv/guidelinesc.htm

Centers for Disease Control and Prevention. (2022). *Table 1. Recommended adult immunization schedule for ages 19 years or older, United States, 2022.* https://www.cdc.gov/vaccines/schedules/hcp/imz/adult.html

Centers for Disease Control and Prevention. (2022, July). *About heart disease*. https://www.cdc.gov/heartdisease/about.htm

Centers for Disease Control and Prevention. (n.d). *What are the risk factors for lung cancer?* https://www.cdc.gov/cancer/lung/basic_info/risk_factors.htm

Eckel, R. H., Jakicic, J. M., Ard, J. D., de Jesus, J. M., Houston Miller, N., Hubbard, V. S., Lee, I.-M., Lichtenstein, A. H., Loria, C. M., Millen, B. E., Nonas, C. A., Sacks, F. M., Smith, Jr., C, S., Svetkey, L. P., Wadden, T. A., & Yanovski, S. Z. (2014). 2013 AHA/ACC guideline on lifestyle management to reduce cardiovascular risk: A report of the American College of Cardiology/American Heart Association task force on practice guidelines. *Circulation, 129*(25 Suppl. 2), S76–S99. https://doi.org/10.1161/01.cir.0000437740.48606.d1

Goff, D. C., Lloyd-Jones, D. M., Bennett, G., Coady, S., D'Agostino, R. B., Gibbons, R., Greenland, P., Lackland, D. T., Levy, D., O'Donnell, C. J., Robinson, J. G., Schwartz, J. S., Shero, S. T., Smith, Jr., C, S., Sorlie, P., Stone, P., & Wilson, P. W. F. (2014). 2013 ACC/AHA guideline on the assessment of cardiovascular risk: A report of the American College of Cardiology/American Heart Association Task Force on Practice guidelines. *Circulation, 129*(25 Suppl. 2), S49–S73. https://doi.org/10.1161/01.cir.0000437741.48606.98

Hesse, B. W., Gaysynsky, A., Ottenbacher, A., Moser, R. P., Blake, K. D., Chou, W. -Y. S., Vieux, S., & Beckjord, E. (2014). Meeting the healthy people 2020 goals: Using the health information national trends survey to monitor progress on health communication objectives. *Journal of Health Communication, 19*, 1497–1509. https://doi.org/10.1080/10810730.2014.954084

Jensen, M. D., Ryan, D. H., Apovian, C. M., Ard, J. D., Comuzzie, A. G., Donato, K. A., Hu, F. B., Hubbard, V. S., Jakicic, J. M., Kushner, R. F., Loria, C. M., Millen, B. E., Nonas, C. A., Pi-Sunyer, F. X., Stevens, J., Stevens, V. J., Wadden, T. A., Wolfe, B. M., & Yanovski, S. Z. (2014). 2013 AHA/ACC/TOS guideline for the management of overweight and obesity in adults: A report of the American College of Cardiology/American Heart Association Task Force on Practice Guidelines and the Obesity Society. *Circulation, 129*(25 Suppl. 2), S102–S138. https://doi.org/10.1161/01.cir.0000437739.71477.ee

Mazzone, P. J., Silvestri, G. A., Souter, L. H., Caverly, T. J., Kanne, J. P., Katki, H. A., Wiener, R. S., & Detterbeck, F. C. (2021). Screening for lung cancer: CHEST guideline and expert panel report. *Chest, 160*(5), 427–494. https://doi.org/10.1016/j.chest.2021.06.063

Moody, T. E., Spraitzar, C. L., Eisenhart, E., & Tully, S. (2017). The American urological association's prostate cancer screening guideline: Which cancers will be missed in average-risk men aged 40 to 54 years? *Reviews in Urology, 19*(2), 106–112. https://doi.org/10.3909/riu0748

National Cancer Institute. (2019, March 1). *HPV and cancer*. https://www.cancer.gov/about-cancer/causes-prevention/risk/infectious-agents/hpv-fact-sheet#q2

National Center for Health Statistics. (2017). *Leading causes of death*. https://www.cdc.gov/nchs/fastats/leading-causes-of-death.htm

Oeffinger, K. C., Fontham, E. T. H., Etzioni, R., Herzig, A., Michaelson, J. S., Shih, Y. -C. T., Walter, L. C., Church, T. R., Flowers, C. R., LaMonte, S. J., Wolf, A. M. D., DeSantis, C., Lortet-Tieulent, J., Andrews, K., Manassaram-Baptiste, D., Saslow, D., Smith, R. A., Brawley, O. W., Wender, R., & American Cancer Society, . (2015). Breast cancer screening for women at average risk: 2015 guideline update from the American Cancer Society. *Journal of the American Medical Association, 314*(15), 1599–1614. https://doi.org/10.1001/jama.2015.12783

Office of the Surgeon General. (2014). *The health consequences of smoking—50 years of progress: A report of the surgeon general*. U.S. Department of Health and Human Services. https://www.surgeongeneral.gov/library/reports/50-years-of-progress/full-report.pdf

Qaseem, A., Lin, J. S., Mustafa, R. A., Horwitch, C. A., Wilt, T. J., & for the Clinical Guidelines Committee of the American College of Physicians. (2019). Screening for breast cancer in average-risk women: A guidance statement from the American College of Physicians. *Annals of Internal Medicine, 170*, 547–560. https://doi.org/10.7326/M18-2147

Qaseem, A., Snow, V., Sherif, K., Aronson, M., Weiss, K. B., & Owens, D. K. (2007, April 3). Screening mammography for women 40 to 49 years of age: A clinical practice guideline from the American College of Physicians. *Annals of Internal Medicine, 146*(7), 511–515. https://doi.org/10.7326/0003-4819-146-7-200704030-00007

Scarinci, I. C., Garcia, F. A. R., Kobetz, E., Partridge, E. E., Brandt, H. M., Bell, M. C., & Castle, P. E. (2010). Cervical cancer prevention: New tools and old barriers. *Cancer, 116*(11), 2531–2542. https://doi.org/10.1002/cncr.25065

Smith, R. A., Andrews, K., Brooks, D., DeSantis, E. C., Fedewa, S. A., Lortet-Tieulent, J., Manassaram-Baptiste, D., Brawley, O. W., & Wender, R. C. (2016). Cancer screening in the United States, 2016: A review of current American Cancer Society guidelines and current issues in cancer screening. *CA: A Cancer Journal for Clinicians, 66*, 95–114.

U.S. Preventive Services Task Force. (2018). *Final recommendation Statement: Cervical cancer: Screening*. https://www.uspreventiveservicestaskforce.org/uspstf/recommendation/cervical-cancer-screening

U.S. Preventive Services Task Force. (2018). *Final recommendation Statement: Coronary heart disease: Screening with electrocardiography*. https://www.uspreventiveservicestaskforce.org/uspstf/recommendation/cardiovascular-disease-risk-screening-with-electrocardiography

U.S. Preventive Services Task Force. (2018). *Final recommendation Statement: Weight loss to prevent obesity-related morbidity and mortality in adults: Behavioral interventions*. https://www.uspreventiveservicestaskforce.org/Page/Document/UpdateSummaryFinal/obesity-in-adults-interventions

U.S. Preventive Services Task Force. (2018). *Final recommendation statement: Cardiovascular disease risk: Screening with electrocardiography*. www..uspreventiveservicestaskforce.org/uspstf/recommendation/cardiovascular-disease-risk-screening-with-electrocardiography

U.S. Preventive Services Task Force. (2019). *Final recommendation statement: Human immunodeficiency virus (HIV) infection: Screening*. https://www.uspreventiveservicestaskforce.org/uspstf/recommendation/human-immunodeficiency-virus-hiv-infection-screening

U.S. Preventive Services Task Force. (2019). *Final recommendation Statement: Abdominal aortic aneurysm: Screening*. https://www.uspreventiveservicestaskforce.org/Page/Document/UpdateSummaryFinal/abdominal-aortic-aneurysm-screening

U.S. Preventive Services Task Force. (2019). *Final recommendation Statement: Chlamydia and Gonorrhea: Screening*. https://www.uspreventiveservicestaskforce.org/uspstf/recommendation/chlamydia-and-gonorrhea-screening

U.S. Preventive Services Task Force. (2020). *Final recommendation Statement: Hepatitis C Infection in adolescents and adults: Screening*. https://www.uspreventiveservicestaskforce.org/uspstf/recommendation/hepatitis-c-screening

U.S. Preventive Services Task Force. (2021a). *Final recommendation Statement: Prostate Cancer: Screening*. https://www.uspreventiveservicestaskforce.org/uspstf/recommendation/prostate-cancer-screening

U.S. Preventive Services Task Force. (2021b). *Final recommendation Statement: Lung cancer: Screening*. https://www.uspreventiveservicestaskforce.org/uspstf/recommendation/lung-cancer-screening

U.S. Preventive Services Task Force. (2021c). *Final recommendation Statement: Colorectal cancer: Screening*. https://www.uspreventiveservicestaskforce.org/uspstf/recommendation/colorectal-cancer-screening

U.S. Preventive Services Task Force. (2021d). *Final recommendation Statement: Prediabetes and type 2 diabetes mellitus: Screening*. https://www.uspreventiveservicestaskforce.org/uspstf/recommendation/screening-for-prediabetes-and-type-2-diabetes

U.S. Preventive Services Task Force. (2021e). *Final Recommendation Statement: High blood pressure in adults: Screening*. https://www.uspreventiveservicestaskforce.org/Page/Document/UpdateSummaryFinal/high-blood-pressure-in-adults-screening

U.S. Preventive Services Task Force. (2021f). Final recommendation statement: Asymptomatic carotid artery stenosis: Screening. Recommendation: Asymptomatic Carotid Artery Stenosis: Screening | United States Preventive Services Taskforce (uspreventiveservicestaskforce.org)

U.S. Preventive Services Task Force. (2021g). *Final recommendation statement: Tobacco smoking cessation on adults, including pregnant persons: interventions*. www.uspreventiveservicestaskforce.org/uspstf/recommendation/tobacco-use-in-adults-and-pregnant-women-counseling-and-interventions

U.S. Preventive Services Task Force. (2022). *Final Recommendation statement: Statin use for the primary prevention of cardiovascular disease in adults: Preventive Medication*. www.uspreventiveservicestaskforce.org/uspstf/recommendation/statin-use-in-adults-preventive-medication

Wender, R., Fontham, E. T., Barrera, E., Colditz, G. A., Church, T. R., Ettinger, D. S., Etzioni, R., Flowers, C. R., Gazelle, S., Kelsey, D. K., LaMonte, S. J., Michaelson, J. S., Oeffinger, K. C., Shih, Y.-C. T.,

Sullivan, D. C., Travis, W., Walter, L., Wolf, A. M. D., Brawley, O. W., & Smith, R. A. (2013). American Cancer Society lung cancer screening guidelines. *CA: A Cancer Journal for Clinicians, 63*(2), 106–117. https://doi.org/10.3322/caac.21172

Wilt, T. J., Harris, R. P., & Qaseem, A. (2015). Screening for cancer: Advice for high-value care from the American College of Physicians. *Annals of Internal Medicine, 162*(10), 718–725. https://doi.org/10.7326/M14-2326

Wolf, A. M., Fontham, E. T., Church, T. R., Flowers, C. R., Guerra, C. E., LaMonte, S. J., Etzioni, R., McKenna, M. T., Oeffinger, K. C., Shih, Y.-C. T., Walter, L. C. Andrews., S, K., Brawley, O. W., Brooks, D., Fedewa, S. A., Manassaram-Baptiste, D., Siegel, R. L., Wender, R. C., & Smith, R. A. (2018). Colorectal cancer screening for average-risk adults: 2018 guideline update from the American Cancer Society. *CA: A Cancer Journal for Clinicians, 68*, 250–281. https://doi.org/10.3322/caac.21457

Wolf, A. M., Wender, R., Etzioni, R., Thompson, I., D'Amico, A., Volk, R., Brooks, D. D., Dash, C., Guessous, I., Andrews, K., DeSantis, C., Smith, R., & American Cancer Society Prostate Cancer Advisory Committee, . (2010). American Cancer Society guideline for the early detection of prostate cancer: Update 2010. *CA: A Cancer Journal for Clinicians, 60*, 70–98. https://doi.org/10.3322/caac

HEMODYNAMIC MONITORING DEVICES

Nicole Cavaliere

Disclosure: Healthcare equipment is continuously developing. It is the responsibility of the provider to stay abreast to new products and evolving technology. The provider must ensure that the products they choose are validated with sufficient, unbiased evidence, and are safe for patient care. This author does not promote or recommend any particular product. This chapter is strictly an overview of current technology at the time of this writing.

OVERVIEW OF CONDITION

Hemodynamic instability is one of the leading causes of admission to the ICU. Hemodynamic collapse, considered to be any instability in a patient's blood pressure (BP), can lead to inadequate arterial blood flow to organs. It often results from a mismatch between oxygen demand and oxygen consumption, which leads to tissue hypoxia and cell death. Patients who experience hemodynamic instability are at risk of organ damage and possibly death.

Hemodynamic instability requires physiologic and mechanical support to ensure there is adequate cardiac input and output, or BP. The goal of the critical care provider is to quickly identify the type of hemodynamic collapse present and to treat the condition appropriately to improve survival. See Box IV.1 for a list of definitions and abbreviations commonly used in reference to hemodynamic monitoring equipment.

INDICATIONS

In the past, providers have followed vital signs, such as heart rate (HR), BP, and decreased urine output (UOP), to determine if shock is present. Unfortunately, these symptoms develop late in the disease process, and alterations in these vital signs can occur due to a myriad of causes. This makes diagnosis difficult and delayed.

Many providers are now searching for new technologies to aid the diagnosis of cardiovascular collapse. This chapter will outline many devices that will assist the provider in identifying specific parameters related to hemodynamic instability.

NONINVASIVE MONITORING

Noninvasive hemodynamic monitoring may be indicated in patients who are stable but still require monitoring, patients who are prone to infections, or patients and their families who do not desire invasive lines. There are no inherent precautions for noninvasive monitoring. There are several different types of noninvasive hemodynamic monitoring devices that may be used.

Transthoracic Echocardiography

Transthoracic echocardiography (TTE) provides information on:
A. Left ventricular function.
B. Right ventricular function.
C. Inferior vena cava (IVC) dimensions.

Measurements that can be obtained through this type of monitoring include preload, cardiac output (CO), ejection fraction, and IVC compressibility, which can be calculated as a measurement determining fluid status.

Noninvasive Pulse Contour Analysis

Noninvasive pulse contour analysis is performed through the use of devices that calculate stroke volume

---

BOX IV.1   EQUIPMENT DEFINITIONS AND ABBREVIATIONS

Calibration refers to the process of modifying equipment to ensure optimal precision and accuracy of measurements.

Calibrated devices perform continuous measurements and should be recalibrated at frequent intervals to ensure accuracy.

Noncalibrated devices use patient demographics, such as age and ideal body weight, to derive and determine measurements. *Note:* When using noncalibrated devices, the provider is responsible for understanding that the accuracy of these products diminishes when preload, afterload, or contractility is significantly altered, such as in cases of high vasopressor support or significant cardiovascular collapse.

Commonly used abbreviations:

CO, cardiac output
CI, cardiac index
SV, stroke volume
SVV, stroke volume variance
PPV, pulse pressure variance
CVP, central venous pressure
SVR, systemic vascular resistance

(SV) and/or CO from analysis of the arterial pressure waveform. This analysis of the arterial pressure waveform is completely noninvasive. It may be achieved through noninvasive finger pressure that tracks changes in the intra-arterial wall.

Devices

Several different devices can be used to achieve noninvasive pulse contour analysis. Many of these devices use photoplethysmography via a finger probe. Once in use, the devices can estimate CO/cardiac index (CI), SV, stroke volume variance (SVV), systemic vascular resistance (SVR), and pulse pressure variance (PPV), and can provide continuous BP monitoring. Although these devices have variable accuracy, they are sometimes indicated for use in patients undergoing moderate- to high-risk surgeries who may not have an arterial line and in patients where determining fluid responsiveness is informative.

Thoracic Bioimpedance And Thoracic Bioreactance

Thoracic bioimpedance is a noninvasive form of monitoring that uses skin electrodes to send a high-frequency current across the thorax and measures the amplitude of that current against the returning current. This form of monitoring estimates ventricular ejection fraction, SV, HR, and CO.

Thoracic bioreactance is an advancement on bioimpedance. This form of monitoring measures the phase shift in voltage through four electrodes that send alternating voltage of known frequency through the thorax. Sensors then calculate time delay, referred to as phase shift. Thoracic bioreactance devices can measure SV, stroke volume index (SVI), CO/CI, and total peripheral resistive index.

Estimated Continuous Cardiac Output Monitoring

Estimated continuous CO monitoring determines CO by pulse oximetry and pulse wave transit time, and can also incorporate pulse oximetry and EKG signals. This is a noncalibrated system.

Passive Leg Raise

Fluid responsiveness can also be determined using a passive leg raise. This simple bedside test involves a leg raise that, by way of gravity, will return an estimated 150 to 300 mL of blood back to the heart. Changes in BP and HR should be analyzed by the healthcare provider to determine if the patient would respond to fluid administration.

Ultrasonography

Ultrasonography is another form of noninvasive monitoring that can be used to evaluate volume status. To assess the IVC, the probe in ultrasound is held in the subcostal longitudinal view (see Figure IV.1). An average IVC is approximately 1.5 to 2.5 cm in diameter. If the IVC diameter is less than 1.5 cm, this may indicate volume depletion. In trauma, a diameter less than 1.0 cm is likely related to hemorrhage. If the IVC is greater than

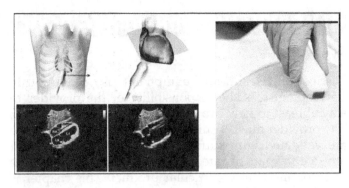

FIGURE IV.1   Subcostal window to visualize inferior vena cava.

Source: Reproduced with permission from Mayo Foundation for Medical Education and Research.

2.5 cm, then the patient likely will not respond to more fluids as this diameter suggests fluid overload.

It is also important to be aware of IVC compressibility. The IVC typically collapses 50% during inspiration. A collapse less than 50% typically suggests fluid overload. A collapse greater than 50% typically suggests intravascular volume depletion.

Ultrasonic Cardiac Output Monitoring

Ultrasonic CO monitoring can be used to calculate the aortic and pulmonary outflow tracts to estimate CO. It is important to note that patients with structural heart disease may provide false values. Clinical correlation is warranted and more invasive testing may be indicated for further evaluation. Values obtained in this form of monitoring are:

A. CO/CI.

B. SV.

C. SVR.

D. HR.

MINIMALLY INVASIVE MONITORING

Forms of minimally invasive monitoring use some combination of noninvasive and invasive monitoring to provide the most accurate information about the patient's hemodynamic status with the most minimal use of invasive devices possible. For example, the pulmonary artery catheter (PAC), an invasive centrally placed catheter, was used to provide critical information. It has been replaced largely by waveform analysis using an arterial catheter, which is considered minimally invasive. Minimally invasive monitoring is preferred over invasive monitoring whenever appropriate.

Esophageal Doppler (Transesophageal Echocardiogram)

Esophageal Doppler (transesophageal echocardiogram [TEE]) is a Doppler device that is placed into the midesophagus to obtain ultrasound views of the heart from within the body. Some TEE devices allow for frequent or continuous monitoring and allow the provider to visualize heart chambers, valves, blood flow, and any abnormalities that may exist. These abnormalities may include pericardial effusion or wall motion abnormalities. TEE also allows the provider to measure blood flow velocity, CO, and ejection fraction.

Devices

Several devices can be used for TEE that calculate the SV, and subsequently the CO, from measuring the arterial pulse pressure via an indwelling arterial catheter. Values obtained are:

A. CO/CI.
B. HR.
C. SV.
D. SVR.
E. SVV.

Using an indwelling arterial catheter for TEE allows providers to obtain measurements by estimating the SV by measuring the area under the curve of the systolic phase. This is a noncalibrated measurement that obtains the following:

A. CO/CI.
B. SV.
C. HR.
D. PPV.
E. SVV.

Other devices determine SV, and subsequently CO, by measuring the area under the curve of the entire cardiac cycle, both systolic and diastolic. These are calibrated devices that deliver predetermined amounts of lithium chloride to the patient through a central or peripheral line. The remaining concentration of lithium is then measured at the arterial catheter site. Values obtained using these devices are:

A. CO/CI.
B. SV.
C. HR.
D. SVR.
E. SVV.

Minimally Invasive Pulse Contour Analysis

Several types of minimally invasive devices can calculate SV and/or CO from analysis of the arterial pressure waveform. The devices use proprietary algorithms to calculate pressure–volume relationships based on SVR, arterial compliance, and/or aortic impedance from the arterial line waveform (Figure IV.2). Most of these devices provide loose accuracy when patients become significantly unstable.

Transpulmonary Thermodilution

Transpulmonary thermodilution is the method of injecting cold saline into a central access point and measuring the change in temperature at the arterial access point. Calculations used in this method are derived from the thermodilution equation, which is:

$$CO = \frac{\{(Tb - Ti) \times K\}}{\left\{\int_0^\infty \Delta Tb(t)dt\right\}}$$

where Tb is blood temperature, Ti is injectate temperature, and K is computed constant.

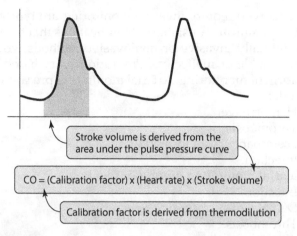

FIGURE IV.2 Example of minimally invasive pulse contour analysis.

CO, cardiac output.

Devices

Several devices can be used to achieve transpulmonary thermodilution to obtain the following values:

A. CO/CI.
B. HR.
C. SV.
D. SVR.
E. SVV.
F. PPV.
G. Global end diastolic volume (GEDV), which can estimate preload.
H. Intrathoracic blood volume (ITBV).
I. Pulmonary vascular permeability index (PVPI).
J. Global ejection fraction (GEF).

Ultrasound Flow Dilution

The final minimally invasive form of monitoring is ultrasound flow dilution, which can be used to measure CO. This can be achieved using a machine that calculates CO via transpulmonary ultrasound dilution technology by measuring changes in blood ultrasound velocity and blood flow after saline injection. The device requires a central line and arterial line, as well as an extracorporeal arteriovenous (AV) loop tube set. This calibrated device obtains the following values:

A. CO/CI.
B. SV/SVI.
C. Total ejection fraction.
D. SVR/Systemic Vascular Resistance Index (SVRI).
E. Total end diastolic volume index.
F. Central blood volume index.

INVASIVE MONITORING

Invasive monitoring is a relative term that typically includes central vein access and arterial monitoring, but can also refer to devices on a continuum. For instance, a radial arterial line is technically an invasive procedure, but is considered minimally invasive when compared with the placement of a brachial arterial line. Central lines are invasive, but less invasive than PACs when used with noninvasive cardiac monitoring devices.

Patients who require invasive monitoring are typically hemodynamically unstable with indications that the use of minimally invasive or noninvasive methods would be unreliable or ineffective. Precautions vary based on the form of monitoring. Arterial monitoring precautions include:

A. Hemorrhage.

B. Thrombosis.

C. Pseudoaneurysm formation.

D. Infection.

Central monitoring precautions include:

A. Infection.

B. Damage to surrounding structures.

C. Thrombosis.

D. Arterial puncture.

Central Venous Pressure Monitoring

Central venous pressure (CVP) is the measurement of the pressure of the right atrium. In this form of monitoring, CVP is obtained from a central venous catheter that is placed in the subclavian or internal jugular vein and terminates in the superior vena cava at the right atrium. Although CVP is commonly used as a marker of fluid status, many studies have shown that CVP does not correlate to circulating blood volume and that CVP cannot predict fluid responsiveness in many clinical scenarios. Therefore, CVP monitoring is not useful in guiding fluid management in most cases; however, it should be noted that CVP monitoring could guide management of the right ventricle and prove beneficial in patients who have right ventricular dysfunction from either myocardial infarct or pulmonary embolism.

Pulmonary Artery Catheter

A PAC is a flow-directed catheter that is fed through a central venous introducer. The catheter is guided through the introducer to the right atrium, through the right ventricle, and to the pulmonary artery. At one point, this device was the gold standard tool for measurement of fluid status, but its use has recently fallen out of favor. Many studies have found no mortality benefits with the use of PAC, and some studies even show a risk of increasing mortality. Many reports have shown misinterpretation of data and user error as leading to the inaccuracy of the values obtained. For these reasons, less invasive tools are now being utilized more frequently. However, PAC can still be a beneficial measurement tool in right ventricular heart failure or pulmonary hypertension. Values obtained with this form of monitoring are:

A. CVP.

B. Pulmonary artery pressure (PAP).

C. Pulmonary artery occlusion pressure (PAOP).

EVALUATION AND RESULTS

Use of hemodynamic monitoring should be tailored and interpreted carefully for each patient. Critically ill patients may have confounding factors that make absolute interpretations difficult. Noninvasive monitoring may be limited by patient cooperation or body habitus. Invasive monitoring may be limited by poor circulation or misplacement of lines. It is essential that the healthcare provider provide careful interpretation in each individual case.

CLINICAL PEARLS

When using hemodynamic monitoring devices, the advanced practice provider (APP) should keep the following in mind:

A. Positioning is the key to optimal visualization in noninvasive monitoring using echocardiography.

B. Arterial lines may become dampened if the BP is very low. However, this may also be caused by air pockets in the transducer. Flushing the lines may resolve this issue.

C. Always use optimal view on the monitor.

D. Invasive monitoring can provide significant information about the patient's condition, but information must be interpreted with caution.

BIBLIOGRAPHY

Bender, J. S., Smith-Meek, M. A., & Jones, C. E. (1997). Routine pulmonary artery catheterization does not reduce morbidity and mortality of elective vascular surgery: Results of a prospective, randomized trial. *Annals of Surgery, 226,* 229–237. https://doi.org/10.1097/00000658-199709000-00002

CNSystems Medizintechnik. (n.d). *CNAP monitor 500 HD.* http://www.cnsystems.com/products/cnap-monitor-500

Hadian, M., & Pinsky, M. (2006). Evidence-based review of the use of the pulmonary artery catheter: Impact data and complications. *Critical Care, 10*(Suppl. 3), S8. https://doi.org/10.1186/cc4834

Ilies, C., Bauer, M., Berg, P., Rosenberg, J., Hedderich, J., Bein, B., Hin, J., & Hanss, R. (2012). Investigation of the agreement of a continuous non-invasive arterial pressure device in comparison with invasive radial artery measurement. *British Journal of Anaesthesia, 108,* 202–210. https://doi.org/10.1093/bja/aer394

Marik, P. E. (2013). Noninvasive cardiac output monitors: A state-of the-art review. *Journal of Cardiothoracic Vascular Anesthesia, 27,* 121–134. https://doi.org/10.1053/j.jvca.2012.03.022

Marik, P. E., Baram, M., & Vahid, B. (2008). Does central venous pressure predict fluid responsiveness? A systematic review of the literature and the tale of seven mares. *Chest, 134*(1), 172–178. http://www.sciencedirect.com/science/article/pii/S0012369208601634

Mimoz, O., Rauss, A., Rekik, N., Brun-Buisson, C., Lemaire, F., & Brochard, L. (1994). Pulmonary artery catheterization in critically ill patients: A prospective analysis of outcome changes associated with catheter-prompted changes in therapy. *Critical Care Medicine, 22,* 573–579. https://doi.org/10.1097/00003246-199404000-00011

Monnet, X., & Teboul, J. L. (2015). Minimally invasive monitoring. *Critical Care Clinics, 31,* 25–42. https://doi.org/10.1016/j.ccc.2014.08.002

Murdoch, S. D., Cohen, A. T., & Bellamy, M. C. (2000). Pulmonary artery catheterization and mortality in critically ill patients. *British Journal of Anaesthesia, 85,* 611–615. https://doi.org/10.1093/bja/85.4.611

Rajaram, S. S., Desai, N. K., Kalra, A., Gajera, M., Cavanaugh, S. K., Brampton, W., & Rowan, K. (2013). Pulmonary artery catheters for adult patients in intensive care. *Cochrane Database of Systematic Reviews, 2013*(2), CD003408. https://doi.org/10.1002/14651858.CD003408.pub3

Renner, J., Grünewald, M., & Bein, B. (2016). Monitoring high-risk patients: Minimally invasive and non-invasive possibilities. *Best Practice & Research Clinical Anaesthesiology, 30,* 201–216. https://doi.org/10.1016/j.bpa.2016.04.006

Richard, C., Warszawski, J., Anguel, N., Deye, N., Combes, A., Barnoud, D., & Teboul, J.-L. (2003). Early use of the pulmonary artery catheter and outcomes in patients with shock and acute respiratory distress syndrome. *Journal of the American Medical Association, 290,* 2713–2720. https://doi.org/10.1001/jama.290.20.2713

Roth, S., Fox, H., Fuchs, U., Schulz, U., Costard-Jäckle, A., Gummert, J. F., Horstkotte, D., Oldenburg, O., & Bitter, T. (2018). Noninvasive pulse contour analysis for determination of cardiac output in patients with chronic heart failure. *Clinical Research in Cardiology, 107*, 395–404. https://doi.org/10.1007/s00392-017-1198-7

Sangkum, L., Liu, G. L., Yu, L., Yan, H., Kaye, A. D., & Liu, H. (2016). Minimally invasive or noninvasive cardiac output measurement: An update. *Journal of Anesthesia, 30*, 461–480. https://doi.org/10.1007/s00540-016-2154-9

Saugel, B., Cecconi, M., Wagner, J. Y., & Reuter, D. A. (2015). Noninvasive continuous cardiac output monitoring in perioperative and intensive care medicine. *British Journal of Anaesthesia, 114*, 562–575. https://doi.org/10.1093/bja/aeu447

Shah, M. R., Hasselblad, V., Stevenson, L. W., Binanay, C., O'Connor, C. M., Sopko, G., & Califf, R. M. (2005). Impact of the pulmonary artery catheter in critically ill patients. *Journal of the American Medical Association, 294*, 1664–1670. https://doi.org/10.1001/jama.294.13.1664

Vincent, J. L., Rhodes, A., Perel, A., Martin, G. S., Della Rocca, G., Vallet, B., & Singer, M. (2011). Clinical review: Update on hemodynamic monitoring—a consensus of 16. *Critical Care, 15*, 229. https://doi.org/10.1186/cc10291

TELEMEDICINE IN ACUTE CARE

Kristen L. Talvacchia and Lewis J. Kaplan

INTRODUCTION

Healthcare evolution is driven by novel discoveries, including advanced technology, guiding both routine and acute care interventions. One such advance is digital platform-driven oversight and care, better known as telemedicine or telehealth. Telemedicine links healthcare professionals remote from one another to support integrated patient care using digital, video, and voice communications. The COVID-19 pandemic was a significant driver in the evolution of telemedicine in acute care as both consultants and family members were often outside of the acute care facility. Moreover, the need for telemedicine consultation—in particular addressing critical care—highlighted resource limitations, including that of specialty-trained clinicians. Sending staff and equipment to disaster areas to help render care is a reasonable option for crises of limited size and duration—neither was the case with the COVID-19 pandemic, which continues to stress hospital resources and staff. Instead, telemedicine is a powerful tool to remotely deliver essential clinical expertise to resource-limited facilities and avoid physical resource deployment. Due to the flexibility of telemedicine, platforms, and capabilities, a variety of acute care domains are readily supported using remote clinician assessment, consultation, guidance, and when linked across an accessible electronic health record (EHR), intervention (Figure IV.3).

DOMAINS OF TELEMEDICINE IN ACUTE CARE

Telestroke

Acute stroke assessment and care have been transformed by introducing highly effective but time-sensitive therapies. Therefore, rapid assessment and decision-making are key in engaging high efficacy, but also potentially high-risk therapeutics. Facilities without routine access to stroke-focused clinicians (including rural and critical access hospitals) may experience delays in deciding what therapy to pursue. Telestroke programs remotely connect those facilities and their patients with stroke experts to aid in diagnosis and treatment decision-making (including patient transfer). Telestroke consultation also helps set expectations for the family if they are present. Importantly, telestroke consultation may occur in the absence of any other telemedicine program using stand-alone devices. While telestroke management leverages an inpatient or outpatient (ED) clinician to effect bedside care in conjunction with a remote specialist, so too does telepsychiatry.

Telepsychiatry

Like telestroke, telepsychiatry provides consultation but can also render acute cognitive behavioral therapy or emergency psychiatric care. Not all EDs are staffed with emergency medicine-trained clinicians, nor are all

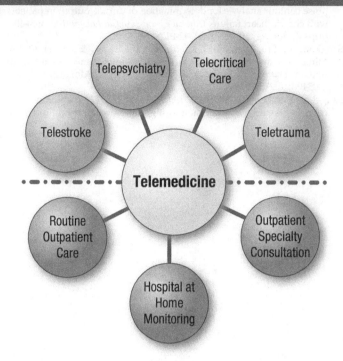

FIGURE IV.3 Telemedicine applications. This graphic depicts current domains of telemedicine that include acute care (top) and nonacute care (bottom). It is anticipated that other applications will arise, all of which remain part of telemedicine. Of note, routine care that is undertaken as part of remote management is variably termed telehealth.

staffed with advanced practice providers (APPs) trained in mental health either. Moreover, a psychiatrist may not be available in person during the evening or night hours, even in major medical centers. Telepsychiatry can fill the void when acute psychiatric consultation and management are required but a psychiatrist is not present. Telepsychiatry can assist in determining if a patient needs an inpatient stay (voluntary or involuntary) or can be discharged. Rapid evaluation and decision-making reduces ED occupancy and time to disposition—key aspects of reducing ED overcrowding. In addition, telepsychiatry can assist in determining a coordinated discharge plan, including engagement with outpatient mental health care and support services. Telemedicine may also support complex care such as that which occurs in the ICU.

Telecritical Care

Telemedicine deployed in the ICU was initially popularized as tele-ICU; it is now known as telecritical care since critical care occurs in locations outside the traditional ICU. Novel ICUs erected in cafeterias and de novo structures in parking lots during COVID-19 clearly demonstrated this aspect of telecritical care. Telecritical care allows specialty-trained clinicians (e.g., physicians, APPs, nurses) to remotely monitor critically ill patients, identify changes in physiology, assess lab and radiology data, and intervene in conjunction with the bedside team to improve care. Since only ~50% of all U.S. facilities are staffed with a trained intensivist, telecritical care can help fill a vast staffing gap, especially during a crisis. While it is easier to provide a remote physician or APP to help guide decision-making and care, the bedside critical care nurse is not remotely replaceable. Instead, critical care nurses who provide telecritical care services offer oversight and remote monitoring when the primary nurse is engaged with another patient or in a different room during an emergency. Using a team-based approach, telecritical care programs can concomitantly cover ICU patients at multiple facilities. Telecritical care services ideally provide access to the EHR, in-room monitors, and a high-resolution digital camera and screen for two-way real-time communication and patient assessment. Such arrangements can be accomplished using a hardwired system or a mobile platform such as that for telestroke or telepsychiatry consultation.

Teletrauma

The majority of American College of Surgeons Committee on Trauma state-verified level 1 trauma centers are located in urban spaces. Level 2 and 3 centers are more disseminated, but rural and critical access facilities may be quite remote from major trauma centers. Therefore, patients who present with complex or evolving injuries to nontrauma centers may benefit from rapid consultation by an injury expert to decide on an initial management approach as well as transport method and priority. Such consultation may drive temporizing surgical care at the initial facility (e.g., splenectomy, packing, temporary abdominal wall closure) while transport is being arranged to the facility whose faculty provides consultation. Evolving technology may support ongoing consultation during transport as well. Currently, platforms used principally for social media may afford real-time video linkage during operation or transportation. However, such an approach lacks EHR integration, may encounter issues with personal health information protection, and relies on a smartphone or tablet that is not regulated by facility software or intrusion policies and packages.

PLATFORMS

Multiple platforms may enable an acute care facility to enhance care using telemedicine. The selection of a particular platform may be influenced by patient volume, acuity, local resource complement, and finances. There are three general platform approaches:

A. Continuous care: Monitoring patients without interruption for a predetermined portion of a day (e.g., from 6 p.m. to 6 a.m.) or all day; nighttime coverage is the dominant approach. This approach typically utilizes an operation center known as the "hub" that houses all of the required equipment for the remote team. Team members must travel to the hub to engage in remote care.

B. Episodic care: Intermittent and short-term care that occurs throughout the day on a predetermined schedule. Episodic care may target times when communication is essential (e.g., during patient rounds and change of shift reports). This may occur from within a hub but is not required to do so.

C. Responsive care: Consultative care that is unscheduled and in response to an alert or specific request (e.g., common with telestroke or telepsychiatry). This care generally occurs outside of a hub and often occurs using an individual clinician's desktop or institution-supplied mobile device.

SYSTEM APPROACHES
Hub and Spoke

A centralized program that links multiple outlying sites through a central location is known as a "hub and spoke" structure. The monitoring center is geographically fixed and often aligned with and staffed by individuals from a tertiary or quaternary care facility. The spoke facilities may be part of an established health network but need not be administratively aligned. Continuous patient monitoring, especially during the evening and nighttime 12-hour periods, is typical for this system structure. Even systems with an in-house fellow or intensivist may use this model for oversight and to guide care when the in-house team is engaged in emergency care and cannot address other patients in the ICU. Remote clinician-guided intervention is clearly aided by two-way (visual and vocal) communication capability with the in-room team. The remote team may be engaged using an emergency call trigger or having electronically generated alerts direct their attention to a specific patient.

Decentralized

A decentralized telemedicine structure is commonly referred to as a point-to-point system. Unlike the hub and spoke model, a decentralized approach typically delivers episodic or responsive care. It is important to note that some hub and spoke systems deploy continuous care for the ICU and a point-to-point approach for services like telestroke. Given this model's ability to be mobile, it may be ideally positioned for disaster care that occurs outside of a hardwired ICU. Decentralized care approaches may not always offer the ability to enter information into the EHR that is active at the patient's initial care site. Accordingly, an EHR agnostic platform has been developed within the National Emergency Tele-Critical Care Network for such use.

STAFFING

Early telemedicine solely deployed physicians as remote care partners. Given the multidimensional and multiprofessional care permeating medicine, particularly critical care, staffing now includes APPs and critical care nurses alongside a technical expert in continuous care models. Telemedicine physicians are commonly board-certified in critical care medicine (or neurocritical care) and come from parent specialties, including internal medicine, pulmonary medicine, anesthesiology, surgery, emergency medicine, or neurology; other disciplines are less commonly represented. At least 5 years of bedside critical care experience is generally required for APPs and RNs. Advanced certification, such as the Critical Care Registered Nurse (CCRN) certificate, is usually necessary for RNs.

Hub and spoke models typically staff their rosters from existing faculty and employee pools using either full-time or per-diem salary models. This approach links the remote team with the bedside team using shared experiences and preexisting personal relationships; this model is intuitively embraceable. Alternatively, staffing may be outsourced to another facility or independent agency. No clearly superior approach is identified with regard to patient-level outcomes.

BENEFITS

Telemedicine benefits are identifiable in five distinct areas: Staffing, care quality, patient safety, guideline and protocol compliance, and communication. The SARS-CoV-2 pandemic underscored how a tiered staffing model that linked non-ICU clinicians with seasoned ICU clinicians could help a facility address patient surge. Telecritical care is ideal for expanding the available pool of intensivists to help support the tiered staffing approach. Alternative staffing approaches were fundamentally important during the COVID-19 pandemic when the intensivist pool was reduced due to acute illness. Expanded team-based coverage and specialist consultation enhance specialty healthcare access and can improve care quality by reducing variations in care. Additionally, telemedicine can help align patient care needs with facility capability by more precisely directing transfers into tertiary or quaternary care centers when needed.

Care standardization is a critical aspect in reducing medical errors and improving value as well as safety. Nonetheless, guideline and protocol adoption is often less than ideal due to a variety of individual factors as well as practice barriers. Telemedicine evaluation of the evidence to practice gap coupled with the ability to address that gap helps ensure compliance with the current evidence-based recommendations. Guidelines such as those addressing venous thromboembolism prophylaxis, sepsis/septic shock, acute respiratory distress syndrome (ARDS) ventilation, and ICU liberation are ideally suited to telemedical surveillance and repair in conjunction with the bedside team to decrease ICU and ventilator length of stay, delirium, disordered consciousness, and mortality.

Furthermore, telemedicine can enable communication between staff and patient families. This aspect of telemedicine does not require a remote team but instead uses a digital platform to link the bedside team with the family; many of these platforms are used for educational conferences or committee-related work. It is not uncommon for patients' family members to live far away—especially if the patient is transferred to a tertiary or quaternary facility for specialty care—or have competing commitments (e.g., work, childcare) that keep them from traveling to the hospital for clinical updates during the typical workday. Virtual family conferences increase family satisfaction, strengthen trust for clinicians, and reduce stress and conflict between clinicians and family members, all while keeping them updated regarding their loved ones. This approach also supports having timely goals-of-care discussions so that teams engage in goal-concordant care.

FUTURE IMPLICATIONS

While healthcare systems have expanded their use of telemedicine in diverse spaces, including home-based monitoring, training within this evolving healthcare remains sparse. Instead, clinicians who engage in acute care telemedicine provide remote care as a small portion of their clinical practice and do so without specific training other than that which addresses equipment use. Other elements relevant for providing remote care include data science and data visualization approaches to interrogating care volume, quality, successes, and failures. Telemedicine appears underrepresented in nursing, APP, as well as physician preclinical and clinical training programs. Such education would be ideal to support how bedside teams work with remote teams and how individuals prepare to serve as part of a remote team. Indeed, one could envision telemedicine as its own subspecialty within each parent discipline.

Telecritical care is often engaged during the evening and nighttime hours within a hub and spoke model. While the RNs often view their hub work as one of their shifts, many APPs and physicians come to the hub after working their day job, leaving them somewhat fatigued throughout their telecritical care shift. Such fatigue may increase symptoms of burnout syndrome, an untoward syndrome for which critical care practitioners commonly rank near the apex of the list compared with all other medical specialties. Instead, a novel approach appears to be warranted. The remote aspect of telemedicine allows healthcare systems to take advantage of differences in global time zones. If the hub team is located in a geographic location and time zone that is 12 hours apart from the site that needs to be monitored, the hub team can provide care during their daytime, which coincides with the evening and night hours for the bedside staff. This model has been deployed using a hub team in Australia and a care site in southeastern United States. The benefit of having a well-rested and actively engaged hub team cannot be overstated.

Acute care telemedicine remains poised for further expansion and hinges on expanding monitoring sites, clinicians interested in providing such remote care, and specific training to do so. Technology-driven innovation will undoubtedly enhance how telemedicine further shapes care within and without the acute care facility. It is time to begin to train clinicians of all specialties in telemedicine so that it is no longer viewed as a unique care approach, but is instead embraced as an expected aspect of integrated care.

BIBLIOGRAPHY

Canfield, C., Perez-Protto, S., Siuba, M., Hata, S., & Udeh, C. (2022). Beyond the nuts and bolts: Tele-critical care patients, workflows, and activity patterns. *Telemedicine and e-Health, 28*(1), 73–83. https://doi.org/10.1089/tmj.2020.0452

Gibson, N. A., Arends, R., & Hendrickx, L. (2021). Tele-U to tele-ICU: Telehealth nursing education. *Critical Care Nurse, 41*(5), 34–39. https://doi.org/10.4037/ccn2021109

Herasevich, V., & Subramanian, S. (2019). Tele-ICU technologies. *Critical Care Clinics, 35*(3), 427–438. https://doi.org/10.1016/j.ccc.2019.02.009

Hiddleson, C., Buchman, T., & Coiera, E. (2019). Turning "Night into day": Challenges, strategies, and effectiveness of re-engineering the workflow to enable continuous electronic intensive care unit collaboration between Australia and U.S. *Health Informatics*, 281–287. https://doi.org/10.1007/978-3-030-16916-9_16

Khurrum, M., Asmar, S., & Joseph, B. (2020). Telemedicine in the ICU: Innovation in the critical care process. *Journal of Intensive Care Medicine, 36*(12), 1377–1384. https://doi.org/10.1177/0885066620968518

Kleinpell, R., Moss, M., Good, V. S., Gozal, D., & Sessler, C. N. (2020). The critical nature of addressing burnout prevention. *Critical Care Medicine, 48*(2), 249–253. https://doi.org/10.1097/ccm.0000000000003964

Pamplin, J. C., Scott, B. K., Quinn, M. T., Little, J. R., Goede, M. R., Pappas, P. A., Jolly, B. T., Hipp, S. J., Colombo, C. J., & Davis, K. L. (2021). Technology and disasters: The evolution of the national emergency tele-critical care network. *Critical Care Medicine, 49*(7), 1007–1014. https://doi.org/10.1097/ccm.0000000000005001

Pun, B. T., Balas, M. C., Barnes-Daly, M. A., Thompson, J. L., Aldrich, J. M., Barr, J., Byrum, D., Carson, S. S., Devlin, J. W., Engel, H. J., Esbrook, C. L., Hargett, K. D., Harmon, L., Hielsberg, C., Jackson, J. C., Kelly, T. L., Kumar, V., Millner, L., Morse, A. … Ely, E. W. (2019). Caring for critically ill patients with the ABCDEF bundle. *Critical Care Medicine, 47*(1), 3–14. https://doi.org/10.1097/ccm.0000000000003482

Subramanian, S., Pamplin, J. C., Hravnak, M., Hielsberg, C., Riker, R., Rincon, F., Laudanski, K., Adzhigirey, L. A., Moughrabieh, M. A., Winterbottom, F. A., & Herasevich, V. (2020). Tele-critical care: An update from the society of critical care medicine tele-ICU committee. *Critical Care Medicine, 48*(4), 553–561. https://doi.org/10.1097/ccm.0000000004190

Tumma, A., Berzou, S., Jaques, K., Shah, D., Smith, A. C., & Thomas, E. E. (2022). Considerations for the implementation of a telestroke network: A systematic review. *Journal of Stroke and Cerebrovascular Diseases, 31*(1), 106171. https://doi.org/10.1016/j.jstrokecerebrovasdis.2021.106171

Weiss, B., Paul, N., Balzer, F., Noritomi, D. T., & Spies, C. D. (2021). Telemedicine in the intensive care unit: A vehicle to improve quality of care? *Journal of Critical Care, 61*, 241–246. https://doi.org/10.1016/j.jcrc.2020.09.036

TRANSITIONAL CARE

Amy Blake

INTRODUCTION

Care transitions are receiving widespread focus in academia, clinical practice, executive, and regulatory forums. The Hospital Readmissions Reduction Program, created under the Affordable Care Act (ACA) in 2012, has imposed financial penalties for higher-than-expected readmissions for acute myocardial infarction, heart failure, pneumonia, chronic obstructive pulmonary disease, and total hip and knee arthroplasties. Higher-than-expected readmissions come with additional costs and can be associated with increased mortality and poor outcomes. This has inspired institutions to focus on the development of programs dedicated to improving a patient's transition from one setting to another.

Healthcare can appear to be fast-paced, fragmented, and confusing to both the lay observer and to those who participate in healthcare delivery. Understanding how the various branches of healthcare situate themselves among the kaleidoscope of options available to a consumer can be a challenge. Navigating a patient's healthcare path is a complex process that is becoming a specialty unto itself. Finding the safest, most cost-effective continuum is currently one of healthcare's hottest topics.

CARE TRANSITIONS DEFINED

Efforts to define transitional care have focused on determining a set of actions to minimize known risks, such as fragmentation, poor communication, and poor coordination, that can lead to unfavorable outcomes. Fragmentation of care has been associated with increased hospital readmissions. The 2003 position statement from the American Geriatrics Society defined transitional care as a set of actions designed to ensure the coordination and continuity of healthcare as patients transfer between different locations or between different levels of care within the same location. Representative locations include, but are not limited to, the following:

A. Hospitals.
B. Postacute: Long-term acute care (LTAC) and subacute rehabilitation facilities.
C. Long-term care (LTC) facilities.
D. Assisted living facilities.
E. Primary and specialty care offices.
F. The patient's home.

In this definition, transitional care is based on several factors that encompass both the sending and the receiving aspects of care, including:

A. Comprehensive plan of care.
B. The availability of healthcare practitioners who are well-trained in chronic care and have current, clearly communicated information about the patient's problems, goals, preferences, and clinical status.

C. Defined logistical arrangements, education of the patient and the family, and coordination among all health professionals involved in the transition.

Naylor and Keating noted in 2008 that transitional care encompasses a broad range of time-limited services designed to:

A. Ensure healthcare continuity.
B. Avoid preventable poor outcomes.
C. Ensure timely transfer of patients from one level of care to another or from one type of setting to another.

Communication as Cornerstone

It is important to remember that no matter the exact definition, the cornerstone of effective transitional care is communication. Communication must be embedded in an easily accessible platform throughout each phase of the continuum to allow for effective coordination and delivery of appropriate care. Lack of communication leads to poor understanding of priorities, fragmentation, unnecessary duplication of tests, and, at times, omission of important follow-up. The Society for Post-Acute and Long-Term Care Medicine stresses that communication is key to improving care transitions between nursing facilities and acute care hospital settings. Specific recommendations include the following:

A. Information about the patient, including medications, problem list, and plan of care, should be collected through the hospital stay and be available well in advance of any transfer.
B. Professionals involved in the care of LTC patients and other frail, at-risk patients should actively work with other relevant professionals and each site of care to create and improve policies and procedures that assure timely and accurate communication.
C. When possible, information about transfers should be communicated from professional to professional in different sites of care.
D. The sending and receiving professionals should have reliable contact information for each other.

When considering transitional care, it is also important to remember that transitions occur not only from setting to setting, but also from provider to provider. For example, an older adult patient with a history of morbid obesity, obstructive sleep apnea, and diastolic heart failure could be hospitalized after a fall for an acute hip fracture. The patient may undergo repair, have their diuretic held for mild acute kidney injury, experience elevated blood pressure due to pain, and transition to a skilled rehab center to focus on strength and mobility. In the new setting, the patient will be at risk should a chronic comorbidity decompensate, thus potentially shifting the balance and priorities of care. This shifting continuum will recur in a dynamic fashion among all settings from the hospital to postacute care, to home, and back again as a different condition demands priority.

INTERIM RISKS IN TRANSITIONAL CARE

Multiple transitions through different settings with different providers and managing shifting priorities caused by dynamic comorbidities leave a multitude of avenues for fragmentation and care breakdown. Interim risks include several different factors.

Medication Changes and Errors

Medication errors are a common area of communication breakdown. Medication lists are reconciled numerous times from setting to setting, and new changes and formulary substitutions are accommodated. Forster et al. (2003) estimate that approximately one in five patients experience adverse drug events in the weeks following hospitalization, and up to one-third of these adverse events are considered to be preventable or ameliorable. Medications with higher rates of adverse effects include:

A. Antibiotics.
B. Corticosteroids.
C. Cardiovascular medications.
D. Anticoagulants.
E. Antiepileptics.
F. Analgesic medications, including narcotics.
G. Time-limited therapies with unspecified duration.

New, changed, and discontinued medications should be clearly noted in the discharge summary along with important reasons for the change, such as an adverse reaction or complication that prompted the change.

Unclear Follow-Up Instructions

Unclear follow-up instructions are another common area of risk in transitional care. Incompletely communicated instructions for follow-up care and pending or incomplete diagnostic and laboratory studies leave abundant space for important aspects of care to fall through the cracks. A higher margin for miscommunication exists in patients with long hospitalizations, during which multiple specialists see the patient and order multiple diagnostic tests. Strategies to increase communication of follow-up instructions include the following:

A. Important diagnostic studies, procedures, and lab values should be clearly documented in discharge instructions along with pending results that require follow-up.
B. Providers whom a patient should follow up with should also be clearly documented along with contact information.
C. Information regarding durable medical equipment (DME) required at discharge, such as noninvasive ventilators (continuous positive airway pressure [CPAP], bilevel positive airway pressure [BiPap], average volume assure pressure support [AVAP]), should be included along with settings and the equipment provider's name and contact number. It is helpful to include whether the equipment is rented or if the patient requires a qualification process or further testing in order to have the equipment at home.

1. Example: If a patient with respiratory failure requires BiPap or AVAP at home, they require special qualification processes in order to have a home machine. A skilled nursing facility (SNF) may rent an interim machine for the patient, but if care is not taken to qualify and attain approval for the equipment a patient could ultimately end up at home without a crucial noninvasive ventilator, rendering them at high risk for readmission from hypercapnic respiratory failure.

Poorly Communicated or Unaddressed Advance Directives

Poorly communicated or unaddressed advance directives and code status put a patient at risk for treatments and resuscitation they may have decided for or against. It is important for the advanced practice provider (APP) to take the following actions:

A. Ensure a discussion has taken place regarding advance directives and the identification of a healthcare proxy or durable power of attorney for healthcare.
B. Ensure that each patient is asked about a living will or similar document. This document describes in detail the patient's wishes with regard to resuscitation, hospitalization, treatment goals and limits, and a healthcare proxy.
C. The goal of advance directives is to provide the patient autonomy in decisions regarding the manner and location of death as well as *relieving family burden and conflict* while the older individual is *mentally competent* to do so.

1. The Five Wishes Form is useful to guide choices. The Five Wishes Form is a document that assists individuals in making preferences and care wishes in the case of an emergency or incapacity. This form will help the designated decision-maker to make informed choices on the patient's behalf. The form asks the patient to indicate the following:
   a. The person I want to make care decisions for me when I cannot.
   b. The kind of medical treatment I want or do not want.
   c. How comfortable I want to be.
   d. How I want people to treat me.
   e. What I want my loved ones to know.

2. Many states have a MOST form (Medical Orders for Scope of Treatment) or a POLST form (Physician Order for Life-Sustaining Treatment). The exact type of form varies from state to state. The APP should become familiar with the form used in their own state. This is a legal document that specifies the type of care a person would like in their final year of life and provides orders, signed by a provider, whereas the advance directive provides general wishes.

D. Clearly communicate a patient's advance directive desires and code status in the discharge summary and ensure the appropriate MOST or POLST forms are completed before transfers take place.

Complex Problem Lists

Problem lists are specified in the discharge summary by priority. Recall that priorities remain dynamic and can shift unexpectedly. Clearly delineate primary and secondary problem lists with the associated plan, if helpful. Consider the following notes that may appear in the chart of the aforementioned patient:

Primary Dx:
A. Acute hip fracture s/p (status post) open reduction and internal fixation (ORIF): Continue physical therapy/occupational therapy.
B. Acute kidney injury, mild: Home doses of Lasix and lisinopril held for creatinine bump to 2.0 from baseline of 1.3. Monitor creatinine closely and restart when closer to baseline.
C. Hypertension stable on beta-blockers, note angiotensin-converting enzyme (ACE) inhibitor and diuretic on hold secondary to #2.
D. Pain management: Vicodin every 4 to 6 hours as needed.
E. Diastolic heart failure. Stable. Continue beta-blockers. Typically diuretic-dependent: Restart loop diuretic and ACE inhibitor when able. Monitor daily weight and fluid balance closely.
F. Obstructive sleep apnea: Postop course complicated by hypercapnic and hypoxic respiratory failure, patient's continuous positive airway pressure (CPAP) was upgraded to bilevel positive airway pressure (BiPap). Continue BiPap at 14/8 with 3 L of oxygen bleed-in at hemorrhagic stroke. Qualifications for home machine completed. Follow up with Dr. Smith of Pulmonary.

Consider the scenario that a receiving facility is out of Vicodin, and no one is immediately available to substitute a pain medication. The patient's blood pressure elevates from pain over the next 24 to 48 hours in the setting of diastolic heart failure. The information regarding the patient's heart failure was not communicated since it was "stable." The patient's family is happy the patient is finally out of the hospital and brings the patient all of their favorite drinks and a ham dinner. The information pertaining to the patient's history of diuretic dependence and temporary cessation of diuretic and angiotensin-converting enzyme (ACE) inhibitor therapy was not clearly communicated. The patient is at risk for decompensated heart failure, hypertensive urgency, and pulmonary edema. Clear communication is key. Ideally, a clear, well-constructed problem list might appear as in Table IV.9.

Varying Medical Record Systems

Different providers have privileges allowing access to different medical record systems, whether they are electronic medical records (EMRs) or paper-based. Different facilities and offices can have many different brands of EMRs. Unless there is a functional unifying accessible electronic medical system that is capable of pulling from all of these varied systems and documents, chances are limited that a provider will view a complete, up-to-date picture of a patient's plan of care. This makes communication an ongoing challenge.

Geriatric Needs

Frail, older adult patients are routinely transferred from setting to setting multiple times, often with a sense of urgency. This vulnerable population may have limited ability to communicate their needs, expectations, complex comorbidities, and recent circumstances, let alone navigate the overwhelming continuum of healthcare they are experiencing. They remain at risk for poor outcomes and decompensation from a variety of transitional risk perspectives. It is of vital importance for the APP to consider these challenges when providing transitional care to geriatric patients and to consider the special communication needs of these patients to ensure continuity of care.

ACTIONS TO MITIGATE RISKS IN TRANSITIONAL CARE

It cannot be stated enough: Good communication is the cornerstone of improving care transitions. However, communication in a fast-paced world is often more difficult in reality than postulated. Phone calls can go unanswered or result in return calls that arrive outside of a crucial evaluation window. Messages logged and passed via computer can be brief and lackluster in clarifying complexity, and messages passed via word of mouth may not ultimately reach the assessing provider. Such messages may not even contain the originally communicated content. Faxes may not transmit. Routine texting is not Health Insurance Portability and Accountability Act (HIPAA)-compliant. Complete medical records may not arrive with a patient or in a timely manner. EMR systems may not communicate with each other. Many states have made progress in this area by implementing statewide EMR housing systems. Secure texting platforms are now available; however, they may not be uniformly utilized by all systems, organizations, or providers in a community.

Bridging Gaps

Specific actions have been recommended to bridge the known gaps in transitional care. Strategies focused on population health are being trialed, such as placing a hospitalist in postacute and LTC settings. Specialists such as cardiologists, pulmonologists, and wound care experts are being deployed to postacute settings to enhance and direct the care of patients with congestive heart failure, chronic obstructive pulmonary disease, and complex wounds.

The Care Transitions Intervention

Another approach is referred to as the care transitions intervention. This nationally recognized program is led by Eric Coleman from the University of Colorado. Within this program, Coleman developed four pillars, also called *domains*, of transitional care interventions. These pillars are:
A. Medication self-management.
B. Maintenance of a personal health record.
C. Close follow-up with a primary care provider.

TABLE IV.9 PROBLEM LIST

Current Problem	Diagnosis	Tracking
Diastolic heart failure	2D echo (date): Preserved EF, grade 2 diastolic dysfunction	Ongoing
OSA	On CPAP at home prior to admission	Ongoing
Acute on chronic hypercapnic respiratory failure	Upgraded to BiPap postop, discharged on same	
AKI, mild	Restart ACE and loop diuretic as able	Ongoing
HTN	Continue BB, restart ACE as able or add other agent if SBP >140/80	Ongoing
Hip fracture status post ORIF (date)	Continue PT/OT	
Pain management	Continue Vicodin, gabapentin	Ongoing

2D, two-dimensional; ACE, angiotensin-converting enzyme; AKI, acute kidney injury; BiPap, bilevel positive airway pressure; CPAP, continuous positive airway pressure; EF, ejection fraction; HTN, hypertension; ORIF, open reduction and internal fixation; OSA, obstructive sleep apnea; OT, occupational therapy; PT, physical therapy; SBP, systolic blood pressure.

D. Identification of red flags that should prompt evaluation.

When implemented, the program is led by a transitions coach who oversees the transition of the patient from hospitalization to home. The coach identifies patient goals and assists in the development of self-management skills. In summary, the key components of a successful transitional care plan involve the following:

A. Firming up the pitfalls that can lead to poor outcomes.

B. Providing uniformity across the continuum of settings.

C. Paying close attention to medication reconciliation and delineating any medication changes or substitutions.

D. Developing clear, legible discharge templates that identify important features of the hospitalization, including:

    1. Pertinent diagnostic and laboratory tests.

    2. Pending diagnostic and laboratory tests.

    3. Future plan of care.

    4. Providers involved in the hospitalization and the providers that are needed for follow-up.

E. Clearly defining and continuously reviewing goals of care, advance directives, and code status in every setting.

This approach implements evidence-based practices that utilize dedicated, focused transitional providers to improve outcomes and reduce hospitalizations. Providers armed with evidence-based strategies can do the following:

A. Bridge the information and communication gap between settings.

B. Set goals among patients and the healthcare team.

C. Educate patients and families to self-manage.

D. Simultaneously provide complex monitoring, evaluation, and early intervention for decompensating dynamic comorbidities.

BILLING FOR TRANSITIONAL CARE

Transitional care billing codes were introduced in 2013 to reimburse for services centered around the provision of continuity of care services for the first 30 days after discharge from an inpatient or partial hospitalization back into the community. What does this mean? There are several components required to meet transitional care billing requirements; keep in mind they are updated periodically. This is intended as a brief overview.

To qualify, a patient must be discharged from an inpatient or partial hospitalization. These stays are defined by the Centers for Medicare & Medicaid Services (CMS) as:

A. Inpatient acute care or psychiatric hospital stay.

B. Inpatient rehabilitation (LTAC) stay.

C. SNF or LTC stay.

D. Hospital observation stay.

E. Partial hospitalization at a community mental health center.

Returning to the community includes home, domiciliary, nursing home, and assisted living facilities.

A. Two cognitive processing therapy (CPT) codes for transitional services are available. They are set apart by level of decision-making complexity and allowable face-to-face visit range. Services for these codes are allowable via telehealth.

    1. CPT code 99495.

        a. Moderate medical complexity.

        b. Face-to-face visit within 14 calendar days.

    2. CPT code 99496.

        a. High medical complexity.

        b. Face-to-face visit within 7 days.

    3. Other components include but are not limited to:

        a. An interactive patient or caregiver contact via phone, email, or face-to-face with 2 business days of discharge by a provider or qualified healthcare professional.

        b. Comprehensive medication reconciliation and management (completed no later than the date of the face-to-face visit).

        c. Review of discharge information and pertinent diagnostic tests, treatments, necessary follow-up and community service communication, facilitation, and/or referrals.

        d. Education of patient and caregivers.

MOVING FORWARD

Future efforts in transitional care should seek to integrate and improve care across continuums instead of in isolated circumstances and settings. Such efforts will reduce stress and increase the health and well-being of our society as a whole. Population health strategies that focus on medical home models and transitional care management are exciting alternatives to fragmented traditional care. Medical homes without walls and telemedicine also provide promising alternatives by bringing advanced care providers and technology into the patient's home. Advances in unified, accessible health information databases will also improve care and reduce unnecessary duplication and overuse of health services. Advanced practice studies should include focus on the broadened responsibility and complex communication skills required to advance transitional care and in doing so increase the satisfaction of patients and providers alike.

BIBLIOGRAPHY

Aging With Dignity. (2011). *Five wishes*. https://fivewishes.org/docs/default-source/default-document-library/product-samples/fwsample.pdf?sfvrsn=2

American Medical Directors Association. (2010). *Transitions of care in the long-term care continuum clinical practice guideline*. Author. https://www.nhqualitycampaign.org/files/Transitions_of_Care_in_LTC.pdf

Bixby, M. B., & Naylor, M. D. (2010). The transitional care model (TCM): Hospital discharge screening criteria for high risk older adults. *Medsurg Nursing, 19*(1), 62–63.

CMS Medicare Learning Network. (2022). *Transitional care management services*. Author. (MLN908628).

Cohen-Mekelburg, S., Rosenblatt, R., Gold, S., Scherl, E., Burakoff, R., Steinlauf, A., & Unruh, M. (2018). Fragmented care is prevalent among IBD hospitalizations and is associated with worse outcome. *Gastroenterology, 154*(1 Suppl.), S101. https://doi.org/10.1053/j.gastro.2017.11.239

Coleman, E. A. (2001, November 2). *Infusing true person centered care into improving the quality of transitional care*. Paper presented at Transitions of Care: Improving Care Across Settings, Cincinnati, OH: *Greater Cincinnati Health Council*

Coleman, E. A. (2003). Falling through the cracks: Challenges and opportunities for improving transitional care for persons with continuous complex care needs. *Journal of the American Geriatrics Society, 51*(4), 549–555. https://doi.org/10.1046/j.1532-5415.2003.51185.x

Forster, A. J., Murff, H. J., Peterson, J. F., Gandhi, T. K., & Bates, D. W. (2003). The incidence and severity of adverse events affecting patients after discharge from the hospital. *Annals of Internal Medicine, 138*(3), 161–167. https://doi.org/10.7326/0003-4819-138-3-200302040-00007

Jencks, S. F., Williams, M. V., & Coleman, E. A. (2009). Rehospitalizations among patients in the Medicare fee-for-service program. *The New England Journal of Medicine, 360*(14), 1418–1428. https://doi.org/10.1056/NEJMsa0803563

Jha, A. K., Joynt, K. E., Orav, E. J., & Epstein, A. M. (2012). The long-term effect of premier pay for performance on patient outcomes. *The New England Journal of Medicine, 366*(17), 1606–1615. https://doi.org/10.1056/NEJMsa1112351

Joynt, K. E., & Jha, A. K. (2012). Thirty-day readmissions—truth and consequences. *The New England Journal of Medicine, 366*(15), 1366–1369. https://doi.org/10.1056/NEJMp1201598

Naylor, M. D., Aiken, L. H., Kurtzman, E. T., Olds, D. M., & Hirschman, K. B. (2011). The importance of transitional care in achieving health reform. *Health Affairs, 30*(4), 746–754. https://doi.org/10.1377/hlthaff.2011.0041

Naylor, M. D., & Keating, S. A. (2008). Transitional care. *American Journal of Nursing, 108*(Suppl. 9), 58–63. https://doi.org/10.1097/01.NAJ.0000336420.34946.3a

Nelson, J., & Pulley, A. (2015). Transitional care can reduce hospital readmissions. *American Nurse Today, 10*(4). https://www.americannursetoday.com/transitional-care-can-reduce-hospital-readmissions

University of Pennsylvania School of Nursing. (n.d.). *Transitional care model*. http://www.nursing.upenn.edu/ncth/transitional-care-model/index.phpblank

ACUTE CARE BILLING

Dawn Carpenter

INTRODUCTION

Hospitals rely on adult gerontology acute care nurse practitioners' (AGACNPs) clinical documentation to support hospital billing. Hospitals commonly contract with group practices to hire AGACNPs to work within the hospital. Thus, ensuring the highest level of reimbursement for the hospital yields higher reimbursement, which in turn can indirectly support the cost of AGACNPs' salary.

Clear, direct, and comprehensive documentation delineates the higher levels of acuity seen in acutely and critically ill patients. Documenting completely and thoroughly including a comprehensive list of all active primary and secondary problems and complications are key to providing holistic patient care. Clinical documentation MUST support the billing claims to avoid the risk of fraudulent billing. AGACNPs will spend significant amount of time documenting the care that is provided. Thus, becoming proficient at documentation is essential to effective and efficient coding and billing by the hospital.

Additionally, hospitals seek to hire AGACNPs who have experience with billing; thus, documentation and billing are key skills to learn and refine while in clinical rotations. Be sure to speak with preceptors regularly about how they bill for their services. Students can also practice billing while still in school by applying these billing concepts in their electronic clinical documentation program such as Typhon.

The Centers for Medicare & Medicaid Services (CMS) is commonly the largest payor system for hospital services. The CMS sets specific rules and regulations regarding documentation requirements and reimbursement for patients covered by Medicare and Medicaid. Many other insurance carriers tend to follow these trends set forth by the CMS. Thus, documentation standards should consistently meet the CMS requirements. Failure to meet the documentation standards will result in insurance denials for claims that are submitted. In short, documentation matters greatly!

HOSPITAL VERSUS GROUP PRACTICE BILLING

Different coding systems exist for hospitals and group practice to bill for care and services. Hospitals bill insurance for the care of the patients whose diagnoses are coded into diagnosis-related groups (DRGs) and the technical components of procedures, whereas group practices bill insurances for the professional services when providers evaluate and manage patients, as well as for the professional service to perform surgery and procedures (Figure IV.4).

Hospital Billing

Hospitals use the International Classification of Diseases (ICD), 10th Edition to describe clinical conditions. These clinical conditions are then grouped into DRGs. DRGs are patient classification structure that relates the type of patients a hospital treats (i.e., its case mix) to the costs incurred by the hospital. Hospitals also bill for the technical components of procedures. This billing covers the costs of the procedural space, technology required to complete the procedure, and any overhead costs for electricity, staff, and so forth to be able to perform procedures. Examples of the technical components include cardiac catheterizations, endoscopies, and all operations in the operating rooms. These procedures are denoted by the procedural classification system (PCS).

International Classification of Diseases, 10th Revision, Clinical Modification Codes

The ICD, 10th Revision, Clinical Modification codes are a series of alphanumeric coding to describe a disease state. These codes represent patients' diagnoses and problems. These codes are used for both professional billing and hospital billing. A simplified sample demonstrates the formatting of the coding:

A01 – (Disease)
- A01.0 (Disease) of the lungs
  - ◆ A01.01 … simple
  - ◆ A01.02 … complex
- A01.020 … affecting the trachea
- A01.021 … affecting the cardiopulmonary system
  - ◆ A01.021A … initial encounter
  - ◆ A01.021D … subsequent encounter
  - ◆ A01.021S … sequela

These codes are increasingly being built directly into electronic health records (EHR) for ease of use and clarity. The AGACNP, along with the residents and attendings, is responsible for building and maintaining an accurate problem list and clarifying details in the assessment and plan section of the history and physical (H&P) and progress notes. The hospital's coding specialists will routinely request additional or clarifying data to enhance the specificity. These requests are commonly called clinical documentation inquiries (CDI). The query seeks additional information or clarification. The clinician determines the answer to these queries and documents it in the notes. Be sure to respond promptly to these queries as they help document specific details as are pertinent. Accurate and detailed documentation is good for the patients and the institution.

Diagnosis-Related Groups

The ICD-10 codes from an admission encounter are compiled and assigned into a DRG of similar conditions that consume comparative hospital resources and length of stay. DRGs take into consideration illness severity, comorbid conditions, and mortality risk to calculate reimbursement.

A simple analogy of this is a healthy young adult admitted with pneumonia paid based on "simple

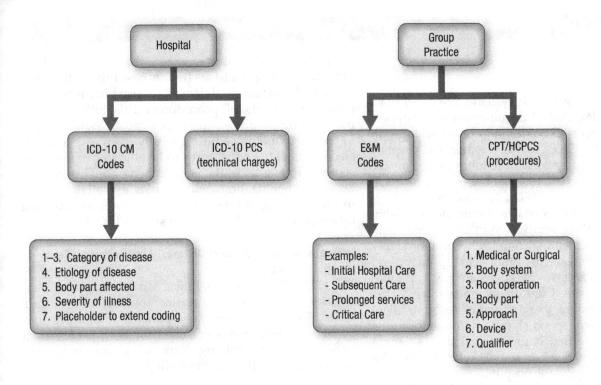

FIGURE IV.4 Overview of hospital and group practice coding.

CPT, Current Procedural Terminology; E&M, evaluation and management; HCPCS, Healthcare Common Procedure Coding System; ICD-10 CM, International Classification of Diseases, 10th Edition, Clinical Modification; PCS, Procedure Coding System.

pneumonia" and reimbursed at a lower rate than a medically complex patient who has diabetes, heart disease, hyperlipidemia, chronic kidney disease, and recent myocardial infarction (MI), which would fall into the category "simple pneumonia with complication or comorbidity (CC) or major complication or comorbidity (MCC)." The latter case would be reimbursed at a higher rate due to the number of resources and medications needed to care for this patient during the hospital stay. In short, accurate and detailed documentation makes a difference in reimbursement!

Case Mix Index

The case mix index (CMI) measures the severity of illness or complexity of the inpatient population. The calculation is an average of the relative weights of all DRGs of a hospital over time periods. The higher the CMI, the more complex the hospital population, with higher acuity levels and greater utilization of resources. Provider documentation of comorbid conditions and complications enhances the CMI. The CMI is linked to hospital reimbursements. Thus, accuracy and completeness of documentation translate into greater hospital revenue.

Hospital reimbursement is critical as many hospitals contract with group practices for services such as critical care services. The hospital pays the group practice, which in turn allows the group practice to pay their employees, including the nurse practitioners' (NPs) salaries. Thus, to ensure NPs' salaries are covered, it is imperative NPs provide exemplary documentation in the medical records to enhance the CMI.

Technical Charges

Hospitals can also bill for technical charges, which are charges for use of hospital facilities. Technical charges include overhead, room and board, nursing care, equipment, and so forth. Examples include the technical component of performing a heart catheterization. The physician would bill for their skills in performing and interpreting the procedure, whereas the hospital would bill the technical charge for the cath lab room and equipment, including fluoroscopy and catheters, nurses, technicians, and so forth, for the procedure.

Group Practice Billing

Group practices bill for professional services provided by providers, including physician, NP, and physician assistants. Professional billing is determined by the Current Procedural Terminology (CPT) codebook and the Healthcare Common Procedure Coding System (HCPCS) book. These codebooks have specific codes for procedures as well as evaluation and management (E&M) codes. E&M codes are used to bill for hospital admissions, discharges, critical care time, daily or subsequent care, and so forth.

A critical detail that AGACNPs need to know is whether they are hired by the hospital or group practice. AGACNPs who are hired by a group practice are able to bill for their professional services, whereas AGACNPs who are hired directly by the hospital are unable to bill for professional services. This distinction may not be immediately clear as many AGACNPs who work within the hospital walls may in fact be hired by the group practice and then subsequently contracted by the hospital to work within the hospital.

AGACNPs should clarify whether the expectation is to bill for professional services or whether their role is to solely support the department for economic efficiency and to enhance patient outcomes. If this has not been made clear up front, the AGACNP should ask. The practice manager will know the answer to this question. Many hospitals do hire the NPs directly to provide support to surgical service lines. This AGACNP then frees up the surgeons to operate more and see more new patients, which can then maximize surgeons' and physicians' productivity and subsequently augments revenue and reduce costs. The costs of preoperative and postoperative care are included in a 90-day global period; thus, services related to surgeries cannot be billed separately during this global period.

Healthcare Common Procedure Coding System

The HCPCS coding system is a system of codes for providers to submit billing claims for healthcare services to insurance companies in a consistent method. HCPCS includes two sets of codes: HCPCS level I and HCPCS level II. HCPCS level I codes are the CPT codes used to submit claims to payers for procedures and services performed by providers, hospitals, clinics, and laboratories. HCPCS level II codes are the procedure codes set for medical equipment suppliers for medical devices, supplies, medications, transportation services, and so forth. HCPCS level I codes for procedures and E&M services commonly used by AGACNPs are discussed in the following:

International Classification of Diseases, 10th Edition Procedure Coding System Codes

The ICD-10 Procedure Coding System (PCS) codes are the codes used to bill for procedures. The codes detail the specifics of anatomy, type of procedure, technique, and devices used. Box IV.2 outlines the components of the PCS codes.

Common bedside procedures performed by AGACNPs include suturing, central venous catheter insertion, arterial line insertion, paracentesis, thoracentesis, intubations, chest tube insertions, and so forth.

BOX IV.2 COMPONENTS OF THE INTERNATIONAL CLASSIFICATION OF DISEASES, 10TH EDITION PROCEDURE CODING SYSTEM CODES

Section relates to the type of procedure.
Body system.
Root operation specifies the objective of the procedure.
Body part is the specific body part/system on which the procedure is performed.
Approach is the technique used to reach the site of the procedure.
Device specifies any device that remains after the procedure has been completed.
Qualifier provides additional information about the procedure.

AGACNPs hired by group practices will be expected to bill for these procedures. Templated notes in the EHR can help ensure all documentation requirements are included in the procedure notes.

Evaluation and Management

E&M codes are the codes used for providers to bill insurance companies for their professional services to diagnose and treat patient conditions. Inpatient AGACNPs commonly bill for observation care, initial hospital care, subsequent hospital care, critical care time, prolonged services, and discharges. Initial hospital care is billed for at the time of admission to inpatient hospital admission. Each of these is addressed in specific sections further in this chapter.

Inpatient Admission

The severity of illness and the intensity of services that are required need to justify the need for an acute inpatient level of care. To qualify for inpatient status, the AGACNP should expect the patient to require hospital care that spans at least two midnights. While AGACNPs can perform the admission process, the CMS still requires a physician certify that inpatient hospital services are reasonable and medically necessary. Medical necessity for inpatient care is determined by:
A. The clinician's assessment of the patient.
B. Current medical needs.
C. Severity of signs and symptoms.
D. Risk of something medically adverse happening.
E. Need for and availability of diagnostic studies.
F. Whether Medicare deems a procedure to require inpatient care.

Observation Status

Observation status equates to an outpatient status. Observation status represents clinically appropriate short-term services. Observation status requires *one* of the following:
A. Diagnostic evaluation (e.g., rule out MI).
B. Acute treatment and evaluation of this treatment (e.g., observe for drug reaction).
C. Monitoring for event (e.g., arrhythmia).
D. Recovery (e.g., from drug/alcohol ingestion).

Once deemed observation status, further data from the assessment, treatments, or reassessments will guide the decision whether patients require ongoing treatment with a full inpatient admission or be able to be discharged. This determination is frequently made within the first 24 hours; however, the decision can be made up to 48 hours and still qualify as observation. At the 48-hour mark, the determination to discharge or admit to inpatient must be made. This is unofficially known as the "two-midnight rule." A patient who stays beyond two midnights and continues to require hospital level of care then qualifies for inpatient admission status.

DOCUMENTATION REQUIREMENTS

In the nursing world, "If it's not documented, it's not done." However, in the NP role, the phrase "if it's not documented, it's not reimbursable" applies. The key to demonstrating superior patient outcomes and securing maximal reimbursement is detailed and specific documentation. Thorough and comprehensive documentation supports billing and reduces the risk of fraud.

The documentation requirements for both observation and inpatient care are similar. Four main elements are needed to bill E&M codes. These four elements are history, physical exam (PE), medical decision-making (MDM) complexity, and time (Tables IV.10–IV.14). The majority of the history required for initial observation and hospital care is either detailed or comprehensive as outlined in the following section. Note the details for each level and time for each level vary by specific codes.

History and Physical Examination

Specific components and the amount of details of history and PE are essential elements of a thorough documentation. Patients who are of observation status or are admitted require comprehensive history and PE. Get in the habit of always being thorough in the documentation to consistently provide high-quality care that is billable at the highest

levels. Table IV.11 provides the specific details required for detailed and comprehensive history and PE documentation. This table may be used while writing notes in clinical and working. EHRs are established to meet these markers to help ensure all the metrics required to bill the highest levels are met. Do not skip sections of the EHR or overly simplify customized note templates or these elements will be missed.

Medical Decision-Making

Three elements are required to determine MDM. Presenting problem points, data complexity points, and risk of complication encompass the overall MDM (see Table IV.12). Problem points and complexity data points are elaborated upon in Table IV.13. The MDM score is the average of two out of the three areas. As an example: A patient scores 2 points for complexity data points and high complexity for presenting problem points; the average is moderate complexity for the overall MDM. Most hospitalized patients are moderate or high complexity MDM. Each of the problem points and data points is elaborated upon in Table IV.13, while risk stratification is elaborated upon in Table IV.14.

TABLE IV.10 SAMPLE OF EVALUATION AND MANAGEMENT DOCUMENTATION

Level	History	PE	MDM	Time	E&M
	Problem-focused	Problem-focused	Straightforward		99XXX
	Expanded problem-focused	Expanded problem-focused	Low		99XXX
	Detailed	Detailed	Moderate		99XXX
	Comprehensive	Comprehensive	High		99XXX

E&M, evaluation and management code; MDM, medical decision-making; PE, physical exam.

TABLE IV.11 HISTORY AND PHYSICAL EXAM ELABORATION

History		Physical Exam	
Detailed	**Comprehensive**	**Detailed**	**Comprehensive**
Chief complaint	Chief complaint	At least 12 bullet points from any organ system	At least 2 bullet points from each of 9 organ systems
Four HPI elements or the status of three chronic or inactive problems	Four HPI elements or the status of three chronic or inactive problems	Organ systems	
–	–	Constitutional Eyes Ears/nose/mouth/throat Neck Respiratory Cardiovascular Chest	Abdomen Genitourinary Lymphatic Musculoskeletal Integumentary Neurologic Psychiatric
2–9 systems in ROS	10 systems in ROS		
≥1 element of PFSH	Complete all 3 of PFSH		

HPI, history of present illness; PFSH, past family social history; ROS, review of systems.

TABLE IV.12 MEDICAL DECISION-MAKING ELABORATION

Overall MDM	Presenting Problem Points	Complexity of Data Points	Risk of Complication and/or Morbidity/Mortality
Straightforward	1	1	Minimal
Low complexity	2	2	Low
Moderate complexity	3	3	Moderate
High complexity	4	4	High

MDM, medical decision-making.

TABLE IV.13 PROBLEM POINTS AND DATA POINTS ELABORATION

Problem Points		Data Points	
Problem	Points	Data	Points
Self-limited or minor (max 2)	1	Review/order laboratory tests	1
Established problem/stable or improving (these may be multiplied by the number of problems being treated)	1	Review/order radiology test	1
Established problem, worsening (these may be multiplied by the number of problems being treated)	2	Review/order medical test	1
New problem, no additional workup planned (highest level is 3 no matter how many problems)	3	Discuss test with the performing provider	1
New problem, additional workup planned (highest level is 3 no matter how many problems)	4	Independent review of image, tracing, or specimen	2
		Decision to obtain old records	1
		Review and summarize old records	2

Most patients who are admitted have a new problem with additional workup needed; thus, they score four problem points. Most AGACNPs will review the patient's chart, labs, radiology, and other diagnostic testing and discuss with an attending physician, thus garnering a minimum of four data points. Risk of complication and/or morbidity/mortality is determined by the risk related to the disease process that is anticipated between the current encounter and the next encounter (see Table IV.14). Patients who are admitted to observation meet moderate risk and those who are admitted must meet high level of risk.

Time

AGACNPs can bill by the amount of time spent in an encounter; however, additional caveats exist. New AGACNPs will naturally take longer in encounters until they become proficient. Therefore, AGACNPs who choose to use time as the billing factor need to document this time in the patient's EHR. This documentation MUST support, in ample detail, the nature of the

encounter. Selection of the code must be based on total face-to-face time for the encounter. Additionally, the EHR needs to demonstrate sufficient detail to justify the code. Thus, it is recommended to adhere to the history, PE, and MDM requirements to bill the E&M codes, as well as document the time in the note.

In summary, the elements that need to be thoroughly documented in every note to bill for E&M services include the history, PE, medical decision-making, and time. Get in the habit of always documenting comprehensive history and PE so the highest level of billing can be secured. Documenting the specific level of complexity of decision-making helps support the billing as well.

INITIAL HOSPITAL CARE

The term *initial hospital care* refers to the H&P note documenting the care required for hospital admission or observation. To bill initial hospital care, all three of the history, PE, and MDM are required to be met across the board or the time requirement (Table IV.15).

TABLE IV.14   RISK ELABORATION

Minimal	Lowest level of risk possible; not for inpatients
	Requires one element in any of the three categories:
	Presenting problem
	  ■ One self-limiting or minor problem
	Diagnostic procedures/tests, for example:
	  ■ CXR, EKG, EEG, UA
	  ■ Ultrasound, echo
	Management, for example:
	  ■ Rest, elastic bandages, superficial dressings

Low	Second lowest level of risk; low-risk patients are generally quite healthy
	Requires one element in any of the three categories:
	Presenting problem
	  ■ One stable chronic illness
	  ■ Acute, uncomplicated illness or injury
	Diagnostic procedures/tests, for example:
	  ■ Physiologic tests not under stress (e.g., PFTs)
	  ■ Noncardiovascular imaging studies with contrast
	  ■ Superficial needle biopsies
	  ■ ABGs
	Management, for example:
	  ■ Over-the-counter medications
	  ■ Minor surgery with no identified risk factors
	  ■ Physical or occupational therapy
	  ■ IV fluids without additives

Moderate	Second highest risk level; required for level 2 hospital progress note
	Requires one element in any of the three categories:
	Presenting problem
	  ■ One or more chronic illness with mild exacerbation or progression
	  ■ Two or more stable chronic illnesses
	  ■ Undiagnosed problem with uncertain prognosis
	  ■ Acute illness with systemic symptoms (e.g., pyelonephritis, pneumonitis, colitis)
	  ■ Acute complicated injury (e.g., head injury with brief loss of consciousness)
	Diagnostic procedures/tests, for example:
	  ■ Physiologic tests under stress (e.g., cardiac stress test)
	  ■ Diagnostic endoscopies with no identified risk factors
	  ■ Deep needle or incisional biopsies
	  ■ Cardiovascular imaging studies with contrast and no identified risk factors (e.g., arteriogram, cardiac catheterization)
	  ■ Obtain fluid from body cavity (e.g., lumbar puncture, thoracentesis, paracentesis)
	Management, for example:
	  ■ Minor surgery with identified risk factors
	  ■ Elective major surgery with no risk factors
	  ■ Prescription drug management
	  ■ Therapeutic nuclear medicine
	  ■ IV fluids with additives
	  ■ Closed treatment of fracture or dislocation without manipulation

High	Highest level of risk; required for level 3 admission
	Requires one element in any of the three categories:
	Presenting problem
	  ■ One or more chronic illness with severe exacerbation or progression
	  ■ Acute or chronic illness or injuries which pose a threat to life or bodily function (e.g., multiple trauma, acute MI, pulmonary embolism, severe respiratory distress, peritonitis, acute kidney injury)
	Diagnostic procedures/tests, for example:
	  ■ Cardiovascular imaging studies with contrast with identified risk factors
	  ■ Cardiac EP testing
	  ■ Diagnostic endoscopies with identified risk factors
	Management, for example:
	  ■ Elective major surgery with identified risk factors
	  ■ Emergency major surgery
	  ■ Parenteral controlled substances
	  ■ Drug therapy requiring intensive monitoring for toxicity
	  ■ Decision not to resuscitate or to de-escalate care due to poor prognosis

ABGs, arterial blood gas; CXR, chest x-ray; echo, echocardiogram; EP, electrophysiology; IV, intravenous; MI, myocardial infarction; PFTs, pulmonary function tests; UA, unstable angina.

TABLE IV.15   DOCUMENTATION ELEMENTS FOR BILLING INITIAL HOSPITAL CARE

Level	History	PE	MDM	Time (Minutes)	E&M
1	Detailed	Detailed	Straightforward/low	30	99221
2	Comprehensive	Comprehensive	Moderate	50	99222
3	Comprehensive	Comprehensive	High	70	99223

E&M, evaluation and management code; MDM, medical decision-making; PE, physical exam.

INITIAL OBSERVATION CARE

To bill for initial observation care, all three of the history, PE, and MDM must be met across the board or time (Table IV.16).

INITIAL OBSERVATION WITH DISCHARGE ON SAME DATE OF SERVICE

To bill an initial observation and discharge on the same date of service requires all three of the history, exam, and MDM to be met across the board or time (Table IV.17).

SUBSEQUENT CARE

Subsequent care is the term used to depict the sequential days of hospitalization and is documented in daily progress notes. Subsequent care requires two of the three of the history, PE, and MDM criteria to be met or time, or can be based on time if greater than 50% of the time spent at the bedside is spent coordinating care (Table IV.18).

SUBSEQUENT OBSERVATION

Subsequent observation care requires two of the three of the history, exam, and MDM to be met or time (Table IV.19).

CRITICAL CARE

Critical care codes are time-based billing and are used for any life-, limb-, or organ-saving interventions. Critical care time can be provided in a variety of settings, not just for patients within ICUs. Any patient who is hemodynamically unstable, have life-threatening arrhythmias or arrhythmias that cause the patient to be symptomatic (i.e., chest pain, shortness of breath, hypotension), or have respiratory distress, hypoxia, symptomatic hypercarbia, active bleeding, or changes in mental status qualifies for critical care time regardless of physical location. CMS guidance offers that to qualify as critical care, failure to initiate urgent interventions for these situations could likely result in clinically significant or life-threatening deterioration.

The AGACNP should record the total time spent evaluating, managing, and documenting such activities. This time includes time spent reviewing the chart, performing history and PE, interpreting laboratory and diagnostic testing, considering differential diagnoses, consulting with expert clinicians, creating and executing a management plan, and documenting this care.

Time spent can also be at the bedside, discussing the case with staff, documenting the medical record, and time spent with family members (or MDM) discussing specific treatment issues and making clinical decisions such as do not intubate (DNI) or do not resuscitate (DNR) status. During this time, the NP must devote their full attention to this particular patient. Critical care time specifically EXCLUDES any time spent performing procedures that are billed for separately.

The two codes for billing critical care time are 99291 for the first hour, but may be billed after the halfway threshold has been met at 30 minutes, and 99292 for each additional 30 minutes beyond the initial hour, and may be billed once the halfway threshold has been met at 75 minutes. Multiple 99292 can be billed for a date of service provided the patient's status remains tenuous or continues to have evolving changes in their condition. Time that is EXCLUDED from critical care is time spent in performing procedures, daily family updates, and professional services for interpretation of diagnostic testing.

While NPs routinely interpret EKGs and chest x-rays (CXRs), the cardiologists and radiologists are the qualified experts who provide the "official" interpretation and will bill the professional services for these and other diagnostic testing. Daily family updates are expected elements of the routine care that is provided. That being said, formal family meetings, specifically where patient care decisions are made, can be included as critical care time. Decisions such as making the patient DNR or withdrawing life-sustaining interventions are also considered billable time.

Critical care services can additionally be billed on the same day as initial or subsequent hospital care, if the patient has a change in clinical condition and the critical care time was provided after the previous E&M code was billed. Additionally, critical care time may be billed in addition to a surgical procedure that has a global surgical period, if the critical care time is unrelated to the surgical procedure. Examples include managing septic shock, hypoxia, acute kidney injury, and arrhythmias, as long as the management is not part of the routine surgical care or managing complications related to the surgical procedure.

These services need to be medically necessary and separate and distinct from the previous services. AGACNPs should document and report a "modifier 25"

TABLE IV.16   DOCUMENTATION ELEMENTS FOR BILLING INITIAL OBSERVATION CARE

Level	History	PE	MDM	Time (Minutes)	E&M
1	Detailed	Detailed	Straightforward/low	30	99218
2	Comprehensive	Comprehensive	Moderate	50	99229
3	Comprehensive	Comprehensive	High	70	99220

E&M, evaluation and management code; MDM, medical decision-making; PE, physical exam.

TABLE IV.17   DOCUMENTATION ELEMENTS FOR BILLING INITIAL OBSERVATION WITH DISCHARGE ON SAME DATE OF SERVICE

Level	History	PE	MDM	Time (Minutes)	E&M
1	Detailed	Detailed	Straightforward/low	40	99234
2	Comprehensive	Comprehensive	Moderate	50	99235
3	Comprehensive	Comprehensive	High	55	99236

E&M, evaluation and management code; MDM, medical decision-making; PE, physical exam.

TABLE IV.18   DOCUMENTATION ELEMENTS FOR BILLING SUBSEQUENT CARE

Level	Patient	History	PE	MDM	Time (Minutes)	E&M
1	Stable or improving	Problem-focused	Problem-focused	Straightforward/low	15	99231
2	Inadequate response to treatment or minor complication	Expanded problem-focused	Expanded problem-focused	Moderate	25	99232
3	Unstable or has significant complication or a significant new problem	Detailed	Detailed	High	35	99233

E&M, evaluation and management code; MDM, medical decision-making; PE, physical exam.

TABLE IV.19   DOCUMENTATION ELEMENTS FOR BILLING SUBSEQUENT OBSERVATION

Level	Patient	History	PE	MDM	Time (Minutes)	E&M
1	Stable or improving	Problem-focused	Problem-focused	Straightforward/low	15	99224
2	Inadequate response to treatment or minor complication	Expanded problem-focused	Expanded problem-focused	Moderate	25	99225
3	Unstable or has significant complication or a significant new problem	Detailed	Detailed	High	35	99226

E&M, evaluation and management code; MDM, medical decision-making; PE, physical exam.

on the claim when reporting critical care services when a prior E&M code has been billed for that day.

PROLONGED SERVICES

Prolonged service codes are used when coordinating care is time-consuming. E&M code 99356 requires an additional 60 or more minutes of time spent face to face with the patient beyond the E&M code for the day. Each additional increment of 30 or more minutes (beyond the first hour) can be billed using code 99357.

To be successfully reimbursed for prolonged services, the NP must record several additional elements in the daily progress note. The AGACNP must record the time they went into and out of the patient's room, including start and stop time. Additionally, the AGACNP must describe the care and coordination or discussion that occurred for each entry into the patient's room. Specific items CANNOT be billed as prolonged services, including time spent reviewing the chart, discussions with residents or nursing staff that is not directly face-to-face contact with the patient, awaiting diagnostic results, or managing changes in the patient's condition. Of note, Medicare specifically states: "While Medicare recognizes the effort that goes into prolonged services, it doesn't expect to see the codes used very often." These codes are frequently scrutinized and may trigger an audit if used too recurrently.

DISCHARGES

All discharges can be billed; however, they have different E&M codes depending on whether they were admitted as inpatient or observation. Patients who are admitted and discharged on the same day have one set of codes. Another code is used for patients who are admitted to observation and discharged on different days. Patients who are admitted and discharged on the same calendar date use codes 99234, 99235, and 99236, as listed in Table IV.17. Patients who are admitted to observation and discharged on a different day use code 99217. Inpatient discharges are further delineated by less than or greater than 30 minutes. Inpatients who are discharged in less than 30 minutes use code 99238, while patients whose discharge takes longer than 30 minutes use code 99239. Note that specific time must be documented and the services that were performed on the day of discharge specified. Patients who die are also considered discharges; thus, these same discharges codes may be used for patients who die and the time spent should be included in the death summary.

GLOBAL PERIOD

The global period is broadly defined as a period of time whereby routine care associated with the procedure cannot be billed. The initial consultation, by a surgeon, to determine the need for major surgery is not included in the global period. This decision-making visit should be billed separately for major surgical procedures. Once a decision has been made to perform surgery, certain care is encompassed in the payment for that surgery. Minor procedures have a 10-day postoperative period, whereas major procedures have a 90-day postoperative period. Typically, the day of the procedure is not a separately billable visit. Thus, the total global period is 11 days for minor procedures. For major procedures, the day prior to and the day of the procedure are included in the global period. Thus, for major procedures the total global time period is 92 days.

Care that is specifically *included* in the global period includes:

A. Preoperative visits after the decision to operate is made.
B. Intraoperative services which are a usual and necessary part of the surgical procedure.
C. All medical or surgical care needed, by the surgeon, in the postoperative period, including care of surgical complications (which do not require return trips to the operating room).
D. Follow-up visits during the postoperative period that are related to the surgery.
E. Usual postoperative pain management.
F. Management of wound care, including dressing removal or changes, incisional care, and removal of packing.
G. Removal of any sutures and staples, tubes, drains, or wires, casts, or splints.
H. Insertion, maintenance, and removal of urinary catheters.
I. Management of peripheral intravenous catheters and nasogastric and/or rectal tubes, and changes or removal of tracheostomy tubes.

Care that is specifically *excluded* in the global period includes:

A. Services of other surgeons or physicians specifically related to the surgery (unless the surgeon and another physician agree that transfer of care is required. This agreement should be documented in the discharge summary or EHR).
B. Care not related to the surgical procedure.
C. Treatment for an underlying condition or additional treatment that is not part of usual recovery from the surgery.
D. Diagnostic testing or procedures, including diagnostic radiologic procedures.
E. Obviously distinct surgical procedures that are needed in the postoperative period and are not considered reoperations or care for surgical complications.
F. Treatment for postoperative complications requiring a return trip to the operating room.
G. A second procedure is payable separately if a more extensive procedure is required because a more conservative approach fails.
H. Immunosuppressive therapy for organ transplantation
I. Critical care services (CPT codes 99291 and 99292) which are unrelated to the surgery.

SPLIT OR SHARED BILLING

Split or shared services are E&M codes for services provided by both an NP or a physician assistant and a physician. The AGACNP and the physician must be hired in the same group and work in a facility. These services may be provided in both face-to-face and nonface-to-face format. The visit is billed by the provider who provides the substantive portion—the history, PE, and MDM—of the visit. For critical care, time must be more than half of the total time. This applies to new and established patients, as well as initial, subsequent, and prolonged services. The EHR must readily identify which two individuals performed the services. Each provider should document their respective time in the note. Additionally, the provider, who has provided the substantive portion of care and is billing the services, needs to sign and date the notes.

TELEHEALTH SERVICES

The CMS has expanded and extended the temporary billing and payment for telehealth services, which accelerated during the COVID-19 pandemic. Telehealth services is defined as multimedia communications that include both audio and video transmissions that allow for two-way, real-time, interactive communication between the provider and the patient. The CMS is regularly reassessing and revising telehealth services. For example, geographic restrictions were removed, and the CMS is expanding telehealth service to include audio only for mental health services in limited circumstances and now requires a face-to-face visit annually. The current regulations are in place until December 31, 2023.

CODING AND BILLING TIPS

A. Get to know the coding specialist for the department. Take time to meet them and ask questions. They are there to educate and support you and answer questions.
B. Promptly respond to coders' clinical queries or requests for additional clarification.
C. Discuss who and what will be billed with the attending of record on a daily basis.
D. Be sure to attend mandatory training requirements. Come with questions and examples to discuss.

REIMBURSEMENT

The CMS sets the rules and regulations for documentation requirements and reimbursement for patients covered by Medicare. Many private insurance carriers tend to follow these trends set forth by the CMS. The CMS is commonly the insurance which covers the greatest number of hospitalized patients, thus making it the largest source of hospitals' payors. The term *payor mix* comprises compilation and ratio of payors' sources. The CMS, private insurances, and patients who self-pay comprise the payor mix.

NPs are reimbursed at 85% of the physicians. The historical reason given for this discrepancy is that physicians have higher student loans, are responsible for paying for the overhead costs of the practice site, have higher premiums for malpractice insurance, and care for more complex patients.

Numerous national nursing organizations continue to lobby at the state and national levels for equitable pay for equitable and value-based services. Please be sure to join a national organization, such as the American Association of Nurse Practitioners (AANP), and your state NP association to stay abreast of state and local advocacy.

The most important element an AGACNP can do to ensure the highest reimbursement for services rendered is to ensure complete documentation in the EHR. The number one reason for insurance denial is missing or incomplete information. Partner with the billing expert in the department who can review documentation and help augment the accuracy and details of your notes. Accurate documentation can help prevent insurance company audits, which can result in having to pay back overpayments for services and associated penalties.

MEDICARE ACCESS AND CHIP REAUTHORIZATION ACT

The Medicare Access and CHIP Reauthorization Act (MACRA) is a law that was created to change reimbursement from a fee-for-service model to a program of payment that promotes quality of care and value based on performance measures. There are two ways for organizations to participate in quality payment programs: Merit-based incentive payments (MIPS), which provide performance-based bonus payment adjustments; or alternative payment models (APMs), where incentive payment can be earned for engagement in innovative payment models. These programs enroll institutions, not the individual AGACNP. AGACNPs need to have a basic understanding of these programs, at their respective organizations, as these programs are drivers of organizational change, to enhance the care that is being delivered.

SUMMARY

Learning to document well to support maximal billing requires attention to detail, along with practice and repetition. Coaching by the billing specialist is key to mastering these skills. Take time to build a relationship with the coding and billing specialist of the department and meet with them regularly. Be sure to promptly respond to clinical queries, preferably on the same day.

BIBLIOGRAPHY

American Academy of Pediatrics. (2018). *Specific criteria must be met to use prolonged services codes.* AAP News. https://publications.aap.org/aap news/news/13575?autologincheck=redirected

The American Health Information Management Association. (2022). *Observation Status or Inpatient Admission—Guidance for Physicians.* https://library.ahima.org/doc?oid=59565#.YqnyNBPMI1I

Carpenter, D. (2022). *Fast facts for the adult-gerontology acute care nurse practitioner.* Springer Publishing Company.

Centers for Medicare & Medicaid Services. (2015). *MACRA: What is a MACRA?* https://www.cms.gov/Medicare/Quality-Initiatives-Patient-Assessment-Instruments/Value-Based-Programs/MACRA-MIPS-and-APMs/MACRA-MIPS-and-APMs

Centers for Medicare & Medicaid Services. (2018). *Are you a hospital inpatient or outpatient?* Author. https://www.medicare.gov/sites/default/files/2018-09/11435-Are-You-an-Inpatient-or-Outpatient.pdf

Centers for Medicare & Medicaid Services. (2019, October 2019). *Design and development of the Diagnosis Related Group (DRG) PBL-038.* https://www.cms.gov/icd10m/version37-fullcode-cms/fullcode_cms/Design_and_development_of_the_Diagnosis_Related_Group_(DRGs).pdf

Centers for Medicare & Medicaid Services. (2021). *Calendar Year (CY) 2022 Medicare physician fee schedule final rule.* https://www.cms.gov/newsroom/fact-sheets/calendar-year-cy-2022-medicare-physician-fee-schedule-final-rule

Centers for Medicare & Medicaid Services. (2022a). *Medicare claims processing manual chapter 12 - Physicians/Nonphysician Practitioners*. https://www.cms.gov/regulations-and-guidance/guidance/manuals/downloads/clm104c12.pdf

Centers for Medicare & Medicaid Services. (2022b). *MS-DRG classifications and software*. https://www.cms.gov/Medicare/Medicare-Fee-for-Service-Payment/AcuteInpatientPPS/MS-DRG-Classifications-and-Software

Centers for Medicare & Medicaid Services. (2022c). *Quality payment program*. https://www.cms.gov/Medicare/Quality-Payment-Program/Quality-Payment-Program

CMS Medicare Learning Network. (2018). *Global surgery booklet*. https://www.cms.gov/outreach-and-education/medicare-learning-network-mln/mlnproducts/downloads/globalsurgery-icn907166.pdf

CMS Medicare Learning Network. (2021). *Evaluation and management services guide*. https://www.cms.gov/outreach-and-education/medicare-learning-network-mln/mlnproducts/downloads/eval-mgmt-serv-guide-icn006764.pdf

Dean, S. M., Gilmore-Bykovskyi, A., Buchanan, J., Ehlenfeldt, B., & Kind, A. J. (2016). Design and hospital wide implementation of a standardized discharge summary in an electronic health record. *The Joint Commission Journal on Quality and Patient Safety, 42*(12), 555–AP511. https://doi.org/10.1016/S1553-7250(16)30107-6

Hazelwood, A. (2006). *ICD-9 CM to ICD-10 CM: Implementation Issues and Challenges. The American health information management association*. https://library.ahima.org/doc?oid=59978#.YuEVei-B3-Y

Sanderson, A. L., & Burns, J. P. (2020). Clinical documentation for intensivists: The impact of diagnosis documentation. *Critical Care Medicine, 48*(4), 579–587. https://doi.org/10.1097/CCM.0000000000004200

CASE SCENARIOS ANSWER KEY

CHAPTER 3

CARDIAC CARE

1. C) Use of tobacco. The only modifiable risk factor is tobacco use as it represents a behavior that can be reduced or eliminated with lifestyle modifications. Moreover, smoking is the primary preventable cause of morbidity and mortality in the United States. Data from the World Health Organization also show that after abstaining from smoking for 1 year, one's risk of cardiovascular disease decreases by 50%. Age, sex, and family history are important factors when assessing a patient's risk of developing heart disease; however, they are non-modifiable with behavior change.

2. C) New systolic murmur. In a patient with suspected acute coronary syndrome, the presence of a new systolic murmur is concerning and signifies the potential for cardiac compromise. Although this finding does not denote a specific pathology, it is most commonly associated with papillary muscle dysfunction, significant mitral regurgitation, or a ventricular septal defect, where any of these abnormalities can result in urgent hemodynamic instability. Patients with acute coronary syndrome may have a carotid bruit when auscultating the carotid arteries. This finding signifies the presence of turbulent blood flow secondary to atherosclerosis in the carotid arteries but does not signal an urgent change in cardiovascular status. The presence of a xanthoma, a yellow deposit on the skin, and a corneal arcus, a white-appearing ring at the cornealscleral junction, can occur in patients with atherosclerosis, which is a risk factor for ischemic heart disease; however, these physical examination findings are not cause for emergent concern.

3. B) Non-ST-segment elevation myocardial infarction (NSTEMI). Based on this patient's presenting signs and symptoms and diagnostic test results, the most likely diagnosis is an NSTEMI. The patient's history is significant for modifiable (i.e., tobacco use) and non-modifiable risk factors (i.e., age, sex, family history) for ischemic disease. Additionally, the discomfort is characterized as pressure-like, radiating to the left arm, and exertional, which are hallmark findings in acute coronary syndrome. When evaluating the objective findings, the EKG does not reveal any ST-segment elevations; this would be indicative of an ST-segment elevation myocardial infarction (STEMI). This patient's EKG findings of ST-segment depressions can occur secondary to unstable angina or an NSTEMI as a marker of ischemia;

however, the concomitantly elevated cardiac biomarker (troponin) solidifies the diagnosis of an NSTEMI. Pericarditis can also present with chest pain; however, it is often characterized as pleuritic and positional (worsening when supine and improved when leaning forward) and a pericardial friction rub can sometimes be appreciated on physical examination. Although there can be elevated troponins in the setting of pericarditis (secondary to inflammation not myocardial necrosis), the most common EKG changes are diffuse ST-segment elevations.

4. B) Vasodilator. Given this patient's presenting signs and symptoms that are concerning for acute coronary syndrome, it is imperative that an antiplatelet (e.g., 324 mg of oral aspirin) is administered promptly. This class of medications works by preventing the formation of clots in the vasculature, which is an important step in the management of acute coronary syndrome. Fibrinolytic therapy, a class of medications used to dissolve clots, should be avoided in patients without evidence of an ST-segment elevation myocardial infarction (STEMI) as the risks of this medication, such as significant bleeding, outweigh the benefits. Vasodilators, like nitroglycerin, are first-line therapy in patients with acute coronary syndrome, as they reduce anginal pain and lower blood pressure/myocardial oxygen demand; however, in this scenario, the patient's blood pressure is somewhat low, and to avoid the risk of hemodynamic compromise this medication would not be the initial treatment of choice. One can consider the use of opioids, like morphine, for patients with acute coronary syndrome who report persistent chest pain despite the use of antiplatelet and vasodilating agents; however, in this scenario, it would not be the initial treatment of choice and has the potential to cause worsening hypotension.

CHAPTER 4

ACUTE ABDOMEN

1. D) All of the above. Mr. N's pain centers in the mid/upper abdomen, which can help zero in on the differential diagnosis (DD). The most common causes of this type of pain are acute ischemia, abdominal aortic aneurysm (AAA), myocardial infarction (MI), acute appendicitis, inflammatory bowel disease (IBD), gastroenteritis, and peptic ulcer disease (PUD). Several are very unlikely. AAA and MI are rare in this age group, and in the absence of vomiting or diarrhea gastroenteritis is unlikely. Acute ▶

ischemia is unlikely given the absence of pain out of proportion. He reports this is the first time he has experienced the symptoms, making IBD unlikely. Therefore, the remaining DD options are appendicitis, PUD, bowel obstruction, and pancreatitis. It could be argued that a must-not-miss diagnosis for this patient would be an MI, so obtaining an EKG is a simple way to evaluate this possibility. As he is neither hypotensive nor experiencing abdominal distention, the remaining DD list is set to explore.

2. A) Complete blood count (CBC) and CT of the abdomen. Obtaining a CBC to evaluate for the presence or absence of infection is an important part of this workup. Continued observation with reexamination, a surgery consult, and abdominal CT scan with and without contrast are appropriate in this patient who is presenting as if he has appendicitis.

3. D) Notify surgery of the exam findings. Migration of pain to the right lower quadrant (RLQ) suggests appendicitis due to parietal peritoneal inflammation. Less likely considerations are Crohn's disease, diverticulitis, or colon cancer, which are unlikely in the patient's age group. This symptom complex, including pain migration and intensification, is highly suggestive of appendicitis. Once CT is complete, another call to surgery with an update on exam and CT results would be appropriate.

4. C) Expand differential to consider pregnancy, pelvic inflammatory disease (PID), and ovarian pathology. If the patient were a woman, one would consider pregnancy, PID, and ovarian pathology (such as ruptured ovarian cyst, ruptured ectopic pregnancy, or ovarian torsion).

PANCREATITIS

1. C) Calcium <8 mg/dL. Calcium <8 mg/dL that develops over the course of 48 hours becomes part of the Ranson criteria. It is not taken into account at admission. The other criteria are recorded in the Ranson score at the time of admission.

2. D) The overall mortality is less than 1%. The mortality for pancreatitis has remained unchanged at 10% for decades.

PEPTIC ULCER DISEASE

1. B) Esophagogastroduodenoscopy (EGD). The most accurate diagnostic test with sensitivity and specificity >90% in diagnosing peptic and duodenal ulcers is EGD.

2. C) Nonsteroidal anti-inflammatory drugs (NSAIDs). NSAIDs are associated with the incidence of ulcer disease and should be discontinued. They do not aid in the eradication of *Helicobacter pylori* infection.

CHAPTER 5

ACUTE KIDNEY INJURY

1. D) Rosuvastatin. Statins are identified as a common cause of medication-induced rhabdomyolysis. Potential mechanisms include vasoconstriction within the kidney and ischemic tubular injury, cast formation, and

myoglobin-induced direct tubular toxicity. A urine dipstick positive for blood in the absence of red blood cells (RBCs) and elevated creatine kinase (CK) and myoglobin levels are frequent findings. CK levels greater than 40,000 U/L are associated with an increased risk of acute kidney injury (AKI). A urine dipstick can be positive for blood because the peroxidase agent reacts with heme, contained in both hemoglobin and myoglobin, leading to a false-positive test for the presence of blood.

BENIGN PROSTATIC HYPERTROPHY

1. B) Alpha-blocker such as tamsulosin. The alpha-1-adrenergic receptor blockers are considered the first-line therapy for benign prostatic hypertrophy (BPH). This patient has presumed BPH as from his above lower urinary tract symptoms (LUTS) and urinary retention. An alpha-blocker will help relax the smooth muscle of the prostate and bladder neck. Beta-blockers are not known to help with BPH. The patient is constipated, so a bowel regimen may help by releasing pressure off of the bladder by the distended bowel so that the bladder can empty better. However, it will not effectively treat BPH. Phosphodiesterase-5 inhibitors can be used but are seldom first line unless the patient also reports erectile dysfunction.

CHRONIC KIDNEY DISEASE

1. C) 3b. Stage 3b is an estimated glomerular filtration rate (eGFR) range between 30 and 44, moderate to severe kidney damage. The goal is to treat blood pressure and diabetes, as well as to avoid any further damage to the kidneys, for example, avoidance of nephrotoxic medications.

2. D) Renin-angiotensin-aldosterone system (RAAS) inhibitor and sodium glucose cotransporter-2 (SGLT-2) inhibitor. Therapy to slow the rate of progression in proteinuric patients with chronic kidney disease is centered on treating the patient with either an angiotensin-converting enzyme (ACE) inhibitor or an angiotensin receptor blocker (ARB). A reduction in urinary protein excretion has been found to slow chronic kidney disease (CKD) progression. In addition, such patients may benefit from treatment with SGLT2 inhibitors.

HEMATURIA

1. D) CT urogram. The best answer is CT urogram. This study will determine if there is any kidney stones or masses of the genitourinary (GU) tract. A CT urogram is a multiphasic contrasted CT scan of the abdomen and pelvis. The first phase is a dry CT, which will reveal any stones in the kidneys or ureter. The second phase is with contrast, which will identify renal masses. The third phase is a delayed phase, which allows for contrast excretion by the kidneys and will identify filling defects in the collecting system, which may be concerning for upper tract urothelial tumors. Although checking a hepatic function panel may be helpful in determining any indication of liver disease that may cause increased bleeding, the patient has no other symptoms of liver disease, making this less likely. A renal ultrasound may identify renal masses but may not identify ureteral stones or tumors. Checking a serial hemoglobin and hematocrit will help determine if the patient needs blood transfusion, but will not help with diagnosis and treatment of the hematuria.

HYPERCALCEMIA

1. A) Ectopic synthesis of calcitriol from the lymphoma. Ectopic synthesis of calcitriol from the lymphoma is the most likely mechanism of this patient's hypercalcemia.

HYPERKALEMIA

1. B) Intravenous (IV) calcium gluconate. IV calcium gluconate is the first step in management.

HYPERMAGNESEMIA

1. B) Hypermagnesemia. Hypermagnesemia is the most common etiology of the patient's symptoms.

HYPERNATREMIA

1. C) IV D5W. IV D5W is the most appropriate in vitro fertilization (IVF) as first-line management of hypernatremia.

HYPERPHOSPHATEMIA

1. C) Acute phosphate nephropathy. Acute appendicitis is the most likely diagnosis.

HYPOCALCEMIA

1. B) Order 3 g calcium gluconate IV now, check EKG to assess QT interval, and order ionized calcium level now and to repeat after IV infusion. This is acute hypocalcemia most likely caused by tissue consumption of calcium due to infection and sepsis. The patient had a normal calcium level 2 months ago. Replace calcium urgently to avoid the side effects of hypocalcemia. Always check EKG for acute changes. Always repeat calcium as ionized calcium to ensure adequate replacement. Vitamin D and parathyroid hormone (PTH) assessment is not an acute measure, but rather part of chronic calcium management associated with secondary hypocalcemia.

HYPOKALEMIA

1. D) Potassium chloride 40 mEq IV one-time dose, then repeat the serum potassium level after the infusion is complete and daily, and start potassium 20 mEq PO once a day. This patient has past and ongoing renal and gastrointestinal (GI) losses of potassium that need to be urgently replaced due to severely low potassium level and hypokalemia symptoms. Calculate the current total extracellular potassium deficit as extracellular fluid volume (ECFV) × *desired* serum potassium (4.0 or 4.5 mEq/L) – ECFV × serum potassium (mEq/L). The desired potassium level is at least 4 mEq/L. ECFV = total body water [0.6 × weight (kg)] × ⅓. Thus, immediate ECFV potassium deficit is [4.0 mmol/L–2.5] × [(90 kg × 0.6) × 0.26] = 1.4 × [54 × 0.26] = 1.5 × 14.04 = 19.656 mmol/L or 20 mEq, delivered intravenously.

However, the patient has been losing potassium chronically, so she also has intracellular depletion. She also has ongoing losses. You need to give more than 20 mEq IV now due to ongoing losses and start daily replacement for intracellular and ongoing losses. Always monitor potassium levels frequently during replacement to avoid overcorrection.

2. B) Continue potassium chloride 20 mEq PO once a day. The patient still has hypokalemia but is now asymptomatic and is now losing less potassium. Calculate the current total extracellular potassium deficit as extracellular fluid volume (ECFV) × *desired* serum potassium (4.0 or 4.5 mEq/L) – ECFV × serum potassium (mEq/L). The desired potassium level is at least 4 mEq/L. ECFV = total body water [0.6 × weight (kg)] × ⅓. Thus, ECFV potassium deficit is [4.0 mmol/L–3.1] × [(90 kg × 0.6) × 0.26] = 0.9 × [54 × 0.26] = 0.9 × 14.04 = 12.6 mmol/L or 13 mEq. She also has ongoing losses so you need to give more than 13 mEq. Always monitor potassium levels frequently during replacement to avoid overcorrection.

HYPOMAGNESEMIA

1. D) Hypomagnesemia. Hypomagnesemia is associated with symptoms such as cramping or spasms, often carpal-pedal. Hypomagnesemia is associated with alcoholism and seen in association with hypokalemia.

2. A) Order intravenous (IV) magnesium 6 g now to infuse over 8 hours. This is a critically low magnesium level associated with hypokalemia and requires IV replacement because oral magnesium replacement is unpredictably absorbed. The magnesium level is less than 1 mg/dL due to high-dose diuretic use and is associated with hypokalemia, indicating 4–8 g IV replacement should be ordered. This must be infused slowly over 8 to 12 hours because magnesium is distributed very slowly and the excess will be excreted by the kidneys if infused quickly. Always repeat magnesium levels after infusions and repeat as indicated.

HYPONATREMIA

1. B) 3% sodium 100-mL bolus now over 20 minutes, then reassess both serum sodium and neurologic exam; may repeat ×2 if still symptomatic and if sodium level has not improved by 4 to 6 mEq/L from baseline. This is acute severe hyponatremia with moderately severe symptoms, which indicates emergency treatment. The patient is solute-depleted due to vomiting and diuretics with preserved total body water. Sodium should be acutely replaced to improve symptoms to target sodium increased by 5% or by 4 to 6 mEq/L. Monitor sodium levels frequently to avoid overcorrection too quickly; never raise the sodium faster than by 10 mEq/L the first day or 8 mEq/L on subsequent days for acute hyponatremia.

HYPOPHOSPHATEMIA

1. A) Sodium phosphate 40 mmol IV once over 6 hours. Repeat serum phosphorous level every day with labs. Replace phosphorous now with sodium phosphate because potassium (as part of the basic metabolic panel) is normal. The initial recommended dose for hypophosphatemia in a 90-kg patient is 14.4 (0.16 mmol/kg) to 22.5 (0.25 mmol/kg) mmol, but this patient is symptomatic and unable to wean from the vent. In this case, you can use up to 45 mmol (0.5 mmol/kg). Give this as a one-time dose slowly over 4 to 6 hours and redose as indicated based on repeated serum phosphorous levels.

METABOLIC ACIDOSIS

1. A) Gastrointestinal (GI) loss such as vomiting. GI loss is associated with loss of bicarbonate. The other options occur due to excess acid.

2. A) Hyperventilation. Acidosis is a strong stimulant to the respiratory center in the medulla. It triggers hyperventilation in an effort to normalize acidotic levels. Hypoventilation is associated with metabolic alkalosis. Confusion and anxiety do not serve as compensatory responses to acidosis.

NEPHROLITHIASIS

1. D) CT of the abdomen/pelvis, without IV contrast. A noncontrast CT scan of the abdomen looking for possible nephrolithiasis commonly follows a stone protocol and is the "gold standard" for evaluating possible kidney stones. The sensitivity of CT in detecting kidney stones is the highest of all radiologic tests, in part because kidney stones have a distinctly different composition compared with the surrounding tissue and absorb considerably more radiation and so are easily identified without the need for contrast. Since kidney stones absorb so much radiation, this allows for the overall use of lower radiation exposure (30 mAs or lower, compared with standard CT of 100 mAs); hence, the term *stone protocol* is used when ordering the test. Besides the lack of need for intravenous (IV) contrast to visualize the kidney stones, in this particular case the patient's elevated serum creatinine level (1.8) puts him at risk for a contrast-induced acute kidney injury (AKI) if IV contrast dye would be used. A renal ultrasound would be a good alternative choice if there was a concern for radiation exposure, for instance in a pregnant female. Ultrasonography also makes use of the tangible differences between stones and the surrounding tissue to visualize any stones present. Besides the lack of radiation exposure, ultrasound also has an advantage in that it provides for a portable or bedside exam versus a fixed CT scanner. Overall, however, ultrasounds are currently less sensitive and specific than CT imaging in detecting and sizing stones. A standard radiologic kidney, ureter, bladder (KUB) film uses radiation to expose a stone, but in a single plane versus multiple/three-dimensional (3D) planes compared with a CT exam, and therefore the sensitivity and specificity are much lower. Consequently, it is not as good at providing the exact location of the stones, although for patients with known stones it can be utilized for serial documentation and monitoring purposes.

PROSTATITIS

1. B) Order a CT scan of the pelvis. Order a CT scan of the pelvis to rule out a prostatic abscess. The patient is on day 3 of appropriate, culture-specific antibiotics,r

and is not responding well to treatment. He also had a recent procedure which should raise suspicion for abscess. A renal/bladder ultrasound would not likely diagnose a prostatic abscess. However, a transrectal ultrasound would identify abscess/collection if CT imaging is not available. At this time, adding vancomycin is not needed based on his current urine cultures and may increase future antibiotic resistance. Repeating another urine culture is a good choice for fever workup but not likely to change treatment plan.

PYELONEPHRITIS

1. D) Gentamicin. The patient is exhibiting symptoms of acute pyelonephritis based on the presence of white blood cell (WBC) casts in the urine. There is also presence of nitrites in her urine, which is most likely indicative of a gram-negative bacterial organism. Vancomycin and ampicillin cover mostly gram-positive organisms. Macrobid is an oral antibiotic that does not penetrate the kidney well. Gentamicin will cover the suspected gram-negative organism that is most likely causing this patient's infection.

URINARY INCONTINENCE

1. C) Bladder ultrasound/postvoid residual. A basic metabolic panel would reveal acute kidney injury but would not determine the cause of the patient's incontinence. A CT scan of the abdomen/pelvis could rule out bladder or kidney stones, but the patient's history is not indicative of calculus. A cystoscopy may eventually be warranted but is not cost-effective. The best choice is bladder ultrasound/postvoid residual. This would be easy to obtain and will rule out overflow incontinence due to possible bladder outlet obstruction.

DYSURIA

1. D) Fosfomycin 3 g orally as a single dose. The patient should be presumed pregnant until a confirmed repeat negative urine pregnancy test. Bactrim and nitrofurantoin are to be avoided during the first trimester of pregnancy. Ciprofloxacin is pregnancy category C and should be avoided during pregnancy. Fosfomycin as a single dose is safe during pregnancy and is a first-line antibiotic for treatment of a urinary tract infection.

CHAPTER 6

UNRESPONSIVENESS AFTER CARDIAC ARREST

1. B) Load with Keppra. This is a typical presentation of anoxic brain injury. Once the airway is secured, CT of the head should be performed to rule out underlying hemorrhage. It is common for the initial CT of the head to be normal, but after several days it may show brain edema with loss of gray/white matter differentiation. For this reason, MRI of the brain is not necessary at the time of admission. Jerking movements are suspicious for a clinical seizure, aborted by Ativan, so the next appropriate step would be to load with an antiepileptic drug (AED) such as Keppra. Continuous EEG should be ordered but should not delay medical management of seizure. Targeted temperature management is appropriate, but the patient is already hypothermic, so there is no need to initiate targeted temperature management (TTM), but rather continue for a 24-hour period before rewarming.

BRAIN DEATH

1. B) Order ancillary brain death testing. This scenario shows the progression of anoxic brain injury complicated by status epilepticus leading to suspected brain death. It is common for the initial CT of the head to be normal, but after several days it may show brain edema with loss of gray/white matter differentiation. EEG confirmation of termination of status epilepticus and no further seizure activity despite being off midazolam and ketamine infusions suggest additional antiepileptics are not required. An MRI of the brain without contrast is not the appropriate study as it does not evaluate cerebral blood flow to confirm brain death. Repeating the clinical brain death exam is likely to be inconclusive in this situation. The most appropriate next step would be to order ancillary brain death testing to confirm the diagnosis.

FOUR DAYS OF HEADACHE

1. B) Admit to the hospital for IV antiemetics, dihydroergotamine, and steroids. This case scenario is typical for status migrainosus. This is defined by a migraine attack, with or without aura, that is unremitting for greater than 72 hours and with pain and/or associated symptoms that are debilitating. In general, status migrainosus can be managed on an outpatient basis with prescriptions for nausea, pain, and sleep. However, if there is intractable pain or vomiting, IV hydration, dihydroergotamine (DHE), and steroids are indicated and best achieved by admission to the hospital. DHE is safe to give in this patient as the last triptan dose was greater than 24 hours prior to presentation. Ketorolac and diphenhydramine are a good start to try to abort the migraine in the ED; however, this patient demonstrates signs and symptoms of dehydration and at this point would benefit from a higher level of care and not be discharged home. Lumbar puncture is not indicated as there are no signs of infection or raised intracranial pressure. 100% oxygen is used as an abortive treatment for cluster headache.

INTRAPARENCHYMAL HEMORRHAGE

1. C) Initiate strict blood pressure control and start nicardipine drip as needed. The priority intervention in this patient is to achieve strict blood pressure control; the recommended range would be systolic blood pressure (SBP) <140. The use of nicardipine drip or clevidipine drip is as needed. The goal of strict blood pressure control is to reduce the risk of hemorrhagic expansion. A repeat CT of the head should be performed within 6 hours of admission in order to assess the stability of the hemorrhage. Seizure prophylaxis is not routinely recommended for patients with cerebellar hemorrhages, but should be considered if witness or clinical suspicion of seizures is present. Neurosurgery should be consulted for surgical evaluation, but given the patient's neurologic exam this can be done on a routine basis.

RIGHT-SIDED HEMIPLEGIA

1. B) Order CT of the head with CT angiography (CTA) of the head and neck. In this scenario, CT of the head should be done immediately since stroke is in the differential diagnosis. If there is no hemorrhage, intravenous (IV) tissue plasminogen activator (tPA) can be started immediately if there are no exclusion criteria. Noncontrast CT of the head should be followed immediately by a CT angiogram of the head and neck to look for a large cerebral vessel occlusion to determine if there is a role for mechanical thrombectomy. Given the patient's National Institutes of Health Stroke Scale (NIHSS) score and history of atrial fibrillation, but being off anticoagulation, there is high suspicion for a large vessel occlusion from a cardioembolic source. Lab draw should not delay CT imaging and can be done after the patient returns from the scanner. MRI of the brain would take too long to determine life-saving interventions such as tPA and thrombectomy. Although the patient is in atrial fibrillation, his rate is less than 120 and he is hemodynamically stable and therefore does not need IV metoprolol, which would be used to treat atrial fibrillation (Afib) with rapid ventricular response (RVR).

STATUS EPILEPTICUS

1. B) Initiate a midazolam drip. This is a common scenario of status epilepticus as a complication of anoxic brain injury. Jerking movements are suspicious for a clinical seizure, treated with an appropriate dose of lorazepam and levetiracetam load without resolution. This should prompt the practitioner to progress to the next tier of treatment, and in this case a midazolam drip would be the best option. Continuous EEG should be ordered but should not delay medical management of seizure. Targeted temperature management is appropriate, but the patient is already hypothermic, so there is no need to initiate targeted temperature management (TTM), but rather continue for a 24-hour period before rewarming. Further evaluation with an MRI of the brain with or without contrast may be helpful with prognostication, but is not a priority intervention in a patient that is clinically unstable.

TRANSIENT LEFT FACE AND ARM WEAKNESS

1. C) Admit to the hospital for further workup of a suspected transient ischemic attack (TIA). This patient presented with symptoms of a right middle cerebral artery (MCA) stroke, which resolved in less than 24 hours, consistent with TIA. She has multiple risk factors for TIA and is at high risk for stroke in the coming days. She should be admitted to the hospital for further workup, including CT of the head, MRI of the brain, vessel imaging, and lab work. She should be started on antiplatelet and anticholesterol medications. She should be counseled on lifestyle changes, including smoking cessation. While complex migraine can cause stroke-like symptoms, the patient's headache is mild and she does not have a history of migraine. As her symptoms resolved by the time she arrived at the ED, she would not meet the criteria for tissue plasminogen activator (tPA). CT of the head alone is not sufficient for TIA workup.

CHAPTER 7

CARDIAC ARREST

1. C) Catheters are associated with higher rates of deep vein thrombosis (DVT) than surface cooling devices. Catheters are associated with higher rates of DVT than surface cooling devices.

CHAPTER 8

ADRENAL INSUFFICIENCY

1. C) Adrenocorticotrophic hormone (ACTH). ACTH will differentiate between primary AI (PAI) and secondary or tertiary causes. PAI is the only type that will lead to elevated ACTH levels. This is due to the increased demand from the pituitary (ACTH) for the adrenal gland to produce cortisol and the adrenal gland is not working due to an autoimmune destruction. Cortisol levels remain low and ACTH levels rise, typically at least 2× the normal. Cortisol levels, results of the stimulation test, and signs and symptoms can be similar in all types of adrenal insufficiency.

2. D) Use of fludrocortisone. The use of fludrocortisone is essential for most patients with primary adrenal insufficiency (PAI) due to the loss of aldosterone production in addition to steroids. This can be evaluated by checking serum aldosterone, sodium, and potassium. Patients who need mineralocorticoid treatment will have a low serum aldosterone, low sodium, and high potassium levels.

3. E) All of the above. All of these conditions put patients at higher risk for adrenal insufficiency (AI), and clinicians should remain attuned to the possibility, especially if they present with signs/symptoms consistent with AI.

4. A) Hydrocortisone is generally preferred for most patients. Hydrocortisone is generally the preferred medication for most patients due to the physiologic similarity to endogenous insulin production (short half-life). Patients can take it twice a day with higher doses in the morning and lower doses in the afternoon to mimic a normal circadian rhythm. Patients should use the lowest dose possible while maintaining normal metabolism. If patients are taking the equivalent of endogenous steroid replacement, they will not be at excess risk for bone loss or diabetes, assuming other risk factors are not present.

DIABETES MELLITUS: TYPE 1

1. C) Weight loss and ketonuria. Type 1 diabetics present with recent history of unintentional weight loss and ketonuria. Type 2 diabetics typically endorse uncontrolled weight gain and do not have the presence of ketonuria on admission.

2. C) Greater than or equal to 6.5. In addition to a fasting glucose test greater than 126 mg/dL and a 2-hour oral glucose test greater than 200 mg/dL, a hemoglobin A1C (HgA1C) of 6.5 or greater will confirm the diagnosis of diabetes mellitus.

3. B) Insulin. The mainstay of treatment for type 1 diabetes is tight serum glucose control with insulin. Type 1 diabetes cannot be controlled with oral medications (e.g., metformin) and diet modifications, as it is possible in some patients with type 2 diabetes.

4. B) The 50/50 Rule. Insulin administration for type 1 diabetics should follow the 50/50 Rule: 50% of the daily required insulin is administered as a basal dose (long-acting insulin) dose and the remaining 50% of the daily required insulin intake is to be administered in three equal prandial doses with meals (short-acting insulin).

DIABETES MELLITUS: TYPE 2

1. B) Absence of ketones in unstable angina (UA). Type 2 diabetes and type 1 diabetes can appear similar on presentation; however, the absence of ketones detected in UA is suggestive of type 2 diabetes. Type 1 diabetics typically present with ketonuria.

2. B) Greater than 50%. 90% to 95% of all cases of diabetes in the United States are type 2 diabetes.

3. B) Metformin. Metformin is in a class of medications called biguanides and is considered the first-line treatment for newly diagnosed type 2 diabetes.

4. C) Rule of 15. The Rule of 15: Consume 15 g of carbohydrates every 15 minutes until glucose is above 70 mg/dL (e.g., ½ cup soda, ½ cup juice, glucose gel, glucose tablets).

DIABETIC KETOACIDOSIS

1. A) Anion gap metabolic acidosis. Diabetic ketoacidosis is diagnosed by the triad of urine analysis with a large amount of ketones, hyperglycemia, and anion gap metabolic acidosis.

2. B) IV fluids and insulin glucose tolerance test (GTT). After identifying diabetic ketoacidosis (DKA) as the cause of the patient's condition, the mainstays of treatment are intravenous fluids and insulin diabetic ketoacidosis test (GTT). Additionally, treat the underlying cause and correct electrolyte imbalances. In this case, the underlying cause is a viral illness.

3. A) Adults with type 1 diabetes. Diabetic ketoacidosis (DKA) is predominantly seen in adults with type 1 diabetes under the age of 45 years old. Adults under the age of 45 years with type 2 diabetes are the second most common population to present with DKA.

4. D) Greater than 250 mg/dL. Serum glucose levels of 250 mg/dL are indicative of diabetic ketoacidosis (DKA). Some DKA patients can have a serum glucose as high as 800 mg/dL, but this is rare. Serum glucose greater than 600 mg/dL is typically indicative of a hyperglycemic hyperosmolar state (HHS) diagnosis.

HYPERGLYCEMIC HYPEROSMOLAR STATE

1. C) Dilantin. Dilantin or phenytoin can inhibit endogenous insulin secretion. Patients taking Dilantin are at a rare but increased risk of developing hyperglycemic hyperosmolar state (HHS).

2. A) Blood glucose (BG) >800 and no ketones present in urinalysis. Diabetic ketoacidosis (DKA) rarely presents with a serum glucose level >800, and ketonuria is a hallmark feature of DKA. The fact that this patient's serum glucose was 957 mg/dL and there was no evidence of ketonuria point to a diagnosis of hyperglycemic hyperosmolar state (HHS).

3. C) Large volume fluid replacement, insulin glucose tolerance test (GTT), electrolyte repletion. In hyperglycemic hyperosmolar state (HHS), it is critical to replete fluid volume at the same time as using insulin in these patients, as insulin without concomitant vigorous fluid replacement increases the risk of shock. HHS patients can have as much as 10-L fluid deficit. Electrolytes should be repleted and checked routinely every 2 to 4 hours.

4. C) Develops over days to week. The development of hyperglycemic hyperosmolar state (HHS) is typically secondary to infection, cerebrovascular accident (CVA), myocardial infarction (MI), trauma, or alteration in/starting new medications. The condition slowly develops over days to week prior to a change in level of consciousness.

METABOLIC SYNDROME

1. A) Insulin resistance syndrome. Despite being a known type 2 diabetic who has been regularly taking insulin, the patient has developed metabolic syndrome or insulin resistance syndrome. This patient is at increased risk of developing cardiovascular disease.

2. A) Blood pressure (BP) 172/86, fasting glucose 200, diabetes mellitus type 2 (DM2). Metabolic syndrome is confirmed when a patient presents with three or more criteria: Waist circumference greater than 40 in. in men, greater than 35 in. in women; triglyceride level of 150 mg/dL; high-density lipoprotein (HDL) below 40 mg/dL in men and below 50 mg/dL in women; blood pressure above 130/85 mmHg; and fasting glucose greater than 100 mg/dL.

3. A) Diet and lifestyle modifications. In some incidence of metabolic syndrome, the addition of medications can reduce the risk of developing type 2 diabetes. However, the first-line treatment is diet and lifestyle modifications aimed at weight loss and increased activity.

4. D) >65 years old. The risk of metabolic syndrome increases with age.

PHEOCHROMOCYTOMA

1. A) Paroxysmal symptoms. Paroxysmal symptoms are a key finding in pheochromocytoma. Weight loss is common. Hyperthyroidism would be a very rare cofinding, although the symptoms overlap and the patient should be screened. Generally, symptoms do not improve with rest since they are hormonally driven (not stress related).

2. A) Discuss changing her medications for a time period before hormonal testing is completed. The patient is on three different medications that can interfere with the catecholamine test. If there is high suspicion for pheochromocytoma and the situation is more urgent, then abdominal CT scan can be done first. Typically, if prudent to wait, the best approach would be to change her medications for a time period (2 weeks) and then order plasma or urine metanephrines in the outpatient setting. If this patient is admitted for another reason, then the workup should be deferred to the outpatient setting.

3. A) Patients require both beta-adrenergic and alpha-adrenergic blockade to prevent severe hypertension or cardiopulmonary crisis perioperatively. Combined alpha- and beta-adrenergic blockade is standard treatment for pheochromocytoma to avoid perioperative hypertensive crisis that can be caused by unopposed beta-blockade.

PREDIABETES

1. B) Prediabetes. The patient's elevated body mass index (BMI), undiagnosed obstructive sleep apnea (OSA), hypertension, and lab results are all indicative of a diagnosis of prediabetes. Fortunately, this patient required admission to the hospital for catheterization and was able to be diagnosed and seen by endocrinology services and diabetes education team.

2. A) Diet and lifestyle modifications. Treating cardiovascular risks (hypertension [HTN], hyperlipidemia [HLD]), weight loss, increased activity, improved nutrition, and healthy sleep habits can reduce the risk of prediabetes progressing to type 2 diabetes.

3. B) Body mass index (BMI) ≥25 kg/m². Patients with a BMI ≥25 kg/m² have up to 24% chance of developing type 2 diabetes within 5 years.

4. B) Metformin. Metformin, in addition to weight loss and lifestyle modifications, may reduce the risk of type 2 diabetes mellitus in prediabetes patients by up to 30%.

THYROID DISORDER: EUTHYROID SICK SYNDROME

1. B) Consult endocrinology. A consult for endocrinology service is required for urgent evaluation and should not be treated by advanced practice provider (APP) alone. Treatment is not straightforward in the absence of a diagnosis of primary hypothyroidism.

2. C) Euthyroid sick syndrome. The working diagnosis for this patient is euthyroid sick syndrome or nonthyroidal illness syndrome, given the recent major surgery and prolonged critical illness, with no evidence of primary or secondary thyroid dysfunction.

3. A) Treat and manage underlying illness. Thyroid replacement is rarely indicated and could cause further complications and increased mortality. Repeat thyroid tests, as an outpatient, 2 to 3 months after complete recovery.

4. D) 2 to 3 months after recovery. Repeat testing should be avoided as the treatment for euthyroid sick syndrome is to treat the underlying disease and the levels are not expected to return to the patient's normal until 2 to 3 months after complete recovery from the underlying illness and hospitalization.

THYROID DISORDER: HYPERTHYROIDISM

1. B) Thyroid storm. Diagnosed in patients presenting with anxiety, delirium, and altered level of consciousness. These symptoms, in the presence of significantly elevated free triiodothyronine (FT3) and free thyroxine (FT4), require immediate attention with a thioamide.

2. A) Dantrolene. Dantrolene is the treatment for malignant hyperthermia and is not a treatment for hyperthyroidism. Malignant hyperthermia is a rare life-threatening emergency that occurs as a reaction to anesthesia. Hyperthyroidism which progresses to thyroid storm under anesthesia can be mistaken for malignant hyperthermia.

3. C) Graves disease. Graves disease is an autoimmune disorder in which thyroid-stimulating hormone (TSH) receptor antibodies stimulate the overproduction of thyroid hormone and thyroid gland growth.

4. A) Tracheal compression by goiter. Tracheal compression by goiter would warrant further CT and anesthesia evaluation for concerns of difficult intubation and airway compromise.

THYROID DISORDER: HYPOTHYROIDISM

1. C) Thyroid-stimulating hormone (TSH). The patient's TSH is significantly elevated, which is indicative of hypothyroidism.

2. D) Levothyroxine. The standard of care for treatment of hypothyroidism is levothyroxine. This medication has a long half-life, a low side effect profile, easily absorbed, and is relatively cost-effective.

3. D) 1 hour before breakfast. For maximum absorption, levothyroxine should be taken on an empty stomach with no food for 1 hour after ingestion and no other supplements for 4 hours after ingestion.

4. C) Every 6 weeks. Lab values should be monitored every 6 weeks until acceptable thyroid-stimulating hormone (TSH) levels have been reached. Once a patient has achieved a safe and stable TSH level, the testing can be pushed out to every 3 to 6 months.

THYROID DISORDER: MYXEDEMA COMA

1. C) Myxedema coma. Given a medical history of hypothyroidism, prolonged hospitalization, infection, surgery secondary to trauma, and the patient's inability to maintain compliance with taking her levothyroxine, there is a high suspicion for myxedema coma given the acute change in clinical condition.

2. B) IV thyroid hormone. The gold standard for treatment of myxedema coma is intravenous (IV) thyroid hormone replacement, in coordination with slow rewarming via a rewarming blanket and IV fluids.

3. E) All of the above. All of these factors put patients at higher risk for developing myxedema coma. However, the incidence is rare.

4. A) Concomitant adrenal insufficiency. Due to lack of circulating thyroid hormone, patients with myxedema coma can experience adrenal insufficiency. This must be addressed and treated for best outcomes. Adrenal insufficiency is treated with intravenous (IV) administration of hydrocortisone every 8 hours until resolved.

THYROID DISORDER: THYROID STORM

1. C) Thyroid storm. The patient's lab values for free T4 and free T3 are exceeding normal lab values. The higher than normal thyroid hormone values, in addition to agitation, anxiety, and lethargy, are concerning for thyroid storm, which requires immediate treatment.

2. B) Burch–Wartofsky Point Scale (BWPS). The BWPS is a tool used to determine true thyroid storm and other biochemical thyrotoxicosis. A higher score (>45) is indicative of thyroid storm; a score of 25 to 44 can be suggestive of imminent storm; a score of <25 rules out thyroid storm.

3. D) Propylthiouracil (PTU). PTU is a thionamide that blocks the conversion of free T4 to T3.

4. A) Thyroidectomy. The definitive treatment is thyroidectomy following the resolution of acute thyrotoxicosis.

CHAPTER 9

BIPOLAR DISORDER

1. C) Bipolar disorder. The most important diagnosis to rule out is bipolar I. Many factors in this case suggest mania, including the roommate thinking she is out of control, poor intake associated with poor sleep for the past 3 days, and signs of paranoia, which could indicate mania associated with psychosis. Dehydration is often common in bipolar mania as patients are goal-oriented and may not be able to take care of self-care needs such as eating, drinking, or bathing. It is important to recognize the potential for activation of underlying bipolar when treated with antidepressant medications, especially selective serotonin reuptake inhibitors (SSRIs). The appropriate course of action in this case would include discontinuation of the SSRI, hydration, and lab monitoring for electrolyte imbalance and/or substance use/intoxication. It is important to know that if mania resolves after SSRI is discontinued, then it is likely not bipolar I, rather mania induced by medication and/or substance. However, if it persists, the patient would likely meet the criteria for bipolar I and this would be her first manic episode.

CHAPTER 10

COLITIS: INFECTIVE

1. A) Complete blood count (CBC), comprehensive metabolic panel (CMP), stool polymerase chain reaction (PCR). The patient is exhibiting signs of severe disease, with more than 7 days of symptoms, and meeting systemic inflammatory response syndrome (SIRS) criteria. CT of the abdomen may be helpful in ruling out complications. More than 82% of community-acquired clinical documentation inquiries (CDI) have some form of healthcare exposure other than hospitalization.

2. B) Bolus patient with IV fluids and trend lactate and vital signs (VS). The patient is meeting systemic inflammatory response syndrome (SIRS) criteria with elevated heart rate (HR) and respiratory rate, and sepsis protocol should be initiated. SIRS is likely is due to dehydration and not bacteremia, but blood cultures ×2 should be drawn before specific antibiotic treatment is started.

3. A) Loperamide. Treatment for severe *Clostridioides difficile* should include all but loperamide.

4. D) Take the entire course of vancomycin and return to primary care provider (PCP) if symptoms recur. Recurrence rates with clinical documentation inquiries (CDI) are high, even with community-acquired CDI (28%). Antidiarrheals may lead to toxic megacolon with CDI. Retesting is not recommended in patients who are asymptomatic.

ENCEPHALITIS

1. A) Lumbar puncture (LP). Neuroimaging is indicated prior to LP in patients with Glasgow Coma Scale (GCS) score <12, focal neurologic signs, presence of papilledema, and new or uncontrolled seizures. These findings could indicate the presence of a space-occupying lesion. LP in the presence of a space-occupying lesion may result in brain herniation and death. The initial neuroimaging choice is a noncontrast head CT. If the CT shows no acute processes, an LP can be performed for cerebrospinal fluid (CSF) sampling. MRI and PET scans are time-consuming and may delay the needed treatment. They may be performed at a later date to confirm suspected diagnosis but are not the initial diagnostic tests.

2. C) Broad-spectrum antibiotics plus acyclovir should be started once cerebrospinal fluid (CSF) results are obtained. Based on the patient's presentation and history, the suspected diagnosis is a neuroinfection, likely encephalitis. Treatment should not be delayed until CSF results are returned as outcomes are worse when treatment is delayed. Broad-spectrum antibiotics *plus* acyclovir (to cover for possible herpes simplex virus [HSV] encephalitis) should be started empirically. Medications are tailored once the results are available. Not all patients with encephalitis will need a hemicraniectomy, so neurosurgery consultation at this time is not indicated. The patient does not need to be placed on contact isolation.

INFLUENZA

1. D) No. She is presenting too late to place her on the recommended therapies for influenza, and a positive test would not change my targeted therapy. Targeted influenza treatments need to be started within 48 hours of symptom onset and provide maximum efficacy when started within 30 hours. The exception to this would be a medically complex patient with significant symptoms after consultation with an infectious disease provider. This patient does not fit this category. Therefore, testing this patient would not change management, and supportive care is best used.

2. D) No. She is outside of the recommended window to begin antivirals for influenza. This patient presents outside of the window of within 48 hours of symptom onset and therapy should not be started.

3. A) Yes. Her reported symptoms of adverse reaction are mild and do not represent a medical contraindication to influenza vaccination. All individuals over the age of 6 months should receive the influenza vaccine unless they have had a severe allergic reaction to prior influenza vaccine (this does not include minor flu-like symptoms) or a severe allergic reaction to egg proteins if receiving the live attenuated vaccine (nasal). Also of note, immunocompromised patients, pregnant women, and patients 50 years of age or older should not receive live attenuated vaccine.

4. B) She may have acute seroconversion given her recent multiple partners and should be tested for HIV based on her social history inquiry. Cytomegalovirus (CMV) mostly occurs in immunocompromised individuals. The patient is not sick enough based on this presentation to warrant a respiratory panel and admission to the hospital. She is out of the season for West Nile virus and her presentation is not consistent with this diagnosis. Acute seroconversion should be considered and HIV testing may be warranted. This typically presents similarly to an acute viral illness. She has had several new partners and would be at risk for this diagnosis.

MENINGITIS

1. C) Turbid appearance, white blood cell (WBC) 2,000/mm³ (predominantly neutrophils), protein 250 mg/dL, glucose 20 mg/dL. The suspected diagnosis is bacterial meningitis based on presentation and history. Cerebrospinal fluid (CSF) results in option C are consistent with bacterial meningitis. Option A is a normal CSF result. Option B is consistent with viral meningitis. Option D is consistent with a fungal meningitis.

2. C) Empiric treatment should include coverage for *Listeria monocytogenes*. The suspected diagnosis is bacterial meningitis. The patient presents with fever, headache, nuchal rigidity, and lethargy, all four classic signs of bacterial meningitis. Although only 45% will have all four of these findings, at least two of the findings will be present in 95% of patients with bacterial meningitis. Empiric antibiotics should be started within 1 hour to prevent significant morbidity and mortality associated with delay in treatment. The patient is older than 60 years however and so the causative organism is more likely to be *Listeria monocytogenes*. Therefore, coverage must include ceftriaxone, vancomycin *and* ampicillin for *L. monocytogenes*. Coverage of all close contacts is only necessary if the causative organism is *Neisseria meningitidis*, and with absence of petechial rash it is unlikely. Supportive care is appropriate for viral meningitis, not bacterial meningitis.

NECROTIZING FASCIITIS

1. A) *Streptococcus pyogenes*. Among the choices, only *S. pyogenes (group A streptococci)* is known to cause necrotizing fasciitis. Three other pathogens are also known, including *Staphylococcus aureus* and *Clostridium per-fringens*. *Ornithodoros moubata* transmits African swine fever. It is not associated with necrotizing fasciitis. Neither *Listeria* or *Leishmania* are associated with necrotizing fasciitis.

2. C) Immediate surgical debridement. The only known cure for necrotizing fasciitis is surgical debridement. Mortality increases exponentially based on delay of surgery. Antibiotics are important in survival but are not as effective as surgery. Antibiotics alone cannot treat necrotizing fasciitis.

OSTEOMYELITIS

1. D) Secondary disease. The index of suspicion for osteomyelitis should be higher in patients with underlying conditions, including poorly controlled diabetes mellitus, neuropathy, peripheral vascular disease, chronic or ulcerated wounds, history of recent trauma, sickle cell disease, history of implanted orthopedic hardware, or history or suspicion of intravenous drug use.

2. C) *Staphylococcus aureus*. Methicillin-sensitive *S. aureus* is the most frequently identified pathogen across all types of osteomyelitis, followed by *Pseudomonas aeruginosa* and methicillin-resistant *S. aureus*. Microbial causes of osteomyelitis in adults may originate from distance foci of infection, such as skin abscesses or endocarditis, indwelling vascular catheters, or injection drug use.

3. A) Back pain. A diagnosis of osteomyelitis should be considered in any patient with acute onset or progressive worsening of musculoskeletal pain accompanied by constitutional symptoms such as fever, malaise, lethargy, and irritability.

4. B) Erythrocyte sedimentation rate (ESR). Initial laboratory evaluation should include a complete blood count, ESR, C-reactive protein, and blood cultures.

PERITONITIS

1. C) CT angiography (CTA). CTA is ordered as at this point the patient is not showing signs or symptoms of sepsis. The patient's only concerning objective sign is hypoxia. Pain medicine was decreased to oral Tylenol and the patient was tolerating pain. The patient's newly prescribed Eliquis was held for surgery. The patient has no tachycardia; he was started on metoprolol, so tachycardia is unlikely, but there is concern for postoperative pulmonary embolism (PE).

2. B) No. Although the patient's labs and vital signs have been stable for 3 days, his clinical condition is gradually deteriorating and he now has an elevated right hemidiaphragm. He has elevated blood glucose and is hypothermic. The patient is unlikely to meet systemic inflammatory response syndrome (SIRS) criteria due to oxygen supplementation, beta-blocker therapy, and ongoing PO antibiotic treatment.

3. D) Uptitrate antibiotic therapy. Increase antibiotic therapy. Clinically, the patient shows secondary peritonitis, with firm abdomen and increasing pain with palpation and movement. The patient has elevated blood glucose and hypothermia and continuing elevated white blood cell (WBC). The patient should be started on ceftizone 2 g daily and Flagyl.

SYSTEMIC INFLAMMATORY RESPONSE SYNDROME/BACTEREMIA/SEPSIS

1. A) Initiate epinephrine IV for hypotension when IV crystalloids have failed to resuscitate. Based on the International Guidelines for Management of Sepsis and Septic Shock (2021), norepinephrine, not epinephrine, is the drug of choice to use in septic shock. Broad-spectrum antimicrobials, not beta-lactams, are recommended to start with, and enteral, not parenteral, nutrition is the method of feeding that is recommended if the patient is unable to take oral feedings. In addition, the question asks for definitive treatment, which in this case would be a surgical consult for incision and drainage of the wound.

RIGHT KNEE PAIN

1. B) Rheumatoid disease. Patients with rheumatoid disease, including rheumatoid arthritis, are at increased risk of septic arthritis than the general population due to joint damage and immunosuppression.

2. D) Prothrombin time (PT) and partial thromboplastin time (PTT). Aspiration of synovial fluid is the criterion and "gold standard" for diagnosis. White blood cell (WBC) count with differential, Gram stain, and culture are important in making the diagnosis of septic arthritis.

3. C) *Staphylococcus aureus*. The most common cause of septic arthritis is *S. aureus*, which accounts for 52% of cases. Many are a result of staphylococcal infection or transient bacteremia from skin or mucous membrane sources.

4. A) Vancomycin. Vancomycin is generally the initial antibiotic used especially in areas where methicillin-resistant *Staphylococcus aureus* (MRSA) is increased. If the patient is immunocompromised or an intravenous (IV) drug abuser, then vancomycin plus third-generation cephalosporin is recommended.

TUBERCULOSIS

1. B) INH + rifampin (RIF) + pyrazinamide (PZA) + EMB for 2 months. Based on the Infectious Diseases Society of America (IDSA) guidelines, this patient is categorized as in the intensive phase and the four-drug combination is recommended for 2 months because new tuberculosis cases worldwide may be caused by organisms that are resistant to isoniazid (INH) alone. It is recommended to follow susceptibilities, and if it is found that the active organism is susceptible to INH then ethambutol (EMB) can be discontinued.

CHAPTER 12

ANEMIA

1. A) Chronic blood loss associated with nonsteroidal anti-inflammatory drug (NSAID) use. Given the insidious nature of the patient's symptoms and regular use of NSAIDs, the most likely cause of the patient's ▶

symptoms is chronic blood loss associated with gastro-intestinal bleeding.

2. A) Anemia associated with renal insufficiency and B) An undiagnosed gastrointestinal (GI) malignancy. The most likely differential diagnoses include anemia associated with renal disease. The patient's age and history of diabetes increase the risk of renal insufficiency. The likelihood of malignancy increases with age, and GI malignancy may be associated with chronic blood loss with insidious onset of anemia symptoms.

3. B) Making sure the patient is hemodynamically stable before planning any procedures. The patient's history of coronary artery disease and new onset of chest pain put him at increased risk for an acute cardiac event. Before any invasive procedure, the provider should assess for hemodynamic stability.

4. A) Adequate iron stores, B) Renal function, C) Risk factors for venous thrombosis, and D) Risk factors for stroke. All of the options are correct. For adequate red blood cell production to occur, the body's iron stores must be adequate. Renal function plays a role in the ability to produce endogenous erythropoietin and may influence the dose needed. Erythropoiesis-stimulating factors have been associated with increased risk of thrombosis; therefore, the provider should assess for preexisting risk factors for thrombotic events.

BLEEDING DIATHESES

1. B) Immune thrombocytopenic purpura. Immune thrombocytopenic purpura (ITP) is a result of antibodies that cause excessive platelet destruction. Primary ITP is an autoimmune disorder in which platelets are destroyed or platelet formation is inhibited. Secondary ITP may occur in association with autoimmune disease or chronic infection. Thrombotic thrombocytopenia purpura (TTP) occurs in combination with hemolytic anemia, renal insufficiency, fever, and neurologic changes. von Willebrand disease is a hereditary disorder and lack of family history of bleeding disorder makes this diagnosis less likely. Antiphospholipid antibody syndrome is associated with hypercoagulability and does not cause excessive bleeding.

2. A) TTP often presents with fever, renal failure, and hemolytic anemia. Thrombotic thrombocytopenia purpura (TTP) typically presents with concomitant fever, hemolytic anemia, low platelet count, as well as renal dysfunction and neurologic abnormalities. It can occur in individuals with autoimmune diseases and HIV infection as well as during pregnancy. Onset is abrupt and concomitant thrombosis can lead to significant complications.

3. A) Ibuprofen, C) Methotrexate, and D) Aspirin. Ibuprofen and aspirin are nonsteroidal anti-inflammatory drugs (NSAIDs) and are widely recognized as medications that can increase risk of bleeding. Methotrexate, a chemotherapeutic agent used in treatment of autoimmune disorders, is associated with bone marrow suppression and may increase risk of thrombocytopenia.

4. A) Monitor for changes in menstrual flow and report them to her healthcare provider and B) Notify her dentist about her condition before having any invasive procedures. The patient should continue to self-monitor for evidence of bleeding and notify her provider about any changes that signal a recurrence of thrombocytopenia. She should notify all of her healthcare providers about her condition, and any invasive procedures should be coordinated with her primary care providers to assess the risk of bleeding. There is no need for antibiotic prophylaxis with isolated thrombocytopenia. Prolonged sitting is a risk factor for deep vein thrombosis (DVT) and not a major concern with thrombocytopenia.

COAGULOPATHIES

1. A) Factor V Leiden. Factor V Leiden is a hereditary factor associated with risk of thrombosis.

2. A) An undiagnosed malignancy, B) Antiphospholipid antibodies, C) Coagulopathy associated with oral contraceptive use, and D) Thrombocytosis. An undiagnosed malignancy, such as breast cancer in an adult female, should be considered. Antiphospholipid antibodies syndrome is among the most common acquired coagulopathies and should be considered. Oral contraceptive increases risk of clotting, so a thorough review of the patient's medications is warranted. Thrombocytosis can be identified easily with complete blood count (CBC) and should be included in the differential diagnosis.

3. B) Myocardial infarction. Superior vena cava (SVC) occurs as a result of occlusion by a clot or external compression of the SVC. Arterial thrombosis in an extremity would result in pallor and coolness rather than warmth, erythema, and edema. Myocardial infarction may be a result of thrombus in a coronary artery.

4. A) Avoid prolonged immobility as this can increase risk of deep vein thrombosis (DVT), B) Maintain a healthy weight because obesity increases risk of blood clots, and C) Be sure to keep follow-up appointment with her provider for ongoing assessment. Immobility even with anticoagulation can increase the risk of clotting and should be avoided. Obesity increases the risk of clotting as well so achieving and maintaining a healthy weight should be encouraged. Ongoing evaluation of the patient's condition and monitoring the effectiveness of treatment are essential for safe care of patients receiving anticoagulant therapy. Regular follow-up should be encouraged. Individuals receiving anticoagulation therapy are at risk of bleeding and should use caution when engaging in activities that pose risk of injury. Providers should assess patients' activity level to identify potential risks.

DEEP VEIN THROMBOSIS

1. B) Venous stasis. The patient in the scenario has just returned from traveling on a long trans-oceanic flight. This type of travel is associated with venous stasis. Obesity further contributes to venous stasis.

2. B) Unilateral lower extremity edema, C) Recent orthopedic surgery, D) Recent prolonged travel with dependent lower extremities, and E) History of malignancy. Lower extremity deep vein thrombosis (DVT) most often presents with unilateral edema. Risk factors for DVT include malignancy, recent surgery, and prolonged travel.

3. A) Cellulitis and B) Lymphedema. Both cellulitis and lymphedema can present with unilateral edema. Peripheral arterial disease is less likely to present with edema. The likelihood of chronic venous insufficiency is low with no history of vascular problems.

4. A) Bleeding gums, B) Tarry stool, and C) Sudden onset of lightheadedness. Bleeding gums and tarry stools are obvious signs of bleeding. A sudden onset of lightheadedness can also be a symptom of active bleeding and patients should seek medical attention. A change in appetite is nonspecific and does not warrant immediate attention.

SICKLE CELL CRISIS

1. A) Infection, B) Dehydration, C) Excessive physical exertion, and D) Cigarette smoking. Infection, dehydration, tobacco smoke, and excessive exertion can all precipitate an acute pain episode in patients with sickle cell disease (SCD).

2. D) Patient-controlled analgesics allowing the patient to have control over when he receives the opioid analgesic and provide adequate relief. The patient is requiring medication with increased frequency to relieve his symptoms. As-needed doses are often insufficient to control severe pain. Regular intermittent dosing or continuous infusion with patient-controlled analgesia (PCA) at adequate dose and frequency provides the most even dosing and allows for optimal pain control.

3. D) Use of distraction techniques. Nonsteroidal anti-inflammatory drugs (NSAIDs) including ketorolac can contribute to impaired renal function in individuals with sickle cell disease. Application of ice may contribute to sickling of red blood cells (RBCs). Exchange transfusion is not indicated in most cases. Distraction techniques can contribute to pain relief and do not contribute to the side effects associated with opioid medications.

4. A) He should be advised to take a laxative on a regular basis to reduce risk of opioid-induced constipation, B) He should be advised to continue to drink sufficient amounts of liquids to maintain optimal hydration, and D) He should follow up with his primary care provider to make sure he is kept up to date on immunizations. Constipation is a frequent side effect of opioids, and patients taking opioids on a regular basis should take a laxative regularly to avoid constipation. Adequate hydration is a key component of health maintenance for individuals with sickle cell disease (SCD). Many patients with SCD have chronic pain at baseline and require opioids to carry out day-to-day activities. Abrupt cessation of opioids may cause acute withdrawal symptoms. Infection is often a trigger for acute pain episodes and patients should receive recommended immunizations to reduce risk of vaccine-preventable infections.

CHAPTER 13

ALTERED MENTAL STATUS

1. B) MRI of the brain with and without contrast. The next best test after CT of the head would be MRI of the brain with and without contrast. This can help differentiate between malignancy and infection (although not always). If malignancy, the MRI can detect if there are additional smaller lesions not seen on CT, which would suggest metastatic etiology. MRI also helps with neurosurgical planning if indicated. While continuous EEG should be performed during admission to evaluate for subclinical seizures, this is not the priority. If the patient did have evidence of rhythmic movements on exam in the ED, she should be treated clinically with a benzodiazepine. Given the history of twitching and temporal location of the tumor, she should be started on an antiepileptic drug (AED). CT of the chest, abdomen, and pelvis is helpful if there is suspicion for metastasis from a primary source, but is not the priority. One might expect to see enlarged lymph nodes or lesions in other organs such as lung and liver. This study should be done with contrast. CT angiogram of the head and neck is not clearly indicated in this case. The hypodense region in the left temporal lobe is due to vasogenic edema (swelling) from the tumor. The smaller hypodensity in the thalamus may represent an area of acute ischemia (stroke) but this would be due to mass effect from the tumor/swelling and not from an occlusion of the blood vessel from a clot.

CERVICAL CANCER

1. C) HPV 16 and 18. Most cases of cervical cancer are attributable to human papillomavirus (HPV) infection. The most common HPV types are 16, 18, 31, 33, 35, 45, 52, and 58. HPV 16 accounts for approximately 50% of cases and HPV 18 for 20%.

2. B) Rash. Recurrence rates for even stage I cervical cancer can range between 10% and 20%. During survivorship care, counseling should include review of common symptoms seen in recurrence since 46% to 95% of patients present with symptoms including vaginal bleeding or discharge, abdominal/pelvic pain, leg symptoms (lymphedema or pain), urinary symptoms, cough, and weight loss.

ENDOMETRIAL CANCER

1. A) Low body mass index (BMI). Typically with endometrial cancer, excess of endogenous (obesity) or exogenous estrogen without adequate opposition by a progestin is a main risk factor. Low BMI does not correlate with excess estrogen.

2. B) Postmenopausal bleeding. In endometrial cancer, the cardinal symptom is abnormal uterine bleeding. Most patients are diagnosed at an early stage, when the disease is still confined to the uterus.

OVARIAN CANCER

1. B) Genetic testing. The National Comprehensive Cancer Network recommends genetic testing for personal history of epithelial ovarian cancer at any age, regardless of family history. Several ovarian cancer ▶

susceptibility genes have been identified, which include *BRCA1, BRCA2 (primarily)*, other genes in the homologous recombination pathway, and mismatch repair genes associated with Lynch syndrome (hereditary nonpolyposis colorectal cancer).

2. A) Hysterectomy/bilateral salpingo-oophorectomy (BSO)/debulking. With imaging showing treatment response or a complete response, the next step would usually be hysterectomy/BSO/debulking to no residual disease. Adjuvant chemotherapy is needed after neoadjuvant chemotherapy.

HEAD AND NECK CANCER

1. History should evaluate for decline related to mucositis side effects. Include a 24-hour recall of the volume of food and liquids the patient is able to consume and the barriers to eating (trismus, mastication, xerostomia, pain, etc.), as well as volume of alcohol use and tobacco use. Assess pain level, medications currently being taken for pain, and adequacy, as well as current oral care management. Assess for signs of early sepsis due to mucositis, and which multidisciplinary team the patient has been referred to and attended consultations with as recommended (e.g., nutrition, speech therapy).

2. He may likely be developing treatment-related fatigue, dermatitis, and unmanaged chemotherapy-induced nausea and vomiting. Combined side effects and daily treatments make it difficult for patients to sleep and recover. This often leads to decline in overall performance status, falls, and need for more social support at home. For this reason, multidisciplinary approach and team management care are key to avoid treatment delays in this cancer population.

3. Start saline or baking soda rinse before and after meals and before going to bed. Encourage good oral hygiene. Discuss options for alcohol and tobacco cessation. Create a pain management plan or consult pain management as symptoms will likely continue and can worsen through treatment and up to 2 to 4 weeks following completion of radiation care. Consult speech therapy for swallow evaluation to ensure no aspiration. Consult nutrition. If oral intake does not improve, discuss plan for percutaneous endoscopic gastrostomy (PEG) tube placement. Rule out early sepsis and treat any other underlying infections.

4. Opioids, gabapentin, doxepin, and oral anesthetics (diphenhydramine/lidocaine/antacid mouthwash).

ACUTE LEUKEMIAS

1. D) M5: Acute monocytic leukemia. The bone marrow biopsy results showed monocytoid blasts and immature monocytes (blast equivalents) which, according to the French–American–British (FAB) classification system, are consistent with acute monocytic leukemia. Patients with this type of leukemia often have 80% monoblasts, promonocytes, and monocytes, as well as extramedullary disease and abnormalities in chromosome 11q. In addition, the CT scan showed widespread lymphadenopathy, which is consistent with extramedullary disease.

2. C) Poor risk. Per the results of this patient's bone marrow, he has more than three chromosomal abnormalities, which we call a "complex karyotype," as well as −7/monosomy 7, multiple translocations involving chromosome 3, and a high-level MECOM (EVI1) rearrangement. These results indicate poor risk disease. Overexpression of MECOM (EVI1) contributes to disease progression and an aggressive phenotype correlating with poor clinical outcomes in myeloid malignancies. Patients in this category, unfortunately, do not respond well to standard chemotherapy. When patients do respond, they do not have a durable remission and relapse quickly. Patients with a MECOM rearrangement have a significantly lower overall survival.

3. B) White blood cell (WBC) count of 208 K/mcL. Although all of the laboratory values mentioned are out of normal range, a WBC count over 100 K/mcL in a patient with acute myeloid leukemia (AML) with peripheral blasts is an oncologic emergency and needs to be treated immediately. Hyperleukocytosis, especially in a patient with AML, can lead to leukostasis, causing impairment of microvascular perfusion (inadequate oxygen delivery to the body's cells), and eventually end organ damage. Patients must undergo reduction of the WBC count with chemotherapy (most common), leukapheresis, or hydroxyurea. Leukostasis has a very high mortality rate if left untreated.

4. A) Periodic monitoring of minimal/measurable residual disease (MRD) on bone marrow aspirate (BMA) or peripheral blood (PB) by flow cytometry, cytogenetic/fluorescent in situ hybridization (FISH) testing, or molecular diagnostics (next generation sequencing [NGS] or polymerase chain reaction [PCR]) depending on treatment. The patient has a diagnosis of acute monocytic leukemia. Following treatment with chemotherapy and/or targeted therapy, the patient will require a bone marrow aspiration with or without biopsy, including cytogenetic analysis, molecular testing, and flow cytometry. Timing of this testing depends on the type of treatment the patient is receiving and the expectations of response. Although some patients with acute myeloid leukemia (AML) may require a lumbar puncture (LP) depending on their risk category, it would not be helpful to obtain weekly LPs on this patient. Monthly MRIs of the brain are not necessary and would neither be helpful nor cost-effective in this scenario. Supportive care, while necessary in all patients with leukemia, would not help directly monitor response. We can use this to monitor the patient's transfusion requirements, which if lower could predict bone marrow aspirate (BMA) response.

CHRONIC LEUKEMIA

1. B) Thoracentesis for diagnostic and/or therapeutic purposes. Given persistent pleural effusion and association with pleural effusions and dasatinib, thoracentesis with fluid analysis should be performed to evaluate etiology. Typically, pleural fluid will be exudative with lymphocyte predominance if dasatinib-related. Once ▶

other causes are ruled out, consider altering treatment (dose-reduce or change tyrosine kinase inhibitors [TKIs]).

2. A) At baseline, 7 days after initiation of therapy, and then periodically. Nilotinib is known to cause QTc prolongation. EKG monitoring for nilotinib should be at baseline, 7 days after starting, and then periodically, especially with addition to or adjustment of QTc-prolonging agents.

3. D) Check BCR-ABL1 every 3 months; once BCR-ABL1 is ≤1%, continue to monitor every 3 months for 2 years and then every 3 to 6 months. As you have changed therapy, monitoring should return to the recommended monitoring as if you started initial therapy in order to ensure ongoing response to therapy. Bone marrow aspiration and biopsy are no longer indicated for monitoring of disease response. In this scenario, referral for allogeneic stem cell transplant would not be recommended as there is no confirmed loss of response to therapy.

4. C) Check a BCR-ABL1 kinase domain mutation analysis. If there is a loss of response to therapy, there would be high concern for tyrosine kinase inhibitor (TKI)-resistant disease, which can be evaluated by a BCR-ABL1 kinase domain mutation analysis. The patient should continue on nilotinib while awaiting test results. If TKI-resistant disease is confirmed, treatment should then be changed and the patient should be referred for allogeneic stem cell transplant.

MYELODYSPLASTIC SYNDROMES

1. C) Further labs studies: Peripheral smear, iron studies, ferritin, B₁₂, folate, serum erythropoietin, thyroid studies. Evaluate for other causes of pancytopenia, including nutritional or metabolic causes.

2. A) Referral to a hematologist/oncologist for bone marrow biopsy/aspirate and further follow-up. The patient should be referred to a hematologist/oncologist for a bone marrow biopsy and aspirate. A bone marrow biopsy will show the cellularity and architecture. The aspirate is needed to obtain detailed cellular morphology and evaluation of percent of blasts. The aspirate is sent for cytogenetics, flow cytometry, fluorescent in situ hybridization (FISH), and next generation sequencing (NGS).

3. C) MDS with single-lineage dysplasia (MDS-SLD). There is evidence of only a single mutation and therefore it would be classified as myeloproliferative disorder (MDS) with single-lineage dysplasia.

4. A) Darbepoetin with transfusion support as needed. Starting a patient with myeloproliferative disorder (MDS) on darbepoetin has been shown to improve hemoglobin levels and reduce transfusion needs in 40% to over 60% of patients, with an overall duration of 18 to 24 months.

MYELOPROLIFERATIVE NEOPLASMS

1. D) All of the above. Fatigue (cytopenias), weight loss (malignant process), and abdominal fullness (splenomegaly) are all common presenting complaints in myeloproliferative neoplasm (MPN).

2. A) Flushed face. Flushed face or plethora is a common physical finding in myeloproliferative neoplasm (MPN).

3. D) All of the above. Complete blood count (CBC) would be helpful in detecting cytopenias, bone marrow biopsy would detect fibrosis, and abdominal ultrasound would confirm splenomegaly. In this case, positive findings would support a diagnosis of myeloproliferative neoplasm (MPN), specifically myelofibrosis.

4. D) All of the above. Depending on risk stratification, all could be appropriate next steps for a patient with myelofibrosis (MF).

LUNG CANCER

1. D) Interventional radiology biopsy. The National Comprehensive Cancer Network (NCCN) guidelines recommend high-risk nodules >8 mm with predisposing factors such as smoking history should undergo biopsy. PET/CT is also an option for further evaluation of a concerning nodule but is not a diagnostic procedure.

2. B) MRI of the brain and PET/CT. The National Comprehensive Cancer Network (NCCN) guidelines recommend further evaluation with PET/CT and MRI of the brain to rule out metastatic disease due to lung cancers' high risk of spread.

3. C) Smoking history. The risk of lung cancer linked to smoking is up to 91% for squamous cell carcinoma histologies.

4. B) False. Much evidence exists to suggest that older adults with good functional status can tolerate combination chemotherapy in the treatment of lung cancer. Chronological age alone should not dictate treatment options.

NON-HODGKIN LYMPHOMA

1. B) Night sweats, fatigue, unintentional weight loss. B symptoms refer to symptoms of fever >38°C, drenching night sweats, fatigue, and weight loss of >10% in the last 6 months. Chest pain, dyspnea, and facial swelling are more concerning for superior vena cava (SVC) syndrome, not B symptoms. Nontender cervical lymphadenopathy is also concerning for lymphoma but may have other etiologies as well and is not defined as B symptoms.

2. C) Chemotherapy or radiation. Treatment for superior vena cava (SVC) syndrome is often chemotherapy and/or radiation. If a thrombus is present and symptoms are severe, stenting may be a treatment option. Thoracentesis can be considered for pleural effusions, but is not an appropriate first-line therapy. Nebulizers and oxygen may help with symptoms, but will not treat SVC syndrome. Surgery is not an appropriate first-line therapy for SVC syndrome.

3. D) Core biopsy. A core biopsy or excisional lymph node biopsy is essential to making an accurate histologic diagnosis. A fine needle aspiration (FNA) is often not adequate to make a diagnosis of lymphoma. MRI could be considered to rule out complications such as spinal cord compression, but will not make a definitive diagnosis of lymphoma. PET scan is useful for staging ▶

and should be considered, but will not make a definitive diagnosis. If the patient is stable, a biopsy should be obtained prior to starting treatment with steroids or radiation.

4. A) HIV and hepatitis panel. Non-Hodgkin lymphoma (NHL) has been associated with HIV and immunocompromised status. Hepatitis B or C can be reactivated by some of the treatment options given for lymphoma and should be tested prior to initiating chemotherapy. Given the patient's remote history of intravenous (IV) drug use, these studies are especially important in this patient. There is no indication for blood cultures in this patient. Thyroid studies and lipid panel are not critical to obtain prior to initiating chemotherapy.

MULTIPLE MYELOMA

1. A) MRI of lumbar spine. Conservative management would not be an ideal choice since the patient has a history of osteoporosis and his back pain is increasing. There is concern for pathologic fracture due to his history of osteoporosis and there is no recent injury to explain his back pain. Compression fractures are typically diagnosed by lateral x-rays of the vertebral column.

2. B) Low-dose, whole-body CT scan if no concern for spinal cord compression. The patient's neurologic exam is normal and there is no concern for spinal cord compression. However, the lytic lesions and pathologic compression fractures are concerning for multiple myeloma. Low-dose, whole-body CT scan is the study of choice to detect osteolytic disease per the International Myeloma Working Group.

3. C) Lab work for multiple myeloma workup: Complete blood count (CBC) with differential, comprehensive metabolic panel (CMP), serum protein electrophoresis with immunofixation electrophoresis (SPEP/IFE), 24-hour urine protein electrophoresis with immunofixation electrophoresis (UPEP/IFE), serum free light chain assay (kappa and lambda), serum immunoglobulin levels (IgA, IgG, IgM, IgD, IgE), beta-2 microglobulin, lactate dehydrogenase (LDH). Both serum and urine must be studied for presence of a monoclonal protein.

4. A) Refer to hematology for bone marrow biopsy. The patient has multiple myeloma. He has a monoclonal protein in his serum, along with the associated CRAB criteria (hypercalcemia, renal insufficiency, anemia, and bone lesions).

SARCOMA

1. C) Core needle biopsy. Core needle biopsy is essential in sarcomas. Often, fine needle aspiration (FNA) does not contain enough tissue for the pathologist to determine the specific type of sarcoma. Core needle biopsy can also have enough tissue to send for additional genomic testing. One would not do an excisional biopsy on such a large sarcoma as it would compromise too much healthy tissue and be impossible to remove intact.

2. B) CT of the chest with intravenous (IV) contrast. CT of the chest with IV contrast is critical to determine if lung metastasis is present. It likely would not change the plan of care, but it would change the goal from curative to palliative.

3. A) Present the case at the multidisciplinary sarcoma tumor board. Present at the multidisciplinary sarcoma tumor board with presence of an orthopedic oncologist, radiation oncologist, pathologist, radiologist, and medical oncologist to review the case in depth. Discuss pathology, location of tumor, and involving vessels and nerves that would be affected should surgery and radiation take place. You determine the tumor is very extensive and the best chance to give the patient function of his extremity would be to shrink and kill the tumor with neoadjuvant chemotherapy first.

4. D) Doxorubicin (Adriamycin)/ifosfamide (Ifex). Doxorubicin (Adriamycin)/ifosfamide (Ifex) is most likely to shrink and kill the patient's sarcoma.

SKIN CANCER

1. D) Basal cell carcinoma. This is likely a basal cell carcinoma (BCC) based on the classic appearance of a nonhealing sore. BCC is the most common cancer.

2. A) Most basal cell carcinoma (BCCs) have an excellent prognosis. Most BCCs have an excellent prognosis when identified and managed early. You will refer the patient to dermatology for further assessment and management. You reassure the patient that this has been caught early and anticipate a positive outcome.

CHAPTER 14

BACK PAIN

1. B) Straight leg raise test. The straight leg raise test is the most helpful test in detecting lumbosacral nerve root compression such as lumbar disc herniation. The log roll test is the most specific test to assess hip pain and integrity of the hip joint. It is used to identify potential hip pathology such as labral tears. The Spurling maneuver test is used to diagnose cervical radiculopathy whether neck pain is due to cervical nerve compression. The Hoffman reflex is a test that providers use to examine the reflexes of the upper extremities with a high correlation with cervical dysfunction. This is a quick test for possible spinal cord compression from a lesion on the spinal cord or another underlying nerve condition.

2. A) Concern for malignancy. Concern for malignancy due to age 50 or older, unexplained weight loss, pain unrelieved by bedrest, and pain lasting more than a month. The patient's vital signs are not concerning for infection, as well as her medical history. She had no previous or recent history of trauma, which would not predispose her to a compression fracture. She has a neurologic problem that needs further investigation.

3. A) CT myelogram. When metallic devices are present, such as a pacemaker, CT myelogram is the most useful imaging to aid in diagnosis. Metallic device is contraindicated in MRI scan. Plain x-ray films will not offer any ▶

guidance in diagnosis. A bone scan is a test that uses nuclear imaging to diagnose a number of bone conditions, including bone metastasis, bone fracture, and bone infection.

4. C) Metastatic carcinoma of the breast. Breast cancer most commonly metastasizes to the bone and has a particular affinity with the spine. The bone is the most common site of metastasis, with osseous metastases developing in 8% of all patients with breast cancer and 69% of patients with advanced breast cancer disease.

COMPARTMENT SYNDROME OF THE LOWER LEG

1. B) Take off Ace wrap dressing. The best next course of action is to take off any constrictive dressing, such as an Ace wrap, to restore circulation and tissue perfusion. You need to check the international normalized ratio (INR) before you can potentially turn off the heparin drip to see if it is elevated, which predisposes the patient to bleeding. Elevating the leg and applying ice therapy can lead to worsening of symptoms.

2. D) Pulselessness. Pulselessness is a late finding and can lead to poor acute coronary syndrome (ACS) outcome. As intracranial pressure (ICP) rises, a loss of limb pulses indicates a decline in arterial perfusion. An absolute indication for fasciotomy is an arterial ischemic time greater than 4 hours. Poikilothermia, pain out of proportion, and pallor are early signs and symptoms of ACS.

3. A) Stryker pressure monitoring device. Stryker pressure monitoring device is the best way to measure limb intracranial pressure (ICP). Delta pressure can be used to measure ICP but is not the preferred method. Creatinine kinase (CK) is a laboratory test to measure myoglobinuria due to rhabdomyolysis present in acute coronary syndrome (ACS). There is no alpha pressure measured in ACS.

4. C) 30 mmHg or above. An intracranial pressure (ICP) of 30 mmHg or above is the correct measurement and corresponds to an acute compartment syndrome diagnosis. The other measurements are too low and are erroneous measurements for ICP.

JOINT PAIN

1. A) Ultrasound-guided hip aspiration for synovial fluid analysis. Due to this condition being less than 6 weeks in duration (acute) and the nature of the underlying pathologic process being inflammatory, aspiration and analysis of synovial fluid including cell count are always indicated in acute monoarthritis or when an infectious or crystal-induced arthropathy is suspected. Options B, C, and D are all imaging techniques that are better appropriate when the patient presents with a history of trauma, suspected chronic infection, progressive disability, or when a baseline assessment is desired for what appears to be a chronic process.

2. C) Patient should try to lose weight as a way of relieving joint pain. Weight loss is suggested to lessen strain on joints. Option A is incorrect because nonsteroidal anti-inflammatory drug (NSAID) therapy is contraindicated in patients with kidney disease due to the

possibility of worsening renal insufficiency. Option B is incorrect because even though the patient has diabetes his recent hemoglobin A1C (HgA1C) shows that his diabetes is controlled on his current regimen. Option D is wrong because low-impact aerobic exercise, and not high-impact, is suggested when a patient presents with joint pain.

3. B) Gout. The presence of uric acid crystals in synovial fluid analysis confirms gout arthropathy. Option A, pseudogout, is consistent with calcium pyrophosphate dihydrate crystals. Options C and D are incorrect due to the presence of crystals and white blood cell (WBC) less than 50,000/mcL. Inflammatory fluid has an increased white count between 2,000 and 50,000/mcL but no crystals, and septic fluid is usually purulent with a WBC of greater than 50,000/mcL.

OSTEOARTHRITIS

1. C) Previous injury. Although options A and D are also risk factors for the patient developing osteoarthritis (OA), they are modifiable and the patient should be encouraged to lose weight and educated on supportive care while at work. Hyperlipidemia is not a risk factor for OA.

2. C) X-ray of the right knee. An x-ray of the right knee is the most appropriate initial imaging. Knee radiographs should be performed with the patient standing to reveal the extent of joint space narrowing of the tibiofemoral joint. Although MRI and CT scan would be highly sensitive in diagnosing osteoarthritis (OA), these would not be first line. If the patient had effusion on her physical exam, a joint aspiration would be useful to rule out other pathology, such as gout or pseudogout; however, normal results of the patient's joint aspiration would only be supportive.

3. A) Acetaminophen. Acetaminophen should be the patient's first line as long as she does not have liver disease. Naproxen nonsteroidal anti-inflammatory drugs (NSAIDs) are effective in treating joint pain in patients with osteoarthritis (OA); however, given the patient's use of apixaban, she should be advised to avoid these as they cause increased risk of bleeding. The use of opioids is not indicated as first line and should be avoided as they have high risk of toxicity, somnolence, respiratory depression, falls, and high potential for addiction. Glucosamine, alone or in combination, is no better than placebo in reducing pain in patients with knee or hip.

RHEUMATOID ARTHRITIS

1. D) Elevated anticitrullinated protein/peptide antibody (ACPA). Although all of the options are likely to be found in the lab work of someone with rheumatoid arthritis (RA), elevated ACPA is the most specific to support the diagnosis of RA.

2. B) RF can be falsely positive in those with other autoimmune disease (e.g., celiac disease). Rheumatoid factor (RF) can also be found among those with acute infection, older adults (even healthy), and patients with other autoimmune diseases.

3. C) Heavy alcohol use. Methotrexate is still recommended as the first-line treatment for rheumatoid arthritis by the American College of Rheumatology, unless contraindications (e.g., frequent alcohol use, preexisting liver disease) are present.

4. A) NSAIDs, unlike DMARDs, do not inhibit progression of structural joint damage in those suffering from RA. Both nonsteroidal anti-inflammatory drugs (NSAIDs) and disease-modifying antirheumatic drugs (DMARDs) can improve symptoms of rheumatoid arthritis (RA); however, DMARDs, as their name suggests, can hinder the progression of joint disease in those with RA.

SPONDYLOARTHROPATHIES

1. B) X-rays including anteroposterior (AP) of the pelvis and lumbar spine. Radiographic features of ankylosing spondylitis (AS) include bilateral symmetric sacroiliitis, with initial sclerosis progressing to erosive changes and/or fusion of the sacroiliac joints. Spinal involvement may include squaring of the vertebral bodies and/or show a classic "bamboo" spine appearance. If radiographic evidence is not seen, an MRI may be more sensitive to early changes. Synovial fluid analysis of the hips or bloodwork with elevated C-reactive protein (CRP) and erythrocyte sedimentation rate (ESR) may give us some information on an inflammatory reaction taking place, but generally do not correlate with disease activity. Urinalysis or urine culture positive for chlamydia may be more diagnostic of reactive arthritis and not AS.

2. D) Nonsteroidal anti-inflammatory drug (NSAID) therapy. Treatment of ankylosing spondylitis (AS) begins with NSAIDs, which have been shown to provide rapid relief of inflammatory back pain. A positive response to NSAID therapy is helpful in diagnosing AS. Outpatient physical therapy or antitumor necrosis factor (anti-TNF) therapy can be used as adjunctive therapy or a second-line agent after NSAID use. Oral corticosteroids in conventional dosages are of little value in the treatment of AS.

3. A) Human leukocyte antigen (HLA)-B27. There is a greater than 50% prevalence of the HLA-B27 gene in ankylosing spondylitis (AS) even though there are no specific diagnostic tests for spondyloarthropathies. Absence of rheumatoid factor helps support AS diagnosis. Only about 10% of patients have anticyclic citrullinated peptide (anti-CCP) antibodies. Elevated levels of uric acid are associated with psoriatic arthritis.

SYSTEMIC LUPUS ERYTHEMATOSUS

1. D) ANA, DsDNA, Smith, ribonucleoprotein (RNP), SSA/SSBA, and complements, alongside CBC and CMP. Having a full panel will help clarify the diagnosis and expedite a referral to a rheumatology; simply ordering an antinuclear antibody (ANA) is not enough to diagnose systemic lupus erythematosus (SLE) and can create anxiety on the patient and family.

2. D) 20 to 60 mg. It will depend on the severity of the patient's symptoms—if mild, such as fatigue and joint pain alone, the patient can be started on nonsteroidal anti-inflammatory drugs (NSAIDS); if fever, weight loss, rashes, and swelling are present, the clinician can start the patient on prednisone at doses of 20 to 60 mg daily.

3. B) Works with the rheumatologist to treat complications of treatment and uses preventive care. The role of the primary care is complex and includes treatment of complications of treatment such as hypertension, hyperlipidemia, diabetes, and osteoporosis. Continuous communication with the rheumatologist will facilitate care and increase compliance with medications.

VASCULITIS

1. B) Henoch–Schönlein purpura (immunoglobulin A [IgA] vasculitis). The patient's age is appropriate for onset. It is preceded by a recent strep throat infection, which is common in overall presentation (approximately 50% of cases). The patient also has palpable purpura described on physical exam.

2. D) Biopsy. A biopsy (usually skin biopsy) can help reveal leukocytoclastic vasculitis with immunoglobulin A (IgA) deposition, which is a key characteristic of Henoch–Schönlein purpura.

3. C) Nonsteroidal anti-inflammatory drugs (NSAIDs) and Tylenol. This is the best initial treatment for Henoch–Schönlein purpura (HSP). If pain becomes refractory or more severe in nature, then corticosteroids can be used.

4. B) Small vessel. This is the correct answer given that the answers to the preceding questions are all indicative of Henoch–Schönlein purpura, which is a condition under the small vessel vasculitis classification system.

CHAPTER 15

DERMATOLOGY

1. A) Drug reaction dermatitis. The patient did not report a history of new exposure, product, or drug. Drug eruption dermatitis typically presents as a generalized exanthematous or morbilliform eruption (erythematous maculopapular eruption), unlikely to be localized to the lower extremity.

2. B) Cellulitis. Cellulitis misdiagnosis is common and has been associated with the unnecessary use of oral antibiotics, unnecessary hospitalization, increased healthcare costs, and potential for patient harm.

3. B) Triamcinolone 0.1% ointment. Topical steroids are indicated for erythema, pruritus, vesiculation, and oozing. Petroleum-based topical corticosteroids such as triamcinolone ointment or fluocinolone ointment without additives are best to minimize the risk of sensitization. High- to mid-potency corticosteroids in an ointment formulation are applied to the affected area of the skin once or twice daily for 1 to 2 weeks.

CHAPTER 16

DELIRIUM

1. D) Medical intervention. If an individual presents needing urgent medical care that is reflective of delirium, it is important to treat the underlying cause or condition that is contributing to it. It is important that the provider educate the patient's family about the signs of delirium.

DEMENTIA

1. D) Donepezil and memantine. Cholinesterase inhibitors such as donepezil, galantamine, and rivastigmine can be used in the management of dementia, with all being used to treat mild to moderate dementia. All three medications possess the same mechanism of action. However, memantine is an uncompetitive antagonist of the N-methyl-D-aspartate (NMDA) type of glutamate receptor, which can be used in the management of moderate to severe Alzheimer disease.

FALLS

1. E) All of the above. It appears that the patient's fall may have resulted from malnutrition, so nutritional evaluation and resource support to help with food insecurity are both essential. Medication safety is unknown at this point, so medication reconciliation by a pharmacist would evaluate this and help with readiness for discharge to home. Finally, evaluation by physical therapy and occupational therapy will help with recovery from injury and assess any mobility or functional issues to facilitate safety at home.

URINARY INCONTINENCE

1. D) All of the above. All of these interventions are appropriate to support the patient with the urinary incontinence and the associated skin breakdown she is experiencing. Frequent opportunities for toileting will allow her to empty her bladder; mobility aids and transfer assistance will support her with ambulation to the toilet; and barrier cream will help prevent further skin breakdown due to moisture.

CHAPTER 17

CHEST TRAUMA

1. C) Placement of thoracostomy tube (chest tube). A pneumothorax occurs when air is forced into the pleural space. Air in the pleural space with no means of escape causes a collapse of the lung on the affected side. Immediate treatment involves elimination of the air collection and reexpansion of the affected lung. This can be done with needle decompression or placement of a thoracoscopy tube.

2. B) Flail chest. Flail chest is defined as fractures of two or more adjacent ribs in two or more places. It is often described as paradoxical movement of the chest wall, impacting breathing mechanics and overall gas exchange.

3. D) Cardiac tamponade. Pericardial tamponade is a life-threatening condition that occurs when blood, fluid, or air accumulates in the pericardium, restricting cardiac activity and interfering with cardiac output. Symptoms may evolve within minutes to an hour after injury. Classic presentation includes the Beck's triad (hypotension, distended jugular veins, and muffled heart sounds).

4. C) Tension pneumothorax. Tension pneumothorax develops when air becomes trapped in the pleural cavity under positive pressure. As air accumulates and creates increased pressure in the chest, it can cause displacement of the mediastinal structures (to the opposite, unaffected side). This can lead to reduced blood flow to the heart and lead to compromise of cardiopulmonary function.

INTRACRANIAL PENETRATING TRAUMA

1. C) Blood that has not been drained using traditional tube thoracostomy. Retained hemothorax is blood that has not been drained by traditional chest tube management and often requires intrapleural instillation of fibrinolytic therapy or may require surgical intervention.

2. D) Hemodynamic instability with blood pressure (BP) less than 90 and heart rate (HR) greater than 120. Hemodynamic instability is one of the indicators of need for possible emergent surgical intervention. The goal of treatment is aimed at hemorrhage control while maintaining adequate perfusion and oxygenation for the patient.

3. B) Urban dwelling, young males. Groups at higher risk of penetrating thoracic trauma include young adult males and males over 65 years old (often suicide attempts), inner city residents, individuals in lower income brackets, and those with history of suicide attempts or substance use.

4. B) High-energy injuries. Firearm injuries/gunshots are often considered high-energy mechanisms and tend to cause more injury when compared with other forms of penetrating injury, such as stab wound and impalement.

PENETRATING INTRACRANIAL INJURIES

1. B) A quick, simple, and objective assessment of neurologic exam. The Glasgow Coma Scale is a quick and objective measure of level of consciousness.

2. D) Less than 8. A Glasgow Coma Scale (GCS) score of 8 or less is considered coma. These patients should be intubated for airway protection.

3. B) MAP-intracranial pressure (ICP). Cerebral perfusion pressure (CPP) is the net pressure gradient that drives oxygen delivery to cerebral tissue. Measured in millimeters of mercury (mmHg), it is the difference between the mean arterial pressure (MAP) and the ICP. A normal CPP range is between 60 and 80 mmHg.

$$CPP = MAP-ICP.$$

It is an important assessment tool when considering extracranial factors such as changes in blood volume or arterial pressure, which can result in increased brain swelling and ischemia. Careful management and treatment of the traumatic brain-injured patient using the CPP can result in decreased risk of secondary ischemia to the brain tissue.

4. C) High-energy, high-velocity injuries. Penetrating intracranial injuries are considered high-energy, high-velocity injuries that cause extensive damage as the object enters the body. The blast effect can be as high as 30 to 40 times the diameter of the bullet. With any injury to the brain, there is an increased risk of seizure activity.

A 32-YEAR-OLD IN A MOTOR VEHICLE CRASH

1. A) Hypovolemic. Hypovolemic shock occurs when there is significant fluid loss causing intravascular volume depletion. Causes of this fluid loss range anywhere from hemorrhage, nausea/vomiting/diarrhea, burns, diabetes insipidus, and ascites, to poor oral intake. Tachycardia, hypotension, pale/cool/clammy skin, flat jugular veins, and abdominal tenderness are signs of volume depletion and should prompt the provider to suspect that this patient who had sustained blunt abdominal trauma is experiencing hypovolemic shock.

SPINAL CORD INJURIES

1. B) American Spinal Injury Association (ASIA). ASIA uses a letter grading scale to describe the severity of the injury. The more severe the injury, the less likely a recovery will occur. The scale ranges from ASIA A (most severe) to ASIA E (normal).

2. D) Respiratory effort. The level and degree of spinal cord injury can impact spontaneous breathing.

3. C) Flaccidity (loss of muscle tone) and loss of reflexes that occur immediately after spinal cord injury. Spinal shock refers to the flaccidity (loss of muscle tone) and loss of reflexes that occur immediately after injury. Neurogenic shock results in the loss of vasomotor tone and sympathetic innervation to the heart.

4. B) Classification of spinal cord injury (SCI). Spinal cord injury without radiographic abnormality (SCIWORA) refers to evidence of SCI on clinical exam without radiographic evidence of injury.

TRAUMATIC BRAIN INJURY

1. C) Ensure correct placement of endotracheal tube. Confirmation of proper endotracheal tube placement should be completed on all patients at the time of intubation and with any patient movement.

2. A) Prevent secondary injury. Prevention of secondary injury by maintaining adequate oxygenation and perfusion to brain tissue is the primary goal in severe brain injury treatment.

3. A) Start antibiotic therapy immediately. Adding antiseizure medication for prophylaxis is considered protective and should be started in the first 1 to 2 hours after identification of traumatic brain injury (TBI).

4. C) Nausea, vomiting, and headache. Symptoms of concussion may include headache, nausea, vomiting, dizziness, photophobia, and lethargy.

SECTION IV

END OF LIFE

1. D) All of the above are important considerations. It is important to consider the setting where the news will be delivered as well as what will be said. During the interview, the advanced practice provider (APP) should sit down with the patient, maintain eye contact, and effectively manage time constraints and interruptions.

2. C) "What do you understand about what brought you into the hospital?" During the interview, open-ended questions should be used to ask the patient what they understand about the disease process.

NORMAL LABORATORY VALUES

ABIM LABORATORY TEST REFERENCE RANGES: JANUARY 2019

Laboratory Tests	Reference Ranges
1,25-Dihydroxyvitamin D(1,25-Dihydroxycholecalciferol), serum	See vitamin D metabolites
17-Hydroxyprogesterone, serum	
Female, follicular	<80 ng/dL
Female, luteal	<285 ng/dL
Female, postmenopausal	<51 ng/dL
Male (adult)	<220 ng/dL
5-Hydroxyindoleacetic acid, urine	2–9 mg/24 hr
6-Thioguanine, whole blood	230–400 pmol/8 × 10 RBCs
ANC	2,000–8,250/mcL
25-Hydroxyvitamin D (25-Hydroxycholecalciferol), serum	See vitamin D metabolites
ACE, serum	8–53 U/L
Acid phosphatase, serum	
Prostatic fraction	0.1–0.4 unit/mL
Total	0.5–2.0 (Bodansky) units/mL
ACTH, plasma	10–60 pg/mL
aPTT	25–35 sec
ADAMTS13 activity	>60%
Albumin, serum	3.5–5.5 g/dL
Albumin, urine	<25 mg/24 hr
Albumin to creatinine ratio, urine	<30 mg/g
Aldolase, serum	0.8–3.0 IU/mL
Aldosterone, plasma	
Supine or seated	Up to 10 ng/dL
Standing	<21 ng/dL
Low sodium diet (supine)	Up to 30 ng/dL
Aldosterone, urine	5–19 mcg/24 hr

(continued)

ABIM LABORATORY TEST REFERENCE RANGES—JANUARY 2019 (CONTINUED)

Laboratory Tests	Reference Ranges
Alkaline phosphatase, bone-specific	5.6–18.0 mcg/L for premenopausal women
Alkaline phosphatase, serum	30–120 U/L
AAT, serum	150–350 mg/dL
Alpha-2-antiplasmin activity, plasma	75%–115%
Alpha-amino nitrogen, urine	100–290 mg/24 hr
Alpha-fetoprotein, serum	<10 ng/mL
Amino acids, urine	200–400 mg/24 hr
Aminotransferase, serum alanine (ALT, SGPT)	10–40 U/L
Aminotransferase, serum aspartate (AST, SGOT)	10–40 U/L
Ammonia, blood	40–70 mcg/dL
Amylase, serum	25–125 U/L (80–180 [Somogyi] units/dL)
Amylase, urine	1–17 U/hr
Androstenedione, serum	Female: 30–200 ng/dL; male: 40–150 ng/dL
Anion gap, serum	7–13 mEq/L
Antibodies to double-stranded DNA	0–7 IU/mL
Anticardiolipin antibodies	
IgG	<20 GPL
IgM	<20 MPL
Anticyclic citrullinated peptide, antibodies	<20 units
Antideoxyribonuclease B	<280 units
Anti-F-actin antibodies, serum	1:80 or less
Antihistone antibodies	<1:16
Anti-LKM antibodies	<1:20
Antimitochondrial antibodies	1:5 or less
Antimyelin-associated glycoprotein antibody	<1:1,600
Antimyeloperoxidase antibodies	<1 U
Antinuclear antibodies	1:40 or less
Antismooth muscle antibodies	1:80 or less
Antistreptolysin O titer	<200 Todd units
Antithrombin activity	80%–120%
Antithyroglobulin antibodies	<20 U/mL
Antithyroid peroxidase antibodies	<2.0 U/mL
Antitissue transglutaminase antibodies	See tissue transglutaminase antibody

(continued)

ABIM LABORATORY TEST REFERENCE RANGES—JANUARY 2019 (*CONTINUED*)

Laboratory Tests	Reference Ranges
Arterial blood gas studies (patient breathing room air)	
pH	7.38–7.44
$PaCO_2$	38–42 mmHg
PaO_2	75–100 mmHg
Bicarbonate	23–26 mEq/L
Oxygen saturation	95% or greater
Methemoglobin	0.5%–3.0%
Ascorbic acid (vitamin C), blood	0.4–1.5 mg/dL
Ascorbic acid, leukocyte	16.5 ± 5.1 mg/dL of leukocytes
(1,3)-Beta-D-glucan, serum	<60 pg/mL
Beta subunit chorionic gonadotropin, urine	<2 mIU/24 hr
Beta-2-glycoprotein I antibodies	
IgG	<21 SGU
IgM	<21 SMU
Beta-hydroxybutyrate, serum	<0.4 mmol/L
Beta-2-microglobulin, serum	0.54–2.75 mg/L
Bicarbonate, serum	23–28 mEq/L
Bilirubin, serum	
Total	0.3–1.0 mg/dL
Direct	0.1–0.3 mg/dL
Indirect	0.2–0.7 mg/dL
Bleeding time (template)	<8 min
BUN, serum or plasma	8–20 mg/dL
B-type natriuretic peptide, plasma	<100 pg/mL
C peptide, serum	0.8–3.1 ng/mL
Calcitonin, serum	Female: 5 pg/mL or less; male: 10 pg/mL or less
Calcium, ionized, serum	1.12–1.23 mmol/L
Calcium, serum	8.6–10.2 mg/dL
Calcium, urine	Female: <250 mg/24 hr; male: <300 mg/24 hr
Carbohydrate antigens, serum	
CA 19–9	0–37 U/mL
CA 27–29	<38.0 U/mL
CA 125	<35 U/mL

(continued)

ABIM LABORATORY TEST REFERENCE RANGES—JANUARY 2019 (*CONTINUED*)

Laboratory Tests	Reference Ranges
Carbon dioxide content, serum	23–30 mEq/L
Carboxyhemoglobin, blood	<5%
Carcinoembryonic antigen, plasma	<2.5 ng/mL
Carotene, serum	75–300 mcg/dL
Catecholamines, plasma	
Dopamine	<30 pg/mL
Epinephrine	
Supine	<50 pg/mL
Standing	<95 pg/mL
Norepinephrine	
Supine	112–658 pg/mL
Standing	217–1,109 pg/mL
Catecholamines, urine	
Dopamine	65–400 mcg/24 hr
Epinephrine	2–24 mcg/24 hr
Norepinephrine	15–100 mcg/24 hr
Total	26–121 mcg/24 hr
CD4 T-lymphocyte count	530–1,570/mcL
Cell count, CSF	
Leukocytes (WBCs)	0–5 cells/mcL
Ceruloplasmin, serum (plasma)	25–43 mg/dL
Chloride, CSF	120–130 mEq/L
Chloride, serum	98–106 mEq/L
Chloride, urine	
Spot	mEq/L; varies
24-hr measurement	mEq/24 hr; varies with intake
Cholesterol, serum	
Total	
Desirable	<200 mg/dL
Borderline-high	200–239 mg/dL
High	>239 mg/dL
High-density lipoprotein	
Low	Female: <50 mg/dL; male: <40 mg/dL

(continued)

ABIM LABORATORY TEST REFERENCE RANGES—JANUARY 2019 (*CONTINUED*)

Laboratory Tests	Reference Ranges
Low-density lipoprotein	
Optimal	<100 mg/dL
Near-optimal	100–129 mg/dL
Borderline-high	130–159 mg/dL
High	160–189 mg/dL
Very high	>189 mg/dL
Cholinesterase, serum (pseudocholinesterase)	0.5 or more pH units per hour
Packed cells	0.7 or more pH units per hour
Chorionic gonadotropin, beta-human (beta-hCG), serum	Female, premenopausal nonpregnant: <1.0 U/L; female, postmenopausal: <7.0 U/L; male: <1.4 U/L
Chromogranin A, serum	<93 ng/mL
Citrate, urine	250–1,000 mg/24 hr
Clotting time (Lee–White)	5–15 min
Coagulation factors, plasma	
Factor I (fibrinogen)	200–400 mg/dL
Factor II (prothrombin)	60%–130%
Factor V (accelerator globulin)	60%–130%
Factor VII (proconvertin)	60%–130%
Factor VIII (antihemophilic globulin)	50%–150%
Factor IX (plasma thromboplastin component)	50%–150%
Factor X (Stuart factor)	60%–130%
Factor XI (plasma thromboplastin antecedent)	60%–130%
Factor XII (Hageman factor)	60%–130%
Factor XIII	57%–192%
Cold agglutinin titer	>1:64 positive
Complement components, serum	
C3	100–233 mg/dL
C4	14–48 mg/dL
CH50	110–190 units/mL
Copper, serum	100–200 mcg/dL
Copper, urine	0–100 mcg/24 hr
Coproporphyrin, urine	50–250 mcg/24 hr
Cortisol, free, urine	4–50 mcg/24 hr

(*continued*)

ABIM LABORATORY TEST REFERENCE RANGES—JANUARY 2019 (*CONTINUED*)

Laboratory Tests	Reference Ranges
Cortisol, plasma	
8:00 a.m.	5–25 mcg/dL
4:00 p.m.	<10 mcg/dL
1 hour after cosyntropin	18 mcg/dL or greater
Overnight suppression test (1 mg)	<1.8 mcg/dL
Overnight suppression test (8 mg)	>50% reduction in cortisol
Cortisol, saliva, 11 p.m.midnight	<0.09 mcg/dL
C-reactive protein, serum	0.8 mg/dL or less
C-reactive protein (high sensitivity), serum	Low risk: <1.0 mg/L; average risk: 1.0–3.0 mg/L; high risk: more than 3.0 mg/L
Creatine kinase, serum	
Total	Female: 30–135 U/L; male: 55–170 U/L
MB isoenzymes	<5% of total
Creatine, urine	Female: 0–100 mg/24 hr; male: 0–40 mg/24 hr
Creatinine clearance, urine	90–140 mL/min
Creatinine, serum	Female: 0.50–1.10 mg/dL; male: 0.70–1.30 mg/dL
Creatinine, urine	
Spot	mg/dL; varies
24-hr measurement	15–25 mg/kg body weight/24 hr
Cyclosporine, whole blood (trough)	
Therapeutic	100–200 ng/mL
0–3 months posttransplantation	150–250 ng/mL
More than 3 months posttransplantation	75–125 ng/mL
D-dimer, plasma	<0.5 mcg/mL
DHEA-S, serum	Female: 44–332 mcg/dL; male: 89–457 mcg/dL
Delta-aminolevulinic acid, serum	<20 mcg/dL
Digoxin, serum	Therapeutic: 1.0–2.0 ng/mL (<1.2 ng/mL for patients with heart failure)
Dihydrotestosterone, serum	Adult male: 25–80 ng/dL
Dopamine, plasma	<30 pg/mL
Dopamine, urine	65–400 mcg/24 hr
D-xylose absorption (after ingestion of 25 g of D-xylose)	
Serum	25–40 mg/dL
Urinary excretion	4.5–7.5 g during a 5-hr period

(*continued*)

ABIM LABORATORY TEST REFERENCE RANGES—JANUARY 2019 (*CONTINUED*)

Laboratory Tests	Reference Ranges
Electrolytes, serum	
Sodium	136–145 mEq/L
Potassium	3.5–5.0 mEq/L
Chloride	98–106 mEq/L
Bicarbonate	23–28 mEq/L
Epinephrine, plasma	
Supine	<110 pg/mL
Standing	<140 pg/mL
Epinephrine, urine	<20 mcg/24 hr
Erythrocyte count	4.2–5.9 million/mcL
Erythrocyte sedimentation rate (Westergren)	Female: 0–20 mm/hr; male: 0–15 mm/hr
Erythrocyte survival rate (Cr)	T½ = 28 d
Erythropoietin, serum	4–26 mU/mL
Estradiol, serum	
Female, follicular	10–180 pg/mL
Midcycle peak	100–300 pg/mL
Luteal	40–200 pg/mL
Postmenopausal	<10 pg/mL
Male	20–50 pg/mL
Estriol, urine	>12 mg/24 hr
Estrogen receptor protein	Negative: <10 fmol/mg protein
Estrone, serum	10–60 pg/mL
Ethanol, blood	<0.005% (<5 mg/dL)
Coma level	More than 0.5% (more than 500 mg/dL)
Intoxication	0.08%–0.1% or greater (80–100 mg/dL or greater)
Euglobulin clot lysis time	2–4 hr at 37.0°C
Everolimus, whole blood (trough)	Therapeutic: 3.0–8.0 ng/mL
Factor XIII, B subunit, plasma	60–130 U/dL
Fecal fat	<7 g/24 hr
Fecal nitrogen	<2 g/24 hr
Fecal pH	7.0–7.5
Fecal potassium	<10 mEq/L
Fecal sodium	<10 mEq/L

(*continued*)

ABIM LABORATORY TEST REFERENCE RANGES—JANUARY 2019 (*CONTINUED*)

Laboratory Tests	Reference Ranges
Fecal urobilinogen	40–280 mg/24 hr
Fecal weight	<250 g/24 hr
Ferritin, serum	Female: 11–307 ng/mL; male: 24–336 ng/mL
Fibrin(ogen) degradation products	<10 mcg/mL
Fibrinogen, plasma	200–400 mg/dL
Fibroblast growth factor-23, serum	30–80 RU/mL
Flecainide, serum	Therapeutic: 0.2–1.0 mcg/mL
Folate, red cell	150–450 ng/mL of packed cells
Folate, serum	1.8–9.0 ng/mL
Follicle-stimulating hormone, serum	
Female, follicular/luteal	2–9 mIU/mL (2–9 U/L)
Female, midcycle peak	4–22 mIU/mL (4–22 U/L)
Female, postmenopausal	>30 mIU/mL (>30 U/L)
Male (adult)	1–7 mIU/mL (1–7 U/L)
Children, Tanner stages 1, 2	0.5–8.0 mIU/mL (0.5–8.0 U/L)
Children, Tanner stages 3, 4, 5	1–12 mIU/mL (1–12 U/L)
Free kappa light chain, serum	3.3–19.4 mg/L
Free kappa to free lambda light chain ratio, serum	0.26–1.65
Free lambda light chain, serum	5.7–26.3 mg/L
Fructosamine, serum	175–280 mmol/L
Gamma globulin, CSF	6.1–8.3 mg/dL
Gamma-glutamyl transpeptidase, serum	Female: 8–40 U/L; male: 9–50 U/L
Gastric secretion	
Basal acid analysis	10–30 units of free acid
Basal acid output	Female: 2.0 ± 1.8 mEq of HCl/hr; male: 3.0 ± 2.0 mEq of HCl/hr
Maximal output after pentagastrin stimulation	23 ± 5 mEq of HCl/hr
Gastrin, serum	<100 pg/mL
Gentamicin, serum	Therapeutic: peak 5.0–10.0 mcg/mL; trough: <2.0 mcg/mL
Glucose, CSF	50–75 mg/dL
Glucose, plasma (fasting)	70–99 mg/dL
Glucose-6-phosphate dehydrogenase, blood	5–15 units/g of hemoglobin
Glycoprotein subunit, serum	<1 ng/mL
Growth hormone, serum	

(continued)

ABIM LABORATORY TEST REFERENCE RANGES—JANUARY 2019 (*CONTINUED*)

Laboratory Tests	Reference Ranges
At rest	<5 ng/mL
Response to provocative stimuli	>7 ng/mL
Haptoglobin, serum	83–267 mg/dL
Hematocrit, blood	Female: 37%–47%; male: 42%–50%
Hemoglobin A1C	4.0%–5.6%
Hemoglobin, blood	Female: 12–16 g/dL; male: 14–18 g/dL
Hemoglobin fractionation	
HbA	96%–98%
HbA2	1.5%–3.5%
HbF	<1%
Hemoglobin, plasma	<5.0 mg/dL
Heparin–anti-factor Xa assay, plasma	0.3–0.7 IU/mL (therapeutic range for standard [unfractionated] heparin therapy)
Heparin–platelet factor 4 antibody, serum	Positive: >0.4 optical density units
Hepatic copper	25–40 mcg/g dry weight
Hepatic iron index	<1.0
Histamine excretion, urine	20–50 mcg/24 hr
Homocysteine, plasma	5–15 µmol/L
Hydroxyproline, urine	10–30 mg/m of body surface/24 hr
Immature platelet fraction	1%–5% of platelet count
Immune complexes, serum	0–50 mcg/dL
Immunoglobulins, serum	
IgA	90–325 mg/dL
IgE	<380 IU/mL
IgG	800–1,500 mg/dL
IgM	45–150 mg/dL
Immunoglobulin free light chains, serum	
Kappa	3.3–19.4 mg/L
Lambda	5.7–26.3 mg/L
Kappa to lambda ratio	0.26–1.65
Insulin, serum (fasting)	<20 µU/mL
IGF-1 (somatomedin-C), serum	
Ages 16–24	182–780 ng/mL

(*continued*)

ABIM LABORATORY TEST REFERENCE RANGES—JANUARY 2019 (*CONTINUED*)

Laboratory Tests	Reference Ranges
Ages 25–39	114–492 ng/mL
Ages 40–54	90–360 ng/mL
Ages 55 and older	71–290 ng/mL
Iodine, urine	
Spot	mcg/L; varies
Iron, serum	50–150 mcg/dL
Iron-binding capacity, serum (total)	250–310 mcg/dL
Lactate, arterial blood	<1.3 mmol/L (<1.3 mEq/L)
Lactate, serum or plasma	0.7–2.1 mmol/L
Lactate, venous blood	0.6–1.8 mEq/L; 6–16 mg/dL
Lactate dehydrogenase, serum	80–225 U/L
Lactic acid, serum	6–19 mg/dL (0.7–2.1 mmol/L)
Lactose tolerance test, GI	Increase in plasma glucose: >15 mg/dL
Lead, blood	15–40 mcg/dL
Lead, urine	<80 mcg/24 hr
Leukocyte count	4,000–11,000/mcL
Segmented neutrophils	50%–70%
Band forms	0%–5%
Lymphocytes	30%–45%
Monocytes	0%–6%
Basophils	0%–1%
Eosinophils	0%–3%
Lipase, serum	10–140 U/L
Lipoprotein(a), serum	Desirable: <30 mg/dL
Lithium, plasma	
Therapeutic	0.6–1.2 mEq/L
Toxic level	>2 mEq/L
LH, serum	
Female, follicular/luteal	1–12 mIU/mL (1–12 U/L)
Female, midcycle peak	9–80 mIU/mL (9–80 U/L)
Female, postmenopausal	>30 mIU/mL (>30 U/L)
Male (adult)	2–9 mIU/mL (2–9 U/L)
Children, Tanner stages 1, 2, 3	<9.0 mIU/mL (< 9.0 U/L)

(continued)

ABIM LABORATORY TEST REFERENCE RANGES—JANUARY 2019 (*CONTINUED*)

Laboratory Tests	Reference Ranges
Children, Tanner stages 4, 5	1–15 mIU/mL (1–15 U/L)
Lymphocyte subsets	
CD3	900–3,245/mcL
CD4	530–1,570/mcL
CD8	430–1,060/mcL
CD19	208–590/mcL
Magnesium, serum	1.6–2.6 mEq/L
Magnesium, urine	14–290 mg/24 hr
Mean corpuscular hemoglobin	28–32 pg
Mean corpuscular hemoglobin concentration	33–36 g/dL
Mean corpuscular volume	80–98 fL
Mean platelet volume	7–9 fL
Metanephrines, fractionated, plasma	
Metanephrine	<0.5 nmol/L
Normetanephrine	<0.9 nmol/L
Metanephrines, fractionated, 24-hr urine	
Metanephrine	<400 mcg/24 hr
Normetanephrine	<900 mcg/24 hr
Myoglobin, serum	<100 mcg/L
Norepinephrine, plasma	
Supine	70–750 pg/mL
Standing	200–1,700 pg/mL
Norepinephrine, urine	0–100 mcg/24 hr
Normetanephrine, fractionated, plasma	<0.9 nmol/L
Normetanephrine, fractionated, 24-hr urine	<900 mcg
N-telopeptide, urine	Female: 11–48 nmol BCE/mmol creatinine; male: 7–68 nmol BCE/mmol creatinine
NT-pro-BNP, serum or plasma	If eGFR >60 mL/min/1.73 m
18–49 years of age	Heart failure unlikely: 300 pg/mL or less; high probability of heart failure: 450 pg/mL or greater
50–75 years of age	Heart failure unlikely: 300 pg/mL or less; high probability of heart failure: 900 pg/mL or greater
Older than 75 years of age	Heart failure unlikely: 300 pg/mL or less; high probability of heart failure: 1,800 pg/mL or greater; If eGFR <60 mL/min/1.73 m
18 years of age or older	High probability of heart failure: 1,200 pg/mL or greater

(*continued*)

ABIM LABORATORY TEST REFERENCE RANGES—JANUARY 2019 (*CONTINUED*)

Laboratory Tests	Reference Ranges
Osmolality, serum	275–295 mOsm/kg H_2O
Osmolality, urine	38–1,400 mOsm/kg H_2O
Osmotic fragility of erythrocytes	Increased if hemolysis occurs in over 0.5% NaCl; decreased if hemolysis is incomplete in 0.3% NaCl
Osteocalcin, serum	Male: 11.3–35.4 ng/mL; female: 7.2–27.9 ng/mL
Oxalate, urine	<40 mg/24 hr
Oxygen consumption	225–275 mL/min
Oxygen saturation, arterial blood	95% or greater
Parathyroid hormone, serum	
C-terminal	150–350 pg/mL
Intact	10–65 pg/mL
Intact (dialysis patients only)	Target: 130–585 pg/mL
Parathyroid hormone-related protein, serum	<1.5 pmol/L
Partial thromboplastin time (activated)	25–35 sec
pH, urine	4.5–8.0
Phenolsulfonphthalein, urine	At least 25% excreted by 15 min; 40% by 30 min; 60% by 120 min
Phenytoin, serum	Therapeutic: 10–20 mcg/mL
Phosphatase (acid), serum	
Total	0.5–2.0 (Bodansky) units/mL
Prostatic fraction	0.1–0.4 unit/mL
Phosphatase (alkaline), serum	30–120 U/L
Phospholipids, serum (total)	200–300 mg/dL
Phosphorus, serum	3.0–4.5 mg/dL
Phosphorus, urine	500–1,200 mg/24 hr
Platelet count	150,000–450,000/mcL
PFA-100	
Collagen–epinephrine closure time	60–143 sec
Collagen–ADP closure time	58–123 sec
Platelet survival rate (Cr)	10 d
Potassium, serum	3.5–5.0 mEq/L
Potassium, urine	
Spot	mEq/L; varies
24-hr measurement	mEq/24 hr; varies with intake
Prealbumin, serum	16–30 mg/dL

(continued)

ABIM LABORATORY TEST REFERENCE RANGES—JANUARY 2019 (*CONTINUED*)

Laboratory Tests	Reference Ranges
Pregnanetriol, urine	0.2–3.5 mg/24 hr
Pressure (opening; initial), CSF	70–180 mm CSF (70–180 mm H_2O)
Procalcitonin, serum	Less than or equal to 0.10 ng/mL
Progesterone, serum	
Female, follicular	0.02–0.9 ng/mL
Female, luteal	2–30 ng/mL
Male (adult)	0.12–0.3 ng/mL
Proinsulin, serum	3–20 pmol/L
Prolactin, serum	<20 ng/mL
Prostate-specific antigen, serum	ng/mL; no specific normal or abnormal level
Protein C activity, plasma	65%–150%
Protein C antigen, plasma	70%–140%
Protein catabolic rate, urine	Goal: 1.0–1.2 g/kg/24 hr
Protein S activity, plasma	57%–131%
Protein S antigen, plasma	
Total	60%–140%
Free	60%–130%
Protein, urine	
Spot	mg/dL; varies
24-hr measurement	<100 mg/24 hr
Protein, CSF total	15–45 mg/dL
Protein, serum	
Total	5.5–9.0 g/dL
Albumin	3.5–5.5 g/dL
Globulin	2.0–3.5 g/dL
Alpha-1	0.2–0.4 g/dL
Alpha-2	0.5–0.9 g/dL
Beta	0.6–1.1 g/dL
Gamma	0.7–1.7 g/dL
Protein to creatinine ratio, urine	<0.2 mg/mg
Prothrombin time, plasma	11–13 sec
Pyruvic acid, blood	0.08–0.16 mmol/L
Quinidine, serum	Therapeutic: 2–5 mcg/mL

(*continued*)

ABIM LABORATORY TEST REFERENCE RANGES—JANUARY 2019 (CONTINUED)

Laboratory Tests	Reference Ranges
RDW	9.0–14.5
Red cell mass	Female: 22.7–27.9 mL/kg; male: 24.9–32.5 mL/kg
Renin activity (angiotensin-I radioimmunoassay)	
Peripheral plasma	
Normal diet	
Supine	0.3–2.5 ng/mL/hr
Upright	0.2–3.6 ng/mL/hr
Low-sodium diet	
Supine	0.9–4.5 ng/mL/hr
Upright	4.1–9.1 ng/mL/hr
Diuretics + low-sodium diet	6.3–13.7 ng/mL/hr
Renal vein concentration	Normal ratio (high:low): <1.5
Reptilase time	10–12 sec
Reticulocyte count	0.5%–1.5% of red cells
Reticulocyte count, absolute	25,000–100,000/mcL
Rheumatoid factor (nephelometry)	<24 IU/mL
Rheumatoid factor, latex test	1:80 or less
Ristocetin cofactor activity of plasma	50%–150%
Russell viper venom time, dilute	33–44 sec
Salicylate, plasma	Therapeutic: 20–30 mg/dL
Sex hormone-binding globulin	Female, nonpregnant: 18–144 nmol/L; male: 10–57 nmol/L
Sodium, serum	136–145 mEq/L
Sodium, urine	
Spot	mEq/L; varies
24-hr measurement	mEq/24 hr; varies with intake
Specific gravity, urine	1.002–1.030
Sperm density	10–150 million/mL
Sweat test for sodium and chloride	<60 mEq/L
T3 resin uptake	25%–35%
T-lymphocyte count, CD4	530–1,570/mcL
Tacrolimus, whole blood (trough)	Therapeutic: 5–15 ng/mL (for transplant patients: 10.0–15.0 ng/mL [0–3 months posttransplantation]; 5.0–10.0 ng/mL [more than 3 months posttransplantation])
Testosterone, bioavailable, serum	Female, age 18–69 years: 0.5–8.5 ng/dL

(continued)

ABIM LABORATORY TEST REFERENCE RANGES—JANUARY 2019 (*CONTINUED*)

Laboratory Tests	Reference Ranges
Testosterone, free, serum	Male: 70–300 pg/mL
Testosterone, serum	Female: 18–54 ng/dL; male: 291–1,100 ng/dL
Theophylline, serum	Therapeutic: 8–20 mcg/mL
Thrombin time	17–23 sec
Thyroid function studies	
T3 resin uptake	25%–35%
Thyroglobulin, serum	<20 ng/mL
Thyroidal iodine (I) uptake	5%–30% of administered dose at 24 hr
TSH, serum	0.5–4.0 μU/mL (0.5–4.0 mU/L)
TSI	<130%
Thyroxine-binding globulin, serum	12–27 mcg/mL
Thyroxine index, free (estimate)	5–12
Thyroxine (T4), serum	
Total	5–12 mcg/dL
Free	0.8–1.8 ng/dL
Triiodothyronine (T3), serum	
Total	80–180 ng/dL
Reverse	20–40 ng/dL
Free	2.3–4.2 pg/mL
Tissue transglutaminase antibody, IgA (by chemiluminescence method)	<20 AU
Tissue transglutaminase antibody, IgA (by ELISA)	<4.0 U/mL
Tissue transglutaminase antibody, IgG (by chemiluminescence method)	<20 AU
Tissue transglutaminase antibody, IgG (by ELISA)	<6.0 U/mL
Total protein, CSF	15–45 mg/dL
Transaminase, serum glutamic oxaloacetic (SGOT)	See aminotransferase, serum aspartate (AST, SGOT)
Transaminase, serum glutamic pyruvic (SGPT)	See aminotransferase, serum alanine (ALT, SGPT)
Transferrin saturation	20%–50%
Transferrin, serum	200–400 mg/dL
Triglycerides, serum (fasting)	
Optimal	<100 mg/dL
Normal	<150 mg/dL
Borderline-high	150–199 mg/dL

(continued)

ABIM LABORATORY TEST REFERENCE RANGES—JANUARY 2019 (*CONTINUED*)

Laboratory Tests	Reference Ranges
High	200–499 mg/dL
Very high	>499 mg/dL
Troponin I, cardiac, serum	0.04 ng/mL or less
Troponin T, cardiac, serum	0.01 ng/mL or less
Tryptase, serum	<11.5 ng/mL
Urea clearance, urine	
Standard	40–60 mL/min
Maximal	60–100 mL/min
Urea nitrogen, blood	8–20 mg/dL
Urea nitrogen, urine	12–20 g/24 hr
Uric acid, serum	3.0–7.0 mg/dL
Uric acid, urine	250–750 mg/24 hr
Uroporphyrin, urine	10–30 mcg/24 hr
Vanillylmandelic acid, urine	<9 mg/24 hr
Venous oxygen content, mixed	14–16 mL/dL
Venous studies, mixed, blood	
pH	7.32–7.41
PCO_2	42–53 mmHg
PO_2	35–42 mmHg
Bicarbonate	24–28 mEq/L
Oxygen saturation (SvO_2)	65%–75%
Viscosity, serum	1.4–1.8 cp
Vitamin A, serum	
Adult	32.5–78.0 mcg/dL
Pediatric, age 1–2 years (retinol)	20–43 mcg/dL
Vitamin B_{12}, serum	200–800 pg/mL
Vitamin D metabolites, serum	
1,25-Dihydroxyvitamin D (1,25-Dihydroxycholecalciferol)	15–60 pg/mL
25-Hydroxyvitamin D (25-Hydroxycholecalciferol)	30–60 ng/mL
Vitamin E, serum	
Adult	5.5–17.0 mg/L
Pediatric, age 1–2 years (alpha-tocopherol)	2.9–16.6 mg/L

(*continued*)

ABIM LABORATORY TEST REFERENCE RANGES—JANUARY 2019 (*CONTINUED*)

Laboratory Tests	Reference Ranges
Volume, blood	
Plasma	Female: 43 mL/kg body weight; male: 44 mL/kg body weight
Red cell	Female: 20–30 mL/kg body weight; male: 25–35 mL/kg body weight
von Willebrand factor antigen, plasma	50%–150%
Zinc, serum	75–140 mcg/dL

AAT, alpha-1 antitrypsin; ABIM, American Board of Internal Medicine; ACE, angiotensin-converting enzyme; ACTH, adrenocorticotrophic hormone; ADP, adenosine diphosphate; ALT, alanine aminotransferase; ANC, absolute neutrophil count; anti-LKM, anti-liver-kidney microsomal; aPTT, activated partial thromboplastin time; AST, aspartate aminotransferase; beta-hCG, beta-human chorionic gonadotropin; BUN, blood urea nitrogen; CA, carbohydrate antigen; Cr, creatinine; CSF, cerebrospinal fluid; DHEA-S, dehydroepiandrosterone sulfate; eGFR, estimated glomerular filtration rate; ELISA, enzyme-linked immunosorbent assay; GI, gastrointestinal; HCl, hydrochloric acid; IgA, immunoglobulin A; IgE, immunoglobulin E; IGF-1, insulin-like growth factor 1; IgG, immunoglobulin G; IgM, immunoglobulin M; LH, luteinizing hormone; NT-pro-BNP, N-terminal-pro-B-type natriuretic peptide; $PaCO_2$, partial pressure of carbon dioxide in arterial blood; PaO_2, partial pressure of oxygen in arterial blood; PCO_2, partial pressure of carbon dioxide; PO_2, partial pressure of oxygen; PFA, platelet function analysis; RBC, red blood cell; RDW, red cell distribution width; SGOT, serum glutamic oxaloacetic transaminase; SGPT, serum glutamic pyruvic transaminase; SvO_2, venous oxygen saturation; TSH, thyroid-stimulating hormone; TSI, thyroid-stimulating immunoglobulin; WBCs, white blood cells.

Source: Reproduced with permission from the American Board of Internal Medicine. Retrieved from https://www.abim.org//media/ ABIM%20Public/ Files/pdf/exam/laboratory-reference-ranges.pdf.

INDEX